Essentials of

Cardiopulmonary Physical Therapy

Essentials of
Cardiopulmonary
Physical Therapy

Second Edition

Ellen A. Hillegass, EdD, PT, CCS

Adjunct Faculty
Department of Physical Therapy
Emory University
Saint Joseph's Hospital of Atlanta
Atlanta, Georgia

Cardiovascular and Pulmonary Consultant

H. Steven Sadowsky, MS, RRT, PT, CCS

Associate Clinical Professor
School of Physical Therapy
Texas Woman's University
Denton, Texas

Physical Therapist
Department of Rehabilitation Services
Presbyterian Hospital of Dallas
Dallas, Texas

W.B. SAUNDERS COMPANY
A Harcourt Health Sciences Company
Philadelphia   London   New York   St. Louis   Sydney   Toronto

W.B. SAUNDERS COMPANY
A Harcourt Health Sciences Company

The Curtis Center
Independence Square West
Philadelphia, Pennsylvania 19106

Library of Congress Cataloging-in-Publication Data

Essentials of cardiopulmonary physical therapy / [edited by] Ellen A. Hillegass,
H. Steven Sadowsky.—2nd ed.

p. cm.

Includes bibliographical references and index.

ISBN 0-7216-7288-4

1. Cardiopulmonary system—Diseases—Physical therapy.   I. Hillegass, Ellen
   A.   II. Sadowsky, H. Steven

RC702.E88 2001   616.1′062—dc21   00-056293

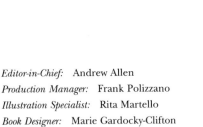

Editor-in-Chief: Andrew Allen
Production Manager: Frank Polizzano
Illustration Specialist: Rita Martello
Book Designer: Marie Gardocky-Clifton

ESSENTIALS OF CARDIOPULMONARY PHYSICAL THERAPY   ISBN 0-7216-7288-4

Printed in the United States of America.

Last digit is the print number: 9   8   7   6   5   4   3   2   1

Contributors

Rhonda N. Barr, MA, PT, CCS

Adjunct Associate, The University of Iowa; Clinical Specialist, Department of Rehabilitation Therapies, The University of Iowa Hospitals and Clinics, Iowa City, Iowa

Pulmonary Rehabilitation

Lawrence Cahalin, MA, PT, CCS

Clinical Associate Professor, Physical Therapy, Sargent College, Boston University, Boston, Massachusetts

Cardiac Muscle Dysfunction, Pulmonary Medications

Peggy Clough, MA, PT

Supervisor, Physical Therapy Division, University of Michigan Health System, University Hospital, Ann Arbor, Michigan

Restrictive Lung Dysfunction

Meryl Cohen, MS, PT, CCS

Instructor, Division of Physical Therapy, University of Miami School of Medicine, Coral Gables, Florida; Adjunct Instructor, Massachusetts General Hospital, Institute of Health Professions, Boston, Massachusetts

Cardiovascular Medications

Anne Mejia Downs, PT, CCS

Adjunct Faculty, Division of Physical Therapy, University of North Carolina; Cardiopulmonary Specialist, University of North Carolina Hospitals, Chapel Hill, North Carolina

Thoracic Organ Transplantation: Heart, Heart-Lung, and Lung

Susan L. Garritan, MA, PT, CCS

Supervisor, Cardiopulmonary Physical Therapy, New York University Medical Center, New York, New York

Chronic Obstructive Pulmonary Diseases

Kate Grimes, MS, PT, CCS

Clinical Assistant Professor, Massachusetts General Hospital Institute of Health Professions, Boston, Massachusetts

Cardiovascular Medications

Ellen A. Hillegass, EdD, PT, CCS

Adjunct Faculty, Department of Physical Therapy, Emory University; Saint Joseph's Hospital of Atlanta, Atlanta, Georgia; Cardiovascular and pulmonary consultant

Cardiovascular Diagnostic Tests and Procedures, Electrocardiography, Cardiovascular and Thoracic Interventions, Cardiopulmonary Assessment, Therapeutic Interventions in Cardiac Rehabilitation and Prevention

Eugene McColgon, PT, CCS

Program Director, Cardiac Rehabilitation, James A. Haley Veterans Hospital, Tampa, Florida

Ischemic Cardiac Conditions

Erica Nixon, BS, PT

Physical Therapist III, Physical Therapy, University of Michigan Hospitals, Ann Arbor, Michigan

Treatment of Acute Cardiopulmonary Conditions

Peg Pashkow, MEd, PT

President and CEO, HeartWatchers International, Inc., Honolulu, Hawaii

Outcome Measures: Reimbursement Issues and Documentation

H. Steven Sadowsky, MS, RRT, PT, CCS

Associate Clinical Professor, School of Physical Therapy, Texas Woman's University, Denton; Physical Therapist, Department of Rehabilitation Services, Presbyterian Hospital of Dallas, Dallas, Texas

Anatomy of the Cardiovascular and Respiratory System, Cardiovascular and Respiratory Physiology, Ischemic Cardiac Conditions, Pulmonary Diagnostic Tests and Procedures, Cardiovascular and Thoracic Interventions, Monitoring and Life-Support Equipment, Pulmonary Medications

Alexandra Sciaky, MS, PT, CCS

Clinical Faculty, Department of Physical Therapy, University of Michigan-Flint, Flint; Cardiopulmonary Clinical Specialist and Coordinator of Clinical Education, Physical Therapy, University of Michigan Hospitals, Ann Arbor, Michigan

Treatment of Acute Cardiopulmonary Conditions

Jill Stockford, BS, PT

Physical Therapist III, Physical Therapy, University of Michigan Hospitals, Ann Arbor, Michigan

Treatment of Acute Cardiopulmonary Conditions

William C. Temes, MS, PT, OCS

Faculty/Board of Directors, North American Institute of Orthopaedic Manual Therapy; Director, Healthsouth, Eugene, Oregon

Therapeutic Interventions in Cardiac Rehabilitation and Prevention

Tammy Versluis-Burlis, MHS, PT, CCS

Instructor, Program in Physical Therapy, Washington University at St. Louis, School of Medicine, St. Louis, Missouri

Thoracic Organ Transplantation: Heart, Heart-Lung, and Lung

Joanne Watchie, MA, PT, CCS

Part-time Faculty Member, Mount Saint Mary's College; Physical Therapist, USC University Hospital, Los Angeles, California

Cardiopulmonary Implications of Specific Diseases

Preface

Those aspects of physical therapy commonly referred to as "cardiopulmonary physical therapy" are recognized as fundamental components of the knowledge base and practice base of all entry-level physical therapists. Although intended primarily for physical therapists, we know that the first edition of the *Essentials of Cardiopulmonary Physical Therapy* has been useful to practitioners in various disciplines who teach students or who work with patients who suffer from primary and secondary cardiopulmonary dysfunction. We believe that this second edition can also be used by all practitioners who teach students and work with patients.

This second edition of *Essentials of Cardiopulmonary Physical Therapy* has been revised and expanded. There are now six sections: *Anatomy and Physiology; Pathophysiology; Diagnostic Tests and Procedures; Surgical Interventions, Monitoring, and Support; Pharmacology;* and *Cardiopulmonary Assessment and Intervention.* These divisions were chosen in an effort to present the information in what we, the editors, believe to be an orderly progression that facilitates a more thorough understanding of the subject matter. It is our firm belief that the cardiovascular and pulmonary systems should be considered together, as they are related to each other and not separate entities. The anatomy, physiology, and assessment and aspects of the cardiovascular and pulmonary systems are therefore discussed jointly, stressing further their interaction. Pathophysiology, pharmacology, and interventions in the outpatient setting are separate topics because of the quantity of material required to cover all aspects. We have attempted to consider the span of the life cycle in all discussions.

We believe that all physical therapy professionals should choose treatment interventions that address the specific problems identified from a thorough patient assessment, and we have provided a comprehensive assessment chapter and separate intervention chapters based upon the patient setting. Since the publication of the first edition of *The Guide to Physical Therapy Practice,* and although *The Guide* continues to be a work in progress, students and professionals are referred to it for specific diagnostic groupings and lists of assessment tools and intervention procedures. *The Guide* should be used in conjunction with this text in both educational and clinical settings.

Chapter 1 of *Essentials of Cardiopulmonary Physical Therapy,* second edition, presents the developmental and maturational anatomy of the traditional cardiovascular and respiratory systems. Chapter 2 details the basic physiology underlying the "oxygen transport system." Chapters 3 through 7 examine the pathophysiology associated with cardiovascular ischemia (Chapter 3), myocardial dysfunction (Chapter 4), restrictive pulmonary conditions (Chapter 5), chronic obstructive pulmonary conditions (Chapter 6), and other disease processes that have cardiopulmonary implications (Chapter 7). Chapters 8 through 10 describe cardiovascular and pulmonary diagnostic tests and procedures, whereas Chapter 11 presents cardiovascular and thoracic surgical interventions. Since the field of cardiovascular and pulmonary assessment and treatment continually evolves, a new chapter is included for needed information on heart and lung transplantation (Chapter 12). The monitoring and life-support equipment commonly employed in the assessment and treatment of patients with cardiovascular and pulmonary disorders are found in Chapter 13. Pharmacology is discussed in separate chapters with cardiovascular medications in Chapter 14 and pulmonary medications in Chapter 15. Assessment of the patient with cardiopulmonary dysfunction is presented in Chapter 16, followed by three chapters on interventions used in cardiopulmonary conditions. Chapter 17 presents a thorough discussion of treatment in the acute care setting, whereas Chapters 18 and 19 present information on therapeutic interventions for the cardiovascular patient in the outpatient setting (Chapter 18) and during pulmonary rehabilitation (Chapter 19). The text ends with a dynamic new chapter on outcome measures and includes information on documentation and reimbursement.

Whenever possible, we have striven to provide case studies to exemplify the material being presented. Terms that are of particular relevance or that have clinical significance have been highlighted in **bold** throughout the text. These words and abbreviations are then presented with a brief definition in the Glossary.

No matter how well you understand the material in this book, it will not make you a master clinician, skilled in the assessment and treatment of cardiovascular and pulmonary disorders. To become even a minimally competent clinician, you will have to practice physical therapy under the tutelage of an experienced clinician. *Essentials of Cardiopulmonary Physical Therapy* cannot provide you with everything there is to know about the assessment and treatment of cardiovascular and pulmonary disorders. It *will* provide the essentials as the title indicates. We believe that in the ever-evolving realm of patient care learning is a continuous process, and technology and treatment are forever improving; therefore, this text provides clinicians as well as educators with the most current information at the time of publication.

Acknowledgments

Following the publication of the first edition of the *Essentials of Cardiopulmonary Physical Therapy,* we, the editors, celebrated only briefly, realizing that the field was changing fast and that a second edition would soon be needed. We started early to develop our ideas for changes, and we have been fortunate to have a vast array of experts to assist us in making this second edition a reality. We would like to sincerely thank all those clinicians, students, patients, and faculty members, and all other colleagues who provided feedback on this text through the use of the first edition in their courses or everyday practices. Special gratitude is extended to each of the contributors—who are also dear friends and great colleagues. They strengthened this second edition with their expertise and willingness to meet our deadlines. Some special colleagues deserve to be recognized. They challenge others with their knowledge and expertise and keep us current in their specialty areas of cardiovascular and pulmonary rehabilitation and include Claire Rice, Andy Ries, and Joanne Watchie.

We would like to thank all our loved ones who provided their love and patience while we editors spent long days and nights on this project. Finally, we extend our heartfelt thanks to Peg Waltner, our developmental editor, for sticking with this revision process and encouraging us to complete all of our tasks.

Contents

6 CARDIOPULMONARY ASSESSMENT AND INTERVENTION

1

Anatomy and Physiology

1

Anatomy of the Cardiovascular and Respiratory Systems

H. Steven Sadowsky

INTRODUCTION

This chapter reviews the structure of the cardiovascular and respiratory systems. There is no single best manner in which to describe these systems. A fundamental assumption must be made, namely, that the reader already possesses some knowledge of the material that is presented in more detail in later sections. The order of presentation that follows, therefore, is an artificial convenience for which some indulgence is requested.

CARDIOVASCULAR AND RESPIRATORY SYSTEM DEVELOPMENT

Embryonic and Fetal Cardiovascular System

Although the precise details of the developmental process are not entirely clear, it is known that early in the third week of gestation the first blood cells and vessels start to form in several different areas.[1-8] In the yolk sac and the base of the body stalk, small and essentially spherical groups of cells—the **blood islands**—develop. The outermost cells of these islands flatten to form the vascular endothelium, and the innermost cells convert into primitive red corpuscles. The isolated blood-containing spaces coalesce to form a network of blood vessels. Angioblastic tissues in the chorion and the chorionic end of the body stalk form solid strands that contain a few rod-shaped nuclei. Each strand, then, develops into one or two nucleated hemoglobin-containing cells and blood vessels. From these earliest blood vessels, buds grow, become canalized, and are converted into new vessels. Developing vessels meld with vessels from adjacent areas to join the evolving embryonic vascular network.

The first indication of the forming heart can be seen at about the eighteenth day of embryonic maturation when two **endocardial heart tubes** have been formed. By about the twenty-first or twenty-second day of gestation, these tubes fuse to form a single **heart tube.** At about the twenty-third day of gestation, the surrounding pericardial cavity elongates, and the **truncus arteriosus, bulbus cordis, ventricle, atrium,** and **sinus venosus** can be distinguished within the heart tube. Simultaneously, a **myoepicardial mantle** is formed from a thickening of the splanchnic mesenchyme around the heart tube. This myoepicardial mantle differentiates into the **myocardium** and the **epicardium** of the heart. The inner endocardial tube becomes the epithelial lining of the heart, called the **endocardium.**

Initially although fairly straight, by about the twenty-fourth day of gestation, the heart tube has grown so rapidly that it bends upon itself, the bulbus cordis forming a right limb and the ventricle a left limb of a U-shaped **bulboventricular loop** (Fig. 1–1). At first, the primitive heart has only one atrium and one ventricle. However, these

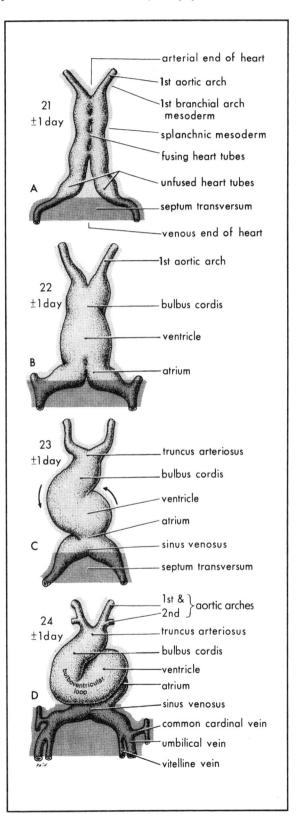

Figure 1–1. Ventral views of the developing heart during the fourth week of gestation. *A* and *B* show fusion of the heart tubes. *C* and *D* show the bending of the single heart tube as the primitive heart grows within a confined space, finally folding upon itself and forming the bulboventricular loop. (From Moore KL. Before We Are Born: Essentials of Embryology and Birth Defects, 3rd ed. Philadelphia, WB Saunders, 1989, p 205.)

chambers begin to be partitioned during the middle of the fourth week of gestation when **endocardial cushions** in the dorsal and ventral walls of the atrioventricular canal grow toward each other and fuse, dividing the single atrioventricular canal into *right* and *left* **atrioventricular canals.**

At about the middle of the fourth week of gestation, the atrium starts to separate into right and left atria with the sequential growth of two septa. First, a crescent-shaped membrane grows from the dorsocranial wall of the primitive atrium toward the endocardial cushions, forming the **septum primum.** As the septum primum advances, the two atria communicate through a diminishing **foramen primum.** Fortunately, the dorsal aspect of the septum deteriorates to create a new right-to-left shunt, through the **foramen secundum,** prior to the end of the fifth week of gestation. Near the end of the eighth gestational week, the **septum secundum** grows from the ventrocranial wall of the atrium on the right side of the septum primum. This septum eventually covers the foramen secundum; the opening in the septum secundum is called the **foramen ovale.** The septum primum forms a valve for the foramen ovale. Before birth, the foramen ovale permits most of the blood entering the right atrium to pass into the left atrium. After birth, the foramen ovale normally closes, and the septum becomes a complete partition.

The left horn of the sinus venosus becomes the **coronary sinus,** and the right horn is incorporated into the wall of the right atrium. A remnant of the right part of the primitive atrium persists as the rough portion of the atrium and the **right auricle.** The terminal portion of the *primitive pulmonary vein* is incorporated into the wall of the left atrium as the left atrium expands. Also, a portion of the left part of the primitive atrium is retained in the left atrium as the **left auricle.**

The bulbus cordis and the truncus arteriosus are divided into the **aorta** and **pulmonary trunk** by a spiral **aorticopulmonary septum** during the fifth gestational week when *bulbar* and *truncal ridges* fuse. Because of the spiral orientation of the aorticopulmonary septum, the pulmonary trunk twists around the ascending aorta. This effect is believed to be a consequence of the force produced by the flow of blood from the developing ventricles.

The primitive ventricle begins dividing into right and left ventricles at the end of the fourth gestational week with the development of the **interventricular septum** in the floor of the ventricle near its apex. The interventricular septum grows toward the fused endocardial cushions, closing the resultant **interventricular foramen** at about the end of the seventh week. After closure, the pulmonary trunk communicates with the right ventricle and the aorta with the left ventricle, essentially completing cardiac development.

Fetal Circulation

Oxygenated blood is delivered to the fetus from the placenta by way of the **umbilical vein** attachment to the **inferior vena cava.** Approximately one half of this umbilical blood bypasses the liver via the **ductus venosus.** After passing through the inferior vena cava, the blood enters the right atrium. Because the inferior vena cava also receives blood from the lower limbs, abdomen, and pelvis of the fetus, the blood entering the right atrium is not as well oxygenated as that in the umbilical vein.

Blood from the inferior vena cava is primarily directed through the foramen ovale to the left atrium by the inferior border of the septum secundum. In the left atrium, the blood is mixed with a small amount of deoxygenated blood that is returning from the lungs via the pulmonary veins. From the left atrium, blood passes into the left ventricle and leaves the heart via the ascending aorta. Therefore, the coronary arteries, the head and neck, and the upper limbs receive relatively well-oxygenated blood.

A small amount of oxygenated blood originally from the placenta remains in the right atrium and is mixed with blood from the **superior vena cava** and the coronary sinus before passing into the right ventricle. This blood exits via the pulmonary trunk, most of it passing through the ductus arteriosus into the aorta. Very little blood passes on to the lungs prior to birth. The blood pumped into the aorta circulates through the body and eventually returns via the vena cava.

Circulation in the Newborn

Major circulatory adjustments occur at birth and are due to the cessation of fetal circulation through the placenta and the beginning of gas exchange in the lungs. Occlusion of the placental circulation causes blood pressure to fall in the inferior vena cava and right atrium of the newborn. Likewise, aeration of the lungs is accompanied by a significant fall in pulmonary vascular resistance, a marked increase in pulmonary blood flow, and a thinning of the walls of the pulmonary arteries. Subsequent to the increased pulmonary blood flow, the pressure in the left atrium rises above that of the right atrium. This presses the septum primum against the septum secundum, closing the foramen ovale.

Embryonic and Fetal Respiratory System

Development of the respiratory system begins during the fourth week of gestation[1, 5, 7–10] when the **laryngotracheal groove** forms in the caudal end of the ventral wall of the pharyngeal floor. Shortly thereafter, a **laryngotracheal diverticulum** separates from the pharynx and grows caudally to partition the foregut into the **esophagus** and **laryngotracheal tube.**

The **larynx** forms from the proximal endoder-

Clinical Notes: Fetal Changes at Birth

As a result of the systemic circulatory changes that occur at birth, several fetal structures are transformed:

- The intra-abdominal portion of the umbilical vein becomes the *ligamentum teres,* which passes from the umbilicus to the left branch of the portal vein.
- The ductus venosus eventually becomes the *ligamentum venosum,* which passes through the liver from the left branch of the portal vein to the inferior vena cava.
- Most intra-abdominal portions of the umbilical arteries become the *medial umbilical ligaments.*
- The proximal parts of these arteries persist as the *superior vesical arteries* supplying the superior part of the urinary bladder.
- The foramen ovale normally closes functionally at birth, and anatomic closure occurs later with the adhesion of the septum primum to the left margin of the septum secundum.
- The ductus arteriosus eventually becomes the *ligamentum arteriosum,* which passes from the left pulmonary artery to the arch of the aorta (anatomic closure generally occurs by the third postnatal month).

mal lining of the laryngotracheal tube and the fourth and sixth pairs of branchial arches. The endodermal lining distal to the larynx in the central laryngotracheal tube forms the epithelium and glands of the **trachea,** while the surrounding splanchnic mesenchyme forms the tracheal cartilage, connective tissue, and muscle. The inferior end of the laryngotracheal tube forms a **lung bud.**

The lung bud divides into two **bronchial buds** that ultimately differentiate into the bronchi and lungs, as shown in Figure 1–2. Right and left **primary bronchi** grow from the bronchial buds and subdivide into **secondary bronchi.** Three secondary bronchi arise from the right primary bronchus: the superior secondary bronchus supplies the upper lobe of the lung; the inferior secondary bronchus continues on to supply the lower lobe, but first gives off a middle secondary bronchus to the middle lobe. The left primary bronchus gives rise to two secondary bronchi that supply the superior and inferior lobes of the left lung. The ensuing development of the lung often is divided into four stages, or periods.

Pseudoglandular Period (weeks 5 to 17). As the secondary bronchi continue to develop, they progressively branch and bifurcate until, by the seventh week of gestation, there are ten segmental bronchi—the **bronchopulmonary segments**—in the right lung and eight or nine in the left lung. The splanchnic mesenchyme surrounding the developing bronchi eventually gives rise to the supportive cartilaginous plates, the bronchial smooth muscle and connective tissue, and the pulmonary connective tissue and capillaries.

Canalicular Period (weeks 16 to 25). Because the upper segments of the lung develop faster than the lower ones, this period of development overlaps the pseudoglandular period. But it is during this phase that about 17 orders of branches develop. The most distal bronchioles—the **terminal bronchioles**—each yield two or more **respiratory bronchioles,** each of which, in turn, divides into as many as six **alveolar ducts.** Toward the end of the canalicular period, the alveolar ducts begin to develop **terminal sacs,** complete with capillary loops.

Terminal Sac Period (week 24 to birth). Additional terminal sacs—**pulmonary alveoli**—continue to develop along with their attendant blood and lymphatic capillary networks during this period of development. The type II alveolar epithe-

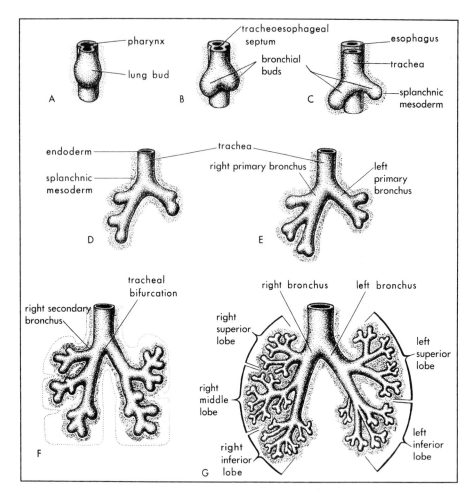

Figure 1-2. Ventral views showing the successive stages of development of the bronchi and lungs during the fourth to eighth weeks of gestation: *A* to *D*, 4 weeks; *E,* 5 weeks; *F,* 6 weeks; *G,* 8 weeks. (From Moore KL. Before We Are Born: Basic Embryology and Birth Defects. 3rd ed. Philadelphia, WB Saunders, 1989, p 162.)

lial cells begin to produce **surfactant** at about 28 weeks.

Alveolar Period (late fetal period to 7 or 8 years). The numbers of pulmonary alveoli increase toward their adult level; about one sixth to one eighth of the adult number of alveoli are present at birth.

Ventilation in the Newborn

The lung of the fetus is not collapsed in utero; rather, it is filled with an ultrafiltrate of plasma roughly equal in volume to the functional residual capacity of the lung in the newborn (between 25% and 40% of the total lung capacity).[1, 5, 9, 10] This liquid is about 100 times more viscous than air, and although such viscosity poses a problem, it also keeps the radius of curvature at the air-liquid

interface relatively large. As will be discussed in Chapter 2, this enlarged radius of curvature reduces both the surface tension forces resisting inflation and the tendency of the airways toward collapse.

Obviously, if the newborn is to breathe and if efficient gas exchange is to occur, the lungs must be rapidly cleared of the fluid that occupies them. As the neonate passes through the vagina, about a

Clinical Notes: Fetal Chest Movement

Although the fetus exhibits bursts of regular ventilatory-like chest movement interspersed with periods of seeming apnea, these intrauterine ventilatory movements are not a necessity for normal lung development, and a regular rhythmic pattern is probably not established before birth.

third of the fluid in its lungs is squeezed out. During the first few breaths approximately one half of the remaining fluid is absorbed into the capillaries, and the other half is removed by the pulmonary lymphatics.

The newborn's central and peripheral chemoreceptors are strongly stimulated because the fetus is made hypoxemic and hypercapnic as a result of drastically impaired placental gas exchange during the birth process. Moreover, the neonate is no longer isolated from tactile, thermal, visual, and other stimuli. This combination of stimuli results in the initiation of ventilation within moments of birth. Nonetheless, the first few breaths do not uniformly expand the alveoli because airway resistance is not homogeneous and some of the alveoli remain filled with fluid. Thus, although the lungs contain a small volume of air after the first breath, subsequent inhalations require decreasing transpulmonary pressures because successively reduced impedances are encountered until normal residual volume is attained. Pulmonary surfactant is a necessary requisite for the maintenance of patent alveoli at the new lower transpulmonary pressures.

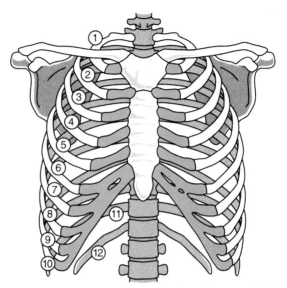

Figure 1–3. Anterior view of the thoracic cage with the costal cartilages highlighted. (Modified from Evans A, Patterson P, Riley D, Sutherland S. Human Anatomy: An Illustrated Laboratory Guide. San Francisco, Regents of the University of California, 1982, Fig. 1.)

THORAX

In addition to providing a skeletal framework for the attachment of the muscles of ventilation, the thorax houses the lungs and mediastinum; the mediastinum houses the heart. As will become evident later in this chapter, the thorax is intimately involved in the ventilatory process.

Thoracic Cage

The thoracic cage (Fig. 1–3) is conical at both its superior and inferior aspects and somewhat kidney-shaped in its transverse aspect. The skeletal boundaries of the thorax are the 12 thoracic vertebrae dorsally, the ribs laterally, and the sternum ventrally. The *thoracic inlet,* or upper margin of the thoracic cage, is bounded by the first thoracic vertebra posteriorly, the superior border of the manubrium anteriorly, and the first ribs laterally. The *thoracic outlet* is bounded by the twelfth thoracic vertebra posteriorly, by the seventh through tenth costal cartilages anteriorly, and the eleventh and

twelfth ribs laterally. The outlet is closed by the diaphragm, which forms the floor of the thoracic cavity.

The *thoracic vertebrae* increase in size as one descends the vertebral column. The anterior surfaces of the vertebrae are highly convex, the posterior surfaces slightly concave. The spinous processes are typically long and directed downward enough to overlap at least the succeeding vertebra. In the lower thoracic area, however, the spinous processes shorten and broaden, becoming more like the lumbar vertebrae. The transverse processes are long and heavy, projecting posteriorly and upwardly as well as laterally; at the end of each is a facet for articulation with the tubercle of a rib.

The *ribs,* although considered "flat" bones, curve forward and downward from their posterior vertebral attachments toward their costal cartilages. The first seven ribs attach via their costal cartilages to the sternum and are called the **true ribs** (also the vertebrosternal ribs); the lower five ribs are termed the **false ribs**—the eight, ninth, and tenth ribs attach to the rib above by their costal cartilages (the vertebrochondral ribs), and the eleventh and twelfth ribs end freely (the vertebral ribs). The true ribs increase in length from above downward, while the false ribs decrease in length from above downward.

Clinical Notes: Thoracic Vertebrae

- The first, ninth, tenth, eleventh, and twelfth thoracic vertebrae are not typical of the others. The body of the first thoracic vertebra is similar to that of the cervical vertebrae (being wider transversely than the typical thoracic vertebrae) and has an entire articular facet for the head of the first rib and a demifacet for the cranial half of the head of the second rib.
- The ninth thoracic vertebra typically has one demifacet cranially, but may occasionally have a second set of demifacets caudally. When it has two sets of demifacets, the tenth has demifacets on its cranial aspect only.
- The tenth thoracic vertebra usually has one entire articular facet, which encroaches the lateral surface of the pedicle.
- The eleventh thoracic vertebra begins the transition in shape toward the lumbar vertebrae. It has one entire articular facet, located principally on the pedicles, for the head of the eleventh rib. The transverse processes are rudimentary and without facets because there is no articulation with the tubercle of the eleventh rib.
- The twelfth thoracic vertebra is similar to the eleventh, but differs at its inferior articular surfaces, which are directed more laterally, like those of the lumbar vertebrae.

Except as noted below, each rib typically has a vertebral end separated from a sternal end by the body or shaft of the rib. The *head* of the rib (at its vertebral end) is distinguished by a twin-faceted surface for articulation with the facets on the bodies of two adjacent thoracic vertebrae. The cranial facet is smaller than the caudal, and a crest between these permits attachment of the interarticular ligament.

The *neck* is the 1-inch long portion of the rib extending laterally from the head; it provides attachment for the anterior costotransverse ligament along its cranial border. The *tubercle* at the junction of the neck and the body of the rib consists of an articular and a nonarticular portion. The articular part of the tubercle (the more medial and inferior of the two) has a facet for articulation with the transverse process of the inferiormost vertebra to which the head is connected. The nonarticular part of the tubercle provides attachment for the ligament of the tubercle.

The *shaft* or *body* of the rib is simultaneously bent in two directions and twisted about its long axis, presenting two surfaces (internal and external) and two borders (superior and inferior). A *costal groove*, for the intercostal vessels and nerve, extends along the inferior border dorsally but changes to the internal surface at the angle of the rib. The sternal end of the rib terminates in an oval depression into which the costal cartilage makes its attachment.

The **sternum** comprises three parts:

The **manubrium** articulates with the clavicles, the first and second ribs, and the body of the sternum.

The *body* articulates with the second through seventh ribs, the manubrium, and the xiphoid process.

The **xiphoid process** articulates with the seventh rib and the body of the sternum.

Mediastinum

The space between the pleurae from the vertebral surfaces to the sternum and from the thoracic inlet to the diaphragm at the thoracic outlet is occupied by the **mediastinum.** As seen in Figure 1–4, the mediastinum may be separated into superior and inferior divisions for description. The **superior division** extends from the thoracic inlet above, downward to a line running from the lower bor-

Clinical Notes: Ribs

- The first, second, tenth, eleventh, and twelfth ribs are unlike the other, more typical ribs. The first rib is the shortest and most curved of all the ribs. Its head is small and rounded and has only one facet for articulation with the body of the first thoracic vertebra. The sternal end of the first rib is larger and thicker than it is in any of the other ribs.
- The second rib, although longer than the first, is similarly curved. The body is not twisted. There is a short costal groove on its internal surface posteriorly.
- The tenth through twelfth ribs each have only one articular facet on their heads. The eleventh and twelfth ribs have no necks or tubercles and are narrowed at their free anterior ends. The twelfth rib may sometimes be even shorter than the first rib.

Figure 1–4. Right lateral view of the mediastinum. The superior division contains the trachea, the arch of the aorta, the common carotid and subclavian arteries, and the upper portion of the esophagus. The inferior division is subdivided into anterior, middle, and posterior compartments. The anterior compartment contains the ascending aorta and the inferior portion of the thymus. The middle compartment contains the heart. The posterior compartment contains the thoracic aorta and the lower portion of the esophagus. (Adapted from Philo R, Bosner MD, LeMaistre A, et al. Guide to Human Anatomy. Philadelphia, WB Saunders, 1985, p 161.)

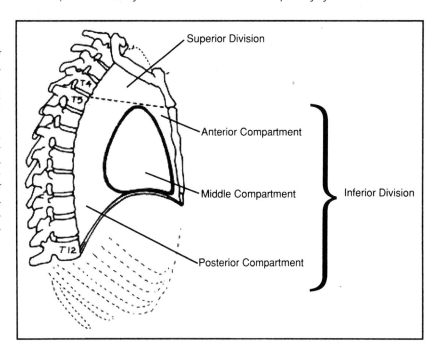

der of the fourth thoracic vertebra to the lower border of the manubrium; it contains the thymus, the trachea, the arch of the aorta, and the esophagus. The **inferior division,** extending below this line downward to the diaphragmatic closure of the thoracic outlet, is further divided into anterior, middle, and posterior compartments by the **pericardium.** The pericardium is a fibroserous sac, which encloses the heart.

The **anterior compartment** lies between the sternum and the pericardium; it contains the ascending aorta. The **middle compartment** of the inferior division is bounded by the pericardium, containing the heart and the large vessels entering or exiting it. The **posterior compartment** lies posterior to the pericardium and the diaphragm and anterior to the bodies of the fifth through twelfth thoracic vertebrae; it contains the esophagus and thoracic aorta. Knowledge of the structure of the mediastinum is important in the interpretation of chest x-rays.

RESPIRATORY SYSTEM

The respiratory system includes the bony thorax, the muscles of ventilation, the upper and the lower airways, and the pulmonary circulation. The many functions of the respiratory system include gas exchange, fluid exchange, maintenance of a relatively low volume blood reservoir, filtration, and metabolism, and they necessitate an intimate and exquisite interaction of these various components. Because the thorax has already been discussed, this section will deal with the muscles of ventilation, the upper and lower airways, and the pulmonary circulation. Respiratory physiology will be presented in Chapter 2.

Muscles of Ventilation

Ventilation of the lungs results from the coordinated interaction of the muscles of the neck, thorax, and abdomen. Note that the specific timing of muscular actions is debatable because the type and extent of activity probably changes with the magnitude of the ventilatory effort.[11] Nonetheless, there is general agreement as to which muscles constitute the primary and major accessory inspiratory groups.

Primary Inspiratory Muscles

The **diaphragm** is a musculotendinous dome that forms the floor of the thorax; its skeletal attachments arise from a tripartite (sternal, costal, and lumbar) origin to converge into a central tendon at the apex of the dome:

The sternal portion arises from the posterior aspect of the xiphoid process.

The costal portion arises from interdigitations with the transverse abdominal muscle, from the inner surfaces of the costal cartilages and the adjacent areas of the last six ribs bilaterally.

The lumbar portion arises via two aponeurotic arches, the medial and lateral lumbocostal arches (arcuate ligaments), and from the lumbar vertebrae by means of a right crus and a left crus. The crura blend with the anterior longitudinal ligament of the vertebral column and are attached to the anterior surfaces of the lumbar vertebral bodies and intervertebral disks— first three on the right, first two on the left. The medial lumbocostal arch extends from the body of the first or second lumbar vertebra to the front of the transverse process of the first lumbar vertebra. The lateral lumbocostal arch extends from the transverse process of the first lumbar vertebra to the tip and lower border of the twelfth rib.

During normal ventilatory effort (with the lower ribs fixed), the diaphragm contracts from its crural and rib attachments to pull the central tendon down and forward. In so doing, the domed shape of the diaphragm is largely maintained until the abdominal muscles end their extensibility, halting the downward displacement of the abdominal viscera, essentially forming a fixed platform beneath the central tendon. The central tendon then becomes a fixed point against which the muscular fibers of the diaphragm contract to elevate the lower ribs and thereby push the sternum and upper ribs forward. The right hemidiaphragm meets more resistance than the left (because the liver underlies the right hemidiaphragm, the stomach the left) during its descent; it is therefore more substantial than the left.

The level of the diaphragm varies considerably depending on body position and depth of ventilation.[12-15] In the supine position, both hemidiaphragms rest high in the thorax and their normal inspiratory excursion is greatest in this position. In the upright position, the level and excursion of the diaphragm is intermediate; in the sitting posi-

tion the diaphragm is lower and its excursion is smaller. In the side-lying position the hemidiaphragms are unequal in their positions: the uppermost side drops to a lower level and has less excursion than that in the sitting position; the lowermost side rises higher in the thorax and has a greater excursion than in the sitting position. In quiet breathing, the diaphragm normally moves about $\frac{2}{3}$ inch; with maximal ventilatory effort the diaphragm may move from $2\frac{1}{2}$ to 4 inches.

Accessory Inspiratory Muscles

Eleven pairs of **intercostal muscles** occupy the intercostal spaces, connecting adjoining ribs. The exact action of the intercostal muscles remains something of a controversy because all the following actions have been reported: as a group they elevate the ribs during inspiratory effort; the external intercostals elevate and the internal intercostals depress the ribs; they act in concert to prevent "bulging" or "sucking in" of the intercostal spaces during ventilation; and they also may act primarily as postural muscles. Perhaps the apparent discrepancy is simply a function of the type and extent of activity that ensues with varying magnitudes of the ventilatory effort.[11] Regardless, the skeletal attachments of the external, internal, and innermost intercostal muscles are as described here:

- *External intercostals.* Each muscle passes obliquely upward and backward from the upper border of one rib to the lower border of the rib above, and extends forward from the tubercle of the rib nearly to the costochondral junction, where it is continued as an aponeurosis—the *external intercostal membrane*—to the sternum.
- *Internal intercostals.* Each muscle passes obliquely upward and forward from the upper border of one rib to the floor of the costal groove of the rib above, and extends backward from the sternum to the posterior costal angle, where it is continued as an aponeurosis—the *internal intercostal membrane*—to blend with the superior costotransverse ligament.
- *Innermost intercostals.* These muscles attach to the internal aspects of two adjacent ribs, running in the same direction as the internal intercostals. They occupy the middle half of the ribs, being

separated from the internal intercostals by the intercostal nerves and vessels, and are not well formed in the upper thoracic level.

The **sternocleidomastoid** arises by two heads (sternal and clavicular, from the medial part of the clavicle), which unite to extend obliquely upward and laterally across the neck to the mastoid process.

The **scalene muscles** lie deep to the sternocleidomastoid, but may be palpated in the posterior triangle of the neck.

- Anterior scalene muscle passes from the anterior tubercles of the transverse processes of the third or fourth to the sixth cervical vertebrae, attaching by tendinous insertion into the first rib.
- Middle scalene muscle arises from the transverse processes of all the cervical vertebrae to insert onto the first rib (posteromedially to the anterior scalene the brachial plexus and subclavian artery pass between anterior scalene and middle scalene).
- Posterior scalene muscle arises from the posterior tubercles of the transverse processes of the fifth and sixth cervical vertebrae, passing between the middle scalene and levator scapulae, to attach onto the second or third rib.

The **trapezius** (upper fibers) muscle arises from the medial part of the superior nuchal line on the occiput and the ligamentum nuchae (from the vertebral spinous processes between the skull and the seventh cervical vertebra) to insert onto the distal third of the clavicle.

The **pectoralis major** arises from the medial third of the clavicle, from the lateral part of the anterior surface of the manubrium and body of the sternum, and from the costal cartilages of the first six ribs to insert upon the lateral lip of the crest of the greater tubercle of the humerus.

The **pectoralis minor** arises from the second to fifth or the third to sixth ribs upward to insert into the medial side of the coracoid process close to the tip.

The **serratus anterior** arises from the outer surfaces of the upper eight or nine ribs to attach along the costal aspect of the medial border of the scapula.

The **latissimus dorsi** arises from the spinous processes of the lower six thoracic, the lumbar, and the upper sacral vertebrae, from the posterior aspect of the iliac crest, and slips from the lower three or four ribs to attach to the intertubercular groove of the humerus.

The **serratus posterior superior** passes from the lower part of the ligamentum nuchae and the spinous processes of the seventh cervical and first two or three thoracic vertebrae downward into the upper borders of the second to fourth or fifth ribs.

The **quadratus lumborum** extends from the iliac crest (and the transverse processes of the lumbar vertebrae between) upward to the twelfth rib.

The **iliocostalis** muscles form the most lateral division of the erector spinae.

- **Iliocostalis lumborum** extends from the sacrum, the iliac crest, and the spinous processes of most of the lumbar and the lower two thoracic vertebrae, upward to the lower borders of the last six or seven ribs as far laterally as their angles.
- **Iliocostalis thoracis** reaches from the upper borders of the lower six ribs medial to the insertion of the iliocostalis lumborum up to the upper six ribs.
- **Iliocostalis cervicis** passes medial to the iliocostalis thoracis from the angles of the upper six ribs to insert into the transverse processes of the fourth, fifth, and sixth cervical vertebrae.

Pleurae

A membranous serous sac—the **pleura**—covers each lung (Fig. 1–5). The pleura covering the surface of each lung is called the **visceral pleura** and is inseparable from the tissue of the lung, invaginating to adhere to all surfaces of the lung. The pleura covering the inner surface of the chest wall, the exposed part of the diaphragm, and the mediastinum is called the **parietal pleura.** The parietal pleura is frequently described with reference to the anatomic surfaces it covers: the portion lining the ribs and vertebrae is named the *costovertebral pleura;* the portion over the diaphragm is the *diaphragmatic pleura;* the portion covering the uppermost aspect of the lung in the neck is the *cervical pleura;* and that overlying the mediastinum is called the *mediastinal pleura.* Parietal and visceral pleurae blend with one another where they come together to enclose the root of the lung. Normally

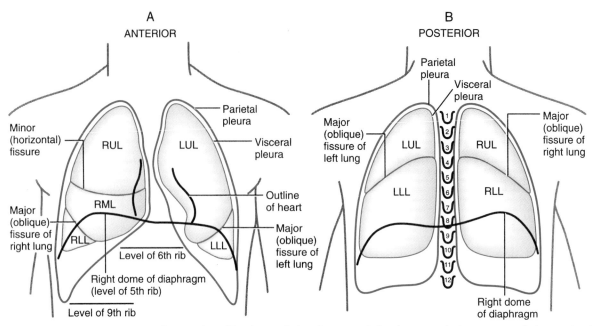

Figure 1-5. Anterior (*A*) and posterior (*B*) views of the fissures of the lungs and the extent of the parietal pleura. (Redrawn from Kersten LD. Comprehensive Respiratory Nursing: A Decision Making Approach. Philadelphia, WB Saunders, 1989, p 8.)

the pleurae are in intimate contact during all phases of the ventilatory cycle, being separated only by a thin serous film. The potential space between the pleurae is called the **pleural space.**

The parietal pleura receives its vascular supply from the intercostal, internal thoracic, and musculophrenic arteries. Venous drainage is accomplished by way of the systemic veins in the adjacent parts of the chest wall. The bronchial vessels supply the visceral pleura.

Lungs

The lungs are located on either side of the thoracic cavity, separated by the mediastinum. Each lung lies freely within its corresponding pleural cavity, except where it is attached to the heart and trachea by the root and pulmonary ligament. The substance of the lung—the **parenchyma**—is normally porous and spongy in nature. The surfaces of the lungs are marked by numerous intersecting lines, which indicate the polyhedral (secondary) lobules of the lung. The lungs are basically cone-shaped and are described as having an apex, a base, three borders, and two surfaces.

The apex of each lung is situated in the root of the neck, its highest point being about 1 inch above the middle third of each clavicle. The base of each lung is concave, resting on the convex surface of the diaphragm, which separates the left lung from the left lobe of the liver, the fundus of the stomach, and the spleen and separates the right lung from the right lobe of the liver. The inferior border of the lung separates the base of the lung from its costal surface; the posterior border separates the costal surface from the vertebral aspect of the mediastinal surface; the anterior border of each lung is thin and overlaps the front of the pericardium. Additionally, the anterior border

Clinical Notes: Pleural Nerves

The parietal pleura receives somatosensory nerve fibers, but the visceral pleura does not. The intercostal nerves supply the costal and peripheral diaphragmatic pleura; the phrenic nerve supplies the mediastinal and central diaphragmatic pleura. Thus, irritation of the intercostally innervated pleura may result in the referral of pain to the thoracic or abdominal walls, and irritation of the phrenic supplied pleura can result in referred pain in the lower neck and shoulder.

of the left lung presents a **cardiac notch.** The costal surface of each lung conforms to the shape of the overlying chest wall. The medial surface of each lung may be divided into vertebral and mediastinal aspects. The vertebral aspect contacts the respective sides of the thoracic vertebrae and their intervertebral disks, the posterior intercostal vessels, and nerves. The mediastinal aspect is notable for the *cardiac impression;* this concavity is larger on the left than the right lung to accommodate the projection of the apex of the heart toward the left. Just posterior to the cardiac impression is the **hilus,** where the structures forming the root of the lung enter and exit the parenchyma. The extension of the pleural covering below and behind the hilus from the root of the lung forms the **pulmonary ligament.**

Hila and Roots

The point at which the nerves, vessels, and primary bronchi penetrate the parenchyma of each lung is called the **hilus.** The structures entering the hila of the lungs and forming the roots of each of the lungs are the principal bronchus, the pulmonary artery, the pulmonary veins, the bronchial arteries and veins, the pulmonary nerve plexus, and the lymph vessels (Fig. 1–6). They lie next to the vertebral bodies of the fifth, sixth, and seventh thoracic vertebrae. The right root lies behind the superior vena cava and a portion of the right atrium, below the end of the azygos vein; the left root lies below the arch of the aorta and in front of the descending thoracic aorta. The pulmonary ligament lies below the root; the phrenic

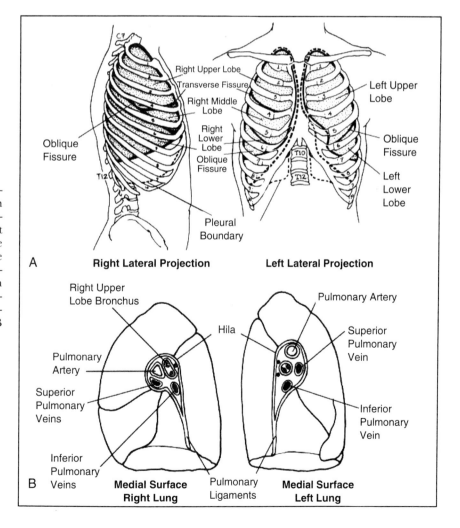

Figure 1–6. *A,* Lateral and anterior views of the lungs through the rib cage at functional residual capacity, showing the extent of the pleurae and the relative positions of the lungs. *B,* The medial view of the lungs demonstrates hilar structures. (Redrawn from Philo R, Bosner MS, LeMaistre A, et al. Guide to Human Anatomy. Philadelphia, WB Saunders, 1985, pp 156, 158.)

nerve and the anterior pulmonary plexus lie in front of the root; the vagus nerve and posterior pulmonary plexus lie behind the root.

Fissures and Lobes

The upper and middle lobes of the right lung are separated from the lower lobe by the **oblique (major) fissure** (Figs. 1–5 and 1–6). Starting on the medial surface of the right lung at the upper posterior aspect of the hilus, the oblique fissure runs upward and backward to the posterior border at about the level of the fourth thoracic vertebra, it then descends anteroinferiorly across the anterior costal surface to intersect the lower border of the lung about 5 inches from the median plane, and then passes posterosuperiorly to rejoin the hilus just behind and beneath the upper pulmonary vein. The middle lobe is separated from the upper lobe by the **horizontal (minor) fissure,** which joins the oblique fissure at the midaxillary line at about the level of the fourth rib and runs horizontally across the costal surface of the lung to about the level of the fourth costal cartilage; on the medial surface, it passes backward to join the hilus near the upper right pulmonary vein. The left lung is divided into upper and lower lobes by the *oblique fissure,* which is somewhat more vertically oriented than that of the right lung; there is no horizontal fissure.

Pulmonary Vessels

There are actually two vascular systems serving the lungs: the *pulmonary circulation* delivers deoxygenated blood to the lungs and returns oxygenated blood to the heart, and the *bronchial circulation* delivers the nutrient blood supply to the lungs.

Pulmonary Circulation

The number of pulmonary arteries and veins going to and from the terminal respiratory units of each lung is set at birth.[16–18] However, the number of vessels within the terminal respiratory units at birth is markedly less than after the first 10 years of life (their development paralleling that of new primary lobules).

Other changes to the pulmonary arteries occur during growth as well. During gestation, all arterial branches of the pulmonary circulation have relatively thick walls because of the large amount of smooth muscle in their medial layers. Following birth (with the normal lowering of pulmonary vascular resistance) the distal arteries rapidly become thinner until, by the age of 4 months, they closely resemble those of adult lungs (with respect to muscular content and distribution).[19]

The **pulmonary trunk,** the **right** and **left pulmonary arteries,** and their principal branches down to the (secondary) lobular level are considered to be elastic arteries; the intralobular arteries are of the muscular type. Nonetheless, the muscular arteries have very thin muscular layers (not exceeding 5% of the external diameter of the vessel, except in pathologic conditions). The **pulmonary arterioles** have a partial muscular layer near their origins, but this tapers away until the vessel wall consists of only thin endothelium and elastic lamina.[20, 21] The **pulmonary capillaries** form an intermeshed network in the walls and septa of the alveolar ducts and alveoli. The **pulmonary veins** drain the pulmonary capillaries, from which they coalesce to form larger branches, until ultimately coming into proximity with the pulmonary arteries as two pulmonary veins from each lung. The pulmonary veins serve as a relatively low volume reservoir for the left ventricle, normally obviating the minor fluctuations in right ventricular stroke volume that occur as a result of ventilatory effort.

The right pulmonary artery gives off a large branch to the upper lobe before entering the hilus of the right lung. The continuation of the right pulmonary artery passes between the upper lobe and continuing mainstem bronchi toward the oblique fissure, where it gives branches to the middle and lower lobes. The left pulmonary artery crosses anterior to the left mainstem bronchus toward the posterolateral aspect of the hilus; upon entering the lung, it gives off branches first to the upper lobe segments and then to the lower lobe segments. Although the pulmonary veins and arteries closely parallel the main divisions of the bronchi, they assume different relationships at the segmental level. Generally, the pulmonary arteries accompany the bronchi in their segmental divisions. The coalescing tributaries of the pulmonary veins, however, run between the bronchopulmonary segments. In this manner, the tributaries drain adjacent segments and each segment is drained by more than one vein. The variation in the subsegmental branching of the bronchi, arteries, and veins is considerable, the veins being the most variable and the bronchi the least.

Bronchial Circulation

The bronchial arteries vary significantly in their number and origin. There is typically one right bronchial artery, arising from the right intercostal, right subclavian, or internal mammary artery. Two left bronchial arteries often arise directly from the upper thoracic aorta. The number of branches entering the root of each lung is variable, but upon entry, they distribute themselves within the connective tissue surrounding the bronchi in a peribronchial plexus that accompanies each subdivision of the airways down to the level of the terminal bronchioles. Near the terminal bronchioles, the bronchial arterioles form a network of capillaries that anastomose readily with the capillaries of the pulmonary circulation. Total bronchial blood flow to both lungs is estimated to be about 1% to 2% of the cardiac output.

The bronchial veins are frequently considered in two parts: the **deep (distal) bronchial veins** and the **superficial (proximal) bronchial veins.** The deep bronchial veins begin as a network around the terminal bronchioles and form tributaries (sometimes referred to as bronchopulmonary veins) that join the pulmonary veins. The superficial bronchial veins (true bronchial veins) are formed from tributaries originating around the segmental and lobar bronchi and from pleural branches near the hilus. These bronchial veins drain into the azygos, hemiazygos, or intercostal veins, the blood ultimately reaching the vena cava and returning to the right atrium. Although not directly measured in humans, it is estimated that about 25 to 33% of the bronchial arterial supply is returned to the right atrium via the true bronchial veins, and two thirds to three quarters is returned to the left atrium via the pulmonary veins.[22, 23] The relationship of the bronchial and pulmonary circulations is symbiotic. Thus, if the perfusion pressure of one system changes, there is a concomitant oppositely directed change in the other. The benefit of this reciprocal relationship should be immediately apparent—preservation of viability when either circulation is impaired by disease.[24]

A third circulatory system in the lungs—the lymphatic circulation—must also be considered.

The lymphatic circulation drains excess fluids from the interstitial spaces and serves as a pathway for the elimination of particulate matter and microorganisms that reach the alveoli. The pulmonary lymphatics reside in the pleural, interseptal, and peribronchiovascular connective tissue spaces, where lymphatic capillaries form extensive plexuses. Although further discussion will not be made here, the importance of the lymphatic system should not be overlooked; for a detailed discussion, the reader is referred to Leak and Jamuar.[25]

Upper Respiratory Tract

The upper respiratory tract (upper airways, Fig. 1–7) extends from the nasal and oral orifices to the false vocal cords in the larynx.

Nose

The nose is a conglomerate of bone and hyaline cartilage. The nasal bones (right and left), the frontal processes of the maxillae, and the nasal part of the frontal bone combine to form the bony framework of the nose. The septal, lateral, and major and minor alar cartilages combine to form the cartilaginous framework of the nose. The periosteal and perichondral membranes blend to connect the bones and cartilages to one another.

A small slip of muscle—the *procerus muscle*—originating as a continuation of the occipitofrontalis, attaches to the fascia covering the lower part of the nasal bone and the upper part of the lateral nasal cartilage (this is the muscle that "wrinkles" the skin of the nose). The *nasalis muscles* (the muscles that flare the anterior nasal aperture) arise lateral to the nasal notch of the maxilla and spread over the bridge of the nose to form a joint aponeurosis with the procerus (the transverse part), in addition to attaching to the alar cartilages (the alar part). The *depressor septi muscle* runs from the maxilla above the central incisor tooth to the nasal septum; together with the nasalis, it flares the nostrils. Skin covers the external nose.

Nasal Cavity

The **nasal cavity** is a wedge-shaped passageway, divided vertically into right and left halves by the

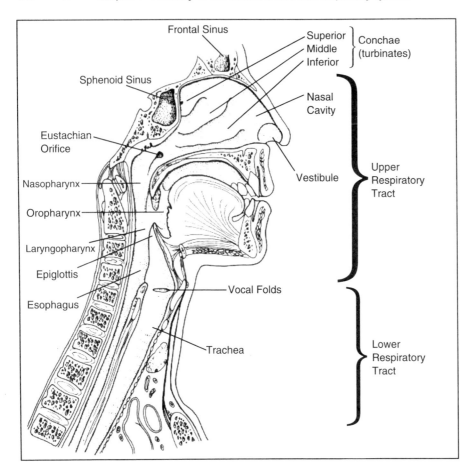

Figure 1–7. Sagittal section through the head and neck showing the upper respiratory tract and the superior aspect of the lower respiratory tract. (Redrawn from Philo R, Bosner MS, LeMaistre A, et al. Guide to Human Anatomy. Philadelphia, WB Saunders, 1985, p 76.)

nasal septum and compartmentalized by the **paranasal sinuses** (Fig. 1–8). Opening anteriorly via the **nares** (nostrils) to the external environment, the nasal cavity blends posteriorly with the nasopharynx. The two halves are essentially identical, having a floor, medial and lateral walls, and a roof divided into three regions—the vestibule, the olfactory region, and the respiratory region. The primary respiratory functions of the nasal cavity include air conduction, filtration, humidification, and temperature control; it also plays a role in the olfactory process.

The palatine process of the maxilla (anterior three fourths) and the horizontal part of the palatine bone (posterior one fourth) form the floor of the nasal cavity. The medial wall is formed by the nasal septum. Three **nasal conchae** project into the nasal cavity from the lateral wall toward the medial wall; they are named the superior, middle, and inferior conchae. The roof is made up of frontonasal, ethmoidal, and sphenoidal parts that correspond to the bones that form each part.

The **vestibule of the nasal cavity** extends from the nares backward and upward about $\frac{2}{3}$ inch to the **limen nasi** (which corresponds to the upper limit of the lower nasal cartilage). The vestibule is lined with skin containing many coarse hairs and sebaceous and sweat glands. Mucous membrane lines the remainder of the nasal cavity. Figure 1–9 depicts examples of some selected types of mucosal coverings in the upper and lower respiratory tracts.

The **olfactory region of the nasal cavity** is distinguished by the specialized mucosa overlying it in the area of the superior concha, the roof, and upper aspect of the septum opposite the superior concha. This pseudostratified olfactory epithelium is thicker than the respiratory mucosa covering the respiratory region of the nasal cavity and is composed of ciliated receptor cells, nonciliated sustentacular cells, and basal cells.

The rest of the nasal cavity is considered the **respiratory region.** This area, and the paranasal sinuses, is lined with a mixture of columnar or

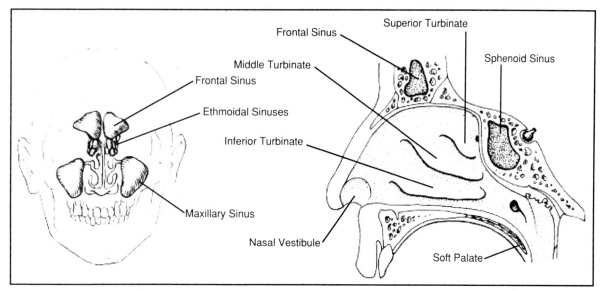

Figure 1-8. The nasal cavity, the nasopharynx, and the paranasal sinuses. (Redrawn from Philo R, Bosner MS, LeMaistre A, et al. Guide to Human Anatomy. Philadelphia, WB Saunders, 1985, pp 77–78.)

pseudostratified ciliated epithelial cells, goblet cells, nonciliated columnar cells with microvilli, and basal cells. Serous and mucous glands, which open to the surface via branched ducts, underlie the basal lamina of respiratory epithelium.[26-28]

The submucosal glands and goblet cells secrete an abundant quantity of mucus over the mucosa of the nasal cavity, making it moist and sticky. Turbulent airflow, created by the conchae, causes inhaled dust and other particulate matter, larger than about 10 μm, to "rain out" onto this sticky layer, which is then moved by ciliary action backward and downward out of the nasal cavity into the nasopharynx at an average rate of about 6 mm per minute.[29, 30]

The **paranasal sinuses**—*frontal, ethmoidal, sphenoidal,* and *maxillary*—vary widely in their size and shape from person to person. Their exact function is unknown and they will not be considered further here.

Pharynx

The **pharynx** is a musculomembranous tube about 5 to 6 inches long having an upper limit that corresponds with the basal surface of the skull and a lower limit that corresponds with a line extending from the sixth cervical vertebra to the lower border of the cricoid cartilage. The pharynx con-

sists of three parts: the nasopharynx, the oropharynx, and the laryngopharynx. These parts will be described briefly; consideration of the muscles of the pharynx exceeds the scope of this chapter.

Nasopharynx

The **nasopharynx** is a continuation of the nasal cavity, beginning at the posterior nasal apertures and continuing backward and downward. Its roof and posterior wall are continuous; its lateral walls are formed by the openings of the eustachian tubes; and its floor is formed by the soft palate anteriorly and the pharyngeal *isthmus* (the space between the free edge of the soft palate and the posterior wall of the pharynx), which marks the transition to the oropharynx. The epithelium of the nasopharynx is composed of ciliated columnar cells.

Oropharynx

The **oropharynx** extends from the soft palate and pharyngeal isthmus superiorly to the upper border of the epiglottis inferiorly. Anteriorly, it is bounded by the oropharyngeal isthmus (which opens into the mouth) and the pharyngeal part of the tongue. The posterior aspect of the orophar-

SQUAMOUS

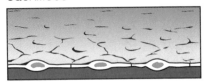

including
mesothelium–lining coelomic surfaces;
endothelium–lining vascular channels.
Structural variants include continuous,
discontinuous, and fenestrated endothelia.

CUBOIDAL

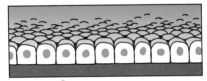

COLUMNAR

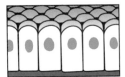

Without surface
specialization

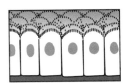

With microvilli
(brush/striated border)

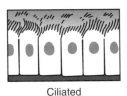

Ciliated

Figure 1-9. Types of cells composing the mucosal lining of the upper and lower respiratory tracts. (Modified from Williams PL, Warwick R, Dyson M, Bannister LH [eds]. Gray's Anatomy. 37th ed. New York, Churchill Livingstone, 1989, p 52.)

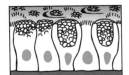

Glandular

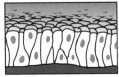

Pseudostratified
(distorted columnar)

STRATIFIED
CUBOIDAL/COLUMNAR

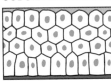

TRANSITIONAL

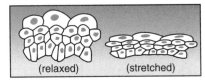

(relaxed)   (stretched)

ynx is at the level of the body of the second cervical vertebra and upper portion of the body of the third cervical vertebra. The epithelium in the oropharynx is composed of stratified squamous cells.

level of the lower portion of the third, the bodies of the fourth and fifth, and the upper portion of the body of the sixth cervical vertebrae. The epithelium in the laryngopharynx is composed of stratified squamous cells.

Laryngopharynx

The **laryngopharynx** extends from the upper border of the epiglottis to the inferior border of the cricoid cartilage and the esophagus. The laryngeal orifice and the posterior surfaces of the arytenoid and cricoid cartilages form the anterior aspect of the laryngopharynx. The posterior aspect is at the

Larynx

A cartilaginous framework composed of the thyroid, cricoid, and epiglottic cartilages, and the paired arytenoid, cuneiform, and corniculate cartilages forms the **larynx**. It extends anteriorly from the laryngopharynx, between the great vessels of the neck, downward to the trachea (with which it is continuous). The position of the larynx depends upon the age and sex of the individual, being opposite the third to sixth cervical vertebrae in the adult male and somewhat higher in adult females and children. In infants up to about 1 year of age, the highest part of the larynx is a little above the level of the upper aspect of the dens. Further consideration of the structure or the musculature of the larynx is beyond the scope of this chapter.

The cavity of the larynx, extending from the laryngeal inlet to the lower border of the cricoid cartilage, may be divided into three parts: upper, middle, and lower. The vestibular folds separate the upper and middle parts; the vocal folds separate the middle and lower parts.

The laryngeal inlet angles downward from front to back because the anterior wall of the larynx is much longer than the posterior wall; the upper edge of the epiglottis marks its anterior aspect; the **aryepiglottic folds,** formed in the mucosal tissue stretching between the sides of the epiglottis and the apex of the arytenoid cartilage, form its lateral borders; the posterior margin is formed by the mucous membrane stretching between the arytenoid cartilages. The laryngeal vestibule extends from the inlet to the vestibular folds. The vestibular folds are thick folds of mucous membrane covering the vestibular ligament, a fibrous band of tissue stretched between an anterior attachment at the angle of the thyroid cartilage just below the level of the epiglottic cartilage, extending to the anterolateral surface of the arytenoids posteriorly.

The middle part of the laryngeal cavity is the smallest, extending from the *rima vestibuli* (the fissure between the vestibular folds) to the *rima glottidis* (the fissure between the vocal folds, commonly called the **glottis**). A fusiform recess, known as the *sinus of the larynx,* lies between the vestibular and vocal folds. A small pouch—the *saccule of the larynx*—extends upward from the anterior aspect of the sinus. Many mucous glands open into the saccule, which is enclosed in a fibrous capsule receiving a few muscular fasciculi from the thyroepiglottic muscle. The muscles squeeze the sac, expelling its mucus secretions onto the surfaces of the vocal folds, lubricating and nourishing them. The vocal folds are thin folds of mucous membrane stretched between the middle angle of the thyroid cartilage to the vocal processes of the arytenoid cartilages. The epithelial covering of

stratified squamous cells is so closely bound to the elastic *vocal ligament* (a continuation of the cricothyroid ligament) that there is no submucosal layer or blood vessels.

The lower part of the laryngeal cavity extends from the vocal folds to the lower border of the cricoid cartilage.

Lower Respiratory Tract

The lower respiratory tract extends from the level of the true vocal cords in the larynx to the alveoli within the lungs (Fig. 1–10). Generally, the lower respiratory tract may be divided into two parts: the *tracheobronchial tree*, or *conducting airways*, and the *acinar* or *terminal respiratory units* (Fig. 1–10A and C). As noted earlier, the basic structure of the cartilaginous conducting airways is complete at the time of birth; additional branching does not occur. In fact, although the extent of the process is controversial, the number of nonrespiratory bronchioles may actually decrease, due to their conversion by alveolarization into respiratory units, up to the age of 3 years.[31, 32]

Tracheobronchial Tree— Conducting Airways

The conducting airways are not directly involved in the exchange of gases in the lungs; they simply conduct air to and from the respiratory units. Airway diameter progressively decreases with each succeeding generation of branching, starting at about 1 inch in diameter at the trachea and reaching 1 mm or less at the terminal bronchioles. The cartilaginous rings of the larger airways give way to irregular cartilaginous plates, which become smaller and more widely spaced with each generation of branching, until they disappear at the bronchiolar level.[5, 33] There may be as many as 16 generations of branching in the conducting airways from the mainstem bronchi to the terminal bronchioles (Fig. 1–11).[34]

Trachea. From the lower margin of the cricoid cartilage, the trachea is a tube (about 4 to $4\frac{1}{2}$ inches long and about 1 inch in diameter) extending downward along the midline of the body. As it enters the thorax, it passes behind the left bra-

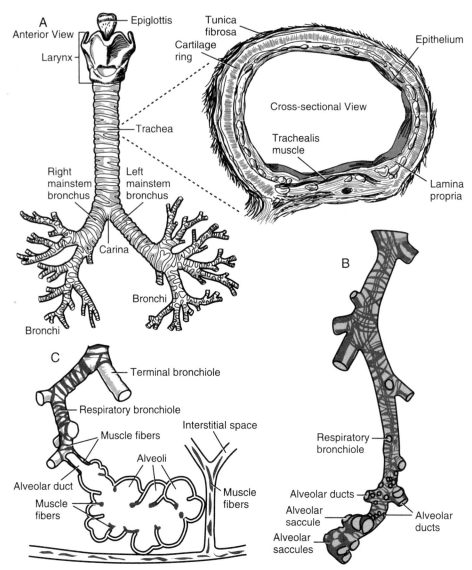

Figure 1–10. The lower respiratory tract. *A,* The trachea in anterior and cross-sectional views. (Redrawn with permission from Clemente CD. Gray's Anatomy. 30th ed. Philadelphia, Lea & Febiger, 1985, pp 1377–1378.) *B,* The general distributional scheme of the smaller airways. (Redrawn from Romanes R. Cunningham's Textbook of Anatomy. 11th ed. London, Oxford University Press, 1972, p 496. By permission of Oxford University Press.) *C,* The gross organization of the alveoli and the intimate intertwining meshwork of the capillaries, elastic fibers, and smooth muscle. (Redrawn from Nagaishi C. Functional Anatomy and Histology of the Lung. Baltimore, University Park Press, 1972, p 245.)

chiocephalic vein and artery and the arch of the aorta. At its distal end, the trachea deviates slightly to the right of midline before bifurcating into right and left mainstem bronchi. Between 16 and 20 incomplete rings of hyaline cartilage occupy the anterior two thirds of the tracheal circumference, forming a framework for the trachea. Two or more cartilages are often joined together partly or completely. Fibrous and elastic tissues and smooth muscle fibers complete the ring posteriorly. The first and last tracheal cartilages differ somewhat from the others: the first is broader and is attached by the cricotracheal ligament to the lower border of the cricoid cartilage, and the last is thicker and broader at its middle, where it projects a hook-shaped process downward and backward from its lower border—the **carina**—between the two mainstem bronchi.

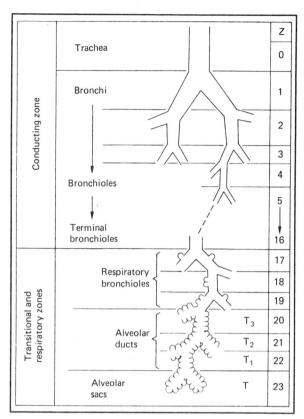

Figure 1-11. Generational structure of the airways in the human lung. (Reproduced with permission from Weibel ER, Taylor CR. Design and structure of the human lung. In: Fishman AP [ed]. Pulmonary Diseases and Disorders. 2nd ed. New York, McGraw-Hill, 1988, p 13.)

Mainstem and Lobar Bronchi. The right mainstem bronchus is wider and shorter than its left counterpart, and it diverges at about a 25-degree angle from the trachea. It passes laterally downward behind the superior vena cava for about 1 inch before giving off its first branch—the **upper (superior) lobe bronchus**—and entering the root of the right lung. About 1 inch farther, it gives off its second branch—the **middle lobe bronchus**—from within the oblique fissure. Thereafter, the remnant of the mainstem bronchus continues as the **lower (inferior, basal) lobe bronchus.**

The left mainstem bronchus leaves the trachea at an angle of about 40 to 60 degrees and passes below the arch of the aorta and behind the left pulmonary artery, proceeding for a little more than 2 inches before it enters the root of the left lung before giving off the *upper* (superior) *lobe bronchus* and continuing on as the *lower* (inferior, basal) *lobe bronchus.* The left lung has no middle lobe, which is a major distinguishing feature in the general architecture of lungs.

Segmental and Subsegmental Bronchi. Each of the lobar bronchi gives off two or more segmental bronchi; an understanding of their anatomy is essential to the appropriate assessment and treatment of pulmonary disorders (Fig. 1–12). The right upper lobe bronchus divides into three segmental bronchi about $\frac{1}{2}$ inch from its own origin: the first—the **apical segmental bronchus**—passes superolaterally toward its distribution in the apex of the lung; the second—the **posterior segmental bronchus**—proceeds slightly upward and posterolaterally to its distribution in the posteroinferior aspect of the upper lobe; the third—the **anterior segmental bronchus**—runs anteroinferiorly to its distribution in the remainder of the upper lobe. The right middle lobe bronchus divides into a **lateral segmental bronchus,** which is distributed to the lateral aspect of the middle lobe, and a **medial segmental bronchus** to the medial aspect. The right lower lobe bronchus first gives off a branch from its posterior surface—the **superior segmental bronchus**—which passes posterosuperiorly to its distribution in the upper portion of the lower lobe. Then, after continuing to descend posterolaterally, the lower lobe bronchus yields the **medial basal segmental bronchus** (distributed to a small area below the hilus) from its anteromedial surface. The next offshoots from the lower lobe bronchus are the **anterior basal segmental bronchus,** which continues its descent anteriorly, and a very small trunk that almost immediately splits into the **lateral basal segmental bronchus** (distributed to the lower lateral area of the lower lobe) and the **posterior basal segmental bronchus** (distributed to the lower posterior area of the lower lobe).

The left upper lobe bronchus extends laterally from the anterolateral aspect of the left mainstem bronchus before dividing into correlates of the right upper and middle lobar bronchi. However, these two branches remain within the left upper lobe because there is no left middle lobe. The uppermost branch ascends for about $\frac{1}{3}$ inch before yielding the **anterior segmental bronchus,** then continues its upward path as the **apicoposterior segmental bronchus** before subdividing further into its subsegmental distribution. The caudal branch descends anterolaterally to its distribution

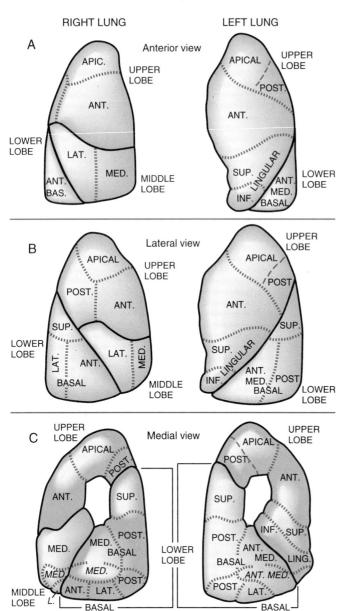

Figure 1–12. Anterior (*A*), lateral (*B*), and medial (*C*) views of the bronchopulmonary segments as seen projected to the surface of the lungs. (Redrawn from Waldhausen JA, Pierce WS [eds]. Johnson's Surgery of the Chest. 4th ed. Chicago, Year Book Medical Publishers, 1985, pp 64–65.)

in the anteroinferior area of the left upper lobe—a region called the **lingula.** This lingular bronchus divides into the **superior lingular** and **inferior lingular segmental bronchi.**

The left lower lobe bronchus descends posterolaterally for about $\frac{1}{3}$ inch before giving off the superior segmental bronchus from its posterior surface (its distribution is similar to that of the right lower lobe superior segmental bronchus). After another $\frac{1}{2}$ to $\frac{2}{3}$ inch, the lower lobe bronchus splits in two: the anteromedial division is called the **anteromedial basal segmental bronchus,** and the pos-

terolateral division immediately branches into the **lateral basal** and **posterior basal segmental bronchi.** The distributions of these segmental bronchi are similar to those of their right lung counterparts.

Many anatomists stop the naming of the segmental branches of the upper division of the left upper lobe at the apicoposterior bronchus, but many others identify its first dichotomous branches as the apical and posterior segmental bronchi. Similarly, the anteromedial basal segmental bronchus of the left lower lobe may be described as separate anterior basal and medial basal segmental bronchi arising from a common trunk. This lack of agreement should not seriously hamper an understanding of the basic segmental distribution of the conducting airways.

Segmental bronchi in both lungs ramify within self-contained, functionally independent bronchopulmonary segments. The bronchopulmonary segments are surrounded by visceral pleura, thus forming distinctly compartmentalized ventilatory units (the importance of this compartmentalization will become clearer in later chapters dealing with pathologic states and treatment interventions). The segmental bronchi continue to repeatedly branch downward to bronchiolar size until ultimately a **lobular bronchiole** enters the **secondary lobule.**

Topographic Relationships. Topographic (ballpark) boundaries for the bronchopulmonary segments of each lung are as follows:

UPPER LOBE

1. Anterior segment (right or left)
   - Upper border: clavicle
   - Lower border: a horizontal line at the level of the third intercostal space (ICS), or fourth rib, anteriorly
2. Apical segment (R) or apical aspect, apicoposterior segment (L)
   - Anteroinferior border: clavicle
   - Posteroinferior border: a horizontal line at the level of the upper lateral border of the spine of the scapula
3. Posterior segment (R) or posterior aspect, apicoposterior segment (L)
   - Upper border: a horizontal line at the level of the upper lateral border of the spine of the scapula
   - Lower border: a horizontal line at, or approximately 1 inch below, the inferomedial aspect of the spine of the scapula

MIDDLE LOBE (R) OR LINGULA (L)

   - Upper border: a horizontal line at the level of the third ICS, or fourth rib, anteriorly
   - Lower and lateral borders: the oblique fissure (a horizontal line at the level of the sixth rib anteriorly) extending to the anterior axillary line; from the anterior axillary line, angling upward to approximately the fourth rib at the posterior axillary line

   - The midclavicular line separates the medial and lateral segments of the right middle lobe
   - A horizontal line at the level of the fifth rib, anteriorly, separates the superior and inferior lingular segments

LOWER LOBE

1. Superior (basal) segment (right or left)
   - Upper border: a horizontal line at, or approximately 1 inch below, the inferomedial aspect of the spine of the scapula
   - Lower border: a horizontal line at, or approximately 1 inch above, the inferior angle of the scapula
2. Posterior (basal) segment (right or left)
   - Upper border: a horizontal line at, or approximately 1 inch above, the inferior angle of the scapula
   - Lateral border: a "plumb line" bisecting the inferior angle of the scapula
   - Lower border: a horizontal line at the level of the tenth ICS, posteriorly
3. Lateral (basal) segment (right or left)
   - Upper border: a horizontal line at, or approximately 1 inch above, the inferior angle of the scapula
   - Medial border: a "plumb line" bisecting the inferior angle of the scapula
   - Lateral border: the midaxillary line
   - Lower border: a horizontal line at the level of the tenth ICS, posteriorly
4. Anterior (basal) segment (R) or anterior aspect, anteromedial (basal) segment (L)
   - Upper border: the oblique fissure (a horizontal line at the level of the sixth rib anteriorly, extending to the anterior axillary line; from the anterior axillary line, angling upward to approximately the fifth rib at the midaxillary line
   - Lateral border: the midaxillary line

Primary and Secondary Lobules of the Lung. Pyramid-shaped secondary lobules are the smallest portions of the lung surrounded by a discrete connective tissue septum; they are about $\frac{1}{3}$ to $\frac{2}{3}$ inch in size (Fig. 1–13).[35, 36] Within the secondary lobule, each of the lobular bronchioles immediately divides into five or six **terminal bronchioles,** which in turn subdivide into one to three **respiratory bronchioles.** The respiratory bronchioles mark the transition point from **conducting air-**

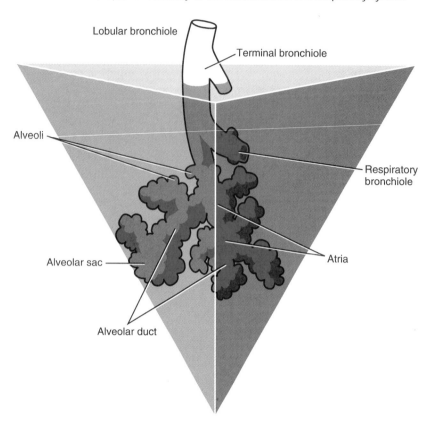

Figure 1–13. The pyramid-shaped secondary lobule arises from a lobular bronchiole. Secondary lobules are the smallest portion of the lung (about one to two thirds of an inch) surrounded by a connective tissue septum. The lung tissue supplied by a first-order alveolar duct, together with its vessels and nerves, is sometimes called the primary lobule. There may be as many as 50 primary lobules within a secondary lobule.

ways to **respiratory airways.** Although there is some disagreement regarding the nomenclature down to the level of the terminal bronchiole, there is not much disagreement regarding the terminology used to describe the airways distal to this point.

Bronchial Epithelium. The epithelium of the upper regions of the conducting airways is pseudostratified and, for the most part, ciliated. The epithelium of the terminal and respiratory bronchioles is single-layered and more cuboidal in shape, and many of the cells are nonciliated. The lamina propria, to which the epithelial basal lamina is attached, contains, throughout the length of the tracheobronchial tree, longitudinal bands of elastin that spread into the elastin network of the terminal respiratory units. The framework thus created is responsible for much of the elastic recoil of the lungs during expiration. At least eight types of cells have been identified in the bronchial epithelium of the human lung.

The most abundant types of cells in the bronchial epithelium are the *ciliated cells.* Ciliated cells are found in all levels of the tracheobronchial tree down to the level of the respiratory bronchioles. As will be discussed elsewhere, the cilia projecting from their luminal surfaces are intimately involved in the removal of inhaled particulate matter from the airways via the "mucociliary escalator" mechanism.

Two of the bronchial epithelial cells are mucus-secreting: the **mucous cells** and **serous cells.** Mucous cells, formerly called goblet cells, are normally more numerous in the trachea and large airways, becoming less numerous with distal progression until they are infrequently found in the bronchioles. Serous cells are much less numerous than mucous cells and are confined predominantly to the extrapulmonary bronchi. Both types of cells are nonciliated, although both exhibit filamentous surface projections.

Ovoid undifferentiated **basal cells** are located on the basement membrane, and are responsible for the characteristic pseudostratified appearance of the bronchial epithelium. They are most numerous in the epithelium of the extrapulmonary bronchi, although they may be found as far as the bronchioles. Basal cells have no specific function other than to differentiate as needed for the replacement of superficial ciliated or mucous cells. **Intermediate cells** are derived from the basal cells and form a pseudolayer over them. The intermediate cells elongate as they differentiate into ciliated or mucous cells.

Brush cells are also nonciliated, but have a distinct brushlike border of microvilli on their luminal surfaces. The function of brush cells is not clearly understood. However, the presence of pinocytotic vesicles at the base of the microvilli is believed to indicate a role in liquid absorption.

The **Clara cells** are found mostly in the terminal airways. These nonciliated cells may be recognized by their cytoplasmic luminal projections and contain secretory granules and lamellar bodies. The Clara cells have been postulated to be a ciliated or brush cell progenitor as well as a source of materials present in surfactant.[37-40]

The least abundant epithelial cell types are **Kulchitsky's cells,** which are similar to specialized endocrine cells of the gastro-entero-pancreatic system. Because they store and secrete amines, Kulchitsky cells have been included in the APUD (amine and amine precursor, uptake, and decarboxylation) category of the endocrine system.[41, 42] A possible role in regulation of airway or capillary luminal size in response to acute hypoxia has been suggested for aggregations of apparently innervated Kulchitsky's cells—neuroepithelial bodies—in the bronchial and bronchiolar mucosa.[43]

Two additional cell types normally occur in the bronchial epithelium but are migratory in nature. The **globular leukocytes** have numerous filopodia and are thought to derive from mast cells. **Lymphocytes** are the second non-native cells found in the mucosa. Both cell types are thought to have immunologic functions.

A characteristic feature of the submucosal layer underlying the bronchial epithelium is the presence of **bronchial glands,** which are quite numerous in the medium-sized bronchi, becoming less prevalent distally until they are absent in the bronchioles. Submucosal bronchial glands are believed to be parasympathetically innervated and are composed of several cell types, including serous cells, mucous cells, duct cells, lymphocytes, myoepithelial cells, mast cells, and Kulchitsky's cells.[44] The glands are shaped somewhat like a dual-bulbed vase with an inverted, funnel-like exit duct at the top; the two "bulbs" are lined with mucous and serous cells.[45, 46] The material that reaches the bronchial lumen from the bronchial glands is a combination of the secretions of the mucous and serous cells.

Terminal Respiratory (Acinar) Units

The **respiratory bronchioles,** which exhibit small lateral outpouchings—**alveoli**—that provide an accessory respiratory surface, open into one to three **alveolar ducts** that lead via expanded **atria** into **alveolar sacs.** The number of alveolar outpouchings increases dramatically with distal progression into the alveolar sacs. Various authors call the lung tissue supplied by a first-order alveolar duct, together with its vessels and nerves, the primary lobule,[47, 48] acinus,[49, 50] or terminal respiratory unit.[51, 52] There may be as many as 50 primary lobules within a secondary lobule.

Alveoli. The normal mature lungs contain an average of about 300 million alveoli, each of which is extremely small (between 200 to 300 μm in diameter). The total mean alveolar surface area is estimated to be about 143 ± 4 m[2].[53, 54] The walls of the alveoli consist of a thin epithelial layer over a connective tissue sublayer. The walls of the adjacent alveoli abut one another much like the pieces of a three-dimensional jigsaw puzzle, sandwiching the connective tissue and its associated vasculature between the epithelial layers. The **interalveolar septum** thus formed is composed of the alveolar epithelium, the capillary endothelium, and the interstitial space. Insofar as the proportion of cell types that compose the parenchyma of normal adult lungs, alveolar epithelium accounts for about 24% of the cell types, capillary endothelium about 30%, macrophages about 9.5%, and interstitial cells the remaining 36%.[55, 56] The interalveolar septa are interrupted by channels called the **pores of Kohn** as well as by **Lambert's canals,** which are postulated to account for significant collateral alveolar ventilation.[52, 57-60]

Alveolar Epithelium. The alveolar epithelium consists of two primary cell types (Fig. 1–14). **Type I (squamous) pneumocytes,** which cover about 93% of the alveolar surface and account for approximately 8.3% of the total cells of the parenchyma, have very thin, broad extensions projecting from their central bodies.[39, 55] Type I cells contain

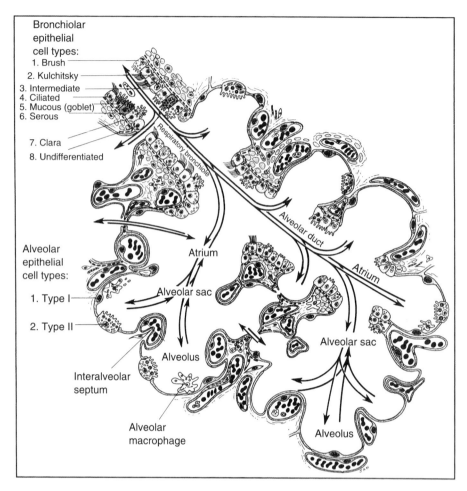

Bronchiolar
epithelial
cell types:
1. Brush
2. Kulchitsky
3. Intermediate
4. Ciliated
5. Mucous (goblet)
6. Serous
7. Clara
8. Undifferentiated

Respiratory bronchiole

Alveolar duct

Atrium

Atrium

Alveolar
epithelial
cell types:

1. Type I
2. Type II

Alveolar sac

Alveolar sac

Alveolus

Interalveolar
septum

Alveolar
macrophage

Alveolus

Figure 1-14. A cross-sectional view of the terminal respiratory unit showing the bronchiolar and alveolar epithelial cell types. (From Williams PL, Warwick R, Dyson M, Bannister LH [eds]. Gray's Anatomy. 37th ed. New York, Churchill Livingstone, 1989, p 1280.)

few cytoplasmic organelles, such as mitochondria. **Type II (granular) pneumocytes** account for approximately 16% of the total cells composing the parenchyma, but occupy only about 7% of the alveolar surface because of their small, cuboidal shape.[39, 55] The importance of the type II cells rests in their location (in the "corners" of the alveoli) and their function. Type II pneumocytes are believed to be the primary producers of the phospholipid film **surfactant.** Surfactant consists mostly of dipalmitoyl-lecithin, a surface-active substance that acts to lower the surface tension of the alveoli as their size decreases during expiration and increases the surface tension of the alveoli as their size increases during inspiration. This activity will be considered further in Chapter 2. The capillary endothelium is a very thin layer of simple squamous cells. These cells perform many nonrespiratory functions (e.g., clearance of emboli and

thrombi, exchange of liquids and solutes) in addition to their gas exchange role. Because the capillaries are interwoven throughout the interstitial space, a meshwork of intercommunicating capillaries is formed.

Alveolar-Capillary Septum (Membrane). As may be seen in Figure 1–15, two distinct portions of the alveolar-capillary membrane are readily identifiable. The thin portion of the septum is where the two basement membranes come into direct contact, giving the appearance of being fused together. This is the primary site for gas exchange, the distance across the membrane being about 0.5 μm.[61, 62] The thick portion is an area where the two basement membranes are separated by an interstitial space filled with fibrocollagenous fibers and rare fibroblasts. Although some gas exchange occurs here, this is the primary site for liquid and solute exchange in the lung.

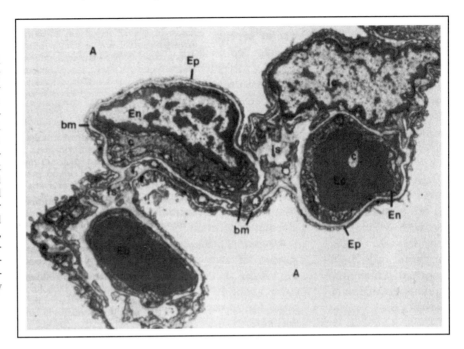

Figure 1–15. Cross-sectional electron micrograph showing the alveolar capillary membrane of the normal human parenchyma. Air in the alveolar lumina (A) is separated from the erythrocytes (Ec) in the capillaries (C) by epithelial cells (Ep), basement membranes (bm), endothelial cells (En), and the interstitial space (is). (From Dantzker DR. Cardiopulmonary Critical Care. 2nd ed. Philadelphia, WB Saunders, 1991, p 6. Micrograph courtesy of Theodore F. Beals, MD, Department of Pathology, University of Michigan.)

Innervation of the Lungs

Nerve Fibers. The lungs are invested with a rich supply of afferent and efferent nerve fibers and specialized receptors.[31, 63, 64] Parasympathetic fibers are supplied, by preganglionic fibers from the vagal nuclei via the vagus nerves, to ganglia around the bronchi and blood vessels. Postganglionic fibers innervate the bronchial and vascular smooth muscle, as well as the mucous cells and submucosal bronchial glands. The parasympathetic postganglionic fibers from thoracic sympathetic ganglia innervate essentially the same structures. Posterior and anterior pulmonary plexuses are formed by contributions from the postganglionic sympathetic and parasympathetic fibers at the roots of the lungs. Generally, stimulation of the vagus nerve results in bronchial constriction, dilation of pulmonary arterial smooth muscle, and increased glandular secretion. Stimulation of the sympathetic nerves causes bronchial relaxation, constriction of pulmonary arterial smooth muscle, and decreased glandular secretion.

Pulmonary Plexuses. The pulmonary plexuses lie anterior and posterior to the bronchial and vascular structures in the roots of the lungs; the anterior pulmonary plexus is much smaller than the posterior. Nerves from the plexuses form networks around the branches of the bronchi and the pulmonary and bronchial vessels. Branches from the vagus nerves and the deep cardiac plexus form the **anterior pulmonary plexus;** the left anterior plexus receives additional fibers from the superficial cardiac plexus. Branches from the vagus nerves, from the deep cardiac plexus, and from the second and fifth thoracic sympathetic ganglia form the posterior pulmonary plexus; the left posterior plexus also receives branches from the left recurrent laryngeal nerve.

CARDIOVASCULAR SYSTEM

The cardiovascular system consists of the blood vessels and the heart and has the primary function of the transportation of extracellular fluid (blood) to all parts of the body. The blood vessels form a conduit network, and the heart provides the force to circulate the blood through it. This chapter confines itself to a consideration of the structure of the heart and the principal blood vessels within the thorax, although the peripheral vascular system is also a major component of the total cardiovascular system.

Blood Vessels

In addition to the *anatomic names* for the vessels of particular dimension and position—*arteries, arterioles, capillaries* or *sinusoids, venules,* and *veins*—a functional classification for the vessels should also be considered (see Fig. 1–16).

Functions of the Vessels

The large arteries leaving the heart, and their principal branches, contain a significant amount of elastic tissue in their walls (elastic arteries) that serves to change the intermittent contractions of the heart into a smoother, albeit pulsatile, flow of blood. The smaller arterial branches, although still exhibiting elasticity, contain increasing amounts of nonstriated muscle in their walls (muscular arteries). The controlled contraction or relaxation of these muscular walls permits a variable distribution of the overall blood flow to the other organ systems in accordance with their fluctuating physiologic needs. Thus, the elastic and muscular arteries may collectively be thought of as *distributing vessels.*

The muscular walls of the arterioles and precapillary sphincters provide an even more delicate control of the flow of blood through the various tissues. These vessels are also the primary source of the peripheral resistance to blood flow and may, therefore, be referred to as *resistance vessels.* As will be discussed in more detail in Chapter 2, these vessels, together with the volume of cardiac output, determine the arterial blood pressure.

Because the exchange of gases, nutrients, metabolic products, and other substances occurs across the walls of the capillaries, sinusoids, and postcapillary venules, they may be collectively referred to

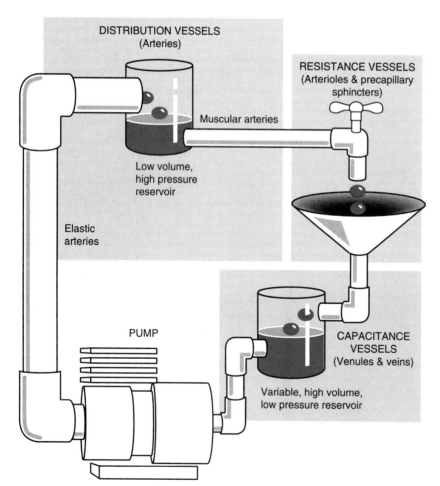

Figure 1–16. Functional depiction of the vascular system as distribution, resistance, and capacitance vessels.

as *exchange vessels.* The larger venules and veins form a large, variable-volume, and low-pressure reservoir referred to as the *capacitance vessels.*

Structure of the Vessels

It is generally accepted that despite dimensional and ultrastructural differences in the various parts of the system, one common structural component is ubiquitous—a single layer of smooth endothelial cells. Furthermore, all vessels larger than a capillary present zones of organized tissue that surround their endothelial lining. Although the organization of these zones varies with respect to the function of the vessels, three zones are recognized in the vessel walls. From the outside inward, they are named the **adventitia,** the **media,** and the **intima.** Figure 1–17 illustrates these structural features of typical arteries and veins.

The outermost zone of the vessel wall, the adventitia, is a connective tissue coat with a primarily longitudinal organization. The larger vessels are supplied by their own nutrient blood vessels, the **vasa vasorum,** which permeate the adventitia to supply it and the outer part of the media. The rest of the vessel (or smaller vessels) obtains its nutritional supply by means of diffusion from the blood in the lumen of the vessel. A fenestrated *external elastic lamina* underlies the adventitia. The media, a circumferentially organized fibromuscular zone, lies between the external elastic lamina and the *internal elastic lamina.* In the coronary arteries, a thick layer of longitudinal muscle and fibrous tissue abuts the internal elastic lamina. This structure is thought to permit the vessels to accommodate the significant length changes that occur throughout the cardiac cycle. The intima is a single layer of longitudinally oriented endothelial cells, which rests on a delicate layer of subendothelial connective tissue.

Because venous pressure is so much lower, there are fewer muscle cells and elastic fibers in the media of the veins. Therefore, the major difference between the veins and the arteries lies in the comparative weakness of the media of the veins. Furthermore, most veins have valves that prevent the retrograde flow of blood (as shown in Fig. 1–18).

Reference is frequently made to the great vessels, which are the vena cavae (superior and inferior), the pulmonary trunk, right and left pulmonary arteries, and the aorta.

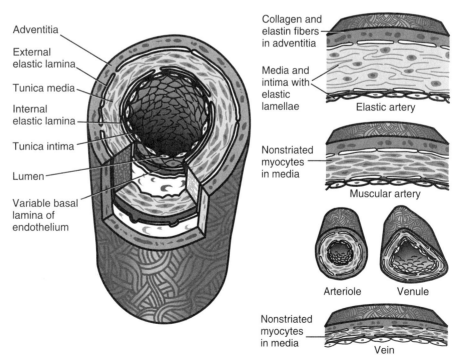

Figure 1–17. The principal structural features of the larger blood vessels. (Redrawn from Williams PL, Warwick R, Dyson M, Bannister LH [eds]. Gray's Anatomy. 37th ed. New York, Churchill Livingstone, 1989, p 685.)

Adventitia
External elastic lamina
Tunica media
Internal elastic lamina
Tunica intima
Lumen
Variable basal lamina of endothelium

Collagen and elastin fibers in adventitia
Media and intima with elastic lamellae
Elastic artery

Nonstriated myocytes in media
Muscular artery

Arteriole   Venule

Nonstriated myocytes in media
Vein

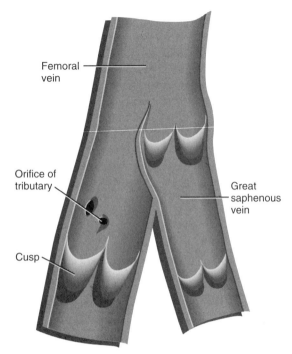

Figure 1-18. Valves inside the upper portions of the great saphenous and femoral veins, illustrated here at approximately two thirds their natural size. (Redrawn from Williams PL, Warwick R, Dyson M, Bannister LH [eds]. Gray's Anatomy. 37th ed. New York, Churchill Livingstone, 1989, p 691.)

Heart

The relationship of the heart to the anterior thoracic wall depends upon the size of the individual and the position of the body. Nonetheless, the average projections are seen in Figure 1–19. Clinically, the **base of the heart** is related to the second intercostal space parasternally. The **apex of the heart** projects into the fifth intercostal space at the midclavicular line. A radiograph of the chest (Fig. 1–20) shows the right atrium, the superior vena cava, the aortic knob, the left pulmonary artery, the left atrial appendage, and the left ventricle. About one third of the heart lies to the right of the midline; two thirds are to the left.

The heart is contained in a **pericardial sac** within the mediastinum. The pericardial sac actually consists of an outer sac, the **fibrous pericardium,** and a double-layered inner sac, the **serous pericardium.** The fibrous pericardium is a bag of collagenous fibrous tissue, the mouth of which blends with the adventitia of the great vessels as they enter and exit the heart. The bottom of this bag is attached to the central tendon and to a small portion of the left half of the diaphragm.

A closed sac surrounding the heart and lining the fibrous pericardium, the serous pericardium consists of a *visceral* and a *parietal layer.* The visceral layer, also known as the **epicardium,** intimately covers the heart and the great vessels from which it is reflected to form the parietal layer lining the fibrous pericardium. Where the visceral layer covers the great vessels, it forms two tubes. The aorta and the pulmonary trunk are enclosed in one of the tubes; the superior and inferior vena cavae and the pulmonary veins are enclosed in the second tube, forming a cul-de-sac, known as the *oblique sinus,* behind the left atrium. The space formed between the aorta and the pulmonary trunk is called the *transverse sinus.*

External Features

Topology. The heart has a pyramidal shape and lies obliquely in the chest behind the body of the sternum and the adjoining costal cartilages

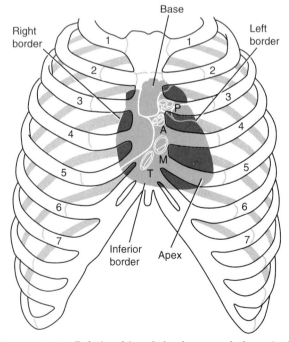

Figure 1-19. Relationship of the heart and the principal valves to the overlying rib cage. A, aortic valve; M, mitral valve; P, pulmonary valve; T, tricuspid valve.

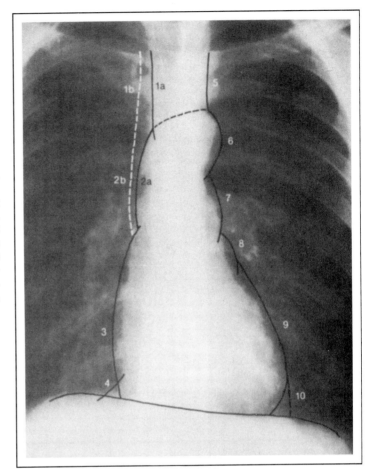

Figure 1-20. A normal mediastinal profile as seen on a posteroanterior radiograph of the chest. 1, Superior vena cava as in a young adult and as in the elderly; 2, ascending aorta as in a young adult and as in the elderly; 3, right atrium; 4, inferior vena cava (not always seen); 9, left ventricle; 10, cardiac fat pad (not always seen). (From Kersten LD. Comprehensive Respiratory Nursing: A Decision Making Approach. Philadelphia, WB Saunders, 1989, Fig. 15–35, p 428.)

and ribs. The base of the pyramid faces posteriorly and toward the right, forming the *anatomic base* of the heart. The apex of the pyramid points anteriorly and toward the left, forming the *anatomic apex* of the heart. Because of this oblique orientation, and because the pyramid is somewhat distorted, precise definition of its surfaces and intervening margins becomes problematic. Furthermore, terminology arising from widespread clinical usage obfuscates the issue of nomenclature. Throughout the remainder of this description, an attempt will be made to follow the official terminology, with its common clinical correlate in parentheses. Thus, the heart may be described as having a *base (posterior surface)* and an *apex; upper, inferior (acute),* and *left (obtuse) margins;* and *sternocostal (anterior), diaphragmatic (inferior), right,* and *left (pulmonary) surfaces.*[65]

Figure 1–21 illustrates the basal and diaphragmatic surfaces of the heart. As may be seen, all the great veins enter the heart at its base, which is formed principally by the *left atrium* but includes the *right atrium* to the right margin of the heart (do not confuse this anatomic base of the heart with the clinical base, referred to during auscultation, as underlying the parasternal area at the second intercostal space). The area of the heart from the base to the apex is the *diaphragmatic surface,* which is composed, chiefly, of the *left ventricle.* Passing between the *inferior vena cava* and the right margin of the heart, the **coronary sulcus** separates the left atrium from the left ventricle (where the specialized cells of the **coronary sinus** are located) as it courses upward toward the left (obtuse) margin of the heart.

Figure 1–22 illustrates the sternocostal (anterior) surface of the heart. Upon crossing the left (pulmonary) surface of the heart, the coronary sulcus may be seen as it passes between the *left auricle* and the left ventricle to end at the root of

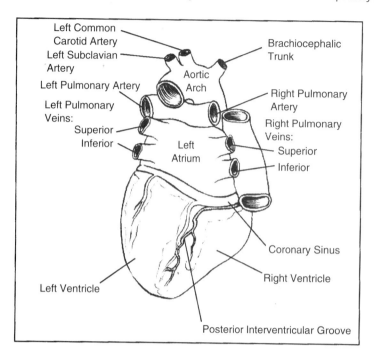

Figure 1–21. View of the diaphragmatic (posterior) surface of the heart, illustrating the external features. (Redrawn from Philo R, Bosner MS, LeMaistre A, et al. Guide to Human Anatomy. Philadelphia, WB Saunders, 1985, p 166.)

the *pulmonary trunk*. The coronary sulcus may also be seen here as it passes from the root of the aorta to separate the right atrium from the right ventricle on its way toward the inferior vena cava.

The **anterior interventricular sulcus** is shown separating the right from the left ventricles.

Cardiac Vessels. The aorta is described in sections for convenience. Within the fibrous pericar-

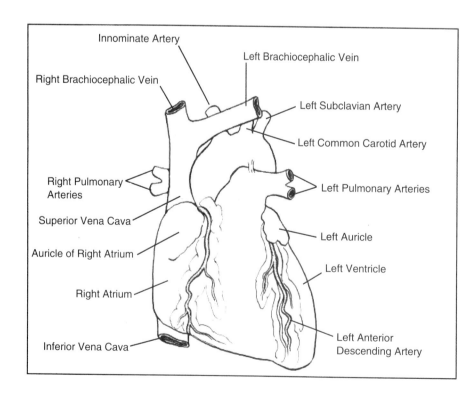

Figure 1–22. View of the sternocostal (anterior) surface of the heart, illustrating the external features. (Redrawn from Philo R, Bosner MS, LeMaistre A, et al. Guide to Human Anatomy. Philadelphia, WB Saunders, 1985, p 165.)

dium, the **ascending aorta** begins at the base of the left ventricle and is about 2 inches long. From the lower border of the third costal cartilage at the left of the sternum, it passes upward and forward toward the right as high as the second right costal cartilage. The aorta exhibits three dilatations above the attached margins of the cusps of the aortic valve at the root of the aorta—the **aortic sinuses** (of Valsalva). The sinuses extend beyond the level of the free borders of the cusps, as indicated by the *supravalvular ridge.* The coronary arteries (Fig. 1–23) open near the supravalvular ridge from the sinuses of their origin; the left is typically a little lower than the right. The **arch of**

the aorta continues from about the level of the second costosternal articulation in an upward, backward, and leftward orientation, arching to pass in front of the trachea on its downward turn along the left side of the fourth thoracic vertebral body and proceeding to the level of the left second costal cartilage, from which point it is known as the **descending aorta.** Three branches typically arise from the upper aspect of the arch: the **brachiocephalic trunk** (innominate artery), the **left common carotid artery,** and the **left subclavian artery.**

The **right coronary artery** arises from the right anterolateral surface of the aorta and passes be-

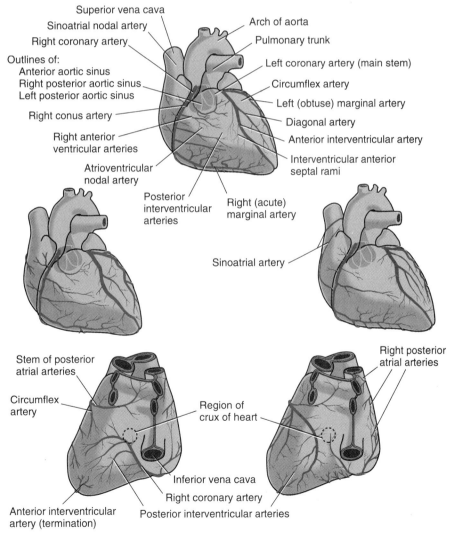

Figure 1–23. Typical distributions of the right and left coronary arteries. (Redrawn from Williams PL, Warwick R, Dyson M, Bannister LH [eds]. Gray's Anatomy. 37th ed. New York, Churchill Livingstone, 1989, pp 728–729.)

tween the auricular appendage of the right atrium and the pulmonary trunk, typically giving off a *branch to the sinus node* and yielding two or three *right anterior ventricular rami* as it descends into the coronary sulcus to curve around the right (acute) margin of the heart into the posterior aspect of the sulcus. As the right coronary artery crosses the right margin of the heart, it gives off the **right (acute) marginal artery** before continuing as far as the posterior interventricular sulcus, where it usually turns to supply the diaphragmatic surfaces of the ventricles as the **posterior interventricular (posterior descending) artery.** In about 70% of hearts, an *atrioventricular nodal artery* is given off just before the posterior interventricular artery.[66]

The **left coronary artery** originates from the left anterolateral aspect of the aorta and generally, while still behind the pulmonary trunk, splits into two smaller branches, the anterior interventricular and circumflex arteries (in about 35% of hearts, a sinoatrial artery is given off at this point).[67, 68] The **anterior interventricular (anterior descending) artery** traverses the anterior interventricular groove to supply sternocostal aspects of both ventricles. In its course, the anterior interventricular artery gives off right and left anterior ventricular and anterior septal branches. The larger left anterior ventricular branches vary in number from two to nine, the first being designated the **diagonal artery.** The **circumflex artery** runs in the coronary sulcus between the left atrium and ventricle, crosses the left margin of the heart, and usually continues to its termination, just short of the junction of the right coronary and the posterior interventricular arteries. In many instances, as the circumflex artery crosses the left margin of the heart it gives off a large branch that supplies this area—the **left marginal (obtuse) artery.**

The right coronary artery is the primary supply route for blood to the majority of the right ventricle and the posterior portion of the left ventricle in 80 to 90% of human hearts. Less typically, instead of the right coronary artery, it is a continuation of the circumflex artery that yields the posterior interventricular arterial branches and the branch to the atrioventricular node, constituting a so-called *left dominant* coronary arterial system. Ascribing dominance to either of the coronary arteries implies that the dominant artery provides the majority of the blood supply to the tissues of the heart. In about 50% of hearts, more blood

flow is attributable to the right coronary artery than the left; in about 30% of hearts the blood flow is equally distributed between the two coronary arteries; and in 20%, the left coronary artery supplies the dominant blood flow.

The *pulmonary trunk* runs upward and backward (first in front of, and then to the left of the ascending aorta) from the base of the right ventricle; it is about 2 inches in length. At the level of the fifth thoracic vertebra, it splits into right and left pulmonary arteries. The **right pulmonary artery** runs behind the ascending aorta, superior vena cava, and upper pulmonary vein, but in front of the esophagus and right primary bronchus to the root of the lung. The **left pulmonary artery** runs in front of the descending aorta and the left primary bronchus to the root of the left lung. It is attached to the arch of the aorta by the ligamentum arteriosum.

The pulmonary veins, unlike the systemic veins, have no valves. They originate in the capillary networks and join together to ultimately form two veins—a **superior** and an **inferior pulmonary vein**—from each lung, which open separately into the left atrium.

The **superior vena cava** is about 3 inches long from its termination in the upper part of the right atrium opposite the third right costal cartilage to the junction of the two brachiocephalic veins. The **inferior vena cava** extends from the junction of the two common iliac veins, in front of the fifth lumbar vertebra, passing through the diaphragm to open into the lower portion of the right atrium. The vena cavae have no valves.

The cardiac veins will be considered as three groups: the coronary sinus and its supplying veins, the anterior cardiac veins, and the thebesian veins. Most of the veins of the heart drain into the **coronary sinus,** which runs in the posterior aspect of the coronary sulcus and empties through the valve of the coronary sinus, a semilunar flap, into the right atrium between the opening of the inferior vena cava and the tricuspid valve. As shown in Figure 1–24, the **small** and **middle cardiac veins,** the **posterior vein of the left ventricle,** the **left marginal vein,** and the **great cardiac vein** feed the coronary sinus.

The *anterior cardiac veins* are fed from the anterior part of the right ventricle. They originate in the subepicardial tissue, crossing the coronary sulcus as they terminate directly into the right

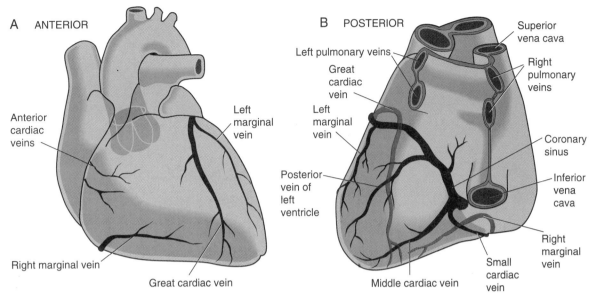

Figure 1–24. Anterior (*A*) and posterior (*B*) views of typical distributions of the major cardiac veins.

atrium. The **right marginal vein** runs along the right border of the heart and usually opens directly into the right atrium. Occasionally, it may join the small cardiac vein.

The **thebesian veins** (venae cordis minimae) vary greatly in their number and size. These tiny veins open into all the cavities of the heart, but are most numerous in the right atrium and ventricle, occasional in the left atrium, and rare in the left ventricle.

Internal Features

Right Atrium. The chamber of the right atrium (Fig. 1–25*A*) consists of two parts: (1) a smooth-walled posterior part, and (2) a thin-walled, trabecular anterior part. A muscular ridge, the *crista terminalis,* separates the two parts as it passes in front of and along the right side of the superior vena caval orifice from the upper part of the atrial septum, extending downward to the right side of the inferior vena caval orifice, and connects to the right side of the valve of the inferior vena cava. Muscular ridges, the **pectinate muscles,** run from the crista terminalis across the anterior wall, forming an interconnected network of tissue that continues into the superior part of the atrium. This upper anterior part of the chamber forms a small, muscular, conical appendage—the

auricle—which projects toward the left to overlap the right side of the root of the ascending aorta. The trabeculated free wall of the atrium is a vestige of the embryonic right atrium.

The superior vena cava enters the right atrium, without a valve, in the upper posterior region. The inferior vena cava opens into the lowest part of the atrium near the interatrial septum, its orifice being associated with the *valve of the inferior vena cava.* The coronary sinus opens into the right atrium between the inferior vena cava and the atrioventricular orifice; a thin *valve of the coronary sinus* guards its orifice. The valves of the inferior vena cava and the coronary sinus are inconsistent and are remnants of the embryonic right venous valve.

The posteromedial wall of the atrium is formed by the **interatrial septum.** Above and to the left of the inferior vena caval orifice, on the lower central portion of the septal wall, is an ovoid depression—the **fossa ovalis.**

Tricuspid Valve Apparatus. The atrioventricular valves cannot be considered as isolated structures; each is, instead, an integrated complex of several structures: the valvular orifice and its associated annulus, the valve leaflets, the chordae tendinae, and the papillary muscles (which are addressed with their associated ventricle).

The orifice of the tricuspid valve (Fig. 1–25*A*) is more a transition into the valvular leaflets than

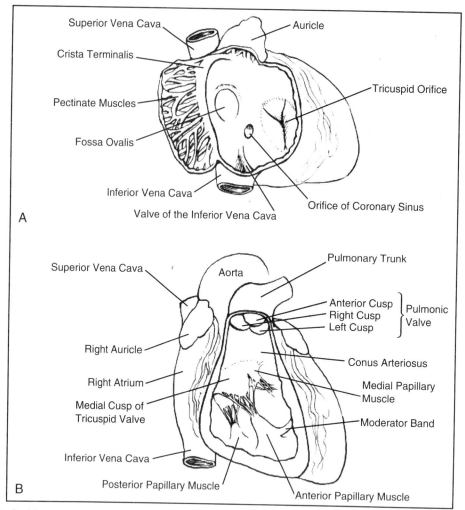

Figure 1–25. Inside view of the right atrium (*A*) and right ventricle (*B*). (Redrawn from Philo R, Bosner MS, LeMaistre A, et al. Guide to Human Anatomy. Philadelphia, WB Saunders, 1985, pp 166–167.)

a distinct demarcation between the atrial walls and the bases of the leaflets. As such, the orifice is apparent only after dissection of the leaflets. To complicate matters further, the shape of the orifice has been variously described as circular, ovoid, or almost triangular; if the naming of the valve leaflets were any indication, it would seem that the consensus tends toward the triangularity of the orifice. Clearly, the age, health status, and method of preparation of the specimen have influenced the description of the valve opening.

Some texts suggest that the orifices of the ventricular inflow and outflow tracts are surrounded by uniform collagenous rings to which the bases of the valve leaflets are attached. However, the annulus of the tricuspid valve is little more than a to-

ken of connective tissue that varies greatly in its deposition at different regions of the circumference of the orifice. The tricuspid annulus is joined, as are the annuli of the other inflow and outflow orifices, to a dense, membranous, and collagenous framework of tissue—the fibroelastic skeleton—which lies roughly in the plane of the coronary sulcus. Although the tricuspid atrioventricular orifice and the tissues making up the annulus do not actually lie in a singular plane, their approximate orientation is almost vertical at about 45 degrees to the sagittal plane.

There are typically three *valve leaflets* (thus, the name of the valve), named the *septal,* the *anterior* (posterolateral), and the *posterior,* that correspond to similarly named sectors of attachment at the

Clinical Notes: Classes of Chordae

There are five primary classes of chordae: *fan-shaped, rough zone, free edge, deep,* and *basal*.[69] The radiating branches of the fan-shaped chordae project outward from a single stem, attaching to the margins of the interleaflet commissures. Rough chordae also arise from a single stem, but split into three filaments: one attaches at the free margin of the leaflet, another attaches to the ventricular aspect of the leaflet at the boundary of the rough region, and the third attaches to some intermediate position. Free edge chordae are single strands that usually arise from the papillary muscle and attach near the middle of the scalloped free margin of a leaflet. The deep chordae attach to the more peripheral parts of the rough region and even to the clear region. Basal chordae arise directly from the ventricular wall to insert into the basal regions of the leaflets.

orifice. The leaflets present three distinct topographic and histologic regions: the *basal region,* extending about 0.1 inch from the basal attachment of the leaflet, is vascularized and relatively thick, and is often invested with some atrial myocardial cells; the *clear region* is thin and smooth, almost translucent, with few attachments of chordae; the *rough region* is thickened and roughened, especially on the ventricular side, receiving the insertions of most of the chordae tendinae. The chordae tendinae are fibrous collagenous cords: the **true chordae** span the gap between the papillary muscles and the valve leaflets, and the **false chordae** pass from the papillary muscles to one another or the ventricular walls.

Right Ventricle. The right ventricle (Fig. 1–25B), like the right atrium, may be considered in two parts: (1) a posteroinferior inflow tract, which contains the tricuspid valve, and (2) an anterosuperior outflow tract, from which the pulmonary trunk arises. The *supraventricular crest* marks the transition between these portions superiorly, and anteroinferiorly near the apex of the ventricle, the *septomarginal trabecula* (also known as the *moderator band*) forms the boundary. The cavity of the right ventricle is crescent-shaped in transverse section.

The walls of the inflow tract are heavily trabeculated, especially so at the apical aspect. These **trabeculae carnae** form irregular muscular ridges or bands of variable thickness, which project into the cavity of the ventricle. Some of the trabeculae are simple ridges, others are fixed to the septal or ventricular walls only by their ends, and still others, the **papillary muscles,** are attached only at their bases to the walls of the ventricle, their apices extending into the ventricular cavity and becoming continuous with the **chordae tendinae.** The chordae tendinae are collagenous cords that, with the papillary muscles, are part of the tricuspid valve. The *anterior papillary muscle* is fairly consistent in its origin from the inferior aspect of the moderator band. The *posterior papillary muscle* arises at the apical ventriculoseptal juncture. The *medial* or *septal papillary muscle(s)* are variable and less prominent.

The outflow tract of the right ventricle (**conus arteriosus** or **infundibulum**) has only a few trabeculae, the subpulmonic region being smooth-walled. It is possible that these smooth walls increase the velocity of the ventricular stroke volume during systole. The outflow tract is a vestige of the embryonic bulbus cordis.

Pulmonary Valve. The plane of the pulmonary valve (Figs. 1–25B and 1–26) faces superiorly, toward the left, and slightly backward, lying somewhat anterior and superior to the other principal valves. There are three *cusps* attached at their convexities to the thickened, triple-scalloped, fibrous annulus at the junction of the pulmonary

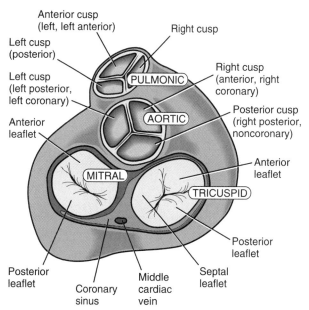

Figure 1–26. Nomenclature for the leaflets and cusps of the principal valves of the heart.

trunk and the right ventricle. The cusps of the valve are named anterior (left, left anterior), left (posterior), and right. The *Nomina Anatomica* names of the cusps relate to the embryonic positions of the cusps prior to the leftward rotation of the heart. The names in parentheses relate to the approximate *in situ* positions of the cusps in the normal adult heart.

Left Atrium. Although the volume of the left atrium (Fig. 1–27A) is smaller than that of the right, the atrial walls are much thicker. The essentially smooth cavity and walls are largely formed by the proximal parts of the pulmonary veins that are assimilated during the development of the atrium. The pulmonary veins open into the upper aspect of the posterior surface of the left atrium; typically, there are two on each lateral border. There

may occasionally be three pulmonary veins joining on the right; sometimes, there is only one on the left.

The generally smooth septal surface of the atrium presents an irregularly curved impression — the *valve of the foramen ovale*—that corresponds to the embryonic septum primum, covering the ostium secundum. The left upper anterior portion of the atrium constricts slightly at its union with the *left auricle,* which is longer and narrower than the right auricle. Pectinate muscles cover the inner surface of the auricle. With careful inspection, numerous openings of the thebesian veins, which allow blood to return directly from the myocardium, may be found on the walls of the atrium.

The *left atrioventricular orifice* is smaller than that of the triscuspid orifice. It lies almost vertically in the left anteroinferior aspect of the atrium at 45 degrees to the sagittal plane. Although almost in the same plane as the tricuspid orifice, the mitral orifice lies more superiorly and posteriorly; in relation to the aortic valve, it is posteroinferior and offset to the left.

Mitral Valve Apparatus. Much of the description of the tricuspid valve apparatus is applicable to the *mitral valve* apparatus (Figs. 1–26 and 1–27A). Like the triscuspid annulus, the mitral valve annulus is not a continuous ring of fibrous tissue; it becomes continuous with the laminae fibrosae of the valve leaflets and varies greatly in the consistency of its deposition. The annuli will be discussed further in a later consideration of the fibroskeleton of the heart.

There are typically two mitral valve leaflets.[70, 71] However, these may more correctly be viewed as a continuous curtain, with several indentations (receiving the fan-shaped chordae) along the free edge, circumscribing the entire mitral orifice. Two of the indentations are deep and typically present in consistent positions—the anterolateral and posteromedial commissures—which give the appearance of dividing the curtain into an *anterior* and a *posterior leaflet.* The anterior (anteromedial, aortic, septal) leaflet of the mitral valve has no basal zone, the clear region extending to the annulus. The posterior (ventricular, mural, posterolateral) leaflet has the same basal, clear, and rough zones as those described with the tricuspid leaflets.

The chordae tendineae are generally the same as those of the tricuspid apparatus. However, the true chordae may be divided into commissural and

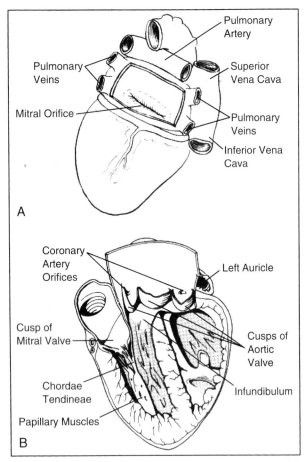

Figure 1–27. Inside view of the left atrium (*A*) and left ventricle (*B*). (Redrawn from Philo R, Bosner MS, LeMaistre A, et al. Guide to Human Anatomy. Philadelphia, WB Saunders, 1985, pp 168–169.)

leaflet categories. The *leaflet chordae* of the anterior leaflet are rough zone chordae with specialized variants—the *strut chordae*. The leaflet chordae of the posterior leaflet include rough zone, fan-shaped, and basal chordae. The *commissural chordae* arise from their corresponding papillary muscles. The branches of the posteromedial commissural chordae are longer and thicker than the anterolateral ones. The papillary muscles will be considered in the discussion of the left ventricle.

Left Ventricle. The almost conical left ventricle (Fig. 1–27*B*) is longer and narrower than the right ventricle. The walls of the left ventricle are about three times thicker than those of the right, and the transverse aspect of the cavity is almost circular. In contrast to the inflow and outflow orifices of the right ventricle, those of the left are located adjacent to one another, being separated only by the anterior leaflet of the mitral valve and the common fibrous ridge to which it and the left and posterior cusps of the aortic valve are attached.

The interventricular septum forms the anterolateral wall of the left ventricle and is about the same thickness as the rest of the ventricle except near the aortic valve. The *limbus marginalis* makes a clear demarcation between the muscular septum and a rounded, thin, collagenous area—the *membranous septum*—immediately below the right and posterior cusps of the aortic valve. The trabeculae carneae of the left ventricle are more stout than those of the right ventricle, but present the same three types. They are particularly dense toward the apex of the ventricle.

The two papillary muscles of the left ventricle are quite variable in their appearance, being anywhere from long and thin to short and stubby, sometimes even bifurcating at their tips. The *anterior* (anterolateral) *papillary muscle* arises from the sternocostal wall of the ventricle; the *posterior* (posteromedial) *papillary muscle* from the diaphragmatic wall. The chordae tendinae have previously been discussed, but they extend from the tips and margins of the apical third of the papillary muscles to attach to the mitral leaflets. The outflow tract of the left ventricle is smooth, becoming increasingly fibrous in its terminal aspect—the *aortic vestibule*.

Aortic Valve. The aortic valve (Fig. 1–26) shares many structural features with the pulmonic valve, having three semilunar cusps attached at their bases to a fibrous annulus, and three dilatations **(sinuses of Valsalva)** in the aortic wall that correspond to the cusps. The aortic valve lies anterosuperior and to the right of the mitral valve, facing superiorly, toward the right and somewhat anteriorly.

The aortic annulus is made up of three semicircular fibrocollagenous thickenings or scallops joined to encircle the junction of the aortic vestibule and the aorta like a three-pronged crown, the prongs of which are directed toward the apex of the heart. The lamina fibrosa of the semilunar valvular cusps fuses with the tissue of the luminal aspect of the arches of each of the crown points. The annular arches thus form triangular intervals between the cusps that are fused with the fibrous walls of the aortic vestibule.

The **semilunar cusps** of the aortic valve are thicker at their basal attachments than along their free edges, except that at the midpoints of the free edges there are nodular, fibrous thickenings—the *nodules of Arantius*. On either side of the nodules, just inward from the free edge, the lamina fibrosa becomes quite thin—the *lunules*—and is often fenestrated. The aortic surfaces of the cusps are rougher than the ventricular surfaces. The naming of the cusps of the aortic valve can easily be confusing because there are three different systems for doing so; all three names are provided in Figure 1–26.

The aortic sinuses are larger than those of the pulmonary trunk, extending upward well beyond the free edge of each cusp to terminate at the *supravalvular ridges*. As noted previously, the two coronary arteries usually open near these ridges.

Fibroskeleton

The myocardial cells are intimately invested with, and everywhere enveloped by, connective tissue that is greatly variable in its organization in different areas of the heart. As has been alluded to in the foregoing discussions of the annuli of the principal valvular orifices, a complex framework of dense and membranous collagen—the **fibroskeleton of the heart** (Fig. 1–28)—is recognizable as an intricate, malleable, three-dimensional continuum.[5, 72]

The annuli of the atrioventricular valves have already been described as essentially coplanar and

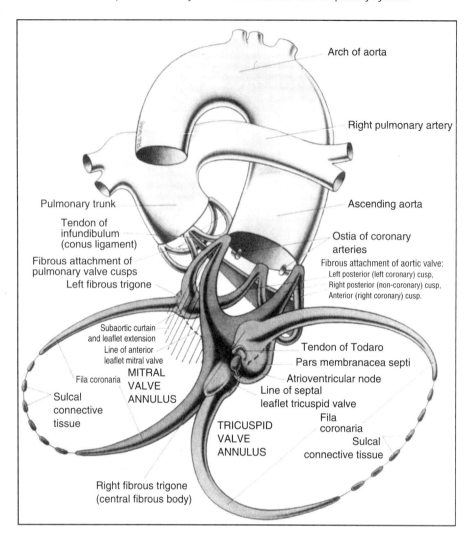

Arch of aorta

Right pulmonary artery

Pulmonary trunk

Ascending aorta

Tendon of infundibulum (conus ligament)

Fibrous attachment of pulmonary valve cusps

Left fibrous trigone

Ostia of coronary arteries

Fibrous attachment of aortic valve:
Left posterior (left coronary) cusp,
Right posterior (non-coronary) cusp,
Anterior (right coronary) cusp.

Subaortic curtain and leaflet extension

Line of anterior leaflet mitral valve

Fila coronaria

MITRAL VALVE ANNULUS

Sulcal connective tissue

Tendon of Todaro

Pars membranacea septi

Atrioventricular node

Line of septal leaflet tricuspid valve

Fila coronaria

TRICUSPID VALVE ANNULUS

Sulcal connective tissue

Right fibrous trigone (central fibrous body)

Figure 1–28. The fibroskeleton and valvular annuli of the heart. (From Williams PL, Warwick R, Dyson M, Bannister LH [eds]. Gray's Anatomy. 37th ed. New York, Churchill Livingstone, 1989, p 716.)

at 45 degrees to the sagittal plane, facing toward the apex of the heart. Likewise, the aortic valve annulus was described as facing superiorly, to the right and somewhat anteriorly, lying anterosuperior and to the right of the mitral annulus. Notwithstanding their disparate orientations, these three annuli are interconnected by a basal collagenous framework. Although situated at a distance, anterosuperior, and almost at a right angle to the aortic annulus, the pulmonary annulus is connected to the aortic annulus (and thereby to the atrioventricular annuli) by a tendinous band—the *tendon of the conus arteriosus* (conus ligament).

The fibroskeleton serves to maintain the position of the heart within the pericardium by providing a platform of attachment for the myocardium, valve cusps, and leaflets; it also separates (from an electrophysiologic standpoint) the atrial from the ventricular musculature. The fibroskeleton may be viewed as projecting outward from the three scallops of the centrally located aortic annulus. The aortic end of the tendon of the conus arteriosus blends into the tissue, forming the scallop of the right (anterior) aortic cusp at its nadir. At the low point of the left (left posterior) cusp scallop, the connective tissue thickens to form the *left fibrous trigone* and provides attachment for part of the anterior leaflet of the mitral valve. From its posterolateral aspect, the left fibrous trigone continues as the anterolateral arm of the mitral annulus—the *filum coronarium*. The nadir of the posterior (right posterior) scallop yields the most prominent collagenous aggregation—the *central fibrous body* (right fibrous trigone). The ellipsoid mass of the central body structurally links to the aortic, mitral, and tricuspid annuli: it continues into the second filum coronarium of the mitral annulus; it provides the base for both fila coronaria of the tricuspid annulus; posterosuperiorly, it extends, as the *tendon of Todaro,* into the right atrial wall, curving toward the medial aspect of the valve of the inferior vena cava where it marks the position of the atrioventricular node; anteriorly, it blends with the membranous septum of the aortic vestibule.

Cardiac Muscle

The following description, a distillation of the work of many others, is by no means a definitive, or universally accepted, model. Nonetheless, it is offered in the hope that it will facilitate, rather than obfuscate, the visualization of the muscle pathways. The cardiac muscle fibers may be conveniently divided into those of the atria and those of the ventricles; these being separated by the fibrous annuli. The atrial muscle fibers are arranged in two layers: superficial fibers, which pass over both atria; and deep fibers, which are confined to each atrium.[73, 74] The superficial fibers cross the anterior aspect of the atria most distinctly, and appear as a thin sheet transversely across the bases of the atria. Looped deep fibers cross each atrium, connecting to the atrioventricular annuli. Annular deep fibers surround the auricles and encircle the vena caval orifices and the fossa ovalis.

The muscle fibers of the ventricles are more complex than those of the atria; both superficial and deep layers have been described, but the deep layers are less circumscribed in the ventricles than in the atria.[75, 76] The strata of the superficial layer include (1) fibers that pass from the conus tendon, curve across the diaphragmatic surface, traverse leftward across the anterior interventricular groove, swirl into a vortex around the apex of the heart, and finally pass back upward into the papillary muscles of the left ventricle; (2) fibers from the tricuspid annulus that cross the diaphragmatic surface of the right ventricle to the sternocostal surface where they pass under the fibers from the conus tendon, across the anterior interventricular groove, wind around the cardiac apex, and terminate in the posterior papillary muscle of the left

ventricle; (3) fibers that cross the posterior interventricular groove from the mitral annulus to pass into the papillary muscles of the right ventricle. The deep ventricular layers begin in the papillary muscles of one ventricle and cross the septum to end in the papillary muscles of the other ventricle; the outermost layers of one become the innermost of the other (see Fig. 1–29). Beginning at the medial papillary muscle of the right ventricle, the outermost layer of deep muscle fibers circles around the right ventricle, crosses the interventricular septum (becoming the innermost layer), and blends with the superficial fibers from the tricuspid annulus to jointly form the posterior papillary muscle of the left ventricle. The second (middle) layer of deep muscle fibers spirals outward from the anterior papillary muscle to cross the septum, where it joins the superficial fibers from the anterior aspect of the conus tendon, and continues to the left ventricular side of the septal wall. The third layer of fibers, innermost of the right ventricular deep fibers, departs the posterior papillary muscle, crosses the septum (becoming the outermost layer), encircles the left ventricle to mesh with the superficial fibers from the posterior aspect of the conus tendon, together forming the anterior papillary muscle of the left ventricle.

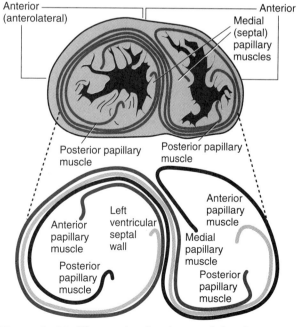

Figure 1–29. The overlapping layers of the deep ventricular muscle fibers.

Structure of the Cardiac Cells

Cardiac muscle is structurally and physiologically different from both skeletal and smooth muscle.[5, 77-79] It is made up of tracts of striated muscle cells—**myocytes**—and intervening connective tissue. Each cell has a single, centrally located nucleus and a discrete plasma membrane separated by sarcoplasm. The individual cells may split at their ends into branches that impinge upon adjacent cells, giving the appearance of a syncytial network, but this impression has been shown to be structurally incorrect. Each cardiac myocyte is striated in an organizational manner that is identical to that of skeletal muscle (although less conspicuous), with A, I, Z, and H bands (see Fig. 1–30). The pattern of actin and myosin filaments is also similar to that of skeletal muscle, but they are not grouped into distinctive myofibrils. The transverse tubule system is also present, but unlike in skeletal muscle (where it penetrates the cell at the A-I band junction), it penetrates cardiac muscle at the Z band. The sarcoplasmic reticulum is less abundant than in skeletal muscle.

Each cardiac myocyte possesses an intrinsic, spontaneous rhythm—**myogenic rhythm**—which may be neurally influenced in accordance with functional demand. The rate of this rhythmic depolarization and repolarization in individual myocytes is slower than that of the heart as a whole and slower in the ventricles than in the atria. For simplicity, these cells may be thought of as working myocytes. Their rhythmicity is normally synchronized by other specialized conducting myocytes. These conducting myocytes may be subdivided into **nodal, transitional,** and **Purkinje myocytes,** accumulating in a regional network of nodes and tracts. There is general agreement regarding the principal parts of the specialized conduction system of the heart, but some aspects remain debatable.[80-82]

Nodal myocytes contain few myofibrils and have an atypical sacrotubular system. They are present in clusters in both the sinoatrial and atrioventricular nodes. Transitional myocytes are not as wide as regular working myocytes, but are otherwise similar. They, too, are found in the nodes, extending into the atrioventricular bundle and the principal branches of the conducting system. Purkinje myocytes are wider and shorter than regular working myocytes, contain fewer myofibrils and more mito-chondria, and have larger intercalated disks. They are found on the terminal branches of the conduction system.

Specialized Conduction System

As mentioned earlier, the parts of the conducting system (Fig. 1–31) are the **sinoatrial (sinus) node,** the **atrioventricular node,** the **common atrioventricular bundle,** the **left** and **right bundle branches,** and the **Purkinje fibers.** Additional, and still debatable, components include the *interatrial, internodal,* and *accessory atrioventricular tracts or bundles.*

The sinoatrial (sinus or SA) node is situated in the crista terminalis at the junction of the superior vena cava and right atrium. Its name reflects its embryonic origin at the junction of the sinus venosus and the primitive atrium. The SA node is generally described as being a flattened ellipsoid about 10 to 20 mm long, 3 mm wide, and 1 mm thick. An artery of the SA node (mentioned earlier) traverses the length of the node. Nodal myocytes occupy the central region of the SA node, being circumferentially organized around the nodal artery. Transitional myocytes surround the nodal myocytes, and numerous Purkinje myocytes are located around the margins of the SA node. The sinus node is normally the pacemaker of the heart. Excitation of the atrial myocardium is initiated by the nodal myocytes. That conduction is slowed along the transitional myocytes, speeds up again along the Purkinje myocytes, and finally spreads by excitation-contraction coupling between the atrial working myocytes.[5, 83]

The atrioventricular (AV) node lies in the right atrial septal wall immediately posterior to the attachment of the septal leaflet of the tricuspid valve, just above the orifice of the coronary sinus (as noted previously, it is almost surrounded by the tendon of Todaro). It, too, is shaped like a flattened ovoid, approximately 7 to 8 mm long, 1 mm wide, and 3 mm high. Posteriorly, the AV node projects into the atrial septum, where it forms the nodal crest. The anteroinferior aspect of the node, which is closely associated with the central fibrous body, continues into the common AV bundle. Nodal myocytes occupy a small area inside the AV node, especially near the central fibrous body. The bulk of the node is composed of transi-

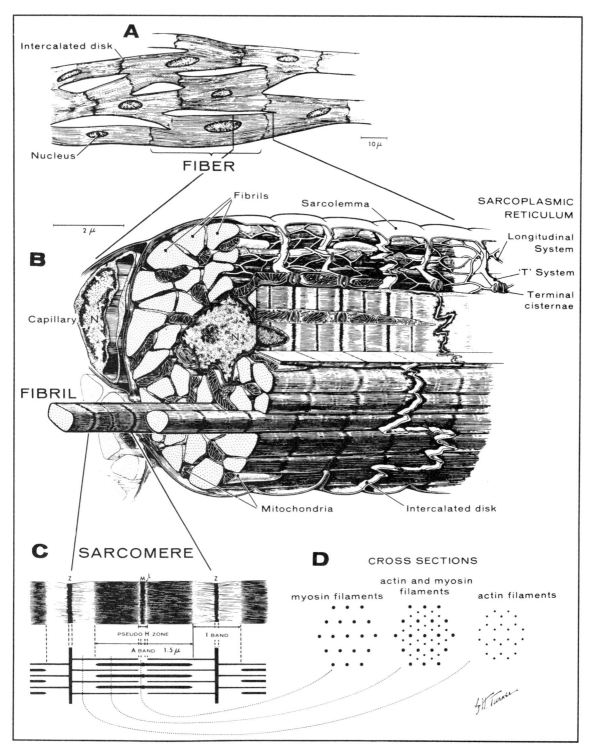

Figure 1–30. Cardiac muscle fibers as viewed under the light microscope and the electron microscope. (From Braunwald E, Ross J, Sonnenblick EH. Mechanisms of contraction of the normal and failing heart. N Engl J Med 277:794, 1967. Reprinted with permission of the New England Journal of Medicine.)

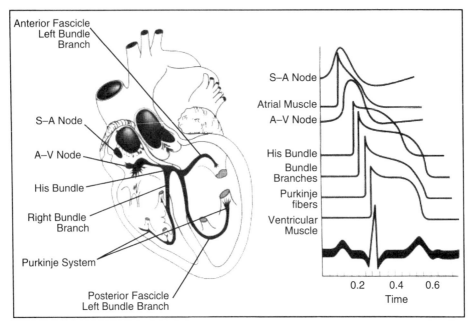

Figure 1–31. The specialized conduction system of the heart and tracings of typical transmembrane action potentials for specific portions of the system illustrate the relative contributions made to the summated electrical activity displayed in an electrocardiogram. (Adapted from Ganong WF. Review of Medical Physiology. 15th ed. Norwalk, CT, Appleton & Lange, 1991, p 505.)

tional myocytes, but Purkinje myocytes cover its outer margins, receiving the terminal branchings of the internodal tracts and continuing into the AV bundle.

The AV bundle (bundle of His) rapidly narrows from its origin at the anteroinferior pole of the AV node, enters a channel through the central fibrous body to the posteroinferior margin of the membranous septum of the aortic vestibule, and reaches the crest of the muscular interventricular septum. A narrow, rounded right bundle branch splits off at this point toward the right ventricular apex where it enters the septomarginal trabecula and passes to the anterior papillary muscle. Upon reaching the anterior papillary muscle, the right bundle branch divides into a fine network of fibers that take a recurrent path toward the right ventricular base (the Purkinje fibers). The left bundle branch leaves the left margin of the common bundle as a flattened sheet of fascicles that arch across the muscular septum to diverge at the left ventricular apex into anterior and posterior sheets that pass to the anterior and posterior papillary muscles, respectively. From the papillary muscles, the two sheets form complex networks of fibers that take recurrent paths toward the left ventricular

base. The common bundle is made up of mostly transitional myocytes, but as its distal aspect is approached it assumes the character of Purkinje myocytes.

Although several investigators have proposed the existence of special routes of impulse transmission between the SA and AV nodes and to distal portions of the atrial musculature, the existence of such pathways remains controversial.[84–96] These pathways are composed of a mixture of ordinary working cells and Purkinje cells.

The anterior internodal tract leaves the anterior aspect of the sinus node near the superior vena cava and passes posteromedially to the anterior margin of the interatrial septum. A few fibers branch off at this point to spread out into the left atrial walls (Bachmann's bundle) before the remainder continue their descent posteriorly along the right side of the septum and divide into terminal fascicles at the AV node.

The middle internodal tract (Wenckebach's bundle) leaves the SA node from its posterosuperior aspect, passes behind the orifice of the superior vena cava, reaching and crossing the interatrial septum to finally break up around the AV node.

The posterior internodal tract (Thorel's bundle) exits from the posteroinferior part of the SA node, continues through the crista terminalis and the valve of the inferior vena cava, proceeding to the posterior margin of the AV node.

Last, accessory atrioventricular bundles (Kent bundles) have been postulated as an explanation for various arrhythmias. These bundles may be present at any point around the atrioventricular annuli.

Innervation of the Heart

In addition to the specialized conducting system, the rate and strength of the cardiac rhythm are mediated by an extrinsic nerve supply. This extrinsic influence results from afferent and efferent fibers of the autonomic nervous system. The parasympathetic fibers arrive from branches of the vagus nerve and sympathetic fibers from rami of the sympathetic trunk. Preganglionic vagal fibers arise in the medulla from the nucleus ambiguus, reticular nuclei, and possibly the dorsal nucleus of the vagus, reaching the cardiac plexuses without interruption. The preganglionic sympathetic fibers arise from neurons in the lateral gray column of the first five or six cranial segments of the thoracic spinal cord, ending in the cervical and third and fourth thoracic sympathetic ganglia, from which the postganglionic fibers leave as cardiac nerves to proceed to the heart. Upon reaching the heart, the sympathetic cardiac nerves and the parasympathetic vagal cardiac branches form a mixed cardiac plexus.

The **cardiac plexus** is situated at the base of the heart and is divided into the closely associated superficial (ventral) and deep (dorsal) parts. The plexus contains several ganglia. The **superficial cardiac plexus** lies below the arch of the aorta, anterior to the right pulmonary artery. It is formed by the cardiac branch of the superior cervical ganglion of the left sympathetic trunk and the lower of the two cervical cardiac branches of the left vagus. The superficial part of the plexus gives branches to the deep part of the plexus, to the right coronary plexus, and to the left anterior pulmonary plexus.

The **deep cardiac plexus** lies in front of the bifurcation of the trachea, above the pulmonary trunk, but behind the aortic arch. The cardiac nerves from the cervical and upper thoracic ganglia of the sympathetic trunk and the cardiac branches of the vagus and recurrent laryngeal nerves form the deep cardiac plexus. A right half of the deep part of the plexus passes in front and behind the right pulmonary artery; those fibers passing behind the pulmonary artery give some filaments to the right atrium and then continue, forming part of the left coronary plexus; those passing in front of the pulmonary artery give a few filaments to the right anterior pulmonary plexus before going on to form a part of the right coronary plexus. The left half of the deep part of the cardiac plexus is connected with the superficial part of the plexus, giving filaments to the left atrium and to the left anterior pulmonary plexus before continuing, forming the greater portion of the left coronary plexus. The **left coronary plexus** accompanies the left coronary artery, giving branches to the left atrium and ventricle. The smaller **right coronary plexus** accompanies the right coronary artery, giving branches to the right atrium and ventricle.

References

1. Moore KL, Persaud TVN. Before We Are Born: Essentials of Embryology and Birth Defects. 5th ed. Philadelphia, WB Saunders, 1998.
2. Fishman MC, Chien KR. Fashioning the vertebrate heart: Earliest embryonic decisions. Development 124:2099, 1997.
3. Tanaka M, Izumo S. Overview of the molecular mechanisms of cardiac development. Heart Vessels Suppl:1–6, 1997.
4. Rudolph AM. Developmental biology of the heart: Is there a role for the physiologist? Semin Perinatol 20:589–595, 1996.
5. Gray H, Williams PL, Bannister LH. Gray's Anatomy: The Anatomical Basis of Medicine and Surgery. 38th ed. New York, Churchill Livingstone, 1995.
6. Alyn IB, Baker LK. Cardiovascular anatomy and physiology of the fetus, neonate, infant, child, and adolescent. J Cardiovasc Nurs 6:1–11, 1992.
7. Johnson KE, Slaby FJ. Anatomy: Review for New National Boards. Alexandria, VA, J&S Publishing Co, 1992.
8. Evans JA. Aberrant bronchi and cardiovascular anomalies. Am J Med Genet 35:46–54, 1990.
9. Price WA, Stiles AD. New insights into lung growth and development. Curr Opin Pediatr 8:202–208, 1996.
10. Hume R, Conner C, Gilmour M. Lung maturation. Proc Nutr Soc 55:529–542, 1996.
11. Basmajian JV, De Luca CJ. Muscles Alive: Their Functions Revealed by Electromyography. 5th ed. Baltimore, Williams & Wilkins, 1985.
12. Farkas GA, Cerny FJ, Rochester DF. Contractility of the ventilatory pump muscles. Med Sci Sports Exerc 28:1106–1114, 1996.
13. Gierada DS, Curtin JJ, Erickson SJ, et al. Diaphragmatic

motion: Fast gradient-recalled-echo MR imaging in healthy subjects. Radiology 1995;194:879–884.

14. Cohen E, Mier A, Heywood P, et al. Excursion-volume relation of the right hemidiaphragm measured by ultrasonography and respiratory airflow measurements. Thorax 49:885–889, 1994.

15. Houston JG, Angus RM, Cowan MD, et al. Ultrasound assessment of normal hemidiaphragmatic movement: relation to inspiratory volume. Thorax 49:500–503, 1994.

16. Hislop A, Reid L. Pulmonary arterial development during childhood: Branching pattern and structure. Thorax 28:129–135, 1973.

17. Robertson B. The intrapulmonary arterial pattern in normal infancy and in transposition of the great arteries. Acta Paediatr Scand Suppl:7–36, 1968.

18. Robertson B. The normal intrapulmonary arterial pattern of the human late fetal and neonatal lung. A microangiographic and histologic study. Acta Paediatr Scand 56:249–264, 1967.

19. Hislop A, Howard S, Fairweather DV. Morphometric studies on the structural development of the lung in Macaca fascicularis during fetal and postnatal life. J Anat 138:95–112, 1984.

20. Haworth SG. Development of the normal and hypertensive pulmonary vasculature. Exp Physiol 80:843–853, 1995.

21. Zeltner TB, Burri PH. The postnatal development and growth of the human lung. II. Morphology. Respir Physiol 67:269–282, 1987.

22. Murata K, Itoh H, Todo G, et al. Bronchial venous plexus and its communication with pulmonary circulation. Invest Radiol 21:24–30, 1986.

23. Beyers JA. Radiological features of normal and abnormal pulmonary blood flow. S Afr Med J 55:881–884, 1979.

24. Suga K, Matsunaga N, Nishigauchi K, et al. Radionuclide angiography and ventilation/perfusion studies in two patients with systemic arterial supply to the basal segment of the left lung. Clin Nucl Med 22:526–531, 1997.

25. Leak LV, Jamuar MP. Ultrastructure of pulmonary lymphatic vessels. Am Rev Respir Dis 128:S59–65, 1983.

26. Helfferich F, Viragh S. Histological investigations of the nasal mucosa in human fetuses. Eur Arch Otorhinolaryngol Suppl 1:S39–42, 1997.

27. Lund VJ. Nasal physiology: Neurochemical receptors, nasal cycle, and ciliary action. Allergy Asthma Proc 17:179–184, 1996.

28. Mygind N, Winther B. Light- and scanning electron-microscopy of the nasal mucosa. Acta Otorhinolaryngol Belg 33:591–602, 1979.

29. Richerson HB. Lung defense mechanisms. Allergy Proc 11:59–60, 1990.

30. Janson-Bjerklie S. Defense mechanisms: Protecting the healthy lung. Heart Lung 12:643–649, 1983.

31. Sparrow MP, Weichselbaum M, McCray PB. Development of the innervation and airway smooth muscle in human fetal lung. Am J Respir Cell Mol Biol 20:550–560, 1999.

32. Tschanz SA, Burri PH. Postnatal lung development and its impairment by glucocorticoids. Pediatr Pulmonol Suppl 16:247–249, 1997.

33. Berend N, Woolcock AJ, Marlin GE. Relationship between bronchial and arterial diameters in normal human lungs. Thorax 1979;34:354–358.

34. Weibel ER. Morphometry of the human lung: the state of the art after two decades. Bull Physiopathol Respir (Nancy) 15:999–1013, 1979.

35. Corcoran HL, Renner WR, Milstein MJ. Review of high-resolution CT of the lung. Radiographics 12:917–939; discussion 940–941, 1992.

36. Gurney JW. Pathophysiology of obstructive airways disease. Radiol Clin North Am 36:15–27, 1998.

37. Nakajima M, Kawanami O, Jin E, et al. Immunohistochemical and ultrastructural studies of basal cells, Clara cells and bronchiolar cuboidal cells in normal human airways. Pathol Int 48:944–953, 1998.

38. Strayer MS, Guttentag SH, Ballard PL. Targeting type II and Clara cells for adenovirus-mediated gene transfer using the surfactant protein B promoter. Am J Respir Cell Mol Biol 18:1–11, 1998.

39. Jeffery PK, Gaillard D, Moret S. Human airway secretory cells during development and in mature airway epithelium. Eur Respir J 5:93–104, 1992.

40. Mason RJ. Surfactant synthesis, secretion, and function in alveoli and small airways. Review of the physiologic basis for pharmacologic intervention. Respiration 51:3–9, 1987.

41. Gail DB, Lenfant CJ. Cells of the lung: Biology and clinical implications. Am Rev Respir Dis 127:366–387, 1983.

42. Becker KL, Silva OL. Hypothesis: The bronchial Kulchitsky (K) cell as a source of humoral biologic activity. Med Hypotheses 7:943–949, 1981.

43. van Lommel A, Lauweryns JM, Marcus M, Vertommen JD. Neuroepithelial bodies in relatively mature lungs: An investigation in prenatal and newborn lambs. Acta Anat 153:203–209, 1995.

44. Widdicombe JG. Neuroregulation of the nose and bronchi. Clin Exp Allergy 26 (suppl 3):32–35, 1996.

45. Nadel JA. Role of enzymes from inflammatory cells on airway submucosal gland secretion. Respiration 58:3–5, 1991.

46. Nadel JA. Role of airway epithelial cells in the defense of airways. Prog Clin Biol Res 263:331–339, 1988.

47. Miller WS. The Lung. 2nd ed. Springfield, IL, Charles C Thomas, 1947.

48. Ryan SF. The structure of the primary lung lobule. Ann Clin Lab Sci 3:147–155, 1973.

49. Hislop A, Reid L. Development of the acinus in the human lung. Thorax 29:90–94, 1974.

50. Berend N, Rynell AC, Ward HE. Structure of a human pulmonary acinus. Thorax 46:117–121, 1991.

51. Ten Have-Opbroek AA. The development of the lung in mammals: an analysis of concepts and findings. Am J Anat 162:201–219, 1981.

52. Scarpelli EM. The alveolar surface network: A new anatomy and its physiological significance. Anat Rec 251:491–527, 1998.

53. Colebatch HJ, Ng CK. Estimating alveolar surface area during life. Respir Physiol 88:163–170, 1992.

54. Zeltner TB, Caduff JH, Gehr P, et al. The postnatal development and growth of the human lung. I. Morphometry. Respir Physiol 67:247–267, 1987.

55. Crapo JD, Barry BE, Gehr P, et al. Cell number and cell characteristics of the normal human lung. Am Rev Respir Dis 126:332–337, 1982.

56. Mercer RR, Russell ML, Crapo JD. Alveolar septal structure in different species. J Appl Physiol 77:1060–1066, 1994.

57. Menkes H, Traystman R, Terry P. Collateral ventilation. Fed Proc 38:22–26, 1979.

58. Delaunois L. Anatomy and physiology of collateral respiratory pathways. Eur Respir J 2:893–904, 1989.

59. Bastacky J, Goerke J. Pores of Kohn are filled in normal lungs: low-temperature scanning electron microscopy. J Appl Physiol 73:88–95, 1992.

60. Topol M. Collateral respiratory pathways of pulmonary acini in man. Folia Morphol 54:61–66, 1995.

61. Schneeberger EE. Structural basis for some permeability properties of the air-blood barrier. Fed Proc 37:2471–2478, 1978.

62. West JB, Tsukimoto K, Mathieu-Costello O, Prediletto R. Stress failure in pulmonary capillaries. J Appl Physiol 70: 1731–1742, 1991.

63. Fox B, Bull TB, Guz A. Innervation of alveolar walls in the human lung: An electron microscopic study. J Anat 131: 683–692, 1980.

64. Richardson JB. The innervation of the lung. Eur J Respir Dis Suppl 117:13–31, 1982.

65. Message MA, Anderson RH. Towards a new terminology for clinical anatomy, with special reference to the heart. Clin Anat 9:317–329, 1996.

66. Abuin G, Nieponice A. New findings on the origin of the blood supply to the atrioventricular node. Clinical and surgical significance. Tex Heart Inst J 25:113–117, 1998.

67. Krauss D, Carter JE Jr, Feldman T. Anomalous connection between the sinus node artery and the A-V node artery. Cathet Cardiovasc Diagn 29:236–239, 1993.

68. Anderson KR, Ho SY, Anderson RH. Location and vascular supply of sinus node in human heart. Br Heart J 41:28–32, 1979.

69. Towne WD. Classification of chordae tendineae. Circulation 47:209, 1973.

70. van Rijk-Zwikker GL, Delemarre BJ, Huysmans HA. Mitral valve anatomy and morphology: Relevance to mitral valve replacement and valve reconstruction. J Cardiovasc Surg 9: 255–261, 1994.

71. Walmsley R. Anatomy of human mitral valve in adult cadaver and comparative anatomy of the valve. Br Heart J 40: 351–366, 1978.

72. Coelho R, Pannu HS, Thakurta SG, et al. Ruptured aneurysm sinus of Valsalva and Gerbode defect with severe tricuspid and aortic regurgitation. A case report and its surgical correction. J Cardiovasc Surg (Torino) 38:531–533, 1997.

73. Cabrera JA, Sanchez-Quintana D, Ho SY, et al. The architecture of the atrial musculature between the orifice of the inferior caval vein and the tricuspid valve: The anatomy of the isthmus. J Cardiovasc Electrophysiol 9:1186–1195, 1998.

74. Wang K, Ho SY, Gibson DG, Anderson RH. Architecture of atrial musculature in humans. Br Heart J 73:559–565, 1995.

75. Lunkenheimer PP, Redmann K, Scheld H, et al. The heart muscle's putative "secondary structure." Functional implications of a band-like anisotropy. Technol Health Care 5:53–64, 1997.

76. Schmid P, Niederer P, Lunkenheimer PP, Torrent-Guasp F. The anisotropic structure of the human left and right ventricles. Technol Health Care 5:29–43, 1997.

77. Labeit S, Kolmerer B. Titins: Giant proteins in charge of muscle ultrastructure and elasticity [see comments]. Science 270:293–296, 1995.

78. Kim HD, Kim DJ, Lee IJ, et al. Human fetal heart development after mid-term: Morphometry and ultrastructural study. J Mol Cell Cardiol 24:949–965, 1992.

79. Vye MV. The ultrastructure of striated muscle. Ann Clin Lab Sci 6:142–151, 1976.

80. Denes P, Ezri MD. Clinical electrophysiology—A decade of progress. J Am Coll Cardiol 1:292–305, 1983.

81. Perry RS, Illsley SS. Basic cardiac electrophysiology and mechanisms of antiarrhythmic agents. Am J Hosp Pharm 43:957–974, 1986.

82. Pollard AE, Barr RC. The construction of an anatomically based model of the human ventricular conduction system. IEEE Trans Biomed Eng 37:1173–1185, 1990.

83. Taccardi B, Lux RL, Ershler PR, et al. Anatomical architecture and electrical activity of the heart. Acta Cardiol 52:91–105, 1997.

84. Ho SY, Kilpatrick L, Kanai T, et al. The architecture of the atrioventricular conduction axis in dog compared to man: its significance to ablation of the atrioventricular nodal approaches. J Cardiovasc Electrophysiol 6:26–39, 1995.

85. Waller BF, Gering LE, Branyas NA, Slack JD. Anatomy, histology, and pathology of the cardiac conduction system—Part VI. Clin Cardiol 16:623–628, 1993.

86. Waller BF, Gering LE, Branyas NA, Slack JD. Anatomy, histology, and pathology of the cardiac conduction system—Part V. Clin Cardiol 16:565–569, 1993.

87. Waller BF, Gering LE, Branyas NA, Slack JD. Anatomy, histology, and pathology of the cardiac conduction system—Part IV. Clin Cardiol 16:507–511, 1993.

88. Waller BF, Gering LE, Branyas NA, Slack JD. Anatomy, histology, and pathology of the cardiac conduction system—Part III. Clin Cardiol 16:436–442, 1993.

89. Waller BF, Gering LE, Branyas NA, Slack JD. Anatomy, histology, and pathology of the cardiac conduction system: Part II. Clin Cardiol 16:347–352, 1993.

90. Waller BF, Gering LE, Branyas NA, Slack JD. Anatomy, histology, and pathology of the cardiac conduction system: Part I. Clin Cardiol 16:249–252, 1993.

91. Kafer CJ. Internodal pathways in the human atria: a model study. Comput Biomed Res 24:549–563, 1991.

92. Anderson RH, Ho SY, Smith A, Becker AE. The internodal atrial myocardium. Anat Rec 201:75–82, 1981.

93. Hoffman BF. Fine structure of internodal pathways. Am J Cardiol 44:385–386, 1979.

94. Wenckebach KF. Beitrage zur Kenntnis der menschlichen Herztätigkeit. Anat Physiol 3:53, 1908.

95. Thorel C. Über den Aufbaum des Sinusknoten und seine Verbindung mit der Cava superior und den Wenckenbachschen Bündeln. Munch Med Wochenschr 57:83, 1910.

96. Bachman G. The inter-auricular time interval. Am J Physiol 41:309, 1916.

2

Cardiovascular and Respiratory Physiology

H. Steven Sadowsky

INTRODUCTION

The lungs primarily function to exchange gas between the blood and atmospheric air, while the heart primarily functions to pump blood through the vascular system. This chapter is intended to introduce the normal physiologic considerations that underlie these vital processes. After a very brief discussion of the basic units of measurement used to describe respiratory and cardiovascular function, the components of the autonomic nervous system are reviewed. Then, the specific functions of the respiratory and cardiovascular systems are presented.

BASIC UNITS OF MEASURE

In clinical practice, the clinician is often simultaneously faced with several alternative units of measure. For example, in cardiovascular medicine, pressures are frequently reported in terms of millimeters of mercury (mm Hg), whereas in pulmonary medicine, pressures are frequently reported in terms of centimeters of water (cm H_2O). The Système International (SI) units pascals and kilopascals (Pa and kPa, respectively) are also being applied. Table 2–1 presents conversion factors for changing from one unit to another. Throughout this chapter, the units of measure will be presented as they are commonly reported in the clinical setting.

THE AUTONOMIC NERVOUS SYSTEM

The **autonomic nervous system** comprises all the afferent and efferent nerves through which the viscera are innervated.[1] This section will consider the efferent pathways to the various blood vessels, heart, larynx, trachea, bronchi, and lungs. Structurally, the autonomic nerves are characterized by a two-neuron chain: the cell body of the primary (preganglionic) neuron lies within the brain stem or spinal cord, and sends its axon to synapse with outlying secondary (postganglionic) neurons. Autonomic efferent signals are carried to the viscera via two essentially antagonistic subdivisions of the autonomic nervous system, the **sympathetic** and the **parasympathetic** divisions (Fig. 2–1).

The preganglionic neuronal axons of the sympathetic nerves leave the spinal cord via the ventral roots of the spinal nerves from the first thoracic to the third or fourth lumbar vertebrae (T1

Table 2-1
Basic Units of Measure and Examples of Derived Units and Conversion Factors

BASIC UNITS	MEASUREMENT	SYMBOL
mole	amount of a substance	mol
ampere	electric current	A
meter	length	m
candela	luminous intensity	cd
kilogram	mass	kg
kelvin	temperature	K
second	time	s

DERIVED UNITS		
square meter	area	m^2
cubic meter	volume	m^3
meter per second	velocity	$m \cdot s^{-1}$
meter per second per second	acceleration	$m \cdot s^{-2}$
newton	force	N or $kg \cdot m \cdot s^{-2}$
pascal	pressure	Pa or $N \cdot m$
joule	work (energy)	J or $kg \cdot m^2 \cdot s^{-2}$
watt	power	W or $J \cdot s^{-1}$ or $kg \cdot m^2 \cdot s^{-3}$

TO CONVERT	TO	MULTIPLY BY
mm Hg	kPa	0.133
mm Hg	cm H_2O	1.36
cm H_2O	kPa	0.098
cm H_2O	mm Hg	0.735
kPa	mm Hg	7.519
kPa	cm H_2O	10.225

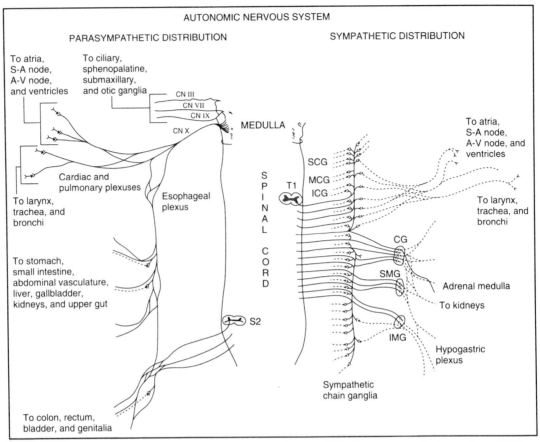

Figure 2–1. Sympathetic and parasympathetic efferent pathways. SCG, Superior cervical ganglion; MCG, middle cervical ganglion; ICG, inferior cervical ganglion; CG, celiac ganglion; SMG, superior mesenteric ganglion; IMG, inferior mesenteric ganglion.

to L3 or L4). They pass into the paravertebral sympathetic ganglion chains, most ending on the cell bodies of the postganglionic neurons. Axons of some of the postganglionic neurons reach the viscera via various sympathetic nerves; others reenter the spinal nerves via the gray rami from the chain ganglia to be distributed in the areas supplied by those spinal nerves. The superior, middle, and stellate ganglia in the cranial extension of the sympathetic chain give off the postganglionic sympathetic nerves to the blood vessels of the head. The adrenal medulla is a sympathetic ganglion with postganglionic neurons that are specialized for secretion directly into the bloodstream.

Parasympathetic innervation of the vasculature and other viscera of the head is carried via cranial nerves III (oculomotor), VII (facial), and IX (glossopharyngeal); that of the thorax and upper abdomen via cranial nerve X (vagus); and that of the pelvic region via the second and third (occasionally, also the first and fourth) sacral spinal nerves. About 75% of all parasympathetic nerve fibers are in the vagus nerves. Parasympathetic preganglionic fibers end on short postganglionic neurons located on or near the targeted visceral structures.

Neurotransmitters

The sympathetic and parasympathetic nerve fibers secrete one of two transmitter substances at the various synaptic junctions, **acetylcholine** and **norepinephrine.** Acetylcholine-secreting fibers are referred to as **cholinergic;** those secreting norepinephrine are called **adrenergic.** All the preganglionic fibers of the parasympathetic and sympathetic divisions, and the postganglionic neurons of the parasympathetic division, are cholinergic. Most of the postganglionic sympathetic neurons are adrenergic, although the postganglionic sympathetic fibers to the sweat glands, the piloerector muscles, and a few blood vessels are cholinergic. This fact will be important in later discussions of pharmacologic activity (see Chapters 14 and 15).

Acetylcholine is synthesized in the terminal endings of cholinergic fibers, mostly outside the axoplasmic vesicles in which it is ultimately stored until its release. Once acetylcholine has been secreted at the cholinergic nerve ending, it is metabolized by **acetylcholinesterase.** This is the same process by which acetylcholine is eliminated from the neuromuscular junctions of skeletal nerves in the peripheral nervous system. Norepinephrine synthesis starts in the axoplasm, but is completed inside the axoplasmic vesicles of the terminal nerve endings. After secretion by the terminal nerve endings, most norepinephrine is reabsorbed into the nerve endings themselves; some diffuses away from the release site into the surrounding interstitial fluid and eventually into the blood; and the remainder is metabolized by other enzymes (either **monoamine oxidase** (MAO), at the synaptic cleft, or by **catechol-*O*-methyl transferase** (COMT), which is present diffusely throughout all tissues). Before acetylcholine or norepinephrine can actually stimulate a response, each must first bind to a specific receptor site on the cell membrane of an effector organ.

Neurotransmitter Receptors

Typically, neurotransmitter receptors are portions of proteins that extend from the outer surface of the cell membrane, penetrating through it, to the interior of the cell. When the transmitter substance binds with the receptor, there is often a conformational change in the receptor protein that excites or inhibits cellular activity. Alterations of cellular activity occur as a result of a change in the permeability of the cell membrane to one or more ions, or by activation or deactivation of an enzyme (second messenger) attached to the end of the receptor on the inside of the cell. Although there are several types of postsynaptic receptors, this discussion is confined to three of them: the cholinergic, adrenergic, and **dopaminergic.** The

general locations and typical responses for these neurotransmitter receptor types are summarized in Table 2–2.

There are two categories of cholinergic receptors: **muscarinic** and **nicotinic.** Muscarinic receptors are located at the interfaces between the postganglionic neurons and the effector cells of all parasympathetic terminal synapses and some specialized sympathetic postganglionic cholinergic branches (e.g., to some blood vessels). Nicotinic receptors are found at the junctions between the preganglionic and postganglionic neurons of both branches of the autonomic nervous system and at the neuromuscular junctions of skeletal muscle fibers in the peripheral nervous system.

There are also two categories of adrenergic receptors: **alpha** and **beta.** Based on the sensitivity of these receptors to different endogenous and exogenous agents, each adrenergic receptor subcategory is further subdivided. The alpha receptors are divided into two subtypes.[2] *Alpha*$_1$ receptors are primarily located on visceral and vascular smooth muscle. *Alpha*$_2$ receptors are primarily located on the presynaptic terminals of certain adrenergic synapses, where they serve to modulate norepinephrine release. Norepinephrine and epinephrine have different effects in exciting the alpha and beta receptors. The beta receptors have recently been expanded to include four sub-types.[3, 4] *Beta*$_1$ receptors are principally located in cardiac and renal tissues. *Beta*$_2$ receptors are found mostly in the smooth muscle of certain vascular beds and the bronchioles. *Beta*$_3$ receptors are primarily located on adipocytes. The existence of the *beta*$_4$ subtype remains controversial.

Dopaminergic receptors constitute another class of neurotransmitter receptors within the sympathetic branch of the autonomic nervous system. There are several subclasses of dopaminergic receptors located throughout the body (e.g., in the adrenal glands, blood vessels, carotid bodies, intes-

> ### Clinical Note: Medications and the Autonomic Nervous System
> The clinician must be very knowledgeable about the autonomic nervous system because of the impact of various medications, including alpha and beta blockers and stimulants, on the autonomic nervous system. (See Chapter 15 for discussion of medications.)

Table 2-2

Locations and Typical Responses of Some Cardiovascular, Pulmonary, and Renal Autonomic Neurotransmitter Receptors

NEUROTRANSMITTER	TYPE OF RECEPTOR	LOCATION	RESPONSE
Cholinergic			
	Muscarinic	Smooth muscle of lungs and bronchioles	Contraction
		Cardiac muscle	Decreased rate of contraction
	Nicotinic	Autonomic ganglia	Mediates postganglionic neuronal transmission
Adrenergic			
	Alpha$_1$	Vascular smooth muscle	Contraction
	Alpha$_2$	Special CNS inhibitory synapses	Decreased sympathetic discharge
		Peripheral adrenergic presynaptic terminals	Modulates norepinephrine release
		Fat cells	Decreased lipolysis
	Beta$_1$	Atria, SA node, AV node	Increased rate and force of contraction
		Ventricles	Decreased rate and force of contraction
		Kidney	Increased renin secretion
		Fat cells	Increased lipolysis
	Beta$_2$	Bronchiolar smooth muscle	Dilation
		Skeletal muscle and hepatic vascular smooth muscle	Dilation
		Skeletal muscle and hepatic cells	Increased metabolic rate
Dopaminergic		Renal arterioles	Dilation at low dosage Contraction at high dosage

tines, heart, parathyroid glands, and kidneys and urinary tract).[5] This discussion considers the cardiac muscle, renal vascular, and peripheral vascular influences of the dopaminergic receptors. In the heart, dopaminergic receptors contribute to the modulation of cardiac output; in the kidneys, they regulate renal hemodynamics and electrolyte and water transport, as well as renin secretion; and in the blood vessels, they contribute to the modulation of vasomotor tone.

THE GAS TRANSPORT SYSTEM

To satisfy the gas exchange needs of the body, the cardiovascular and respiratory systems are functionally integrated as a single **gas transport system** for the support of cellular respiration (Fig. 2-2). The respiratory system moves gas to and from the alveoli (**ventilation**) and provides for the passage

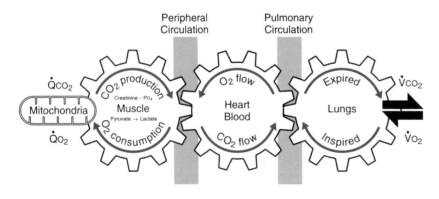

Figure 2-2. The interdependence of the musculoskeletal, respiratory, and cardiovascular systems is well illustrated as interdigitating gears, forming a single gas transport system, which supports cellular respiration. QO_2 and QCO_2 are the respective portions of perfusion related to O_2 and CO_2. (Redrawn with permission from Wasserman K, Hansen JE, Sue DY, Whipp BJ. Principles of Exercise Testing and Interpretation. Philadelphia, Lea & Febiger, 1987, p 2.)

of oxygen and carbon dioxide across the alveolar-capillary interface (**diffusion**). The cardiovascular system contributes by transporting dissolved and bound gases to and from the lungs and the cells in the blood (**perfusion**). The various cells of the body ultimately drive the gears of the gas transport system by means of oxygen consumption and carbon dioxide production in the utilization of metabolic substrates (**respiration**).

Ventilation

Ventilation of the lungs—the movement of air into and out of the lungs—is accomplished by means of the coordinated interaction of the respiratory muscles, the rib cage, and the lungs. Together, the respiratory muscles and the rib cage constitute the chest wall. Although the actions of the musculoskeletal system are generally analyzed in terms of force, length, and velocity, the force-length and force-velocity relationships of the respiratory system are inferred from measurements of pressure (implying force), volume (implying length), and flow (implying velocity).

Chest Wall Motion

The diaphragm, intercostals (internal, external, and innermost), abdominals, and several accessory muscles (e.g., sternocleidomastoids, scalenes, trapezii, quadratus lumborum) are the ventilatory muscles. Although the specific interactions of these muscles during inspiration remain a topic of controversy, most investigators would agree that the contributions of the intercostal/accessory and abdominal muscles are necessary for the proper displacement of the chest wall. For example, consider the breathing efforts of a patient with a spinal cord injury resulting in quadriplegia (e.g., C5–C7 injury): on inspiration, the diaphragm would contract, lifting and expanding the rib cage, thus decreasing intrathoracic pressure and initiating airflow into the lungs. However, because the intercostal/accessory and abdominal muscles are paralyzed, there would be no resistance to the resultant inward pull on the supra-, inter-, or subcostal tissues; likewise, there would be no resistance to the downward displacement of the abdominal contents. Consequently, the supra-, inter-, and subcostal tissues would be sucked inward and the abdomen would be pushed outward as the diaphragm descended. Clearly, the efficacy of the inspiratory effort would be minimized. Figure 2–3 contrasts the chest wall and abdominal motions that would be anticipated in a healthy person and in a quadriplegic patient.

The ribs normally function as levers when acted upon by the respiratory muscles. The fulcrum of each rib is located just lateral to the costotransverse articulation, such that when the shaft of the rib is elevated the neck of the rib is depressed. Small movements at the vertebral ends of the ribs result in much greater movements at the anterior

Figure 2-3. Normal chest wall and abdominal movements during inhalation to total lung capacity are contrasted with the chest wall and abdominal movements that occur as a result of quadriplegia arising from spinal cord injury.

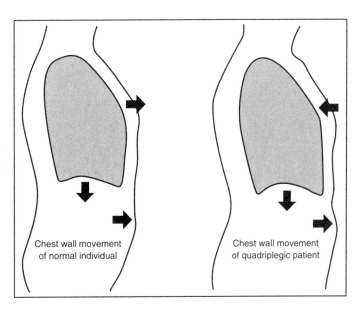

Chest wall movement
of normal individual

Chest wall movement
of quadriplegic patient

ends. The anteroposterior diameter of the thorax is first increased when the anterior ends of true ribs (most especially ribs three to six) are elevated secondary to the backward rotation of their necks, lifting the sternum forward and upward. This is, however, a minimal motion and soon the middle part of the shaft of the ribs is elevated, increasing the transverse diameter of the thorax. The costovertebral and costotransverse joints, as well as the movements of the ribs with inspiration, are illustrated in Figure 2–4. The seventh through tenth ribs primarily increase the transverse diameter of the thorax because there is only slight rotation of their necks and, therefore, their anterior ends move very little. The shaft of these ribs is elevated by an outward (lateral) and backward (posterior) movement. Any distortion of this normal movement, as might occur in extreme obesity or in kyphoscoliosis, would impair chest wall mechanics. Likewise, because the diaphragm and abdominal musculature are integral parts of the thorax, any condition (elevation of the diaphragm, spasticity of the abdominal muscles) that reduces their free movement also impairs chest wall mechanics. Because the lungs normally fill the chest so that the visceral and parietal pleurae are in contact, the lungs act in unison with the chest wall and can be thought of as a pump which may be characterized by its mechanical properties, e.g., elastic, flow-resistant, and inertial.

Lung Volumes

Before considering the mechanical properties of the lungs, it will be helpful to consider the *static*

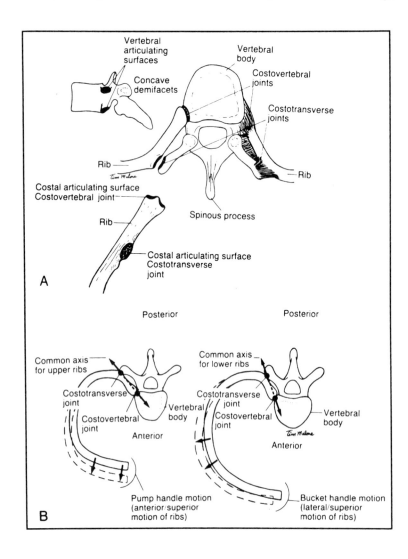

Figure 2–4. *A,* Typical costovertebral and costotransverse joints. The "pump handle" and "bucket handle" motions of the ribs during inspiration are illustrated in *B.* (From Norkin CC, LeVangie PK. Joint Structure and Function. A Comprehensive Analysis. 2nd ed. Philadelphia, F.A. Davis, 1992, pp 182–183.)

Clinical Note: Functional Anatomy of the Chest

Assessment of the chest wall configuration and integrity of the thoracic musculature is important to determine the impact of the functional anatomy on the individual's respiratory physiology.

volumes of the lungs (Fig. 2–5).[6–8] Spirometric and other tests of pulmonary function are discussed in Chapter 10. The volume of air normally inhaled and exhaled with each breath during quiet breathing is called the **tidal volume** (VT). The additional volume of air that can be taken into the lungs beyond the normal tidal inhalation is called the **inspiratory reserve volume** (IRV). The additional volume of air that can be let out beyond the normal tidal exhalation is called the **expiratory reserve volume** (ERV). The volume of air that remains in the lungs after a forceful expiratory effort is called the **residual volume** (RV). The **inspiratory capacity** (IC) is the sum of the tidal and inspiratory reserve volumes; it is the maximum amount of air that can be inhaled after a normal tidal exhalation. The **functional residual capacity** (FRC) is the sum of the expiratory reserve and residual volumes; it is the amount of air remaining in the lungs at the end of a normal tidal exhalation. The importance of FRC cannot be overstated; it represents the point at which the forces tending to collapse the lungs are balanced against the forces tending to expand the chest wall. The **vital capacity** (VC) is the sum of the inspiratory reserve, tidal, and expiratory reserve volumes; it is the maximum amount of air that can be exhaled following a maximum inhalation. The **total lung capacity** (TLC) is the maximum volume to which the lungs can be expanded; it is the sum of all the pulmonary volumes.

The amount of air moved into or out of the lungs per unit time is called the **minute ventilation** ($\dot{V}E$); it equals the product of the tidal volume and the respiratory rate. For example, if an individual were breathing at a frequency of 15 breaths per minute with a tidal volume of 400 mL, the inspired minute ventilation ($\dot{V}I$) would be 6000 ml · min^{-1}. The expired $\dot{V}E$ is normally slightly less than the $\dot{V}I$ because the metabolic production of carbon dioxide ($\dot{V}CO_2$) is less than the metabolic consumption of oxygen ($\dot{V}O_2$).

Dead Space

By recalling the anatomic relationships of the upper and lower respiratory tracts, it will be obvious that not all of the air that is inhaled reaches the alveoli. The volume of gas that occupies the nonrespiratory conducting airways is called the *anatomic dead space volume* (VD; normally about 150

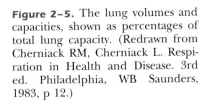

Figure 2–5. The lung volumes and capacities, shown as percentages of total lung capacity. (Redrawn from Cherniack RM, Cherniack L. Respiration in Health and Disease. 3rd ed. Philadelphia, WB Saunders, 1983, p 12.)

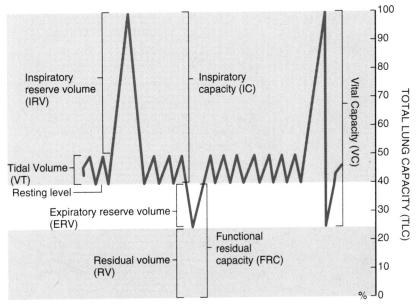

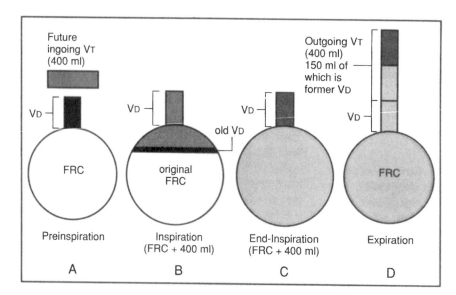

Figure 2-6. One respiratory cycle, demonstrating the distribution of a normal tidal volume (VT) and showing the effect of dead space (VD) on alveolar ventilation.

mL). To illustrate the dead space volume, Figure 2–6 depicts the tidal nature of the respiratory cycle. Panel A shows an individual at FRC, with the existing VD shown in black. In Panels B and C, the individual inhales a volume of 400 mL; the existing VD and 250 mL of the incoming VT are mixed with the FRC, and 150 mL of the VT becomes the new VD. Then, in Panel D, the ensuing exhalation pushes the VD out of the airways, along with 250 mL of the expired tidal volume, into the environment (the last 150 mL of which remains in the airways as a new VD).

Distribution of Gas

It is important to realize that not all regions of the normal lung are ventilated equally.[9-11] In the upright position, for example, the force created by the weight of the lungs makes the pressure near the base of the lungs less negative than that at the apices. Consequently, the bases of the lungs are relatively compressed at FRC and, hence, have a greater potential for expansion on inspiration than the apical (already relatively expanded) portions. There is, therefore, a continuum of ventilation within the lungs that is position-dependent. In the upright position, the bases of the lungs have a larger change in volume and a smaller resting volume than the apices; therefore, their ventilation is greater (Fig. 2–7). In the supine position, these differences disappear, and apical and basal ventila-

tion become equal. However, the ventilation of the posterior (lowermost) aspects of the lungs becomes greater than that of the anterior (uppermost) aspects. Likewise, in the side-lying position, the dependent (lowermost) lung is better ventilated.

Mechanical Properties

It should be no great revelation, at this point, that the gas transport system is made of elastic materials. This means that by its structural nature, its constituent parts try to pull themselves back to their original shapes whenever they are stretched. At FRC, the elastic recoil of the lungs (pulling inward) is balanced by the elastic recoil of the chest wall (pulling outward); these opposing forces generate a subatmospheric pressure of approximately 5 cm H_2O in the pleural space (the pleural pressure; Ppl). Keep in mind that the actual Ppl varies according to where it is measured, becoming more negative (subatmospheric) as the apices of the lungs are approached (in the upright position). At FRC, this negative intrapleural pressure holds the lungs inflated at a volume greater than would be observed if they were removed from the chest cavity while pulling the chest wall "down" to a volume that is less than would be observed if the chest wall were opened. For example, if an individual were medically paralyzed (e.g., given a neuromuscular blocking agent), positioned to rest in a

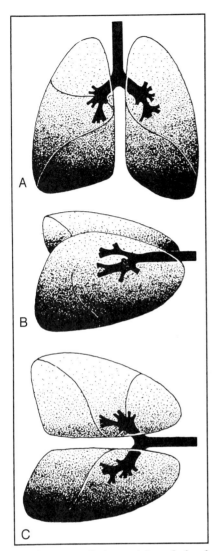

Figure 2–7. Because of the weight of the lungs, the pressure near the lowermost aspects of the dependent portions is greater (more positive, less negative) than that at the uppermost aspects. Thus, a continuum of ventilation is created within the lungs, and gas is preferentially distributed to the dependent areas. Erect (*A*), supine (*B*), and side-lying (*C*) positions are shown. (From Shapiro BA, Harrison RA, Cane RD, Templin R. Clinical Application of Blood Gases. 4th ed. Chicago, Year Book Medical Publishers, 1989, p 24.)

semi-Fowler's position, and given positive pressure breaths from a mechanical ventilatory assistance device, it would be a simple matter to inflate the lungs to TLC and then incrementally deflate them until RV was reached.

By measuring the alveolar pressure (P_A), the P_{pl}, and the atmospheric (barometric) pressure (P_B), the *transmural pressures* of the lungs, the chest wall, and the entire respiratory system could be calculated. As long as there is no movement of air into or out of the lungs, the pressure within the airways, from the mouth (P_m) or nose to the alveoli, is the same as the atmospheric pressure. The difference, then, between the pressure in the airways (atmospheric) and the pleural pressure (atmospheric −5 cm H_2O) is the pressure difference across the lung (the **transpulmonary pressure**; P_L). To illustrate, consider the lungs within the chest wall as if they were one balloon inside another as shown in Figure 2–8. In this simple balloon-within-a-balloon model of the lungs and rib cage, there are transmural pressures across the lungs ($P_L = P_A − P_{pl}$), across the chest wall ($P_W = P_{pl} − P_B$), and across the entire respiratory system ($P_{rs} = P_A − P_B$). Each of these pressures is crucial to the quantification of the distensibility of the respiratory system. Clearly, even this representation presents many complexities; imagine the complexity of 300 million balloons (alveoli) within the chest wall!

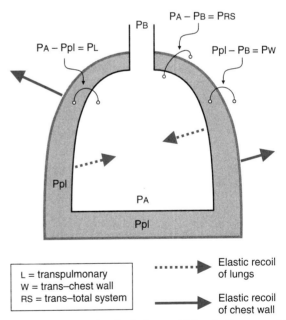

| L = transpulmonary |
| W = trans–chest wall |
| RS = trans–total system |

⋯⋯▶ Elastic recoil of lungs

──▶ Elastic recoil of chest wall

Figure 2–8. In a simple balloon-within-a-balloon model of the lungs and chest wall, only three transmural pressures—across the inner balloon (P_L), across the outer balloon (P_W), and across both balloons (P_{RS})—must be considered. Imagine the complexity that arises with two lungs and 300 million alveoli. (Adapted from Mines AH. Respiratory Physiology. 2nd ed. New York, Raven Press, 1986, p 21.)

Compliance

The **elastance** of a material is a measure of the stiffness of the material. With respect to the gas transport system, the amount of stretch on the elastic walls is measured by change in volume; the force exerted by the walls as they try to return to their original volume is measured by change in pressure. Thus, the elastance of the walls of the gas transport system may be defined as the change in pressure divided by the change in volume. Clinically, however, it is the **compliance** of the heart, the blood vessels, or the lungs that is of concern. Compliance is the inverse of elastance; it is a measure of the distensibility of a material:

$$\text{Compliance} = \frac{\text{change of volume } (\Delta V)}{\text{change of pressure } (\Delta P)}$$

Recall from physics that the forces acting to restore a material to its original shape are proportional to the amount of stretch applied to them. Moreover, the amount of the material being stretched will affect the total force that is generated. For example, if two springs, each made from the same material, but one twice as big as the other, were stretched by equal amounts, the bigger spring would generate the greater force; even though the springs are made of a material having the same elastance, there is more of the material in the larger spring. Therefore, to better describe the elastance of the material, the force exerted is divided by the cross-sectional area of the object being stretched, yielding the *stress* or *tension* (σ). In the case of alveoli, which are essentially spherical, the tension forces ($\sigma \times$ circumference) tending to collapse the spheres must be balanced by the pressure forces inside the spheres (P $\times$ area of the sphere) tending to expand them, if alveolar collapse is to be avoided. Thus, by equating the tension and pressure forces, dividing by π, and rearranging (a little magic, smoke, and mirrors), the formula for Laplace's law for a sphere is derived: $P = 2\sigma/r$.[12, 13] It must be pointed out that this equation assumes that the only pressure acting on the walls is the pressure inside the sphere, but this is true only if there is no force pushing back at the wall from the outside. Thus, the pressure calculated from the preceding equation is actually the pressure across the wall (the transmural pressure), which is the pressure inside the sphere minus the pressure outside the sphere.

From the volume-pressure curves shown in Figure 2–8, it may be seen that the lungs have a low compliance initially (starting from TLC), but after deflating by about 17% their compliance is approximately $0.2\ \text{L} \cdot \text{cm}\ H_2O^{-1}$ until FRC is reached; below RV, their compliance is very high. The compliance of the chest wall between TLC and FRC also remains fairly constant at about $0.2\ \text{L} \cdot \text{cm}\ H_2O^{-1}$, but the chest wall gets stiffer between FRC and RV. The respiratory system as a whole has a relatively low compliance near TLC (like the lungs) and between FRC and RV (like the chest wall), but the compliance in the midrange is higher, being about $0.1\ \text{L} \cdot \text{cm}\ H_2O^{-1}$, which indicates that the total system is about twice as stiff as either of its parts.

Surface Tension

Although the elastic characteristics of the lung tissue itself play a role in lung compliance, the **surface tension** at the air-liquid interface on the alveolar surface has a greater influence. Anyone who has ever attempted to separate two wet microscope slides by lifting (not sliding) the top slide from the bottom has firsthand experience with the forces of surface tension. As an example of the effect of surface tension in a curved structure, consider the transmural pressures needed to maintain an alveolus open at FRC: if we assume that at FRC there is a representative alveolus with a surface tension of 75 dynes/cm and a radius of 50×10^{-4} cm, the pressure $= 2\sigma/r = 2(75\ \text{dynes/cm}) \div (50 \times 10^{-4}\ \text{cm}) = 30 \times 10^3\ \text{dynes/cm}^2$. Converting dynes/cm^2 to cm H_2O (1 cm H_2O = 980 dynes/cm^2), the calculated pressure needed to maintain an alveolus open at FRC is about 31 cm H_2O. This calculation suggests that the transmural pressures required to keep the alveoli open should be much greater than those actually observed (Fig. 2–9). Something must, therefore, be acting to decrease the alveolar surface tension in the lungs.

For example, consider two alveoli of different sizes, one at either end of a bifurcated respiratory bronchiole (see Fig. 2–10A); because of the size difference, the smaller alveolus must have a higher pressure than the larger alveolus if the surface tension of each is the same. In order to keep the

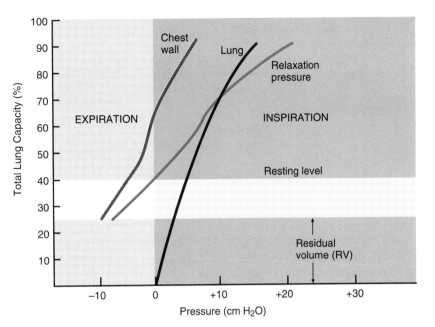

Figure 2-9. Volume versus transmural pressure curves for the chest wall in isolation, the lungs in isolation, and the total system. (Redrawn from Cherniack RM, Cherniack L. Respiration in Health and Disease. 3rd ed. Philadelphia, WB Saunders, 1983, p 17.)

air in the smaller alveolus from emptying into the larger, a surface-active agent is needed to decrease the overall surface tension of the alveoli in order to lower wall tension in proportion to the radius of the alveolus (Fig. 2-10B). Moreover, it must do so almost in anticipation of diminishing alveolar size. Only if such a surface-active agent were present could alveoli with different radii coexist in the lungs.

The surface-active agent in the human lung that performs this function is called **surfactant.** Pulmonary surfactant is not composed of a single class of

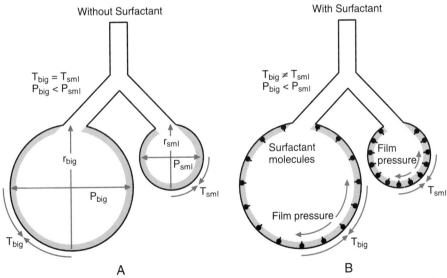

Figure 2-10. Two pairs of unequally filled alveoli arranged in parallel illustrate the effect of a surface-active agent. One pair of alveoli is shown without surfactant (A) and the other is shown with surfactant (B). In the alveoli without surfactant, if T_{sml} were the same as T_{big}, P_{sml} would have to be many times greater than P_{big}; otherwise, the smaller alveolus would empty into the larger one. In the alveoli with surfactant, T_{sml} is reduced in proportion to the radius of the alveolus, which permits P_{sml} to equal P_{big}. Thus, alveoli of different radii can coexist. Refer to the text for details.

Clinical Note: Surfactant

Surfactant is often thought of as being similar to the film found in soapy bubbles mix.

molecules but, rather, is a collection of interrelated macromolecular lipoprotein complexes that differ in composition, structure, and function.[14] Nonetheless, the principal active ingredient of surfactant is dipalmitoyl phosphatidyl choline (DPPC). The structure of the surfactant molecule is such that it presents a nonpolar end of fatty acids (two palmitate residues) that is insoluble in water and a smaller, polar end (a phosphatidyl choline group) that dissolves readily in water.[15, 16] Surfactant, therefore, orients itself perpendicularly to the surface in the alveolar fluid layer; its nonpolar end projecting toward the lumen. If surfactant were uniformly dispersed throughout the alveoli, its concentration at the air-fluid interface would vary in accordance with the surface area of any individual alveolus. Thus, the molecules would be compressed in the smaller alveoli, as depicted in Figure 2–10B. Compressing the surfactant molecules increases their density and builds up a film pressure that counteracts much of the surface tension at the air-fluid interface. The rate of change in the surface tension resulting from compression of the surfactant molecules as the alveolus gets smaller is faster than the rate of change of the decreasing alveolar radius so that a point is rapidly reached in which the pressure in the small alveolus equals the pressure in the big alveolus.

Unfortunately, if the alveolus were to remain smaller permanently, the surfactant molecules would begin to be squeezed out of the surface and the surface tension would gradually rise. Therefore, maintenance of a constant surface area (as with constant volume breathing) could result in a gradual increase of alveolar surface tension, leading to the collapse of smaller alveoli. Fortunately, we normally sigh periodically and the result is a spreading out of the surfactant molecules (for reasons not well understood, there is also an increase in the number of surfactant molecules at the air-liquid interface).

Resistance to Gas Flow

When the respiratory muscles contract to expand the chest wall, the air in the lungs is decompressed, PA becomes subatmospheric, and PB pushes air into the lungs down a pressure gradient. When the respiratory muscles relax, the chest wall recoils back to FRC, compressing the air in the lungs; PA is raised above PB and air moves out of the lungs along a pressure gradient. At relatively low flow rates, gas travels parallel to the walls of the airways in a laminar flow pattern; at high flow rates, the parallel flow of gas is disrupted, and turbulent flow results (Fig. 2–11). Generally, the pressure required to make gas flow through the airways under laminar flow conditions is proportional to the flow rate of the gas, whereas under turbulent conditions it is proportional to the square of the flow rate. Thus, relaxation and longer, slower breaths are important for patients suffering from pulmonary disease.

Along with several other factors (e.g., the density of the gas, the average velocity of the gas, the radius of the airway, and the viscosity of the gas), the flow pattern of the gas in the airways dramati-

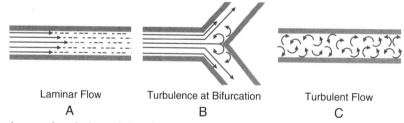

Laminar Flow
A

Turbulence at Bifurcation
B

Turbulent Flow
C

Figure 2–11. Laminar and turbulent airflow in the airways. *A,* At low flow rates, air flows in a laminar pattern and the resistance to airflow is proportional to the flow rate. *B,* At airway bifurcation, eddy formation creates a transitional flow pattern. *C,* At high flow rates, when a great deal of turbulence is created, the resistance to airflow is proportional to the square of the flow rate. (Redrawn from West JB. Respiratory Physiology—The Essentials. 2nd ed. © 1979, Williams & Wilkins, Baltimore, p 103.)

cally influences resistance to the gas flow. *Resistance to airflow* (Raw) is expressed as the pressure difference between alveolar and atmospheric pressure (ΔP) divided by airflow ($\dot{V}$):

$$\text{Raw} = \frac{\Delta P}{\dot{V}}$$

Lung volume also influences Raw because as the lungs expand during inhalation, the caliber of the bronchi and bronchioles is increased. Conversely, at low lung volumes the small airways may close completely. The variation in Raw that occurs with changes in lung volume is shown in Figure 2–12.

To demonstrate the compliance, flow resistance, pressure, and volume characteristics of the lungs, consider the following scenario. Assume that the simplified respiratory system depicted in Figure 2–13 represents the lungs of an individual breathing 20 times per minute; the measured lung compliance (C_L) is 0.2 L · cm^{-1} H$_2$O, and Raw is 2.0 cm · sec · L^{-1} H$_2$O. Panel A depicts FRC just prior to inspiration. There is no gas flow, and therefore PB = PA and the intrapleural pressure is -5 cm H$_2$O (representing the pressure created by the opposing recoil forces of the lungs and the chest wall). Panel B depicts the pleural and alveolar pressures at FRC plus 500 (ΔV) mL with an inspiratory flow rate of 1.5 L · min^{-1}. The values shown were derived by knowing that PA must be lower than PB. Thus, we can calculate that

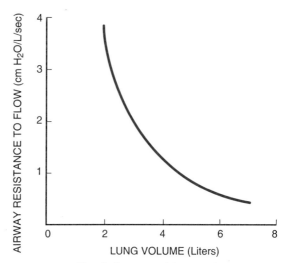

Figure 2–12. The influence of lung volume on resistance to airflow in the lungs.

$$
\begin{aligned}
\text{PB} - \text{PA} &= \text{V/sec} \times \text{Raw} \\
&= 1.5 \text{ L} \cdot \text{sec}^{-1} \times 2 \text{ cm} \cdot \text{sec} \cdot \text{L}^{-1} \text{ H}_2\text{O} \\
&= 3 \text{ cm H}_2\text{O}
\end{aligned}
$$

Therefore, PA = -3 cm H$_2$O (the alveolar pressure necessary to achieve a flow rate of 1.5 L · min^{-1} against a resistance of 2.0 cm · sec · L^{-1}). At FRC, PL was $+5$ cm H$_2$O, and it must increase as the lung volume increases during inspiration. Because the amount of the change in lung volume (FRC + 500 mL) and the lung compliance

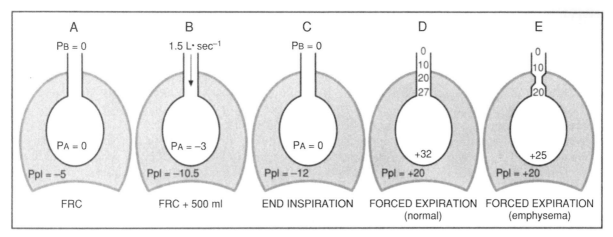

Figure 2–13. The compliance, flow resistance, pressure, and volume characteristics of the lungs at different stages of the respiratory cycle. Refer to the text for details. PB, Barometric pressure; PA, alveolar pressure; Ppl, pleural pressure; FRC, functional residual capacity.

$(0.2 \ L \cdot cm^{-1})$ are known, the change in transpulmonary pressure can be calculated as follows:

$$\Delta PL = \Delta V \div CL = 0.5 \ L \div 0.2 \ L \cdot cm^{-1} \ H_2O$$
$$= 2.5 \ cm \ H_2O$$

If the initial PL was 5 cm H_2O, it has increased by 2.5 cm H_2O and is 7.5 cm H_2O at a volume of FRC + 500 mL. Based on PL = PA − Ppl, the new Ppl is −10.5 cm H_2O. Panel C depicts end inspiration when there is no airflow and the Ppl = −12 cm H_2O. (What is the volume at end inspiration?) Panel D demonstrates a situation of forced expiration from end inspiration in a person with normal lungs. The expiratory muscles have generated an intrapleural pressure of +20 cm H_2O, which when added to the transpulmonary pressure, yields an alveolar pressure of +32 cm H_2O that moves air along a pressure gradient out of the lungs. Keeping in mind that Panels A through D depict the kind of pressure and volume changes that occur normally, now consider Panel E. Panel E presents the same situation as that depicted in Panel D, but in a person with severe emphysema. The expiratory muscles again generate an intrapleural pressure of +20 cm H_2O, but because the lungs are excessively compliant, the alveolar pressure is only +25 cm H_2O. Air begins to flow out of the lungs, but a point is reached at which flow becomes dependent only on the lung volume and the forced expiratory effort collapses the airways. The significance of this obstructive effect is discussed in Chapter 6 and the pulmonary function tests that may be used to identify it are presented in Chapter 10.

Diffusion

Diffusion, which is the passive tendency of molecules to move from an area of high concentration to an area of lower concentration, is responsible for the passage of oxygen and carbon dioxide between the alveoli and the pulmonary capillary blood. In order for O_2 molecules to get in and CO_2 molecules to get out, they must pass through gas, tissue, and liquid.

With each breath, the linear velocity of the gas in the upper airways is very high, but it becomes less and less as the cross-sectional area of airways increases with successive branching. The magnitude of change in cross-sectional area from the trachea to the alveolar ducts is astounding, being a factor of about 5000. Airflow is effectively stopped beyond the alveolar ducts because the linear velocity of the gas molecules at that point is on the order of only about 0.4 mm · sec^{-1} during normal resting inspiratory effort. Therefore, gas molecules must diffuse through the gaseous medium within the alveoli in order to cross the small distances separating the alveolar ducts and the alveolar surface lining to effect gas exchange. According to *Graham's law*, the relative rates of diffusion for two gases in a gaseous medium (the air already in the lungs) vary inversely as the square roots of their densities. More simply stated, the rate of diffusion of two gases is inversely proportional to the ratios of their molecular weights. For example, this relationship can be used to calculate relative diffusion rates for O_2 and CO_2:

$$\frac{\text{rate of diffusion of } CO_2}{\text{rate of diffusion of } O_2} =$$
$$\frac{\sqrt{MW \ O_2}}{\sqrt{MW \ CO_2}} = \frac{\sqrt{32}}{\sqrt{44}} = 0.85$$

The gaseous diffusion of CO_2 is 85% as rapid as the gaseous diffusion of O_2. The question arises, therefore, of just how much time it takes for new inhaled gas to come into equilibrium with the gas already present in the lungs. Because the average alveolar diameter is only about 0.1 mm, it would take only about 0.0005 second for the gases to come into equilibrium.[17, 18] Hence, any differences in the diffusion rates of O_2 and CO_2 are normally eliminated in a fraction of a second. However, if alveolar diameters were to be enlarged (as occurs in emphysema) and diffusion distances were to become greater, the diffusion times for the gas molecules would also be increased.

The rate of gas transfer across the alveolar-capillary membrane is directly proportional to the tissue area and inversely proportional to the thickness of the tissue. Moreover, the molecular weight of the gas and its solubility in the liquid are factors. Therefore, the amount of gas actually diffusing through the gas-blood barrier and across the alveolar-capillary membrane is proportional to the area available for diffusion (A), a diffusibility constant that expresses the relationship of the molecular weight and the solubility of the gas (d) and the driving pressure ($P_1 - P_2$), and is inversely proportional to the thickness of the tissues (T). These relationships are described in *Fick's law*.[19, 20]

$$\dot{V} = (d)\left(\frac{A}{T}\right)(P_1 - P_2)$$

Do not forget that diffusion depends on a concentration difference. The concentration of a gas in a gaseous medium is directly proportional to the partial pressure of the gas. In a liquid medium, the concentration is directly proportional to the partial pressure of the gas times its solubility in that liquid. The partial pressure of each gas in any system may be thought of as the pressure that the gas would exert if it were alone in the system. The contribution of an individual gas to the total pressure exerted by a mixture of gases is dependent upon the percentage of the total that the individual gas occupies *(Dalton's law)*. For example, in the Earth's atmosphere nitrogen (N_2) composes 79% of the constituent gases; O_2 makes up 20.93%; CO_2 is about 0.03%; and all other gases make up about 0.04%. If these atmospheric gases were at standard conditions of temperature and pressure, and dry (STPD; 0°C, a pressure of 760 mm Hg, and no water vapor pressure), the partial pressure of O_2 (PO_2) would simply be the product of the atmospheric pressure (PB) and the fraction of O_2:

$$PO_2 = 760 \text{ mm Hg} \times 0.2093 = 159.06 \text{ mm Hg}$$

However, in the real world, inspired gases are rarely completely dry. When the partial pressure of the water vapor is known, it becomes a relatively straightforward process to convert from a volume expressed in terms of STPD to ambient temperature and pressure, saturated with water vapor (ATPS), or to body temperature and ambient atmospheric pressure, saturated with water vapor (BTPS). For example, at sea level and with a typical body temperature of 37°C, water vapor exerts a partial pressure of 47 mm Hg.[17, 21, 22] Thus, the PO_2 in the trachea would be calculated as follows:[21, 22]

$$760 \text{ mm Hg} - 47 \text{ mm Hg} = 713 \text{ mm Hg}$$
$$713 \text{ mm Hg} \times 0.2093 = 149 \text{ mm Hg}$$

Henry's law allows us to calculate the concentration of a gas in a liquid if its partial pressure and solubility coefficient are known. The solubility coefficient for O_2 in a watery solution is about $0.03 \text{ mL } O_2 \cdot \text{mm Hg} \cdot L^{-1}$ and for CO_2 about $0.7 \text{ mL } CO_2 \cdot \text{mm Hg} \cdot L^{-1}$. It is clear that CO_2 is about 23 times more soluble than O_2. By combining Graham's and Henry's laws, we can see that O_2 diffuses about 15% more rapidly than CO_2 through a gas, but only about 5% as rapidly through a liquid. To illustrate the importance of this fact, consider the effect of pulmonary edema on the exchange of gases across the alveolar-capillary membrane—the acquisition of O_2 will be hindered to a greater extent than the elimination of CO_2.

Oxygen Transport

Oxygen diffuses through the pulmonary alveolar-capillary membrane and is then carried to the tissues in two forms: (1) physically dissolved in the plasma and (2) chemically bound to **hemoglobin** (Hb) in the erythrocytes (Fig. 2–14*A*).

Dissolved Oxygen

As previously discussed, the amount of O_2 that can physically dissolve in the plasma is determined by its solubility and is directly proportional to its partial pressure in the plasma. Thus, if the arterial PO_2 (Pa_{O_2}) were 100 mm Hg, there would be 3 mL of O_2 dissolved in each liter of the blood. If this small amount of oxygen were the only source of O_2 available to the body, a tremendous blood flow would be needed just to supply the body's resting requirements for oxygen. For example, if the body's requirement for O_2 at rest were $3.5 \text{ mL} \cdot kg^{-1} \cdot min^{-1}$, a person weighing 65 kg would need about $228 \text{ mL} \cdot min^{-1}$ of O_2; with only

---

Clinical Note: Diffusion in Pulmonary Edema

Clinically, the blood gas values often seen in individuals with pulmonary edema are a decreased PO_2 and normal PCO_2 demonstrating the severe hypoxemia resulting from the diffusion interference.

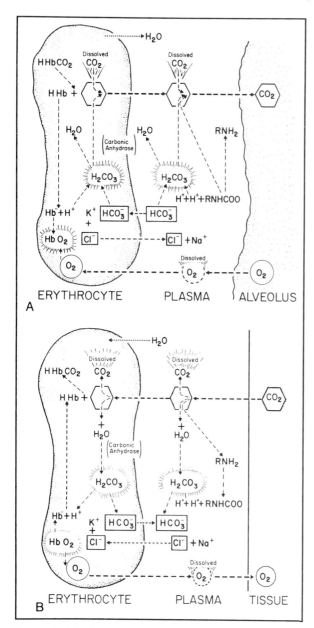

Figure 2–14. Gas exchange at the alveolar-capillary interface (A) and at the capillary-tissue interface (B). (Adapted from Cherniack RM, Cherniack L. Respiration in Health and Disease. 3rd ed. Philadelphia, WB Saunders, 1983, p 77.)

be another, more efficient, means by which oxygen is carried to the tissues of the body.

Oxygen Bound to Hemoglobin

The hemoglobin (Hb) molecule, found inside erythrocytes, is made up of four *heme* groups attached to a *globin* molecule. Heme is formed when a ferrous ion covalently binds to the four nitrogens on the pyrrole group of a *porphyrin* ring (four pyrrole groups cyclically linked by methylene bridges). The globin molecule is formed by a combination of four amino acid chains (two alpha and two beta) that contain imidazole nitrogen groups that are capable of covalently bonding with metal ions. The heme groups are believed to bind to the globin molecule by a fifth bond. Thus, the ferrous ion in each heme has a sixth covalent bond available to bind with oxygen (if it is available) or with an imidazole nitrogen group in the polypeptide chains of the globin molecule.

Because of hemoglobin's ability to reversibly bind to oxygen, the blood's carrying capacity for oxygen is significantly increased. For example, in the adult male, there are normally about 147 g of Hb in each liter of blood, and this amount of hemoglobin can carry about 197 mL O_2.[22, 23] If hemoglobin were the only source for the delivery of O_2, the 65-kg person from the previous example would need to circulate only about 1.2 L of blood per minute to meet the body's demand for O_2.

Oxyhemoglobin Dissociation Curve

The *oxyhemoglobin dissociation curve* (Fig. 2–15) describes the relationship between the amount of O_2 bound to Hb and the partial pressure of O_2 with which the Hb is in equilibrium.[24–26] Clinically, this is referred to as the percentage of saturation of hemoglobin. Under ideal conditions (blood pH = 7.4, body temperature = 37°C, [Hb] = 147 g · L^{-1}), less than 10% of the O_2 dissociates from the Hb as PO_2 falls 40 mm Hg, from 100 to 60 mm Hg. However, nearly 60% of the O_2 is

3 mL of O_2 available per liter of blood, about 76 L of blood per minute would need to be circulated to meet the body's resting demand for O_2 (remember, normal cardiac output is only about 5 L of blood per minute at rest). Clearly, there must

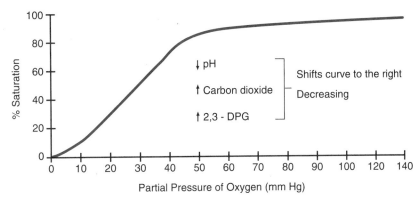

Figure 2–15. The oxyhemoglobin dissociation curve. Note that in the "flat" portion of the curve (80 mm Hg, and above), a change in Pa_{O_2} of as much as 20 mm Hg does not appreciably alter the hemoglobin saturation. However, in the "steep" portion of the curve (below 60 mm Hg), relatively small changes in saturation result in large changes in the Pa_{O_2}. pH = the logarithm of the reciprocal of hydrogen ion concentration; DPG = diphosphoglycerate.

dissociated from the Hb as PO_2 falls another 40 mm Hg, from 60 to 20 mm Hg. Decreasing the pH (increasing acidemia) of the blood from the normal value of 7.40 to 7.30 shifts the hemoglobin dissociation curve downward and to the right an average of about 7 to 8%; in contrast, alkalemia shifts the curve to the left. Increasing the concentration of CO_2 in the tissue capillary beds displaces oxygen from the hemoglobin, delivering the O_2 to the tissues at a higher PO_2 than would otherwise occur. In conditions of prolonged hypoxemia (lasting longer than a few hours), the amount of 2,3-diphosphoglycerate (2,3-DPG; a phosphate compound present in the blood in varying concentrations under different conditions) in the blood is increased, resulting in a rightward shift in the hemoglobin dissociation curve. Increasing the temperature of the tissue, as happens normally in exercising muscle, also results in a shift of the hemoglobin dissociation curve to the right. The result of these rightward shifts is a decreased hemoglobin affinity for oxygen. Although a rightward shift in the hemoglobin dissociation curve can be beneficial, the reader is cautioned that the range of variability normally tolerated by the body is relatively narrow—rapid fluctuations in pH or core temperature are not at all well tolerated.

Total Oxygen Content

The total amount of oxygen attached to hemoglobin and dissolved in plasma is represented by the arterial oxygen content (Ca_{O_2}), which is calculated as follows:

$$Ca_{O_2} = \left[\underbrace{(Pa_{O_2})(0.003)}_{\text{amount dissolved}} \right] + \left[\underbrace{(1.34)(\% \text{ sat})(Hb)}_{\text{amount bound}} \right]$$

where the constant 0.003 is the Bunsen solubility coefficient for O_2 in plasma at BTPS; 1.34 (mL O_2/g Hb) represents the experimentally determined capacity of hemoglobin to carry O_2; % sat represents the percentage of hemoglobin actually bound with O_2 and is analytically determined; Hb represents the hemoglobin content of the blood, expressed as grams of hemoglobin per 100 mL blood, normally 12 to 16 g/100 mL.[21, 23] The adequacy of tissue oxygenation depends on the relationship between O_2 and hemoglobin. Hence, the hematocrit (the packed cell volume of the blood) is probably the single most influential component in determining the oxygen-carrying capacity of the blood.

Carbon Dioxide Transport

Carbon dioxide diffuses through the tissue-capillary membrane and is then carried to the lungs in three forms: (1) physically dissolved; (2) bound to proteins as carbamino compounds; and (3) in bicarbonate (Fig. 2–14B).

Carbon Dioxide in the Plasma

Once CO_2 has diffused across the tissue-capillary membrane, some CO_2 physically dissolves in the plasma, some forms carbamino compounds and H^+ ions by binding to the amine groups of plasma proteins, and some is hydrated to H_2CO_3, which dissociates into HCO_3^- and more H^+ ions. The H^+ ions freed by the formation of carbamino compounds and the dissociation of H_2CO_3 are buffered to a large extent by the plasma proteins (see Acid-Base Balance, later in this chapter). Most of the CO_2, however, diffuses through the plasma and into the erythrocytes.

Carbon Dioxide in the Erythrocytes

Once carbon dioxide has diffused into the red blood cell, some is again dissolved into the cytoplasm. Some of the CO_2 forms carbamino hemoglobin and H^+ ions by binding to the amine groups of hemoglobin. The remainder of the CO_2 is hydrated in the erythrocytes because there is an abundance of *carbonic anhydrase* to catalyze the hydration process and because there is a tremendous source of Hb to buffer the H^+. Thus, as the blood passes through the tissues, the vast majority (about 90%) of the CO_2 taken up is converted to HCO_3^- and H^+ ions in the erythrocytes. However, because Hb buffers the H^+ ions, and because the HCO_3^- ions diffuse out of the erythrocytes and into the plasma, accumulation of these by-products of the hydration process is negligible. The influx of HCO_3^- ions into the plasma from the erythrocytes causes a countermovement of Cl^- ions into the erythrocytes. This exchange of HCO_3^- into the plasma and Cl^- into erythrocytes is called the *chloride shift*. Additionally, the increased concentrations of HCO_3^- and Cl^- ions within the erythrocytes make them hypotonic with respect to the plasma fluid. Hence, water moves into the erythrocytes, causing them to swell. For this reason, the hematocrit of venous blood is slightly greater than that of arterial blood.

The reader should keep in mind that the binding of H^+ ions and O_2 to the Hb molecule is a reciprocal process. That is, the binding of H^+ to Hb reduces the strength of the O_2 bonds, shifting the oxyhemoglobin dissociation curve to the right (Bohr shift); likewise, as the Hb deoxygenates, it binds the H^+ more strongly and becomes a weaker acid (Haldane effect).[27] The result of these reciprocal changes is that Hb is able to change its pK (the pH at which equal amounts of acid and basic forms are present), thus minimizing the pH changes of the blood as gas exchange occurs.

Pulmonary Perfusion

The distribution of blood within the pulmonary circulation is dependent on three primary factors: (1) gravity; (2) right ventricular stroke volume (the amount of blood ejected from the right ventricle per unit time); and (3) the pulmonary vascular resistance.

Gravity

In the normal person standing upright, the distance from the top of the lungs to the bottom of the lungs averages about 30 cm.[23] If the pulmonary artery enters each lung at its midpoint, the pulmonary artery pressure would have to be at least 15 cm H_2O in order to get blood flow to the top of the lungs. For this reason, blood preferentially flows through the gravity-dependent regions of the lungs. However, although the normal mean pulmonary arterial pressure is about 10 to 20 mm Hg, there is not normally a total absence of blood flow at the tops of the lungs.

A three-zone model is widely used to describe the effects of gravity on pulmonary perfusion (Fig. 2–16).[23, 28] Zone 1, at the apex of each lung, is the least gravity-dependent region and is an area of potentially no blood flow. Zone 3, at the base of each lung, is the gravity-dependent region and receives almost constant blood flow. Zone 2, the intermediate area of each lung, receives varyingly intermittent blood flow. Whether or not there is blood flow in zone 2 is normally determined by the difference between pulmonary arterial and alveolar pressures. Generally, the greater the right ventricular stroke volume, the greater the pulmonary artery pressure. Normally, then, as cardiac output increases, zone 3 extends farther up each lung.

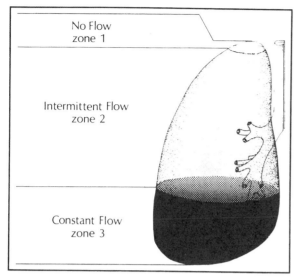

Figure 2–16. The distribution of pulmonary blood flow is gravity dependent. In the upright lung the lowermost portions of the lung are preferentially perfused. (From Shapiro BA, Harrison RA, Cane RD, Templin R. Clinical Application of Blood Gases. 4th ed. Chicago, Year Book Medical Publishers, 1989, p 25.)

Pulmonary Vascular Resistance

Unlike the systemic vascular system, the pulmonary vascular system tends to react in a passive manner to changes in pressure. Nonetheless, the pulmonary arterioles are capable of generating significant increases in resistance to pulmonary blood flow.

Ventilation-Perfusion Interactions and Shunts

The composition of the alveolar gas depends upon the balanced interaction of alveolar gas flow and pulmonary capillary blood flow. The alveolar gas flow is referred to as the **alveolar ventilation** ($\dot{V}A$); the pulmonary blood flow is referred to as **pulmonary perfusion** ($\dot{Q}$). Normally, the lungs receive about 4 L · min^{-1} of alveolar ventilation and about 5 L · min^{-1} of blood flow—hence, $\dot{V}A/\dot{Q}$. As we already know, the $\dot{V}A$ is not equally distributed throughout the lungs, being about 2.5 times greater at the bases than the apices. Similarly, the distribution of $\dot{Q}$ in the lungs is uneven, but $\dot{Q}$

is about six times greater at the bases than at the apices. Overall, however, the ratio of alveolar ventilation to pulmonary capillary blood flow is 0.8. Thus, although alveolar concentrations vary during the breathing cycle, the mean PA_{O_2} is about 102 mm Hg and the mean PA_{CO_2} is about 40 mm Hg. Furthermore, because a greater amount of oxygen is taken out of the alveolar gas than carbon dioxide is added, the expired VT is actually slightly less that the inspired VT.

Because blood flow is not distributed evenly to all parts of the lung, it is possible that some parts of the lung may actually be perfused even though they are not ventilated. Such an excess of perfusion is called a *right-to-left shunt* because the blood passes from the right to the left side of the heart without participating in gas exchange. Likewise, it is possible that some parts of the lung may be ventilated, although they receive no blood flow. Such an excess of ventilation is called **physiologic dead space** because the alveolar gas cannot participate in gas exchange. Under normal conditions, neither extreme right-to-left shunting of blood nor physiologic dead space occurs. However, many alveoli have $\dot{V}A/\dot{Q}$ ratios above or below the typical ratio of 0.8. For this reason, and because there is a small percentage of direct venous return to the left atrium (the bronchial and the thebesian veins), the partial pressure of oxygen in the arterial blood (Pa_{O_2}) is about 12 mm Hg less than the partial pressure of oxygen in the alveoli. Thus, a Pa_{O_2} of 90 mm Hg in a normal person breathing air at sea level is common.

Cellular Respiration

Within the cells, food, under the influence of several enzymes, reacts chemically with oxygen to produce energy (Fig. 2–17). Five percent or less of the overall energy metabolism of the cell occurs in the cytoplasm of the cell. The vast majority of energy is derived from the formation of **adenosine triphosphate** (ATP) within the mitochondria. Pyruvic acid, free fatty acids, and most amino acids are transformed into the intermediate compound acetyl coenzyme A (acetyl-CoA), which is, in turn, acted upon by other enzymes in the **tricarboxylic acid cycle** (the Krebs cycle) and split into carbon dioxide and hydrogen ions.[29, 30] The hydrogen ions eventually combine with oxygen to form H_2O in a

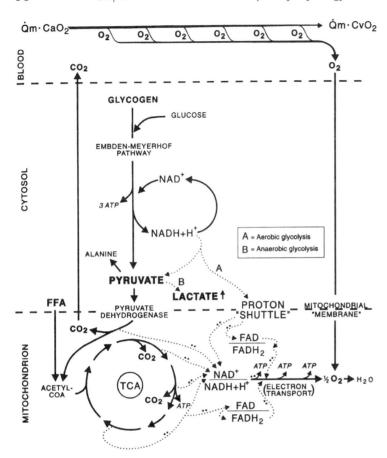

Figure 2–17. Cellular respiration. Refer to text for details. ATP = Adenosine triphosphate; FFA = free fatty acids; NAD$^+$ = nucleosidase; NADH = nicotinamide adenine dinucleotide; TCA = tricarboxylic acid (Krebs) cycle. (Reprinted with permission from Wasserman K, Hensen JE, Sue DY, Whipp BJ. Principles of Exercise Testing and Interpretation. Philadelphia, Lea & Febiger, 1987, p 12.)

process of **oxidative phosphorylation.**[31] The final step of this process is commonly referred to as the *electron transport chain.* The production of CO_2 and utilization of O_2 constitutes cellular respiration.

Even when there is insufficient oxygen available for the cellular oxidation of glucose to continue, small amounts of energy can still be released by the glycolytic breakdown of glucose to pyruvic acid and H$^+$, which are combined with NAD$^+$ to form NADH and H$^+$. These glycolytic by-products react with one another to form lactic acid, which diffuses out of the cells into the extracellular fluids, thus allowing the glycolytic reaction to continue for a few minutes longer.

Acid-Base Balance

Metabolically produced acids are largely eliminated from the body via the lungs in the form of CO_2 because the major blood acid, carbonic acid (H_2CO_3), is volatile. That is, it can chemically vary between a liquid and gaseous state. The other blood acids (dietary acids, lactic acids, and keto acids) are regulated by the kidneys and the liver.[32, 33] The measurement of arterial oxygen or carbon dioxide tension and hydrogen ion concentration for assessment of acid-base balance and oxygenation status are commonly accomplished by means of laboratory analysis of arterial blood gases (ABGs). Generally, an ABG report contains the pH, the Pa_{CO_2}, the Pa_{O_2}, and the HCO_3^- and base excess (BE) values for the sample analyzed. A detailed discussion of acid-base balance and arterial blood gases is presented in Chapter 10.

Control of Breathing

Unlike the muscle of the heart, the respiratory muscles are totally dependent upon impulses from the brain; breathing ceases if the spinal cord is cut above the level of the phrenic nerves (C3–C5). Although influenced by several nonchemical mechanisms, breathing is regulated by changes in arterial PO_2, PCO_2, and H^+ ion concentration. Moreover, although breathing is largely an automatic process, it may also be voluntarily controlled. Thus, there are two separate neural mechanisms that regulate breathing. Efferent output from the cerebral cortex to the motor neurons of the respiratory musculature is carried via the corticospinal tracts and effects voluntary control of breathing. Automatic efferent output, emanating from the pons and the medulla, to the motor neurons of the respiratory musculature is carried in the white matter of the spinal cord between the lateral and ventral corticospinal tracts. Inspiratory fibers terminate on the phrenic motor neurons in the ventral horns of the spinal cord from C3 to C5 and on the external intercostal motor neurons in the ventral horns throughout the thoracic spinal cord. Expiratory fibers terminate principally on the internal intercostal motor neurons in the ventral horns throughout the thoracic spinal cord. The motor neurons of the inspiratory and expiratory muscles are reciprocally innervated with the notable exception that the phrenic axons remain active for a brief portion of the expiratory phase. This activity is postulated to "brake the lung's elastic recoil."[34, 35]

There are two basic types of brain stem respiratory neurons: those that are active during inspiration and those that are active during expiration. Most of the inspiratory neurons increase their discharge rates during inspiration, and most of the expiratory neurons increase their rates of discharge during expiration, but some of the neurons discharge at decreasing frequencies, and others maintain a consistently high rate of discharge during inspiration or expiration.

The classical **respiratory center** of the brain stem is, in actuality, two groups of neurons located in the medulla (Fig. 2–18).[36] A dorsal group of neurons, the *dorsal respiratory group,* is located in and near the nucleus of the tractus solitarius and is composed mostly of inspiratory neurons. A long, columnar ventral group of neurons, the *ventral respiratory group,* is located in the ventrolateral medulla extending through the nucleus ambiguus and the nucleus retroambiguus and is composed of expiratory neurons at either end with inspiratory neurons interspersed centrally. Present knowledge of the mechanism responsible for rhythmic respiratory effort is sparse, but several models for the central respiratory pattern generator have been postulated.[37] Lung transplantation studies have demonstrated that neither the dorsal nor the

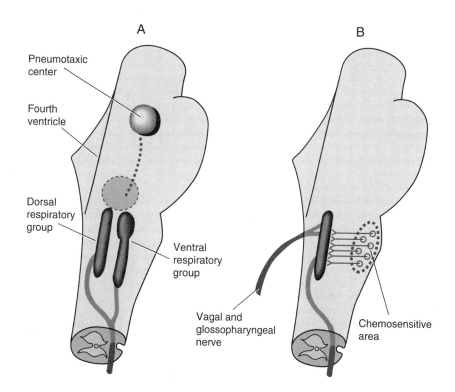

Figure 2–18. The "respiratory center" is located bilaterally in the medulla and pons of the brain stem (*A*). Input from the central and peripheral chemosensitive and peripheral proprioceptive receptors moderates the dorsal respiratory group of neurons (*B*). (Redrawn from Guyton AC. Textbook of Medical Physiology. 8th ed. Philadelphia, WB Saunders, 1991, pp 445–446.)

A

Pneumotaxic center

Fourth ventricle

Dorsal respiratory group

Ventral respiratory group

B

Vagal and glossopharyngeal nerve

Chemosensitive area

ventral respiratory groups of neurons is required for the generation of automatic breathing effort[38] (see Chapter 12).

There are also inspiratory and expiratory neurons in the medial parabrachial and Kölliker-Fuse nuclei of the dorsolateral pons that are active during both phases of breathing in the *pneumotaxic center*. The normal function of the pneumotaxic center is unknown. However, because damage to this area results in a slower rate of breathing with a greater tidal volume, it is believed to play a role in the alternation of inspiratory and expiratory effort.

Chemical and Nonchemical Mediation of Ventilation

Chemoreceptors in the carotid and aortic bodies and in the medulla are sensitive to changes in arterial PCO_2, H^+ ion concentration, or PO_2. The carotid bodies, located near the bifurcation of the common carotid artery bilaterally, and the aortic bodies (of which there are at least two), located near the arch of the aorta, are surrounded by fenestrated sinusoidal capillaries. Studies in cats suggest that some of the cells are closely associated with glossopharyngeal afferent axons and that these cells may be responsible for sensing O_2 tension.[39] Quite possibly, the aortic bodies, which are less well understood than the carotid bodies, may have a greater role in responding to H^+ ion concentration. Afferent fibers from the carotid bodies make their way to the medulla via carotid sinus and glossopharyngeal nerves, and afferent fibers from the aortic bodies travel in the vagi (see Fig. 2–19).

Other chemoreceptors in the medulla are located near the dorsal and ventral respiratory groups of neurons (see Fig. 2–18). These chemoreceptors monitor the H^+ ion concentration of the cerebrospinal fluid. Carbon dioxide in the cranial arteries readily passes the blood-brain barrier into the interstitium of the brain and the cerebrospinal fluid where it is rapidly hydrated. The H_2CO_3 dissociates and the resultant H^+ ions elevate the local concentration, lowering the pH (increasing acidity) and triggering an increase in ventilatory rate. This mechanism is responsible for increasing the minute ventilation when arterial PCO_2 becomes elevated.

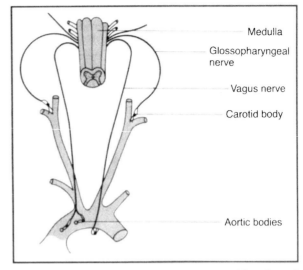

Figure 2–19. Afferent input from the carotid and aortic bodies is carried via the glossopharyngeal and vagus nerves. (From Guyton AC. Textbook of Medical Physiology. 8th ed. Philadelphia, WB Saunders, 1991, p 448.)

Both unmyelinated and myelinated vagal fibers carry impulses from receptors in the bronchi and lungs to the dorsal respiratory group of neurons in the medulla.[40] The unmyelinated fibers are C fibers, which are commonly associated with the *juxtacapillary (J) receptors*. The J receptors are stimulated by hyperinflation of the lungs and respond by causing periods of apnea interspersed with rapid breathing, bradycardia, and hypotension. The receptors supplied by myelinated fibers are further categorized as slowly adapting and rapidly adapting. The slowly adapting receptors are probably distributed in the interstitium along the airways among the smooth muscle cells. Stimulation of these receptors results in shortening of inspiration. The rapidly adapting receptors are distributed among the epithelial cells of the airways in the interstitium. Stimulation of these receptors in the trachea results in coughing, mucus secretion, and bronchoconstriction; stimulation in the lung may result in hyperpnea. The function of additional nonchemical afferent fibers from proprioceptors, from the limbic system and hypothalamus, and from the baroreceptors has been implied from the results of experiments that studied the effects of active and passive joint movement, pain and emotional stimuli, and blood pressure on breathing.

Clinical Note: Stimulation of J Receptors

Hyperpnea is often present in pleural effusion and pulmonary edema, two conditions in which the J receptors are often stimulated.

CARDIOVASCULAR SYSTEM

The primary function of the cardiovascular (circulatory) system is the transportation and distribution of essential substances to the tissues of the body and the removal of the by-products of cellular metabolism. The heart provides the principal force that pushes blood through the vessels of the pulmonary and systemic circuits. However, in the case of the systemic circuit, the recoil of the arterial walls during diastole, skeletal muscle compression of veins during exercise, and negative thoracic pressure during inspiration also move the blood in a forward direction. The pulmonary circuit receives the entire output of the right ventricle with each cardiac cycle, but the systemic circuit is an arrangement of several different circuits in parallel (Fig. 2–20).

Table 2–3		
Representative Intracellular and Interstitial Ionic Concentrations for Myocardial Muscle Cells		
ION	INTRACELLULAR CONCENTRATION (mM)	INTERSTITIAL CONCENTRATION (mM)
K^+	147	4.5
Na^+	12	145
Ca^{2+}	10^{-4}	2
Cl^-	4	112

Electrical Properties of Myocytes

The unique properties of the myocardial cell membrane are responsible for differences in the ionic composition of the intracellular and interstitial fluids. Table 2–3 lists representative values for the intracellular and interstitial concentrations of the principal ions of concern.[21, 41, 42] Although there are almost equal numbers of positively and negatively charged ions on either side of the cell membrane, there are slightly more negatively

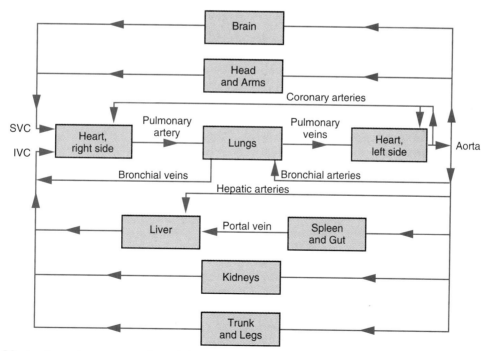

Figure 2–20. A schematic representation of the pulmonary and systemic vascular beds. SVC, Superior vena cava; IVC, inferior vena cava.

charged ions inside than outside the cell, creating a negative charge on the inside. Thus, the **resting membrane potential** for myocardial cells is about −85 mV (the minus sign is used by convention to signify that the inside of the cell is negative in relation to the outside).

Forces Acting on Ions

In general terms, an ion moves across a cell membrane because it is drawn by a difference in charge and concentration. Because of the difference in the concentration of ions inside and outside the cell, an ion tends to move along its concentration gradient (from an area of higher concentration to one of lower concentration). Likewise, because the inside of the cell is negative with respect to the outside, there is an electrical gradient along which an ion moves in accordance with its valence. The membrane potential at which these two forces come into equilibrium (E_{ion}) is expressed in units of millivolts (mV) and is calculated by the Nernst equation*:

$$E_{ion} = -61.5 \log \frac{\text{concentration inside cell}}{\text{concentration outside cell}}$$

In other words, E_{ion} represents how much an ion is drawn to move. However, whether an ion can move across the cell membrane depends on the membrane's permeability (g) to the ion. The product of membrane potential and membrane permeability is an expression of the *flux* for a given ion.

Thus far, this discussion has considered only the membrane equilibrium potential for individual ions. Of course, a cell membrane is actually permeable to several ions concurrently.[43] Ions may cross the hydrophobic membrane of the myocyte only via protein-lined *channels*. Although there are many ion-selective channels across the myocytic cell membrane, only the most notable are mentioned here. The transmembrane potential (V_m), which depends on the intra- and extracellular ion

concentrations $[K^+]$, $[Cl^-]$, $[Ca^{2+}]$, and $[Na^+]$ as well as their conductances or permeability (g_K, g_{Cl}, g_{Ca}, and g_{Na}), is described by the Goldman constant-field equation:

$$V_m = -61.5 \log \frac{g_k[K^+]_{out}}{g_k[K^+]_{in}} + \frac{g_k[Na^+]_{out}}{g_k[Na^+]_{in}} + \frac{g_k[Cl^-]_{out}}{g_k[Cl^-]_{in}} + \frac{g_k[Ca^{2+}]_{out}}{g_k[Ca^{2+}]_{in}}$$

The implication of this equation is that the membrane permeability plays a larger role in determining ionic flux than the concentration difference.[44, 45]

Active transport is the means by which cells move ions against their electrochemical gradients. This process either uses ATP to supply the energy or couples the transport of one ion against its gradient with the movement of another ion down its gradient. For example, because the permeability of the cell membrane to Na^+ is very low at rest, there is very little influx of Na^+ into the cell. Nonetheless, it is the small inward flux of Na^+ that makes the inside of the resting cell membrane slightly less negative than the predicted membrane equilibrium potential for potassium (E_K). Were it not for a metabolic pump that constantly evicts Na^+ in exchange for K^+, the steady inward leak of Na^+ would gradually depolarize the cell. However, because this *sodium-potassium pump* moves both ions against their concentration and electrostatic gradients, energy is required. The pump eliminates Na^+ and brings in K^+ in a ratio of 3:2, using ATP as the power source. The *sodium-calcium antiporter* uses the potential energy of Na^+ as it diffuses down its electrochemical gradient to move Ca^{2+} against its gradient and out of the cell. The *calcium pump* uses ATP to pump Ca^{2+} out of the cell.

As may be seen in Figure 2–21, the depolarization of fast responding myocytes results from the controlled passage of Na^+, K^+, Cl^-, and Ca^{2+} ions across the cell membrane and lasts about 2 ms. When the cell membrane potential suddenly changes to a less negative state, a sequence of opening and closing of ion channels is initiated. This sequence is called an **action potential.** Unlike the action potential of skeletal muscle, this depolarization is followed by a plateau phase that lasts about 200 ms. The rapid depolarization, phase 0, is the result of rapid Na^+ influx resulting from a

---

*In deriving the expression "−61.5," the ion in question was assumed to be univalent and positive; in the case of multivalent ions, the expression should be divided by the valence number. Furthermore, if the ionic valence is negative, the sign of the expression becomes positive.

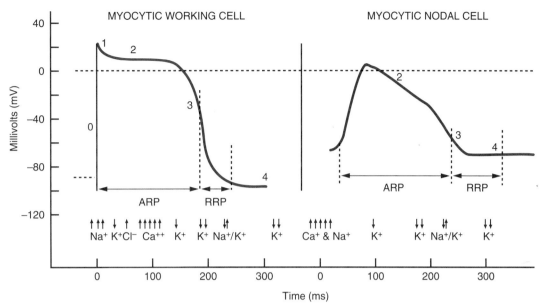

Figure 2-21. A typical action potential in a fast response (working cell) and a slow response (nodal cell) myocyte. In addition to indicating the absolute refractory period (ARP) and the relative refractory period (RRP) for each type of cell, the relative ionic flux is also shown along the bottom of the graphs. (Modified from Berne RM, Levy MN. Cardiovascular Physiology. 6th ed. Chicago, Mosby–Year Book, 1992, p 6.)

sudden increase in membrane permeability to Na^+. When V_m is suddenly changed to the threshold level, the characteristics of the cell membrane alter dramatically. Na^+ moves into the cell via specific fast channels which are controlled by two types of "gates." One gate, the *activation gate,* opens as V_m becomes less negative; the other, the *inactivation gate,* closes the channel as V_m becomes less negative. At resting membrane potential, the activation gates are closed and the inactivation gates are open. Because anything that makes V_m less negative tends to open the activation gates, thus activating the fast Na^+ channels, they are said to be "voltage-gated" channels. The entry of Na^+ inside the cell reverses some of the internal negativity; the resultant further diminution of V_m augments the inward Na^+ flux and opens more activation gates. Finally, V_m passes the threshold, and the remaining activation gates open initiating phase 0 of the action potential. As Na^+ rushes into the cell, the charge inside the cell becomes positive—the *overshoot*—and the inactivation gates start to close. Whereas the opening of the activation gates occurs in about 0.2 ms or less, closure of the inactivation gates takes about 1 ms. Once closed, the inactivation gates "inactivate" the fast Na^+ channels. The inactivation gates remain

closed until about midway through phase 3 when the cell has partially repolarized.

The initial rapid repolarization, phase 1, is due to the closure of the Na^+ channels, Cl^- influx, and K^+ efflux. Transient outward (K_{to}) channels are activated because the interior of the cell is positively charged and because the internal K^+ concentration gradient is so high.

The plateau, phase 2, is the result of the prolonged opening of voltage-gated Ca^{2+} channels. There are two types of Ca^{2+} channels in the cardiac cells, long-lasting (L-type) and transient (T-type). The L-type Ca^{2+} channels are abundantly more plentiful than the T-type and are activated during phase 0 when V_m reaches about -10 mV. The T-type Ca^{2+} channels are activated at more negative potentials than the L-type and their activation duration time is very much shorter. Although their activation duration is less than L-type Ca^{2+} channels, the T-type Ca^{2+} channels are not blocked by calcium channel–blocking drugs. The Ca^{2+} entering the cell throughout phase 2 is involved in *excitation-contraction coupling.*[46, 47]

The long-lasting, slow Ca^{2+} influx during phase 2 is offset by a K^+ efflux. The so-called inwardly rectified K^+ current, mediated via K_1 channels, results from a decrease in g_K for K^+ ions and serves to balance the slow inward currents of Ca^{2+} and Na^+ during phase 2.

Final repolarization, phase 3, is the result of closure of the Ca^{2+} channels and prolonged opening of at least three voltage-gated K^+ channels. The K_{to} channels are more prominent in the atrial myocytes than in the ventricular myocytes. They permit outward K^+ current to exceed the slow inward Ca^{2+} current early in phase 2. The delayed rectifier (K) channels are slowly activated near the end of phase 0. They allow outward K^+ current to gradually increase throughout phase 2. The K_{K1} (inwardly rectified) channels progressively increase their conductance for K^+ allowing the outward K^+ current to increase and accelerate repolarization.

Unlike fast-response action potentials, which consist of three primary components (a spike, a plateau, and a period of repolarization), slow-response action potentials lack a spike. Nodal myocytes, located principally in the sinoatrial (SA) and atrioventricular (AV) nodes, are typical of slow-response fibers. Depolarization in these fibers results from a slow inward Ca^{2+} and Na^+ current through the Ca^{2+} channels. The ionic exchanges in phases 0 and 2 in the slow-response fibers closely resemble those of phase 2 in the fast-response fibers.

Automaticity and Rhythmicity

An ability to initiate its own depolarization—**automaticity**—and the regularity with which such pace-making activity occurs—**rhythmicity**—are intrinsic traits of the heart. As noted in Chapter 1, different types of myocytes are dispersed throughout the heart tissue. Typical working myocytes compose the bulk of the tissue. The other myocytes—nodal, transitional, and Purkinje—make up the specialized conduction system of the heart and serve as pacemaker cells having a recognized hierarchy of rhythmicity. Nodal myocytes exhibit the highest rates of rhythmicity, but have the slowest impulse conduction rates. Transitional myocytes have a slower rhythmicity, but conduct impulses about twice as fast as nodal cells. Purkinje cells conduct impulses about eight times faster than nodal myocytes, but have a very low rate of rhythmicity. Working myocytes have about the same conduction velocity as transitional myocytes, but exhibit the trait of rhythmicity only under abnor-

mal conditions. The proportion of nodal, transitional, and Purkinje cells within the various regions of the specialized conduction system generally dictates the hierarchy of rhythmicity.

Normally, those cells with the highest intrinsic rates of rhythmicity override and pace the cells lower in the hierarchy. Under certain conditions *ectopic pacemakers,* or *ectopic foci,* can initiate a depolarization wave. This can occur if (1) the rhythmicity of the ectopic pacemaker is enhanced, (2) the rhythmicity of higher-order pacemakers is inhibited, and (3) the conduction path from the higher-order pacemakers to the ectopic focus is blocked.

In the nodal myocytes of the SA node, the movement of at least three different ions across the cell membrane is responsible for the instability of the phase 4 membrane potential and hence for automaticity (Fig. 2–22). The movement of Na^+ into the cell, via specific channels that differ from the fast Na^+ channels, contributes to a lessening of the negativity of the cell's membrane potential. This slow Na^+ channel is activated during repolarization, as the membrane potential becomes more negative. The more negative the membrane potential becomes, the greater the activation of the slow Na^+ channels.

The second ion contributing to the phase 4 membrane potential instability is Ca^{2+}. Mediated by the T-type Ca^{2+} channels toward the end of phase 4, the influx of Ca^{2+} destabilizes the membrane potential of the cell. These channels, too, are activated as the membrane potential becomes more negative during repolarization.

The third ion involved in the process of diastolic depolarization is K^+. Its influence comes not from an actual influx or efflux, but rather from the gradual diminution of the efflux of K^+ via the K^+ channel throughout phase 4. As a consequence, the opposition of outward K^+ current to the depolarizing influences of the two inward moving ions decreases.

Clinical Note: Ectopic Beats

Ectopic beats may be palpated in the pulse and should be monitored. In addition, ectopic beats may not be controlled with antiarrhythmic medications and should not be assumed to be absent when an individual is taking these medications. Some antiarrhythmic medications are prorhythmic.

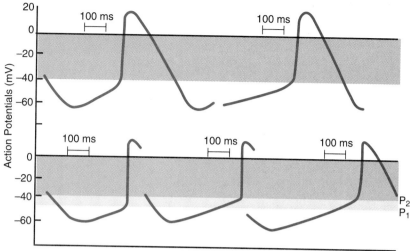

Figure 2–22. Three mechanisms of slowing the discharge frequency of pacemaker cells. In the upper portion of the diagram, the time to onset of phase 0 in the tracing on the right is greater than that on the left because depolarization during phase 4 is prolonged. In the lower portion of the diagram, the threshold potential of the middle tracing is less negative than that of the tracing on the left. Consequently, the time to onset of phase 0 is prolonged. A similar prolongation of the time to onset of phase 0 is achieved by making the resting potential more negative for the tracing on the right. (Redrawn from Berne RM, Levy MN. Cardiovascular Physiology. 6th ed. Chicago, Mosby–Year Book, 1992, p 28.)

Automaticity in the AV node is probably mediated the same way as for the SA node. In the Purkinje fibers, the T-type Ca^{2+} channels are not involved. Thus, the phase 4 membrane potential instability is mediated by the imbalance between the slow Na^+ channels and the gradually deactivating K channels. Additionally, autonomic neurotransmitters can play a role in automaticity by altering ionic currents across the cell membranes. The collective summation of the action potentials of the myocytes is graphically depicted in the electrocardiograph (ECG). The ECG, its importance, and its interpretation are discussed in Chapters 8 and 9.

Myocardial Excitation-Contraction Coupling

The mechanism by which the action potential causes myofibrillar contraction is called **excitation-contraction coupling.**[48-50] The cycle of muscle contraction is actually begun with a "primed" crossbridge—that is, an ATP molecule is hydrolyzed to adenosine diphosphate (ADP) and inorganic phosphate, allowing the crossbridge to bind weakly with an actin monomer (Fig. 2–23A). As an action potential is spread from cell to cell via the gap junctions, it is also transmitted to the innermost surfaces of the cell along the membranes of the T tubules. As noted earlier, during phase 2 of the action potential, the Ca^{2+} channels are activated, and membrane permeability to Ca^{2+} is increased. The Ca^{2+} entering the cell triggers the release of Ca^{2+} ions previously bound to the sarcoplasmic reticulum. The free Ca^{2+} within the cell binds to the troponin-C subunit of the troponin complex (Fig. 2–23B). When the Ca^{2+} binds to troponin-C, the stereochemistry of the troponin complex is changed and the troponin-I subunit is removed as a cover from the myosin binding site on the actin (thin) filament. Consequently, the crossbridges from the myosin (thick) filament are attracted to the active sites of the actin filament. It is postulated that this actin-myosin binding changes the attractive forces between the head of the crossbridge and its arm. This attraction pulls the head toward the arm, thus dragging the actin filament with it (Fig. 2–23C to E). Once the head is pulled to its arm, the actin-myosin bond is broken and the head is free to return to its original position (Fig. 2–23A). Each crossbridge is independent of the others, so the more crossbridges that can bind with the actin filaments, the greater the force of contraction.

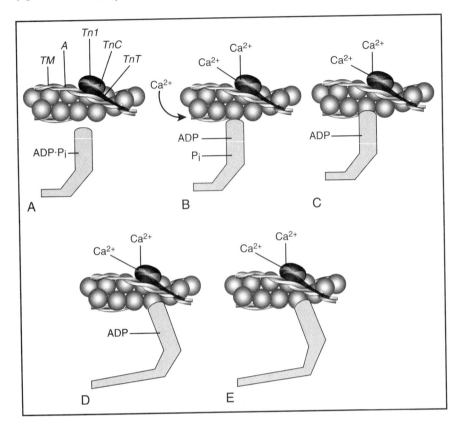

Figure 2–23. The cycle of muscle contraction is the result of a series of chemical and electrical events. A myosin crossbridge is shown at different stages of the contraction cycle. TM = tropomyosin; A = actin; Tn1 = troponin-I; TnC = troponin-C; TnT = troponin-T. *A,* A weakly bound, but "primed" crossbridge is ready for activation. *B,* The muscle has been activated (action potential elicits Ca^{2+} release from the sarcoplasmic reticulum), and the crossbridge binds strongly with actin. *C* to *E,* The actin-myosin binding changes the attractive forces between the head of the crossbridge and its arm. This attraction pulls the head toward the arm, thus dragging the actin filament with it.

At the end of phase 2, the Ca^{2+} channels close and the sarcoplasmic reticulum reaccumulates Ca^{2+} via an ATP-driven calcium pump. Simultaneously, the Na^+-Ca^{2+} antiporter in the cell membrane is also removing Ca^{2+} from the cell. Troponin-I is phosphorylated and the Ca^{2+} binding with troponin-C is inhibited, allowing the troponin complex to return to its original shape, thus recovering the myosin binding site on the actin filament. Muscular contraction ceases until the next action potential.

The Cardiac Cycle

The period from the beginning of one heartbeat to the beginning of the next is called the **cardiac cycle.** Selected events during the cardiac cycle are depicted in Figures 2–24 and 2–25. Beginning with an action potential in the SA node, a depolarization wave is spread through both atria, to the AV node, and then, through the His-Purkinje complex, into the ventricles. However, because of the nature of the specialized conduction system, the impulse is delayed for about 0.1 second in the upper two thirds of the AV node. This allows the atria to contract (a result of excitation-contraction coupling) and pump an additional volume of blood into the ventricles—an atrial "kick." Then, the ventricles provide the primary force to move blood through the vascular system.

The cardiac cycle may be further divided into two periods: **systole** and **diastole.** Systole is the period of ventricular contraction; diastole is the period of ventricular relaxation. Left-sided pressure and volume, ECG, and phonocardiographic events associated with the cardiac cycle are illustrated in Figure 2–25. Closure of the tricuspid and mitral valves generates the first heart sound (S_1), signaling the onset of ventricular systole, and is shown on the phonocardiographic tracing just after the peak of the R wave on the ECG tracing. In early ventricular systole, the ventricular volume remains unchanged despite a rapid rise in ventricular pressure. This **isovolumic contraction** occurs until the aortic valve opens, at which time the **ventricular ejection phase** *begins.* The retrograde bulging of the mitral valve into the left atrium is responsible for the rise in atrial pressure seen during the isovolumic ventricular contraction, the *c*

Figure 2–24. The mechanical events of the cardiac cycle shown in relation to the electrical events of the electrocardiogram. In late diastole, just prior to the P wave, the ventricles are filling passively. At about the time that the P wave ends, the atria contract to eject up to about 30% of the end-diastolic ventricular volume. A period of isovolumic ventricular contraction begins very shortly after the onset of the QRS complex. Ventricular ejection coincides with the early portion of the ST segment.

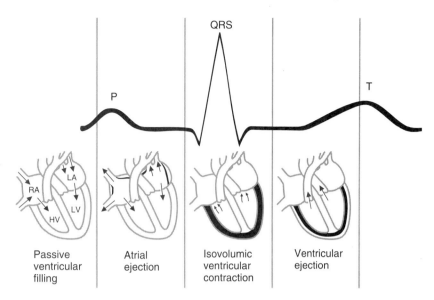

wave. Ventricular ejection continues until the aortic valve closes, terminating systole and generating the second heart sound (S₂). Immediately following aortic valve closure, there is a phase of **isovol-umic relaxation,** which continues until the mitral valve opens when ventricular pressure falls below atrial pressure. The rise in atrial pressure indicated by the *v wave* of the atrial pressure tracing is

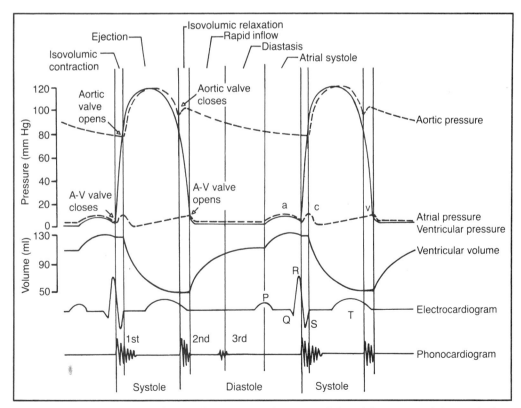

Figure 2–25. The events of the cardiac cycle, showing changes in left atrial pressure, left ventricular pressure, aortic (systemic) pressure, ventricular volume, electrocardiogram, and phonocardiogram. (From Guyton AC. Textbook of Medical Physiology. 8th ed. Philadelphia, WB Saunders, 1991, p 102.)

probably brought about by the relative negative pressure resulting from ventricular relaxation. Once the mitral valve opens, ventricular volume begins rising as the ventricle passively fills during the **rapid-filling phase.** Immediately after the rapid-filling phase is the slow-filling phase, also called **diastasis,** which continues until atrial systole. Atrial systole is indicated on the atrial pressure tracing as the *a wave.* These same events are essentially mirrored on the right side of the heart.

Preload, Afterload, and Contractility

The same physical principles and equations discussed with respect to the behavior of gases in the bronchi and lungs are applicable to a consideration of the behavior of blood in the cardiovascular system. Blood pressure in the aorta is very high and pulsatile in comparison with that in the capillaries and venules. As blood moves from the venules into the small veins, large veins, and vena cavae, the blood pressure increases but remains essentially nonpulsatile. The rate of blood flow (velocity) diminishes across the circulatory tree (from aorta to vena cavae). Although arteries are often viewed as large vessels (especially the aorta), the actual cross-sectional area of the arterioles, capillaries, and venules is many times greater because there are so many more of them. Because of the very compliant walls of the venous component of the circulatory tree, the percentage of the total blood volume that is contained in the venous circulation is several times greater than that contained in the arterial circulation. Figure 2–26 graphically depicts each of these general relationships throughout the systemic circulation.

Blood flow ($\dot{Q}$) is generally expressed in units of mL · min⁻¹ or L · min⁻¹. The normal total blood flow in an adult male at rest is about 5.6 L · min⁻¹; in women, it is about 10 to 20% less. For general purposes, it may be easier to consider a non-gender-specific value of 5 L · min⁻¹ as a representative average value of the amount of blood ejected into the aorta each minute, called the **cardiac output.** The similar amount of blood flowing from the veins into the right atrium per minute is called the **venous return.** The amount of blood ejected from the ventricles with each systolic contraction is called the **stroke volume.**

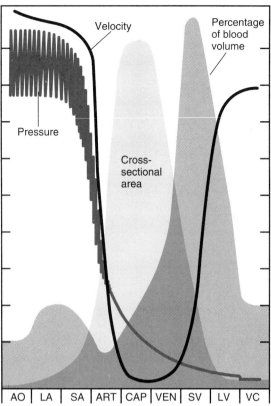

Figure 2–26. The relationships among pressure, velocity of blood flow, cross-sectional area, and capacity of the blood vessels of the systemic circulation. Note the inverse relationship between velocity and cross-sectional area. AO, Aorta; LA, large arteries; SA, small arteries; ART, arterioles; CAP, capillaries; VEN, venules; SV, small veins; LV, large veins; VC, vena cavae. (Redrawn from Berne RM, Levy MN. Cardiovascular Physiology. 6th ed. Chicago, Mosby–Year Book, 1992, p 3.)

Essentially, three factors interact to influence the stroke volume of each ventricular systole:

- **Preload,** which is the amount of tension on the muscle before it contracts
- **Afterload,** which is the load against which the muscle exerts its contraction
- **Contractility,** which includes other changes in stroke volume that are not attributable to either the preload or afterload

Preload is generally described in terms of the end-diastolic volume and end-diastolic pressure, which are the determinants of the tension on the ventricular walls (recall LaPlace's law); up to a point, a larger end-diastolic tension tends to produce a larger stroke volume. Preload is determined by the distensibility of the cardiac muscle as well as the venous return. Afterload is generally described in terms of the resistance that the ventricle must work against. The two major determinants of afterload are aortic valve compliance (and in effect subaortic compliance) and systemic arterial pressure. An elevated systemic arterial pressure provides greater resistance for the left ventricle, as does aortic valve stenosis. Contractility is an ill-defined concept and is affected by the integrity of cardiac muscle and therefore the force of contraction as well as the velocity of contraction.[51, 52] A greater force of contraction is observed in an individual with increased ventricular wall thickness and a velocity of contraction that allows an effective contraction/relaxation cycle. When the velocity of contraction of the heart is greater than 120 beats per minute, the force of contraction actually decreases because of the lack of sufficient time to relax and completely fill with volume prior to the next contraction.

The left ventricular pressure-volume diagram in Figure 2–27 illustrates the concept of *ventricular elastance.* Because the ventricle is an elastic container, the pressure and the volume of blood in the ventricle determine its elastance. The diastolic

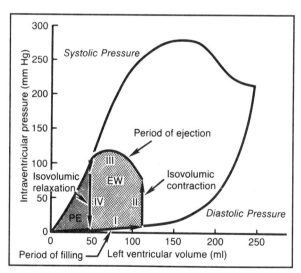

Figure 2–27. The relationship of left ventricular systolic and diastolic pressure and volume curves. The diastolic pressure does not rise significantly and, in fact, is relatively independent of ventricular volumes below 150 ml. However, at volumes greater than 150 ml, the diastolic pressure rises rapidly and retards the flow of blood into the ventricle. The highlighted arrows labeled I to IV show the changes in intraventricular volume and pressure during a typical cardiac cycle. (From Guyton AC. Textbook of Medical Physiology. 8th ed. Philadelphia, WB Saunders, 1991, p 105.)

curve is developed by incrementally filling the ventricle with blood and measuring the diastolic pressure immediately before ventricular contraction begins. The systolic curve is derived by preventing the ejection of blood from the ventricle and measuring the maximal systolic pressure that is achieved at incremental volumes of filling.

The magnitude of the rise in diastolic pressure during ventricular filling, which results from the incoming blood, depends on the elastance of the ventricle. Any increase in ventricular elastance means it takes a greater increase in pressure to add a given volume of blood to the ventricle. The diastolic pressure curve in Figure 2–27 shows that diastolic volumes of up to about 150 mL result in minimal ventricular pressure changes; thus, blood can flow readily from the atrium into the ventricle. However, above 150 mL, the diastolic pressure increases rapidly. The ventricular pressure curve shows that the systolic pressure increases rapidly with progressively increasing ventricular volumes above approximately 160 mL. Thereafter, the pressure drops off rapidly because the actin and myosin filaments are not optimally overlapping. According to LaPlace's law, more force will be required to eject a given volume from the ventricle if it is enlarged from overfilling.

The inclusion of the normal left ventricular pressure-volume loop in Figure 2–27 shows that the elastance of the ventricle increases progressively from its minimum during diastole to its maximum at the end of systole. If elastance did not continue to increase after the opening of the aortic valve, the ventricular pressure would fall and the aortic valve would close. Thus, the larger the end-systolic elastance, the greater the stroke volume.

Figure 2–28 illustrates how changes in preload, afterload, and contractility affect stroke volume. Loop *n* shows a normal ventricular pressure-volume loop for one contraction, with the end-diastolic volume equal to 125 mL. A 25-mL increase in venous return increases the end-diastolic volume to 150 mL for the next contraction, as shown by loop *p*. If the end-systolic pressure and contractility remain unchanged, the end-systolic volume for loops *n* and *p* is the same. Thus, the stroke volume increased from 75 mL to 100 mL, which mirrors the increase in venous return. In an oversimplified manner, this is an example of the Frank-Starling law, which says that if venous return increases, the stroke volume will increase by the same amount, so that the cardiac output will equal

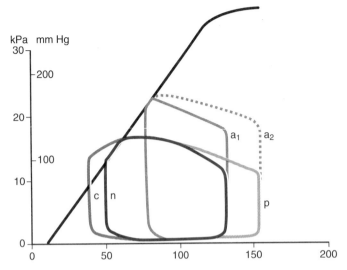

Figure 2–28. The effect of changes in preload, afterload, and contractility on the stroke volume of the left ventricle. (Refer to text for details.)

the venous return. For many years, this self-regulating (not dependent on neural or hormonal influences) property of cardiac muscle was attributed to the amount of overlap between actin and myosin filaments. However, it is now known that two mechanisms are responsible. First, the sensitivity of the thin filaments for Ca^{2+} is enhanced as the sarcomere lengthens. Therefore, more actin-myosin crossbridges can form at the same $[Ca^{2+}]$ in the cytoplasm. Second, as sarcomere length is increased, more Ca^{2+} enters the cytoplasm.

If, as in the case of hypertension, which increases afterload, the ventricle has to generate a higher end-systolic pressure, the stroke volume will be reduced. In Figure 2–28, loop n is a normal ventricular pressure-volume loop for one contraction, showing a normal end-systolic pressure of about 112 mm Hg (15 kPa). The effect of a sudden increase in systemic (aortic) blood pressure on the next contraction is indicated by loop a_1. Although the end-diastolic volumes of loops n and a_1 are the same, it takes a higher ventricular pressure in loop a_1, 150 mm Hg (20 kPa), to push the aortic valve open because of the elevated aortic pressure. Because the contractility is the same, the maximal systolic elastance will also be the same so that loop a_1 intersects the end-systolic pressure-volume curve at a point above and to the right of loop n. Therefore, the end-systolic volume is increased to 75 mL, instead of 50 mL, and the stroke volume is reduced from 75 mL to 50 mL. However, this effect is transient because if the venous return is unchanged, the subsequent diastole will deliver another 75 mL of blood to the ventri-

cle. The resultant new end-diastolic volume will be 150 mL, which is 50 mL more than normal. The increased end-diastolic volume increases the ensuing stroke volume as seen in loop a_2. The net result is an eventual return of stroke volume to a "normal" 75 mL, despite an increase in both the end-diastolic and end-systolic volumes. With hypertension, the ventricle is working harder to pump a normal cardiac output, leaving little reserve capacity for situations in which an increased cardiac output might be necessary.

If contractility is increased, the stroke volume can increase, even though end-diastolic volume and aortic pressure are unchanged. Loop c shows just such a case, in which stroke volume has increased to 85 mL. Clinically, however, it is more common for an increase in contractility to be the compensatory result of the body's effort to maintain a normal stroke volume in the face of an increased aortic pressure or a decreased end-diastolic volume. Anything that increases contractility is said to have a *positive inotropic* effect. On the other hand, the most common example of decreased contractility is a failing heart.

Clinical Note: Increasing Contractility of the Heart

Individuals with a failing heart and decreased contractility are often started on positive inotropic agents, including lanoxin. Although these medications may improve the cardiac contractility, the contractility does not usually achieve normal stroke volume levels.

Cardiac Reflexes

Several of the rapid-acting nervous system mechanisms that have roles in arterial pressure control also influence the heart rate.[53, 54] The **baroreceptor reflexes** are probably the most readily recognized. These stretch receptors are located in the walls of almost all the large arteries, although they are particularly plentiful in the walls of the internal carotid arteries, superior to the carotid bifurcation, in an area called the **carotid sinuses** and in the walls of the arch of the aorta. The baroreceptors are stimulated only at pressures in excess of 60 mm Hg, peaking in activity at about 180 mm Hg.[21] The resultant reflex has two basic effects: (1) vasodilatation, via inhibition of the vasomotor centers of the medulla; and (2) decreased heart rate and strength of contraction, via vagal stimulation. The *Bainbridge reflex* is an atrial stretch reflex that causes changes in heart rate.[55] It is elicited when the right atrial pressure rises sufficiently to distend the right atrium. The Bainbridge reflex causes an increase in the heart rate if the heart is beating at normal rates, but it causes a decrease in the heart rate if the heart is beating at high rates. The *chemoreceptor reflex* manifests itself predominantly as an increase in the depth and rate of ventilation in response to a lack of oxygen, but it also influences heart rate. When ventilatory stimulation is mild, the heart rate usually decreases, but when ventilatory stimulation is pronounced, the heart rate usually increases. Respiratory variation in heart rate is observable in most individuals; typically, there is an acceleration in heart rate during inspiration and a deceleration during expiration (there is an apparent increase in sympathetic activity on inhalation, whereas vagal activity increases on exhalation).

Resistance to Flow and Control of Flow

In Figure 1–16, the arterioles have been labeled as resistance vessels and given the look of a spigot and faucet. The arterioles are portrayed in this way because, just as the opening or closing of a spigot on a faucet controls flow, the changing of arteriolar resistance will control the flow of blood to each of the body's individual capillary beds. With respect to the flow of blood through the various blood vessels, the determinants of resistance are described by Poiseuille's law, which says that the resistance to flow of a fluid through a tube depends on the viscosity of the fluid, the length of the tube, and the fourth power of the radius of the tube:

$$R = \frac{8\eta l}{\pi r^4}$$

where R is the resistance to flow; η is the viscosity of the fluid, which in the case of blood will be reflected by the fraction of the blood that is cells (normally 0.38 in females and 0.45 in males); l is the length of the vessel, which usually doesn't vary much over the short term; and r is the radius of the tube, the most important factor. So in very general terms $\dot{Q}$ is proportional to r^4. Thus, a small change in the radius of the tube will produce a large change in the flow through the tube. Because of the anatomic arrangement and distribution of the blood vessels, they may be thought of as exerting resistances to flow in both series and parallel. Thus, the total resistance through the vessels arranged in series is the sum of the resistances through the individual vessels; and the total resistance through the vessels arranged in parallel is less than any of the individual resistances. In addition to the Frank-Starling principle, three additional factors play a role in controlling the radii of arterioles:

- Local metabolic needs
- Locally released vasoactive substances
- The central nervous system

The best explanation of the mechanism for local regulation suggests that the degree of arteriolar smooth muscle contraction depends on the concentration of fuels (substrates) and metabolic wastes (metabolites) in the interstitial fluid immediately surrounding the arteriole. Basically, when fuels are in short supply or when wastes are accumulating, the arterioles are prompted to dilate, thus increasing blood flow to deliver more fuel and carry away accumulated wastes. Alternatively, when fuel is in abundant supply and the concentration of wastes is low, blood flow is decreased, thereby obviating any excess cardiac output. The specific substrates and metabolites that link metabolism and smooth muscle tone are not known. Foremost among the potential candidates for the role is adenosine, a by-product of the breakdown of ATP that is able to pass readily into the extracellular fluid. Other candidates include CO_2, H^+, NO, insulin, and inorganic phosphates.[56-58]

Other locally mediated control mechanisms that are not directly concerned with substrate supply or metabolite elimination are also active in the regulatory process of blood flow. For example, when antigens are detected by the immune system, mast cells in the connective tissue or basophils in the blood release histamine. Histamine first binds with receptors on the preganglionic sympathetic terminals, thus inhibiting the release of norepinephrine, and it also binds with receptors inside the arterioles on their endothelial membranes. The endothelial cells then produce *endothelium-derived relaxing factor* (EDRF), which diffuses out of the arterioles to the smooth muscles and causes vasodilation.

Local metabolic control of arteriolar resistance accounts for the needs of the cells in the immediate vicinity of the individual vascular bed affected. However, the central nervous system takes into account how the flows to each of the many vascular beds combine to affect the entire body. Table 2–2 summarizes the cardiovascular effects of autonomic sympathetic and parasympathetic activity.

The sympathetic branch of the central nervous system exerts the most important influence on the arterioles. Although the density of the innervation varies from vascular bed to vascular bed, almost all arterioles are innervated by postganglionic sympathetic fibers. The neurotransmitter norepinephrine, released by these postganglionic neurons, binds with the alpha$_1$-adrenoreceptors on the cell membranes of the arterial and arteriolar smooth muscle, resulting in muscular contraction and, thus, increased resistance. In a negative feedback loop that manifests itself when there is an overabundance of norepinephrine, alpha$_2$ receptors in the presynaptic cell membrane will bind with some of the norepinephrine and exert an inhibitory effect on its further release. The arterioles of certain tissues are also innervated by postganglionic fibers of the parasympathetic branch of the nervous system, and to a much lesser extent, parasympathetic stimulation can also play a role in the control of arteriolar resistance. By releasing acetylcholine, the postsynaptic parasympathetic neurons can reduce arteriolar resistance to flow by relaxing arteriolar smooth muscle. Additionally, acetylcholine may play an inhibitory role presynaptically by inhibiting the release of norepinephrine from postganglionic sympathetic neurons.

In addition to the direct neural release of vasoconstricting and vasorelaxing factors, hormonal release into the blood is another way in which the central nervous system can affect arteriolar resistance. For example, in response to low blood volume, the posterior pituitary gland is stimulated to release vasopressin (a potent vasoconstrictor) into the blood. Likewise, as part of a general sympathetic response, the adrenal gland releases the **catecholamines** epinephrine and norepinephrine into the blood. Both catechols bind to alpha receptors on vascular smooth muscle, but epinephrine will preferentially bind to beta$_2$ receptors in those vascular beds that have them. Thus, low concentrations of epinephrine circulating in the blood cause vasodilation because epinephrine binds to beta$_2$ receptors, but high concentrations cause overall vasoconstriction because epinephrine will also bind to alpha receptors if there aren't enough beta$_2$ receptors to accept it.

Clearly, the coordinated interaction between local and central nervous system mediation of arteriolar smooth muscle tone determines the final flow of blood into the vascular beds. Furthermore, this interplay will yield different results in different tissues. The reader is cautioned to keep in mind that alpha and beta receptor functions can be either excitatory or inhibitory. Neither is necessarily associated with excitation or inhibition, but rather with the affinity of the receptor for a particular hormone in a given effector organ.

Once blood enters the capillaries, two mechanisms regulate the exchange of nutrients (O_2, amino acids, glucose) from the blood for wastes (CO_2, urea, etc.) from the cells—diffusion (the same mechanism as was discussed for the exchange of gases at the alveolar-capillary membrane) and filtration. Diffusion may be the principal mechanism, but filtration is important as a means of maintaining the fluid balance between the vascular and extravascular compartments.

Although diffusion across the capillary membrane is governed by the same factors regulating diffusion across the alveolar-capillary membrane, filtration is a bit more complicated. Filtration is the bulk flow of fluids through the tight junctions of the capillary walls and is dependent on how easily water can move through the tight junctions, which is, in turn, dependent on just how "tight" the tight junctions are, and on the pressure gradient from inside the capillary to the interstitial fluid. The pressure gradient has two components: the fluid pressure gradient and the osmotic pressure gradient.

- The *fluid pressure gradient* (hydrostatic pressure gradient) is the difference between the fluid pressure inside the capillary (P_{cap}) and the interstitial fluid ($P_{interstit}$). The blood pressure in the capillary is the same as P_{cap} (P_{cap} = 30 mm Hg, or 4 kPa, at the arteriolar end; 15 mm Hg, or 2 kPa, at the venular end), and $P_{interstit}$ is considered to be 0 (possibly even negative).
- The *osmotic pressure gradient* depends on the concentration of impermeable solutes in the fluid. These are mostly proteins (like albumin) that are much more abundant in the blood than in the interstitial fluid. Thus, the capillary osmotic pressure (P_{cap}, about 25 mm Hg or 3 kPa) is much higher than the interstitial fluid osmotic pressure ($P_{interstit}$, about 2 mm Hg or 0.26 kPa). Because the osmotic pressure gradient is the force tending to attract water, water is pulled toward the higher osmotic pressure.

The balance of these two forces (sometimes called **Starling forces**) is described by the **Starling hypothesis**:

$$\text{filtration or absorption} = k[(P_{cap} + \Pi_{interstit}) - (P_{interstit} + \Pi_{cap})]$$

where P_{cap} is the hydrostatic pressure in capillaries; $P_{interstit}$ is the hydrostatic pressure of interstitial fluid; Π_{cap} is the osmotic pressure of plasma protein (also called oncotic pressure); $\Pi_{interstit}$ is the osmotic pressure of the interstitial fluid; and k is the filtration constant for the capillary membrane. When the equation yields a positive number, filtration occurs; absorption occurs if the sum is negative.[41, 42]

Because the capillary blood pressure decreases from one end of the capillary to the other (greater at the arteriolar end than at the venular end), the filtration rate also changes along the capillary. Normally, capillary blood pressure is greater than plasma osmotic pressure at the arteriolar end, and the plasma osmotic pressure is greater than the capillary blood pressure at the venular end. Figure 2–29 illustrates the pressure gradients across the wall of a muscular capillary.

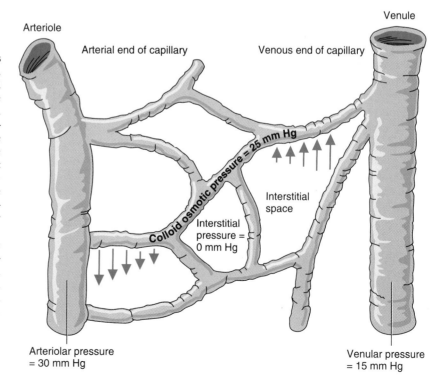

Figure 2–29. Pressure gradients across the wall of a typical capillary. The numbers at the arteriolar and venular ends of the capillary are the respective hydrostatic pressures. Filtration occurs at the arteriolar end of the capillaries because the arteriolar pressure exceeds the sum of the plasma colloid osmotic and the interstitial pressures (35 > 25 + 1). Absorption occurs because the sum of the interstitial and colloid osmotic pressures is greater than the venular pressure (1 + 25 > 15). The arrows indicate the approximate magnitudes of filtration (*outgoing arrows*) or absorption (*incoming arrows*). (Adapted from Ganong WF. Review of Medical Physiology. 15th ed. Norwalk, CT, Appleton & Lange, 1991, p 546.)

Arteriole

Arterial end of capillary

Venule

Venous end of capillary

Colloid osmotic pressure = 25 mm Hg

Interstitial space

Interstitial pressure = 0 mm Hg

Arteriolar pressure = 30 mm Hg

Venular pressure = 15 mm Hg

Some organs have a higher filtration/reabsorption ratio than others. For example, more fluid is filtered out of the liver than is reabsorbed. In contrast, the capillaries of the lungs reabsorb any other fluid that enters the lungs in addition to those fluids filtered. The balance of filtration and reabsorption is greatly influenced by arteriolar resistance. Because the capillaries are connected in series with the arterioles, an increase in arteriolar resistance will lead to a decrease in capillary blood pressure. Lower capillary blood pressure will lead to more reabsorption. For example, after a large blood loss, the baroreflex causes generalized vasoconstriction to maintain blood pressure. The resultant arteriolar constriction and the lowered total plasma volume lead to a lower capillary blood pressure, thus favoring reabsorption.

Edema, which results from fluids leaving the capillaries at a faster rate than they are reabsorbed, can be caused by anything that increases filtration relative to reabsorption or that decreases lymph drainage. For example, pregnancy causes an increase in extracellular fluid volume, which leads to an increase in venous pressure and yields an increase in capillary pressure, thereby increasing filtration pressure.

Summary

- There are two categories of cholinergic receptors: muscarinic and nicotinic. Muscarinic receptors are located at the interfaces between the postganglionic neurons and the effector cells of all parasympathetic terminal synapses. Nicotinic receptors are found at the junction between the preganglionic and postganglionic neurons of both branches of the autonomic nervous system and at the neuromuscular junctions of skeletal muscle fibers in the peripheral nervous system.
- There are two categories of adrenergic receptors: alpha and beta.
- Dopaminergic receptors are a third class of neurotransmitter receptors within the sympathetic branch of the autonomic receptors and are found throughout the body, including the kidneys, heart, intestines, blood vessels, and carotid bodies.
- Ventilation is accomplished by means of the coordinated interaction of the respiratory muscles, the rib cage, and the lungs; therefore, assess-

ment of all three is essential in a comprehensive evaluation.
- The volume of gas that occupies the nonrespiratory conducting airways is called the anatomic dead space volume. This volume increases when an artificial airway is present.
- Compliance (the measure of distensibility of a material), surface tension, diffusion, and resistance to gas flow play roles in the gas transport system and, if not optimal, will affect the respiratory physiology.
- Oxygen diffuses into the capillaries and is carried to tissues either chemically bound to hemoglobin in the erythrocytes or physically dissolved in the plasma.
- Carbon dioxide diffuses through the tissue-capillary membrane and is then carried to the lungs in three forms: physically dissolved in the plasma, bound to proteins as carbamino compounds, and as bicarbonate.
- Chemoreceptors in the carotid and aortic bodies and in the medulla are sensitive to changes in the arterial P_{CO_2}, H^+ ion concentration, or P_{O_2}.
- The heart muscle has an ability to initiate its own depolarization (automaticity) and demonstrates regularity with pacemaking activity (rhythmicity). Under certain conditions (e.g., nicotine or caffeine ingestion, anxiety), ectopic foci can initiate a depolarization wave.
- Three factors interact to influence the stroke volume of each ventricular systole: the amount of tension on the muscle before it contracts (preload), the force of contraction (contractility), and the load against which the muscle exerts its contraction (afterload).
- Baroreceptor reflexes are the stretch receptors located in the walls of most large arteries that respond to increased pressure.
- The Bainbridge reflex is an atrial stretch reflex that causes changes in the heart rate.
- The radii of arterioles are controlled by local metabolic needs, locally released vasoactive substances, and the central nervous system.

References

1. The autonomic nervous system: structure, function and development. Proceedings of a symposium. Oxford, U.K., 13–15 September 1990. J Auton Nerv Syst 33:91–222, 1991.
2. Piascik MT, Soltis EE, Piascik MM, Macmillan LB. Alpha-adrenoceptors and vascular regulation: Molecular, pharma-

cologic and clinical correlates. Pharmacol Ther 72:215–241, 1996.

3. Kaumann AJ, Molenaar P. Modulation of human cardiac function through 4 beta-adrenoceptor populations. Naunyn Schmiedebergs Arch Pharmacol 355:667–681, 1997.

4. Enocksson S, Shimizu M, Lonnqvist F, et al. Demonstration of an in vivo functional beta 3-adrenoceptor in man. J Clin Invest 95:2239–2245, 1995.

5. Jose PA, Eisner GM, Felder RA. Renal dopamine receptors in health and hypertension. Pharmacol Ther 80:149–182, 1998.

6. Kendrick AH. Comparison of methods of measuring static lung volumes. Monaldi Arch Chest Dis 51:431–439, 1996.

7. Baydur A, Sassoon CS, Carlson M. Measurement of lung mechanics at different lung volumes and esophageal levels in normal subjects: Effect of posture change. Lung 174:139–151, 1996.

8. Brown RA. Derivation, application, and utility of static lung volume measurements. Respir Care Clin North Am 3:183–220, 1997.

9. Suga K, Nishigauchi K, Kume N, et al. Dynamic pulmonary SPECT of xenon-133 gas washout. J Nucl Med 37:807–814, 1996.

10. Ross DJ, Wu P, Mohsenifar Z. Assessment of postural differences in regional pulmonary perfusion in man by single-photon emission computerized tomography. Clin Sci (Colch) 92:81–85, 1997.

11. Puybasset L, Cluzel P, Chao N, et al. A computed tomography scan assessment of regional lung volume in acute lung injury. The CT Scan ARDS Study Group. Am J Respir Crit Care Med 158:1644–1655, 1998.

12. Fowler NO. Law of Laplace. N Engl J Med 285:1087–1088, 1971.

13. Gauthier AP, Verbanck S, Estenne M, et al. Three-dimensional reconstruction of the in vivo human diaphragm shape at different lung volumes. J Appl Physiol 76:495–506, 1994.

14. Hawgood S. Pulmonary surfactant apoproteins: A review of protein and genomic structure. Am J Physiol 257:L13–22, 1989.

15. Lacaze-Masmonteil T. Pulmonary surfactant proteins. Crit Care Med 21:S376–379, 1993.

16. Johansson J, Curstedt T. Molecular structures and interactions of pulmonary surfactant components. Eur J Biochem 244:675–693, 1997.

17. Forster RE. The Lung: Physiologic Basis of Pulmonary Function Tests. 3rd ed. Chicago, Year Book Medical Publishers, 1986.

18. Comroe JH Jr. The lung. Sci Am 214:57–66, 1966.

19. Vidal Melo MF, Loeppky JA, Caprihan A, Luft UC. Alveolar ventilation to perfusion heterogeneity and diffusion impairment in a mathematical model of gas exchange. Comput Biomed Res 26:103–120, 1993.

20. Chang HK. Multicomponent diffusion in the lung. Fed Proc 39:2759–2764, 1980.

21. Guyton AC, Hall JE. Textbook of Medical Physiology. 9th ed. Philadelphia, WB Saunders, 1996.

22. Mines AH. Respiratory Physiology. Raven Press Series in Physiology. 3rd ed. New York, Raven Press, 1993.

23. Shapiro BA, Peruzzi WT. Clinical Application of Blood Gases. 5th ed. Chicago, Mosby–Year Book, 1994.

24. Goodfellow LM. Application of pulse oximetry and the oxy-hemoglobin dissociation curve in respiratory management. Crit Care Nurs Q 20:22–27, 1997.

25. Sims J. Making sense of pulse oximetry and oxygen dissociation curve. Nurs Times 92:34–35, 1996.

26. Dickson SL. Understanding the oxyhemoglobin dissociation curve. Crit Care Nurse 15:54–58, 1995.

27. Grant BJ. Influence of Bohr-Haldane effect on steady-state gas exchange. J Appl Physiol 52:1330–1337, 1982.

28. West JB. Respiratory Physiology—the Essentials. 5th ed. Baltimore, Williams & Wilkins, 1995.

29. Molina P, Burzstein S, Abumrad NN. Theories and assumptions on energy expenditure. Determinations in the clinical setting. Crit Care Clin 11:587–601, 1995.

30. Krebs H. Citric acid cycle: A chemical reaction for life. Nurs Mirror 149:30–32, 1979.

31. Maddaiah VT. Exercise and energy metabolism. Pediatr Ann 13:565–572, 1984.

32. Coleman NJ, Houston L. Demystifying acid-base regulation. Aust Nurs J 5:23–26, 1998.

33. Harrison RA. Acid-base balance. Respir Care Clin North Am 1:7–21, 1995.

34. Neural Control of Breathing: Molecular to Organismal Perspectives. Proceedings of a conference. Madison, Wisconsin, 21–25 July 1996. Respir Physiol 110:69–317, 1997.

35. Bonham AC. Neurotransmitters in the CNS control of breathing. Respir Physiol 101:219–230, 1995.

36. Braman SS. The regulation of normal lung function. Allergy Proc 16:223–226, 1995.

37. Rybak IA, Paton JF, Schwaber JS. Modeling neural mechanisms for genesis of respiratory rhythm and pattern. II. Network models of the central respiratory pattern generator. J Neurophysiol 77:2007–2026, 1997.

38. Iber C, Simon P, Skatrud JB, et al. The Breuer-Hering reflex in humans. Effects of pulmonary denervation and hypocapnia. Am J Respir Crit Care Med 152:217–224, 1995.

39. Donoghue S, Felder RB, Jordan D, Spyer KM. The central projections of carotid baroreceptors and chemoreceptors in the cat: a neurophysiological study. J Physiol (Lond) 347:397–409, 1984.

40. Wang CY, Lai CJ, Kou YR. Inhibitory influence of lung vagal C-fiber afferents on the delayed ventilatory response to inhaled wood smoke in rats. Chin J Physiol 39:15–22, 1996.

41. Ganong WF. Review of Medical Physiology. 19th ed. Stamford, CT, Appleton & Lange, 1999.

42. Berne RM, Levy MN. Cardiovascular Physiology. 7th ed. St. Louis, Mosby, 1997.

43. Rudy Y, Shaw RM. Cardiac excitation: An interactive process of ion channels and gap junctions. Adv Exp Med Biol 430:269–279, 1997.

44. Strieter J, Stephenson JL, Palmer LG, Weinstein AM. Volume-activated chloride permeability can mediate cell volume regulation in a mathematical model of a tight epithelium. J Gen Physiol 96:319–344, 1990.

45. Civan MM, Bookman RJ. Transepithelial Na^+ transport and the intracellular fluids: A computer study. J Membr Biol 65:63–80, 1982.

46. Moore RL, Musch TI, Cheung JY. Modulation of cardiac contractility by myosin light chain phosphorylation. Med Sci Sports Exerc 23:1163–1169, 1991.

47. Katz AM. Regulation of myocardial contractility 1958–1983: An odyssey. J Am Coll Cardiol 1:42–51, 1983.

48. Williams AJ. The functions of two species of calcium channel in cardiac muscle excitation-contraction coupling. Eur Heart J 18(suppl A):A27–35, 1997.

49. Spotlight on excitation-contraction coupling in the mammalian myocardium. International symposium, Leeds, 26–29 July 1992. Proceedings. Cardiovasc Res 27:1700–1886, 1993.

50. Balke CW, Gold MR. Excitation-contraction-relaxation coupling in the normal and failing heart. Heart Dis Stroke 2:150–155, 1993.

51. Westerhof N. Physiological hypotheses—Intramyocardial pressure. A new concept, suggestions for measurement. Basic Res Cardiol 85:105–119, 1990.

52. Zinemanas D, Beyar R, Sideman S. Effects of myocardial contraction on coronary blood flow: An integrated model. Ann Biomed Eng 22:638–652, 1994.
53. Feigl EO. Neural control of coronary blood flow. J Vasc Res 35:85–92, 1998.
54. Hainsworth R. The physiological approach to cardiovascular reflexes. Clin Sci (Colch) 91:43–49, 1996.
55. Zullo MA. Atrial regulation of intravascular volume: observations on the tachycardia-polyuria syndrome. Am Heart J 122:188–194, 1991.
56. Schroeder CA Jr, Chen YL, Messina EJ. Inhibition of NO synthesis or endothelium removal reveals a vasoconstrictor effect of insulin on isolated arterioles. Am J Physiol 276: H815–820, 1999.
57. Meng F, Korompai FL, Lynch DM, Yuan YS. Acetylcholine-induced and nitric oxide-mediated vasodilation in burns. J Surg Res 80:236–242, 1998.
58. Ishizaka H, Kuo L. Acidosis-reduced coronary arteriolar dilation is mediated by ATP-sensitive potassium channels in vascular smooth muscle. Circ Res 78:50–57, 1996.

2

Pathophysiology

3

Ischemic Cardiac Conditions

H. Steven Sadowsky and Eugene McColgon

INTRODUCTION

The current estimate is that at least 58 million Americans have one or more forms of cardiovascular disease.[1] Cardiovascular disease is, in reality, many diseases. The American Heart Association (AHA) considers ischemic (coronary) heart disease, hypertensive disease, rheumatic fever/rheumatic heart disease, and cerebrovascular disease (stroke) to be the major cardiovascular diseases. Of the 15 leading causes of death in the United States in 1996, heart disease continued to rank first. Heart disease was responsible for 31.6% of all deaths in 1996, which represents a 3% decline in the mortality rate from 1995. Nonetheless, the World Health Organization estimates that by 2020, cardiovascular diseases will account for up to 40% of all deaths worldwide.[2]

The clinical presentation of the patient with **coronary artery disease** (CAD), the clinical signs and symptoms caused when the myocardium becomes ischemic, was first, and probably most colorfully, described by Heberden[3] in his lecture on "Disorders of the Breast" in 1772:

There is a disorder of the breast, marked with strong and peculiar symptoms considerable for the kind of danger belonging to it, and not extremely rare, of which I do not recollect any mention among medical authors. The seat of it, and sense of strangling and anxiety, with which it is attended, may make it not improperly be called angina pectoris. Those, who are afflicted with it, are seized while they are walking and most particularly when they walk soon after eating, with a painful and most disagreeable sensation in the breast, which seems as if it would take their life away, if it were to increase or to continue; the moment they stand still, all this uneasiness vanishes.

The prevalence of CAD and its surprising presence in seemingly healthy young men was not fully appreciated until 1953, when Enos and colleagues[4] published the results of the autopsies they performed on soldiers killed in the Korean conflict. The investigation, originally performed to evaluate the role played by different ballistic injuries as a cause of death,[5] found that 77.3% of the 300 soldiers examined (mean age = 22.1 years) had observable blockages of their coronary arteries. In 10 of the men, complete obstruction of one or more coronary arteries was found. This was the first report to suggest that CAD is present for many years before an individual becomes aware of it. As a direct result of the work of Enos and co-workers,[4] the medical community now distinguishes CAD (the presence of an obstruction that limits coronary blood flow but does not significantly inhibit heart muscle function) from **coronary heart disease** (CHD—the presence of an obstruction that causes permanent damage to heart muscle fibers downstream, thus inhibiting heart muscle function).

Enos' report[4] was followed by the now famous Framingham Heart Study.[6] In the course of the original Framingham study, 5209 apparently healthy men and women between the ages of 30 and 62 were followed for 20 years. During that period, the subjects were seen for biennial examinations, which consisted of questionnaires on activity and smoking history, blood chemistry studies, blood pressure measurement, and a resting 12-lead electrocardiogram (ECG). Although no one specific cause of CAD could be identified in the Framingham cohort, several major and minor risk factors for its development were discovered and are discussed later in this chapter.

This chapter presents a detailed description of the anatomy and physiology of normal myocardial perfusion, and a discussion of the pathologic changes that occur in coronary arteries as the result of CAD. The risk factors associated with the development of CHD are presented along with the

Clinical Note: Framingham Heart Study

The Framingham Heart Study provided landmark epidemiologic research that has led to the public and professional acceptance of the role of risk factors in the development and progression of cardiovascular disease.

three major patterns of clinical presentation for CHD—chronic stable angina, unstable angina, and sudden cardiac death.

ANATOMY OF THE CORONARY ARTERIES

Although the anatomy of the coronary arteries has been well understood for several years, in order to fully understand what is known about the coronary atherosclerotic process, a presentation of the normal triple-layered structure of arteries is necessary.[7]

Outer Layer

The outer layer of an artery (**adventitia**) consists chiefly of collagenous fibers, mostly fibroblasts, and provides the basic support structure for the artery (Fig. 3–1). This portion of the artery also houses the vessels that furnish the middle layer of the artery with its blood supply—the **vasa vasorum.**

Middle Layer

The middle layer (**media**) of all arteries (of which the coronary arteries are considered medium-

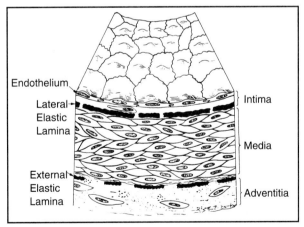

Figure 3–1. Structure of the normal arterial wall, consisting of the adventitia (outer), the media (middle), and the intima (inner) layers. (Reproduced with permission from Ross R, Glomset J. The pathogenesis of atherosclerosis. N Engl J Med 295:369, 1976.)

sized) consists of multiple layers of smooth muscle cells separated from the inner and outer layers by a prominent elastic membrane, or lamina. Through alterations in vasomotor tone, as demands for changes in blood flow to the myocardium are perceived, this muscular layer is responsible for making adjustments to the luminal diameter. These smooth muscle cells are also capable of synthesizing collagen, elastin, and glycosaminoglycans, especially when they react to different physical and chemical stimuli.

Inner Layer

The inner layer (**intima**) consists of an endothelial layer, the basement membrane, and variable amounts of isolated smooth muscle cells as well as collagen and elastin fibers. The boundary of the intima and media is marked by the internal elastic lamina.

The two inner layers of the artery wall have received the most attention with regard to the development of the processes that lead to myocardial ischemia. The arterial endothelium is selectively permeable to macromolecules of the size of a **low-density lipoprotein** (LDL). The concentration of LDL in the lymph of the arterial wall has been found to be approximately one tenth of that in the bloodstream.[8] Although many plasma proteins can enter the artery wall in this concentration, lipoproteins and fibrinogen are particularly likely to accumulate in the intima.[9]

MYOCARDIAL PERFUSION

Before discussing the particulars of myocardial perfusion, it is important to review two basic rules of fluid dynamics. First, all fluids flow according to a pressure gradient, that is, from an area of higher pressure to an area of lower pressure. Second, all fluids follow the path of least resistance. Consequently, if an obstruction is encountered, fluid tends to follow the less resistant path, thereby reducing the fluid volume across the obstruction and decreasing the pressure that would drive the fluid farther down the path beyond the obstruction.

As with all muscle beds, myocardial perfusion occurs primarily during periods of muscle relax-

ation, in this case, during diastole.[10, 11] Figure 3–2 shows the relationship between mean aortic pressure and blood flow in the coronary arteries. Blood flow increases in both the right and left coronary arteries at the onset of systole (first vertical dotted line). When the aortic valve is closed, aortic diastolic pressure is transmitted through the dilated Valsalva sinuses to the openings of the coronary arteries themselves. Throughout diastole the sinuses act as miniature reservoirs, facilitating maintenance of relatively uniform coronary inflow. The pressure generated by the right ventricle during systole is in the range of 15 to 20 mm Hg, whereas the left ventricle produces pressures of 120 mm Hg or higher. Therefore, the occlusive pressure on the right coronary artery terminal vessel is less than that on the left vessel during systole, so there is less difference in blood flow in the right coronary artery between systole and diastole.

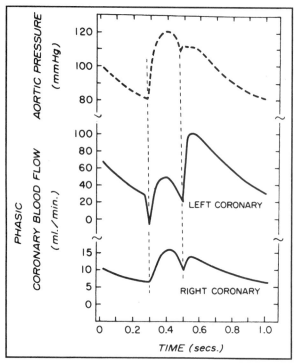

Figure 3–2. The relationship between blood pressure in the aorta (*top*) and blood flow in the left (*middle*) and right (*bottom*) coronary arteries. The first vertical dotted line is the beginning of systole, and the second dotted line is the beginning of diastole. (Reproduced with permission from Boucek R, Morales A, Romanelli R, Judkins M. Coronary Artery Disease: Pathologic and Clinical Assessment. Baltimore, Williams & Wilkins, 1984, p. 132.)

Just as with any other arteries, the coronary arteries distend when blood is forced back into them by the contracting muscle. Inasmuch as the pressure within the coronary arteries is less than that in the aorta, the coronary arteries themselves become reservoirs for the storage of blood. The resultant engorgement provides the initial "pressure head" that drives blood into the myocardium once intramyocardial pressure drops following systole.

An especially important difference between the coronary vascular bed and most others is the presence of anastomotic connections that lack intervening capillary beds (known as **collateral vessels**). In human hearts, the distribution and extent of collateral vessels is quite variable.[12] Under normal conditions, such vessels are generally less[13] than 40 μm in diameter and appear to have little or no functional role. However, when myocardial perfusion is compromised by obstructions that affect major vessels, these collateral vessels enlarge over several weeks, and blood flow through them increases.[14] Given the time to make this adaptation, perfusion via collateral vessels may equal or exceed perfusion via the obstructed vessel.

Major Determinants of Myocardial Blood Flow

- **Diastolic blood pressure** (DBP) is the primary driving force moving blood into the myocardial tissue.
- **Vasomotor tone** (VMT) plays a major role in determining the volume of blood passed along to the tissue by regulating the caliber of the artery. VMT is usually uniform throughout the coronary vascular tree. It aids or opposes diastolic blood pressure.
- **Resistance to flow** (R) is most commonly caused by atherosclerosis. A significant increase in the size and number of collateral vessels decreases total resistance to flow by providing an alternative route for the blood to take around an obstruction.
- **Left ventricular end-diastolic pressure** (LVEDP) is the pressure within the ventricle at end diastole; it causes an occlusive force on the capillary beds of the muscle closest to the pumping chamber, the endocardium.

The entire process can be considered in this relationship:

$$F = DBP + VMT - R - LVEDP$$

where F = flow of blood to the myocardium, DBP = diastolic blood pressure, VMT = vasomotor tone (additive if the vessel is in a dilated state and subtractive if constricted), R = the resistance to flow offered by an obstructive lesion, and LVEDP = left ventricular end-diastolic pressure.

ATHEROSCLEROSIS

The development of **atherosclerosis** is a complex process dependent on the interaction of several risk factors and the sensitivity of the individual to these factors. Atherosclerotic plaques are composed of lipid and thrombus; the relative concentration of each varies widely from individual to individual. In an effort to clarify this process, atherosclerosis is presented here as two processes—"atherosis" and "sclerosis"—that occur within the intima and endothelium of arterial walls. Undoubtedly, one of these components is more prominent than the other in each person who develops this disease. However, in very rare cases (homozygous familial hypercholesterolemia), atherosis is the only cause of the obstructive lesion.

Atherosis

The first detectable lesion of atherosclerosis is the often discussed *fatty streak*, which consists of lipid-laden macrophages and smooth muscle cells. Fatty streaks have been found in the arteries of patients as young as 10 years of age, at the sites where major lesions appear later in life.[15–17]

The development and progression of the fatty streak in humans can be inferred from the findings of animal studies. In such studies, fatty streaks have been found in the lining of the aorta within 12 days of the initiation of a high-fat, high-cholesterol diet. Clusters of monocytes have been found in junctional areas, between endothelial cells, where they accumulate lipid and are known as **foam cells.**[17–19] The subendothelial accumulation of these macrophages constitutes the first stage of fatty streak development. After several months, accumulations of lipid-laden macrophages grow so large that the endothelium is stretched and begins to separate over them. Such endothelial separation exposes the intima-based lesion and the underlying connective tissue to the circulation. Consequently, platelets aggregate and thrombus forms at these locations, a hallmark characteristic of the "sclerotic" phase of atherosclerosis.

Sclerosis

The sclerotic components of the lesions of atherosclerosis are responsible for a reduction of blood vessel compliance. Atherosclerotic intimal lesions that produce symptoms or end-organ damage (ischemia or infarction in the organs fed by the vessel involved) invariably have a major fibrous component. Increased lesion collagen and destruction of medial elastin, in addition to changes in the composition of these fibrous proteins, are important mechanisms underlying sclerosis in atherosclerosis.[20, 21] Pure atherosis (lipid deposition alone), such as that in fatty streaks, does not produce end-organ damage (except with homozygous familial hypercholesterolemia) but may contribute to sclerosis. The exposure of subendothelial structures to the raw material of thrombus formation and the subsequent effect of such exposure on endogenous factors such as endothelium-derived relaxation factor (see later discussion) contribute to the process of sclerosis.

One of the long-standing theories of the development of the atherosclerotic lesion is that of *encrustation*, that is, the formation of an organized "fibrous cap" of thrombi over advanced plaques that have developed on the endothelial lining.[7, 19, 22, 23] Although this theory has never adequately accounted for the exact origin of the lesions, it has always been considered an important part of the process because of findings of extensive thrombus formation on microscopic examination of these plaques. A "response-to-injury" hypothesis has been postulated in an effort to define the initial stages of development of the atherosclerotic plaque.[24–26]

Although the response-to-injury hypothesis does not identify the agent or process responsible for it, investigations of vasospasm have provided some clues to the origin.[27–31] **Platelet-derived growth factor** (PDGF) has been shown to contribute to lesion formation in two ways. First, as the name implies, PDGF stimulates the replication of connective tissue cells in the areas in which it is released. Second, PDGF is a chemoattractant; when released from tissues at the site of endothelial injury, it attracts smooth muscle cells so that they migrate from the media into the intima.[32–34]

VASOSPASM

At the beginning of this century, Sir William Osler was the first to suggest that a basic abnormality existed in the smooth muscle of coronary arteries that were affected by atherosclerosis when he reported to the Royal College of Physicians: "We have, I think, evidence that sclerotic arteries are specially prone to spasm."[35] For the next 50 years, coronary vasospasm was considered only a minor factor in the myocardial blood flow equation. Prinzmetal and colleagues[36] first identified the connection between vasospasm and what they called "variant angina." Variant angina differs from "typical angina" as first described by Heberden[3] in that it is associated with ST-segment elevation instead of depression, occurs at rest (typically in the early morning) instead of during a predictable level of activity, and is not associated with any preceding increase in myocardial oxygen demand. There is also a much stronger anatomic correlation between the ECG leads involved during these attacks and the site of subsequent myocardial infarctions in those patients who went on to have them when compared with the data for patients who experienced exertional angina. This syndrome, which became known as **Prinzmetal's angina,** was similar to typical angina in that it was promptly relieved with nitroglycerin and other vasodilators. Subsequent investigators found that this syndrome was considerably more widespread than had been previously believed, and by 1976 the "proved hypothesis" of a vasospastic nonlesion cause for angina was widely accepted.[37] Nonetheless, the significant prevalence of atherosclerosis in persons suffering Prinzmetal's angina cannot be denied.[38, 39]

It has long been known that hyperplasia of intimal smooth muscle cells is a hallmark of advanced atherosclerosis.[25, 26, 40] It should not be surprising, therefore, that coronary arteries so afflicted would be prone to spasm. Experiments have shown that if the endothelium of the coronary artery is damaged, the intimal smooth muscle constricts instead of relaxing when stimulated.[41, 42] Although exactly what triggers this process continues to be inadequately understood, recent investigations have focused on the interactions of *endothelial-derived relaxation factor* (EDRF), *endothelium-derived hyperpolarizing factor* (EDHF), and *endothelium-derived contracting factor* (EDCF).[43–45]

RISK FACTORS

Researchers and clinicians since the late eighteenth century have pondered the relationship between genetic and behavioral factors and their contribution to the development of coronary atherosclerosis and coronary heart disease. However, it was the Framingham study[6] that first tested these relationships in a long-term, large-scale epidemiologic trial. The American Heart Association has identified several risk factors for coronary heart disease; some of these factors can be changed, although others cannot.[1] Vita and colleagues[46] have suggested that in addition to accelerating the disease process once it is established, risk factors may themselves constitute the "injury" in the response-to-injury hypothesis of Ross and Glomset.[25, 26] Although the presence or absence of significant CAD cannot be determined by any simple arithmetic formula, there is considerable evidence to support the contention that the greater the number of risk factors present, the greater the likelihood that CAD, and ultimately CHD, will be present.[47–51]

Major Risk Factors

The four modifiable major risk factors for coronary heart disease are cigarette/tobacco smoking, high blood pressure (hypertension), high blood cholesterol levels (hypercholesterolemia), and physical inactivity.[1] The three nonmodifiable risk factors are heredity, male sex, and increased age. Each of these risk factors not only has an additive effect on the ability of the other factors to contrib-

ute to the development of CAD and to subsequent CHD, but also exerts a multiplicative effect. Thus, although each modifiable risk factor is discussed individually, it is critical to remember that these factors exist individually only in the isolation of the scientist's laboratory.

Cigarette Smoking

One fifth of all deaths related to heart disease are due to cigarette smoking.[1, 52] Cigarette smoking has been associated with increased risk of cardiovascular disease since 1958.[53] Although no one component of cigarette smoke has been identified as the causative agent for this association, a number of studies have shown how cigarette smoking has a deleterious effect on other known factors involved in the development of atherosclerosis.[54–57] As few as four cigarettes a day increases a smoker's risk of developing CAD and CHD above that of a nonsmoker or an ex-smoker.[58, 59] In comparison to nonsmokers, smokers have been shown to manifest leukocytosis, lower serum **high-density lipoprotein** (HDL) levels, elevated fibrinogen and plasma catecholamine levels, and increased blood pressure.[60, 61] That similar alterations in the risk factor profiles of the preadolescent children of smoking parents have also been observed suggests that cigarette smoking increases the risk of developing CHD in both the smoker and the nonsmoking family members.[62, 63]

Hypertension

Hypertension, or high blood pressure, is known to be one of the most prevalent disease states in America, estimated to be present in 61 million people.[64–66] Hypertension, both systolic (over 140 mm Hg) and diastolic (over 90 mm Hg), is believed to be an independent risk factor for the development of CAD and peripheral and cerebral vascular disease.[67–69] So far, efforts to lower the mobidity and mortality rates associated with hypertension have proved better at reducing stroke than heart attack.[70, 71] Such findings have led some investigators to believe that high blood pressure and coronary vascular disease merely coexist instead of influencing one another in a causal relationship.[72] Nonetheless, the epidemiologic evidence still overwhelmingly points to hypertension as a significant risk factor for the development of CAD.[1, 73, 74]

Elevated Cholesterol

Since the first published results of the Framingham study, the direct link between abnormal levels of cholesterol and the development of CHD has been well established.[75, 76] Several forms of cholesterol have been shown to play a role in atherogenesis: very low density lipoprotein (VLDL), intermediate-density lipoprotein (IDL), LDL, and lipoprotein a (Lpa).[77–79] Direct dietary intake of cholesterol is not the principal influence on the level of cholesterol in the blood. The nutritionally dependent variable most related to increasing levels of blood cholesterol is the amount of saturated fat in the diet.[80–84] The cholesterol-to-saturated fat index (CSI) has proved to be a valuable clinical education tool because it clearly shows the discrepancy between dietary and serum levels of cholesterol.[85–87] From the CSI formula

$$CSI = (1.01 \times g \text{ saturated fat})$$
$$+ (0.05 \times mg \text{ cholesterol})$$

it is clear that the contribution of saturated fat in any particular food item is about 20 times more atherogenic than its cholesterol content. This may be one reason why, although there is a 2% reduction in CHD risk for every 1% reduction in cholesterol level, when cholesterol levels are considered by themselves, there is a significant overlap between individuals who develop CHD and those who do not.[88, 89]

Other studies have documented the importance of HDL as an independent predictor of CHD risk.[90–92] Although the exact mechanism by which increased levels of HDL provide protection from coronary disease is poorly understood, several theories have been proposed. The concept of "reverse cholesterol transport"—bringing free cholesterol from the tissues back to the liver for safe storage—is most often cited.[93–100] The best predictor of risk for developing cholesterol-related blockages in an artery is the ratio of total cholesterol to HDL (CHOL/HDL); a ratio of greater than 4.5 increases an individual's risk of developing atherosclerosis.[101–103] Triglycerides have also become a marker for the development of coronary athero-

sclerosis, particularly when they are associated with low levels of HDL (below 35 mg/dL).[104–106] Therefore, current consensus recommendations call for the following: in the absence of CAD and with less than two risk factors, target levels for LDL cholesterol should be 160 mg/dL; with more than two risk factors, 130 mg/dL; in the presence of CAD, 100 mg/dL. In individuals with hypertriglyceridemia the target level for triglycerides is 200 mg/dL.[80, 107–109]

Physical Inactivity

The role of exercise in the management of CHD has been acknowledged since Morris[110] reported a decreased incidence of myocardial infarction in conductors of British double-decker buses, when compared with drivers. Physical inactivity remains a significant risk factor for developing CHD and is comparable to that observed for high cholesterol, high blood pressure, or cigarette smoking.[1] The Centers for Disease Control and Prevention reported that lack of adequate exercise is the most prevalent risk factor for CHD and that more than 60% of adult Americans do not perform the minimum recommended amount of physical activity.[111–113]

There is more than ample evidence that regular aerobic exercise has a beneficial impact on many CHD risk factors.[114–119] For example: low to moderate intensity exercise has been shown to increase HDL levels by as much as 11 to 28%.[116, 117] Regular aerobic exercise is also known to affect many of the "cornerstones" of CAD development. For example, Katzel and co-workers[120] have shown that aerobic exercise coupled with weight training can yield reductions in plasma triglycerides (TG) of 17% and LDL cholesterol (LDL-C) of 8%, in addition to increasing HDL cholesterol (HDL-C) by 11% (3.7 mg/dL). Some of the lesser-known benefits of long-term endurance training are an increase in fibrinolysis and red blood cell deformability as well as a decrease in platelet aggregability,[121–126] which may be beneficial in preventing initial or subsequent coronary ischemic events. It has been shown that exercise of adequate intensity, duration, and frequency is beneficial in preventing cardiovascular disease and increasing longevity in the healthy population.[119, 123, 127–131]

Minor Risk Factors

The minor or contributing risk factors are not independently significant in predicting the likelihood of an individual's developing CHD. As their name implies, however, they do play a role in its establishment and growth.

Diabetes

Nonenzymatic glycosylation, or the chemical attachment of glucose to proteins without the involvement of enzymes, is known to affect fibrinogen, collagen, antithrombin III, HDL, and LDL, all of which are involved in the evolution of CAD.[132-134] The attachment of glucose to these molecules renders them less sensitive to the enzymes and other substances with which they interact. For example, antithrombin III activity, which normally inhibits excessive blood coagulation, is decreased when it undergoes glycosylation, and fibrinogen is less likely to perform its function of degrading fibrin when so affected. In both these cases, thrombus formation is enhanced. This process may even be the principal cause of basement membrane thickening, long known to be a major tissue change associated with prolonged diabetes (see Chapter 7).

Obesity

Several studies have associated obesity (weight more than 20% above ideal body weight) with the development of CHD.[135-137] This relationship appears to be more significant if the excess body fat is concentrated in the abdomen (central obesity)

as opposed to being more evenly distributed throughout the body.[138, 139] Nonetheless, it is difficult to prove that obesity is an independent risk factor for CAD because it is associated with so many other risk factors, such as hypertension, diabetes, and sedentary lifestyle, for example.

Family History

Family history of CHD, defined as its presence in a parent or sibling, has been shown to be a minor risk factor for the development of CAD.[140-143] With the exception of the familial hypercholesterolemias, no genetic link has been established for CHD; like obesity, the atherogenic contribution of family history is not entirely genetic. Fortunately, the modification of risk factors in subjects with a strong family history of premature coronary disease provides a reduction in overall risk of developing subsequent disease.[144, 145]

Age

Increased age (older than 65) is known to be a risk factor for CHD.[146] Whether older age is an independent pathologic process or simply a consequence of prolonged exposure to the risk factors is less clear. Studies show that interventions on other risk factors have proved to be beneficial in older subsets of patients and have resulted in the reduction of clinical end points, for example, myocardial infarction and symptoms.[147, 148] Also, both patients and subjects without known disease in the young-old and middle-old age groups (ages 67 to 76) have responded to the same extent as young subjects to attempts at risk factor reduction.[149-151]

Although biochemical changes are known to occur as people age—for example, decreased nerve conduction velocity and decreased aerobic enzyme activity—the functional significance of these changes appears to be negligible if they are not complicated by preexisting disease.[152, 153]

> ### Clinical Note: Estrogen Replacement Therapy in CHD
> In the absence of a family history of breast cancer, estrogen replacement is recommended in all peri- and postmenopausal women with a family history of CHD.

Gender

It is a common perception that premenopausal women are "immune" from CHD. Men are six times more likely than women to experience a myocardial infarction before age 55,[91, 154–156] and the overall onset of clinically significant coronary heart disease in women lags 10 years behind that in men.[157–159]

Although it is true that, in general, women experience lower CHD morbidity and mortality rates than men do, this disease still represents a significant health risk to women. Coronary heart disease is the second leading cause of death in all women younger than 45; it is the leading cause of death in black women younger than 45, an age when the majority are still premenopausal.[157, 160–163] In terms of age group, the largest "gain" in either sex during which the greatest increase in CHD occurs is in women aged 55 to 64.[164–166] Once a myocardial infarction occurs, women of all age groups have a higher mortality rate than men. Slightly more women have unrecognized or "silent" myocardial infarctions than men (34% versus 27%), but interestingly, the initial clinical event in women is most often angina, whereas in men it is an acute myocardial infarction. Women who have diabetes are more susceptible to developing CHD than are men.[167–169] Because the gap between CHD incidence in men and women closes between the fifth and sixth decades, it has been argued that menopause plays some nonspecific role in regulating this disease process. It has been found, however, that the risk of developing CHD is no different in women who had natural menopause, were premenopausal, or had "surgical" menopause and were undergoing estrogen replacement therapy. Estrogen is a factor, however, for it was noted that women who had surgical menopause but did not take estrogen replacement therapy did have a significant increase in the incidence of CHD.[160, 170]

Stress

In 1910, Osler[35] described a stereotypic "behavior pattern" for angina patients. It is noteworthy that Osler commented to the Royal College of Physicians that little progress had been made in this area since Heberden's earlier publication. Although the pathogenesis may not have been defined, Friedman and Rosenman[171] related the sense of time urgency and easily aroused hostility to a sevenfold increase in prevalence of CHD—what they termed type A behavior. Therefore, the personality characteristics of hostility and anger may be more descriptive than the traditional term "type A behavior." The identification of what has been termed type A behavior, as an independent risk factor for CHD, is still being debated.[172–174] The exact mechanism by which this predominantly psychological trait increases the risk for the tissue changes of CHD is believed to be related to platelet activation. This contribution to the sclerotic component of CHD is known to be related to increases in levels of catecholamine and platelet-secreted proteins, which have been found in subjects undergoing emotional stress.[175, 176] It is known also that alterations in this type A behavior can reduce morbidity and mortality rates for postmyocardial infarction patients.[99] Additional risk factors for atherosclerotic disease that may or may not have a role in thrombus development or initiation of atherosclerosis include the following:

Infectious agents
Homocysteine
Lipoprotein a
C-reactive protein
Tissue-type plasminogen activator (tPA)
Fibrinogen

Current research is studying these factors to see what role (if any) they play in ischemic conditions. At the time of this publication clear decisions regarding their role had not been made.

Clinical Note: Psychosocial Stress

Psychosocial distress is also associated with increased mortality and morbidity rates after myocardial infarction (MI). In addition, social isolation and depression are associated with a poor prognosis after MI. These findings should emphasize the importance of identifying this risk factor prior to rehabilitation to ensure it is addressed in the total rehabilitation of the patient.

CLINICAL COURSE

The clinical presentation of the patient with CHD typically occurs in one of four ways:

• Sudden cardiac death
• Chronic stable angina
• Unstable angina or infarction
• Cardiac muscle dysfunction (see Chapter 4)

Sudden Cardiac Death

In 20 to 25% of patients with CHD, **sudden cardiac death** (death within 1 hour of onset of symptoms) is the initial presenting syndrome![177] Ventricular fibrillation, leading to cessation of cardiac output, is the usual cause of death. For these patients, prompt delivery of bystander cardiopulmonary resuscitation and entry into the emergency medical system within 10 minutes is their only chance of survival.[178, 179]

Angina

The majority of patients with CHD first seek medical attention because of those "peculiar symptoms" that Heberden[3] described in 1772 as **angina** (old English term for "strangling") pectoris. This sensation, most commonly described as a substernal pressure, can occur anywhere from the epigastric area to the jaw and is described as squeezing, tightness, or crushing. It is now known to be caused by an imbalance in supply and demand of myocardial oxygen.

Chronic Stable Angina

Chronic stable angina, as its name implies, usually has a well-established level of onset. Patients are able to predict reliably those activities that provoke their discomfort; this condition is usually associated with a set level of myocardial oxygen demand. As mentioned earlier, myocardial oxygen demand is closely related to heart rate and systolic blood pressure. By multiplying these values, the so-called *double product* or *rate pressure product,* an index that is useful in correlating functional activities with myocardial capabilities can be obtained. Wall stress, the third determinant of the myocardial oxygen consumption rate (MVO_2), can be accurately measured only with invasive monitoring and is therefore not usually available to the patient performing routine activities.

Patients with stable angina are usually able to bring their symptoms under control by reducing slightly the intensity of the exercise they are performing or by taking sublingual nitroglycerin. Patients have some variability in their tolerance for activity—that is, they have "good days and bad days"—which is probably related to variations in coronary vascular tone, but overall, stable angina is a predictable syndrome.

Unstable Angina

Unstable angina can be defined as the presence of signs or symptoms of an inadequate blood supply to the myocardium in the absence of the demands that usually provoke such an imbalance. The patient who presents with unstable angina or has chronic stable angina that develops an unstable pattern (see later discussion) requires quick recognition and referral for treatment. Although the allied health professional is not responsible for making the diagnosis of unstable angina, he or she may be the person who first detects its presence while following a patient in a cardiac rehabilitation program. It is therefore important for such professionals to have a basic understanding of the mechanisms of unstable angina and know how to detect it.

Patients who have unstable angina are known to have increased morbidity and mortality rates when compared with those who have stable angina, even though the absolute amount of coronary atherosclerosis in both groups is not significantly different.[180, 181] The major physiologic difference between unstable and chronic stable angina is the absence of the need for an increase in myocardial oxygen demand to provoke the syndrome. The notion that imbalances in myocardial blood flow could be related to a primary reduction in oxygen supply without an increase in demand was proved by Chierchia and colleagues.[182] They were able to show that a fall in cardiac vein oxygen saturation always preceded the electrocardiographic or hemodynamic indicators of ischemia in 137 patients who experienced angina while at rest.

Factors That Contribute to Unstable Angina

Several factors have been implicated as contributors to this syndrome. Circadian variations in catecholamine levels (e.g., epinephrine), which increase heart rate and blood pressure; increases in plasma viscosity, known to occur in the first 4 hours of awakening; increases in platelet activation; and pathologic changes in the atherosclerotic plaques themselves have all been proposed as triggers of unstable angina.[183-185]

The atherosclerotic plaque is known to undergo physical changes when a patient is experiencing unstable angina. There are distinct differences in the morphology of atherosclerotic lesions of persons who are experiencing unstable angina compared with that of persons who have stable angina.[186, 187] More recent developments in fiberoptic technology have allowed direct visual inspection of coronary atherosclerotic lesions, thus permitting differentiation of plaques by their appearance.

Because coronary plaque is a dynamic entity and not just a mound of debris, the stability of the disease can be altered quickly. Several clinical clues to the development of unstable angina should alert the health professional to notify a patient's physician:

- Angina at rest
- Occurrence of the patient's typical angina at a significantly lower level of activity than usual
- Deterioration of a previously stable pattern—for

example, discomfort occurring several times a day compared with several times a week
- Evidence of loss of previously present myocardial reserve, such as a drop in blood pressure or increase in heart rate with levels of activity previously well tolerated

Unstable angina should be distinguished from Prinzmetal's or vasospastic angina. Both are most likely to occur in the first few hours of rising, but vasospastic discomfort is usually not as severe and is often relieved with minor activity, whereas unstable angina is not. Patients with vasospastic angina are able to perform high levels of work later in the day without discomfort, but patients with unstable angina are unable to increase their cardiac output significantly without provoking further discomfort, even if their earlier pain has waned.

Up to this point, consideration has been given only to primary prevention schemes. The reader must not lose sight of the fact that although the number of Americans dying from heart disease is decreasing, the number of those living with heart disease is increasing. Primary health care providers must realize that those risk factor modification interventions that have proved so effective for the primary prevention of CAD and CHD are also applicable to secondary prevention. The important role of counseling by clinicians is too often neglected.[52]

NATURAL HISTORY

Although many population and longitudinal studies have been carried out that document the relative importance of single factors or combinations of risk factors, still little is known about the natural history of CHD as it applies to an individual patient.[188, 189] Knowledge of risk factors has allowed the establishment of a model from which relative risk can be approximated, but such tools decrease in value for those who are at either end of the normal distribution of the population. The only "guarantee" that can be offered to the patient with known CHD is that if the factors that caused the disease to be present in the first place remain unchanged, it will progress.

There is some evidence that the progression of

atherosclerotic CHD is not inevitable and, in fact, that it is reversible.[21, 190, 191] More than 50 randomized trials have documented the efficacy and safety of aspirin as an antiplatelet agent and a cardiovascular drug. For patients with ischemic heart disease the range recommended for the prevention of a secondary event, based on strong clinical evidence, is 75 to 160 mg aspirin per day.[192] In addition, the strict control of diabetes also appears to decrease atherosclerotic changes in endothelial and intimal elastin, contributing to beneficial decreases in vessel wall compliance.

Since the Cholesterol Lowering in Atherosclerosis Study,[193, 194] the importance of treating patients pharmacologically to lower cholesterol levels and lessen the risk of developing atherosclerosis is well accepted. There is also clear evidence that aggressive lifestyle modification can elicit significant results without the use of medication.[195] Nonetheless, many general practitioners do not have an aggressive attitude toward the prescription of lipid-lowering interventions, especially when older patients with atherosclerotic lesions are concerned.[196] Perhaps physical therapists should seize the opportunity to incorporate secondary prevention measures for cardiovascular disease into their clinical practices. The establishment of secondary prevention clinics in England resulted in reduced hospital admissions for participants.[197]

Summary

- Coronary heart disease is the most common disease in the industrialized world.
- The presence of coronary heart disease in a given individual is dependent on the presence of any of 10 risk factors for the disease and the susceptibility of the individual to those factors.
  - Cigarette smoking
  - Hypertension
  - Elevated cholesterol levels
  - Physical inactivity
  - Diabetes
  - Obesity
  - Family history
  - Age
  - Gender
  - Stress
- The plaques that obstruct the coronary arteries are a combination of atheroma and thrombus, and they begin to form early in life, probably in the second decade.
- Coronary artery disease remains undetected until it occludes approximately 70% of the original coronary lumen.
- The majority of the risk factors for CAD are modifiable.
- Through control of these risk factors, the progress of CAD can be arrested and in some cases reversed.

CASE STUDIES

Case 1

Mr. H is a 38-year-old white male who, at the age of 30, was experiencing angina with low levels of exertion and was found to have severe obstructions of his left anterior descending (LAD), first diagonal (D1), circumflex (CIRC), first obtuse marginal (OM1), and right coronary arteries (RCA). He underwent five-vessel coronary artery bypass grafting, which relieved his angina. He now has a 2-year history of chronic stable angina, which in the past month has become more frequent, occurring with minimal exertion and occasionally while at rest. Mr. H was admitted to the hospital.

He underwent a repeat cardiac catheterization, which revealed total obstructions of his native proximal LAD, mid-CIRC, and RCA. His venous bypass grafts to his LAD and D1 were also 100% occluded, whereas the grafts to his OM1 and distal RCA were patent.

He has a 20 pack/year (number of packs per day multiplied by the number of years smoked) history of smoking, which he stopped at the time of his bypass surgery. He has a 12-year history of hypertension, which is controlled by medication. He is 67 inches tall and weighs 270 pounds, which is 50 pounds more than he weighed at the time of his bypass surgery. His current blood lipids are cholesterol, 188 mg/dL, triglycerides, 147 mg/dL, HDL, 27 mg/dL, and CHOL/HDL, 6.96 mg/dL. He had been employed as an accountant but stated that he had to quit his job because he was experiencing frequent angina during stressful situations at work. He has never engaged in an organized exercise program.

Study Questions—Case 1

- What is this patient's admitting diagnosis?
- Why did this patient's angina return less than 5 years after bypass surgery?
- Which risk factors did Mr. H modify after his bypass surgery?
- Which risk factors did he not modify after his surgery?

- What lifestyle changes should this patient make to keep his remaining grafts patent?

Case 2

Mr. S is a 65-year-old white male who first experienced chest pressure at rest on September 16. He was admitted to the hospital, and a myocardial infarction was ruled out. While awaiting a diagnostic study, he again had a sudden onset of severe substernal chest pressure, which was associated with ST-segment elevation in his anterior electrocardiogram leads. He was taken for cardiac catheterization, which revealed a complete obstruction of his proximal LAD and a 90% obstruction in his CIRC. His LAD blockage opened to 70% following streptokinase infusion. He went on to have percutaneous transluminal coronary angioplasty of these obstructions, which reduced them to 30%, and he was referred to cardiac rehabilitation.

At the time of admission, he was a 50 pack/year smoker, had poorly controlled hypertension, was 68 inches tall, and weighed 200 pounds. His blood lipids were cholesterol, 181 mg/dL, triglycerides, 139 mg/dL, HDL, 34 mg/dL, and CHOL/HDL, 5.32 mg/dL. He is retired and lives alone; he has never engaged in a regular exercise program.

Study Questions—Case 2

- Which of this patient's risk factors will respond favorably to diet and exercise?
- Which risk factors will not?
- What is his clinical diagnosis during the first few days of his hospitalization?

Case 3

Mr. C is a 56-year-old white male who has a known history of CHD, having had two myocardial infarctions and coronary artery bypass graft surgery in 1988. He was admitted to the hospital on April 13 with a 2-day history of palpitations associated with nausea and vomiting. He was found to be in sustained ventricular tachycardia, which converted to normal sinus rhythm spontaneously. His peak creatine phosphokinase level of 250 mg/dL was 100% from skeletal muscle. His medical history included several admissions to the hospital between 1988 and 1992 for congestive heart failure, and during one of these, his left ventricular ejection fraction was noted to be 22%.

He had been a 75 pack/year smoker but had stopped smoking 15 years earlier. His blood pressure is well controlled at rest but following minimal activity is 230/90 mm Hg. Mr. C is diabetic and requires oral hyperglycemic agents; he is 6 feet tall and weighs 260 pounds. He admits to being "angry" when things do not go as he had planned and in fact has become dependent on diazepam, which he has been taking for 20 years to help with his "hyper" personality. His cur-

rent blood lipids are cholesterol, 208 mg/dL, triglycerides, 240 mg/dL, HDL, 29 mg/dL, CHOL/HDL, 7.17 mg/dL, and glucose level is 145 mg/dL. He is limited by leg fatigue at a workload of less than 5 METs.

Study Questions—Case 3

- Is this patient's cholesterol level significantly elevated?
- Does this patient have a blood lipid problem? If so, what is it?
- What changes in this patient's medication program should be made before he begins cardiac rehabilitation?
- In view of this patient's ejection fraction, should he be considered a candidate for cardiac rehabilitation? Why or why not?

Case 4

Mr. G is a 44-year-old white male who was asymptomatic and apparently healthy until December 19. On that date, he had a sudden onset of severe substernal chest pressure, which radiated to his left shoulder. He was admitted to the hospital and was diagnosed as having an acute anterior myocardial infarction. He was taken to the cardiac catheterization laboratory and underwent emergent percutaneous transluminal coronary angioplasty to his LAD, reducing his blockage from 100% to 30%. The remainder of his hospital stay was uncomplicated.

He has a 60 pack/year history of smoking and was smoking two packs per day at the time of admission to the hospital. Both his father and an older brother had had myocardial infarctions. He is 6 feet tall and weighs 242 pounds. His current blood lipids are cholesterol, 247 mg/dL, triglycerides, 165 mg/dL, HDL, 38 mg/dL, CHOL/HDL, 6.50 mg/dL, and glucose level is 100 mg/dL. His first marriage ended in divorce, and he reports that the onset of his chest discomfort at the time of his myocardial infarction occurred when he was arguing with his second wife about their mutually owned business. He states that because he works 60 to 70 hours per week, he has never participated in a regular exercise program.

Study Questions—Case 4

- What two major risk factors does this patient have for developing more atherosclerosis?
- What two lifestyle changes would increase this patient's HDL level?
- What one aspect of this patient's personality is likely to contribute to the progression of his CHD?

References

1. 1998 Heart and Stroke Statistical Update. Dallas, TX, American Heart Association, 1997.
2. Mortality Patterns—Preliminary Data, United States, 1996. *MMWR* 46:941–944, 1997.

3. Heberden W. An account of a disorder of the breast. *Med Trans R Coll Physicians* 2:59–67, 1786.

4. Enos W, Holmes R, Beyer J. Coronary disease among United States soldiers killed in action in Korea. *JAMA* 152:1090–1093, 1953.

5. Strong JP. Landmark perspective: Coronary atherosclerosis in soldiers. A clue to the natural history of atherosclerosis in the young. *JAMA* 256:2863–2866, 1986.

6. Kannel WB, Castelli WP, Gordon T, McNamara PM. Serum cholesterol, lipoproteins, and the risk of coronary heart disease. The Framingham study. *Ann Intern Med* 74:1–12, 1971.

7. Wissler R. Principles of the pathogenesis of atherosclerosis. In: Braunwald E (ed): *Heart Disease: A Textbook of Cardiovascular Medicine*. 2nd ed. Philadelphia, WB Saunders, 1984.

8. Reichl D. Lipoproteins of human peripheral lymph. *Eur Heart J* 11(suppl E):230–236, 1990.

9. Haberland ME, Fless GM, Scanu AM, Fogelman AM. Malondialdehyde modification of lipoprotein(a) produces avid uptake by human monocyte-macrophages. *J Biol Chem* 267:4143–4151, 1992.

10. Gorlin R. Coronary anatomy. *Major Probl Intern Med* 11:40–58, 1976.

11. Ambrose JA, Tannenbaum MA, Alexopoulos D, et al. Angiographic progression of coronary artery disease and the development of myocardial infarction. *J Am Coll Cardiol* 12:56–62, 1988.

12. Fulton WFM. The coronary arteries: Arteriography, microanatomy, and pathogenesis of obliterative coronary artery disease. Springfield, IL, Charles C Thomas, 1965, pp. 354.

13. Allwork SP. The applied anatomy of the arterial blood supply to the heart in man. *J Anat* 153:1–16, 1987.

14. Schaper W. The physiology of the collateral circulation in the normal and hypoxic myocardium. *Ergeb Physiol* 63:102–145, 1971.

15. Tracy RE, Newman WP 3rd, Wattigney WA, Berenson GS. Risk factors and atherosclerosis in youth autopsy findings of the Bogalusa Heart Study. *Am J Med Sci* 310(suppl 1):S37–41, 1995.

16. Stary H. Evolution of atherosclerotic plaques in the coronary arteries of young adults. *Atherosclerosis* 3:471a, 1983 (abstract).

17. Stary HC. Evolution and progression of atherosclerotic lesions in coronary arteries of children and young adults. *Arteriosclerosis* 9:I19–32, 1989.

18. Srinivasan SR, Radhakrishnamurthy B, Vijayagopal P, Berenson GS. Proteoglycans, lipoproteins, and atherosclerosis. *Adv Exp Med Biol* 285:373–381, 1991.

19. Ross R. The pathogenesis of atherosclerosis—An update. *N Engl J Med* 314:488–500, 1986.

20. Hassig A, Wen-Xi L, Stampfli K. The pathogenesis and prevention of atherosclerosis. *Med Hypotheses* 47:409–412, 1996.

21. Blankenhorn DH, Kramsch DM. Reversal of atherosis and sclerosis. The two components of atherosclerosis. *Circulation* 79:1–7, 1989.

22. Campbell JH, Campbell GR. Cell biology of atherosclerosis. *J Hypertens Suppl* 12:S129–132, 1994.

23. Kinlay S, Ganz P. Role of endothelial dysfunction in coronary artery disease and implications for therapy. *Am J Cardiol* 80:11I–16I, 1997.

24. Karsch KR. Atherosclerosis—Where are we heading? *Herz* 17:309–319, 1992.

25. Ross R, Glomset JA. The pathogenesis of atherosclerosis (second of two parts). *N Engl J Med* 295:420–425, 1976.

26. Ross R, Glomset JA. The pathogenesis of atherosclerosis (first of two parts). *N Engl J Med* 295:369–377, 1976.

27. DiCorleto PE. Cellular mechanisms of atherogenesis. *Am J Hypertens* 6:314S–318S, 1993.

28. Forstermann U, Mugge A, Alheid U, et al. Selective attenuation of endothelium-mediated vasodilation in atherosclerotic human coronary arteries. *Circ Res* 62:185–190, 1988.

29. Ludmer PL, Selwyn AP, Shook TL, et al. Paradoxical vasoconstriction induced by acetylcholine in atherosclerotic coronary arteries. *N Engl J Med* 315:1046–1051, 1986.

30. Marmur JD, Poon M, Rossikhina M, Taubman MB. Induction of PDGF-responsive genes in vascular smooth muscle. Implications for the early response to vessel injury. *Circulation* 86:III53–60, 1992.

31. Nilsson J, Volk-Jovinge S, Svensson J, et al. Association between high levels of growth factors in plasma and progression of coronary atherosclerosis. *J Intern Med* 232:397–404, 1992.

32. Grotendorst GR, Chang T, Seppa HE, et al. Platelet-derived growth factor is a chemoattractant for vascular smooth muscle cells. *J Cell Physiol* 113:261–266, 1982.

33. Krettek A, Fager G, Lindmark H, et al. Effect of phenotype on the transcription of the genes for platelet-derived growth factor (PDGF) isoforms in human smooth muscle cells, monocyte-derived macrophages, and endothelial cells in vitro. *Arterioscler Thromb Vasc Biol* 17:2897–2903, 1997.

34. Marumo T, Schini-Kerth VB, Fisslthaler B, Busse R. Platelet-derived growth factor-stimulated superoxide anion production modulates activation of transcription factor NF-kappa B and expression of monocyte chemoattractant protein 1 in human aortic smooth muscle cells. *Circulation* 96:2361–2367, 1997.

35. Osler W. Second Lumleian lecture on angina pectoris. *Lancet* March 26:839–844, 1910.

36. Prinzmetal M, Ekemecki A, Kennamer R, et al. Angina pectoris. 1. A variant form of angina pectoris. *Am J Med* 27:375–388, 1959.

37. Meller J, Pichard A, Dack S. Coronary arterial spasm in Prinzmetal's angina: A proved hypothesis. *Am J Cardiol* 37:938–940, 1976.

38. Maseri A, Severi S, Nes MD, et al. "Variant" angina: One aspect of a continuous spectrum of vasospastic myocardial ischemia. Pathogenetic mechanisms, estimated incidence and clinical and coronary arteriographic findings in 138 patients. *Am J Cardiol* 42:1019–1035, 1978.

39. Maseri A. Abnormal coronary vasomotion in ischemic heart disease. *J Cardiovasc Pharmacol* 20:S30–31, 1992.

40. Haudenschild CC. Pathogenesis of atherosclerosis: State of the art. *Cardiovasc Drugs Ther* 4(suppl 5):993–1004, 1990.

41. Yasue H, Matsuyama K, Matsuyama K, et al. Responses of angiographically normal human coronary arteries to intracoronary injection of acetylcholine by age and segment. Possible role of early coronary atherosclerosis. *Circulation* 81:482–490, 1990.

42. Okumura K, Yasue H, Matsuyama K, et al. Diffuse disorder of coronary artery vasomotility in patients with coronary spastic angina. Hyperreactivity to the constrictor effects of acetylcholine and the dilator effects of nitroglycerin. *J Am Coll Cardiol* 27:45–52, 1996.

43. Das UN. Can free radicals induce coronary vasospasm and acute myocardial infarction? *Med Hypotheses* 39:90–94, 1992.

44. Abrams J. Role of endothelial dysfunction in coronary artery disease. *Am J Cardiol* 79:2–9, 1997.

45. Vanhoutte PM. Endothelial dysfunction and atherosclerosis. *Eur Heart J* 18(suppl E):E19–29, 1997.

46. Vita JA, Treasure CB, Nabel EG, et al. Coronary vasomotor response to acetylcholine relates to risk factors for coronary artery disease. *Circulation* 81:491–497, 1990.

47. Kannel WB. Some lessons in cardiovascular epidemiology from Framingham. *Am J Cardiol* 37:269–282, 1976.

48. Kannel WB. Contributions of the Framingham Study to the conquest of coronary artery disease. *Am J Cardiol* 62:1109–1112, 1988.

49. Mancia G. The need to manage risk factors of coronary heart disease. *Am Heart J* 115:240–242, 1988.

50. Battegay E, Gasche A, Zimmerli L, et al. Risk factor control and perceptions of risk factors in patients with coronary heart disease. *Blood Press Suppl* 1:17–22, 1997.

51. Goble A, Jackson B, Phillips P, et al. The family atherosclerosis risk intervention study (FARIS): Risk factor profiles of patients and their relatives following an acute cardiac event. *Aust NZ J Med* 27:568–577, 1997.

52. Chronic Disease Notes and Reports. National Center for Chronic Disease Prevention and Health Promotion, Centers for Disease Control and Prevention, U.S. Department of Health and Human Services, 1997, pp 1–36.

53. Hammond EC, Horn D. Landmark article, March 15, 1958: Smoking and death rates—Report on forty-four months of follow-up of 187,783 men. *JAMA* 251:2840–2853, 1984.

54. Heitzer T, Yla-Herttuala S, Luoma J, et al. Cigarette smoking potentiates endothelial dysfunction of forearm resistance vessels in patients with hypercholesterolemia. Role of oxidized LDL. *Circulation* 93:1346–1353, 1996.

55. Lin SJ. Risk factors, endothelial cell turnover and lipid transport in atherogenesis. *Chung Hua I Hsueh Tsa Chih (Taipei)* 58:309–316, 1996.

56. Vogel RA. Coronary risk factors, endothelial function, and atherosclerosis: A review. *Clin Cardiol* 20:426–432, 1997.

57. Veyssier Belot C. [Tobacco smoking and cardiovascular risk] *Rev Med Interne* 18:702–708, 1997.

58. Rosengren A, Wilhelmsen L, Wedel H. Coronary heart disease, cancer and mortality in male middle-aged light smokers. *J Intern Med* 231:357–362, 1992.

59. Wilhelmsen L. Coronary heart disease: Epidemiology of smoking and intervention studies of smoking. *Am Heart J* 115:242–249, 1988.

60. Simon JA, Fong J, Bernert JT Jr, Browner WS. Relation of smoking and alcohol consumption to serum fatty acids. *Am J Epidemiol* 144:325–334, 1996.

61. van de Vijver LP, van Poppel G, van Houwelingen A, et al. Trans-unsaturated fatty acids in plasma phospholipids and coronary heart disease: A case-control study. *Atherosclerosis* 126:155–161, 1996.

62. He Y, Lam TH, Li LS, et al. The number of stenotic coronary arteries and passive smoking exposure from husband in lifelong non-smoking women in Xi'an, China. *Atherosclerosis* 127:229–238, 1996.

63. Moskowitz WB, Mosteller M, Schieken RM, et al. Lipoprotein and oxygen transport alterations in passive smoking preadolescent children. The MCV Twin Study. *Circulation* 81:586–592, 1990.

64. Marwick C. NHANES III health data relevant for aging nation. *JAMA* 277:100–102, 1997.

65. Gillum RF. Coronary heart disease, stroke, and hypertension in a U.S. national cohort: The NHANES I epidemiologic follow-up study. *Ann Epidemiol* 6:259–262, 1996.

66. Sorel JE, Heiss G, Tyroler HA, et al. Black-white differences in blood pressure among participants in NHANES II: The contribution of blood lead. *Epidemiology* 2:348–352, 1991.

67. Redon J, Campos C, Narciso ML, et al. Prognostic value of ambulatory blood pressure monitoring in refractory hypertension: A prospective study. *Hypertension* 31:712–718, 1998.

68. Nielsen WB, Lindenstrom E, Vestbo J, Jensen GB. Is diastolic hypertension an independent risk factor for stroke in the presence of normal systolic blood pressure in the middle-aged and elderly? *Am J Hypertens* 10:634–639, 1997.

69. Rutan GH, Kuller LH, Neaton JD, et al. Mortality associated with diastolic hypertension and isolated systolic hypertension among men screened for the Multiple Risk Factor Intervention Trial. *Circulation* 77:504–514, 1988.

70. Black HR. The coronary artery disease paradox. *Am J Hypertens* 9:2S–10S, 1996.

71. Borhani NO. Risk management in stroke prevention: Major clinical trials in hypertension. *Health Rep* 6:76–86, 1994.

72. Doyle AE. Does hypertension predispose to coronary disease? Conflicting epidemiological and experimental evidence. *Am J Hypertens* 1:319–324, 1988.

73. Waters D, Craven TE, Lesperance J. Prognostic significance of progression of coronary atherosclerosis. *Circulation* 87:1067–1075, 1993.

74. Assmann G, Schulte H. The Prospective Cardiovascular Münster Study: Prevalence and prognostic significance of hyperlipidemia in men with systemic hypertension. *Am J Cardiol* 59:9G–17G, 1987.

75. Olson RE. Discovery of the lipoproteins, their role in fat transport and their significance as risk factors. *J Nutr* 128:439S–443S, 1998.

76. Pekkanen J, Linn S, Heiss G, et al. Ten-year mortality from cardiovascular disease in relation to cholesterol level among men with and without preexisting cardiovascular disease. *N Engl J Med* 322:1700–1707, 1990.

77. Shoji T, Nishizawa Y, Kawagishi T, et al. Atherogenic lipoprotein changes in the absence of hyperlipidemia in patients with chronic renal failure treated by hemodialysis. *Atherosclerosis* 131:229–236, 1997.

78. Chapman MJ, Guerin M, Bruckert E. Atherogenic, dense low-density lipoproteins. Pathophysiology and new therapeutic approaches. *Eur Heart J* 19(suppl A):A24–30, 1998.

79. Frost PH, Havel RJ. Rationale for use of non-high-density lipoprotein cholesterol rather than low-density lipoprotein cholesterol as a tool for lipoprotein cholesterol screening and assessment of risk and therapy. *Am J Cardiol* 81:26B–31B, 1998.

80. Grundy SM, Balady GJ, Criqui MH, et al. When to start cholesterol-lowering therapy in patients with coronary heart disease. A statement for healthcare professionals from the American Heart Association Task Force on Risk Reduction. *Circulation* 95:1683–1685, 1997.

81. Kris-Etherton PM, Krummel D, Russell ME, et al. The effect of diet on plasma lipids, lipoproteins, and coronary heart disease. *J Am Diet Assoc* 88:1373–1400, 1988.

82. Kris-Etherton PM, Krummel D. Role of nutrition in the prevention and treatment of coronary heart disease in women. *J Am Diet Assoc* 93:987–993, 1993.

83. Smith-Schneider LM, Sigman-Grant MJ, Kris-Etherton PM. Dietary fat reduction strategies. *J Am Diet Assoc* 92:34–38, 1992.

84. Srinath U, Jonnalagadda SS, Naglak MC, et al. Diet in the prevention and treatment of atherosclerosis. A perspective for the elderly. *Clin Geriatr Med* 11:591–611, 1995.

85. Connor SL, Gustafson JR, Artaud-Wild SM, et al. The cholesterol/saturated-fat index: An indication of the hypercholesterolaemic and atherogenic potential of food. *Lancet* 1:1229–1232, 1986.

86. Connor SL, Gustafson JR, Artaud-Wild SM, et al. The cholesterol-saturated fat index for coronary prevention: Background, use, and a comprehensive table of foods. *J Am Diet Assoc* 89:807–816, 1989.

87. Artaud-Wild SM, Connor SL, Sexton G, Connor WE. Differences in coronary mortality can be explained by differences in cholesterol and saturated fat intakes in 40 countries but not in France and Finland. A paradox. *Circulation* 88:2771–2779, 1993.
88. Brown WV. Review of clinical trials: Proving the lipid hypothesis. *Eur Heart J* 11 (suppl H):15–20, 1990.
89. Satler LF, Pearle DL, Rackley CE. Reduction in coronary heart disease: Clinical and anatomical considerations. *Clin Cardiol* 12:422–426, 1989.
90. Gordon DJ, Probstfield JL, Garrison RJ, et al. High-density lipoprotein cholesterol and cardiovascular disease. Four prospective American studies. *Circulation* 79:8–15, 1989.
91. Miller M, Mead LA, Kwiterovich PO Jr, Pearson TA. Dyslipidemias with desirable plasma total cholesterol levels and angiographically demonstrated coronary artery disease. *Am J Cardiol* 65:1–5, 1990.
92. Drexel H, Amann FW, Beran J, et al. Plasma triglycerides and three lipoprotein cholesterol fractions are independent predictors of the extent of coronary atherosclerosis. *Circulation* 90:2230–2235, 1994.
93. Verdery RB. Reverse cholesterol transport from fibroblasts to high density lipoproteins: Computer solutions of a kinetic model. *Can J Biochem* 59:586–592, 1981.
94. Berger GM. High-density lipoproteins, reverse cholesterol transport and atherosclerosis—Recent developments. *S Afr Med J* 65:503–506, 1984.
95. Miller NE, La Ville A, Crook D. Direct evidence that reverse cholesterol transport is mediated by high-density lipoprotein in rabbit. *Nature* 314:109–111, 1985.
96. Gwynne JT. High-density lipoprotein cholesterol levels as a marker of reverse cholesterol transport. *Am J Cardiol* 64:10G–17G, 1989.
97. Schmitz G, Bruning T, Williamson E, Nowicka G. The role of HDL in reverse cholesterol transport and its disturbances in Tangier disease and HDL deficiency with xanthomas. *Eur Heart J* 11(suppl E):197–211, 1990.
98. Pieters MN, Schouten D, Van Berkel TJ. In vitro and in vivo evidence for the role of HDL in reverse cholesterol transport. *Biochim Biophys Acta* 1225:125–134, 1994.
99. Assmann G, Schulte H, von Eckardstein A, Huang Y. High-density lipoprotein cholesterol as a predictor of coronary heart disease risk. The PROCAM experience and pathophysiological implications for reverse cholesterol transport. *Atherosclerosis* 124(suppl): S11–20, 1996.
100. Hill SA, McQueen MJ. Reverse cholesterol transport—A review of the process and its clinical implications. *Clin Biochem* 30:517–525, 1997.
101. Kannel WB. Hazards, risks, and threats of heart disease from the early stages to symptomatic coronary heart disease and cardiac failure. *Cardiovasc Drugs Ther* 11(suppl 1):199–212, 1997.
102. Chennell A, Sullivan DR, Penberthy LA, Hensley WJ. Comparability of lipoprotein measurements, total:HDL cholesterol ratio and other coronary risk functions within and between laboratories in Australia. *Pathology* 26:471–476, 1994.
103. Castelli WP, Anderson K. A population at risk. Prevalence of high cholesterol levels in hypertensive patients in the Framingham Study. *Am J Med* 80:23–32, 1986.
104. Krauss RM. Atherogenicity of triglyceride-rich lipoproteins. *Am J Cardiol* 81:13B–17B, 1998.
105. Hodis HN, Mack WJ. Triglyceride-rich lipoproteins and progression of atherosclerosis. *Eur Heart J* 19(suppl A):A40–44, 1998.
106. Castelli WP. The triglyceride issue: A view from Framingham. *Am Heart J* 112:432–437, 1986.
107. McNicoll S, Latour Y, Rondeau C, et al. Cardiovascular risk factors and lipoprotein profile in French Canadians with premature CAD: Impact of the national cholesterol education program II. *Can J Cardiol* 11:109–116, 1995.
108. Stein Y. Comparison of European and USA guidelines for prevention of coronary heart disease. *Atherosclerosis* 110(suppl):S41–44, 1994.
109. Schaefer EJ. New recommendations for the diagnosis and treatment of plasma lipid abnormalities. *Nutr Rev* 51:246–253, 1993.
110. Morris JN, Kagan A, Pattison DC, Gardner MJ. Incidence and prediction of ischaemic heart-disease in London busmen. *Lancet* 2:553–559, 1966.
111. Health risk factor surveys of commercial plan- and Medicaid-enrolled members of health-maintenance organizations—Michigan, 1995. *MMWR Morb Mortal Wkly Rep* 46:923–926, 1997.
112. Prevalence of physical inactivity during leisure time among overweight persons—Behavioral Risk Factor Surveillance System, 1994. *MMWR Morb Mortal Wkly Rep* 45:185–188, 1996.
113. Prevalence of sedentary lifestyle—Behavioral Risk Factor Surveillance System, United States, 1991. *MMWR Morb Mortal Wkly Rep* 42:576–579, 1993.
114. Berg A, Halle M, Franz I, Keul J. Physical activity and lipoprotein metabolism: Epidemiological evidence and clinical trials. *Eur J Med Res* 2:259–264, 1997.
115. Fonong T, Toth MJ, Ades PA, et al. Relationship between physical activity and HDL-cholesterol in healthy older men and women: A cross-sectional and exercise intervention study. *Atherosclerosis* 127:177–183, 1996.
116. Leon AS, Casal D, Jacobs D Jr. Effects of 2,000 kcal per week of walking and stair climbing on physical fitness and risk factors for coronary heart disease. *J Cardiopulm Rehabil* 16:183–192, 1996.
117. Manninen V, Elo MO, Frick MH, et al. Lipid alterations and decline in the incidence of coronary heart disease in the Helsinki Heart Study. *JAMA* 260:641–651, 1988.
118. Wood PD. Physical activity, diet, and health: independent and interactive effects. *Med Sci Sports Exerc* 26:838–843, 1994.
119. Young DR, Haskell WL, Jatulis DE, Fortmann SP. Associations between changes in physical activity and risk factors for coronary heart disease in a community-based sample of men and women: The Stanford Five-City Project. *Am J Epidemiol* 138:205–216, 1993.
120. Katzel LI, Bleecker ER, Rogus EM, Goldberg AP. Sequential effects of aerobic exercise training and weight loss on risk factors for coronary disease in healthy, obese middle-aged and older men. *Metabolism* 46:1441–1447, 1997.
121. Huonker M, Halle M, Keul J. Structural and functional adaptations of the cardiovascular system by training. *Int J Sports Med* 17(suppl 3): S164–172, 1996.
122. Kvernmo HD, Osterud B. The effect of physical conditioning suggests adaptation in procoagulant and fibrinolytic potential. *Thromb Res* 87:559–569, 1997.
123. Ponjee GA, Janssen EM, Hermans J, van Wersch JW. Regular physical activity and changes in risk factors for coronary heart disease: A nine month prospective study. *Eur J Clin Chem Clin Biochem* 34:477–483, 1996.
124. Sasaki Y, Morimoto A, Ishii I, et al. Preventive effect of long-term aerobic exercise on thrombus formation in rat cerebral vessels. *Haemostasis* 25:212–217, 1995.
125. Drygas WK. Changes in blood platelet function, coagulation, and fibrinolytic activity in response to moderate, exhaustive, and prolonged exercise. *Int J Sports Med* 9:67–72, 1988.

126. De Paz JA, Lasierra J, Villa JG, et al. Changes in the fibrinolytic system associated with physical conditioning. *Eur J Appl Physiol* 65:388–393, 1992.

127. Tanaka K, Nakanishi T. Obesity as a risk factor for various diseases: necessity of lifestyle changes for healthy aging. *Appl Human Sci* 15:139–148, 1996.

128. Jako P. [The role of physical activity in the prevention of certain internal diseases]. *Orv Hetil* 136:2379–2383, 1995.

129. Nolte LJ, Nowson CA, Dyke AC. Effect of dietary fat reduction and increased aerobic exercise on cardiovascular risk factors. *Clin Exp Pharmacol Physiol* 24:901–903, 1997.

130. Haskell WL. J.B. Wolffe Memorial Lecture. Health consequences of physical activity: Understanding and challenges regarding dose-response. *Med Sci Sports Exerc* 26:649–660, 1994.

131. Larson EB, Bruce RA. Health benefits of exercise in an aging society. *Arch Intern Med* 147:353–356, 1987.

132. Brownlee M. The pathological implications of protein glycation. *Clin Invest Med* 18:275–281, 1995.

133. Giugliano D, Ceriello A, Paolisso G. Diabetes mellitus, hypertension, and cardiovascular disease: Which role for oxidative stress? *Metabolism* 44:363–368, 1995.

134. Duncan BB, Heiss G: Nonenzymatic glycosylation of proteins—A new tool for assessment of cumulative hyperglycemia in epidemiologic studies, past and future. *Am J Epidemiol* 120:169–189, 1984.

135. Bao W, Srinivasan SR, Valdez R, et al. Longitudinal changes in cardiovascular risk from childhood to young adulthood in offspring of parents with coronary artery disease: The Bogalusa Heart Study. *JAMA* 278:1749–1754, 1997.

136. Colombel A, Charbonnel B. Weight gain and cardiovascular risk factors in the post-menopausal woman. *Hum Reprod* 12(suppl 1): 134–145, 1997.

137. Gensini GF, Comeglio M, Colella A. Classical risk factors and emerging elements in the risk profile for coronary artery disease. *Eur Heart J* 19(suppl A):A53–61, 1998.

138. Anderssen SA, Holme I, Urdal P, Hjermann I. Associations between central obesity and indexes of hemostatic, carbohydrate and lipid metabolism. Results of a 1-year intervention from the Oslo Diet and Exercise Study. *Scand J Med Sci Sports* 8:109–115, 1998.

139. Shaper AG. Obesity and cardiovascular disease. *Ciba Found Symp* 201:90–103, 1996.

140. Akimova EV, Bogmat LF. Premature coronary heart disease: The influence of positive family history on platelet activity in vivo in children and adolescents (family study). *J Cardiovasc Risk* 4:13–18, 1997.

141. Saito T, Nanri S, Saito I, et al. A novel approach to assessing family history in the prevention of coronary heart disease. *J Epidemiol* 7:85–92, 1997.

142. Allen JK, Blumenthal RS. Risk factors in the offspring of women with premature coronary heart disease. *Am Heart J* 135:428–434, 1998.

143. Pohjola-Sintonen S, Rissanen A, Liskola P, Luomanmaki K. Family history as a risk factor of coronary heart disease in patients under 60 years of age. *Eur Heart J* 19:235–239, 1998.

144. Khaw KT, Barrett-Connor E. Family history of heart attack: A modifiable risk factor? *Circulation* 74:239–244, 1986.

145. Barrett-Connor E, Khaw K. Family history of heart attack as an independent predictor of death due to cardiovascular disease. *Circulation* 69:1065–1069, 1984.

146. Neaton JD, Wentworth D. Serum cholesterol, blood pressure, cigarette smoking, and death from coronary heart disease. Overall findings and differences by age for 316,099 white men. Multiple Risk Factor Intervention Trial Research Group. *Arch Intern Med* 152:56–64, 1992.

147. Smith SC Jr. Risk reduction therapies for patients with coronary artery disease: A call for increased implementation. *Am J Med* 104:23S–26S, 1998.

148. Grundy SM, Balady GJ, Criqui MH, et al. Primary prevention of coronary heart disease: Guidance from Framingham: A statement for healthcare professionals from the AHA task force on risk reduction. *Circulation* 97:1876–1887, 1998.

149. Haskell WL, Alderman EL, Fair JM, et al. Effects of intensive multiple risk factor reduction on coronary atherosclerosis and clinical cardiac events in men and women with coronary artery disease. The Stanford Coronary Risk Intervention Project (SCRIP). *Circulation* 89:975–990, 1994.

150. Williams MA. Cardiovascular risk-factor reduction in elderly patients with cardiac disease. *Phys Ther* 76:469–480, 1996.

151. McCann TJ, Criqui MH, Kashani IA, et al. A randomized trial of cardiovascular risk factor reduction: Patterns of attrition after randomization and during follow-up. *J Cardiovasc Risk* 4:41–46, 1997.

152. Morley JE, Reese SS. Clinical implications of the aging heart. *Am J Med* 86:77–86, 1989.

153. Rodeheffer RJ, Gerstenblith G, Beard E, et al. Postural changes in cardiac volumes in men in relation to adult age. *Exp Gerontol* 21:367–378, 1986.

154. Dahlberg ST. Gender difference in the risk factors for sudden cardiac death. *Cardiology* 77:31–40, 1990.

155. Orchard TJ. The impact of gender and general risk factors on the occurrence of atherosclerotic vascular disease in non-insulin-dependent diabetes mellitus. *Ann Med* 28:323–333, 1996.

156. Motro M, Shemesh J. Prevalence of coronary calcification in relation to age, gender and risk factor profile in the insight population. *Br J Clin Pract Suppl* 88:1–5, 1997.

157. Villablanca AC. Coronary heart disease in women. Gender differences and effects of menopause. *Postgrad Med* 100:191–196, 201–202, 1996.

158. Rao AV. Coronary heart disease risk factors in women: Focus on gender differences. *J La State Med Soc* 150:67–72, 1998.

159. Kitler ME. Coronary disease: Are there gender differences? *Eur Heart J* 15:409–417, 1994.

160. Gorodeski GI. Impact of the menopause on the epidemiology and risk factors of coronary artery heart disease in women. *Exp Gerontol* 29:357–375, 1994.

161. Wister AV, Gee EM. Age at death due to ischemic heart disease: Gender differences. *Soc Biol* 41:110–126, 1994.

162. Adams KF Jr, Dunlap SH, Sueta CA, et al. Relation between gender, etiology and survival in patients with symptomatic heart failure. *J Am Coll Cardiol* 28:1781–1788, 1996.

163. Roger VL, Jacobsen SJ, Pellikka PA, et al. Gender differences in use of stress testing and coronary heart disease mortality: a population-based study in Olmsted County, Minnesota. *J Am Coll Cardiol* 32:345–352, 1998.

164. Shumaker SA, Brooks MM, Schron EB, et al. Gender differences in health-related quality of life among post-myocardial infarction patients: Brief report. CAST Investigators. Cardiac Arrhythmia Suppression Trials. *Womens Health* 3:53–60, 1997.

165. Kambara H, Kinoshita M, Nakagawa M, Kawai C. Gender difference in long-term prognosis after myocardial infarction—Clinical characteristics in 1000 patients. The Kyoto and Shiga Myocardial Infarction (KYSMI) Study Group. *Jpn Circ J* 59:1–10, 1995.

166. Behar S, Zion M, Reicher-Reiss H, et al. Short- and long-term prognosis of patients with a first acute myocardial

infarction with concomitant peripheral vascular disease. SPRINT Study Group. *Am J Med* 96:15–19, 1994.

167. Brochier ML, Arwidson P. Coronary heart disease risk factors in women. *Eur Heart J* 19 (suppl A):A45–52, 1998.

168. Lunetta M, Barbagallo A, Attardo T, et al. Coronary heart disease in type 2 diabetic patients: Common and different risk factors in men and women. *Diabetes Metab* 23:230–231, 1997.

169. Frost PH, Davis BR, Burlando AJ, et al. Coronary heart disease risk factors in men and women aged 60 years and older: Findings from the systolic hypertension in the elderly program. *Circulation* 94:26–34, 1996.

170. Dallongeville J, Marecaux N, Isorez D, et al. Multiple coronary heart disease risk factors are associated with menopause and influenced by substitutive hormonal therapy in a cohort of French women. *Atherosclerosis* 118:123–133, 1995.

171. Friedman M, Rosenman RH. Association of specific overt behavior pattern with blood and cardiovascular findings. *JAMA* 169:1286–1296, 1959.

172. Lachar BL. Coronary-prone behavior. Type A behavior revisited. *Tex Heart Inst J* 20:143–151, 1993.

173. Keltikangas-Jarvinen L, Raikkonen K, Hautanen A, Adlercreutz H. Vital exhaustion, anger expression, and pituitary and adrenocortical hormones. Implications for the insulin resistance syndrome. *Arterioscler Thromb Vasc Biol* 16:275–280, 1996.

174. King KB. Psychologic and social aspects of cardiovascular disease. *Ann Behav Med* 19:264–270, 1997.

175. Grignani G, Pacchiarini L, Zucchella M, et al. Effect of mental stress on platelet function in normal subjects and in patients with coronary artery disease. *Haemostasis* 22:138–146, 1992.

176. Markovitz JH, Matthews KA. Platelets and coronary heart disease: Potential psychophysiologic mechanisms. *Psychosom Med* 53:643–668, 1991.

177. Myerburg RJ, Interian A Jr, Mitrani RM, et al. Frequency of sudden cardiac death and profiles of risk. *Am J Cardiol* 80:10F–19F, 1997.

178. Guidelines for cardiopulmonary resuscitation and emergency cardiac care. Emergency Cardiac Care Committee and Subcommittees, American Heart Association. Part IX. Ensuring effectiveness of communitywide emergency cardiac care. *JAMA* 268:2289–2295, 1992.

179. White RD. Optimal access to- and response by public and voluntary services, including the role of bystanders and family members, in cardiopulmonary resuscitation. *New Horiz* 5:153–157, 1997.

180. Hilton TC, Chaitman BR. The prognosis in stable and unstable angina. *Cardiol Clin* 9:27–38, 1991.

181. Brann WM, Tresch DD. Management of stable & unstable angina in elderly patients. *Compr Ther* 23:49–56, 1997.

182. Chierchia S, Brunelli C, Simonetti I, et al. Sequence of events in angina at rest: primary reduction in coronary flow. *Circulation* 61:759–768, 1980.

183. Chasen C, Muller JE. Cardiovascular triggers and morning events. *Blood Press Monit* 3:35–42, 1998.

184. Kristensen SD, Ravn HB, Falk E. Insights into the pathophysiology of unstable coronary artery disease. *Am J Cardiol* 80:5E–9E, 1997.

185. Osborne JA, Stone PH. Recent advances in the understanding and management of stable and unstable angina pectoris and asymptomatic myocardial ischemia. *Curr Opin Cardiol* 9:448–456, 1994.

186. Haft JI, Mariano DL, Goldstein J. Comparison of the histopathology of culprit lesions in chronic stable angina, unstable angina, and myocardial infarction. *Clin Cardiol* 20:651–655, 1997.

187. Thieme T, Wernecke KD, Meyer R, et al. Angioscopic evaluation of atherosclerotic plaques: Validation by histomorphologic analysis and association with stable and unstable coronary syndromes. *J Am Coll Cardiol* 28:1–6, 1996.

188. Rosengren A, Wilhelmsen L, Hagman M, Wedel H. Natural history of myocardial infarction and angina pectoris in a general population sample of middle-aged men: A 16-year follow-up of the Primary Prevention Study, Goteborg, Sweden. *J Intern Med* 244:495–505, 1998.

189. Lewis CE, Raczynski JM, Oberman A, Cutter GR. Risk factors and the natural history of coronary heart disease in blacks. *Cardiovasc Clin* 21:29–45, 1991.

190. Kramsch DM, Blankenhorn DH. Regression of atherosclerosis: Which components regress and what influences their reversal. *Wien Klin Wochenschr* 104:2–9, 1992.

191. Hodis HN. Reversibility of atherosclerosis—Evolving perspectives from two arterial imaging clinical trials: The cholesterol lowering atherosclerosis regression study and the monitored atherosclerosis regression study. *J Cardiovasc Pharmacol* 25:S25–31, 1995.

192. Patrono C. Prevention of myocardial infarction and stroke by aspirin: Different mechanisms? Different dosage? *Thromb Res* 92:S7–12, 1998.

193. Azen SP, Mack WJ, Cashin-Hemphill L, et al. Progression of coronary artery disease predicts clinical coronary events. Long-term follow-up from the Cholesterol Lowering Atherosclerosis Study. *Circulation* 93:34–41, 1996.

194. Blankenhorn DH, Johnson RL, Nessim SA, et al. The Cholesterol Lowering Atherosclerosis Study (CLAS): Design, methods, and baseline results. *Controlled Clin Trials* 8:356–387, 1987.

195. Ornish D, Scherwitz LW, Billings JH, et al. Intensive lifestyle changes for reversal of coronary heart disease. *JAMA* 280:2001–2007, 1998.

196. Strandberg TE, Pitkanen A, Larjo P, et al. Attitude changes of general practitioners towards lowering LDL cholesterol. *J Cardiovasc Risk* 5:43–46, 1998.

197. Campbell NC, Thain J, Deans HG, et al. Secondary prevention clinics for coronary heart disease: Randomised trial of effect on health. *BMJ* 316:1434–1437, 1998.

4

Cardiac Muscle Dysfunction

Lawrence Cahalin

INTRODUCTION

Cardiac muscle dysfunction (CMD) is a term that has gained popularity in describing an apparently common finding in patients with heart and lung disease.[1-3] CMD effectively, yet very simply, describes the most common cause of congestive heart failure (CHF).[2] It is estimated that 2 million or more Americans suffer from CHF and that 400,000 new cases occur yearly, requiring 900,000

106

hospitalizations each year.[4] In addition, years of cardiovascular data compiled in Framingham, Massachusetts, show that the 1% prevalence of CHF in those aged 50 to 59 years increases progressively with advancing age to reach approximately 10% in 80- to 89-year-olds.[5] Individuals with a wide variety of heart and lung diseases very likely will develop CHF at some time during their lives,[3] frequently manifested as **pulmonary congestion** or **pulmonary edema.**[1] This chapter describes the clinical manifestations resulting from CMD and demonstrates how it affects all body systems.

Many of the signs and symptoms of CHF are the result of a "sequence of events with a resultant increase in fluid in the interstitial spaces of the lungs, liver, subcutaneous tissues, and **serous cavities.**"[6] The etiology of CHF is varied, but it is most commonly the result of CMD. Nevertheless, the interdependence and interrelationship between the cardiac and pulmonary systems are evident. In fact, the most common mechanism responsible for pulmonary edema is increased pulmonary capillary pressure, although other factors may contribute to its origin (Table 4–1). Left ventricular failure is the most common cause of such increased pulmonary capillary pressure, which produces the congestion of CHF. Therefore, the term CMD accurately describes the primary cause of pulmonary edema as well as the underlying pathophysiology of CHF because CMD essentially *impairs* the heart's ability to *pump blood* or the left ventricle's ability to *accept blood.*[6]

The heart's ability to accept and pump blood depends upon a number of factors of which the primary variables are presented in the periphery of Figure 4–1. Many of these factors are responsible for CMD and CHF. Conversely, many of them can be used to treat the pathophysiology of CMD and CHF. Examples of this include providing supplemental oxygen to decrease myocardial ischemia, and subsequently improve myocardial contraction or using different body positions to either increase or decrease the return of blood to the heart (such as supine versus sitting positions, respectively). Increased return of blood to the heart due to a supine body position could worsen CMD and CHF in a person with existing CHF and an increased volume of blood in the ventricles, but the same body position might be beneficial for a person with CHF and decreased volume of blood in the ventricles due to aggressive diuresis to remove fluid from the lungs and various parts of the body.[6]

This apparent ambiguity can be better understood by further discussing Figure 4–1B in which the volume of blood in the ventricle of the heart (ventricular end-diastolic volume; VEDV) is plotted against ventricular performance. Excessive VEDV decreases ventricular performance (if extreme, shock can ensue), but lower levels of VEDV tend to improve ventricular performance. However, if the VEDV is inadequate because of decreased body fluid and blood volume or change in body position (both of which may decrease the return of blood to the heart), ventricular performance can worsen. A person with CHF typically has increased VEDV (because of a poorly contracting heart), which can increase further from the increased venous return of a supine position. Other mechanisms can also increase venous return such as increasing venous tone and the pumping action of skeletal muscle. Even a slight increase in the VEDV of a person with CHF may worsen the CMD and CHF.[6]

These examples demonstrate the important role a physical therapist plays in either improving or worsening CMD and CHF. Subsequent sections in this chapter review the many interrelated pathophysiologic mechanisms of CHF as well as the implications they have for physical therapy practice.

HEART FAILURE

As previously mentioned, CHF is the result of a sequence of events that results in increased fluid

Table 4–1

Mechanisms Responsible for Pulmonary Edema

Increased pulmonary capillary pressure
(e.g., left ventricular failure)
Decreased plasma oncotic pressure
(e.g., hypoalbuminemia secondary to multisystem dysfunction)
Increased negativity of interstitial pressure
(e.g., asthma)
Altered alveolar-capillary membrane permeability
(e.g., aspiration of acidic gastric contents or infectious pneumonia)
Lymphatic insufficiency
(e.g., after lung transplant)
Unknown or incompletely understood
(e.g., high altitude, after cardiopulmonary bypass)

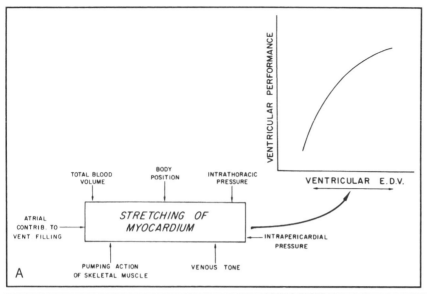

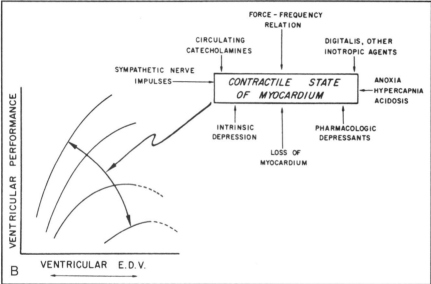

Figure 4–1. *A,* Determinants of myocardial stretching and ventricular performance. The Frank-Starling mechanism is based on adequate "stretch" of the myocardium that produces an increased end-diastolic volume (E.D.V.) and subsequently increases ventricular performance. The major influences that contribute to the stretching of the myocardium are depicted here. *B,* Determinants of myocardial contraction and ventricular performance. The major "contractile" influences affecting ventricular performance are depicted here, and end-diastolic volume (E.D.V) is a major factor. (From Braunwald E, Ross J, Sonnenblick E, et al. Mechanisms of Contraction of the Normal and Failing Heart. 2nd ed. Boston, Little, Brown, 1976.)

in many parts of the body.[6] CHF is often described as a syndrome with many pathophysiologic and compensatory mechanisms that occur in an attempt to maintain an adequate ejection of blood from the ventricle each minute (cardiac output) to the organs and tissues of the body (cardiac index). A description of the various ways CHF is categorized follows.

Right-sided or left-sided CHF simply describes which side of the heart is failing, as well as the side that is initially affected and behind which fluid tends to localize. For example, left-sided heart failure is frequently the result of left ventric-

ular insult (e.g., myocardial infarction, hypertension, aortic valve disease), which causes fluid to accumulate behind the left ventricle. This, in turn, produces an accumulation of fluid in the lungs, liver, abdomen, and ankles (manifestations of right-sided heart failure).[6] Thus, right-sided CHF may occur because of left-sided CHF or because of right ventricular failure (e.g., secondary to pulmonary hypertension, pulmonary embolus, right ventricular infarction). In either case, fluid backs up behind the right ventricle and produces the accumulation of fluid in the liver, abdomen, and ankles, as mentioned earlier.

Low-output CHF is the description most frequently associated with heart failure and is the result of a low cardiac output at rest or during exertion. **High-output CHF** usually results from a volume overload, as may occur in pregnancy, **thyrotoxicosis** (overactivity of the thyroid gland, such as in **Graves' disease**), and renal insufficiency.[6-10] It is important to note that although the term *high-output* implies a greater cardiac output, it is nonetheless still lower than it was before CHF developed.

Systolic versus diastolic heart failure is perhaps the most informative and useful distinction in CHF because optimal cardiac performance is dependent on both proper systolic and diastolic functioning. The impaired contraction of the ventricles during systole that produces an inefficient expulsion of blood is termed *systolic heart failure*. *Diastolic heart failure* is associated with an inability of the ventricles to accept the blood ejected from the atria. Both types are very important in the overall scheme of CHF and often occur simultaneously, as in the patient who suffers a massive anterior myocardial infarction (loss of contracting myocardium, producing systolic heart failure) with subsequent replacement of the infarcted area with nondistensible fibrous scar tissue (which does not readily or adequately accept the blood ejected into the left ventricle from the left atria and produces diastolic heart failure). Despite the various descriptions of CHF just presented, the primary cause of CHF is CMD.

CAUSES AND TYPES OF CARDIAC MUSCLE DYSFUNCTION

The varied causes of CMD can be best classified according to 10 specific processes/causes.[6-8]

• Hypertension
• Coronary artery disease (myocardial infarction/ischemia)
• Cardiac dysrhythmias
• Renal insufficiency
• Cardiomyopathy
• Heart valve abnormalities and congenital/acquired heart disease
• Pericardial effusion or myocarditis

• Pulmonary embolism or pulmonary hypertension
• Spinal cord injury
• Age-related changes

Of these, cardiomyopathy, congenital abnormalities, renal insufficiency, and aging are more commonly associated with *chronic* heart failure, whereas the others are associated with *acute* CHF. As previously described, acute and chronic heart failure can be more specifically described as forward or backward, right-sided or left-sided, low-output or high-output, or systolic or diastolic heart failure.[6]

Hypertension and Coronary Artery Disease

Hypertension and **coronary artery disease** are the most common causes of CMD,[3] which occurs because of dysfunction of the left or right ventricle or both.[11-13] This development was demonstrated in the example given earlier of a patient who, after suffering a massive anterior myocardial infarction, loses a significant amount of strategically located cardiac muscle, subsequently decreasing the performance of the left ventricle; this decrease produces a decreased **ejection fraction** and, in many instances, a decreased physical work capacity.

The increased arterial pressure seen in systemic hypertension eventually produces left ventricular hypertrophy, which is worsened by CMD and CHF. The extremely elevated ventricular and occasionally elevated atrial pressures commonly seen in patients with CMD tend to produce a less effective pump as the myocardial contractile fibers become overstretched, thus increasing the work of each myocardial fiber in an attempt to maintain an adequate cardiac output.[14, 15] Myocardial work continued in this manner eventually produces left ventricular hypertrophy as the contractile fibers adapt to the increased workload.[16, 17] The primary problem with left ventricular hypertrophy is the increased energy expenditure (metabolic cost) required for myocardial contraction because of increased myocardial cell mass.[14, 16, 18] This scenario is typical of that commonly seen in cardiomyopathies.

Treatment of hypertension and coronary artery disease can improve CMD and frequently requires the combination of pharmacologic and nonpharmacologic strategies. The specific treatment of acute myocardial infarction depends on many factors, primarily the presence or absence of CHF, ventricular arrhythmias, recurrent angina, and persistent hypotension.[19] The primary treatments are as follows:

- Oxygen
- Nitroglycerin
- Analgesia
- Electrical defibrillation
- Atropine
- Lidocaine
- Pacemaker
- Thrombolytic agents
- Beta blocker
- Calcium-channel blocker
- Anticoagulant and platelet-inhibitory agents
- Percutaneous transluminal coronary angioplasty
- Intra-aortic balloon counterpulsation and other circulatory assist devices
- Surgical intervention[20]

These therapeutic measures are considered most crucial in the treatment of acute myocardial infarction, and a variety of patient variables dictate which of these treatments should be used. A detailed review of the early management of patients with acute myocardial infarction with an emphasis on patient identification, stratification, and treatment progression has previously been published and provides detailed information regarding the treatment of myocardial infarction.[20]

Postperfusion (postpump) syndrome is a complication associated with cardiopulmonary bypass surgery and essentially represents "organ and subsystem dysfunction."[21] Not only is CMD common after bypass surgery,[22] but abnormal bleeding, inflammatory reactions, renal dysfunction, hemodynamic and metabolic problems (from peripheral and possibly central vasoconstriction), breakdown of red blood cells, and possibly increased susceptibility to infection have all been reported as "damaging effects of cardiopulmonary bypass."[21] The importance of investigating for the presence of any of the previously mentioned complications is emphasized by the following quote "the fact that most patients convalesce normally after cardiopulmonary bypass attests only to patients' abilities to compensate for these damaging effects and not to their absence."[21]

In conclusion, several important risk factors

have been recognized to be associated with the postpump syndrome, including the following:

- Duration of cardiopulmonary bypass greater than 90 to 120 minutes for young infants or 150 minutes for adults
- Patient age
- Presence of preoperative cyanosis
- Perfusion flow rate
- Composition of the **perfusate**
- Oxygenating surface
- Patient temperature during perfusion[21]

Coronary angioplasty has also been associated with a certain degree of myocardial damage or "stunning," the clinical significance of which is still under investigation.[23, 24]

Cardiac Arrhythmias and Renal Insufficiency

Cardiac arrhythmias and **renal insufficiency** can also cause CMD for reasons similar to those given for myocardial infarction.[6] Extremely rapid or slow cardiac arrhythmias or volume overload from abnormal kidney function can impair the functioning of the left or right ventricle, or both, and an overall CMD ensues. Correcting the arrhythmia or decreasing the volume overload can remedy this type of CMD quickly.[25, 26]

Cardiac arrhythmias that produce CMD are the result of prolonged very slow or very fast heart rates and frequently are due to a **sick sinus node syndrome** or heart blocks (producing very slow heart rates), prolonged supraventricular tachycardia (i.e., rapid atrial fibrillation or flutter), or ventricular tachycardia (both tachycardias produce very fast heart rates).[27, 28]

Very slow heart rates or heart blocks are often an adverse reaction or side effect of a specific medication, but when medications are withheld and slow heart rates or a heart block persists, the implantation of a permanent pacemaker is generally performed.[27] This type of CMD is readily amenable to treatment and quite reversible.

Cardiac muscle dysfunction due to very rapid heart rates is also reversible. Rapid atrial fibrillation or flutter can produce CMD and is often easily treated by the administration of verapamil or digoxin[27] (see Chapter 14). If these drugs fail, electrical cardioversion is usually performed, after which rapid heart rates frequently become much more normal as the cyclic "circus movement" propagating the rapid rhythm is disrupted and the sinoatrial node is allowed to resume control of the heart's rhythm.[27] Ventricular tachycardia and fibrillation are life-threatening cardiac arrhythmias, which, if prolonged, rapid, or both, can also produce CMD and death. The treatment of ventricular tachycardia and fibrillation is dependent on the clinical status of the patient and follows the guidelines set forth by the American Heart Association.[27] The use of automatic implantable cardiac defibrillators (AICDs) has been a treatment of choice for patients with recurrent ventricular tachycardia and fibrillation that is unresponsive to antiarrhythmic medications.[28]

Ventricular function is intimately related to cardiac rhythm. Any abnormally fast, slow, or unsynchronized rhythm can impair ventricular and atrial function quickly and progress to CHF and even death.[27] Many patients with CMD have preexisting arrhythmias that must be controlled, typically with medication, but sometimes by other methods (e.g., ablation, AICD)[28] to prevent further deterioration of a muscle that is already compromised.

As previously discussed, acute or chronic renal insufficiency tends to produce a fluid overload, which frequently progresses to CMD and CHF that can often be reversed if it is the only underlying pathophysiologic process. However, other pathophysiologic processes may produce the fluid overload that caused CMD.[29] Therefore, CMD is seldom reversed by the correction of fluid volume alone. Nevertheless, the primary treatment is to decrease the reabsorption of fluid from the kidneys so that more fluid is eliminated (in essence, diuresed).[29] The diuretic most commonly used is furosemide (Lasix), which can be given intravenously or orally. The dosage is dependent on the degree of fluid overload and the desired diuretic effect; furosemide is commonly given orally at a dosage of 20 to 80 mg every 6 to 8 hours.[29] Patients receiving a diuretic such as furosemide in the acute care setting are carefully monitored (hourly measurement of input and output) and frequently undergo titrated doses to achieve the desired effects. There is a certain degree of guesswork associated with the assessment and treatment of fluid overload. However, it appears that **bioimpedance analysis,** a method frequently used to evaluate percentage of body fat and lean body mass, may also be of assistance in assessing fluid volume (total body water).[30] The measurement of total body water may prove to be invaluable in the treatment of patients receiving diuretics so that less guesswork and more objective information can direct the proper dosage of diuretics.

In addition to and as a result of the administration of a diuretic, electrolyte levels are carefully monitored, ensuring that potassium and sodium levels are within the normal range to prevent further retention of fluid from high levels of potassium and sodium or the detrimental effects of low levels (e.g., cardiac arrhythmias and muscle weakness).

Severe renal insufficiency, demonstrating advanced azotemia, is best treated by **dialysis (peritoneal or hemodialysis),** which is designed to

- Remove solutes
- Alter the electrolyte concentration of the extracellular fluid
- Remove as much as 1 L of extracellular fluid per hour[29]

Cardiomyopathy

Individuals with **cardiomyopathy** are often less fortunate than the patients previously discussed because no apparent treatment can reverse the fatal progression of this disease at present (except for **palliative treatment** via cardiac transplantation). Cardiomyopathy is a disease in which the contraction and relaxation of myocardial muscle fibers are impaired.[16] This impaired contractility can result from either primary or secondary causes.[31] The *primary* causes are the result of pathologic processes in the heart muscle itself, which impair the heart's ability to contract. The *secondary* causes of cardiomyopathy are the result of a systemic disease process rather than of pathologic myocardial processes and can be classified according to the systemic disease that subsequently affects myocardial contraction. These diseases are of the following types:

- Inflammatory
- Metabolic
- Toxic
- Infiltrative
- Fibroplastic

- Hematologic
- Hypersensitive
- Genetic
- The result of physical agents
- Acquired (miscellaneous)
- Idiopathic (unknown)[16]

Each secondary cause can be further subdivided, as shown by the classification in Table 4-2.

Cardiomyopathies are also classified from a *functional* standpoint, emphasizing three basic categories:

- Dilated cardiomyopathy
- Hypertrophic cardiomyopathy
- Restrictive cardiomyopathy[16]

Table 4-2
Secondary Causes of Cardiomyopathy

Inflammation
    Viral infection
    Bacterial infection
Metabolic
    Selenium deficiency
    Diabetes mellitus
Toxic
    Alcohol
    Bleomycin
Infiltrative
    Sarcoidosis
    Neoplastic
Fibroplastic
    Carcinoid fibrosis
    Endomyocardial fibrosis
Hematologic
    Sickle cell anemia
    Leukemia
Hypersensitivity
    Cardiac transplant rejection
    Methyldopa
Genetic
    Hypertrophic cardiomyopathy
    Duchenne's muscular dystrophy
Miscellaneous acquired
    Postpartum cardiomyopathy
    Obesity
Idiopathic
    Idiopathic hypertrophic cardiomyopathy
Physical agents
    Heat stroke
    Hypothermia
    Radiation

Adapted from Braunwald E. Heart Disease: A Textbook of Cardiovascular Medicine. 3rd ed. Philadelphia, WB Saunders, 1988, Table 42-1, p 1411.

Dilated cardiomyopathy is characterized by ventricular dilation and cardiac muscle contractile dysfunction. **Hypertrophic cardiomyopathy** is distinguished by inappropriate and excessive left ventricular hypertrophy and normal or even enhanced cardiac muscle contractile function. **Restrictive cardiomyopathy** is identified by marked endocardial scarring of the ventricles, with resulting impaired diastolic filling. Patients often present with a combination of these functional classifications.[16]

As previously discussed, cardiomyopathies can be the result of either primary (due to pathologic changes in heart muscle) or secondary (due to systemic diseases, which subsequently affect heart muscle) causes, which when classified via heart function include dilated cardiomyopathies, hypertrophic cardiomyopathies, and restrictive cardiomyopathies. The cardiomyopathies are distinguished from one another by echocardiographic and myocardial biopsy results.[16]

Dilated Cardiomyopathies

Dilated cardiomyopathies "probably represent a final common pathway that is the end result of myocardial damage produced by a variety of toxic, metabolic, or infectious agents."[16] Possible causes of dilated cardiomyopathies include the following:

- Long-term alcohol abuse
- Systemic hypertension
- A variety of infections
- Cigarette smoking
- Pregnancy
- Carnitine deficiency[16]

These conditions may not be primarily responsible for dilated cardiomyopathy but may act to lower the threshold for its development.

Little is known regarding the further development of dilated cardiomyopathies, but the dilation that occurs in this type of cardiomyopathy, and that sets it apart from hypertrophic cardiomyopathy, appears to be due to myocardial mitochondrial dysfunction.[16] Dysfunction of myocardial mitochondria leads to a lack of energy necessary for proper cardiac function, causing the heart to be a less effective pump.[16] Ineffective pumping increases both the left ventricular end-diastolic volume and pressure, which dilates the left ventricle (and frequently the other heart chambers). Because of inappropriate energy sources, the left ventricle is unable to contract properly or to relax individual muscle fibers in response to increased workload, therefore preventing myocardial hypertrophy but producing ineffective *systolic* (pumping) function.

Hypertrophic Cardiomyopathy

Hypertrophic cardiomyopathy should be thought of as the opposite of dilated cardiomyopathy, both functionally and etiologically. The hypertrophy associated with hypertrophic cardiomyopathy is inappropriate for the applied hemodynamic load and is associated with proper myocardial mitochondrial function. Furthermore, the dysfunction of hypertrophic cardiomyopathy is one of *diastolic* dysfunction, which impairs the filling of the ventricles during diastole.[16] This increases the left ventricular end-diastolic pressure and eventually increases left atrial, pulmonary artery, and pulmonary capillary pressures, all of which cause a hypercontractile left ventricle. The hypercontractile myocardial muscle fibers of hypertrophic cardiomyopathy are frequently disorganized and demonstrate a "quantitative relationship between the extent of cellular disarray and hypertrophic cardiomyopathy because the disorganization of myocardial fibers is far greater in hypertrophic cardiomyopathy than in other disorders (coronary artery disease, congenital heart disease, and cor pulmonale)."[16]

Susceptibility to hypertrophic cardiomyopathy appears to be genetically transmitted as an *autosomal dominant trait.* It has been suggested that the apparent myocardial *isometric* contraction of hypertrophic cardiomyopathy is the result of malaligned myocardial muscle fibers[17] or an abnormal configuration of the interventricular septum in response to a genetic influence.[32] Other causes of hypertrophic cardiomyopathy have been suggested, including abnormal sympathetic stimulation, subendocardial ischemia, and abnormal calcium ion dynamics.[16]

The characteristic findings of hypertrophic cardiomyopathy are rapid ventricular emptying and high ejection fraction, which are the opposite of those found in dilated cardiomyopathy but somewhat similar to those found in restrictive cardiomyopathy.[16]

Restrictive Cardiomyopathy

Restrictive cardiomyopathy, like hypertrophic cardiomyopathy, is a cardiomyopathy of diastolic dysfunction and frequently unimpaired contractile function. Little is known about restrictive cardiomyopathy, but certain pathologic processes, including myocardial fibrosis, hypertrophy, infiltration, or a defect in myocardial relaxation may result in its development.[16]

Implications for Management of Cardiomyopathies

The functional classification of cardiomyopathies just discussed as well as the cardiovascular pathophysiologic changes (i.e., left ventricular hypertrophy and cardiac arrhythmias) all tend to contribute to the progression of CMD, which is managed *initially* by several of the body's *compensatory mechanisms,* of which atrial natriuretic peptide is an important factor.

Unfortunately, research suggests that cardiomyopathy is perhaps much more common than was originally believed. Myopathic change in cardiac and skeletal muscle has been associated with class 3 hypertension and diabetes;[33, 34] it has also been found in individuals with and without skeletal muscle disease[35, 36] and in patients with CHF.[35, 36] These findings have great implications for the health care providers as the aged population increases and newer technologies are used to prolong and sustain life.

The specific treatment of cardiomyopathy is dependent on the underlying cause but in general includes "physical, dietary, pharmacological, mechanical, and surgical intervention."[16] One pharmacologic intervention worth mentioning is beta-adrenergic blockade, which appears to improve symptoms and survival via "(1) negative chronotropic effect with reduced myocardial oxygen demand, (2) reduced myocardial damage due to decreased catecholamines, (3) improved diastolic relaxation, (4) inhibition of sympathetically mediated vasoconstriction, and (5) increase in myocardial beta-adrenoceptor density."[16] These factors are important because they are the basic mechanisms supporting the use of beta blockers for dilated, restrictive, and hypertrophic cardiomyopathies as well as CHF in general, because "treatment is on the same basis as that for heart failure."[16]

Heart Valve Abnormalities

Heart valve abnormalities can also cause CMD, as blocked valves (**valvular stenosis**) or incompetent valves (**valvular insufficiency** due to abnormal or poorly functioning valve leaflets), or both, cause heart muscle to contract more forcefully to expel the cardiac output. This subsequently produces myocardial hypertrophy, which can decrease ventricular distensibility and produce a mild diastolic dysfunction; if prolonged, this dysfunction can lead to more profound diastolic as well as systolic dysfunction.[37] Incompetent valves are frequently associated with myocardial dilation in addition to hypertrophy, because regurgitant blood fills the atria or ventricles forcefully.[37] Atrial dilation often accompanies mitral and tricuspid insufficiency, whereas ventricular dilation accompanies aortic or pulmonary insufficiency. Aortic insufficiency can dilate the left ventricle, while pulmonary insufficiency can dilate the right ventricle. Mitral insufficiency frequently dilates the left atrium, whereas tricuspid insufficiency dilates the right atrium. Such dilation can lengthen individual cardiac muscle fibers in the atria and ventricles to such a degree that myocardial contraction is impaired severely, but frequently the accompanying myocardial hypertrophy prevents such extreme dilation. However, the abnormal hemodynamics from hypertrophy and dilation often produce CMD.[37]

Acute heart valve dysfunction or rupture can cause rapid and life-threatening CMD because a ruptured valve impairs cardiac output and regurgitant blood fills the heart's chambers rather than exiting the aorta.[7] If left untreated, valve rupture will ultimately produce pulmonary edema and eventually death.

Heart valve abnormalities that cause CMD appear to be reversible to a point. If the abnormality persists for too long, cardiac function appears to be permanently impaired.[37] Acute problems such as heart valve rupture can affect proper cardiac muscle function profoundly and as mentioned are fatal if not surgically repaired within a relatively short period. The most common valvular surgeries are valvular replacement, **valvuloplasty** (pressurized reduction of atherosclerotic plaque, similar to angioplasty of the coronary arteries), **valvulotomy** (incision), and **commissurotomy** (incision to separate adherent, thickened leaflets).[37]

Other heart valve conditions can be classified as chronic conditions and include the stenotic and regurgitant abnormalities of the aortic, pulmonary, mitral, or tricuspid valves. Prolonged valvular stenosis or regurgitation affects cardiac function and can eventually lead to CMD, but cardiac function is less likely to return to normal after valvuloplasty or surgical repair or replacement of a chronic valvular condition.[37]

Pericardial Effusion and Myocarditis

Injury to the pericardium of the heart can cause acute *pericarditis* (inflammation of the pericardial sac surrounding the heart), which may progress to **pericardial effusion** occasionally resulting in *cardiac compression* as fluid fills the pericardial sac.[16] Increased fluid accumulation within the pericardial space increases intrapericardial pressure and produces *cardiac tamponade*. Cardiac tamponade is characterized by elevated intracardiac pressures, progressively limited ventricular diastolic filling, and reduced stroke volume.[16] Thus, the mechanism of CMD, which is primarily a diastolic dysfunction (limited ventricular diastolic filling because of cardiac compression), produces a secondary systolic dysfunction. The same sequence of primary diastolic CMD producing secondary systolic CMD occurs in myocarditis.

The prompt treatment of pericarditis with nonsteroidal anti-inflammatory agents (aspirin or indomethacin) or corticosteroids (usually prednisone) frequently prevents pericardial effusion. Treatment of the causative inflammatory process in myocarditis (most commonly viral) should prevent the diastolic and systolic CMD of pericardial effusion and myocarditis.[16] However, patients who do not respond to this therapy must undergo more extensive treatment, including drainage of fluid from the **pericardium (pericardiocentesis)** for pericardial effusion; immunosuppressive, antibiotic, and possibly antiviral agents for myocarditis; and aggressive CHF management (digitalization, diuresis, and afterload or preload reduction) for both pericardial effusion and myocarditis.[16]

Pulmonary Embolism

Cardiac muscle dysfunction from a **pulmonary embolism** is the result of elevated pulmonary artery pressures, which dramatically increase right ventricular work. Right as well as left ventricular failure can occur because of decreased oxygenated coronary blood flow and decreased blood flow to the left ventricle.[38] A similar, but often less extreme, condition occurs in pulmonary hypertension.

An acute pulmonary embolism is also a potentially life-threatening condition. As previously mentioned, the primary CMD resulting from a pulmonary embolism is due to a very high pulmonary artery pressure (because of damaged lung tissue and less area for proper pulmonary perfusion), which increases the work of the right ventricle and eventually produces right-sided heart failure. Left-sided heart failure may accompany right-sided failure because of decreased blood volume and coronary perfusion to the left ventricle, impairing the pumping ability of the heart.[38]

The treatment of a pulmonary embolism consists of the following:

- A thrombolytic agent (typically heparin) to decrease the blood clot
- A sedative to decrease the patient's anxiety and pain
- Oxygen to improve the Pa_{O_2} and decrease the pulmonary artery pressure
- Occasionally an **embolectomy**[38]

Cardiac muscle dysfunction due to a pulmonary embolism occasionally can be reversed (especially if treatment is initiated immediately), but quite frequently some degree of CMD ensues because of infarcted lung tissue, which increases the work of the right ventricle.[38] When such a condition exists, the pulmonary artery pressure rises and may produce pulmonary hypertension. Pulmonary hypertension can often produce CMD by increasing right ventricular work, resulting in right ventricular hypertrophy (and inefficient right ventricular performance). This may reduce the right ventricular stroke volume, thereby decreasing the left ventricular stroke volume and cardiac output.

Spinal Cord Injury

Spinal cord injury also can produce CMD because of cervical spinal cord transection, which "causes an imbalance between parasympathetic and sympathetic control of the cardiovascular system."[39] Several studies have identified pulmonary edema as a frequently fatal complication of cervical spinal cord transection.[40–42]

Transection of the cervical spinal cord prevents sympathetic nervous system information from reaching the cardiovascular system (heart, lung, arterial and venous systems), thus *preventing* the sympathetic-driven changes necessary to maintain cardiac performance (i.e., increased heart rate and force of myocardial contraction, constriction of venous capacitance vessels, or arterial constriction). Lacking these cardiovascular adaptations, patients with spinal cord injuries (who frequently are volume-depleted because of fluid loss from multiple injuries) may develop a specific type of CMD that produces pulmonary edema.[39]

In view of the possibility of volume depletion, it has been recommended that cardiac filling pressures be monitored, that "cardiac preload be increased by giving fluids,"[39] and that construction of a ventricular function curve may be useful in guiding therapy and treatment for patients with spinal cord injuries.[39] It appears, then, that a slightly elevated pulmonary capillary wedge pressure (not exceeding 18 mm Hg) may facilitate optimal cardiac performance in these patients.

Age-Related Changes and Cardiac Muscle Dysfunction

Congenital Abnormalities and Aging

Although distinctly different processes, congenital or acquired heart diseases and the aging process can produce a similar type of CMD, which is often initially well tolerated but, as the dysfunction persists, may become more symptomatic and troublesome. The adaptability of infants and children to extreme conditions is evident in congenital heart disease, which frequently can be managed for many years with specific medications before surgical intervention becomes necessary.[43, 44] The CMD associated with the aging process is initially well tolerated not because of the aged individual's ability to adapt but because the degree of CMD is usually mild. Aging appears to decrease cardiac output by altered contraction and relaxation of cardiac muscle.[45, 46] However, heart disease, hypertension, and other pathologic processes can increase CMD substantially and subsequently can impair functional abilities.[45, 46]

Congenital heart disease is the result of "altered embryonic development of a normal structure or failure of such a structure to progress beyond an early stage of embryonic or fetal development."[43] Approximately 0.8% of live births are complicated by cardiovascular malformations, such as **ventricular septal defect, atrial septal defect, patent ductus arteriosus, coarctation of the aorta, and tetralogy of Fallot.** The two most common cardiac anomalies are the "congenital nonstenotic bicuspid aortic valve and the leaflet abnormality associated with mitral valve prolapse."[43]

Heart disease can also be *acquired* in infancy and childhood. Such disease processes include the following:

- Rheumatic heart disease
- Connective tissue disorders
- **Mucopolysaccharidoses**
- **Hyperlipidemia**
- Nonrheumatic inflammatory diseases (infective myocarditis, infective pericarditis, and **postpericardiotomy syndrome**)
- Primary (endocardial fibroelastosis) and secondary cardiomyopathies (due to glycogen storage disease, neonatal **thyrotoxicosis,** infantile **beriberi,** protein-calorie malnutrition, tropical endomyocardial fibrosis, **anthracycline toxicity, Kawasaki's disease,** and diabetes in mothers)[43]

Although the disease processes are different in acquired and congenital heart disease, the resultant pathophysiologic processes are not unlike those seen in adults with CMD because it is dysfunctional cardiac muscle that eventually produces the clinical signs and symptoms.[43] The primary manifestations are as follows:

- Congestive heart failure
- Cyanosis
- Hepatomegaly
- Acid-base imbalances
- Impaired growth

- Pulmonary hypertension
- Chest pain
- Syncope
- Arrhythmias

Age-Associated Changes in Cardiac Performance

The aging process involves several interrelated pathophysiologic processes, all of which have the potential to impair physical performance, including cardiac function. Although several earlier studies have revealed a reduced cardiac output in the elderly (at rest and with exercise),[47–49] a study that excluded subjects with ischemic heart disease demonstrated no "age effect" on cardiac performance.[50] In this study, the heart rates of the elderly were lower at most workloads, but increased stroke volume apparently compensated for the decreased heart rates and thus maintained cardiac output (cardiac output = heart rate × stroke volume).[50]

However, other age-associated changes, such as increased systolic arterial pressure and decreased aortic distensibility, probably contribute to the mild-to-moderate left ventricular hypertrophy commonly found in the elderly.[51] This hypertrophy preserves left ventricular systolic function but impairs left ventricular diastolic function. Diastolic dysfunction delays left ventricular filling, which is more profound in the presence of hypertension, coronary artery disease, and higher heart rates.[52] Additionally, increased norepinephrine levels (probably because of decreased catecholamine sensitivity) and decreased baroreceptor sensitivity and plasma renin concentrations have been reported in elderly subjects.[45]

These pathophysiologic processes, as well as other confounding variables such as coronary artery disease, exposure to environmental toxins (cigarette smoking, radiation), malnutrition, and other lifestyle habits, must be considered to accurately document the effects of aging on cardiac and exercise performance. Nonetheless, the consensus regarding the cardiovascular aging process is as follows:

- After neonatal development, the number of myocardial cells in the heart does not increase.
- There is moderate hypertrophy of left ventricular myocardium, probably in response to increased arterial vascular stiffness and dropout of myocytes.

- When myocardial hypertrophy occurs, it is *out of proportion to* capillary and vascular growth. The ability of the myocardium to generate tension is well maintained as a result of prolonged duration of contraction and greater stiffness despite a modest decrease in the velocity of shortening of cardiac muscle.
- There is a selective decrease in beta-adrenergic receptor–mediated inotropic, chronotropic, and vasodilating cardiovascular responses with aging.
- Increased pericardial and myocardial stiffness and delayed relaxation during aging may limit left ventricular filling during stress.[46]

The primary cause of the changes associated with aging has been attributed to one or a combination of three theories: the genome, the physiologic, and the organ theories.[46] The genome theories are based on the programming of genes for aging, death, or both, whereas the physiologic theories (cross-linkage theory) are dependent on specific pathophysiologic processes. The organ theories (primarily immunologic and neuroendocrine) may be the most encompassing because immunologic and neurohormonal dysfunction is hypothesized to produce both general and specific aging effects.[46]

Muscular Changes Associated with Aging

The specific changes in skeletal and cardiac muscle are discussed in this section, and a brief review of the effects of exercise training on cardiac and skeletal muscle in the elderly is presented. Table 4–3 provides a useful overview of the effects of aging.

Cardiac Muscle. Animal studies have revealed that the contraction and relaxation times of cardiac muscle are prolonged in aged rats.[53–56] This prolongation "can be attributed to alterations in mechanisms that govern excitation-contraction coupling in the heart,"[46] primarily the increase and decrease of **cytosolic** calcium in the myofilaments. The rate that the sarcoplasmic reticulum pumps calcium is reduced in hearts of older animals and "appears to be a major contributor to the prolonged transient and prolonged time course of cardiac muscle relaxation."[46] The diminished ability of the sarcoplasmic reticulum to

Table 4–3 **Effects of Aging**	
CHANGE DUE TO AGING	**EFFECT**
Decreased vascular elasticity	Increased blood pressure
Left ventricular hypertrophy	Decreased ventricular compliance
Decreased adrenergic responsiveness	Decreased exercise heart rate
Decreased rate of calcium pumped by the sarcoplasmic reticulum	Prolonged time for cardiac muscle relaxation
Prolonged time to peak force of cardiac muscle	Prolonged contraction time of cardiac muscle
Decreased cardiac muscle twitch force	Reduction in the velocity of the cardiac muscle shortening
Decreased rate of ATP hydrolysis	Reduction in the velocity of the cardiac muscle shortening
Decreased myosin ATPase activity	Reduction in the velocity of the cardiac muscle shortening
Diastolic dysfunction	Impaired ventricular filling with potential to increase cardiac preload and congestive heart failure
Decreased lean body mass	Decreased muscle strength and peak oxygen consumption

ATP = adenosine triphosphate.

pump calcium may also be responsible for the following changes observed in elderly animals:

- Prolonged time to peak force and half relaxation time of peak stiffness[57–59]
- Lower muscular twitch force at higher stimulation rates[60]

In addition, the rate of ATP hydrolysis and myosin ATPase activity declines progressively with age. The decline in activity contributes to the reduction in the velocity of shortening as well as the prolonged contraction and relaxation times of cardiac muscle.[46]

In summary, in healthy elderly individuals, exercise cardiac output is, for the most part, maintained by the Frank-Starling mechanism (increasing end-diastolic volume) to increase stroke volume because of lower heart rates in the elderly.

Aged subjects with hypertension are unable to fully utilize the beneficial effects of the Frank-Starling mechanism because of a hypertrophied and noncompliant myocardium and most likely will be unable to maintain exercise cardiac output, as demonstrated in Figure 4–2.[45] Finally, the lower exercise heart rates seen in the elderly are probably mediated by an age-associated decreased responsiveness to beta-adrenergic stimulation.[61]

Skeletal Muscle. Many of the same changes observed in cardiac muscle also occur in the skeletal muscles of elderly persons. However, skeletal muscle change may be more profound than cardiac muscle change in view of the following physiological observations in the elderly: skeletal muscle atrophy,[62] slowed muscle contraction and reduced capacity for twitch potentiation,[63] decreased insulin sensitivity and skeletal muscle enzyme activity,[64] decreased skeletal muscle mitochondrial respiratory chain function,[65] impaired cardiopulmonary (primarily vascular and neurohumoral) receptor reflex activity,[66] increased defects and pseudotumors of the diaphragm,[67] and greater percentage of type I (slow oxidative) fibers.[68, 69] The last finding is im-

> **Clinical Note: Heart Rate and Blood Pressure in the Elderly**
> • Possible resting systolic and diastolic hypertension
> • Possibly blunted or decreased systolic blood pressure during exercise
> • Possible increase in diastolic blood pressure during exercise
> • Possibly lower exercise heart rates

portant and may be one reason that older athletes (masters) are able to perform as well as younger athletes, despite having a lower VO$_{2 max}$.[69] Although this finding is somewhat paradoxical, it exemplifies the importance and benefits of exercise training in the elderly, who seem to benefit from training with an increased endurance and functional capacity (via a greater capillary-to-fiber ratio and improved oxidative skeletal muscle enzyme activity)[69] as well as enhanced psychosocial function.[70] Therefore, exercise training appears to decrease the magnitude of impairments seen in elderly individuals.

Exercise Training in the Elderly

A study of cardiac performance in elderly rats performing long-term exercise has revealed

• A diminution or elimination of the age-associated increase in duration of myocardial contraction and dynamic stiffness
• A modest augmentation of cytochrome oxidase activity in heart muscle
• A diminution or elimination in the progressive decline of myocardial calcium-activated actomyosin ATPase activity[46]

Studies that evaluate changes in cardiac performance of elderly humans during long-term exercise training have been scarce or poorly conducted. However, exercise training adaptations in the elderly have been suggested to include increased joint stability and mobility (via increased muscle and tendon strength), improved neuromuscular coordination, increased flexibility and muscular strength, and the previously mentioned increase in endurance and physical work capacity.[61] In addition, several beneficial effects of exercise training may occur, such as the modification of

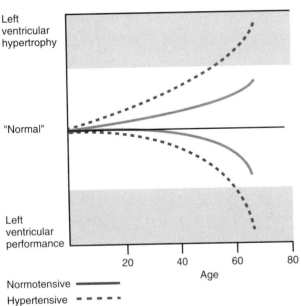

Figure 4–2. The effects of aging and hypertension on cardiovascular performance. Aging is accompanied by an increase in left ventricular mass and a subsequent decrease in left ventricular performance (possibly owing to less distensible myocardium). These changes are partly responsible for the increased incidence of congestive heart failure in the elderly.

coronary risk factors (obesity, hypertension, hyperglycemia, and hyperlipidemia), slowing or delay of mineral loss from bone, enhanced self-confidence and a sense of well-being, and possibly improved cognitive function.[61] "Exercise of almost any kind, suitable in degree and duration . . . can and does play a useful role in the maintenance of both physical and mental health of the aging individual . . . ,"[70] despite the reduction in cardiovascular performance.

EVALUATION OF CARDIAC MUSCLE DYSFUNCTION IN PHYSICAL THERAPY

Cardiac muscle dysfunction can produce observable and measurable signs and symptoms, such as a reduced physical work capacity, which, if thoroughly understood, could help physical therapists determine realistic and obtainable goals for their patients. The goal of this section is to assist the physical therapist in identifying the presence and severity of CMD.

Study of the demographics of CMD in physical therapy have revealed two very important findings.[71] First, physical therapists in all specialty areas, not just those in cardiopulmonary physical therapy, are treating a significant number of patients with CMD. Second, and perhaps most important, many practicing clinicians may be unfamiliar with the specifics of CMD (its presence and effect on patient treatment).

Increasing numbers of persons with CMD and CHF are being treated by physical therapists throughout the United States and abroad in industrialized countries. This increase in the number of patients is due to the greater numbers of the aged population, improved technology (such as **tissue plasminogen activator** and **streptokinase**—anticlotting agents that frequently salvage oxygen-deprived myocardium during an acute myocardial infarction), **percutaneous transluminal coronary angioplasty,** heart and heart-lung transplantation, and newer cardiovascular medications.[3, 7] These improved and innovative technologies have decreased the mortality rate from cardiovascular disease while increasing the morbidity rate in many of those who otherwise would have expired. Physi-

cal therapists are responsible to assess the functional status of these patients and to provide proper treatment to improve the quality of their lives and possibly to lessen the morbidity rate, or provide primary physicians with information to enhance medical therapy.

Characteristics of Congestive Heart Failure

Congestive heart failure is commonly associated with several characteristic signs and symptoms:

- Dyspnea
- Tachypnea
- Paroxysmal nocturnal dyspnea (PND)
- Orthopnea
- Peripheral edema
- Cold, pale, and possibly cyanotic extremities
- Weight gain
- Hepatomegaly
- Jugular venous distention
- Rales (crackles)
- Tubular breath sounds and consolidation
- Presence of an S_3 heart sound
- Sinus tachycardia
- Decreased exercise tolerance or physical work capacity

Only when the dysfunction of the cardiac muscle is so great that the heart's functional compensatory mechanisms are inadequate does CHF occur. Identification of several of the signs and symptoms listed earlier frequently suggests the presence of CHF, but radiologic and occasionally laboratory findings usually confirm the diagnosis and provide a baseline from which to evaluate therapy.[6]

Radiologic Findings in Congestive Heart Failure

Radiologic evidence of CHF is dependent on the size and shape of the cardiac silhouette (evaluating left ventricular end-diastolic volume) as well as the presence of interstitial, perivascular, and alveolar edema (evaluating fluid in the lungs).[6] Interstitial, perivascular, and alveolar edema form the radiologic hallmark of CHF and generally occur when pulmonary capillary pressures (which reflect the left ventricular end-diastolic pressure) exceed 20 to 25 mm Hg.[6] Figure 5–16 shows the presence of pulmonary edema. Pleural effusions (**parenchymal** fluid accumulations) and **atelectasis** (collapsed lung segments) may also be present.

Laboratory Findings in Congestive Heart Failure

Proteinuria; elevated urine specific gravity, blood urea nitrogen (BUN), and creatinine levels; and decreased **erythrocyte sedimentation rates** (because of decreased fibrinogen concentrations resulting from impaired fibrinogen synthesis) are associated with CHF.[6] Frequently, but not consistently, Pa_{O_2} and oxygen saturation levels are reduced and Pa_{CO_2} levels elevated.[34] Liver enzymes, such as serum glutamic-oxaloacetic transaminase (SGOT) and alkaline phosphatase, are often elevated, and **hyperbilirubinemia** commonly occurs, resulting in subsequent **jaundice.**[6] Serum electrolytes are generally normal, but individuals with chronic CHF may demonstrate **hyponatremia** during rigid sodium restriction and diuretic therapy, or **hypokalemia,** which also may be the result of diuretic therapy.[1] **Hyperkalemia** may occur for several reasons but most commonly is due to a marked reduction in the **glomerular filtration rate** (especially if individuals are receiving a potassium-retaining diuretic) or overzealous potassium supplementation (when a non-potassium-retaining diuretic is used).[6]

Symptoms of Congestive Heart Failure

Dyspnea

Dyspnea (breathlessness or air hunger) is probably the most common finding associated with CHF and is frequently the result of poor gas transport between the lungs and the cells of the body. The cause of poor transport at the lungs is often excessive blood and extracellular fluid in the alveoli, producing a shunt "characterized by a reduction of vital capacity as a consequence of the replacement of the air in the lungs with blood or interstitial fluid or both."[6] However, the cause of poor transport at the cellular level may be less apparent. A review of Wasserman and associates' "gas transport mechanisms" (Fig. 4–3) reveals the interrelationship of the lungs, heart, and muscle and shows that inadequate oxygen supply either at rest or during muscular activity undoubtedly increases the frequency of breathing (respiratory rate) or the amount of air exchanged (tidal volume) or both.[72] For this reason, subjects with CHF characteristically complain of easily provoked dyspnea or, in severe cases of CHF, dyspnea at rest.

Paroxysmal Nocturnal Dyspnea

Another common complaint of individuals suffering from CHF is **paroxysmal nocturnal dyspnea (PND),** in which sudden, unexplained episodes of

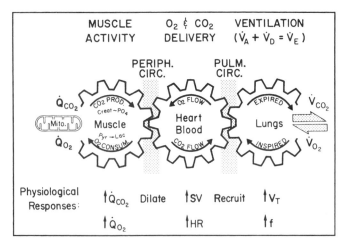

Figure 4–3. Physiologic interdependence of the muscular, cardiopulmonary, and metabolic systems is evident as mitochondrial and metabolic activity are enhanced by the increased physiologic responses of the cardiopulmonary systems. (From Wasserman K, et al. Principles of Exercise Testing and Interpretation. Philadelphia, Lea & Febiger, 1987. Used with permission.)

shortness of breath occur as patients with CHF assume a more supine position to sleep.[6] After a period of time in a supine position, excessive fluid fills the lungs. Earlier in the day, this fluid was shunted to the lower extremities because upright positions and activities permitted more effective minute ventilation (V) and **perfusion** (Q) of the lungs (correcting the V/Q mismatch). During upright activity, the effects of gravity keep the lungs relatively fluid-free, depending on the degree of CHF (which, if severe, would fill the lungs even in upright positions). Individuals suffering from PND frequently place the head of the bed on blocks or sleep with more than two pillows and often find it difficult to breathe with fewer than two pillows. Patients with marked CHF often assume a sitting position to sleep and are sometimes found sleeping in a recliner instead of a bed.[6]

Orthopnea

The term **orthopnea** describes the development of dyspnea in the recumbent position.[6] Sleeping with two or more pillows elevates the upper body to a more upright position and enables gravity to draw excess fluid from the lungs to the more distal parts of the body. The severity of CHF can sometimes be inferred from the number of pillows used to prevent orthopnea. Thus, the terms two-, three-, four-, or more pillow orthopnea indirectly allude to the severity of CHF (e.g., four-pillow orthopnea suggests more severe CHF than two-pillow orthopnea).

Signs Associated with Congestive Heart Failure

Breathing Patterns

A rapid respiratory rate at rest, characterized by quick and shallow breaths, is common in patients with CHF. Such **tachypnea** is apparently not due to hypoxemia (which may or may not be of sufficient magnitude) but rather to stimulation of interstitial **J-type receptors** (stretch receptors in the interstitium). The quick, shallow breathing of tachypnea may assist the pumping action of the lymphatic

vessels, thus minimizing or delaying the increase in interstitial liquid.[73]

A clinical finding observed in many patients with CMD is extreme dyspnea after a change in position, most frequently from sitting to standing. This response appears to be occasionally but inconsistently associated with **orthostatic hypotension** and increased heart rate activity. The orthostatic hypotension and dyspnea (tachypnea) may be the result of (a) lower extremity muscle deconditioning, producing a pooling of blood in the lower extremities when standing, with a subsequent decrease in blood flow to the heart and lungs, which may result in marked dyspnea and increased heart rates; or (b) attenuation of the atrial **natriuretic factor** (release of a regulatory hormone from the atria because of elevated atrial pressure, which produces a brisk **diuresis** to reduce fluid volume), which may suggest advanced atrial distention and poor left ventricular function.[74] It appears that the more pronounced the dyspnea, the more severe the CMD, and vice versa. This pattern of breathing, therefore, is another clinical finding that can be timed (time for the dyspnea to subside) and occasionally measured (blood pressure and heart rate) to document progress or deterioration in patient status.

In addition, frequently associated with CHF is a breathing pattern characterized by waxing and waning depths of respiration with recurring periods of apnea. Although the Scottish physician John Cheyne and the Irish physician William Stokes first observed this breathing pattern in asthmatics and thus coined the term **Cheyne-Stokes respiration,** it has been observed in individuals who are suffering central nervous system damage (particularly those in comas) and in individuals with CMD.[6]

Clinical Note: Breathing in CHF
- Tachypnea
- Resting dyspnea likely
- Dyspnea with exertion likely
- Occasionally dyspnea with positional change with or without orthostatic hypotension
- Waxing and waning depth of breathing (Cheyne-Stokes respiration)

Rales (Crackles)

Carefully obtained subjective information can suggest a specific pathophysiology, but objective information obtained from physical examination frequently confirms one's suspicions. **Rales** are one such objective finding. Pulmonary rales, sometimes referred to as crackles, are abnormal breath sounds that, if associated with CHF, occur during inspiration and represent the movement of fluid in the alveoli and subsequent opening of alveoli that previously were closed because of excessive fluid.[6] A simple analogy of the dynamics (as well as the sound) responsible for rales is the sound heard when a sailboat sail suddenly fills with wind and becomes fully drawn. This sound is produced in the body with the opening of alveoli and airways that previously had no air; after the sound associated with such an opening is transmitted through the tissues overlying the lungs, the characteristic sound of rales is identical to that of hair near the ears being rubbed between two fingers. Rales are frequently heard at both lung bases in individuals with CHF but may extend upward, depending on the patient's position, the severity of CHF, or both. Therefore, auscultation of all lobes should be performed in a systematic manner, allowing for bilateral comparison.

The importance of the presence and magnitude of rales was addressed in 1967 and provided data for the Killip and Kimball classification of patients with acute myocardial infarction.[75] Table 4–4 defines classes I through III, each of which is associated with an approximate mortality rate. Individuals with rales extending over more than 50% of the lung fields were observed to have a far poorer prognosis.

Heart Sounds

Heart sounds can provide a great deal of information regarding cardiopulmonary status but unfortunately are forgotten in most physical therapy examinations. The normal heart sounds include a first heart sound (S_1), which represents closure of the mitral and tricuspid valves, and a second sound (S_2), which represents closure of the aortic and pulmonary valves. The most common abnormal heart sounds are the third (S_3) and fourth

Table 4–4

Killip Classification of Patients with Acute Myocardial Infarction and Approximate Mortality Rate

	DEFINITION	APPROXIMATE MORTALITY RATE (%)
Class I	Absence of rales and S_3 heart sound	8
Class II	Presence of S_3 heart sound or rales in 50% or less of the lung fields	30
Class III	Rales extending over more than 50% of the lung fields	44

(S_4), which occur at specific times in the cardiac cycle as a result of abnormal cardiac mechanics. This can be best understood by viewing Figure 4–4, which displays graphically the normal and abnormal heart sounds and their respective locations in the cardiac cycle. Note that S_3 may be normal in children and young adults.[76] As displayed, S_4 is presystolic, and S_3 occurs during early diastole. Splitting of S_1 and S_2 is also occasionally heard and represents the closure of both the mitral and tricuspid valves in S_1 and the aortic and pulmonary valves in S_2 (Fig. 4–5).

The presence of an S_3 indicates a noncompliant left ventricle and occurs as blood passively fills a poorly relaxing left ventricle that appears to make contact with the chest wall during early diastole.[76] The presence of an S_3 is considered the hallmark of CHF.[77] There are several reasons why the left ventricle may be noncompliant, of which fluid overload and myocardial scarring (via myocardial infarction or cardiomyopathy) appear to be the most common.

The presence of an S_4 represents "vibrations of the ventricular wall during the rapid influx of blood during atrial contraction" from an exaggerated atrial contraction (atrial "kick").[76] It is commonly heard in patients with hypertension, left ventricular hypertrophy, increased left ventricular end-diastolic pressure, pulmonary hypertension, and **pulmonary stenosis.**[76]

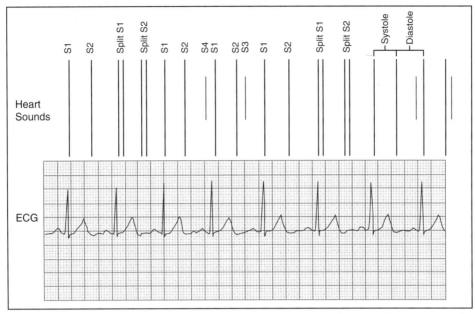

Figure 4–4. The relationship of heart sounds to the electrocardiogram. The physiologic and mechanical events of myocardial activity are depicted. Assessment of the electrocardiogram and heart sounds provides important information about cardiac performance and patient status.

Auscultation of the heart (see Fig. 4–5) may also reveal **adventitious** (additional) sounds, most frequently murmurs. Murmurs not only are common in patients with CMD but also appear to be of great clinical significance. Stevenson and coworkers demonstrated that the systolic murmur of secondary mitral regurgitation was an important marker in the treatment of a subgroup of patients with congestive cardiomyopathy.[78] The patients who benefited from afterload (the resistance to ventricular ejection or peripheral vascular resistance) reduction were those with a very large left ventricle (left ventricular end-diastolic dimension greater than 60 cm) and a resultant **systolic murmur.**[78] This study demonstrated the importance of auscultation of the heart at rest and immediately after exercise in persons with CHF to gain insight into the dynamics of myocardial activity.

Peripheral Edema

Peripheral edema frequently accompanies CHF, but in some clinical situations it may be absent when, in fact, a patient has significant CHF.[6] In CHF, fluid is retained and not excreted because the **pressoreceptors** of the body sense a decreased volume of blood as a result of the heart's inability to pump an adequate amount of blood. The pressoreceptors subsequently relay a message to the kidneys to retain fluid so that a greater volume of blood can be ejected from the heart to the peripheral tissues.[79] Unfortunately, this compounds the problem and makes the heart work even harder, which further decreases its pumping ability. The retained fluid commonly accumulates bilaterally in the dependent extracellular spaces of the periphery.[6] Dependent spaces such as the ankles and pretibial areas tend to accumulate the majority of fluid and can be measured by applying firm pressure to the pretibial area for 10 to 20 seconds, then measuring the resultant indentation in the skin (pitting edema). This is frequently graded as mild, moderate, or severe, or it is given a numerical value, depending on the measured scale (Table 4–5). Peripheral edema can also accumulate in the sacral area (the shape of which resembles the popular fanny packs) or in the abdominal area (ascites).

By using the pitting edema scale to determine the severity and location of peripheral edema (pretibial or sacral, distal or proximal) and obtaining girth measurements of the lower extremities and the abdomen, important information regard-

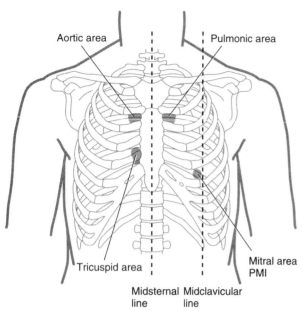

Figure 4–5. Primary auscultatory areas. Auscultation of the heart is performed in a systematic fashion using both the bell and diaphragm of the stethoscope at the indicated sites.

ing patient status can be obtained. However, it should be noted that peripheral edema is a sign that is associated with many other pathologies and does not by itself imply CHF.

Jugular Venous Distention

Jugular venous distention also results from fluid overload. As fluid is retained and the heart's ability to pump is further compromised, the retained fluid "backs up," not only into the lungs but also into the venous system, of which the jugular veins are the simplest to identify and evaluate. The external jugular vein lies medial to the external jugu-

Table 4–5
Pitting Edema Scale

1+	Barely perceptible depression (pit)
2+	Easily identified depression (EID) (skin rebounds to its original contour within 15 sec)
3+	EID (skin rebounds to its original contour within 15–30 sec)
4+	EID (rebound > 30 sec)

lar artery, and with an individual in a 45-degree semirecumbent position, it can be readily measured for signs of distention. Although individuals with marked CHF may demonstrate jugular venous distention in all positions (supine, semisupine, and erect), typically jugular venous distention is measured when the head of the bed is elevated to 45 degrees.[76, 80] The degree of elevation should be noted as well as the magnitude of distention (mild, moderate, severe).

More detailed measurements can be obtained by rotating the head slightly away from the vein being examined; at the point of elevation of the bed at which distention is first observed, pressure should be applied to the external jugular vein just above and parallel to the clavicle for approximately 10 to 20 seconds. This amount of time should allow the lower part of the vein to fill, and after quickly withdrawing the finger that was occluding the vein, the height of the distended fluid column within the vein should be measured. Normally, the level is less than 3 to 5 cm above the sternal angle of Louis. Measurements of the internal jugular vein may be more reliable than those of the external jugular vein. Nonetheless, the highest point of visible pulsation is determined as the trunk and head are elevated and the vertical distance between this level and the level of the sternal angle of Louis is recorded (Fig. 4–6).[73, 76]

Evaluation of the jugular waveforms can also be performed in this position, but catheterization of

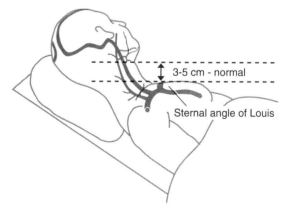

Figure 4–6. Evaluation of venous pressure. Elevated venous pressure frequently represents right-sided and left-sided heart failure, which is characterized by pulmonary congestion and distention of the external jugular vein that is greater than 3 to 5 cm above the sternal angle of Louis.

the pulmonary artery for assessment of pulmonary arterial pressures provides the greatest amount of information. A tremendous amount of information can be projected to a hemodynamic monitor, where the pulmonary artery pressure can be assessed and specific waveforms may be observed. The **A wave** of venous distention from right atrial systole, occurring just before S_1, and the **V wave,** frequently indicating a regurgitant tricuspid valve, are two such examples and are displayed in Figure 4–7.[73, 76] Although the assessment of hemodynamic function via pulmonary artery pressure monitoring is considered an advanced skill, it is relatively simple to interpret the typical intensive care unit monitor and thus obtain important hemodynamic information. Perhaps the most important aspect of such monitoring is identifying the pulmonary artery pressure, which is schematized in Figure 4–7. A mean pulmonary artery pressure greater than 25 mm Hg is the definition of pulmonary hypertension and appears to be associated with a variety of pathophysiologic phenomena (hypoxia, cardiac arrhythmias, and pulmonary abnormalities).[76, 80]

Pulsus alternans (mechanical alteration of the femoral or radial pulse characterized by a regular rhythm and alternating strong and weak pulses) can frequently identify severely depressed myocar-

dial function and CHF in general. This is performed using light pressure at the radial pulse with the patient's breath held in mid*expiration* (to avoid the superimposition of respiratory variation on the amplitude of the pulse).[76] **Sphygmomanometry** can more readily recognize this phenomenon, which commonly demonstrates 20 mm Hg or greater alternating systolic blood pressure. Characteristically, if pulsus alternans exists, a 20 mm Hg or greater decrease in systolic blood pressure occurs during breath holding because of increased resistance to left ventricular ejection. It should be noted that a difference exists between pulsus alternans and **pulsus paradoxus,** which is characterized by a marked reduction of both systolic blood pressure (-20 mm Hg) and strength of the arterial pulse during in*spiration*. Pulsus paradoxus can also be detected by sphygmomanometry[76] and is occasionally seen in CHF. However, it is associated more frequently with cardiac tamponade and constrictive pericarditis primarily due to increased venous return and volume to the right side of the heart, which bulges the interventricular septum into the left ventricle, thus decreasing the amount of blood present in the left ventricle and the amount of blood ejected from it (because of decreased left ventricular volume and opposition to stroke volume from the bulging septum).[76]

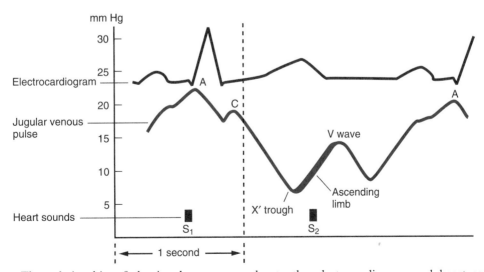

Figure 4–7. The relationship of the jugular venous pulse to the electrocardiogram and heart sounds. The jugular venous pulse (and its various component wave patterns, C, V, and A waves) can be observed in the external jugular vein or via intensive care monitoring (which is often accompanied by an electrocardiogram). The physiologic and mechanical events producing the above wave patterns can be better analyzed by assessing the heart sounds and their respective location in the cardiac and venous pulse cycles.

Changes in the Extremities

Occasionally, the extremities of persons with CHF will be cold and appear pale and **cyanotic.** This abnormal sensation and appearance are due to the increased sympathetic nervous system activation of CHF, which increases peripheral vascular vasoconstriction and decreases peripheral blood flow.[81, 82]

Weight Gain

As fluid is retained, total body fluid volume increases, as does total body weight. Fluctuations of a few pounds from day to day are usually considered normal, but increases of several pounds per day (over 3 lb) are suggestive of CHF in a patient with CMD.[6] Body weight should always be measured from the same scale at approximately the same time of day with similar clothing and before exercise is started.

Sinus Tachycardia

Sinus tachycardia or other tachyarrhythmias may occur in CHF as the pressoreceptors and chemoreceptors of the body detect decreased fluid volume and decreased oxygen levels, respectively.[6] The body attempts (via increased heart rate) to increase the delivery of fluid and oxygen to the peripheral tissues where it is needed. Unfortunately, this attempt, much like the message to the kidneys to retain fluid, only compounds the problem and makes the heart work even harder, which further impairs its ability to pump.

Decreased Exercise Tolerance

Decreased exercise tolerance is ultimately the culmination of all of the preceding pathophysiologies that produce the characteristic signs and symptoms just discussed. It is apparent that as individuals at rest become short of breath, gain weight, and develop a faster resting heart rate, their ability to exercise is dramatically decreased. This effect has been observed repeatedly in patients with CHF and is the result of the interrelationships among the pathophysiologies briefly discussed.[6]

The methods of measuring exercise tolerance in patients with CHF have improved significantly in the past few years, but many investigators still utilize the criteria set forth by the New York Heart Association in 1964.[83] These criteria categorize patients into one of four classes, depending on the development of symptoms and the amount of effort required to provoke them. In short, patients in class I have no limitations in ordinary physical activity, whereas patients in class IV are unable to carry on any physical activity without discomfort. Patients in classes II and III are characterized by slight limitation and marked limitation in physical activities, respectively (Table 4–6).

A great deal of investigation has been done on measuring exercise tolerance, functional capacity, and survival in persons with CHF.[84–94] Peak oxygen consumption measurements have traditionally been used to categorize persons with CHF and numerous studies have shown that persons with lower levels of peak oxygen consumption have poorer exercise tolerance, functional capacity, and survival than persons with greater levels of peak oxygen consumption (Table 4–7).[84–89] A peak oxygen consumption

Table 4–6	
New York Heart Association Functional Classification of Heart Disease	
Class I	Patients with cardiac disease but without resulting limitations of physical activity. Ordinary physical activity does not cause undue fatigue, palpitation, dyspnea, or anginal pain.
Class II	Patients with cardiac disease that results in a slight limitation of physical activity. Patients are comfortable at rest, but ordinary physical activity results in fatigue, palpitations, dyspnea, or anginal pain.
Class III	Patients with cardiac disease that results in a marked limitation of physical activity. Patients are comfortable at rest, but less than ordinary activity causes fatigue, palpitations, dyspnea, or anginal pain.
Class IV	Patients with cardiac disease resulting in an inability to carry on any physical activity without discomfort. Fatigue, palpitations, dyspnea, or anginal pain may be present even at rest. If any physical activity is undertaken, symptoms increase.

Table 4–7
Maximal Exercise Testing—Relationship to Prognosis in Heart Failure

INVESTIGATOR (REFERENCE)	NUMBER OF PATIENTS	PATIENT POPULATION/AGE	MEASUREMENTS	OUTCOMES
Mancini (84)	114	CHF/50 ± 11	Peak VO_2 NYHA PCWP CI	PS with peak VO_2 < 14 mL/kg/min
Cohn (85)	139	CHF/53 ± 13	Peak VO_2 LVEF PNE	PS with low peak VO_2 and LVEF and high PNE
Slazchic (86)	27	CHF/56 ± 12	Peak VO_2 LVEF RVEF PCWP Other hemodynamics	PS with peak VO_2 < 10 mL/kg/min
Likoff (87)	201	CHF/62 ± 10	Peak VO_2 LVEF Type of HD S_3 HS VA NYHA	PS with low peak VO_2 and presence of S_3 HS and ischemic CM
Cohn (88)	1446	CHF/59 ± 8	Peak VO_2 LVEF CTR VA NE	PS with low peak VO_2 and LVEF and high CTR
Aaronson (89)	272	CHF/52 ± 12	Peak VO_2 % predicted peak VO_2	PS with peak VO_2 < 14 mL/kg/min

CHF = congestive heart failure; VO_2 = oxygen consumption; NHYA = New York Heart Association; PCWP = pulmonary capillary wedge pressure; CI = cardiac index; PS = poorer survival; LVEF = left ventricular ejection fraction; PNE = plasma norepinephrine; RVEF = right ventricular ejection fraction; HD = heart disease; CM = cardiomyopathy; S_3 HS = third heart sound; CTR = cardiothoracic ratio; VA = ventricular arrhythmias; NE = norepinephrine.

threshold range of 10 to 14 mL/kg/min appears to exist, below which patients have been observed to have poorer survival.[84–89] In fact, a peak oxygen consumption below this range is frequently used to list patients for cardiac transplantation.[89]

Measurement of the **anaerobic threshold** (or ventilatory threshold) and the "slope of the rate of CO_2 output from aerobic metabolism plus the rate of CO_2 generated from buffering of lactic acid, as a function of the VO_2," as well as the change in oxygen consumption to change in work rate above the anaerobic threshold, appear to be useful and relatively reliable in determining exercise tolerance in patients with CHF.[90–94]

Unfortunately, most physical therapists do not have access to equipment (or training in its use) to measure respiratory gases. However, simple but thorough exercise assessments that evaluate symptoms, heart rate, blood pressure, heart rhythm via electrocardiogram, oxygen saturation via oximetry, and respiratory rate at specific workloads can provide important and useful information to compare patient response from day to day. Examples of such an assessment include treadmill ambulation, bicycle ergometry, hallway ambulation, or gentle calisthenic or strength training. Through this type of assessment, progress or deterioration can be documented and appropriate therapy implemented.

The 6-minute walk test (6'WT) has been found to be a valuable tool when assessing patients with CHF.[95] It appears to provide an insight into the functional status, exercise tolerance, oxygen consumption, and survival of persons with CHF. Although the exercise performed during the 6'WT is considered submaximal, it nonetheless, closely approximates the maximal exercise of persons with CHF and is correlated to peak oxygen consump-

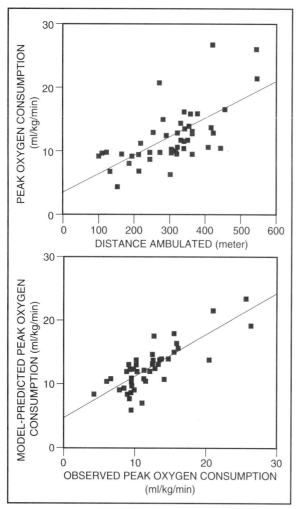

Figure 4–8. Six-minute walk to peak VO_2 regression plot.

tion (Fig. 4–8).[95, 96] Information obtained from the 6'WT has been used to predict peak oxygen consumption (unfortunately with a modest degree of error) and survival in persons with advanced CHF awaiting cardiac transplantation (Table 4–8 and Fig. 4–9). Figure 4–9 demonstrates that patients unable to ambulate greater than 300 m during the 6'WT had poorer short-term survival. Although a relationship between the distance ambulated during the 6'WT and long-term survival was not observed, such a relationship was observed by Bittner et al.[97] In fact, patients unable to ambulate greater than 300 m had poorer long-term survival. Therefore, not only can the cardiopulmonary response and exercise tolerance of a person with CHF be evaluated with

the 6'WT, but a distance of 300 m appears to be important in determining short- and long-term survival. Table 4–9 provides an overview of the relationship among exercise tolerance, oxygen consumption, and several measures of health and functional status.

Several important responses observed during submaximal and maximal exercise testing in patients with CMD include (1) a more rapid heart rate response during submaximal workloads; (2) a lower peak oxygen consumption and oxygen pulse (an indirect measure of stroke volume obtained by dividing the heart rate into oxygen consumption) during submaximal and maximal work; (3) a flat, blunted, and occasionally hypoadaptive systolic blood pressure response to exercise; (4) a possible increase in diastolic blood pressure; (5) electrocar-

Table 4–8
Multivariate Equations for the Prediction of Peak VO_2

1. Distance
   $$Peak\ VO_2 = 0.03 \times distance\ (m) + 3.98$$
   $r = 0.64;\ r^2 = 0.42;\ p < 0.0001;\ SEE = 3.32$

2. Distance + Age + Weight + Height + RPP
   $$Peak\ VO_2 = 0.02 \times distance\ (m) - 0.191 \\ \times age\ (yr) - 0.07 \times wt\ (kg) + 0.09 \\ \times height\ (cm) + 0.26 \times RPP\ (\times 10^{-3}) + 2.45$$
   $r = 0.81;\ r^2 = 0.65;\ p < 0.0001;\ SEE = 2.68$

3. Distance + Age + Weight + Height + RPP + FEV_1 + FVC
   $$Peak\ VO_2 = 0.02 \times distance\ (m) \\ - 0.14 \times age\ (yr) - 0.07 \times wt\ (kg) \\ + 0.03 \times height\ (cm) + 0.23 \times RPP\ (\times 10^{-3}) \\ + 0.10 \times FEV_1(L) \\ + 1.19 \times FVC\ (L) + 7.77$$
   $r = 0.83;\ r^2 = 0.69;\ p < 0.0001;\ SEE = 2.59$

4. Distance + Age + Weight + Height + RPP + LVEF + PAP + CI
   $$Peak\ VO_2 = 0.02 \times distance\ (m) - 0.15 \\ \times age\ (yr) - 0.05 \times wt\ (kg) + 0.04 \\ \times height\ (cm) + 0.17 \times RPP\ (\times 10^{-3}) \\ + 0.03 \times LVEF\ (\%) - 0.04 \times PAP\ (mm\ Hg) \\ + 0.31 \times CI\ (mL/min/m^2) + 8.43$$
   $r = 0.85;\ r^2 = 0.72;\ p = 0.001;\ SEE = 2.06$

r = correlation coefficient; r^2 = coefficient of determination; SEE = standard error of the estimate; RPP = rate-pressure product; LVEF = left ventricular ejection fraction; PAP = pulmonary artery pressure; CI = cardiac index.

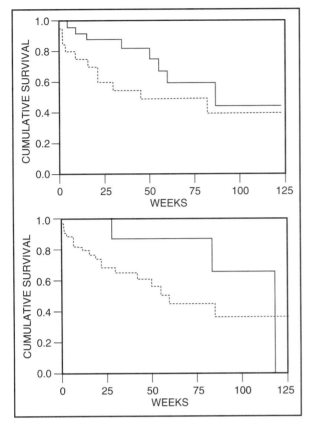

Figure 4–9. Survival curves from 6-minute walk test distance ambulated.

understand quality of life issues used instruments to measure quality of life that were less than comprehensive, such as dyspnea indices and exercise tolerance.[98–100] More comprehensive instruments have been designed and consist primarily of questionnaries that measure specific attributes of life such as socioeconomic factors, psychological status, and function.

One of the earliest such questionnaires was designed by Rector et al. and is titled the Minnesota Living with Heart Failure Questionnaire.[101] This questionnaire (shown in Table 4–10) consists of 21 questions that the patient answers to the best of his or her ability. This self-administered questionnaire appears to be more accurate and reliable with a modest degree of supervision. The Minnesota Living with Heart Failure Questionnaire has been used in several recent studies investigating the effects of various pharmacologic agents in persons with CHF as well as exercise training in CHF and appears useful for measuring quality of life and changes in the quality of life.[102–104] These areas are two very important issues for clinical practice and research, and the information provided by this questionnaire is therefore highly desirable. Other similar questionnaires have been developed, but none have been used as extensively as the Minnesota Living with Heart Failure Questionnaire.

Recently, the Minnesota Living with Heart Failure Questionnaire was used to investigate which variables were of greatest importance in determining the quality of life of elderly persons with CHF. In two seperate studies significant correlates to the quality of life of elderly persons with CHF were identified.[105, 106]

In one study the most powerful predictor of quality of life was quadriceps muscle strength. In this study of 30 elderly persons with CHF (mean age, 72 ± 10 years) poorer quadriceps muscle strength was associated with better quality of life, and persons with greater quadriceps muscle strength had a poorer quality of life.[105] This was a surprising finding and may have been due to altered psychosocial and functional expectations of elderly persons with CHF or the inability of the Minnesota Living with Heart Failure Questionnaire to adequately measure the quality of life of elderly persons with CHF. It is possible that altered psychosocial and functional expectations may have

diographic signs of myocardial ischemia; (6) more easily provoked dyspnea and fatigue, often accompanied by angina; (7) lower maximal workloads when compared with those of subjects without heart disease; and (8) a chronotropic (increased heart rate response) and possibly an inotropic (increased force of myocardial contraction) *incompetence* (resulting in an inability to increase the heart rate or force of myocardial contraction) during exercise in patients with severe coronary artery disease and multisystem disease that may be partially due to an autonomic nervous system dysfunction.[6, 92]

Quality of Life in Congestive Heart Failure

Very little research has been performed in the area of quality of life in CHF. Early attempts to

Table 4–9

Relationships Among Several Functional Classification Schemes Used in Congestive Heart Failure

	NYHA	SAS	CCSFCS	BDI	DFI	O_2CD	6'WT	EX. DUR.	$VO_{2\,max}$	MLWHFQ
NYHA	X									
SAS		X								
CCSFCS			X							
BDI		0.55		X						
DFI[a]					X					
O_2CD		0.42		0.58		X				
6'WT	−0.45	0.47[b]	0.59		0.49		X			
Ex. dur.	−0.54	0.11[c]	−0.64	0.29[c]	0.30[a]	0.02[c]	0.57[d]	X		
$VO_{2\,max}$						0.57[e]			X	
MLWHFQ	0.60[f]									X

NYHA = New York Heart Association Functional Classification Scheme; SAS = Specific Activity Scale; CCSFCS = Canadian Cardiovascular Society Functional Classification Scheme; BDI = Baseline Dyspnea Index; DFI = Dyspnea-Fatigue Index; O_2CD = oxygen cost diagram; 6'WT = 6-minute walk test; Ex. dur. = exercise duration; $VO_{2\,max}$ = maximal oxygen consumption; MLWHFQ = Minnesota Living with Heart Failure Questionnaire.

[a] Although no correlations were developed among these classification schemes, the change in exercise duration after pharmacologic treatment (ACE inhibition via captopril and lisinopril) was correlated to the change in each of the three categories of the DFI (functional impairment, magnitude of task, and pace of task) and the total aggregate score with correlation coefficients of 0.21 to 0.37.

[b] The relationship of the 6'WT to the SAS was also observed to be an indirect relationship with a correlation coefficient of −0.37 (see reference Guyatt CMA, 1985)

[c] The correlation coefficients between these variables were not statistically significant (ex. dur. and SAS $p = 0.47$, ex. dur and BDI $p = 0.06$, and ex. dur. and O_2CD $p = 0.89$).

[d] Guyatt also found a significant correlation between these two variables that was slightly less than that in this table (r = 0.42).

[e] The 6'WT was also found to be able to differentiate between the NYHA classification levels (I–IV) and level of oxygen consumption.

[f] An important finding of the Rector study was the significant correlation (r = 0.80) between a question asked after the MLWHFQ was administered ("Overall, how much did your heart failure prevent you from living as you wanted during the last month?") and the total MLWHFQ score.

produced the results observed because it appears that the longer the duration of CHF, the less the quadriceps muscle strength and the better the quality of life in this elderly cohort. Therefore, elderly persons with CHF who had poorer quadriceps muscle strength appear to have accommodated to decreased activity levels (from the longer duration of CHF) and accepted the lower levels of psychosocial and functional performance associated with CHF. Conversely, elderly persons with CHF and greater quadriceps muscle strength had CHF for a shorter period of time and appeared to be unable to accommodate to the decreased psychosocial and functional status imposed upon them from CHF, and they therefore had a poorer quality of life. Separate analyses of males and females support this hypothesis, but further investigation of these preliminary findings is needed.

In the second study, body weight was the most powerful predictor of quality of life in elderly persons with CHF (mean age, 72 ± 9 years).[106] Patients with lower body weight had better quality of life scores compared to patients who were heavier.[106] These results are not that surprising because lower body weight from proper diet and management of CHF (therapeutic diuresis) allows activities of daily living to be performed with greater ease. Further investigation of quality of life issues in CHF is needed to better understand the effects of various therapies in this growing population.

Summary: Assessment of Cardiopulmonary Status

The signs and symptoms associated with CHF can be ascribed, therefore, to some degree of failure of the several systems that were discussed earlier. Further investigation of the problems in several of

Table 4-10

Content of the Minnesota Living with Heart Failure Questionnaire

These questions concern how your heart failure (heart condition) has prevented you from living as you wanted during the past month. The items listed here describe different ways some people are affected. If you are sure an item does not apply to you or is not related to your heart failure, then circle 0 (No) and go on to the next item. If an item does apply to you, then circle the number rating of how much it prevented you from living as you wanted. Remember to think about ONLY THE PAST MONTH.

Did your heart failure prevent you from living as you wanted during the last month by

	NO	VERY LITTLE			VERY MUCH	
1. causing swelling in your ankles, legs, etc.?	0	1	2	3	4	5
2. making your working around the house or yard difficult?	0	1	2	3	4	5
3. making your relating to or doing things with your friends or family difficult?	0	1	2	3	4	5
4. making you sit or lie down to rest during the day?	0	1	2	3	4	5
5. making you tired, fatigued, or low on energy?	0	1	2	3	4	5
6. making your working to earn a living difficult?	0	1	2	3	4	5
7. making your walking about or climbing stairs difficult?	0	1	2	3	4	5
8. making you short of breath?	0	1	2	3	4	5
9. making your sleeping well at night difficult?	0	1	2	3	4	5
10. making you eat less of the foods you like?	0	1	2	3	4	5
11. making your going places away from home difficult?	0	1	2	3	4	5
12. making your sexual activities difficult?	0	1	2	3	4	5
13. making your recreational pastimes, sports, or hobbies difficult?	0	1	2	3	4	5
14. making it difficult for you to concentrate or remember things?	0	1	2	3	4	5
15. giving you side effects from medications?	0	1	2	3	4	5
16. making you worry?	0	1	2	3	4	5
17. making you feel depressed?	0	1	2	3	4	5
18. costing you money for medical care?	0	1	2	3	4	5
19. making you feel a loss of self-control in your life?	0	1	2	3	4	5
20. making you stay in a hospital?	0	1	2	3	4	5
21. making you feel you are a burden to your family or friends?	0	1	2	3	4	5

Copyright © University of Minnesota, 1986.
Median responses from 83 patients are underlined for each item.
Spearman rank-order correlation between sum of items 1 to 21 and each item.

Clinical Note: Assessment of Cardiopulmonary Status

- Notation of symptoms of CHF (dyspnea, paroxysmal nocturnal dyspnea, and orthopnea)
- Evaluation of pulse and electrocardiogram to determine heart rate and rhythm
- Evaluation of respiratory rate and breathing pattern
- Auscultation of the heart and lungs with a stethoscope
- Evaluation of radiographic findings to determine the existence and magnitude of pulmonary edema
- Performance of laboratory blood studies to determine the Pa_{O_2} and Pa_{CO_2} levels
- Evaluation of the oxygen saturation levels via oximetry
- Palpation for **fremitus** and percussion of the lungs to determine the relative amount of air or solid material in the underlying lung
- Performance of sit-to-stand test to evaluate heart rate and blood pressure (orthostatic hypotension) as well as dyspnea
- Objective measurement of other characteristic signs produced by fluid overload, such as peripheral edema, weight gain, and jugular venous distention
- Assessment of cardiopulmonary response to exercise (e.g., heart rate, blood pressure, electrocardiogram)
- Administration of a questionnaire to measure quality of life

the systems that are affected by CHF is necessary to improve the assessment and treatment of these patients. Specifically, the pathophysiology occurring in the cardiovascular, pulmonary, renal, hepatic, neurohumoral, hematologic, musculoskeletal, nutritional, and pancreatic systems will be reviewed. This will provide a more complete understanding of CMD, including the treatment and progression of patients with CMD.

SPECIFIC PATHOPHYSIOLOGIC CONDITIONS ASSOCIATED WITH CONGESTIVE HEART FAILURE

The pathophysiologic conditions associated with CMD appear to involve eight independent, yet interrelated, systems and one process:

- Cardiovascular
- Renal
- Pulmonary
- Neurohumoral
- Hepatic
- Hematologic
- Musculoskeletal
- Pancreatic
- Nutritional and biochemical factors

The remainder of this section describes and explains each of these factors as they relate to CHF in CMD. Table 4–11 and Figure 4–10 provide an overview of the specific pathophysiologic areas affected by CHF.

Cardiovascular Function

The cardiac disorders that have the potential to produce CMD have been described as the result of "one or more of 12 mechanisms" that produce

---

Table 4–11

Pathophysiologic Conditions Associated with Congestive Heart Failure

PATHOLOGIC SITE	EFFECTS
Cardiovascular	Decreased myocardial performance, with subsequent peripheral vascular constriction to increase venous return (attempting to increase stroke volume and cardiac output) ⇓
Neurochemical	Increased sympathetic stimulation that eventually desensitizes the heart to beta$_1$-adrenergic-receptor stimulation, thus decreasing the heart's inotropic effect ⇓
Renal	Water retention because of decreased cardiac output ⇓
Pulmonary	Pulmonary edema because of a "backup" of blood due to poor cardiac performance and fluid overload ⇓
Hepatic	Possible cirrhosis from hypoperfusion due to an inadequate cardiac output or hepatic venous congestion ⇓
Hematologic	Possible polycythemia, anemia, and hemostatic abnormalities because of a reduction in oxygen transport, accompanying liver disease, or stagnant blood flow in the heart's chambers because of poor cardiac contraction ⇓
Pancreatic	Possible impaired insulin secretion and glucose tolerance as well as the source of a possible myocardial depressant factor ⇓
Nutritional/biochemical	Anorexia that leads to malnutrition (protein-calorie and vitamin deficiencies) and cachexia ⇓
Musculoskeletal	Skeletal muscle wasting and possible skeletal muscle myopathies as well as osteoporosis from inactivity or other accompanying diseases

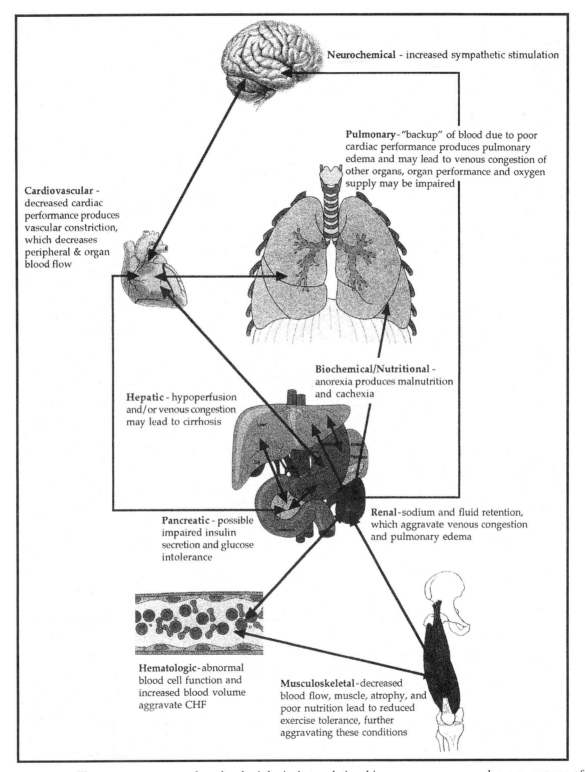

Neurochemical - increased sympathetic stimulation

Pulmonary - "backup" of blood due to poor cardiac performance produces pulmonary edema and may lead to venous congestion of other organs, organ performance and oxygen supply may be impaired

Cardiovascular - decreased cardiac performance produces vascular constriction, which decreases peripheral & organ blood flow

Biochemical/Nutritional - anorexia produces malnutrition and cachexia

Hepatic - hypoperfusion and/or venous congestion may lead to cirrhosis

Renal - sodium and fluid retention, which aggravate venous congestion and pulmonary edema

Pancreatic - possible impaired insulin secretion and glucose intolerance

Hematologic - abnormal blood cell function and increased blood volume aggravate CHF

Musculoskeletal - decreased blood flow, muscle, atrophy, and poor nutrition lead to reduced exercise tolerance, further aggravating these conditions

Figure 4–10. The compensatory and pathophysiologic interrelationships among organs and organ systems affected by congestive heart failure (CHF). (Reprinted from Cahalin I. Physical Therapy 76:516, 1996. With permission of the American Physical Therapy Association.)

CHF primarily via pump failure or secondarily via mechanical complications. Although pump failure (of which myocardial infarction and ischemia are the most common) and mechanical complications can be divided into the primary and secondary causes of CHF, the rationale for both to cause CHF can be understood best by describing the **Frank-Starling mechanism.** The Frank-Starling mechanism was one of the earliest efforts to better understand cardiac muscle relaxation and contraction or, in essence, "the relation between ventricular filling pressure (or end-diastolic volume) and ventricular mechanical activity,"[107] expressed as the volume output of the heart or the stroke volume (cardiac output divided by heart rate because CO = HR × SV).

In the early 1900s, Frank and Starling discovered that the stroke volume is dependent on both diastolic cardiac muscle fiber length and myocardial contractility (force of contraction and heart rate).[108] This relationship can be better understood by studying Figure 4–11, in which left ventricular stroke work is plotted against left ventricular filling pressure. The figure shows that an optimal range of left ventricular filling pressures exists that, when exceeded, decreases left ventricular stroke work considerably.[15, 107] As the left ventricular filling pressure increases, so does the stretch on cardiac muscle fiber during diastole. Taken a step further, the left ventricular filling pressure is representative of the left ventricular end-diastolic volume, which determines the degree of stretch on the myocardium.[107, 108] This is apparent in Figure 4–1, which *also* demonstrates that an optimal range of ventricular end-diastolic volume (or filling pressure) exists, which, if exceeded or insignificant, decreases ventricular performance. In addition, Figure 4–1 shows the major influences that determine the degree of myocardial stretch—atrial contribution to ventricular filling, total blood volume, body position, intrathoracic pressure, intrapericardial pressure, venous tone, and pumping action of skeletal muscle, all of which should be considered when evaluating and treating patients.[15]

The stroke volume was described earlier as the result of the degree of myocardial stretch (or as previously stated, the diastolic cardiac muscle fiber length) as well as that of myocardial contractility. Myocardial contractility is influenced by many variables; the major ones are illustrated in Figure 4–1. These factors include force-frequency relations, circulating **catecholamines, sympathetic** nerve impulses, intrinsic depression, loss of myocardium, pharmacologic depressants, **digitalis** or other **inotropic** agents, anoxia, **hypercapnia,** and acidosis.[15]

Despite these major influences, without adequate diastolic filling (and the "necessary degree of myocardial stretch"), stroke volume remains unchanged. The importance of diastolic filling of the ventricles is apparent in patients who have **pericardial effusion** (i.e., cardiac tamponade) or **myocarditis,** and because of cardiac compression or infectious agents, respectively, are unable to attain adequate diastolic filling. This situation results in a decreased stroke volume that can be hemodynamically significant, producing pulsus paradoxus as well as a **hypoadaptive** systolic blood pressure response to exercise.

The left ventricular end-diastolic pressure is often referred to as the preload. This filling pressure (the pressure in the left ventricle before the ejection of the stroke volume) is analogous to the pulling backward on the rubber band of a slingshot before releasing the rubber band to eject an object. The afterload is the resistance that the stroke volume encounters after it is ejected from

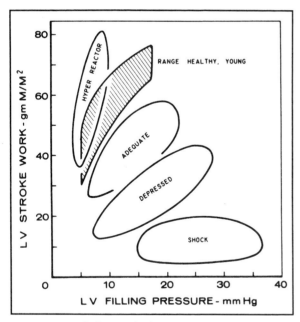

Figure 4–11. Left ventricular (LV) function. Left ventricular performance is dependent on left ventricular filling (utilizing the Frank-Starling mechanism) and the resultant pressure, which, if extensive, dramatically decreases left ventricular work. (From Sodeman WA, Sodeman TM. Sodeman's Pathologic Physiology: Mechanisms of Disease. 7th ed. Philadelphia, WB Saunders, 1985, p 343.)

the left ventricle. The resistance (or afterload), therefore, is essentially the peripheral vascular resistance. Much of the treatment for CMD involves lowering both the preload and afterload of the cardiovascular system.

The left ventricular filling pressure discussed earlier can be closely approximated by the pulmonary capillary wedge pressure, which is frequently monitored in patients in coronary care or intensive care units.[80] Left ventricular systolic performance appears to deteriorate when the pulmonary capillary wedge pressure is greater than 15 to 20 mm Hg. As mentioned earlier, the effects of extremely elevated pressures in the left ventricle decrease ventricular compliance and in the presence of cardiac arrhythmias can impair cardiac performance significantly. This condition is analogous to motor nerve lesions and the subsequent dysfunction of skeletal muscle. Central nervous system activity is needed for proper function of skeletal muscle in much the same way as cardiac muscle function is dependent on proper intrinsic electrical activity (the heart rhythm resulting from the automaticity of cardiac cells).

Atrial Natriuretic Peptide

The increased fluid volume that typically produces increased left ventricular end-diastolic volume "backs up" into the left atrium and likewise produces elevated atrial pressure. The elevated atrial pressure produces significant cardiovascular change and stimulates the release of a specific regulatory hormone, atrial natriuretic peptide (ANP). Atrial natriuretic peptide is released from atrial myocyte granules when atrial pressure or volume exceeds an unknown value (Fig. 4–12).[29]

Once released, ANP binds to receptors in target tissues, such as the aorta, vascular smooth muscle, renal cortex and medulla, and adrenal zona glomerulosa.[29] It then produces a brisk **natriuresis** (excretion of sodium) and diuresis (excretion of water) as well as an increase in the excretion of most other electrolytes (chloride, potassium, calcium, magnesium, and phosphorus).[29] In addition, ANP suppresses secretion of renal renin and aldosterone and release of angiotensin-stimulated aldosterone, which, in effect, attempts to maintain the blood pressure—electrolyte homeostasis.[109] Greater levels of ANP have also been found to be associated with higher morbidity and mortality rates.[110, 111] Although ANP produces these effects to reduce fluid volume, they are only minor forces, which, unfortunately, are no match for the profound fluid retention produced by the kidneys.

Renal Function

The subtle, yet devastating, effects of the renal system in CHF can be appreciated best in Figure 4–13, which outlines the five major steps for the initiation and maintenance of renal sodium reten-

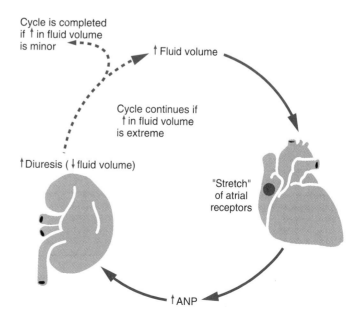

Figure 4–12. Atrial natriuretic peptide (ANP). Elevated vascular volume releases ANP, which increases the glomerular filtration rate (GFR) and facilitates natriuresis and diuresis.

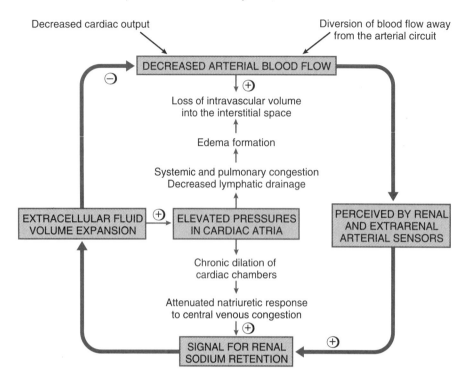

Figure 4-13. Mechanisms of congestive heart failure. Cardiac muscle dysfunction decreases the cardiac output and resultant arterial blood flow, which initiates the cycle illustrated. (From Skorecki KL, Breuner BM. Body fluid homeostasis in congestive heart failure and cirrhosis with ascites. Am J Med 72:323, 1982. With permission from Excerpta Medical Inc.)

tion. As previously mentioned, sodium (and ultimately water) is retained in CHF because of inadequate cardiac output.[14, 18] The arterial system of the body senses, via renal and extrarenal sensors, that the arterial blood flow is inadequate, often because of a poor cardiac output, and initiates a process to retain fluid (to increase arterial blood flow), which is identical to that initiated in **hypovolemic** states.[29] In effect, the kidneys in CHF act like those in an individual with a reduced volume of body fluid.

The subsequent retention of sodium and water are due to several factors:

• Augmented alpha-adrenergic neural activity
• Circulating catecholamines (e.g., epinephrine, norepinephrine)
• Increased circulating and locally produced angiotensin II, which results in renal vasoconstriction, thus decreasing the glomerular filtration rate (GFR) as well as renal blood flow[29]

These effects increase the renal filtration fraction (the ratio of GFR to renal blood flow), which increases the protein concentration in the peritubular capillaries and decreases the postglomerular capillary hydrostatic pressure (increasing renal vascular resistance), thus decreasing the transcapillary

hydraulic pressure gradient.[29] The resulting reduction in peritubular capillary hydrostatic pressure and elevation of peritubular oncotic pressure enhance the peritubular capillary uptake of proximal tubular fluid, thereby increasing the quantity of sodium reabsorbed in the proximal tubule.[112, 113] The reabsorption process and a thorough overview of renal function in CHF are presented in Figure 4-14.

Laboratory findings suggestive of impaired renal function in CHF include increases in BUN or other nitrogenous bodies (**azotemia**) as well as increased blood creatinine levels. This prerenal azotemia is the result of enhanced water reabsorption in the collecting duct, which becomes more pronounced with increased **antidiuretic hormone** (**ADH**) levels and which augments the passive reabsorption of **urea** (the rate of which can be increased with an acute myocardial infarction and by the catabolic state of CHF).[29] An increase in urea production, a decrease in excretion of urine, and an increased BUN may occur even before a decrease in GFR. A decreased GFR is the primary reason for the increased BUN and serum creatinine levels commonly seen in patients with CHF.[29]

In summary, the damaging effect of the renal sodium retention cycle is clearly portrayed in Fig-

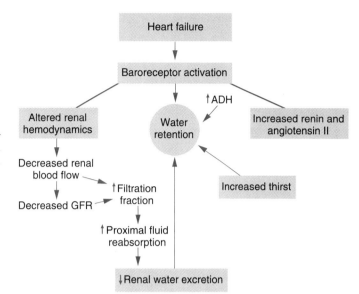

Figure 4-14. Physiologic effects of myocardial failure. Heart failure produces a variety of altered responses that lead to retention of water and often congestive heart failure.

ure 4-13, which demonstrates that if left untreated, the cycle will continue and ultimately lead to death. As previously noted, the extreme overload of fluid produced by the kidneys in CHF exceeds the volume that the left ventricle and eventually the left atrium can maintain, after which the fluid ultimately "backs up" into the lungs and produces CHF. The following section presents the pathophysiology observed when such a condition exists.

Pulmonary Function

As previously mentioned, one of the characteristic signs of CHF is the presence of inspiratory rales during auscultation of the lungs. This review of the pulmonary pathophysiology associated with CHF assists in the understanding of pulmonary edema in general and inspiratory rales in particular.

Pulmonary edema can be **cardiogenic** (hemodynamic) or noncardiogenic (caused by alterations

in the pulmonary capillary membrane) in origin.[6] The differential diagnosis can be made by history, physical examination, and laboratory examination, as shown in Table 4-1. Despite the different origins of pulmonary edema, the "sequence of liquid accumulation"[73] is similar for both and appears to consist of three distinct stages.

Stage 1 of pulmonary edema is unfortunately difficult to detect or quantify because it seems to represent "increased lymph flow without net gain of interstitial liquid."[73] The edema associated with the increased lymph flow may actually improve gas exchange in the lung as more of the small pulmonary vessels are distended. However, if lymph flow continues, pulmonary edema increases, and the airways and vessels become filled with increased amounts of liquid, particularly in the gravity-dependent portions of the lung.[73] This accumulation compromises the small airway lumina, resulting in a mismatch between ventilation and perfusion, which produces hypoxemia and wasted ventilation (stage 2). As a result, the tachypnea of CHF often ensues.[73] In addition, the degree of *hypoxemia* appears to be correlated to the degree of *elevation* of the *pulmonary capillary wedge pressure*.[114]

As lymph flow continues, pulmonary edema increases, increasing the pulmonary capillary wedge pressure and eventually flooding the alveoli. This flooding represents stage 3 pulmonary edema, which significantly compromises gas exchange,

> ### Clinical Note: Laboratory Findings of Impaired Renal Function
> - Increased blood urea nitrogen (BUN)
> - Increased blood creatinine levels (Creat)

producing severe hypoxemia and hypercapnia.[73] In addition, severe alveolar flooding can produce the following: (1) filling of the large airways with blood-tinged foam, which can be expectorated; (2) reductions in most lung volumes (e.g., vital capacity); (3) a right-to-left intrapulmonary shunt; and (4) hypercapnia with acute respiratory acidosis.[73]

Perhaps the most important principle regarding pulmonary edema is that of *"maintaining pulmonary capillary pressures at the lowest possible levels,"*[73] because it has been demonstrated that pulmonary edema can be decreased by more than 50% when pulmonary capillary wedge pressures are decreased from 12 to 6 mm Hg.

The effect of repeated bouts of pulmonary edema (which is common in CHF) upon pulmonary function appears to be profound. In fact, it is believed that more advanced CHF may produce a "global respiratory impairment" that is associated with varying degrees of obstructive and restrictive lung disease.[115, 116] Several measures of pulmonary function have recently been found to be significantly related to the level of dyspnea of persons with advanced CHF (Table 4–12).[117] Mancini and co-workers found similar correlations between dyspnea and pulmonary function of patients with slightly less severe CHF.[118]

Neurohumoral Effects

The neurohumoral system profoundly affects heart function in physiologic (fight-or-flight mechanism)

	PEARSON *r*			
DYSPNEA VARIABLES	FEV$_1$ (%)	FVC (%)	FVC (L)	TLC (L)
Pre-IMT resting dyspnea (N = 14)	−0.60	−0.59	—	—
Pre-IMT exercise dyspnea (N = 14)	−0.57	−0.67	—	—
Post-IMT resting dyspnea (N = 8)	—	—	−0.77	−0.82

Table 4–12

Pearson Product Moment Correlations between Dyspnea and Pulmonary Function

IMT = inspiratory muscle training; FEV$_1$ = forced expiratory volume in 1 second; FVC = forced vital capacity; TLC = total lung capacity.

---

and pathologic states (CMD). In general, the neural effects are much more rapid, whereas humoral effects are slower because the information sent by the autonomic nervous system via efferent nerves travels faster than the information traveling through the vascular system.[119]

Normal Cardiac Neurohumoral Function

Neurohumoral signals to the heart are perceived, interpreted, and augmented by the transmembrane signal transduction systems in myocardial cells.[119] The primary signaling system in the heart appears to be the **receptor–G protein–adenylate cyclase** (RGC) complex as it regulates myocardial contractility. Figure 4–15 illustrates the complexity of this system, which consists of (1) membrane receptors; (2) guanine nucleotide-binding regulatory proteins (the G proteins, which transmit stimulatory or inhibitory signals); and (3) adenylate cyclase, which converts **adenosine triphosphate** (ATP) to **cyclic adenosine monophosphate** (cAMP). Adenylate cyclase is an effector enzyme activated by a receptor agonist, thus enhancing cAMP synthesis. The lower portion of Figure 4–15 shows that increased cAMP synthesis ultimately increases the force of myocardial contraction (the inotropic effect).[119]

Clinical Note: Pulmonary Function in CHF

- Pulmonary edema consists of three stages.
- Stage 1 is difficult to detect.
- Stages 2 and 3 are detectable via auscultation of the lungs which will produce crackles (rales) and an absence of air movement in the lungs (no breath sounds due to consolidation), respectively.
- Greater pulmonary capillary wedge pressures may produce greater levels of hypoxemia, which should be monitored via oximetry and oxygen saturation.
- Repeated bouts of pulmonary edema and hypoxemia worsen pulmonary function and appear to be directly related to a patient's level of dyspnea.

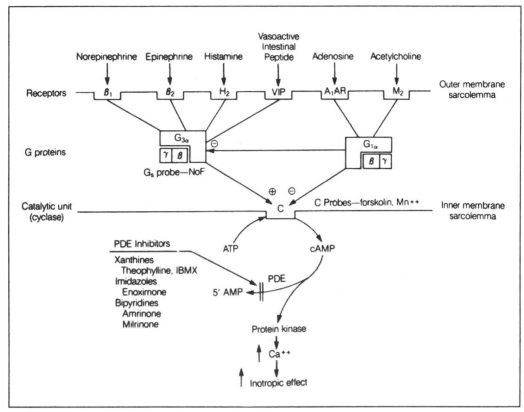

Figure 4–15. Neural control of cardiopulmonary function. The receptor G protein–adenylate cyclase complex and other important receptors, all of which affect the inotropic state of the heart. G_s, G stimulatory protein; G_1, G inhibitory protein; PDE, phosphodiesterase; IBMX, isobutylmethylxanthine; ATP, adenosine triphosphate; cAMP, cyclic adenosine monophosphate.

The top portion of Figure 4–15 shows the receptor agonists responsible for the initial activation of the RGC complex. These agents include norepinephrine, epinephrine, histamine, vasoactive intestinal peptide, adenosine, and acetylcholine.

Although Figure 4–15 shows the complete system, it does not reveal the degree of influence each receptor agonist has on cardiac function. In general, the most influential receptor agonists are the sympathetic neurotransmitters norepinephrine and epinephrine as they relay excitatory autonomic nervous system stimuli to both postsynaptic alpha- and beta-adrenergic receptors (primarily beta for norepinephrine) in the myocardium.[119] Inhibitory autonomic nervous system stimuli are transmitted by the parasympathetic nervous system via the vagus nerve and the neurotransmitter acetylcholine. The adrenergic receptors (alpha$_1$, alpha$_2$, beta$_1$, and beta$_2$) are discussed briefly in the next paragraphs so that Figure 4–15 can be appre-

ciated fully, as well as the neurohumoral changes that accompany CMD.

Alpha-Adrenergic Receptors. Stimulation of **alpha$_1$-adrenergic receptors** appears to activate the phosphodiesterase transmembrane signaling system,[120, 121] which increases **phosphodiesterase** and activates protein kinase, thus marginally increasing the inotropic effect.[122] Conversely, stimulation of **alpha$_2$-adrenergic receptors** activates the inhibitory G protein and inhibits adenylate cyclase, which decreases the inotropic effect.[123]

Beta-Adrenergic Receptors. The importance of the beta-adrenergic pathway cannot be overemphasized because it has been proposed that the heart is a **beta-adrenergic** organ.[124] Two beta-adrenergic receptors have been identified, beta$_1$ and beta$_2$, which are "distinguished by their differing affinities for the agonists epinephrine and norepinephrine." The beta$_2$-adrenergic receptor has a 30-fold greater affinity for epinephrine than for norepinephrine.[125] In brief, beta$_2$-adrenergic receptor stimulation promotes vasodilation of the capillary beds and muscle relaxation in the bronchial tracts, whereas beta$_1$-adrenergic receptor stimulation increases heart rate and myocardial force of contraction.[119]

Guanine Nucleotide-Binding Regulatory Proteins. As briefly discussed, the G proteins transmit stimulatory (G_s) or inhibitory (G_i) signals to the catalytic unit (inner membrane sarcolemma) of myocardial contractile tissue. The stimulatory and inhibiting signals are dependent on a very complex, and only partially understood, mechanism of receptor-mediated activation. Activation depends on several rate-limiting steps, mainly the dissociation of guanosine diphosphate (GDP) in exchange for guanosine triphosphate (GTP) and the action of GTPase enzyme intrinsic to alpha G_s.[119]

Catalytic Unit of Adenylate Cyclase. The activation of adenylate cyclase (and subsequent increase in myocardial force of contraction) is, unfortunately, poorly understood but has been observed to be decreased in patients with CHF. This decrease is the result of "a paradoxical diminution in the function of the RGC complex,"[119] which alters the receptor-effector coupling and "limits the ability of both endogenous and exogenous adrenergic agonists to augment cardiac contractility."[119] The inability of **endogenous** (produced in the body) or exogenous (medications) adrenergic agonists to increase the force of myocardial contraction is frequently seen in patients with CHF, and may be a contributing factor in CMD.[119–129]

Neurohumoral Alterations in the Failing Human Heart

Abnormalities in Sympathetic Neural Function. The sympathetic neural function of the heart is profoundly affected in CHF. The effects are due to abnormal RGC complex function primarily, despite increased concentrations of interstitial (in the interspaces of the myocardium), intrasynaptic, and systemic norepinephrine, which is less effective because of abnormal RGC complex function.[119]

The abnormal RGC complex function in CHF appears to be associated with the insensitivity of

---

> **Clinical Note: Neurohumoral Activity in CHF**
>
> Excessive sympathetic nervous system stimulation occurs in CHF, and because of abnormalities in particular parts of the neurohumoral system, the heart becomes insensitive to beta-adrenergic stimulation which results in a decreased force of myocardial contraction and an inability to attain higher heart rates during physical exertion.

the failing heart to beta-adrenergic stimulation.[119] This insensitivity to beta-adrenergic stimulation is apparently the result of a decrease in beta$_1$-adrenergic receptor density[119] and is very important because the heart contains a ratio of 3.3 to 1.0 beta$_1$- to beta$_2$-adrenergic receptors.[119] In CHF, the ratio decreases to approximately 1.5 to 1.0, producing a 62% decrease in the beta$_1$-adrenergic receptors and no significant increase in beta$_2$ density.[126, 127] Although the number of beta$_2$ receptors does not appear to change in CHF, the beta$_2$ receptor "is partially 'uncoupled' from the effector enzyme adenylate cyclase."[128, 129] This uncoupling only mildly desensitizes the beta$_2$-adrenergic receptors, which *initially* are able to compensate for the decreased number of beta$_1$ receptors by providing substantial inotropic support.[65] The duration of inotropic support appears to be short-lived, and myocardial failure becomes more pronounced.[119]

Liver Function

The fluid overload associated with CHF affects practically all organs and body systems, including liver function. Increased fluid volume eventually leads to hepatic venous congestion, which prevents adequate perfusion of oxygen to hepatic tissues. Subsequent hypoxemia from the hypoperfusion produces a **cardiac cirrhosis,** which is character-

---

> **Clinical Note: Liver Function in CHF**
>
> **Hepatomegaly,** or liver enlargement, is frequently associated with CHF and can be identified readily as tenderness in the right upper quadrant of the abdomen. Patients with long-standing CHF, however, are generally not tender to palpation, although hepatomegaly is frequently present.

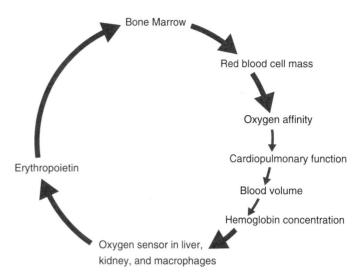

Figure 4–16. Mechanisms of hematologic function. Hematologic function is occasionally disrupted in congestive heart failure and can further impair cardiopulmonary function and patient status.

Hematologic Function

The normal morphology of the blood and blood-forming tissues is frequently disrupted in CHF. The most common abnormality is a secondary **polycythemia** (excess of red corpuscles in the blood), which is due to either a reduction in oxygen transport or an increase in **erythropoietin** production.[130] Erythropoietin is an alpha$_2$-globulin responsible for red blood cell production, and its important role is demonstrated in Figure 4–16. This figure shows that the hypoxia occasionally observed in patients with CHF may stimulate erythropoietin production, which increases not only red blood cell mass, but also blood volume in an already compromised cardiopulmonary system (partly because of fluid volume overload). This potentially vicious circle can progress and cause cardiopulmonary function to deteriorate further.

Clinically, **anemia,** which may be present in some patients with CHF, is a paradox, for when it is severe it can produce CHF independently, but when it precedes CHF, anemia may actually allow for a more efficient and effective cardiac function.[130] Improved cardiac output may occur because blood viscosity is reduced in patients with anemia, which subsequently decreases systemic vascular resistance. Anemia, therefore, acts as an af-terload reducer and may promote an increased cardiac output but at the cost of lower arterial oxygen and oxygen saturation levels as well as increased work for the heart.[130] A term that is frequently applied when such a condition (and others) exists is "a shift in the oxyhemoglobin curve." The curve can be shifted to the right or left but normally follows a pattern depicted in Figure 2–15, which represents a specific percentage of oxygen saturation for a given concentration of arterial oxygen. Oxygen saturation remains relatively stable, with arterial oxygen concentrations greater than 60 mm Hg, but below this level the oxygen saturation drops dramatically. Table 4–13 shows the oxygen saturation levels when arterial oxygen concentrations are less than 60 mm Hg.

Various conditions move this normal curve to the right or left, and these changes subsequently affect the respective oxygen saturation. For example, anemia shifts the curve to the right, representing a lower concentration of arterial oxygen, which moves the critical point of oxygen saturation to 70 mm Hg (therefore, to the right). This means that at levels of less than 70 mm Hg, the level of oxygen saturation decreases dramatically compared with the normal level of 60 mm Hg.

Table 4–13			
Relationship of PaO$_2$ to SaO$_2$			
PaO$_2$ (mm Hg)	40	50	60
SaO$_2$ (%)	70	80	90

Thus, patients with anemia have less reserve before their oxygen stores **desaturate.**[130]

The paradox thus unfolds, and patients with such a condition must be monitored carefully (especially if exercising). A blood transfusion may be given to improve oxygen transport to needed tissues, even though it may further increase the volume overload and potentially worsen the CHF. Therefore, breath sounds, heart rate, blood pressure, and symptoms must be monitored carefully during exercise in patients who have received a transfusion or who are anemic so that adverse reactions or medical emergencies can be prevented.

Also of concern for patients with advanced CMD (or CHF in general) is the state of **hemostasis** (the mechanical and biochemical aspects of platelet function and coagulation), which is frequently disrupted as a result of accompanying liver disease.[6] Normal platelet function is an interrelated process involving a reflex vasoconstriction, formation of platelet plugs, and aggregation of platelets to one another.[131] The aggregation of platelets is an energy-requiring process, which is stimulated by agonists and inhibited by antagonists. The most important stimulants appear to be adenosine diphosphate (ADP), epinephrine, thrombin, and collagen. Inhibition of platelet function to the point at which the platelet count drops below 150,000 cells/μL is termed **thrombocytopenia** and is due to hereditary factors or drugs or often is acquired from systemic disease.[131] Inherited thrombocytopenia is uncommon; however, thrombocytopenia due to drugs is much more common and frequently is an adverse reaction associated with use of aspirin, corticosteroids, antimicrobial agents (penicillins and cephalothins), phosphodiesterase inhibitors (dipyridamole), caffeine, sympathetic blocking agents (beta antagonists), and heparin.[131] Acquired disorders of platelet function are due to systemic disease states or complications arising from a disease. Renal failure frequently leads to **uremia,** which prolongs bleeding time and impairs platelet formation. This is usually corrected by renal dialysis, but patients with chronic CHF may demonstrate a mild-to-moderate level of platelet dysfunction.[131]

Skeletal Muscle Function

Skeletal muscle activity in patients with CHF has been a topic of investigation for many years. Studies have identified skeletal muscle **myopathy** in patients with CHF and in those with CHF and preexisting cardiomyopathy.[132, 133] This section presents information regarding skeletal muscle function when CHF *alone* is present and when CHF is present as a result of a cardiomyopathy. It is essential that the material be presented in this manner because skeletal muscle myopathies are common with cardiomyopathy.[132, 133]

Skeletal Muscle Activity in Congestive Heart Failure without Cardiomyopathy

Unfortunately, the function of skeletal muscle in patients with CHF has been studied far less in patients without cardiomyopathy than in those with cardiomyopathy. However, two studies have evaluated skeletal muscle activity in the presence of CHF without preexisting cardiomyopathy.[132, 133] The first histopathologic study by Shafiq and colleagues examined skeletal muscle in patients with and without **idiopathic** cardiomyopathy.[132] Electromyographic, histochemical, and electron microscopic studies were performed on 15 subjects (four normal subjects, six with CHF and cardiomyopathy, and five with signs and symptoms of CHF but *without* cardiomyopathy). Results revealed no abnormalities in the normal subjects but found a decrease in the average diameters of the type I and type II fibers in the patients with CHF but without cardiomyopathy, and the patients with CHF and cardiomyopathy were found to have three distinct skeletal muscle abnormalities (selective atrophy of type II fibers, pronounced nonselective myopathy, and hypotrophy of type I fibers).[132] Patients with diseases known to affect skeletal muscle (diabetes, collagen vascular disease, and alcoholism) were excluded from the study.

Clinical Note: Hematologic Function in CHF

- Possible polycythemia.
- Possible anemia; if present, oxygen saturation should be monitored.
- Possible hemostasis abnormalities such as thrombocytopenia; monitoring laboratory blood values is recommended.

Lipkin and associates have investigated the abnormalities of skeletal muscle in patients with chronic heart failure.[36] Mean maximal oxygen consumption was very low (11.7 mL · kg^{-1} · min^{-1}), and isometric maximal voluntary contraction of the quadriceps was only 55% (range 31% to 75%) of the predicted value for weight. Eight of the nine biopsies yielded abnormal findings, showing increased intracellular acid phosphatase activity (n = 6), increased intracellular lipid accumulation (n = 4), and atrophy of type I and type II muscle fibers (n = 4).[133] In conclusion, the results of a nuclear magnetic resonance spectroscopy study showed that skeletal muscle fatigue in patients with CHF is associated with intracellular acidosis and **phosphocreatine** depletion,[134] which if prolonged may predispose to myopathic processes.

Skeletal Muscle Activity in Congestive Heart Failure and Cardiomyopathy

Skeletal muscle activity is apparently impaired by chronic CHF as well as by cardiomyopathy. Skeletal muscle abnormalities due to dilated[135–137] and hypertrophic[138–142] cardiomyopathies have been reported previously and have consistently revealed type I and type II muscle fiber atrophy.[135–142]

A detailed study of skeletal muscle abnormalities in patients with hypertrophic and dilated cardiomyopathy was performed by Caforio and coworkers.[35] The ejection fraction of the patients ranged from 20% to 62% with a mean of 41 ± 12%.[143]

Results of the neuromuscular assessment were relatively insignificant, except that (1) all symptomatic patients with dilated cardiomyopathy and one with hypertrophic cardiomyopathy demonstrated a slight **hyposthenia** in the girdles or proximal limbs, and (2) none of the patients had muscular hypotrophy. Electromyographic studies revealed abnormalities typical of **myogenic** myopathy in nine patients (five dilated, four hypertrophic), but none of the patients showed signs of **neurogenic** alteration (i.e., a reduction of nerve conduction velocities or an increase in single motor unit potential duration).[143]

Muscle biopsies consistently detected pathologic changes (primarily mitochondrial abnormalities)

in the type I (slow-twitch) fibers in all nine patients from whom a biopsy was obtained; eight of the biopsies demonstrated increases of atrophy factors. No alteration of type II fibers was observed in any patient.[143]

Caforio and colleagues believe the findings from this study support the hypothesis that skeletal myopathic changes, which are occasionally observed in patients with cardiomyopathy, are of a primary nature rather than a secondary nature (due to congestive heart failure). It is likely that both chronic CHF and cardiomyopathy have profound effects on skeletal muscle activity.

Loss of muscle strength will reduce exercise capacity. At workloads corresponding to 50 and 100% of maximal oxygen consumption in normal subjects, the proportion of maximal muscle force utilized during an isometric contraction is 30 and 50%, respectively. Isometric maximal muscle strength of persons with CHF appears to be reduced to nearly 50% of the value for age-, sex-, and weight-matched control subjects. Loss of muscle strength will result in each muscle fiber operating nearer to its maximal capacity for a given absolute power output. Consequently, the changes in skeletal muscle metabolism that are associated with fatigue might be expected to occur at lower absolute workloads and hence to limit maximal exercise capacity in these patients.[133]

Pancreatic Function

Severe CMD can potentially reduce blood flow to the pancreas "as a consequence of splanchnic visceral vasoconstriction, which accompanies severe left ventricular failure."[144] The reduction in blood flow to the pancreas impairs insulin secretion and glucose tolerance, which are further impaired by increased sympathetic nervous system activity and augmented circulatory catecholamines (inhibiting insulin secretion) that stimulate **glycogenolysis** and elevate blood sugar levels.[145]

Reduced secretion of insulin is of paramount importance because hypoxic and dysfunctional heart muscle depends a great deal on the energy from the metabolism of glucose, which is reduced significantly if insulin secretion is impaired.[144] Ultimately, there is further deterioration of left ventricular function, creating a vicious circle.

Normally, when oxygen is available, the heart obtains 60 to 90% of its energy requirements from the oxidation of free fatty acids, which inhibits glucose uptake, glycolytic flux, and glycogenolysis.[146] The oxidation of free fatty acids increases the production of acetyl coenzyme A (acetyl-CoA), which inhibits pyruvate dehydrogenase and limits carbohydrate metabolism.[146] However, as previously noted, myocardial ischemia (because of the limited supply of oxygen) inhibits the oxidation of free fatty acids and long-chain acyl-carnitine palmitoyl transferase enzyme activity, thus preventing the transport of cytosolic acyl coenzyme A (acyl-CoA) to the mitochondria for oxidation. "Accordingly, intracellular concentrations of acyl-CoA increase and acetyl-CoA content declines."[147]

Increased levels of acyl-CoA produce several deleterious effects on proper cardiac function:

• Increased synthesis of triglycerides, which accumulate in the myocardium
• Inhibition of further formation of CoA esters of fatty acids, limiting oxidation of free fatty acids
• Inhibition of adenine nucleotide translocase, which is important for myocardial energy metabolism because it transports ATP synthesized in the mitochondria to the cytosol[146]

This final inhibition of adenine nucleotide translocase may be a key factor contributing to myocardial dysfunction.[146]

In addition to the previously mentioned changes in metabolism, "the pancreas has also been viewed as the source of a myocardial depressant factor which has been shown to decrease contractility of an isolated papillary muscle preparation."[148, 149]

Finally, CMD and CHF is common in persons with diabetes and is an important risk factor for the development of a cardiomyopathy. Such a relationship clearly identifies the important role nutrition and proper biochemical function have in cardiovascular disease.

Nutritional and Biochemical Aspects

Nutritional concerns are very important when assessing and treating patients with CMD. Stomach and intestinal abnormalities are not uncommon in these patients, who frequently receive many medications with profound side effects.[150] In addition, the interrelated disease processes occurring in other organs because of CMD and CHF frequently produce **anorexia,** which leads ultimately to malnutrition. The primary malnutrition is a protein-calorie deficiency, but vitamin deficiencies have also been observed (folic acid, thiamine, and hypocalcemia-accompanied vitamin D deficiency).[150] These deficient states may simply be the result of decreased intake, but "abnormal intestinal absorption and increased rates of excretion may also contribute."[150]

Protein-calorie deficiency is common in chronic CHF because of cellular hypoxia and hypermetabolism that frequently produces **cachexia** (malnutrition and wasting).[150] A catabolic state may also develop, yielding an excess of urea or other nitrogenous compounds in the blood (**azotemia).** This, as with most organ dysfunction associated with CHF, causes a vicious circle, which, because of gastrointestinal hypoxia and decreased appetite (anorexia) and protein intake, produces cardiac atrophy and more pronounced CMD.[150]

One particular area of concern is thiamine deficiency due to improper nutrition, which can affect this population dramatically. The force of myocardial contraction and cardiac performance in general appear to be dependent on the level of thiamine, and it has been suggested that *"the possibility of thiamine deficiency should be considered in many patients with heart failure of obscure origin."*[9] In addition, patients undergoing prolonged treatment with furosemide (Lasix) (the first drug of choice in the treatment of CHF) have demonstrated significant thiamine deficiency, which may improve with replacement.[151]

Skeletal muscle carnitine deficiency has also been observed in a small population of patients with hypertrophic cardiomyopathy. When carnitine was replenished, cardiac symptoms and echocardiographic parameters apparently improved.[152]

Another biochemical substance that has received much investigation in Europe is coenzyme Q_{10}. A substantial literature supports the supplementation of coenzyme Q_{10} in persons with CHF deficient of this apparently important biochemical component, which appears to have a role in the essential function of mitochondria, antioxidation of heart muscle, and cardiostimulation.[153–157]

These examples demonstrate the interrelatedness of all bodily functions and the importance of a thorough and comprehensive assessment, which is of even greater significance when kidney and liver diseases (frequently accompanying CHF) further complicate a patient's status. Complications associated with renal disease that are specifically related to nutritional aspects of CMD include the following:

- Decreased production of erythropoietin (a hormone synthesized in the kidney that is an important precursor of red blood cell production in bone marrow), causing anemia and possibly less free fatty acid oxidation[158, 159]
- Decreased synthesis of **1,25-dihydroxycholecalciferol,** which may lead to decreased calcium absorption from the gastrointestinal tract,[160] as well as the development of **hyperparathyroidism**[161]
- Impaired intermediary metabolism (impaired **gluconeogenesis** and lipid metabolism, as well as degradation of several peptides, proteins, and peptide hormones including insulin, **glucagon,** growth hormone, and **parathyroid** hormone)[162]

These renal abnormalities can, by themselves, impair liver function (primarily via protein deprivation), which "predisposes to chronic liver disease with a loss of hepatocytes and a decrease in portal venous blood flow."[163] Liver dysfunction further impairs the normal metabolism of many organic and inorganic nutrients, of which three intrahepatic intermediary amino acid metabolic pathways have been identified: the urea cycle, the **phenylalanine-hydroxylase pathway,** and the **trans-sulfuration pathway.**[163]

Although protein deprivation may be a predisposing factor to liver disease, Fischer and colleagues discovered that the aromatic amino acids phenylalanine and tyrosine and the sulfur-containing methionine are elevated, whereas the branched-chain amino acids are depressed in patients with cirrhosis of the liver and **hepatic encephalopathy.**[164, 165] This finding led to the current practice of administering enteral and parenteral products with reduced aromatic amino acids and increased branched-chain amino acids, which many patients with end-stage CHF frequently receive, to patients with liver disease.[163] Thus, the complexity of liver disease alone, not to mention a superimposed CHF and its many complications, makes the patient with CHF a complex challenge.

Clinical Note: Nutritional and Biochemical Aspects of CHF
- Malnutrition may occur in CHF.
- Thiamine and carnitine deficiency should be considered in many patients with CHF of obscure origin.
- Coenzyme Q_{10} is deficient in persons with CHF, and supplementation appears to improve myocardial performance and functional status.

SPECIFIC TREATMENT FOR CONGESTIVE HEART FAILURE

The treatment of CHF, in general, is directed at the underlying cause or causes. The fundamental treatment for CHF involves controlling the pathophysiologic mechanisms responsible for its existence. By improving the heart's ability to pump and reducing the workload and controlling sodium intake and water retention, CHF can be relatively well controlled.[166] These measures are outlined in Table 4–14.

The specific treatments for CHF include the restriction of sodium intake, use of medications (diuretics, digitalis and other positive inotropic agents, dopamine, dobutamine, amrinone, vasodilator therapy, venodilators, angiotensin-converting enzyme inhibitors, and beta-adrenergic blockers), other special measures, and properly prescribed physical activity. These treatments are outlined in Table 4–14, and a brief discussion of each will reveal how the pathophysiology of CHF is affected with each of the following measures.

Dietary Changes and Nutritional Supplementation

Because of the associated dietary and nutritional deficiences, supplementation of vitamins, minerals, and amino acids is often provided to persons with CHF. Vitamins C and E as well as various minerals have shown some promise as important supplements to the diet of persons with CHF.[167–170]

Dietary changes are also important for persons with CHF and include decreasing sodium intake,

Table 4–14

Outline of Treatment of Chronic Congestive Heart Failure

PROPER PRESCRIPTION OF PHYSICAL ACTIVITY

Decrease or discontinue exhaustive activities

Decrease or discontinue full-time work or equivalent activity, introducing rest periods during the day

Gradual progressive exercise training that fluctuates frequently from day to day

Exercise intensity determined by level of dyspnea or adverse physiologic effort (i.e., angina or decrease in systolic blood pressure)

RESTRICTION OF SODIUM INTAKE

Institute a low-sodium diet

DIGITALIS GLYCOSIDE AND OTHER INOTROPIC AGENTS

Dopamine
Dobutamine
Amrinone

DIURETICS

Moderate diuretic (thiazide)
Loop diuretic (furosemide)
Loop diuretic plus distal tubular (potassium-sparing) diuretic
Loop diuretic plus thiazide and distal tubular diuretic

VASODILATORS OR VENODILATORS

Captopril, enalapril, or combination of hydralazine plus isosorbide dinitrate
Intensification of oral vasodilator regimen
Intravenous nitroprusside

ANGIOTENSIN-CONVERTING ENZYME

Captopril—may prevent cardiac dilation
Enalapril maleate
Lisinopril

BETA BLOCKERS

Metoprolol
Bucindolol
Xamoterol

SPECIAL MEASURES

Dialysis and ultrafiltration
Assisted circulation (intra-aortic balloon, left ventricular assist device, artificial heart)
Cardiac transplantation

fluid restrictions, and eating heart-healthy foods that are low in cholesterol and fat. Such changes have been observed to decrease hospital readmissions in persons with CHF. Also, dietary counseling alone has been found to produce similar reductions in hospital readmissions and to improve patient outcomes.[171, 172]

Pharmacologic Treatment

Diuretics. Diuretics remain the cornerstone of treatment for CHF.[166] As outlined in Table 4–14, moderate diuretics and loop diuretics are commonly used to reduce the fluid overload of CHF by increasing urine flow. Most of these diuretics act directly on kidney function by inhibiting solute (substances dissolved in a solution) and water reabsorption. As previously discussed, furosemide is the most commonly used diuretic, and its principal site of action is the thick ascending limb of Henle's loop, where it inhibits the cotransport of sodium, potassium, and chloride.[166]

Digoxin and Other Positive Inotropic Agents. Digoxin (digitalis) is one of medicine's oldest drugs, and most of the digitalis drugs in use today are steroid glycosides derived from the leaves of the flowering plant foxglove, or *Digitalis purpurea*. Despite its long history, there is still controversy over its use in patients with CHF and normal sinus rhythm.[173–175] However, several studies have demonstrated favorable hemodynamic and clinical responses in selected patients.[176–180] The most significant clinical observations tend to be related to the positive inotropic (increased force of contraction) effect evidenced by an increased left ventricular ejection fraction.[181] In addition, the electrophysiologic effects of digoxin on the heart help control rapid supraventricular arrhythmias (primarily atrial fibrillation or flutter) by increasing the parasympathetic tone in the sinus and atrioventricular nodes, thereby slowing conduction.[181]

Dopamine. Dopamine hydrochloride is a chemical precursor of norepinephrine, which stimulates dopaminergic, beta$_2$-adrenergic, and alpha-adrenergic receptors as well as the release of norepinephrine. This results in increased cardiac output and, at doses greater than 10 μg/kg/min, markedly increased systemic vascular resistance and preload.[27] For this reason, the primary indication for dopamine is hemodynamically significant hypotension in the absence of hypovolemia.[27] Dopamine is also useful for patients with refractory CHF, in which case it is carefully titrated until urine flow or hemodynamic parameters improve. In such patients, the hemodynamic and renal effects of dopamine can be profound, and frequently, it is infused together with nitroprusside or nitroglycerin to counteract the vasoconstricting action. In addition, dopamine is frequently administered (as are dobutamine and amrinone) during and after cardiac surgery to improve low cardiac output states.[27]

Dobutamine. Dobutamine is a **sympathomimetic** amine that stimulates beta$_1$- and alpha-adrenergic receptors in the myocardium, thus providing potent inotropic effects.[182] Like dopamine, dobutamine increases cardiac output, but the peripheral resistance decreases; with the use of dopamine, there is a potentially significant increase in peripheral resistance. For this reason, "dobutamine and moderate volume loading are the treatment of choice in patients with hemodynamically significant right ventricular infarction."[27]

Amrinone. Amrinone is a phosphodiesterase inhibitor that produces rapid inotropic and vasodilatory effects but unfortunately can exacerbate myocardial ischemia if coronary occlusion exists.[183] Amrinone can also cause thrombocytopenia in 2% to 3% of patients as well as a variety of other side effects (e.g., gastrointestinal dysfunction, myalgia, fever, hepatic dysfunction, cardiac arrhythmias). Despite these adverse effects, amrinone is recommended and has proved to be therapeutic for patients with severe CHF that is refractory to diuretics, vasodilators, and other inotropic agents.[184]

Several other phosphodiesterase inhibitors (milrinone, pimobendan, and enoximone) appear to be promising for patients in the previously mentioned category.[185, 186] In particular, an increase in exercise tolerance has been observed with the use of milrinone.[185]

Vasodilators and Venodilators. Vasodilators are given to patients with CHF or CMD to relax smooth muscle in peripheral arterioles and produce peripheral vasodilation that decreases the afterload, lessens the work of the heart, and potentially decreases the degree of CMD.[181] Two important studies have demonstrated a 38%[187] and 31%[188] improvement in survival rates in patients

with classes II to III CHF and class IV CHF, respectively, utilizing hydralazine and isosorbide dinitrate. Isosorbide dinitrate not only dilates peripheral arterioles, but also relaxes smooth muscle in the peripheral vessels and thus produces a venodilation that redistributes "blood volume away from the heart and thereby lowers right and left ventricular filling pressures."[181] This action reduces the preload and afterload, which is of major importance for patients with moderate to severe CMD. The clinical management of patients with CHF and CMD frequently combines vasodilators, venodilators, and angiotensin-converting enzyme inhibitors.

Angiotensin-Converting Enzyme Inhibitors. The combined use of **angiotensin-converting enzyme** inhibitors, vasodilators, and venodilators has been demonstrated to be very effective in reducing symptoms and improving exercise tolerance.[189] The primary mechanism of action of these inhibitors is probably via the reduction of **angiotensin II,** a hormone that causes vasoconstriction,[181] but other less well-defined actions may be responsible for the therapeutic effects of angiotensin-converting enzyme inhibitors in patients with CHF. Other poorly understood mechanisms of such inhibitors include "nonspecific vasodilation with unloading of the ventricle, inhibition of excessive sympathetic drive and perhaps modulation of tissue receptor systems."[181]

A great deal of interest has focused on the "prevention" hypothesis regarding the use of angiotensin-converting enzyme inhibitors and the prevention of progressive CMD (dilation and CHF).[190-193] Notably, captopril may prevent such progressive cardiac dilation.[190, 191]

Beta-Adrenergic Antagonists and Partial Agonists. Perhaps one of the most confusing groups of medications used in treating CHF and CMD is beta-adrenergic blockers. One of the many uses of beta blockers is to lower blood pressure, primarily via a reduction in cardiac output.[181] This reduction in cardiac output is the result of a decrease in heart rate and stroke volume, which causes an increase in end-diastolic volume and end-diastolic pressure (primarily because of a slower heart rate, which allows more time for the ventricles to fill before the next myocardial contraction) but somewhat paradoxically reduces the myocardial oxygen requirement.[189] This paradoxical reduction in oxygen requirement is probably the result of a decrease in sympathetic nervous system stimulation because of beta blocker therapy. Sympathetic (catecholamine-driven) increases in heart rate, force of myocardial contraction, velocity, and extent of myocardial contraction, as well as systolic blood pressure, are prevented by beta blockade.[194–195]

Although the mechanisms of action of beta blocker therapy may appear to be helpful to patients in CHF, the use of these medications is still considered experimental because of a lack of large multicenter controlled studies[181] and because the use of beta blockers may "exacerbate CHF by removing sympathetic support from a diseased myocardium."[196] Several uncontrolled observational studies have suggested that small doses of metoprolol (Lopressor) may be efficacious for some patients with CHF and idiopathic dilated cardiomyopathy.[197–201] These studies have hypothesized that the excessive sympathetic nervous system activity common in CHF further depresses myocardial performance, and that "down-regulation of myocardial beta-adrenergic receptors occurs in heart failure."[181] One placebo-controlled trial did confirm this hypothesis, but other studies utilizing beta blockers with intrinsic sympathomimetic activity (e.g., oxprenolol and pindolol), which provide a slight stimulation of the blocked receptor that preserves adequate beta-adrenergic sympathetic tone and maintains cardiac output, have failed to demonstrate clinical benefit in patients with CHF.[202–204]

Beta blockers with peripheral dilating activity (bucindolol) as well as partial beta agonists (drugs with both beta-adrenergic agonist and beta-blocking activity, i.e., xamoterol) may be much more effective in treating CHF and CMD.[205–208] Partial beta agonists may possibly protect "the heart from down-regulation of beta receptors during the progressive rise in sympathetic activity that presumably occurs in advanced heart failure."[181]

Mechanical and Surgical Treatment

Patients who respond unfavorably to the aforementioned methods of treatment for CHF and CMD and who demonstrate signs and symptoms of se-

vere CHF are frequently managed using several rather extreme methods. As noted in Table 4–14, there are three "special measures" categories for treating CHF and CMD: dialysis and ultrafiltration, assisted circulation, and cardiac transplantation.

Dialysis and Ultrafiltration

The mechanical removal of fluid from the pleural and abdominal cavities of patients with CHF is usually unnecessary, but patients unresponsive to diuretic therapy because of severe CHF or insensitivity to diuretics may be in need of peritoneal dialysis or **extracorporeal ultrafiltration.**[166] The mechanical removal of fluid in patients with acute respiratory distress because of large pleural effusions or diaphragms elevated by ascites (both of which compress the lungs) frequently brings rapid relief of dyspnea. However, mechanical removal of fluid (primarily peritoneal dialysis) may be associated with risk of **pneumothorax,** infection, **peritonitis, hypernatremia, hyperglycemia, hyperosmolality,** and cardiac arrhythmias.[166, 209] Cardiovascular collapse may also occur if too much fluid is removed or if removal takes place too rapidly. It is recommended that no more than 200 mL of fluid per hour be removed and no greater than 1500 mL of pleural fluid be removed during dialysis.[166, 209]

For these reasons as well as for simplicity, cost effectiveness, and long-lasting effects, ultrafiltration has recently been the treatment of choice for patients in need of mechanical fluid removal.[209] Extracorporeal ultrafiltration is a relatively new technique, which removes plasma water and sodium via an ultrafiltrate (a blend of water, electrolytes, and other small molecules with concentrations identical to those in plasma) from the blood by convective transport through a highly permeable membrane. Ultrafiltration can be performed vein-to-vein using an extracorporeal pump or with an arteriovenous approach.[209]

Although hemodynamic side effects (hypotension, organ malperfusion, and hemolysis) are also possible with ultrafiltration, proper monitoring of the rate of blood flow through the filter (rates above 150 mL/min or below 500 mL/hour are tolerated without side effects) as well as right atrial pressure (ultrafiltration should be discontinued when the right atrial pressure falls to 2 or

3 mm Hg)[210] and hematocrit levels (should not exceed 50%) should, for the most part, prevent them.[209]

Assisted Circulation

Several methods of treatment assist the circulation of blood throughout the body. Perhaps the most widely used is intra-aortic balloon counterpulsation via the intra-aortic balloon pump (IABP). The intra-aortic balloon pump catheter is positioned in the thoracic aorta just distal to the left subclavian artery via the right or left femoral artery (Fig. 4–17). Inflation of the balloon occurs at the beginning of ventricular diastole, immediately after closure of the aortic valve. This increases intra-aortic pressure as well as diastolic pressure in general and forces blood in the aortic arch to flow in a retrograde direction into the coronary arteries. This mechanism of action is referred to as *diastolic* augmentation and profoundly improves oxygen delivery to the myocardium.[144] In addition to this physiologic assist (greater availability of oxygen for myocardial energy production) to improve cardiac performance, hemodynamic assistance is also obtained as the balloon deflates just before systole, which decreases left ventricular afterload by forcing blood to move from an area of higher pressure to one of lower pressure to fill the space previously occupied by the balloon.[144] Consequently, the intra-aortic balloon pump causes "a 10 to 20% increase in cardiac output as well as a reduction in systolic and an increase in diastolic arterial pressure with little change in mean pressure. There is also a diminution of heart rate and an increase in urine output."[144] In addition, intra-aortic balloon counterpulsation produces a reduction in myocardial oxygen consumption "and decreased myocardial ischemia and anaerobic metabolism,"[144] all of which are very important in the management of CHF and CMD.

The intra-aortic balloon pump is occasionally used in conjunction with a slightly different but similar treatment called **pulmonary artery balloon counterpulsation (PABC)** in the pulmonary artery versus the thoracic aorta, which is helpful in treating right ventricular and biventricular failure unresponsive to inotropic drugs and the intra-aortic balloon pump alone.[144]

Temporary Left Ventricular Assist Devices

Patients awaiting heart transplantation, or those in whom ventricular function is expected to return, occasionally benefit from prosthetic devices that consist of a flexible polyurethane blood sac and diaphragm placed within a rigid case outside the body (Fig. 4–18). Pulses of compressed carbon dioxide from a pneumatic drive line are delivered between the rigid case and the diaphragm. This provides the force necessary to eject blood that has traveled to the prosthetic device via a cannula inserted into the left ventricle through a Dacron graft into the ascending aorta and finally to the periphery. This device can handle almost all the output from the left side of the heart,[166] providing rest or assistance to the impaired myocardium.

A fully implanted left ventricular assist device (LVAD), similar to the previously discussed pros-

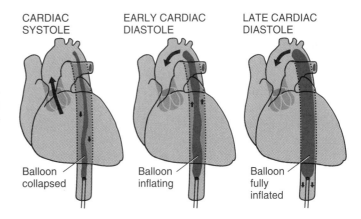

Figure 4–17. The intra-aortic balloon pump. Inflation and deflation of the intra-aortic balloon pump improve diastolic and systolic heart function, respectively.

CARDIAC SYSTOLE   EARLY CARDIAC DIASTOLE   LATE CARDIAC DIASTOLE

Balloon collapsed   Balloon inflating   Balloon fully inflated

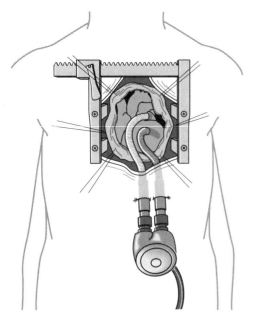

Figure 4–18. Left ventricular assist device. The left ventricular assist device provides myocardial assistance until heart transplantation or corrective measures are taken.

thetic device, that requires no external machinery has been developed.[211] This device, manufactured by the Novacor Corporation, "has an internal computer that serves as a miniaturized controller, with electrical power supplied by a wire buried beneath the skin around the waist"[211] and is activated by inducing a gentle current through the skin. This allows the patient mobility and almost totally eliminates the risk of infection, which is common with the pneumatic-driven devices.

Surgical Treatments

Reparative, reconstructive, excisional, and ablative surgeries are sometimes performed in the treatment of CHF and CMD. Reparative procedures correct cardiac malfunctions such as ventricular septal defect, atrial septal defect, and mitral stenosis and frequently improve cardiac hemodynamics, resulting in improved cardiac performance. Coronary artery bypass graft surgery is probably the most common reconstructive surgery because myocardial ischemia and infarction are the primary causes of CMD and CHF.[212] Its effects are often profound, improving cardiac muscle function and eliminating CHF. Reconstruction of incompetent

heart valves is also common.[21] Excisional procedures, in patients with atrial **myxomas** (tumors) and large left ventricles, are employed less often. The excision of a tumor or **aneurysm** is occasionally performed, and the excised area is replaced with Dacron patches.[21] Ablative procedures are also used less frequently, but for patients with persistent and symptomatic **Wolff-Parkinson-White syndrome** or intractable ventricular tachycardia, ablation (via laser or cryotherapy, etc.) of the reentry pathways appears to be very therapeutic.[21] The surgical implantation of automatic implantable defibrillators has become increasingly common and also appears to be of great therapeutic value for those with ventricular tachycardia that is unresponsive to medications and ablative procedures.[21]

Left Ventricular Muscle Flaps. Although somewhat unusual, the use of muscle flaps (cardiomyoplasty), usually dissected from the latissimus dorsi or trapezius muscle, may be an alternative treatment for a limited number of patients with severe CMD and CHF.[211] The muscle flap is wrapped around the left ventricle and attached to a pacemaker, which stimulates the flap to contract, thus contracting the left ventricle. Many years of animal research have provided procedural treatment protocols and have resulted in the use of muscle flap techniques in approximately 12 human subjects who apparently "carry on a reasonably normal life with adequate exercise tolerance."[211]

The major problem with the use of muscle flaps is muscle fatigue, because skeletal muscle, unlike cardiac muscle, does not have the ability to contract continuously. However, it has been demonstrated that skeletal muscle, after careful training and conditioning, "could adapt itself and assume the functions of the cardiac muscle."[211] This is an area in which physical therapy has the potential to make significant contributions, but further investigation is needed.

Cardiomyoplasty (Partial Left Ventriculectomy—Batista Procedure). Several investigations have shown that the removal of dilated, noncontracting myocardium of persons with CHF and subsequent suturing of remaining viable myocardial tissue decrease the left ventricular chamber size and improve myocardial performance. Improvements in myocardial performance appear to improve the functional status and symptoms of CHF.[213–215]

Cardiac Transplantation. Cardiac transplantation is the last treatment effort for a patient with CHF and CMD because "potential recipients of cardiac transplants must have end-stage heart disease with severe heart failure and a life expectancy of less than one year."[166] Heart transplantation can be **heterologous** (or xenograft, from a nonhuman primate) or more commonly **homologous** (or allograft, from another human).[166] **Orthotopic** homologous cardiac transplantation is performed by removing the recipient's heart, leaving the posterior walls of the atria with their venous connections on which the donor's atria are sutured. In heterotopic homologous cardiac transplantation, the recipient's heart is left intact and the donor heart is placed in parallel, with anastomoses between the two right atria, pulmonary arteries, left atria, and aorta. Heterotopic heart transplantation may be preferable to orthotopic transplantation because if the donor heart is rejected (a primary complicating factor, as are infection and nephrotoxicity secondary to vigorous immunosuppression), the presence of the patient's own heart may improve the likelihood of survival.[166] However, orthotopic heart transplantation is most commonly performed.

A more complete description of cardiac transplantation is provided in Chapter 12, but can be summarized here: "in the absence of rejection, the transplanted heart, which is denervated and lacks autonomic neural control, exhibits normal contractility and contractile reserve," and "as a consequence of this near-normal circulatory response, the transplanted heart permits excellent functional and social and vocational rehabilitation in 90 percent of long-term survivors."[166]

Current Perspectives on Exercise Training

Traditional Exercise Training

Much of the investigation into the issue of CHF and exercise has focused on one of the earlier findings regarding exercise tolerance and anaerobic metabolism. Many patients with CHF apparently have a lower anaerobic threshold than normal individuals, and the resultant anaerobic metabolism becomes the limiting factor (because of lactate acidosis) in exercise performance. The lower anaerobic threshold may be due in part to reduced blood flow to exercising muscles in patients with CHF and is probably the reason that these patients were observed to have a 40% lower exercise capacity than a group of control subjects.[216]

In view of these findings, it seems likely that exercise training should improve the **oxidative capacity** of skeletal muscle, which would reduce lactate production and thereby increase exercise capacity. Three studies have demonstrated such benefits from exercise training in patients with mild-to-moderate CHF (many of whom had cardiomyopathy).[217-219] Perhaps the most detailed study was performed by Sullivan and colleagues, who evaluated the effects of exercise training in patients with chronic heart failure due to left ventricular dysfunction (ejection fraction of $24 \pm 10\%$).[217] After the training period, central hemodynamic and peripheral metabolic adaptations to heart failure were improved, including an increased exercise tolerance and increased $VO_{2\,max}$.[217]

Similar results were also observed in a study of a larger number of subjects (n = 41) with moderately impaired left ventricular function,[218] as well as in a study that utilized **arm ergometry** exercise training alone.[219] The results of this study of 11 patients with a mean left ventricular ejection fraction of $30.1 \pm 9.5\%$ showed an increased work capacity, peak heart rate, peak rate-pressure product, and left ventricular ejection fraction.[219] An important observation in all these studies was that no complications occurred during the exercise training programs, and no further deterioration of ventricular function occurred.

An increase in submaximal oxygen consumption is opposite that seen in normal individuals after exercise training, and the decrease in oxygen consumption seen in normal subjects after exercise training (which is suggestive of improved exercise efficiency) appears to be a training adaptation that is not seen in persons with severe CHF. Although it appears that these patients are less efficient, they are able to perform greater peak workloads and achieve greater peak cardiorespiratory function than prior to exercise training.[220]

An additional factor that was recently considered in exercising persons with CHF is the importance of the relationship between venous return and myocardial performance during exercise. In the early 1980s Foster et al. observed that left ventricular function decreased at maximal exercise and improved immediately after exercise, most likely as a result of decreased venous return from pooling of blood in the lower extremities.[310] Using the above-mentioned concept of improved left ventricular function after exercise is abruptly terminated, a recent exercise training study of persons with severe CHF hypothesized that reductions in venous return and left ventricular end-diastolic pressure may accompany interval exercise training more than during constant, longer duration exercise training and contribute to enhanced training adaptations.[21] Such a possibility appears to exist because significant improvements in cardiorespiratory function were observed after only 3 weeks of such interval exercise training.[21]

Two other studies have demonstrated the importance of a thorough assessment and reassessment as well as an understanding of each patient's disease process to identify specific criteria necessary to promote training effects.[221, 222] Arvan demonstrated that to obtain training effects (for a 12-week training period), patients with left ventricular dysfunction must not exhibit electrocardiographic signs of myocardial ischemia.[221] This finding is not surprising because an individual with left ventricular dysfunction and myocardial ischemia has a poor prognosis from the start.[223] Despite the inability of this group to attain a training effect, routine cardiopulmonary exercise assessments of patients with left ventricular dysfunction can better direct medical therapy and reduce risk factors and *possibly* promote training effects if the exercise training program is performed for an appropriate period of time. As in the study by Coats and colleagues,[238] no complications were reported, but 20 patients were excluded for various reasons (e.g., symptomatic CHF, arrhythmias, severe hypertension). The exclusion of these 20 patients suggests that some patients with left ventricular dysfunction may be inappropriate for exercise training but appropriate for exercise assessments to evaluate symptoms, rhythm, and blood pressure response to varying levels of exertion.[221]

A study by Jugdutt and associates identified patients with left ventricular dysfunction who would benefit least from exercise training.[222] If left ventricular dysfunction was below a specific echocardiographic index of contractility and exercise training was performed, left ventricular function actually deteriorated, decreasing the ejection frac-

tion and functional capacity.[222] These results suggest that initial and follow-up echocardiograms as well as thorough cardiopulmonary exercise assessments must be performed to evaluate patient progression or deterioration.

In summary, based on a large number of studies, exercise assessments and exercise training in patients with poor left ventricular dysfunction can be (1) done safely if patients are thoroughly assessed, (2) quite beneficial (e.g., improve exercise tolerance and awareness of physical capabilities), and (3) invaluable to the primary physician by providing important information that *completes* the physician's assessment and better directs medical therapy. (See Table 4–15 for review of exercise training studies.)[224–256] These concepts are evident in the following quotation:

> *Exercise training appears to be a therapeutic modality that should be considered for patients with ventricular dysfunction related to coronary artery disease. When patients are carefully selected and when exercise training sessions are conducted under close supervision, life-threatening complications of exercise training are infrequent, and favorable physiologic adaptations, most prominently an increase in functional work capacity, occur in most patients. Although only limited data are available, increased levels of physical activity do not appear to have adverse effects on subsequent cardiac mortality or on ventricular function in patients with ventricular dysfunction. In addition, these patients may derive psychologic benefits from participation in exercise training, and the close medical surveillance available in the content of a supervised exercise program may facilitate better clinical decisions concerning pharmacologic therapy, interpretation of symptoms, or the necessity for and timing of operative procedures.[212]*

The end result of such exercise assessments and exercise training is an improved quality of life for patients with CHF.

Exercise Training and Quality of Life

The quality of life of persons with CHF appears to be related to the ability to exercise.[250–260] However, only two recent studies have investigated the effects of exercise training upon the quality of life of persons with CHF.[250, 256] Kavanagh et al.[250] and Keteyian et al.[256] found significant improvements in exercise capacity, symptoms, and quality of life after 24 and 52 weeks of exercise training, respec-

Table 4–15
Review of Exercise Training Studies of Patients with Congestive Heart Failure

AUTHOR	N	Type	EXERCISE TRAINING					MEAN LVEF (%)		COMPLICATIONS	
			Duration	Frequency	Intensity	Training Period	Training Effect	Before Training	After Training	Morbidity	Mortality
Lee	18	W, J, B	20–45 min	2–6x/week	85% HR_{max}	12–42 mo	Positive	35 ± 4	35 ± 6	0	0
Williams	121	?	?	?	?	2–57 mo	Positive	8–26 (n = 14) 30–49 (n = 23) 51–86 (n = 84)	?	?	?
Cody	32	?		4x/week	?	12 mo	Positive	18	?	4	0
Conn	10	B, W/J	35–45 min	3–5x/week	70–80% $VO_{2\,max}$	4–37 mo	Positive	20	?	0	0
Sullivan	16	W, J, B, SC	60 min	3–5x/week	75% $VO_{2\,max}$	4–6 mo	Positive	24 ± 10	Unchanged	4	0
Hoffman	41	?	?	3–7x/week	70–85%	4 mo	Positive	?	?	0	0
Kellerman	11	AE	?	2x/week	90%	36 mo	Positive	30 ± 9.52	?	0	0
Kellerman	11	C	?	2x/week	2.2–7.5 kcal/min	12 mo	Positive	25.5 ± 6.8	?	0	0
Coats	17	B	20 min	5x/week	60–80% HR_{max}	2 mo	Positive	19	?	0	0
Belardinelli*	55	B	40 min	3x/week	60% $VO_{2\,max}$	2 mo	Positive	27	27	3	0
Belardinelli	27	B	30 min	3x/week	40% $VO_{2\,max}$	2 mo	Positive	31 ± 4	33 ± 4	1	0
Squires	20	B, W	30–40 min	4–6x/week	50–60% $VO_{2\,max}$	2 mo	Positive	21 ± 3	?	0	0
Baigrie	17	W	16 min	?	?	4 mo	Positive	21 ± 2	?	?	?
Jette	39	W, J, C, B	30–60 min	5x/week	70–80% HR_{max}	1 mo	Positive	I:24 ± 3.5 II:39 ± 6	28 ± 8 41 ± 9	3 0	0
Meyer	15	B	20–25 min	5x/week	70–80% HR_{max}	1.5 mo	Positive	23 ± 3.2	?	1	1
Hambrecht	22	B	10 min 6x/day for 3 wks; then 40–60 min	7x/week	70% $VO_{2\,max}$	6 mo	Positive	26 ± 9	?	1	1
Kulavuori	20	B	30 min	3x/week	50–60% $VO_{2\,max}$	3 mo	Positive	24 ± 6	?	0	0
Davey	22	B	20 min	5x/week	70–80% HR_{max}	2 mo	Positive	22 ± 8	?	0	0
Koch	25	K	90 min	3x/week	?	3 mo	Positive	26 ± 10	27 ± 10	0	0
Kostis	20	W, B, RW, SC	60 min	3–5x/week	40–60% func. capacity	3 mo	Positive	35 ± 6	32 ± 6	0	0
Meyer	18	B, W	15 min†	3–5x/week	50% $WORK_{max}$†	3 weeks	Positive	21 ± 1	?	0	0
Kavanagh‡	30	W	26–48 min	5x/week	50–60% $VO_{2\,max}$	12 mo	Positive	21 ± 1.5	27 ± 2	4	0
Tyni-Lenne‡	21	B	15 min	3x/week	I:35% $WORK_{max}$ II:70% $WORK_{max}$	2 mo	Positive	28 ± 11	?	0	0
Belardinelli	99	C	40 min	2–3x/week	60% $VO_{2\,max}$	14 mo	Positive	28 ± 6	31 ± 7	10	0

*First study to evaluate the effects of exercise training in patients with diastolic dysfunction.

† Bicycling exercise was performed 5x/week for 15 min in an interval manner with work phases of 30 sec at 50% of the maximal work rate achieved and active recovery phases of 50 sec during which patients pedaled at 15 watts. Walking exercise was performed 3x/week for 10 min in an interval manner with work phases of 60 sec (mean treadmill speed = 2.4 mph) and 60 sec of active recovery (mean treadmill speed = 0.9 mph).

‡ First studies to evaluate the quality of life of persons with heart failure before and after exercise training. Improvements in quality of life and beneficial training effects were observed in both studies.

Codes for type of exercise: W = walking; J = jogging; B = bicycling; RW = rowing; W/J = walking/jogging; SC = stair climbing; AE = arm ergometry; C = calisthenics; K = Koch strength/endurance training device; $VO_{2\,max}$ = maximal oxygen consumption.

LVEF = left ventricular ejection fraction; HR = heart rate.

153

tively. Therefore, in view of limited data, quality of life does appear to be improved after exercise training in persons with CHF.

Nontraditional Exercise Training

Exercise Training During Continuous Intravenous Dobutamine Infusion. Many patients with severe CHF are hospitalized for prolonged periods, receiving continuous IV dobutamine infusion for inotropic support (to improve cardiac muscle contraction) while awaiting cardiac transplantation.[261] Also, it is becoming common practice for patients with severe CHF to occasionally be hospitalized for IV dobutamine infusion ("dobutamine holiday") to transiently improve myocardial performance.[262] Many patients are also being sent home on portable IV dobutamine pumps, and their physical activity is therefore less restricted when the large IV pumps are not used.[263] However, exercise training during continuous IV dobutamine infusion has received little attention.[264]

Individuals receiving inotropic support have only recently been prescribed exercise training programs.[265] Kataoka et al.[264] presented the results of a single case study in which a 53-year-old man with CHF was prescribed an exercise training program while receiving 10 μg/kg/min IV dobutamine (which he had been prescribed for 10 months prior to exercise training). Positive training adaptations were observed without complication and resulted in the patient being weaned from dobutamine.[265] The author has also observed safe and beneficial effects of exercise training during IV dobutamine infusion.[266] Further investigation of exercise training in this patient population is needed.

Exercise Training with Left Ventricular Assist Devices. Particular adjuncts to exercise conditioning in CHF include mechanical support of severe CMD via intra-aortic balloon pumps (IABP) and left or right ventricular assist devices. Although individuals with IABP are limited to breathing exercises and gentle exercise with upper extremities and the noncatheterized leg, individuals with left ventricular assist devices (LVAD) have enjoyed the freedom to exercise with minimal limitation. Improved technology has enabled patients, who otherwise were immobilized because of intra-aortic balloon pump placement or nonmobile

LVAD placement, to become mobile and ambulate with a cart or electric belt system that provides left ventricular assistance via portable pumping of the heart.[267] Patients using LVADs underwent 1173.6 hours of exercise conditioning without major complication and with only four minor complications (3.4 incidents per 1000 patient hours). The four minor complications were quickly corrected and resulted from an acute decrease in pump flow from venous pooling, decreased drive line air volume, and hypovolemia. Improvements in exercise tolerance and functional capacity continued until week 6 of conditioning, after which further improvements were minimal. It has been suggested that delay in cardiac transplantation until 6 weeks of exercise conditioning have been performed may improve postoperative recovery and surgical success.[268]

The reason for a lack of further improvement in exercise tolerance and functional capacity after week 6 was most likely due to the mechanical constraints of the LVAD. Cardiopulmonary exercise testing has demonstrated that LVAD patients demonstrate a modest training effect from chronic exercise training and appear to be limited at maximal exercise by the mechanics of the LVAD.[269] The mechanical constraints of the LVAD appear to prevent maximal levels of exercise from being attained and result in no substantial change in peak oxygen consumption after a mean of 16 weeks of aerobic exercise training. Possible mechanical constraints of the LVAD include flow limitations (10 to 12 L/min), altered cardiovascular function from the mechanically driven cardiac output, and the effects of a 6-lb mass resting below the diaphragm that may alter ventilatory performance. Limited training adaptations may also be due to the same mechanism, but the reductions in submaximal heart rate and blood pressure as well as increases in exercise duration, ventilation, and oxygen consumption at the ventilatory threshold support the benefits that can be attained by exercising patients on LVAD.[269]

Exercise Training During Continuous Positive Airway Pressure Ventilation. Continuous positive airway pressure (CPAP) and bilevel positive airway pressure (BiPAP) have been observed to improve the exercise performance of patients with obstructive lung disease.[270-272] Despite the lack of research on the effect of CPAP or BiPAP upon the exercise performance of patients with

CHF, resting myocardial performance has repeatedly been observed to improve with CPAP in patients with CHF[273-275] and patients with CHF and coexistent obstructive or central sleep apnea.[276-278] The beneficial effect of CPAP upon cardiac performance is postulated to be due to increased intrathoracic pressure, which reduces cardiac preload (by impeding cardiac filling) and afterload (by reducing left ventricular transmural pressure)[273, 274, 278-280] as well as unloading the inspiratory muscles by providing positive pressure ventilation that may increase lung compliance.[275] The effects of CPAP or BiPAP upon exercise performance in patients with CHF are unknown, but several studies cited here have noted an improvement in dyspnea and functional status, and limited pilot work that we have performed suggests an improvement in exercise tolerance and symptoms when BiPAP was used in conjunction with functional and exercise training.[281]

In pilot work, reduced symptoms and improved cardiovascular performance and exercise tolerance have been observed in a single subject case study of a person with muscular dystrophy and severe heart failure.[281] BiPAP allowed this person to perform physical exercise he had been unable to do previously. Also of note in this same patient was the observation of marked pursed-lip breathing while weaning from the BiPAP during bouts of physical exercise. When pursed-lip breathing was performed, the patient's symptoms and exercise tolerance markedly improved.

Ventilatory Muscle Training—Breathing Exercises and Inspiratory and Expiratory Muscle Training

Breathing Exercises. Persons with CHF appear to benefit from breathing exercises.[117, 282] Breathing exercises can be simple or complex and should be provided after a measurement of breathing strength is obtained. Such measurements include the maximal inspiratory pressure (MIP) and the maximal expiratory pressure (MEP), which are frequently measured with a manometer in centimeters of water. After strength measurements are obtained, patients are provided a breathing exercise program at a specific percentage of the MIP or MEP (similar to aerobic exercise training) with a device that resists either inspiration or expiration. The methods of measuring MIP and MEP and implementing a ventilatory muscle training program are provided.[117, 282]

Facilitation of diaphragmatic breathing and inhibition of excessive accessory muscle use may decrease the work of breathing for a person with CHF and in conjunction with pursed-lip breathing may improve respiratory performance and possibly, cardiac performance. Pursed-lip breathing has been shown to be beneficial for persons with COPD by maintaining airway patency via increased positive end-expiratory pressure (PEEP).[283, 284] In view of recent research, the same maintenance of airways from increased PEEP may be helpful for persons with CHF.[118, 285] Furthermore, the increased PEEP and associated increase in intrathoracic pressure from varying degrees of pursed-lip breathing may decrease venous return which could possibly decrease the left ventricular end-diastolic volume and pressure and improve myocardial performance for persons with severe CHF.[286]

In a recent study it was discovered that patients with higher left ventricular end-diastolic volumes demonstrated a greater degree of dyspnea before inspiratory muscle training and a greater percentage improvement in dyspnea after inspiratory muscle training.[285] Although this finding does not fully support the possible effects of pursed-lip breathing upon improving myocardial performance, it does imply that during the expiratory phase of breathing (whether it is through an inspiratory muscle trainer with a narrowed orifice that the mouth is placed over and through which a person expires or with pursed lips) changes may take place that are of benefit to the cardiac and pulmonary systems (Table 4–16).[286]

Expiratory Muscle Training. The majority of studies investigating the effects of expiratory muscle training have involved persons with spinal cord injury or other neurologic disorders. In the majority of these studies expiratory muscle training (performed in a variety of ways but most commonly with weights upon the abdomen and hyperpneic breathing) improved symptoms, functional status, and pulmonary function and reduced pulmonary complications. There is a recent interest in expiratory muscle training of persons with various forms of COPD using PEEP devices but very little literature exists. Likewise, there is little literature regarding expiratory muscle training alone in CHF. A study by Mancini et al. evaluated the effects of inspiratory and expiratory muscle training in CHF and found significant improvements in ventilatory muscle force and endurance, submaximal and

Table 4–16

Key Impairments and Functional Limitations of Congestive Heart Failure and Possible Physical Therapy Interventions

KEY IMPAIRMENTS	PHYSICAL THERAPY INTERVENTION
Dyspnea	Supplemental oxygen, pursed-lip breathing, breathing exercises, ventilatory muscle training
Fatigue	Supplemental oxygen, rest, proper diet and nutrition, pharmacologic agents, individualized gradual progressive exercise training program, patient education

KEY FUNCTIONAL LIMITATIONS	PHYSICAL THERAPY INTERVENTION
Walking	Gait training, strength and aerobic exercise training, balance training
Climbing stairs	Stair stepper exercise, functional exercise training (stair climbing)
Housework and yard-work	Functional activity training
Lifting boxes	Functional activity training
Recreational activities and hobbies	Recreational/hobby training

Physical therapy intervention directed to specific impairments and functional limitations is likely to produce central and peripheral adaptations (cardiovascular, respiratory, and neuromuscular) that should require less cardiac work and subsequently improve the symptoms of congestive heart failure. However, further investigation is necessary to understand if specific training in the listed areas actually improves the symptoms, impairments, and functional limitations of congestive heart failure.

maximal exercise performance, and dyspnea after 3 months of aggressive ventilatory muscle training in eight patients with chronic CHF.[282]

Despite a lack of research in expiratory muscle training alone in CHF, the observations of Mancini et al.[282] and others suggest that expiratory muscle training may be beneficial for persons with CHF by (1) increasing expiratory muscle strength to improve pulmonary function, (2) increasing PEEP to improve airway compliance, and (3) possibly decreasing venous return and the left ventricular end-diastolic volume to improve myocardial performance.[286] These changes may improve the exercise tolerance and functional status of persons with CHF. However, further investigation is needed in this area.

Inspiratory Muscle Training. Inspiratory muscle training has previously been shown to be helpful for patients with pulmonary disease by increasing ventilatory muscle strength and endurance and by decreasing dyspnea, need for medications, emergency room visits, and number of hospitalizations.[287, 288] Recently, individuals with chronic CHF have been found to have poor ventilatory muscle strength,[289-291] and as mentioned earlier, Mancini et al. demonstrated significant improvements in ventilatory muscle strength and endurance, submaximal and maximal exercise capacity, and dyspnea after 3 months of aggressive inspiratory and expiratory muscle training in eight patients with chronic CHF.[282]

Significant improvements in maximal inspiratory and expiratory pressures and degree of dyspnea were recently observed as soon as 2 weeks after ventilatory muscle training was initiated with the Threshold inspiratory muscle trainer at 20% of maximal inspiratory pressure, three times a day, for 5 to 15 minutes (Fig. 4–19).[117] The improvement in ventilatory muscle strength was associated with significantly less dyspnea at rest and with exercise. However, the effects of ventilatory muscle training upon ventilatory muscle endurance, which may be the most important effect of ventilatory muscle training in this patient population, were not evaluated. Nonetheless, improvement in ventilatory muscle strength may decrease the dependency, impairment, and possibly even cost associated with chronic CHF. Increased ventilatory muscle strength may also enhance early postoperative recovery in patients undergoing cardiac transplantation or other cardiac surgery.

Guidelines for Exercise Training

The aforementioned studies that demonstrated improvements in exercise tolerance and patient symptoms were all performed using different methodology; varying modes, intensities, durations, and frequencies of exercise. Specific guidelines for exercise training of patients with CHF are difficult

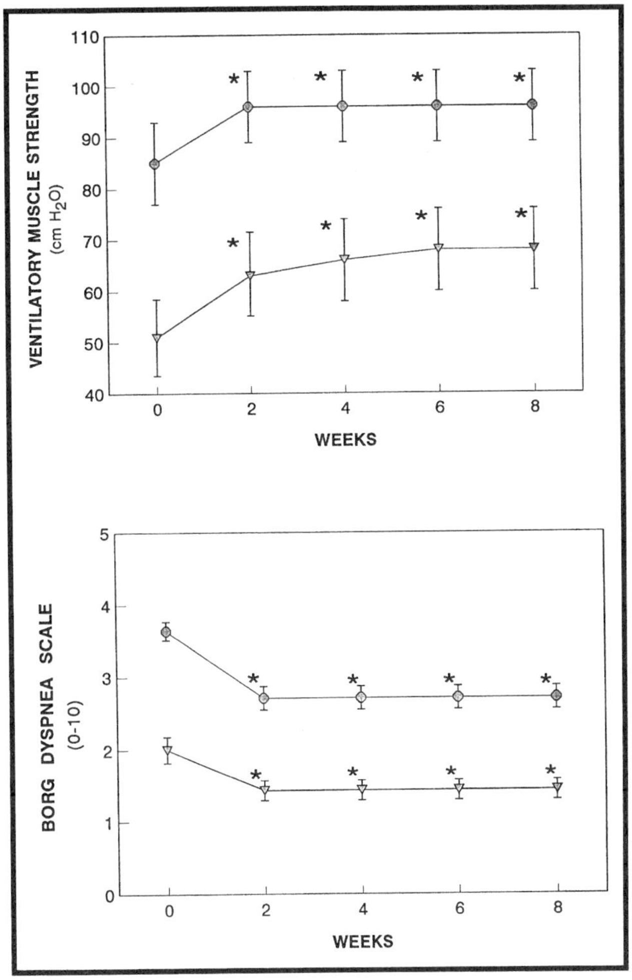

Figure 4-19. *Top,* Maximal inspiratory pressure (triangle) and maximal expiratory pressure (circle) throughout the ventilatory muscle training period. *Bottom,* Dyspnea at rest (triangle) and during submaximal exercise (circle) throughout the ventilatory muscle training period. Asterisks (*) indicate values that are different from baseline values ($p < .05$). (Reprinted from Cahalin LP, Semigran MJ, Dec G. Inspiratory muscle training in patients with chronic heart failure awaiting cardiac transplantation: Results of a pilot clinical trial. Physical Therapy 77:519, 1997. With permission of the American Physical Therapy Association.)

to implement because patient status frequently changes. Despite a lack of specific guidelines for exercising persons with CHF, the U.S. Department of Health and Human Services Agency for Health Care Policy and Research recently outlined the importance of exercise training in treatment of CHF.[292] Exercise training was recommended "as an integral component of the symptomatic management" of persons with CHF "to attain functional and symptomatic improvement but with a potentially higher likelihood of adverse events." This recommendation was based upon significant scientific evidence from previously published investigations that were reviewed by experts in the field of cardiac rehabilitation.[292]

Patients with decompensated (uncontrolled) CHF are typically very dyspneic and therefore should not begin aerobic exercise training until

the CHF is compensated. Specific exercise training guidelines are listed in Table 4-17 and include the attainment of a cardiac index of 2.0 L/min/m² or greater (for invasively monitored patients in the hospital) before aerobic exercise training is implemented and the maintenance of an adequate pulse pressure (not less than a 10 mm Hg difference between the systolic and diastolic blood pressure) during exercise. The development of marked dyspnea and fatigue, S_3 heart sound, or crackles during exercise requires the modification or termination of exercise.[266]

Progression of an exercise conditioning program for patients with CHF can be done as outlined in *Activity Guidelines for Patients Hospitalized with CHF* at the end of this chapter. Although this protocol is designed for hospitalized patients, the same methodology and progression can be applied to patients

Table 4-17

Exercise Training Guidelines for Patients with CHF

I. Relative criteria necessary for the initiation of an aerobic exercise training program: Compensated CHF
   A. Ability to speak without signs or symptoms of dyspnea (able to speak comfortably with a RR <30 breaths/min)
   B. < Moderate fatigue
   C. Crackles present in < one half of the lungs
   D. Resting heart rate <120 bpm
   E. Cardiac index ≥2.0 L/min/m² (for invasively monitored patients)
   F. Central venous pressure <12 mm Hg (for invasively monitored patients)

II. Relative criteria indicating a need to modify or terminate exercise training
   A. Marked dyspnea or fatigue (e.g., Borg rating >3/10)
   B. Respiratory rate >40 breaths/min during exercise
   C. Development of an S_3 heart sound or pulmonary crackles
   D. Increase in pulmonary crackles
   E. Significant increase in the sound of the second component of the second heart sound (P_2)
   F. Poor pulse pressure (<10 mm Hg difference between the systolic and diastolic blood pressure)
   G. Decrease in heart rate or blood pressure of >10 bpm or mm Hg, respectively, during continuous (steady state) or progressive (increasing workloads) exercise
   H. Increased supraventricular or ventricular ectopy
   I. Increase of >10 mm Hg in the mean pulmonary artery pressure (for invasively monitored patients)
   J. Increase or decrease of >6 mm Hg in the central venous pressure (for invasively monitored patients)
   K. Diaphoresis, pallor, or confusion

From Cahalin LP. Heart failure. Phys Ther 76:529, 1996, with permission of the American Physical Therapy Association.

with CHF in outpatient clinics, nursing homes, and their own homes. For most patients, ambulation may be the most effective and functional mode of exercise to administer and prescribe, beginning with frequent short walks and progressing to less frequent, longer bouts of exercise. Occasionally, patients may be so deconditioned that gentle strengthening exercises, restorator cycling, or ventilatory muscle training is the preferred mode of exercise conditioning. As strength and endurance improve, patients can be progressed to upright cycle ergometry or ambulating with a rolling walker.

Because dyspnea is the most common complaint of patients with CHF, the level of dyspnea or Borg rating of perceived exertion appears to be an acceptable method to prescribe and evaluate an exercise program.[212] This is supported by the observation that these subjective indices correlate well with training heart rate ranges in this patient population.[293] Therefore, a basic guideline of increasing the exercise intensity to a level that produces a moderate degree of dyspnea (conversing with modest difficulty, ability to count to 5 without taking a breath, or a Borg rating of 3 on a scale of 10) may be the simplest and most effective method to prescribe exercise for patients with CHF. It also appears to be the most effective method to progress a patient's exercise prescription. The exercise prescription of patients with CHF can be progressed when (1) the cardiopulmonary response to exercise is adaptive (see Table 4-17) and (2) workloads that previously produced moderate dyspnea (e.g., Borg rating of 3/10) produce mild dyspnea (e.g., Borg rating of 2/10) or less.

Finally, the use of heart rate monitoring to determine exercise intensity and progression of an exercise program may be less reliable for patients with CHF, who often suffer from some degree of renal dysfunction. Reduction in maximal heart rate "may be as much as 20 to 40 beats per minute"[294] lower in such patients and frequently is accompanied by a blunted systolic blood pressure response, despite elevated plasma norepinephrine levels. These results may be due to autonomic dysfunction, which is known to exist in this population of patients.[295] However, specific exercise training guidelines can be obtained for each *individual* patient with CHF or CMD by performing a simple exercise assessment. Although heart rate monitoring may be less reliable, it still appears to be a common method for exercise prescription, as is evident in the following statement by Williams:

For patients who can exercise to fatigue without adverse hemodynamic effects or symptoms, we calculate the training range as 60 to 80 percent of the increment between the resting heart rate and the maximal heart rate attained, adding back to the resting heart rate. For patients who develop angina, a fall in left ventricular ejection fraction, an elevation of pulmonary capillary wedge pressure, or a fall in systemic arterial pressure during exertion, we attempt to quantitate the heart rate at which such adverse effects first occur and prescribe the upper limit of subsequent exercise at a level 10 bpm below the heart rate at which such evidence for hemodynamic compromise occurs.[212]

However, more patients with CMD and CHF are being prescribed beta blockers, which often cause little or no change in resting and exercise heart rates. Therefore, the basic guideline of increasing the respiratory rate to a level that allows one to converse comfortably may be the most effective method for prescribing exercise training in patients with CHF ("talk test").[212]

This same principle appears to be useful for determining patient appropriateness for entry into an outpatient cardiac rehabilitation program.[212] Determining the suitability of patients with CHF for exercise training in cardiac rehabilitation programs appears to depend upon the patient performing any level of exertion for several minutes without excessive *dyspnea* or *fatigue* and without adverse *hemodynamic effects, dysrhythmias,* or *evidence of myocardial ischemia.*[212] With this in mind, the following statement summarizes this approach:

> *It is important to emphasize that exercise training of patients with severe ventricular dysfunction does not necessarily involve levels of effort that normal individuals would regard as strenuous. For a person with congestive heart failure whose activities have been limited to sitting in a chair and walking to the bathroom, walking continuously for 15 minutes at 1.5 to 2.0 mph may represent a level of exertion sufficient to induce favorable physiologic adaptations and therefore constitute physical conditioning.*[212]

CONCLUSION

Physical therapists have much to offer patients with CMD, and it is hoped that a sincere effort in understanding and treating these patients will improve their exercise tolerance, functional status, and quality of life. Simple evaluations such as the 6-minute walk test and observing clinical signs and symptoms during exercise sessions appear to be good predictors of exercise tolerance, functional status, and patient prognosis. The information obtained during such evaluations can also be used by

physicians to more objectively implement medical therapy. Traditional and nontraditional exercise training for persons with CHF appear to be valuable and may have greater importance than originally believed. The appropriateness of exercise training and progression of an exercise training program for persons with CHF can be performed with an assessment of dyspnea. Extreme dyspnea is a contraindication for exercise training in CHF, and improvements in dyspnea scores during an exercise training program is evidence of cardiorespiratory improvement and the need for progression of an exercise prescription.

This material demonstrates the widespread occurrence of CMD and the potential role of physical therapy in treatment. Cardiac muscle dysfunction and CHF are disease processes that will continue to challenge physical therapists.

CASE STUDIES

Case 1

This 85-year-old woman had a medical history of coronary artery bypass graft surgery in 1982 to the right coronary artery and left anterior diagonal artery, cholecystectomy, hiatal hernia, gastritis, and peptic ulcer disease. She was admitted 8/9/98 with angina (a myocardial infarction was ruled out) and underwent cardiac catheterization on 8/16/98, which revealed 99% occlusion of the right coronary artery graft, 85% occlusion of the left anterior diagonal artery graft, 95% stenosis of the circumflex artery, moderate mitral regurgitation, dilated left atrium, inferior hypokinesis, and ejection fraction of approximately 30%. Echocardiographic study revealed severe left ventricular hypertrophy with a small left ventricular chamber size, inferior hypokinesis, calcified mitral valve with moderate mitral regurgitation, abnormal left ventricular compliance (left ventricular stiffness), and a dilated left atrium.

The referral for cardiac rehabilitation was written on 8/11/98, at which time the patient was assessed and complained of left scapular pain that increased with deep breathing (different from previous angina and altered with breathing pattern). Physical examination revealed normal sinus rhythm and slightly decreased breath sounds in the left lower lobe. The patient ambulated approximately 250 feet with an adaptive heart rate and blood pressure response, without angina. The patient continued with twice-daily cardiac rehabilitation, increasing the distance ambulated to 800 feet, and underwent a thallium treadmill stress test on 8/13/98. The patient completed 2 minutes 25 seconds of the modified Bruce protocol (attaining a maximal heart rate of 104 bpm, 67% of the age-predicted maximal heart rate), which was terminated because of leg fatigue. The patient experienced no angina and demonstrated no electrocardiographic (ECG) changes consistent with myocardial ischemia. The thallium scan demonstrated moderately severe stress-induced ischemic change in the inferior and septal areas.

Cardiac rehabilitation was performed 8/14/98 through 8/16/98, during which the patient walked 5 to 10 minutes (500 to 1000 feet) with adaptive heart rate and blood pressure responses to exercise, without angina. On 8/17/98, while resting in bed, the patient developed severe angina and dyspnea, which required morphine sulfate, nitroglycerin, and heparin, suggesting impending graft occlusion. In view of these findings, coronary artery bypass graft surgery was repeated on 8/20/98, after which the patient developed numerous complications, requiring intra-aortic balloon pump assistance from which weaning was difficult. In addition, the patient experienced a postoperative anterolateral myocardial infarction as a result of a third-degree heart block that decreased the blood supply to the myocardium, respiratory failure that required full ventilatory support, congestive heart failure, and severe abdominal distention.

The patient's status further deteriorated as she became anemic and was unable to maintain adequate nutritional requirements. However, a radiograph on 8/24/98 revealed no evidence of CHF, and ventilatory measurements demonstrated improved pulmonary function. In addition, hemoglobin and hematocrit levels were slightly increased (10.7 and 29.4, respectively). The patient was extubated on 8/25/98 and began ambulation with nursing on 8/26/98, during which she complained of severe abdominal pain and a feeling of increased abdominal swelling. Because of persistent abdominal pain and distention, an exploratory laparotomy was performed on 8/28/98, resulting in resection of the small bowel.

The patient remained on bedrest for 3 days, after which she began ambulating with nursing. On 9/4/98, the patient ambulated 50 feet with physical therapy, during which she complained of severe dyspnea and mild-to-moderate abdominal discomfort. For this reason, physical therapy discontinued ambulation but continued chest physical therapy and bedside exercise to the upper and lower extremities. However, nursing continued to ambulate the patient approximately four times per day despite her complaints of severe shortness of breath and abdominal discomfort. On 9/6/98 immediately after walking, she developed severe abdominal discomfort associated with nausea and vomiting. Nonetheless, that evening, the patient was ambulated 200 feet, walking approximately 15 minutes, at which time she complained of severe abdominal pain; her respiratory rate was noted to be in the high 50s. On 9/7/98, the patient was again walked approximately 75 feet with a walker and maximal assist of three, at which time she became unresponsive. Physician examination

at this time revealed severe tachypnea and abdominal distention. On 9/10/98, the patient's status further deteriorated with effusion and atelectasis of the left lung base, ischemic bowel, possible abdominal infection, anemia, and azotemia. She expired on 9/11/98.

Discussion

This case study is an example of an 85-year old patient who underwent bypass surgery after the following occurred:

1. She remained asymptomatic during prolonged cardiac rehabilitation exercise assessments with adaptive heart rate and blood pressure responses, but somewhat paradoxically developed angina at rest.
2. A thallium treadmill stress test demonstrated moderately severe ischemic change.
3. A cardiac catheterization revealed occluded grafts to the right coronary artery and left anterior diagonal artery and high-grade occlusion of the circumflex artery, inferior hypokinesis, and depressed ejection fraction (approximately 30%).

Unfortunately, after bypass surgery was performed, the patient developed numerous complications caused primarily by pump failure and improper exercise training that was not appropriately adjusted to the patient's needs. At no time should a patient be ambulated with moderate-to-severe pain (whatever the location or cause), as it most likely represents a pathologic process (in this case, ischemia of the small intestine). In addition, inappropriate responses to exercise training, such as a rapid heart rate or respiratory rate with minimal exercise, must be reassessed and treated before subsequent exercise is performed, or at least changes must be made in the type of exercise performed. Sitting lower extremity exercise would have been much more appropriate for this patient, who demonstrated many interrelated pathophysiologic processes that were exacerbated by improper exercise training and ultimately led to her death.

Case 2

This 64-year-old man was admitted 11/5/98 after returning home from a 5-hour appointment at the University Hospital heart transplant clinic. On his return from the clinic, the patient became increasingly short of breath and fatigued and complained of moderate-to-severe chest pain. He reported to the emergency department, where he was diagnosed with moderate-to-severe CHF and unstable angina, neither of which was present earlier that day during examination at the heart transplant clinic.

The patient's history included hyperlipidemia; previous coronary artery bypass graft surgeries in 1989 and 1994; multiple percutaneous transluminal coronary angioplasties (a total of 15), including dilation of the vein grafts; ischemic cardiomyopathy; mitral regurgitation; peripheral vascular disease; left carotid endarterectomy; and recent anterior myocardial infarction (9/18/98), at which time the following treatments were provided:

10/15/98	Cardiac rehabilitation initiated (approximately 1 month was required to stabilize the patient), at which time patient ambulated 50 feet with an adaptive heart rate response but demonstrated a decrease in systolic blood pressure in response to exercise and complaints of lightheadedness.
10/16/98	Patient seen twice a day, ambulating 100 to 200 feet with moderate dyspnea and a flat heart rate and systolic blood pressure response.
10/18/98	Patient ambulated 500 feet twice a day, at which time he complained of mild nausea but demonstrated a blunted heart rate and systolic blood pressure response.
10/22/98	Patient ambulated 800 feet but complained of mild angina. Nitroglycerin patch increased from 5 to 10 mg/cm.
10/23/98	Patient ambulated 700 feet with adaptive heart rate and systolic blood pressure responses to exercise, without angina.
10/27/98	Patient ambulated 800 feet with adaptive heart rate and systolic blood pressure response, without angina. Patient discharged home with a home exercise program consisting of activities of daily living and home ambulation of 5 to 6 minutes, equivalent to approximately 600 to 800 feet.

Because of the patient's past hospitalization and previous history of diffuse coronary artery disease and ischemic cardiomyopathy with recurrent angina and CHF, he was considered a candidate for cardiac transplantation. However, the 5-hour interview process was apparently more than the patient could tolerate and caused the emergency department admission of 11/5/98. At this time, the patient's hemoglobin was 9.9, hematocrit 25%, BUN 35, and creatinine 1.5. Chest radiograph showed moderately severe CHF, and physical examination revealed jugulovenous distention of 8 cm, with distended and rigid abdomen as well as tenderness over his liver. Auscultation identified moderate-to-severe rales throughout most lobes bilaterally and distant heart sounds with a soft S_3 heart sound. The patient was transferred on 11/8/98 to University Hospital for heart transplantation.

11/9 to 11/15/98	Preoperative assessments and preparation for heart transplantation while awaiting a donor heart. Cardiac rehabilitation treatments were provided twice a day, consisting of baseline measurements of endurance, muscle strength, and pulmonary function during morning sessions and educational and stress reduction classes during afternoon sessions.
11/16/98	Orthotopic heart transplantation performed.
11/18/98	Patient extubated and physical therapy initiated, consisting of gentle passive range of motion to upper and lower extremities.
11/19/98	Passive range of motion repetitions increased and patient encouraged to perform independent lower extremity movements (5 to 10 reps) every hour awake.
11/20/98	Sitting active assist range of motion exercises to the upper and lower extremities and standing pregait activities (weight shifting and plantar flexion).
11/21/98	Ambulation in room (starting with several steps and progressing to 12 feet) and upper extremity wand exercises.
11/22/98	Twice a day ambulation in room, 20 to 30 feet, and 2 minutes of stationary bicycle ergometry.
11/23/98	Patient transferred out of isolation, and ambulation in hallway begun (50 feet).
11/28/98	Ambulation in hallway of 500 feet, and bicycle ergometry for 5 minutes twice a day.
12/2/98	Bicycle ergometry for 10 minutes and independent hallway ambulation.
12/4/98	Bicycle ergometry for 15 minutes. Patient discharged home with instructions to begin phase II cardiac rehabilitation in 3 days.

Case 3

This 69-year-old man had undergone a mitral valve replacement with a porcine Carpentier-Edwards valve in 1993 because of myomatous degeneration. The artificial valve later failed, producing recurrent episodes of CHF and requiring numerous hospitalizations. Cardiac assessment via transesophageal echocardiography revealed moderately severe left ventricular hypertrophy and thickened porcine mitral valve leaflets with "some" prolapse, causing moderate to severe mitral regurgitation with an eccentric jet into the left atrium. Cardiac catheterization showed normal coronary arteries, slightly impaired left ventricular function (ejection fraction of approximately 50%), elevated left ventricular end-diastolic pressure (28 mm Hg), and significant prosthetic mitral insufficiency without stenosis. Soon after a second mitral valve replacement was performed on 5/16/98, he developed adult respiratory distress syndrome (requiring a ventilator and tracheostomy); staphylococcal septicemia; a cerebrovascular accident causing left hemiparesis; and a reduced cardiac output that required an intra-aortic balloon pump, which maintained adequate perfusion except to the distal extremities (right great toe, left second toe, and right index finger). The patient's past medical history otherwise included a bleeding ulcer and left forearm trauma in 1959 that caused a left median nerve injury.

The patient finally recovered and began inpatient cardiac rehabilitation in addition to rehabilitation for his neurologic dysfunction. During inpatient cardiac rehabilitation, the patient progressed slowly at first, performing fewer than 10 repetitions of lower and upper extremity exercises in bed, but soon increased his strength and began to perform the exercises while sitting. He then began ambulating and by week 2 was walking 200 feet without an assistive device but with moderate dyspnea. The patient was then discharged from the hospital and referred to outpatient neurologic rehabilitation, at which time the neurologic physical therapist referred the patient to cardiopulmonary physical therapy services because of marked dyspnea during gait training. The patient was evaluated by cardiopulmonary physical therapy services and was observed to be in moderate CHF, which quickly resolved after the primary physician was contacted and the patient's dosage of Lasix was slightly increased. The patient was then followed by outpatient cardiac rehabilitation, where he slowly progressed to a rather independent and active lifestyle. The following data were obtained during exercise assessments and training sessions, which were initially performed three times per week and gradually decreased to once per week after significant improvement was made.

Patient Assessment

These charts follow the SOAP (subjective data, objective data, assessment, plan) format:

9/26/98
S: Patient reports mild-to-moderate dyspnea during activities of daily living. Community outings have been easier since using the wheelchair, which he frequently pushes (for increased stability) and occasionally sits in (for rest periods).
O: *Weight:* 167.5 lb (up 1.5 lb since 9/24/98)
Meds: potassium 2 qd, Lanoxin 1 qd, Lasix 40 mg bid
RHR: 80 bpm, *PHR:* 110 (bike) and 112 (arms and ambulation)
RBP: 94/70 mm Hg, *PBP:* 110/70 (bike) and 120/70 (arms and ambulation) mm Hg

Appearance: No peripheral edema or jugular venous distention
Auscultation: No S_3 or S_4 heart sounds at rest. Mild-to moderate rales in bilateral lower lobes (left greater than right); intermittent S_3 during exercise
Respiratory rate: Resting, 34 breaths per minute; exercise, 40 to 46 breaths per minute
Vital capacity: 420 L (350 L after exercise)
Bicycle ergometry: 0 watts, 40 rpm × 20 min = 20 min total
Arm ergometry: 0 watts × 32 revolutions, brief rest, 0 watts × 78 revolutions
Ambulation: 1.0 to 1.2 mph, 0% grade, for 2 min without complaint but with ventricular tachycardia versus aberrantly conducted supraventricular beats, because of which ambulation was terminated
A: Occasional to frequent premature ventricular complexes (couplets and triplets) with one 10- to 12-beat salvo of ventricular tachycardia versus aberrantly conducted beats (Fig. 4–20); exercise terminated at this point
P: Case discussed with primary physicians; therapists instructed to continue exercise and to monitor rhythm and symptoms. Information regarding physician discussion and signs and symptoms of ventricular tachycardia relayed to patient and wife.

11/3/98
S: Patient reports slightly increased dyspnea with exercise. No other complaints. Activity is status quo.
O: Weight: 172.8 lb
Meds: Unchanged
RHR: 70 bpm *PHR:* 110 (bike) and 100 (arms) bpm; 110 bpm (ambulation)
RBP: 120/70 (supine), 90/70 (sitting), and 100/70 (standing) mm Hg
PBP: 120/70 (bike), 124/70 (arms), and 110/70 (ambulation) mm Hg
Appearance: No peripheral edema or jugular venous distention.
Auscultation: Moderate rales lower lobes and middle lobes bilaterally.
Respiratory rate: 28 to 30 breaths per minute.
Vital capacity: 500 L (400 L after exercise).
Resting oxygen saturation: 94%.
Exercise oxygen saturation: 92–96%.
Fitron bicycle ergometry: 90 rpm setting (40 rpm) × 10 min, 80 rpm setting (40 rpm) × 5 min = 15 min total
Arm ergometry: 0 watts (500 revolutions) in 15 min
Treadmill ambulation: 1.0–1.2 mph, 0% grade × 2 min, 1.2–1.4 mph, 0% grade × 2 min, 1.6–1.8 mph × 3 min = 7 total min; moderate fatigue and dyspnea
ECG: Less ectopy
A: Patient progressing but still demonstrating chronic rales on auscultation of lungs before exercise.
P: Discuss with primary physicians.

Discussion

This case history demonstrates the interrelatedness of all bodily systems and the use of specialized physical ther-

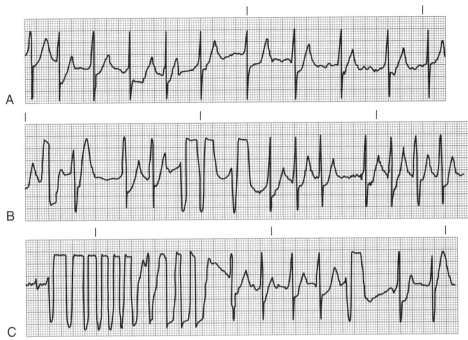

Figure 4-20. Electrocardiogram obtained during an exercise assessment. The single-lead electrocardiograms obtained during an exercise assessment show controlled atrial fibrillation (*A*), atrial fibrillation with frequent premature ventricular contractions or aberrantly conducted beats (*B*), and ventricular tachycardia (*C*).

apy services (neurologic and cardiopulmonary) to facilitate the patient's recovery. In addition, it supports the concept of exercise training in patients with chronic CHF who, although demonstrating only mild left ventricular systolic dysfunction, continue to exhibit signs and symptoms of mild-to-moderate CHF. This was undoubtedly the result of left ventricular diastolic dysfunction as evidenced by the elevated left ventricular end-diastolic pressure and the moderately severe left ventricular hypertrophy.

The patient maintained his increased level of exercise tolerance as the sessions were decreased from three times to once per week. However, shortly thereafter, he reported blood in his stool, which was evaluated by his primary physician, who scheduled a lower gastrointestinal tract test the following week. Unfortunately, the patient died suddenly while sleeping before the test could be performed. Five days earlier during his exercise assessment and training session he demonstrated no signs or symptoms suggestive of cardiac, respiratory, hematologic, or intestinal abnormality. It seems likely because of the "sudden" death that the patient died as a result of a fatal arrhythmia.

Case 4

This 56-year-old man was admitted on 2/22/97 after a cardiac arrest associated with a large anterolateral myocardial infarction that was complicated by recurrent

ventricular tachycardia and CHF. Cardiac rehabilitation was initiated on day 3 of hospitalization, during which increased ventricular ectopy and mild angina with minimal activity prompted an increased dosage of antiarrhythmic (quinidine) and antianginal (nitrates) medications. Chest radiograph revealed only slightly less CHF. Subsequent cardiac catheterization on day 5 revealed 100% occlusion of the left anterior descending artery, 60% occlusion of the right coronary artery, and a large dyskinetic anterolateral wall of the left ventricle with an ejection fraction of 25%.

The patient was treated medically with antiarrhythmics, nitrates, diuretics, and low-dose beta blockers, which significantly decreased the ventricular ectopy and CHF and eliminated the angina during days 6 to 10 after the myocardial infarction. The CHF resolved, and a low-level exercise test performed on day 11 revealed rare to occasional premature ventricular complexes without ventricular tachycardia, fair exercise tolerance (9 minutes of the Sheffield protocol, representing 3 minutes of the Bruce protocol) to a predetermined end point (heart rate of 130 bpm), and hypoadaptive systolic blood pressure response at maximal exercise (from 150/70 to 120/70 mm Hg).

The patient was enrolled in phase II cardiac rehabilitation and participated without angina or significant arrhythmia and with great interest. His primary mode of home exercise training was bicycling for 15 to 30 minutes daily, which he seldom missed, in addition to the three times a week cardiac rehabilitation schedule.

The patient's cardiopulmonary responses to exercise improved, and he began demonstrating signs and symptoms of exercise conditioning, including lower resting heart rate, adaptive blood pressures, and significantly lower exercise heart rates during increased workloads, which were tolerated with less dyspnea and fatigue. After 2 months of home exercise training and cardiac rehabilitation, the patient began bicycling with the SCOR Cardiac Cycling Club during Saturday bicycle rides. He began riding on a tandem bicycle with a physical therapist who continuously monitored the patient's symptoms and heart rate (via a Polar Vantage Heart Rate Monitor) and occasional blood pressures during the 5- to 10-mile rides. On several of the weekend bicycle rides the patient wore a 24-hour Holter monitor, which revealed a well-controlled heart rhythm without significant arrhythmias.

After 1 month of bicycling on a tandem and completing a distance of 20 miles without complaint or complication, it was decided by the primary cardiologist and physical therapist that the patient was safe for independent bicycling, which he performed once a week with the cycling club as well as 4 to 5 days per week as home exercise training. This training routine continued for 4 months, during which no complications occurred. The patient lost approximately 50 pounds and was comfortably bicycling 20 to 50 miles, 4 to 5 days per week. His goal was to participate in an annual 100-mile bicycle ride that was scheduled 2 months later. The patient began increasing his bicycling distance (increased duration versus increased intensity) to an average of 30 to 70 miles, 3 to 4 days per week, and did so comfortably without complication. He began the 100-mile event at 6:00 AM and completed the ride 11 hours later. During the ride, the patient's heart rate and symptoms were monitored intermittently, and he took rests as needed.

He continued to ride an average of 20 miles per day, 3 to 4 times per week, after the 100-mile event, even to the day of his death when he suffered a cardiac arrest several hours after a bicycle ride that coincidentally was approximately 1 year after the 100-mile ride. He considered the 100-mile ride one of his greatest accomplishments.

Discussion

This case history demonstrates (1) that proper exercise progression is essential to cardiac rehabilitation; (2) the importance of exercise training in patients with left ventricular dysfunction; (3) the importance of encouraging exercise that is interesting to the patient, allows goals to be set (100-mile bicycle ride), and provides rewards (camaraderie, increased self-esteem); and (4) the enigma and reality of heart disease in a patient who had progressed so far and done so well, yet still suffered from atherosclerotic heart disease and an increased likelihood of death secondary to an impaired left ventricular function and a history of cardiac arrest and CHF.

Case 5

This 86-year-old man was admitted on 11/25/98 with an acute anterolateral myocardial infarction complicated by rapid atrial fibrillation, occasional short runs of ventricular tachycardia, and mild renal failure. His past medical history included a myocardial infarction in 1990 and a transient ischemic attack several years ago. Chest radiograph on admission revealed mild cardiomegaly and moderate increase in pulmonary vasculature, resulting in a diagnosis of moderate CHF. An echocardiogram performed on 11/26/98 revealed right ventricular and right atrial hypertrophy as well as left ventricular hypertrophy, septal and anterior wall hypokinesis, moderate mitral regurgitation with a dilated left atrium, and mild aortic regurgitation.

The patient's CHF, renal failure, and cardiac arrhythmias were further evaluated and treated, and on 12/3/98 cardiac rehabilitation was initiated. The patient's initial treatment consisted of passive and active upper and lower extremity active range of motion in bed while semisupine and then sitting, which was followed by ambulation (with moderate assist of two) of 3 to 4 steps (from bed to commode) with an adaptive heart rate response and blunted systolic blood pressure response to exercise without significant arrhythmia. The afternoon treatment on 12/3/98 consisted of sitting upper and lower extremity active range of motion exercise, followed by 5 feet of ambulation, requiring minimal assist of two, during which the heart rate and rhythm were adaptive but the systolic blood pressure decreased from 124/62 standing to 86/52 during ambulation, at which time the patient complained of dizziness.

On 12/4/98, the patient ambulated 45 feet in 2½ minutes with minimal assist of two, during which he was asymptomatic, and demonstrated an adaptive heart rate response (60 to 84 bpm) without arrhythmia. Again he experienced a hypoadaptive systolic blood pressure response but of a lesser magnitude (126/74 to 116/64 mm Hg). The same distance was ambulated in the afternoon with a similar response to exercise. On the morning of 12/5/98, the patient ambulated 90 feet in 2½ minutes with an adaptive heart rate response (60 to 102 bpm) and rhythm but with a 30 mm Hg hypoadaptive systolic blood pressure response and complaints of mild dizziness. That afternoon, the patient ambulated approximately 35 feet, at which time he became very dyspneic and diaphoretic and collapsed to the floor.

Electrocardiographic monitoring revealed a very slow normal sinus rhythm of 30 beats per minute and a blood pressure of 60/30 mm Hg. The patient's legs were elevated and atropine was administered. He was further stabilized and the following day underwent cardiac catheterization, which revealed a 90% blockage of the left main coronary artery as well as two 90% occlusions of the left anterior descending artery, a 50% blockage of the circumflex artery, and an 80% occlusion in the right coronary artery. In addition, the patient demonstrated significant mitral regurgitation and a mildly enlarged left ventricle with anteroapical akinesis, an elevated left ventricular end-diastolic pressure, and an ejection fraction of 27%.

Discussion

This case history demonstrates the interrelatedness of all the bodily systems (mild renal failure resulting from CHF that was due to the poorly contracting *hypokinetic* septal and anterior walls of the left ventricle from a myocardial infarction) as well as the effects of myocardial ischemia on cardiac performance. As the patient's exercise was increased, his heart was required to perform more work than it was able to do because the severe 90% blockage in the left main coronary artery decreased the blood flow to the heart. As a result, the myocardium received less blood and became ischemic, and its ability to pump (an ischemic CMD) decreased, which is why the systolic blood pressure repeatedly decreased with progressive exercise.

Case 6

A 29-year-old male with a history of congenital aortic stenosis secondary to a bicuspid valve underwent a valvulotomy (excision of diseased valve) at age 10 because of persistent CHF but recently developed progressive dyspnea and exertional angina. The patient had been evaluated annually since age 10 via echocardiography and exercise interventriculograms. The last evaluation was made approximately 1 year ago, and the patient demonstrated fairly good exercise tolerance without complaint and without a significantly abnormal interventriculogram. However, recently he has developed paroxysmal nocturnal dyspnea and orthopnea and has exhibited a gradual increase in exertional symptoms.

The patient was admitted on 11/26/98 for evaluation of these conditions, and the results of his hospitalization are charted here:

11/26/98	Physical examination showed the following: *Appearance:* Mildly apprehensive and dyspneic with a respiratory rate of 32 breaths per minute. *Pulmonary:* Few crackles (rales) in both bases. *Cardiac:* Precordial thrill; PMI displaced laterally, diffuse and sustained; S_3 with a grade IV/VI holosystolic murmur and grade III/VI decrescendo diastolic murmur. *Laboratory findings:* Prothrombin time 11.8 seconds with a 12-second control.

11/27/98	Two-dimensional echocardiography revealed good left ventricular function but moderate-to-severe aortic stenosis with moderate dilation of the left ventricle.
11/28/98	Cardiac catheterization revealed mild left ventricular hypertrophy with moderate dilation, normal coronary arteries, and moderately severe aortic stenosis with a gradient of 86%.
11/29/98	Aortic valve replacement was performed without complication using a St. Jude prosthetic aortic valve.
12/1/98	Cardiac rehabilitation was initiated, and a chart review revealed a hemoglobin level of 11.1 g/100 mL (reference 14 to 17.7 g/100 mL) and a hematocrit level of 24.3 (reference 40 to 52 vol%). White blood cell count and band cells were elevated, and temperature was 99.5 °F. Radiographic findings revealed clear lungs.
S:	The patient complained of moderate fatigue.
O:	*Auscultation:* Lungs clear with prosthetic valve sounds; possible distant S_3, no S_4, or murmur heard *Heart rate:* 110 (rest) and 120 (exercise) bpm *Blood pressure:* 104/70 (rest) and 110/70 (exercise) mm Hg *Ambulation:* 300 feet in approximately 2 min *Electrocardiogram:* Sinus tachycardia
A:	The patient tolerated exercise well, considering low hemoglobin and hematocrit levels, infection, and complaints of fatigue before exercising. Heart rate, blood pressure, and rhythm responses were adaptive.
P:	Continue twice daily cardiac rehabilitation.
12/3/98	The patient ambulated 800 feet in 6 minutes without complaint and with adaptive heart rate, blood pressure, and rhythm responses to exercise.
12/5/98	Hemoglobin level 13.2 g/100 mL, hematocrit level 28.6, white blood cell count and band cell count decreased to within normal limits, temperature 98.4 °F, and radiograph again reveals clear lungs.

Treatment: The patient ambulated on a treadmill at 1 to 1.4 miles per hour, 0% grade, for 5 minutes without complication or arrhythmia but with complaints of moderate fatigue.

12/6/98 The patient ambulated on a treadmill at 1.4 miles per hour, 0% grade, for 6 minutes, and ascended and descended 20 steps with a blunted heart rate and systolic blood pressure response and complaints of moderate fatigue. *Heart rate:* 120 (rest) and 120 (exercise) bpm
Blood pressure: 100/70 (rest) and 100/70 (exercise) mm Hg. Patient discharged home and instructed to return for occasional cardiopulmonary exercise assessments.

Discussion

This patient was evaluated annually to determine cardiac performance because of a congenital valvular abnormality. These annual assessments were unchanged from previous examinations, but apparently cardiac function rapidly deteriorated within a relatively short period of time and produced signs and symptoms of CHF. This case also presents important hematologic information, such as the role of anticoagulation in patients with valvular abnormalities (prothrombin time at admission was near control) as well as the common reduction of hemoglobin and hematocrit levels in surgically treated patients. This reduction, as well as the increased temperature from infection, produced elevated heart rates and symptoms of fatigue. Although the patient progressed very well during his hospitalization, his limited exercise tolerance (5 to 6 minutes of ambulation at 1 to 1.5 mph, 0% grade) was probably due to his low hemoglobin and hematocrit levels (anemia), which decreased the oxygen-carrying capacity of his blood and produced higher resting and exercise heart rates, thus lowering his threshold for fatigue.

Case 7

The patient was a 32-year-old male with undefined muscular dystrophy, CHF due to poor biventricular function (left ventricular ejection fraction 20%), and marked chronic hypoventilation (Pco_2 112 mm Hg) secondary to ventilatory muscle weakness. The patient also had bradycardia requiring permanent pacemaker implantation (1/98) and was admitted for cardiac transplantation evaluation. The past medical history was significant for muscle weakness noted at age 15 with subsequent multiple biopsies of skeletal muscle (deltoid) which were nondiagnostic of a specific type of muscu-

lar dystrophy. The patient had been hospitalized several times for CHF due to a dilated cardiomyopathy. Myocardial biopsy revealed a severe myopathic process with severe myopathic hypertrophy and vascular degeneration, as well as marked interstitial fibrosis.

Methods

Measurements of electrolytes, blood gases, pulmonary function, body weight, total body water balance (fluid input versus fluid output), chest and diaphragm radiography, electrocardiography, sphygmomanometry, oxygen saturation, exercise tolerance, and ventilatory muscle strength were performed using standard methods. The methods of treatment used in this study included traditional and nontraditional modes of therapy. The sequence of events follows:

5/98 Patient noted exertional dyspnea and pedal edema that progressed to the thigh level immediately after a 4-hour airplane flight.

10/98 Patient admitted for treatment of CHF with diuretics and ACE inhibitors, with relief of symptoms. ECG revealed a ventricular rate of 40 to 50 bpm and a wide QRS complex. Cardiac catheterization revealed normal coronary arteries, biventricular enlargement, and hypokinesis with an estimated left ventricular ejection fraction of 20 to 25%. A modified treadmill exercise test (supported walking) revealed poor exercise tolerance and a maximal heart rate of 85 to 90 bpm. A gated blood pool scan performed on 12/1/98 revealed a reduced left ventricular ejection fraction similar to that estimated at the time of cardiac catheterization.

12/14/98 During an outpatient visit, patient sought advice about initiation of a rehabilitation program. At this time, the patient was noted to be mildly dyspneic and demonstrated 4 to 4⁺ pedal edema. In addition, his pulse was 40 bpm and blood pressure was 140/90 mm Hg. Auscultation revealed clear lungs bilaterally and a soft holosystolic murmur. The ECG was notable for a nodal rhythm with frequent ventricular ectopy and ventricular couplets, as well as an interventricular conduction delay and left axis deviation. Cardiopulmonary rehabilitation was to be initiated at the time of next visit.

1/99   Patient admitted to hospital with CHF for intravenous diuretic therapy (Lasix) and placement of a permanent pacemaker (rate-responsive ventricular pacemaker) with unsuccessful capture of his atria. Patient returned to work with no improvement in functional abilities.

3/3/99   Patient admitted to hospital for treatment of CHF and precardiac transplantation evaluation. Admission medications included captopril 12.5 mg tid, Lasix 80 mg bid, digoxin 0.25 mg qd, Coumadin 2.5/5 mg qd, and potassium chloride.
Arterial blood gases (ABGs) on room air: PA_{O_2} = 60 mm Hg, PA_{CO_2} = 80 mm Hg, pH = 7.39, HCO_3 > 40
Potassium level: 3.9
Pulmonary function tests: FEV_1 1.44 (34%), FVC 1.48 (29%), FEV_1/FVC 0.97, peak flow 6.59 (71%), DL_{CO} 20.4 (64%), KCO (139%)
Impression: Evidence of restrictive lung disease with supernormal KCO and decreased DL_{CO} as well as the elevated FEV_1/FVC ratio, indicating extrinsic compression that may be expected with muscular dystrophy because of poor ventilatory muscle strength. In addition, blood gases drawn at the time of pulmonary function tests demonstrated significant elevation in PCO_2 while patient was supine; this rise was probably related to the upward movement of the abdominal contents, which decreased the downward excursion of the diaphragm and prevented adequate ventilation and perfusion.

3/5/99   *Initial cardiopulmonary rehabilitation evaluation:*
Appearance: Severe peripheral edema (3+) in lower extremities and abdomen
Weight: 86.4 kg
Daily total body balance (TBB) of fluid: +1830 mL
Chest x-ray: Markedly enlarged heart with evidence of pulmonary venous hypertension and interstitial pulmonary edema
Muscle strength: 5/5 without increased tone in all upper extremity muscles except the supraspinatus, infraspinatus, rhomboids, deltoid, biceps, and external/internal rota-

tors, which were all graded at 4−/5 bilaterally
Lower extremity musculature: Hip flexion 4−/5 bilaterally, hip extension 4+/5 bilaterally, thigh adduction 4−/5 with decreased tone bilaterally, otherwise 5/5 without increased tone
Trunk/thoracic movement: Limited secondary to Harrington rod placement (1987) to prevent spinal deformities (kyphoscoliosis) from poor spinal muscle strength
Reflexes: Globally areflexic
Sensory: Intact light touch, pinprick, vibration, and temperature
Cerebellar: Within normal limits
Gait: Significantly compensated, "penguin-like" pattern with predominant hip flexor and hip abductor activity. Patient stabilizes torso and hips with hands in front pockets while manipulating a cane with his right index finger and thumb. Extremely inefficient gait.
12-lead ECG: Intemittent ventricular pacing with a junctional rhythm and premature ventricular complexes; left bundle branch block; extreme left axis deviation.
Single lead ECG: Intermittent paced beats with occasional premature ventricular contractions (PVCs).
Resting heart rate: 73 bpm
Maximal heart rate: 91 bpm
Resting blood pressure: 98/50 mm Hg
Maximal blood pressure: 102/60 mm Hg
Resting oxygen saturation: 94%
Maximal oxygen saturation: 92%
Resting respiratory rate: 18 breaths/min
Maximal respiratory rate: 24 breaths/min
Breathing pattern: Paradoxical breathing after 4 minutes of bicycle ergometry and restorator bicycling
Exercise: Functional activities (sit to stand) and bicycle ergometry, followed by restorator bicycling
Rehabilitation recommendations: Patient to perform restorator (chair bicycle) progressing to bicycling two or three times per day for 2 to 3 minutes (to prevent attaining the threshold for paradoxical breathing), and active range of

motion to the upper and lower extremities

3/7/99   *Chest x-ray:* Unchanged

3/8/99   *Right heart catheterization:* Mean pulmonary capillary wedge pressure 14 mm Hg, mean pulmonary artery pressure 31 mm Hg, mean right atrial pressure 20 mm Hg, cardiac output 5.2 L/min, cardiac index 2.7 L/min/m², ejection fraction 20%.
Weight: 84.1 kg
Potassium level: 3.7

3/10/99   Recurrent ventricular tachycardia.
Weight: 82.7 kg
Potassium level: 4.0

3/11/99   Hypotension secondary to aggressive diuresis and increased dosage of captopril (12.5 mg tid to 25 mg tid), which improved with dobutamine 200 mg and reduction of captopril dose to 12.5 mg tid
Chest x-ray: Mild pulmonary edema

3/12/99   *TBB:* +1883 mL
ABGs on 60% O_2 via face mask:
PA_{O_2} = 182 mm Hg, PcO_2 = 112 mm Hg, pH = 7.27,
HCO_3 > 40
Chest x-ray: Lungs essentially clear
Rehabilitation: None for the past 7 days secondary to medical tests, decompensated CHF, ventricular tachycardia, and hypotension. Gradual return to range of motion exercises and bicycling. Cardiopulmonary response to exercise similar to that on 3/5/99.
Medical therapy update: Theophylline 100 mg bid, Diamox 250 mg qd, and nasal BiPAP initiated (spontaneous/timed breathing mode) with an inspiratory pressure of 8, and an expiratory pressure of 2 for marked marked chronic hypoventilation secondary to ventilatory muscle weakness. Patient no longer considered a candidate for cardiac transplantation because of apparent ventilatory muscle weakness (PcO_2 = 112 mm Hg) and the possibility that the patient would be unable to wean from a ventilator after surgery.

3/13/99   Dobutamine discontinued.
TBB: +406 mL
ABGs (on 1 L O_2):
Sleeping: 60/89/7.34
Supine (awake): 88/97/7.29
Sitting (awake): 69/88/7.36
Bicycle exercise: 79/75/7.39

   Appearance: Severe peripheral edema in lower extremities and abdomen

3/14/99   *TBB:* −792 mL
Rehabilitation: Bicycling for 3 min, 3×/day, and active range of motion exercise to the upper and lower extremities while using BiPAP and 1.0 L of supplemental O_2
Chest x-ray: Minimal pulmonary edema

3/15/99   *Chest x-ray:* Minimal pulmonary edema
TBB: −1622 mL
Weight: 84.1 kg
Potassium level: 4.4

3/16/99   *TBB:* +68 mL
ABGs on 1 L of supplemental O_2:
PA_{O_2} = 72 mm Hg, PA_{CO_2} = 75 mm Hg, pH = 7.42,
HCO_3 > 40

3/17/99   *TBB:* +1522 mL
Rehabilitation: Bicycling and range of motion exercises as previous, without improvement in pulmonary dynamics

3/18/99   *TBB:* +1378 mL
Appearance: Severe peripheral edema in lower extremities
Chest x-ray: Bibasilar atelectasis

3/19/99   *TBB:* + 600 mL
ABGs on 1 L of supplemental O_2:
PA_{O_2} = 91 mm Hg, PA_{CO_2} = 88 mm Hg, pH = 7.28,
HCO_3 > 40
Weight: 83.6 kg
Rehabilitation: Exercise as above, and initial assessment of MIPS and MEPS
Maximal inspiratory pressure (MIP): 50 cm H_2O
Maximal expiratory pressure (MEP): 60 cm H_2O
Ventilatory muscle training initiated at 20% of MIP using the Threshold inspiratory muscle trainer with 1.0 L of supplemental O_2. Ventilatory muscle training exercise prescription: 5 minutes tid before meals.
BiPAP therapy: Applied several times per day to rest the ventilatory muscles and at night during sleep. Inspiratory and expiratory pressures increased to 16 and 6, respectively (spontaneous/timed breathing mode) on 1 L O_2. BiPAP no longer used during exercise.

3/20/99   *TBB:* +600 mL
ABGs on 1.0 L of supplemental O_2:
PA_{O_2} = 88 mm Hg, PA_{CO_2} = 82 mm Hg, pH = 7.30,

$HCO_3 > 40$
Chest x-ray: Clear lungs
Rehabilitation: Exercise as previously noted
MIP: 50 cm H_2O
MEP: 86 cm H_2O
Ventilatory muscle training continued as previously noted. BiPAP continued as before.

3/22/99   *TBB:* −375 mL
ABGs on 1.0 L of supplemental O_2: $PA_{O_2} = 90$ mm Hg, $PA_{CO_2} = 77$ mm Hg, pH = 7.37, $HCO_3 > 40$
Appearance: Severe peripheral edema in lower extremities bilaterally
Weight: 83.2 kg
MIP: 63 cm H_2O
MEP: 100 cm H_2O
Rehabilitation: Bicycling for 2.5 min, 3×/day, and ventilatory muscle training and BiPAP continued as before. Left diaphragm moving slightly better (assessed via palpation).
BiPAP therapy: Spontaneous/timed breathing mode with an expiratory pressure of 6, inspiratory pressure of 18 and 1 L of supplemental O_2.

3/23/99   *TBB:* −1290 mL.
Appearance: Severe peripheral edema in lower extremities bilaterally
Weight: 81.8 kg
Rehabilitation: Bicycling for 3 min, 3×/day, and ambulation of 2.5 feet with moderate assist of two
MIP: 63 cm H_2O
MEP: 100 cm H_2O
Ventilatory muscle training and BiPAP continued as before
ABGs on 1.0 L of supplemental O_2: $PA_{O_2} = 100$ mm Hg, $PA_{CO_2} = 64$ mm Hg, pH = 7.43, $HCO_3 > 40$
Pulmonary function tests (bedside): FEV_1 1.53 L, FVC 1.55 L, PEFR 289 L/min; minimal improvement in PFTs
Fluoroscopy of diaphragm: Movement of both diaphragms with excursion ≥ 50% normal without paradox
Functional status: Patient reports less dyspnea and fatigue and has significantly increased activities of daily living and exercise.

3/24/99   *TBB:* −1000 mL
ABGs on 2.0 L of supplemental O_2: $PA_{O_2} = 120$ mm Hg, $PA_{CO_2} = 71$ mm Hg, pH = 7.39, $HCO_3 > 40$

Rehabilitation: Bicycling as earlier, and ambulation of 5 feet with moderate assist of two and slight paradoxical breathing
Weight: 81.8 kg
Potassium: 4.3

3/25/99   *TBB:* −500 mL
ABGs on 1.0 L of supplemental O_2: $PA_{O_2} = 100$ mm Hg, $PA_{CO_2} = 73$ mm Hg, pH = 7.40, $HCO_3 > 40$
Appearance: Severe peripheral edema in lower extremities bilaterally
Rehabilitation: Exercise as noted earlier, and ambulation of 10 feet with minimal assist of two, without signs of paradoxical breathing. Ventilatory muscle training increased to 25% MIP for 6 minutes tid before meals.

3/27/99   *TBB:* −310 mL
Weight: 82.7 kg

3/29/99   *TBB:* −220 mL
Weight: 83.2 kg
Chest x-ray: Lungs clear
Rehabilitation: Bicycling for 3 min, 3×/day Ventilatory muscle training and BiPAP continued as before.
Heart rate: 102 bpm
Blood pressure: 120/68 mm Hg
ECG: Occasional premature ventricular contractions throughout; ventricular pacing at rest with normal sinus rhythm during exercise (several couplets and one triplet).
Potassium level: 4.2

3/30/99   *TBB:* −425 mL
ABGs on room air: $PA_{O_2} = 68$ mm Hg, $PA_{CO_2} = 58$ mm Hg, pH = 7.41
Weight: 83.6 kg
Potassium level: 4.9
Pulmonary function tests (laboratory): FEV_1 1.19 L (29%), FVC 1.27 L (26%), FEV_1/FVC 94%, peak flow 5.75 L (62%), DL_{CO} 13.6 mL/min/mm Hg (48%), KCO 133% of predicted. *Impression:* Extrathoracic restrictive disease.
Rehabilitation: Bicycling for 5 min, 3×/day, and ambulating 20 feet × 2 with minimal assist of 1. Ventilatory muscle training and BiPAP as noted previously.

3/31/99   *TBB:* + 280 mL
Potassium level: 3.9

4/1/99   *TBB:* + 865 mL
Appearance: Severe peripheral edema in lower extremities bilaterally

Rehabilitation: Bicycling for 3 min, 3×/day. Ventilatory muscle training and BiPAP as before. Ambulation of 20 feet with minimal assist of 1. Patient complains of severe abdominal gas pain which decreased with flatus.
Heart rate: 102 bpm
Blood pressure: 120/70 mm Hg
ECG: Occasional to frequent premature ventricular contractions throughout; no couplets or triplets observed.
Potassium level: 4.2
Sodium: 136

4/2/99
TBB: −800 mL
ABGs on 1.0 L of supplemental O_2*:*
PA_{O_2} = 100 mm Hg, PA_{CO_2} = 64 mm Hg, pH = 7.40
Weight: 84.1 kg
Appearance: Severe peripheral edema in lower extremities bilaterally
Ambulation of 20 feet with standby assistance
Heart rate: 100 bpm
Blood pressure: 120/70 mm Hg
ECG: Occasional premature ventricular contractions throughout; no couplets or triplets.
Potassium level: 4.6
Sodium: 136

4/3/99
Patient transferred to rehabilitation hospital. Medications at time of transfer: Digoxin 0.25 mg qd, Lasix 100 mg po bid, KCl 40 mg qd, Carafate 1 qid, Coumadin 3 mg q hs.

Results

The results of the patient treatments (averaged every 2 days) are shown in Figures 4–21 and 4–22. Arterial blood gases improved as ventilatory muscle strength increased and body weight and TBB decreased (see Fig. 4–21). The cardiovascular performance was relatively consistent during increased levels of exercise and activity (see Fig. 4–22) with rare nonsustained asymptomatic ventricular tachycardia. No complications occurred during the rehabilitation sessions.

Discussion

This case history demonstrates the interdependence of multiple systems as well as the importance of assessing multiple systems during cardiopulmonary rehabilitation. The effects of muscular dystrophy upon cardiac and pulmonary function are evident in this case.[296–299] The increased pulmonary artery pressure during flight (airplane cabins can expose passengers to hypobaric hypoxia equivalent to 8000 feet above sea level) has previously been reported and appears to be the result of

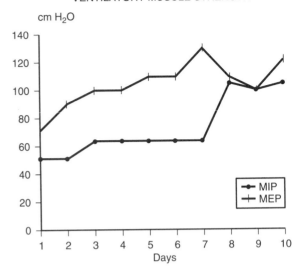

VENTILATORY MUSCLE STRENGTH

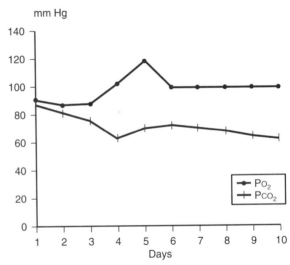

ARTERIAL BLOOD GASES

Figure 4–21. A comparison of these graphs shows that arterial blood gases improved as ventilatory muscle strength increased.

hypoxia, which produces a scenario similar to high-altitude-induced pulmonary hypertension.[299–301] These changes are primarily due to a reduction in pulmonary diffusion as the lower partial pressure of altitude slows the passive diffusion of oxygen and carbon dioxide. The partial pressure, or the diffusion driving force (the difference between the alveolar and venous pressures of oxygen), as it is often referred to, appears to be of primary importance because it is this driving force that saturates hemoglobin with oxygen. For many patients with heart or lung disease, the oxyhemoglobin dissociation curve is unable to compensate for the reduced partial pressure of air flight. This can drastically reduce

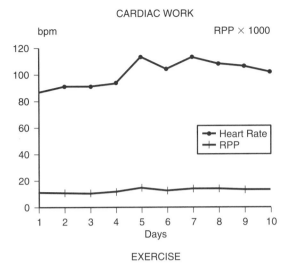

CARDIAC WORK

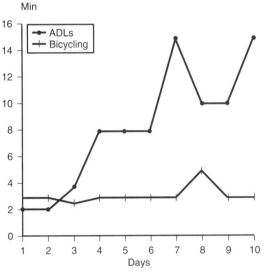

EXERCISE

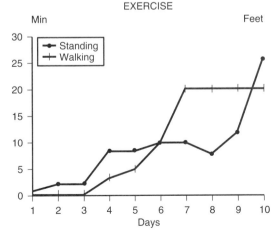

EXERCISE

Figure 4–22. Cardiac work remained relatively stable throughout increasing levels of exercise and activity. ADLs = activities of daily living; RPP = rate pressure product = HR × SBP.

the amount of oxygen saturating hemoglobin and subsequently can produce a vasoconstriction of the blood vessels in the lungs in response to "part of a self-regulatory mechanism for adjusting capillary perfusion to alveolar ventilation."[302] The exact mechanisms for hypoxic pulmonary vasoconstriction is unknown, but it may be due to the local release of histamine or the increased release of calcium into vascular smooth muscle.[302] These mechanisms increase the pressure in the pulmonary arteries and arterioles and produce pulmonary hypertension, which is frequently present in end-stage cardiomyopathies.

The presence of cardiomyopathy with skeletal muscle myopathies has been previously reported.[135–143] The occurrence of cardiomyopathy with muscular dystrophy is reported to be high (50 to 85%). Unfortunately, this patient was afflicted with a severe cardiomyopathy that produced biventricular enlargement and hypokinesis with a left ventricular ejection fraction of approximately 20%. In addition to the cardiomyopathy, this patient also suffered from cardiac conduction system abnormalities. The cardiac dysrhythmias were apparent during the initial cardiopulmonary rehabilitation evaluation on 3/5/99, and a review of the resting 12-lead ECG demonstrated a functional rhythm and left bundle branch block as well as deep Q waves in the lateral and leftward precordial leads (which is characteristic of muscular dystrophy).[303]

Despite aggressive diuretic and ACE-inhibitor therapy, the patient continued to demonstrate signs and symptoms of right-sided heart failure (dyspnea, peripheral edema, etc.). This was most likely due to the patient's poor pulmonary function. The pulmonary function test results of 3/3/99 revealed the severe degree of pulmonary impairment, which was evident from the supernormal KCO and decreased DL_{CO} as well as elevated FEV_1/FVC ratio. These pulmonary function results in this patient strongly suggest the presence of a severe extrinsic compression of the lungs from ventilatory muscle weakness due to muscular dystrophy.[303, 304] Impaired pulmonary function and ventilatory muscle performance were also apparent when the arterial blood gases were drawn on 3/3/99 and 3/13/99. When the patient was placed in a supine position, the PCO_2 was much greater than in more upright positions. More upright positions improved diaphragmatic descent and ventilation and perfusion of the lungs.

Another important finding from the blood gases of 3/13/99 was the improvement in PO_2 and PCO_2 (+14% and −15%, respectively) with bicycle exercise, which was tolerated for approximately 3 minutes, after which the breathing pattern became paradoxical, probably as a result of ventilatory muscle fatigue. The increased ventilation from bicycling decreased the PCO_2 and increased the PA_{O2}. Finally, most of the arterial blood gases demonstrated a pattern of ventilatory failure with respiratory acidosis and metabolic alkalosis.

The specific effects of muscular dystrophy upon the skeletal muscle fibers of the diaphragm and accessory muscles of breathing were significant and life-threatening. Twice during the patient's hospitalization, intubation was strongly recommended, but not performed secondary to (1) the probability of poor weaning from mechanical ventilation in a patient with muscular dystrophy, and (2) the use of BiPAP. BiPAP is a method of noninvasive positive pressure ventilation which has been useful for patients with sleep apnea and more recently as a method to manage patients in respiratory failure without intubation.[273-279] Recently, it has been helpful in the management of acute respiratory failure due to pulmonary edema. For this patient, BiPAP prevented intubation and was used as an adjunct to aerobic exercise and ventilatory muscle training. BiPAP provided the diaphragm with adequate rest periods and, in conjunction with ventilatory muscle training, enabled the inspiratory and expiratory pressures to increase by 110% and 75%, respectively.[270] Ventilatory muscle training has been investigated in persons with muscular dystrophy, but the results have been inconsistent.[306-308]

The benefit of NIPPV in this patient may have been more significant because of CHF. Several studies of patients with CHF have demonstrated significant improvement in cardiac performance that is postulated to be due to increased intrathoracic pressure, which reduces cardiac preload (by impeding cardiac filling) and afterload (by reducing left ventricular transmural pressure).[273, 274] The increased intrathoracic pressure also unloads the inspiratory muscles, which may increase lung compliance.[275] However, no study of exercise performance in heart failure patients using NIPPV has been performed. This case suggests that NIPPV may be beneficial for some patients with CHF.

This case study demonstrates the importance of multiple systems assessment and the result of individualized cardiopulmonary rehabilitation in a patient with muscular dystrophy and cardiopulmonary dysfunction. Diaphragmatic strength and endurance increased substantially and allowed peripheral skeletal muscle conditioning and functional training to be performed which improved the patient's overall function. Such improvements may lead to successful cardiac transplantation in patients with muscular dystrophy (which previously was considered a contraindication for cardiac transplantation).[309] This case history successfully illustrates the following:

1. The effects air flight may have upon patients with cardiopulmonary disease
2. The critical interrelationships among multiple physiologic systems
3. The assessment of multiple physiologic systems
4. The assessment and treatment of the physiologic system upon which other systems are most dependent
5. The effects of progressive exercise conditioning based upon the results of repeated exercise sessions

Summary

- The term *cardiac muscle dysfunction* accurately describes the primary cause of pulmonary edema as well as the underlying pathophysiology, which essentially impairs the heart's ability to pump blood or the left ventricle's ability to accept blood.
- Causes of CMD include (1) myocardial infarction or ischemia, (2) cardiomyopathy, (3) cardiac arrhythmias, (4) heart valve abnormalities, (5) pericardial effusion or myocarditis, (6) pulmonary embolus, (7) renal insufficiency, (8) spinal cord injury, (9) congenital abnormalities, and (10) aging.
- Cardiomyopathy, congenital abnormalities, renal insufficiency, and aging are associated more commonly with chronic heart failure, whereas the other factors tend to cause acute CHF.
- Right-sided or left-sided CHF simply describes which side of the heart is failing, as well as the side initially affected and behind which fluid tends to localize.
- Low-output CHF is the description associated with heart failure and is the result of a low cardiac output at rest or during exertion.
- High-output CHF usually results from a volume overload. The impaired contraction of the ventricles during systole that produces an inefficient expulsion of blood is termed *systolic heart failure*. Diastolic heart failure is associated with an inability of the ventricles to accept the blood ejected from the atria.
- Hypertension and coronary artery disease are the most common causes of CMD.
- Cardiac arrhythmias and renal insufficiency can also cause CMD for reasons similar to those of myocardial infarction.
- Cardiomyopathies are classified from a functional standpoint, emphasizing three categories: dilated, hypertrophic, and restrictive.
- Heart valve abnormalities can also cause CMD as blocked or incompetent valves, or both, cause heart muscle to contract more forcefully to expel the cardiac output.
- Injury to the pericardium can cause acute pericarditis, which may progress to pericardial effusion.
- CMD from a pulmonary embolus is the result of elevated pulmonary artery pressures, which dramatically increase right ventricular work.
- Spinal cord injury can also produce CMD because of cervical spinal cord transection, which causes an imbalance between sympathetic and parasympathetic control of the cardiovascular system.

- Congestive heart failure is commonly associated with several characteristic signs and symptoms, including dyspnea, tachypnea, paroxysmal nocturnal dyspnea, orthopnea, hepatomegaly, peripheral edema, weight gain, jugular venous distention, rales, tubular breath sound and consolidation, presence of an S_3 heart sound, sinus tachycardia, and decreased exercise tolerance.
- Proteinuria; elevated urine specific gravity, blood urea nitrogen, and creatinine levels; and decreased erythrocyte sedimentation rates are associated with CHF.
- Dyspnea is probably the most common finding associated with CHF.
- A rapid respiratory rate at rest, characterized by quick and shallow breaths, is common in patients with CHF.
- The presence of an S_3 heart sound indicates a noncompliant left ventricle and occurs as blood passively fills a poorly relaxing left ventricle.
- The retention of sodium and water is due to

(1) augmented alpha-adrenergic neural activity; (2) circulating catecholamines; and (3) increased levels of circulating and locally produced angiotensin II, resulting in renal vasoconstriction.
- Laboratory findings suggestive of impaired renal function in CHF include increases of BUN as well as blood creatinine levels.
- Pulmonary edema can be cardiogenic or noncardiogenic in origin.
- The most common hematologic abnormality is a secondary polycythemia, which is due to either a reduction in oxygen transport or an increase in erythropoietin production.
- Skeletal muscle abnormalities due to dilated and hypertrophic cardiomyopathies have been reported previously and consistently reveal type I and type II fiber atrophy.
- Severe CMD has the potential to reduce blood flow to the pancreas, which impairs insulin secretion and glucose tolerance.

Activity Guidelines for Patients Hospitalized with CHF*

DAY	STANDARD ACTIVITY REGIMEN	GRADUAL ACTIVITY REGIMEN
1	Commode/chair	Bedrest
2	Room ambulation	Bedrest/gentle active strengthening exercises
3	Hallway ambulation and cycle ergometry ×2 (1–10 min.); MET level goal = 2.0–3.0	Commode/chair/bathroom/restorator cycling/room ambulation/gentle strengthening exercises
4	Independent hallway ambulation ×3 (1–15 min.); MET level goal = 3.0–4.0 Patient adequately ascends/descends two flights of stairs and showers independently; has adequate understanding of home exercise prescription. Outpatient cardiac rehabilitation appointment scheduled. Patient discharged.	Hallway ambulation/restorator or cycle ergometry ×2, ex. duration (1–5 min.); MET level goal = 1.0–2.0 strengthening exercises
5		Hallway ambulation/restorator or cycle ergometry ×2, ex. duration (1–8 min.); MET level goal = 1.5–2.5 strengthening exercises
6		Hallway ambulation/restorator or cycle ergometry ×2, ex. duration (1–10 min.); MET level goal = 2.0–3.0 strengthening exercises
7		Hallway ambulation ×2, ex. duration (1–15 min.); MET level goal = 2.0–4.0 strengthening exercises Patient adequately ascends/descends two flights of stairs and showers independently; has adequate understanding of home exercise prescription. Outpatient cardiac rehabilitation appointment scheduled. Patient discharged.

*Activity protocol is based upon risk stratification (degree of ventricular dysfunction and signs/symptoms) and upon cardiopulmonary response (heart rate no >20 to 30 bpm above resting heart rate without hypoadaptive BP response no >10 to 20 mm Hg decrease) and without significant dysrhythmias or dyspnea. (From Cahalin LP. Heart failure. Physical Therapy 76:530, 1996.)

- The primary malnutrition in CHF is a protein-calorie deficiency, but vitamin deficiencies have also been observed.
- The specific treatments for CHF include restriction of sodium intake, use of medications, and other special measures.
- Many patients with CHF apparently have lower anaerobic thresholds, and the resultant anaerobic metabolism (due to acidosis) becomes the limiting factor in exercise performance.

References

1. The European "Corwin" Study Group. Xamoterol in mild to moderate heart failure: A subgroup analysis of patients with cardiomegaly but no concomitant angina pectoris. Br J Clin Pharmacol 28:67S, 1989.
2. Kannel WB. Epidemiological aspects of heart failure. Cardiol Clin 7:1, 1989.
3. Kannel WB, Belanger AJ. Epidemiology of heart failure. Am Heart J 121:951, 1991.
4. Yancy CW, Firth BG. Congestive heart failure. Dis Month 34:467, 1988.
5. McKee PA, Castelli WP, McNamara PM, et al. The natural history of congestive heart failure: The Framingham Study. N Engl J Med 26:1441, 1971.
6. Braunwald E. Clinical manifestations of heart failure. In: Braunwald E (ed). Heart Disease: A Textbook of Cardiovascular Medicine. Vol. 1. Philadelphia, WB Saunders, 1988, chap 16.
7. Cheng TO. Cardiac failure in coronary heart disease. Am Heart J 120:396, 1990.
8. Hildner FJ. Pulmonary edema associated with low left ventricular filling pressures. Am J Cardiol 44:1410, 1979.
9. Grossman W, Braunwald E. High-cardiac output states. In: Braunwald E (ed). Heart Disease: A Textbook of Cardiovascular Medicine. Vol. 1. Philadelphia, WB Saunders, 1988, chap 25.
10. Perloff JK. Pregnancy and cardiovascular disease. In: Braunwald E (ed). Heart Disease: A Textbook of Cardiovascular Medicine. Vol. 2. Philadelphia, WB Saunders, 1988, chap. 60.
11. Goldberger N, Peled HB, Stroh JA, et al. Prognostic factors in acute pulmonary edema. Arch Intern Med 146:489, 1986.
12. Baigrie RS, Haq A, Morgan CD, et al. The spectrum of right ventricular involvement in inferior wall myocardial infarction. J Am Coll Cardiol 6:1396, 1983.
13. Cintron GB, Hernandez E, Linares E, Aranda JM. Bedside recognition, incidence and clinical course of right ventricular infarction. Am J Cardiol 47:224, 1981.
14. Auchincloss JH, Gilbert R, Morales R, Peppi D. Reduction of trial and error in the equilibrium rebreathing cardiac output method. J Cardiopulm Rehabil 9:87, 1989.
15. Braunwald E, Sonnenblick EH, Ross J Jr. Mechanisms of cardiac contraction and relaxation. In: Braunwald E (ed). Heart Disease: A Textbook of Cardiovascular Medicine. Vol. 1. Philadelphia, WB Saunders, 1988, chap 13.
16. Wynne J, Braunwald E. The cardiomyopathies and myocarditides. In: Braunwald E (ed). Heart Disease: A Textbook of Cardiovascular Medicine. Vol. 2. Philadelphia, WB Saunders, 1988, chap 42.
17. Perloff JK. Pathogenesis of hypertrophic cardiomyopathy: Hypothesis and speculation. Am Heart 101:219, 1981.
18. Braunwald E. Pathophysiology of heart failure. In: Braunwald E (ed). Heart Disease: A Textbook of Cardiovascular Medicine. Vol. 1. Philadelphia, WB Saunders, 1988, chap 14.
19. Pasternak RC, Braunwald E, Sobel BE. Acute myocardial infarction. In: Braunwald E (ed). Heart Disease: A Textbook of Cardiovascular Medicine. Vol. 2. Philadelphia, WB Saunders, 1988, chap 38.
20. American College of Cardiology/American Heart Association Task Force. Guidelines for the early management of patients with acute myocardial infarction. J Am Coll Cardiol 16:249, 1990.
21. Kirklin JW, Blackstone EH, Kirklin JK. Cardiac surgery. In: Braunwald E (ed). Heart Disease: A Textbook of Cardiovascular Medicine. Vol. 2. Philadelphia, WB Saunders, 1988, p 1663.
22. Breisblatt WM, Stein KL, Wolfe CJ, et al. Acute myocardial dysfunction and recovery: A common occurrence after coronary bypass surgery. J Am Coll Cardiol 15:1261, 1990.
23. Klein LW, Kramer BL, Howard E, Lesch M. Incidence and clinical significance of transient creatinine kinase elevations and the diagnosis of non-Q wave myocardial infarction associated with coronary angioplasty. J Am Coll Cardiol 17:621, 1991.
24. Fischell TA, Derby G, Tse TM, Stadius ML. Coronary artery vasoconstriction routinely occurs after percutaneous transluminal coronary angioplasty. A quantitative arteriographic analysis. Circulation 78:1323, 1988.
25. Rabbani LE, Wang PJ, Couper GL, Friedman PL. Time course of improvement in ventricular function after ablation of incessant automatic atrial tachycardia. Am Heart J 121:816, 1991.
26. Holt W, Auffermann W, Wu ST, et al. Mechanism for depressed cardiac function in left ventricular volume overload. Am Heart J 121:531, 1991.
27. American Heart Association. Textbook of Advanced Cardiac Life Support. Dallas, American Heart Association, 1987.
28. Cruz FES, Cheriex EC, Smeets JL, et al. Reversibility of tachycardia-induced cardiomyopathy after cure of incessant supraventricular tachycardia. J Am Coll Cardiol 16:739, 1990.
29. Pastan SO, Braunwald E. Renal disorders and heart disease. In: Braunwald E (ed). Heart Disease: A Textbook of Cardiovascular Medicine. Vol. 2. Philadelphia, WB Saunders, 1988, chap 59.
30. Subramanyan R, Manchanda SC, Nyboer J, Bhatia ML. Total body water in congestive heart failure. A pre and post treatment study. J Assoc Physicians India 28:257, 1980.
31. Abelmann WH. Classification and natural history of primary myocardial disease. Prog Cardiovasc Dis 27:73, 1984.
32. Silverman KJ, Hutchins GM, Weiss JL, Moore GW. Catenoidal shape of the interventricular septum in idiopathic hypertrophic subaortic stenosis: Two dimensional echocardiographic confirmation. Am J Cardiol 49:27, 1982.
33. Zarich SW, Nesto RW. Diabetic cardiomyopathy. Am Heart J 118:1000, 1989.
34. Jermendy G, Khoor S, Koltai MZ, Pogatsa G. Left ventricular diastolic dysfunction in type 1 (insulin-dependent) diabetic patients during dynamic exercise. Cardiology 77:9, 1990.
35. Caforio ALP, Rossi B, Risaliti R, et al. Type 1 fiber abnormalities in skeletal muscle of patients with hypertrophic and dilated cardiomyopathy: Evidence of subclinical myogenic myopathy. J Am Coll Cardiol 14:1464, 1989.

36. Lipkin DP, Jones DA, Round JM, Poole-Wilson PA. Abnormalities of skeletal muscle in patients with chronic heart failure. Int J Cardiol 18:187, 1988.

37. Braunwald E. Valvular heart disease. In: Braunwald E (ed). Heart Disease: A Textbook of Cardiovascular Medicine. Vol. 2. Philadelphia, WB Saunders, 1988, chap 33.

38. Goldhaber SZ, Braunwald E. Pulmonary embolism. In: Braunwald E (ed). Heart Disease: A Textbook of Cardiovascular Medicine. Vol. 2. Philadelphia, WB Saunders, 1988, chap 47.

39. MacKenzie CF, Shin B, Krishnaprasad D, et al. Assessment of cardiac and respiratory function during surgery on patients with acute quadriplegia. J Neurosurg 62:843, 1985.

40. Woolman L. The disturbance of circulation in traumatic paraplegia in acute and late stages. A pathological study. Paraplegia 2:213, 1965.

41. Meyer GA, Berman IR, Doty DB, et al. Hemodynamic responses to acute quadriplegia with or without chest trauma. J Neurosurg 34:168, 1971.

42. Bellamy R, Pitts FW, Stauffer ES. Respiratory complications in traumatic quadriplegia. Analysis of 20 years' experience. J Neurosurg 39:596, 1973.

43. Friedman WF. Congenital heart disease in infancy and childhood. In: Braunwald E (ed). Heart Disease: A Textbook of Cardiovascular Medicine. Vol. 1. Philadelphia, WB Saunders, 1988, chap 30.

44. Borow KM, Braunwald E. Congenital heart disease in the adult. In: Braunwald E (ed). Heart Disease: A Textbook of Cardiovascular Medicine. Vol. 1. Philadelphia, WB Saunders, 1988, chap 31.

45. Moser M. Physiological differences in the elderly. Are they clinically important? Eur Heart J 9(suppl D):55, 1988.

46. Weisfeldt ML, Lakatta KG, Gerstenblith G. Aging and cardiac disease. In: Braunwald E (ed). Heart Disease: A Textbook of Cardiovascular Medicine. Vol. 2. Philadelphia, WB Saunders, 1988, chap 50.

47. Brandfonbrener M, Landowne M, Shock NW. Changes in cardiac output with age. Circulation 12:557, 1955.

48. Strandell T. Circulatory studies on healthy old men. Acta Med Scand 175:1, 1964.

49. Conway I, Wheeler R, Sannerstedt R. Sympathetic nervous activity during exercise in relation to age. Cardiovasc Res 5:577, 1971.

50. Rodeheffer RJ, Gerstenblith G, Becker LC, et al. Exercise cardiac output is maintained with advancing age in healthy human subjects: Cardiac dilatation and increased stroke volume compensate for a diminished heart rate. Circulation 69:203, 1984.

51. Sjorgen AL. Left ventricular wall thickness determined by ultrasound in 100 subjects without heart disease. Chest 60:341, 1971.

52. Gerstenblith G, Fleg JL, Becker LC, et al. Maximum left ventricular filling rate in healthy individuals measured by gated blood pool scans: Effect of age. Circulation 68:91–101, 1983.

53. Capasso JM, Malhotra A, Remily R, et al. Effects of age on mechanical and electrical performance of rat myocardium. Am J Physiol 245:H72, 1983.

54. Lakatta KG, Yin FCP. Myocardial aging: Functional alterations and related cellular mechanisms. Am J Physiol 242:H927, 1982.

55. Bhatnagar GM, Walford GD, Beard ES, et al. ATPase activity and force production in myofibrils and twitch characteristics in intact muscle from neonatal, adult, and senescent rat myocardium. J Mol Cell Cardiol 16:203, 1984.

56. Wei JY, Spurgeon HA, Lakatta KG. Excitation-contraction in rat myocardium: Alterations with adult aging. Am J Physiol 246:H784, 1984.

57. Spurgeon HA, Steinbach MF, Lakatta KG. Chronic exercise prevents characteristic age-related changes in rat cardiac contraction. Am J Physiol 244:H513, 1983.

58. Spurgeon HA, Thorne PR, Yin FCP, et al. Increased dynamic stiffness of trabeculae carneae from senescent rats. Am J Physiol 232:H373, 1977.

59. Yin FCP, Spurgeon HA, Weisfeldt ML, Lakatta KG. Mechanical properties of myocardium from hypertrophied rat hearts. A comparison between hypertrophy induced by senescence and by aortic banding. Circ Res 46:292, 1980.

60. Orchard CH, Lakatta KG. Intracellular calcium transients and developed tensions in rat heart muscle. A mechanism for the negative interval-strength relationship. J Gen Physiol 86:627, 1985.

61. Wenger NK. Exercise for the elderly: Highlights of preventive and therapeutic aspects. J Cardiopulm Rehabil 9:9, 1989.

62. Oertel G. Morphometric analysis of normal skeletal muscles in infancy, childhood and adolescence. An autopsy study. J Neurol Sci 88:303, 1988.

63. Petrella RJ, Cunningham DA, Vandervoort AA, Paterson DH. Comparison of twitch potentiation in the gastrocnemius of young and elderly men. Eur J Appl Physiol 58:395, 1989.

64. Kruszynska YT, Petranyi G, Alberti G. Decreased insulin sensitivity and muscle enzyme activity in elderly subjects. Eur J Clin Invest 18:493, 1988.

65. Cardellach F, Galofre J, Cusso R, Urbano-Marquez A. Decline in skeletal muscle mitochondrial respiration chain function with aging. Lancet 2:44, 1989 (letter).

66. Cleroux J, Giannattasio C, Grassi G, et al. Effects of aging on the cardiopulmonary receptor reflex in normotensive humans. J Hypertens 6(suppl):S141, 1988.

67. Caskey CI, Zerhouni EA, Fishman EK, Rahmouni AD. Aging of the diaphragm: A CT study. Radiology 171:385, 1989.

68. Melichna J, Zauner CW, Havlickova L, et al. Morphologic differences in skeletal muscle with age in normally active human males and their well-trained counterparts. Hum Biol 62:205, 1990.

69. Coggan AR, Spina RJ, Rogers MA, et al. Histochemical and enzymatic characteristics of skeletal muscle in master athletes. J Appl Physiol 68:1894, 1990.

70. White PD. Exercise for the elderly. JAMA 165:70, 1957.

71. Cahalin LP, Wadsworth JB, Fisher DS. Cardiac muscle dysfunction in physical therapy. Cardiopulm Phys Ther J 2:15, 1991.

72. Wasserman K, Hansen JE, Sue DY, Whipp BJ. Principles of Exercise Testing and Interpretation. Philadelphia, Lea & Febiger, 1987.

73. Ingram RH Jr, Braunwald E. Pulmonary edema: Cardiogenic and noncardiogenic. In: Braunwald E (ed). Heart Disease: A Textbook of Cardiovascular Medicine. Vol. 1. Philadelphia, WB Saunders, 1988, chap 18.

74. Moe GW, Canepa-Anson R, Howard RJ, Armstrong PW. Response of atrial natriuretic factor to postural change in patients with heart failure versus subjects with normal hemodynamics. J Am Coll Cardiol 16:599, 1990.

75. Killip T, Kimball JT. Treatment of myocardial infarction in a coronary care unit. A two-year experience with 250 patients. Am J Cardiol 20:457, 1967.

76. Braunwald E. The physical examination. In: Braunwald E (ed). Heart Disease: A Textbook of Cardiovascular Medicine. Vol. 1. Philadelphia, WB Saunders, 1988, chap 2.

77. Chezner MA. Cardiac auscultation: Heart sounds. Cardiology in Practice Sept/Oct:141, 1984.

78. Stevenson LW, Brunken RC, Belil D, et al. Afterload reduction with vasodilators and diuretics decreases mitral

regurgitation during upright exercise in advanced heart failure. J Am Coll Cardiol 15:174, 1990.

79. Skorecki KL, Brenner BM. Body fluid homeostasis in congestive heart failure and cirrhosis with ascites. Am J Med 72:323, 1982.

80. Andreoli KG, Fowkes VH, Zipes DP, Wallace AG. Comprehensive Cardiac Care. 4th ed. St. Louis, CV Mosby, 1979.

81. Constant J. Bedside Cardiology. Boston, Little, Brown, 1985.

82. Guyton AC. The relationship of cardiac output and arterial pressure control. Circulation 64:1079, 1981.

83. Criteria Committee, New York Heart Association, Inc. Diseases of the Heart and Blood Vessels. Nomenclature and Criteria for Diagnosis. 6th ed. Boston, Little, Brown, 1964.

84. Mancini D, Eisen H, Kussmaul W, et al. Value of peak exercise oxygen consumption for optimal timing of cardiac transplantation in ambulatory patients with heart failure. Circulation 83:778–786, 1991.

85. Cohn J, Rector T. Prognosis of congestive heart failure and predictors of mortality. Am J Cardiol 62:25A–30A, 1988.

86. Slazchic J, Massie B, Kramer B, et al. Correlates and prognostic implication of exercise capacity in chronic congestive heart failure. Am J Cardiol 55:1037–1042, 1985.

87. Likoff M, Chandler S, Kay H. Clinical determinants of mortality in chronic congestive heart failure secondary to idiopathic dilated or ischemic cardiomyopathy. Am J Cardiol 59:634–638, 1987.

88. Cohn J, Johnson G, Shabetai R, et al. Ejection fraction, peak exercise oxygen consumption, cardiothoracic ratio, ventricular arrhythmias, and plasma norepinephrine as determinants of prognosis in heart failure. Circulation 87(suppl):VI5–VI16, 1993.

89. Aaronson KD, Mancini DM. Is percentage of predicted maximal exercise oxygen consumption a better predictor of survival than peak exercise oxygen consumption for patients with severe heart failure? J Heart Lung Transplant 14:981–989, 1995.

90. Sullivan MJ, Cobb FR. The anaerobic threshold in chronic heart failure. Relation to blood lactate, ventilatory basis, reproducibility, and response to exercise training. Circulation 81(suppl 11):47, 1990.

91. Tavazzi L, Gattone M, Corra U, De Vito F. The anaerobic index: Uses and limitations in the assessment of heart failure. Cardiology 76:357, 1989.

92. Wasserman K, Beaver WL, Whipp BJ. Gas exchange theory and the lactic acidosis (anaerobic) threshold. Circulation 81(suppl 11):14, 1990.

93. Koike A, Itoh H, Taniguchi K, Marumo F. Relationship of anaerobic threshold (AT) to AVO2/WR in patients with heart disease. Circulation 78(suppl 11):624, 1988 (abstract).

94. Wenger NK. Left ventricular dysfunction, exercise capacity and activity recommendations. Eur Heart J 9(suppl F):63, 1988.

95. Cahalin LP, Mathier MA, Semigran MJ, et al. The six-minute walk test predicts peak oxygen uptake and survival in patients with advanced heart failure. Chest 110:325–332, 1996.

96. Faggiano P, D'Aloia A, Gualeni A, et al. Assessment of oxygen uptake during the six-minute walk test in patients with heart failure [letter]. Chest 111:1146, 1997.

97. Bittner V, Weiner DH, Yusuf S, et al. Prediction of mortality and morbidity with a 6-minute walk test in patients with left ventricular dysfunction. JAMA 270:1702–1707, 1993.

98. Guyatt GH, Thompson PJ, Berman LB, et al. How should we measure function in patients with chronic heart and lung disease? J Chron Dis 38:517–524, 1985.

99. Goldman L, Hashimoto D, Cook EF. Comparative reproducibility and validity of systems for assessing cardiovascular functional class: Advantages of a new Specific Activity Scale. Circulation 64:1227, 1981.

100. Blackwood R, Mayou RA, Garnham JC, et al. Exercise capacity and quality of life in the treatment of heart failure. Clin Pharmacol Ther 48:325–332, 1990.

101. Rector TS, Kubo SH, Cohn JN. Patients' self-assessment of their congestive heart failure: II. Content, reliability and validity of a new measure—The Minnesota Living with Heart Failure Questionnaire. Heart Failure 3:198, 1987.

102. Kavanagh T, Myers MG, Baigrie RS, et al. Quality of life and cardiorespiratory function in chronic heart failure: Effects of 12 months' aerobic training. Heart 76:42–49, 1996.

103. Tyni-Lenne R, Gordon A, Sylven C. Improved quality of life in chronic heart failure patients following local endurance training with leg muscles. J Card Fail 2:111–117, 1996.

104. Guyatt GH. Measurement of health-related quality of life in heart failure. J Am Coll Cardiol 22:185A–191A, 1993.

105. Ball E, Michel T, Cahalin L. Quality of life in elderly heart failure patients is related to quadriceps muscle performance. J Cardiopulm Rehabil 17:329, 1997 (abstract).

106. Cahalin LP, Semigran M, Kacmarek R, et al. Quality of life in elderly heart failure patients is related to lower body weight. Chest 112:95S, 1997.

107. Braunwald E. Assessment of cardiac function. In: Braunwald E (ed). Heart Disease: A Textbook of Cardiovascular Medicine. Vol. 1. Philadelphia, WB Saunders, 1988, chap 15.

108. Parmley WW. Hemodynamic monitoring in acute ischemic disease. In: Fishman AP (ed). Heart Failure. New York, McGraw-Hill, 1978, p 114.

109. Laragh JH. Atrial natriuretic hormone, the renin-aldosterone axis, and blood pressure-electrolyte homeostasis. N Engl J Med 313:1330, 1985.

110. Wallen T, Landahl S, Hedner T, et al. Atrial natriuretic peptides predict mortality in the elderly. J Intern Med 241:269, 1997.

111. Iivanainen AM, Tikkanen I, Tilvis R, et al. Associations between artial natriuretic peptides, echocardiographic findings and mortality in an elderly population sample. J Intern Med 241:261, 1997.

112. Skorecki KL Brenner BM. Body fluid homeostasis in congestive heart failure and cirrhosis with ascites. Am J Med 72:323, 1982.

113. Hostetter TH, Pfeffer JM, Pfeffer MA, et al. Cardiorenal hemodynamics and sodium exaction in rats with myocardial infarction. Am J Physiol 245:H98, 1983.

114. Fillmore SJ, Giumaraes AC, Scheidt AC, Killip T. Blood gas changes and pulmonary hemodynamics following acute myocardial infarction. Circulation 45:583, 1972.

115. Light RW, George RB. Serial pulmonary function in patients with acute heart failure. Arch Intern Med 143:429, 1983.

116. Wright RS, Levine MS, Bellamy PE, et al. Ventilatory and diffusion abnormalities in potential heart transplant recipients. Chest 98:816, 1990.

117. Cahalin LP, Semigran MJ, Dec GW. Inspiratory muscle training in patients with chronic heart failure awaiting cardiac transplantation: Results of a pilot clinical trial. Phys Ther 77:830, 1997.

118. Mancini DM, Henson D, LaManca J, Levine S. Respiratory muscle function and dyspnea in patients with chronic congestive heart failure. Circulation 86:909, 1992.

119. Feldman AM, Bristow MR. The beta-adrenergic pathway in the failing human heart: Implications for inotropic therapy. Cardiology 77(suppl D):1, 1990.

120. Lefkowitz RJ, Caron MG. Adrenergic receptors: Models for the study of receptors coupled to guanine nucleotide regulatory proteins. J Biol Chem 263:4993, 1988.
121. Exton JH. Molecular mechanisms involved in alpha-adrenergic responses. Mol Cell Endocrinol 23:233, 1981.
122. Scholz A, Schaefer B, Schmitz W, et al. Alpha1-mediated positive inotropic effect and inositol triphosphate increase in mammalian heart. J Pharmacol Exp Ther 245:327, 1988.
123. Gilman AG. G proteins: Transducers of receptor-generated signals. Annu Rev Biochem 56:615, 1987.
124. Bristow MR. The beta-adrenergic receptor. Configuration, regulation, mechanism of action. Postgrad Med 29:19, 1988.
125. Bristow MR, Minobe W, Rasmussen R, et al. Alpha$_1$-adrenergic receptors in the non-failing and failing human heart. J Pharmacol Exp Ther 247:1039, 1989.
126. Bristow MR, Ginsburg R, Umans V, et al. Beta$_1$- and beta$_2$-adrenergic receptor subpopulations in nonfailing and failing human ventricular myocardium: Coupling of both receptor subtypes to muscle contraction and selective beta-receptor down-regulation in heart failure. Circ Res 59:297, 1986.
127. Fowler MB, Laser JA, Hopkins GL, et al. Assessment of the beta-adrenergic receptor pathway in the intact failing human heart: Progressive receptor down-regulation and subsensitivity to agonist response. Circulation 74:1290, 1986.
128. Bristow MR, Hershberger RE, Port D, et al. Beta$_1$ and beta$_2$ adrenergic receptor mediated adenylate cyclase stimulation in non-failing and failing human ventricular myocardium. Mol Pharmacol 35:295, 1989.
129. Feldman MA, Copelas L, Gwathney JK, et al. Deficient production of cyclic AMP: Pharmacologic evidence of an important cause of contractile dysfunction in patients with end-stage heart failure. Circulation 75:331, 1987.
130. Rosenthal DS, Braunwald E. Hematological-oncological disorders and heart disease. In: Braunwald E (ed). Heart Disease: A Textbook of Cardiovascular Medicine. Vol. 2. Philadelphia, WB Saunders, 1988, chap 55.
131. Jandl JH. Blood: Textbook of Hematology. Boston, Little, Brown, 1987.
132. Shafiq SA, Sande MA, Carruthers RR, et al. Skeletal muscle in idiopathic cardiomyopathy. J Neurol Sci 15:303, 1972.
133. Poole-Wilson PA. The origin of symptoms in patients with chronic heart failure. Eur Heart J 9(suppl H):49, 1988.
134. Wilson JR, Fink L, Maris J, et al. Evaluation of energy metabolism in skeletal muscle of patients with heart failure with gated phosphorus-31 nuclear magnetic resonance. Circulation 71:57, 1985.
135. Isaacs H, Muncke G. Idiopathic cardiomyopathy and skeletal muscle abnormality. Am Heart J 90:767, 1975.
136. Dunnigan A, Pierpont ME, Smith SA, et al. Cardiac and skeletal myopathy associated with cardiac dysrhythmias. Am J Cardiol 53:731, 1984.
137. Dunnigan A, Staley NA, Smith SA, et al. Cardiac and skeletal muscle abnormalities in cardiomyopathy: Comparison of patients with ventricular tachycardia or congestive heart failure. J Am Coll Cardiol 10:608, 1987.
138. Smith ER, Heffernan LP, Sangalang VE, et al. Voluntary muscle involvement in hypertrophic cardiomyopathy: A study of 11 patients. Ann Intern Med 85:566, 1976.
139. Hootsmans WJM, Meerschwam IS. Electromyography in patients with hypertrophic obstructive cardiomyopathy. Neurology 21:810, 1971.
140. Meerschwam IS, Hootsmans WJM. An electromyographic study in hypertrophic obstructive cardiomyopathy. In: Wolstermolme GEW, O'Connor M, London J, Churchill A (eds). Hypertrophic Obstructive Cardiomyopathy. Ciba Foundation Study Group No. 37. New York, Wiley, 1971.
141. Przybosewki JZ, Hoffman HD, Graff AS, et al. A study of family with inherited disease of cardiac and skeletal muscle. Part 1: Clinical electrocardiographic, echocardiographic, hemodynamic, electrophysiological and electron microscopic studies. S Afr Med J 59:363, 1981.
142. Lochner A, Hewlett RH, O'Kennedy A, et al. A study of a family with inherited disease of cardiac and skeletal muscle. Part 2: Skeletal muscle morphology and mitochondrial oxidative phosphorylation. S Afr Med J 59:453, 1981.
143. Poole-Wilson PA, Buller NP, Lipkin DP. Regional blood flow, muscle strength and skeletal muscle histology in severe congestive heart failure. Am J Cardiol 62:49E, 1988.
144. Massie B, Conway M, Yonge R, et al. Skeletal muscle metabolism in patients with congestive heart failure: Relation to clinical severity and blood flow. Circulation 76:1009, 1987
145. Massie B, Conway M, Yonge R, et al. ^{31}P nuclear magnetic resonance evidence of abnormal skeletal muscle metabolism in patients with congestive heart failure. Am J Cardiol 60:309, 1987.
146. Braunwald E, Sobel BE. Coronary blood flow and myocardial ischemia. In: Braunwald E (ed). Heart Disease: A Textbook of Cardiovascular Medicine. Vol. 2. Philadelphia, WB Saunders, 1988, chap 37.
147. Neely JR, Rovetto MJ, Whitmer JT, Morgan HE. Effects of ischemia on ventricular function and metabolism in the isolated working rat heart. Am J Physiol 225:651, 1973.
148. Lefer AM. Vascular mediators in ischemia and shock. In: Cowley RA, Trump BF (eds). Pathophysiology of Shock, Anoxia, and Ischemia. Baltimore, Williams & Wilkins, 1982.
149. Lefer AM. Pharmacologic and surgical modulation of myocardial depressant factor formation and action during shock. Prog Clin Biol Res 111:111, 1983.
150. Williams GH, Braunwald E. Endocrine and nutritional disorders and heart disease. In: Braunwald E (ed). Heart Disease: A Textbook of Cardiovascular Medicine. Vol. 2. Philadelphia, WB Saunders, 1988, chap 58.
151. Yui Y, Fujiwara H, Mitsui H, et al. Furosemide-induced thiamine deficiency. Jpn Circ J 42:744, 1978.
152. Bautista J, Rafel E, Martinez A, et al. Familial hypertrophic cardiomyopathy and muscle carnitine deficiency. Muscle Nerve 13:192, 1990.
153. Folkers K. Heart failure is a dominant deficiency of coenzyme Q_{10} and challenges for future clinical research on CoQ_{10}. Clin Invest 71:S 51, 1993.
154. Lampertico M, Comis S. Italian multicenter study on the efficacy and safety of coenzyme Q_{10} as adjuvant therapy in heart failure. Clin Invest 71:S 129, 1993.
155. Morisco C, Trimarco B, Condorelli M. Effect of coenzyme Q_{10} therapy in patients with congestive heart failure: A long-term multicenter randomized study. Clin Invest 71:S 134, 1993.
156. Jameson S. Statistical data support prediction of death within 6 months on low levels of coenzyme Q_{10} and other entities. Clin Invest 71:S 137, 1993.
157. Langsjoen PH, Langsjoen PH, Folkers K. Isolated diastolic dysfunction of the myocardium and its response to CoQ_{10} treatment. Clin Invest 71:S 140, 1993.
158. Eschbach JW, Adamson JW. Anemia of end-stage renal disease (ESRD). Kidney Int 28:1, 1985.
159. Eschbach JW, Egrie JC, Downing MR, et al. Correction of the anemia of end-stage renal disease with recombinant human erythropoietin: Results of a combined phase I and II clinical trial. N Engl J Med 316:73–78, 1987.

160. Wilson L, Felsenfeld A, Drezner MK, Llach F. Altered divalent ion metabolism in early renal failure: Role of 1,25(OH)2D. Kidney Int 27:565, 1985.
161. Madsen S, Olgaard K, Ladefoged J. Suppressive effect of 1,25-dihydroxyvitamin D3 on circulating parathyroid hormone in renal failure. J Clin Endocrinol Metab 53:823, 1981.
162. Klahr S. Nonexcretory functions of the kidney. In: Klahr S (ed). The Kidney and Body Fluids in Health and Disease. New York, Plenum Medical Publishing, 1983.
163. Rudman D, Feller AG. Liver disease. In: Brown ML (ed). Present Knowledge in Nutrition. Washington, DC, International Life Sciences Institute-Nutrition Foundation, 1990, chap 46.
164. Fischer JE, Baldessarini R. False neurotransmitters and hepatic failure. Lancet 2:75, 1971.
165. Fischer JE, Funovics JM, Aguirre A, et al. The role of plasma amino acids in hepatic encephalopathy. Surgery 78:276, 1975.
166. Smith TW, Braunwald E, Kelly RA. The management of heart failure. In: Braunwald E (ed). Heart Disease: A Textbook of Cardiovascular Medicine. Vol. 1. Philadelphia, WB Saunders, 1988, chap 17.
167. Burton KP. Evidence of direct toxic effects of free radicals on the myocardium. Free Radic Biol Med 4:15, 1988.
168. Padh H. Vitamin C: Newer insights into its biochemical functions. Nutr Rev 49:65, 1991.
169. Belch JJ, Bridges AB. Oxygen free radicals and congestive heart failure. Br Heart J 65:245, 1991.
170. Gaziano JM. Antioxidant vitamins and coronary artery disease risk. Am J Med 97:18S, 1994.
171. Dracup K, Baker DW, Dunbar SB, et al. Management of heart failure: Counseling, education, and lifestyle modifications. JAMA 272:1442–1446, 1994.
172. Fonarow GC, Stevenson LW, Walden JA, et al. Impact of a comprehensive heart failure management program on hospital readmission and functional status of patients with advanced heart failure. J Am Coll Cardiol 30:725, 1997.
173. Parmley WW. Should digoxin be the drug of first choice after diuretics in chronic congestive heart failure? J Am Coll Cardiol 12:265, 1988.
174. Pitt B. Antagonists viewpoint. J Am Coll Cardiol 12:271, 1988.
175. Mulrow CD, Feussner JR, Velez R. Reevaluation of digitalis efficacy. Ann Intern Med 101:113, 1984.
176. Arnold SB, Byrd RC, Meister W, et al. Long-term digitalis therapy improves left ventricular function in heart failure. N Engl J Med 303:1443, 1980.
177. Lee DC-S, Johnson RA, Gingham JB, et al. Heart failure in outpatients. A randomized trial of digoxin versus placebo. N Engl J Med 306: 699, 1982.
178. Gheorghiade M, St Clair J, St Clair C, Beller GA. Hemodynamic effects of intravenous digoxin in patients with severe heart failure initially treated with diuretics and vasodilators. J Am Coll Cardiol 9:849, 1987.
179. Guyatt GH, Sullivan MD, Fallen EL, et al. A controlled trial of digoxin in congestive heart failure. Am J Cardiol 61:371, 1988.
180. The Captopril-Digoxin Multicenter Research Group. Comparative effects of therapy with captopril and digoxin in patients with mild to moderate heart failure. JAMA 259: 539, 1988.
181. Francis GS. Which drug for what patients with heart failure, and when? Cardiology 76:374, 1989.
182. Leier CV. Acute inotropic support. In: Leier CV (ed). Cardiotonic Drugs: A Clinical Survey. New York, Marcel Dekker, 1986.
183. Rude RE, Kloner RA, Maroko PR, et al. Effects of amrinone on experimental acute myocardial ischemic injury. Cardiovasc Res 14:419, 1980.
184. Taylor SH, Verma SP, Hussain M, et al. Intravenous amrinone in left ventricular failure complicated by acute myocardial infarction. Am J Cardiol 56:29B, 1985.
185. DiBianco R, Shabetai R, Kostuk W, et al. Oral milrinone and digoxin in heart failure: Results of a placebo-controlled, prospective trial of each agent and the combination (abstract). Circulation 76(suppl IV):IV256, 1978.
186. Ruegg J. Effects of new inotropic agents on calcium ion sensitivity of contractile proteins. Circulation 73(suppl 111):78, 1986.
187. Cohn JN, Archibald DG, Ziesche S, et al. Effect of vasodilator therapy on mortality in chronic congestive heart failure. Results of a Veterans Administration cooperative study. N Engl J Med 314:1547, 1986.
188. The CONSENSUS Trial Study Group. Effects of enalapril on mortality in severe congestive heart failure. Results of the cooperative north Scandinavian enalapril survival study (CONSENSUS). N Engl J Med 316:1429, 1987.
189. Massie BM, Packer M, Hanlon JT, Combs DT. Combined captopril and hydralazine for refractory heart failure: A feasible and efficacious regimen. J Am Coll Cardiol 2:338, 1983.
190. Sharpe N, Smith H, Murphy J, Hannon S. Treatment of patients with symptomless left ventricular dysfunction after myocardial infarction. Lancet 1:255, 1988.
191. Pfeffer MA, Lamas GA, Vaughan DA, et al. Effect of captopril on progressive ventricular dilatation after anterior myocardial infarction. N Engl J Med 319:80, 1988.
192. Pfeffer JM, Pfeffer MA, Braunwald E. Hemodynamic benefits and prolonged survival with long-term captopril therapy in rats with myocardial infarction and heart failure. Circulation 75(suppl 1):1149, 1987.
193. Pfeffer MA, Pfeffer JM. Ventricular enlargement and reduced survival after myocardial infarction. Circulation 75(suppl IV):93, 1987.
194. Rutherford JD, Braunwald E, Cohn PF. Chronic ischemic heart disease. In: Braunwald E (ed). Heart Disease: A Textbook of Cardiovascular Medicine. Vol. 2. Philadelphia, WB Saunders, 1988, chap 39.
195. Cahalin LP. Cardiovascular medications. In: Malone T (ed). Physical and Occupational Therapy: Drug Implications for Practice. Philadelphia, JB Lippincott, 1989, chap 3.
196. Goldberg AN. The effects of pharmacological agents on human performance. In: Naughton JP, Hellerstein HK (eds). Exercise Testing and Exercise Training in Coronary Heart Disease. New York, Academic Press, 1973, chap 9.
197. Waagstein F, Hjalmarson A, Varauskas E, Wallentin I. Effect of chronic beta-adrenergic receptor blockade in congestive cardiomyopathy. Br Heart J 37:1022, 1975.
198. Swedberg K, Waagstein F, Hjalmarson A, Wallentin I. Prolongation of survival in congestive cardiomyopathy by beta-receptor blockade. Lancet 1:1374, 1979.
199. Swedberg K, Hjalmarson A, Waagstein F, Wallentin I. Adverse effects of beta blockade withdrawal in patients with congestive cardiomyopathy. Br Heart J 44:134, 1980.
200. Swedberg K, Hjalmarson A, Waagstein F, Wallentin I. Beneficial effects of long-term beta blockade in congestive cardiomyopathy. Br Heart J 44:117, 1980.
201. Engelmeier RS, O'Connell JB, Walsh R, et al. Improvement in symptoms and exercise tolerance by metoprolol in patients with dilated cardiomyopathy: A double-blind, randomized, placebo-controlled trial. Circulation 72:536, 1985.

202. Taylor SH, Silke B. Haemodynamic effects of beta-blockade in ischaemic heart failure. Lancet 2:835, 1981.

203. Binkley PF, Lew RF, Lima N, et al. Hemodynamic-inotropic response to beta-blocker with intrinsic sympathomimetic activity in patients with congestive cardiomyopathy. Circulation 74:1390, 1986.

204. Majid PA, Niznick J, Nishizaki S, et al. Acute hemodynamic and neurohumoral effects of pindolol: A beta adrenoceptor antagonist with high intrinsic sympathomimetic activity in patients with dilated cardiomyopathy. J Cardiovasc Pharmacol 10:309, 1987.

205. Gilbert EM, Anderson JL, Deitchman D, et al. Chronic beta blockade with bucindolol improves resting cardiac function in dilated cardiomyopathy. Circulation 76(suppl IV):IV-358, 1987 (abstract).

206. Pouleur H, Van Mechelen H, Balasim H, et al. Comparisons of the inotropic effects of the beta$_1$ adrenoceptor partial agonists SL 75,177.10 and ICI 118,587 with digoxin in the intact canine heart. J Cardiovasc Pharmacol 6:720, 1984.

207. Rousseau MF, Pouleur H, Vincent MF. Effects of a cardioselective beta$_1$-partial agonist (Corwin) on left ventricular function and myocardial metabolism in patients with a previous myocardial infarction. Am J Cardiol 51:1267, 1983.

208. Kullmer T, Kindermann W, Urhausen A, Hess H. Influence of xamoterol, a partial beta$_1$-selective agonist, on physical performance capacity and cardiocirculatory, metabolic and hormonal parameters. Eur J Clin Pharmacol 34:255, 1988.

209. L'Abbate A, Emdin M, Piacenh M, et al. Ultrafiltration: A rational treatment for heart failure. Cardiology 76:384, 1989.

210. Rimondini A, CipoHa CM, Della BeHa P, et al. Hemofiltration as short-term treatment for refractory congestive heart failure. Am J Med 83:43, 1987.

211. Cardiac Alert 11:6, April 1990.

212. Williams RS. Exercise training of patients with ventricular dysfunction and heart failure. In: Wenger NK (ed). Exercise and the Heart. 2nd ed. Philadelphia, FA Davis, 1985.

213. Bocchi EA, Moreira LFP, Bacal F, et al. Left ventricular regional wall motion, ejection fraction, and geometry changes after partial left ventriculectomy. Circulation 96:I-602, 1997.

214. Vijayanagar R, Weston M, Sears N, et al. Partial left ventriculectomy (PLV) for treatment of end-stage heart disease (ESHD): Evaluation of early experience. Chest 112:48S, 1997.

215. Wong J, Garcia MJ, Starling RC, et al. Alterations in left ventricular wall stress after partial left ventriculectomy surgery. Circulation 96: I-344, 1997.

216. Roubin GS, Anderson SD, Shen WF, et al. Hemodynamic and metabolic basis of impaired exercise tolerance in patients with severe left ventricular dysfunction. J Am Coll Cardiol 15:986, 1990.

217. Cody DV, Denniss AR, Ross DA, et al. Early exercise testing, physical training and mortality in patients with severe left ventricular dysfunction (abstract). J Am Coll Cardiol 1:718, 1983.

218. Sullivan MJ, Higginbotham MB, Cobb FR. Exercise training in patients with severe left ventricular dysfunction: Hemodynamic and metabolic effects. Circulation 78:506–515, 1988.

219. Hoffman A. The effects of training on the physical working capacity of MI patients with left ventricular dysfunction. Eur Heart J 8 (suppl G):43–53, 1987.

220. Belardinelli R, Georgiou D, Cianci G, et al. Exercise training improves left ventricular diastolic filling in patients with dilated cardiomyopathy: Clinical and prognostic implications. Circulation 91:2775–2784, 1995.

221. Arvan S. Exercise performance of the high risk acute myocardial infarction patients after cardiac rehabilitation. Am J Cardiol 62:197, 1988.

222. Jugdutt BI, Bogdon L, Michorowski BL, Kappagoda CT. Exercise training after anterior Q wave myocardial infarction: Importance of regional left ventricular function and topography. J Am Coll Cardiol 12:362, 1988.

223. Epstein SE, Palmeri ST, Patterson RE, et al. Evaluation of patients after acute myocardial infarction: Indications for cardiac catheterization and surgical intervention. N Engl J Med 307:1487, 1982.

224. Franciosa JA, Goldsmith SR, Cohn JN. Contrasting immediate and long-term effects of isosorbide dinitrate on exercise capacity in congestive heart failure. Am J Med 69:59, 1980.

225. Lee AP, Ice R, Blessey R, et al. Long-term effects of physical training on coronary patients with impaired ventricular function. Circulation 60:1519, 1979.

226. Conn EH, Williams RS, Wallace AG. Exercise responses before and after physical conditioning in patients with severely depressed left ventricular function. Am J Cardiol 49:296, 1982.

227. Port S, McEwan P, Cobb FR, et al. Influence of resting left ventricular response to exercise in patients with coronary artery disease. Circulation 63:856, 1981.

228. Litchfield RL, Kerber BE, Benge JW, et al. Normal exercise capacity in patients with severe left ventricular dysfunction: Compensatory mechanisms. Circulation 66:129, 1982.

229. Franciosa JA, Park M, Levine B. Lack of correlation between exercise capacity and indices of resting left ventricular performance in heart failure. Am J Cardiol 47:33, 1981.

230. Letac B, Cribier A, Desplanches JF. A study of left ventricular function in coronary patients before and after physical training. Circulation 56:375, 1977.

231. Williams RS, Conn EH, Wallace AG. Enhanced exercise performance following physical training in coronary patients stratified by left ventricular ejection fraction. Circulation 64:171–186, 1981.

232. Wilson JR, Ferraro N. Exercise intolerance in patients with chronic left heart failure: Relation to oxygen transport and ventilatory abnormalities. Am J Cardiol 51:1358, 1983.

233. Higgenbotham MB, Morris KG, Conn EH, et al. Determinants of variable exercise performance among patients with severe left ventricular dysfunction. Am J Cardiol 51:52, 1983.

234. Greenland P, Chu JS. Effficacy of cardiac rehabilitation services with emphasis on patients after myocardial infarction. Ann Intern Med 109:650, 1988.

235. Greenland P, Chu JS. Cardiac rehabilitation services. Ann Intern Med 109:671, 1988.

236. Kellerman JJ, Shemesh J, Fisman E, et al. Arm exercise training in the rehabilitation of patients with impaired ventricular function and heart failure. Cardiology 77:130–138, 1990.

237. Kellerman JJ, Shemesh J. Exercise training of patients with severe heart failure. J Cardiovasc Pharm 10:S172–S183, 1987.

238. Coats AJS, Adamopoulos S, Radaelli A, et al. Controlled trial of physical training in chronic heart failure. Exercise performance, hemodynamics, ventilation, and autonomic function. Circulation 85:2119–2131, 1992.

239. Belardinelli R, Georgiou D, Scocco V, et al. Low intensity exercise training in patients with chronic heart failure. J Am Coll Cardiol 26:975–982, 1995.

240. Squires RW, Lavie CJ, Brandt TR, et al. Cardiac rehabilitation in patients with severe ischemic left ventricular dysfunction. Mayo Clin Proc 62:997–1002, 1987.

241. Baigre RS, Myers MG, Kavanagh T, et al. Benefits of physical training in patients with heart failure. Can J Cardiol 8(suppl B):107B, 1992 (abstract).

242. Jette M, Heller R, Landrey F, Blumchen G. Randomized 4-week exercise program in patients with impaired left ventricular function. Circulation 84:1561–1567, 1991.

243. Meyer TE, Casadei B, Coats AJS, et al. Angiotensin-converting enzyme inhibition and physical training in heart failure. J Intern Med 230:407–413, 1991.

244. Hambrecht R, Niebauer J, Fiehn E, et al. Physical training in patients with stable chronic heart failure: Effects on cardiorespiratory fitness and ultrastructural abnormalities of leg muscles. J Am Coll Cardiol 25:1239–1249, 1995.

245. Kulavuori K, Toivonen L, Naveri H, Leinonen H. Reversal of autonomic derangements by physical training in chronic heart failure. Eur Heart J 16:490–495, 1995.

246. Davey P, Meyer TE, Coats AJS, et al. Ventilation in chronic heart failure: Effects of physical training. Br Heart J 68:474–477, 1992.

247. Koch M, Douard H, Broustet JP. The benefit of graded physical exercise in chronic heart failure. Chest 101:231S–235S, 1992.

248. Kostis JB, Rosen RC, Cosgrove NM, et al. Nonpharmacologic therapy improves functional and emotional status in congestive heart failure. Chest 106:996–1001, 1994.

249. Meyer K, Samek L, Schwaibold M, et al. Interval training in patients with severe chronic heart failure: Analysis and recommendations for exercise procedures. Med Sci Sports Exerc 29:306–312, 1997.

250. Kavanagh T, Myers MG, Baigrie RS, et al. Quality of life and cardiorespiratory function in chronic heart failure: Effects of 12 months' aerobic training. Heart 76:42–49, 1996.

251. Tyni-Lenne R, Gordon A, Sylven C. Improved quality of life in chronic heart failure patients following local endurance training with leg muscles. J Card Fail 2:111–117, 1996.

252. Keteyian SJ, Levine AB, Brawner CA, et al. A randomized controlled trial of exercise training in patients with heart failure. Ann Intern Med 124:1051, 1996.

253. Cahalin LP, Certo C, LaFiandra M, et al. Exercise training increases the oxygen uptake–work rate relationship in advanced heart failure. Chest 112:49S, 1997.

254. Keteyian SJ, Marks CRC, Brawner CA, et al. Responses to arm exercise in patients with compensated heart failure. J Cardiopulm Rehabil 16:366, 1996.

255. Barlow CW, Qayyum MS, Davey PP, et al. Effect of physical training on exercise-induced hyperkalemia in chronic heart failure: Relation with ventilation and catecholamines. Circulation 89:1144, 1994.

256. Keteyian SJ, Levine TB, Levine AB, Brawner CA. Quality of life and exercise training in patients with heart failure: A randomized trial. Circulation 96:I-84, 1997.

257. Franciosa JA, Park M, Levine TB. Lack of correlation between exercise capacity and indexes of resting left ventricular performance in heart failure. Am J Cardiol 47:33, 1981.

258. Franciosa JA, Ziesche S, Wilen M. Functional capacity of patients with chronic left ventricular failure. Am J Med 67:460, 1979.

259. Jafri SM, Lakier JB, Rosman HS, et al. Symptoms and tests of ventricular performance in the evaluation of chronic heart failure. Am Heart J 112:194, 1986.

260. Blackwood R, Mayou RA, Garnham JC, et al. Exercise capacity and quality of life in the treatment of heart failure. Clin Pharmacol Ther 48:325, 1990.

261. Pickworth KK. Long-term dobutamine therapy for refractory congestive heart failure. Clin Pharm 11:618–642, 1992.

262. Coats AJS, Adamopoulos S. Physical and pharmacological conditioning in chronic heart failure: A proposal for pulsed inotrope therapy. Postgrad Med J 67:S69–S83, 1991.

263. Miller LW. Outpatient dobutamine for refractory congestive heart failure: Advantages, techniques, and results. J Heart Lung Transplant 10:482–489, 1991.

264. Kataoka T, Keteyian SJ, Marks CRC, et al. Exercise training in a patient with congestive heart failure on continuous dobutamine. Med Sci Sports Exerc 26:678–682, 1994.

265. Applefeld MM, Newman KA, Grove WR, et al. Intermittent, continuous outpatient dobutamine infusion in the management of congestive heart failure. Am J Cardiol 51:455, 1983.

266. Cahalin LP. Heart failure. Phys Ther 76:516, 1996.

267. McCarthy PM. HeartMate implantable left ventricular assist device: Bridge to transplantation and future applications. Ann Thorac Surg 59:S46–S51, 1995.

268. Morrone T, Buck L, Catanese K, et al. Early progressive mobilization of left ventricular assist device patients is safe and optimizes recovery prior to cardiac transplant. J Heart Lung Transplant (in press).

269. Buck L, Morrone T, Goldsmith R, et al. Exercise training of patients with left ventricular assist devices: A pilot study of physiologic adaptations. J Cardiopulm Rehabil 17:324, 1997 (abstract).

270. O'Donnell DE, Sanii R, Younes M. Improvement in exercise endurance in patients with chronic airflow limitation using continuous positive airway pressure. Am Rev Respir Dis 138:1510–1514, 1988.

271. Henke KG, Regnis JA, Bye PTP. Benefits of continuous positive airway pressure during exercise in cystic fibrosis and relationship to disease severity. Am Rev Respir Dis 148:1272–1276, 1993.

272. Cahalin L, Cannan J, Prevost S, et al. Exercise performance during assisted ventilation with bi-level positive airway pressure (BiPAP). J Cardiopulm Rehabil 14:323, 1994 (abstract).

273. Baratz DM, Westbrooke PR, Shah PK, Mohsenifar Z. Effect of nasal continuous positive airway pressure on cardiac output and oxygen delivery in patients with congestive heart failure. Chest 102:1397–1401, 1992.

274. Bradley TD, Holloway RM, McLaughlin PR, et al. Cardiac output responses to continuous positive airway pressure in congestive heart failure. Am Rev Respir Dis 145:377–382, 1992.

275. Naughton MT, Rahman MA, Hara K, et al. Effect of continuous positive airway pressure on intrathoracic and left ventricular transmural pressures in patients with congestive heart failure. Circulation 91:1725–1731, 1995.

276. Malone S, Liu PP, Hollway R, et al. Obstructive sleep apnoea in patients with dilated cardiomyopathy: Effects of continuous positive airway pressure. Lancet 338:1480–1484, 1991.

277. Takasaki Y, Orr D, Popkin J, et al. Effect of nasal continuous positive airway pressure on sleep apnea in congestive heart failure. Am Rev Respir Dis 140:1578–1584, 1989.

278. Naughton MT, Liu PP, Benard DC, et al. Treatment of congestive heart failure and Cheyne-Stokes respiration during sleep by continuous positive airway pressure. Am J Respir Crit Care Med 151:92–97, 1995.

279. Pinsky MR, Summer WR, Wise RA, et al. Augmentation of cardiac function by elevation of intrathoracic pressure. J Appl Physiol 54:950, 1983.

280. Pinsky MR, Summer WR. Cardiac augmentation by phasic high intrathoracic pressure support in man. Chest 84:370, 1983.
281. Cahalin L, Zambernardi L, Dec G. Multiple systems assessment during inpatient cardiopulmonary rehabilitation. J Cardiopulm Rehabil 13:344, 1993 (abstract).
282. Mancini DM, Henson D, LaManca J, Levine S. Benefit of selective respiratory muscle training on exercise capacity in patients with chronic congestive heart failure. Circulation 91:320, 1995.
283. Barach AL. Physiologic advantages of grunting, groaning, and pursed-lip breathing: Adaptive symptoms related to the development of continuous positive pressure breathing. Bull NY Acad Med 49:666–673, 1973.
284. Tiep BL, Burns M, Kao D, et al. Pursed lips breathing training using ear oximetry. Chest 90:218–221, 1986.
285. Mancini DM, LaManca J, Donchez L, et al. The sensation of dyspnea during exercise is not determined by the work of breathing in patients with heart failure. J Am Coll Cardiol 28:391–395, 1996.
286. Cahalin LP, Semigran MJ, Dec GW. Author response. Phys Ther 77:1764, 1997.
287. Larson JL, Kim MJ, Sharp JT, et al. Inspiratory muscle training with a pressure threshold breathing device in patients with chronic obstructive pulmonary disease. Am Rev Respir Dis 138:689–696, 1988.
288. Weiner P, Azgad Y, Ganam R, et al. Inspiratory muscle training in patients with bronchial asthma. Chest 102:1357–1361, 1992.
289. McParland C, Krishnan B, Wang Y, et al. Inspiratory muscle weakness and dyspnea in congestive heart failure. Am Rev Respir Dis 146:467–472, 1992.
290. Aubuer M, Trippenbach T, Rousso C. Respiratory muscle fatigue during cardiogenic shock. J Appl Physiol 51:499–504, 1981.
291. Hammond MD, Bauer KA, Sharp JT, Rocha RD. Respiratory muscle strength in congestive heart failure. Chest 98:1091, 1990.
292. Cardiac Rehabilitation. Clinical Practice Guideline, Number 17. U.S. Department of Health and Human Services. Public Health Service. Agency for Health Care Policy and Research. National Heart, Lung, and Blood Institute, 1995.
293. Whaley MH, Brubaker PH, Kaminsky LA, Miller CR. Validity of rating of perceived exertion during graded exercise testing in apparently healthy adults and cardiac patients. J Cardiopulm Rehabil 17:261, 1997.
294. Hagberg JM. Patients with end-stage renal disease. In: Franklin BA, Gordon S, Timmis GC (eds). Exercise in Modern Medicine. Baltimore, Williams & Wilkins, 1989, chap 7.
295. Kettner A, Goldberg AP, Hagberg JM, et al. Cardiovascular and metabolic responses to submaximal exercise in hemodialysis patients. Kidney Int 26:66, 1984.
296. Walton JN, Mastaglia FL (eds). The muscular dystrophies. Br Med Bull 36:105, 1980.
297. Walton JN, Nattrass FJ: On the classification, natural history and treatment of the myopathies. Brain 77:12, 1954.
298. Perloff JK, de Leon AC Jr, O'Doherty D: The cardiomyopathy of progressive muscular dystrophy. Circulation 33:625, 1966.
299. Cullen MJ, Appleyard ST, Bindoff L: Morphologic aspects of muscle breakdown and lysosomal activation. Ann NY Acad Sci 317:440, 1979.
300. Dillard TA, Rosenberg AP, Berg BW: Hypoxemia during altitude exposure: A meta-analysis of chronic obstructive pulmonary disease. Chest 103:422, 1993.
301. Cottrell JJ: Altitude exposures during aircraft flight: Flying higher. Chest 92:81, 1988.
302. Houston CS, Riley RL: Respiratory and circulatory change during acclimatization to high altitudes. Am J Physiol 149:565, 1947.
303. Bensaid J: ECG differentiation of muscular dystrophy types. Am Heart J 125:1820, 1993 (letter).
304. Cotton DJ, Taher F, Mink JT, Graham BL: Effect of volume history on changes in DLCO^{SB}-3EQ with lung volume in normal subjects. J Appl Physiol 73:434, 1992.
305. Crapo RO, Forster RE II: Carbon monoxide diffusing capacity. Clin Chest Med 10:187, 1989.
306. Martin AJ, Stern L, Yeates J, et al: Respiratory muscle training in Duchenne muscular dystrophy. Dev Med Child Neurol 28:314, 1986.
307. Houser CR, Johnson DM: Breathing exercises for children with pseudohypertrophic muscular dystrophy. Phys Ther 51:751, 1971.
308. Collins MN: The effects of inspiratory muscle training on the lung function of children with Duchenne muscular dystrophy. Thesis, Program in Physical Therapy, College of Physicians and Surgeons, Columbia University, 1991.
309. Rees W, Schuler S, Hummel M, et al: Heart transplantation in patients with muscular dystrophy (MD) associated with endstage cardiomyopathy. J Heart Lung Transplant 12:S81, 1992 (abstract).
310. Foster C, Pollock ML, Anholm JD, et al: Work capacity and left ventricular function during rehabilitation after myocardial revascularization surgery. Circulation 69:748–755, 1984.

## 5

Restrictive Lung Dysfunction

Peggy Clough

INTRODUCTION

Pulmonary pathology can be organized and discussed in a number of ways. Within this text pulmonary function abnormalities have been divided into two main categories: obstructive dysfunction and restrictive dysfunction. If the flow of air is impeded, the defect is obstructive. If the volume of air or gas is reduced, the defect is **restrictive.** Although this organization of pulmonary pathology may in some ways clarify the discussion, it must be remembered that a number of diseases and conditions result in both obstructive and restrictive lung impairment. This chapter discusses those pathologies and interventions that result in restrictive lung dysfunction.

ETIOLOGY

Restrictive lung dysfunction (RLD) is an abnormal reduction in pulmonary ventilation. Lung expansion is diminished. The volume of air or gas moving in and out of the lungs is decreased.[1]

Restrictive lung dysfunction is not a disease. In fact, this dysfunction may result from many different diseases arising from the pulmonary system or almost any other system in the body. It can also result from trauma or therapeutic interventions, such as radiation therapy or the use of certain drugs.

PATHOGENESIS

Three major aspects of pulmonary ventilation must be considered to understand the pathophysiology of RLD. They are compliance of both the lung and the chest wall, lung volumes and capacities, and the work of breathing (Fig. 5–1).

Compliance

Pulmonary compliance encompasses both lung and chest wall compliance. It is the physiologic link that establishes a relationship between the pressure exerted by the chest wall or the lungs and the volume of air that can be contained within the lungs.[1] With RLD chest wall or lung compliance, or both, is decreased.

As discussed in Chapter 2, a decrease in compliance of the lungs indicates that they are becoming stiffer and thus more difficult to expand. It takes a greater **transpulmonary pressure** to expand the lung to a given volume in a person with decreased lung compliance.[2] If the amount of pressure used to move air into the lungs is constant, the volume of air would be decreased in the person with decreased lung compliance. The pressure-volume or compliance curve is shifted to the right (Fig. 5–2 and discussion of compliance in Chapter 2, Fig. 2–9). A chest wall low in compliance limits thoracic expansion and therefore lung inflation even if the lung has normal compliance.

Because pulmonary compliance is decreased in RLD, resistance to lung expansion is increased. In other words, decreased pulmonary compliance requires an increase in pressure just to maintain adequate lung expansion and ventilation. This means the patient has to work harder just to move air into the lungs.

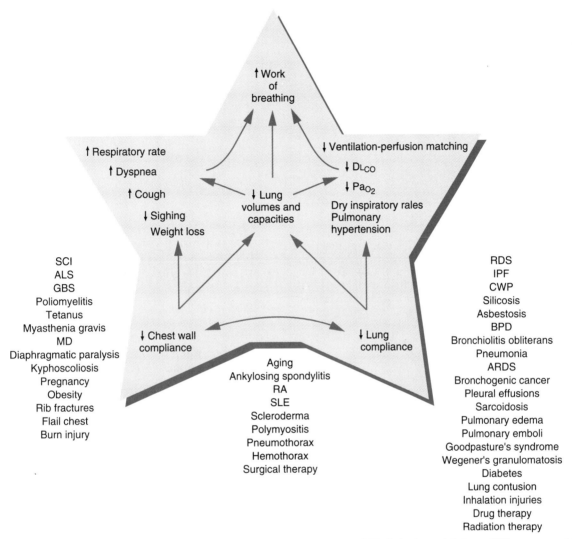

Figure 5–1. Interactive star diagram in restrictive lung dysfunction. SCI, Spinal cord injury; ALS, amyotrophic lateral sclerosis; GBS, Guillain-Barré syndrome; MD, muscular dystrophy; RA, rheumatoid arthritis; SLE, systemic lupus erythematosus; RDS, respiratory distress syndrome; IPF, idiopathic pulmonary fibrosis; CWP, coal workers' pneumoconiosis; BPD, bronchopulmonary dysplasia; ARDS, adult respiratory distress syndrome; DL$_{CO}$, diffusing capacity of the lungs for carbon monoxide; Pa$_{O_2}$, arterial partial pressure of oxygen.

Lung Volumes

Restrictive lung dysfunction eventually causes all the lung volumes and capacities to become decreased. Because the distensibility of the lung is decreased, the **inspiratory reserve volume** (IRV) is diminished. **Tidal volume** (VT) is the volume of air or gas normally moved in and out of the lungs at rest. Although the body tries to preserve the tidal volume in RLD, the compliance gradually decreases and the work of breathing increases; thus the tidal volume decreases. The **expiratory reserve volume** (ERV) is the volume of air or gas that can be exhaled following a normal exhalation. No matter the etiology, RLD effects a reduction in the ERV; this reduction is particularly pronounced if a decrease in lung compliance is the principal etiologic factor. The **residual volume** (RV) is usually decreased, but with some causes of RLD (spinal cord injury, amyotrophic lateral sclerosis, and other neuromuscular disorders) it may be increased. This results in decreasing the dynamic

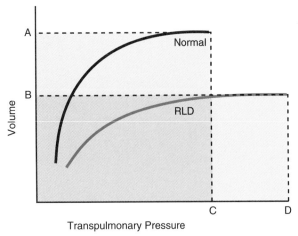

Figure 5-2. Compliance curve. This diagram shows how the lung compliance curve is shifted down and to the right in restrictive lung dysfunction (RLD). Total lung capacity (TLC) in RLD (B) is less than normal (A). The amount of transpulmonary pressure needed to achieve TLC in RLD (D) is greater than that needed to achieve a normal TLC (C). (From Weinberger SE. Principles of Pulmonary Medicine. Philadelphia, WB Saunders, 1986, p 120.)

lung volumes. The most marked decreases in lung volumes are seen in the IRV and ERV.

Because all lung volumes are decreased with RLD, all lung capacities are also decreased. **Total lung capacity** (TLC) and **vital capacity** (VC) are the two most common **spirometric measurements** used in the identification of RLD (Fig. 5-3). Decreases in TLC and **functional residual capacity** (FRC) are a direct result of a decrease in lung

compliance. At TLC the force of the inspiratory muscles is balanced by the inward elastic recoil of the lung. Because the recoil pressure is increased if lung compliance is decreased, this balance occurs at a lower volume, and thus the TLC is diminished. At FRC the outward recoil of the chest wall is balanced by the inward elastic recoil of the lung. Because this elastic recoil is increased, the balance is achieved at a lower lung volume and so the FRC is decreased (Fig. 5-4).[2]

Work of Breathing

With RLD the work of breathing is increased. The respiratory system normally finely tunes the respiratory rate and the VT to minimize the mechanical work of breathing. As previously mentioned, a greater transpulmonary pressure is required to achieve a normal VT. The result is that the patient's work of breathing is increased and a new equilibrium, with a decreased VT and an increased respiratory rate, is sought in an effort to reduce energy expenditure. However, if the respiratory rate is too high, energy is wasted in overcoming airway resistance and in ventilating the anatomic dead space. Furthermore, if the tidal volume is larger than required, energy is wasted overcoming the natural recoil of the lung and in expanding the chest wall. Anything that increases airway resistance, increases flow rates, or decreases lung or chest wall compliance increases the work of breathing. In RLD both lung and chest wall compliance and lung volumes may decrease. These

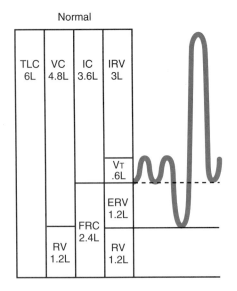

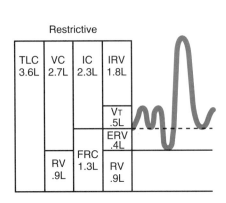

Figure 5-3. Lung volumes and capacities. Comparison between normal and restrictive lung dysfunction. TLC, Total lung capacity; VC, vital capacity; RV, residual volume; IC, inspiratory capacity; FRC, functional residual capacity; IRV, inspiratory reserve volume; VT, tidal volume; ERV, expiratory reserve volume.

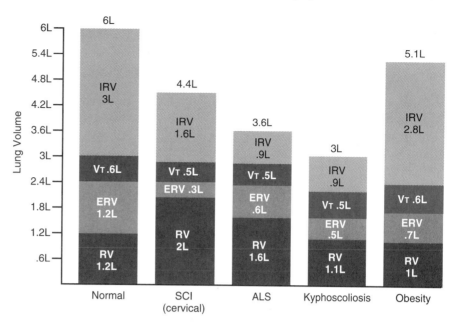

Figure 5–4. Examples of lung volumes in different restrictive impairments. IRV, Inspiratory reserve volume: V_T, tidal volume; ERV, expiratory reserve volume; RV, residual volume; SCI, spinal cord injury; ALS, amyotrophic lateral sclerosis.

changes can significantly change the work of breathing.[3] To overcome the decrease in pulmonary compliance, the respiratory rate is usually increased; the normal inspiratory muscles, especially the diaphragm, work harder; and the accessory muscles of respiration, the scaleni and the sternocleidomastoid (see Chapters 1 and 2), are recruited to assist in expanding the thorax.[4] These additional efforts require additional oxygen (O_2) expenditure. In normal persons at rest, the body uses less than 5% of the oxygen consumption per minute ($\dot{V}O_2$) or 3 to 14 mL $O_2 \cdot min^{-1}$ to support the work of breathing.[3, 5] With RLD the percentage of $\dot{V}O_2$ needed to support the work of breathing can reach and exceed 25%.[3, 5] This change is usually very insidious as the RLD progresses and is countered by the concurrent decrease in activity seen in these patients. Although the respiratory muscle pump is very resistant to fatigue, these patients can experience respiratory muscle fatigue, overuse, and failure as RLD progresses.

CLINICAL MANIFESTATIONS

Signs

Six classic signs often indicate and are always consistent with RLD. The first is **tachypnea** or an increased

respiratory rate. Because the inspiratory muscles have to work so hard to overcome the decreased pulmonary compliance, an involuntary adjustment is made to increase the respiratory rate and decrease the volumes so that the minute ventilation is maintained. Early in the course of RLD there may be *overcompensation,* with the respiratory rate increasing to the point that minute ventilation is increased and alveolar hyperventilation occurs, resulting in greater exhalation of carbon dioxide (CO_2).

Ventilation-perfusion mismatching, an invariable finding in RLD, leads to the second classic sign: **hypoxemia.** This mismatching may be due to changes in the collagenous framework of the lung, scarring of capillary channels, distortion or narrowing of the small airways, compression from tumors within the lung or bony abnormalities of the chest wall, or a variety of other causes. Even if patients are not hypoxemic at rest, they may quickly become hypoxemic with exercise.

The third classic sign of RLD is **decreased breath sounds** with dry inspiratory **rales** (velcro crackles), which are thought to be caused by **atelectatic** alveoli opening at end-inspiration and are most often heard at the bases of the lungs.

The fourth and fifth classic signs are apparent from pulmonary function testing. The decrease in **lung volumes** and **capacities,** determined by spirometry, is the fourth classic sign of RLD. The fifth classic sign is the decreased **diffusing capacity** (DL_{CO}). This arises as a consequence of a widening of the interstitial spaces due to scar tissue, fibrosis of the capillaries, and ventilation-perfusion abnormalities. In RLD the DL_{CO} has been measured at less than 50% of predicted.[6]

The sixth classic sign usually apparent with RLD is **cor pulmonale.** This right-sided heart failure is due to hypoxemia, fibrosis, and compression of the pulmonary capillaries, which leads to pulmonary hypertension. The rise in pressure in the pulmonary circulation increases the work of the right ventricle. Because the pulmonary capillary bed is fibrotic it is also less able to distend to handle the ordinary increase in cardiac output expected with exercise. Therefore, during exercise hypoxemia may occur earlier or be more pronounced. Other signs include a decrease in chest wall expansion and possible **cyanosis** or **clubbing** (Table 5–1).

Symptoms

Three hallmark symptoms are usually experienced with RLD. The first is **dyspnea** or shortness of breath. This symptom typically manifests itself with exercise, but as RLD progresses, dyspnea at rest may also be experienced. The second symptom and the one that usually brings the patient into the physician's office is an irritating, dry, and nonproductive **cough.** The third hallmark symptom of RLD is the **wasted, emaciated appearance** these patients present as the disease progresses. With the work of breathing increased as much as 12-fold over normal, these individuals are using caloric requirements similar to those necessary for running a marathon 24 hours a day.[3] Additionally, because breathing is such hard work and eating makes breathing more difficult, these patients usually are not eager to eat and often report a decrease in appetite. Because their energy expenditure is up and their caloric intake is down, they are very often in a continual weight loss cycle, which becomes more severe as the RLD progresses.

TREATMENT

Treatment interventions for RLD are discussed briefly for each disease and traumatic or therapeutic entity that can result in its appearance. Generally, however, if the etiologic factors that are caus-

Table 5-1	
Signs and Symptoms of Restrictive Lung Dysfunction	
SIGNS	**SYMPTOMS**
Tachypnea	Dyspnea
Hypoxemia	Cough
Decreased lung volumes	Weight loss
Decreased diffusing capacity	Muscle wasting
Decreased breath sounds	
Altered chest radiograph (often reticulonodular pattern)	
Pulmonary hypertension	

ing RLD are permanent (**spinal cord injury**) or progressive (**idiopathic pulmonary fibrosis**), the treatment consists primarily of supportive measures. Supportive interventions include supplemental oxygen to support the arterial partial pressure of oxygen (Pa_{O_2}), antibiotic therapy to fight secondary pulmonary infection, measures to promote adequate ventilation and prevent the accumulation of pulmonary secretions, and good nutritional support. However, if the changes that are causing the RLD are acute and reversible (**pneumothorax**) or chronic but reversible (**Guillain-Barré syndrome**), the treatment consists of specific corrective interventions (e.g., chest tube placement) as well as supportive measures (e.g., temporary mechanical ventilation) to assist the patient to maintain adequate ventilation until the patient is again able to be independent in this activity.

MATURATIONAL CAUSES OF RESTRICTIVE LUNG DYSFUNCTION

Abnormalities in Fetal Lung Development

- **Agenesis** is the total absence of the bronchus and the lung **parenchyma.** Unilateral agenesis is rare.[7]
- **Aplasia** is the development of a rudimentary bronchus without the development of the normal lung parenchyma. This condition is also rare.[7]
- **Hypoplasia** is the development of a functioning

although not always normal bronchus with the development of reduced amounts of lung parenchyma. This developmental abnormality is much more common and may affect one lung or one lobe of a lung. It is often present in infants born with a large diaphragmatic hernia and displaced abdominal organs.[7]

Clinical Manifestations

Depending on the amount of lung parenchyma lost, these infants can be asymptomatic or can exhibit severe pulmonary insufficiency. The pulmonary impairment is restrictive in that the volumes are decreased even though the lung compliance may be normal.

Respiratory Distress Syndrome

Respiratory distress syndrome (RDS), also known as **hyaline membrane disease** (HMD), is a disorder of prematurity or lack of complete lung maturation in the human fetus. It usually takes 36 weeks of normal gestation to achieve lung maturity in the fetus. Infants born with a gestational age less than 36 weeks often exhibit respiratory distress and may develop the full complement of signs and symptoms associated with RDS.[8]

Etiology

Insufficient maturation of the lungs is the cause of RDS, and it is usually linked directly to the gestational age of the fetus at birth. The incidence of RDS in infants with a gestational age of 26 to 28 weeks at birth is approximately 75%.[8] In contrast, the incidence of RDS in infants with a gestational age of 36 weeks at birth is less than 5%.[8] Other factors that seem to contribute to the development of RDS are gender, race, and diabetes in the mother. Premature male infants are more at risk to develop RDS than premature female infants. White premature infants have a greater incidence of RDS than black premature infants. Fetal lung maturation is delayed in pregnant women with diabetes, so infants born of diabetic mothers are at increased risk of developing RDS. Worldwide, 1% of infants are affected by RDS.[8] In the United States RDS is seen in approximately 50,000 infants each year.[9]

Pathophysiology

RDS is caused primarily by abnormalities in the **surfactant system** and inadequate surfactant production. Structural abnormalities, such as alveolar septal thickening, within the immature lung may also contribute to the pathophysiology of this syndrome. The surfactant dysfunction causes the overall retractive forces of the lung to be greater than normal, which decreases lung compliance; increases the work of breathing; and leads to progressive diffuse **microatelectasis,** alveolar collapse, increased ventilation-perfusion mismatching, and impaired gas exchange. In addition, alveolar epithelial and endothelial permeability are abnormal in the immature lung. Therefore, when these premature infants are mechanically ventilated without sufficient normal surfactant, the bronchiolar epithelium is disrupted. This leads to pulmonary edema and the generation of hyaline membranes. Further, because the proximal and distal airways in the infant are very compliant and the alveoli may be less compliant owing to atelectasis and the formation of hyaline membrane, the mechanical ventilator pressures used can disrupt, dilate, and deform the airways. Mechanical ventilator pressures can also cause air leaks, **tension pneumothorax,** and extensive pulmonary interstitial emphysema.

Another cause of decreased gas exchange is the often severe pulmonary hypertension evident in infants with RDS. These infants have hypoxemia and are acidotic, both of which cause vasoconstriction. This response is exaggerated in the infant and causes severe pulmonary hypertension, increased ventilation-perfusion mismatching, and decreased gas exchange. RLD may be complicated further by persistent *patency of the ductus arteriosus,* resulting in a left-to-right shunt within the infant's heart. The patent ductus arteriosus increases pulmonary pressures and blood flow and could allow plasma proteins to leak into the alveolar space, causing pulmonary edema and further interfering with surfactant function.

Complications common in infants with RDS include intracranial hemorrhage, sepsis, pneumonia, pneumothorax, pulmonary hemorrhage, and pulmonary interstitial emphysema. This syndrome can also result in the development of **bronchopulmonary dysplasia.** Recovery in RDS is usually preceded by an abrupt unexplained diuresis.[8]

Clinical Manifestations

Signs

Pulmonary Function Tests. Infants with RDS have an increased respiratory rate, decreased lung compliance, and decreased lung volumes, particularly FRC and VC. The work of breathing is greatly increased.[9]

Chest Radiograph. The lung parenchyma of infants with RDS has a fine **reticulogranular pattern** (homogeneous ground-glass appearance).[9, 10] If the RDS is severe, air bronchograms are prominent, and the **cardiothymic silhouette** becomes indistinct owing to severe diffuse microatelectasis.

Arterial Blood Gases. There is a marked decrease in the Pa_{O_2}. The arterial partial pressure of carbon dioxide (Pa_{CO_2}) is increased, and the pH is decreased or acidotic. Ventilation-perfusion mismatching is prominent. Dead space ventilation is increased, whereas alveolar ventilation is decreased.

Breath Sounds. An *expiratory grunt* is the most common abnormal breath sound associated with RDS. The diffuse atelectasis may also cause rales and decreased breath sounds.[9]

Cardiovascular Findings. Infants may experience bradycardia. There may also be cerebral, pulmonary, or intraventricular hemorrhage as a result of the exaggerated changes in vascular pressures due to the hypoxemia and **acidemia.**

Symptoms. The infant's respiratory pattern is usually rapid and very labored, with significant intercostal, sternal, and substernal retractions. Nasal flaring and grunting are common. Infants with RDS often are cyanotic, and their crying is decreased in volume and strength.[9]

Treatment

Beginning in the late 1980s and early 1990s **surfactant replacement therapy** has become the treatment of choice for these infants. Early intervention is extremely important and the surfactant replacement therapy is most effective when started within the first 2 hours of life. The earlier the intervention, the shorter and more benign the course of the disease. The artificial surfactant is given as a liquid suspension in saline and delivered to the infant by aerosol via endotracheal intubation. The results of this therapeutic intervention are immediate reduction in oxygen requirements, a major decrease in pulmonary complications such as pneumothoraces or pulmonary interstitial emphysema, and rapid weaning from mechanical ventilation, often within 12 to 24 hours.[9] Death in RSD is now almost entirely limited to infants of 24 to 26 weeks gestation weighing 500 to 800 g at birth.[9] Although administration of artificial surfactant has proved effective in decreasing the morbidity and mortality rates of RSD, studies are continuing to determine the best surfactant formulation and therapy regimen.

If the infant does not adequately respond to surfactant administration, then the infant, if large enough, may be treated with extracorporeal membrane oxygenation (ECMO) or nitric oxide administration delivered in the inspiratory gas to cause pulmonary vasodilation.[9]

An alternative to treatment of RDS is prevention of the disease by maternal/fetal treatment with corticosteroids. Administration of corticosteroids to the mother before delivery can accelerate fetal lung maturation by stimulating surfactant synthesis, inducing changes in the elastic properties of the fetal lung, stimulating alveolarization, and decreasing the permeability of the airway and alveoli epithelium.[8, 9]

Normal Aging

Maturation of the various body systems is a natural process that takes place throughout a lifetime. Normal aging usually refers to physiologic changes that occur with regularity in the majority of the population and can therefore be predicted. Physiologic changes that commonly are considered part of the aging process can begin as early as 20 years of age.[11]

Etiology

The normal aging process in the pulmonary system is very slow and insidious, and because we have great ventilatory reserves the changes are often not felt functionally until the sixth or seventh decade of life.[12] Universally, the normal aging process in the lungs is complicated by the fact that throughout life the lungs have had to cope with the external environment. Environmental factors that affect the aging process include general pollution, noxious gases, specific occupational exposures, inhaled drug use, and of course cigarette smoking.[11]

Physiology

The compliance of the pulmonary system starts to decrease at about age 20 and decreases approximately 20% over the next 40 years.[11] Maximum voluntary ventilation decreases by 30% between the ages of 30 and 70.[11] Vital capacity also drops by about 25% between 30 and 70 years of age.[12] However, as stated previously, although some changes start as early as the second and third decades of life, functional status often is not affected until the sixth and seventh decades.

The control of ventilation undergoes significant change. The peripheral chemoreceptors are not as responsive to hypoxia, and the central receptors are not as responsive to acute **hypercapnia.** These changes mean that the ventilatory response mediated by the central nervous system is significantly depressed.[3, 8] The normal Pa_{O_2} in a 70-year-old is 75, a measurement that is not interpreted as hypoxia by the central nervous system.[11]

The thorax undergoes a number of changes, including decalcification of the ribs, calcification of the costal cartilages, arthritic changes in the joints of the ribs and vertebrae, dorsal thoracic kyphosis, and increased anteroposterior diameter of the chest (barrel chest). The effects of these changes combine to decrease the compliance of the chest wall and increase the work of breathing. Oxygen consumption in the respiratory muscles is increased, causing an increase in the minute ventilation. The strength and endurance of the inspiratory muscles gradually diminishes. This results in a decreased maximal ventilatory effort.[3] The forced expiratory volume in 1 second (FEV_1) is reduced by about 40 mL per year.[11]

The lung tissue itself shows enlargement of the air spaces owing to enlargement of the alveolar ducts and terminal bronchioles. The alveolar surface area and the alveolar parenchymal volume are decreased. The alveolar walls become thinner, and the capillary bed incurs considerable loss, with an increase in ventilation-perfusion mismatching. Distribution of inspired air and pulmonary blood flow becomes less homogeneous with age. Diffusing capacity is therefore reduced, and physiologic dead space is increased.[11]

The static elastic recoil of the alveolar tissue decreases, which means that alveolar compliance is increased and the lungs do not empty well. The lung compliance curve is shifted to the left in the elderly. Thus, although TLC may not change with age, RV increases and dynamic volumes therefore decrease[11, 12] (Fig. 5–5).

Closing volumes are increased, which results in early closure of the small airways, particularly in the dependent lung regions. By approximately age 55 small airways are closed at or above FRC in the supine position. In the upright position, with the attendant increase in FRC, this change occurs at approximately age 70.[11]

Of course, normal concomitant aging changes take place in the cardiovascular system, including a decrease in maximum heart rate and cardiac output. These changes combine with the decreased oxygen exchange capability of the lungs and result in a decrease in the maximum oxygen uptake with exercise and therefore a decrease in the anaerobic threshold. After 50 years of age, the maximum oxygen uptake usually declines at a rate of 0.45 mL/kg/min for each year.[3, 8]

Ventilation during sleep is altered in the elderly. **Electroencephalographic** (EEG) studies have shown that total nocturnal sleep time is shorter with more frequent and longer nocturnal awakenings in the elderly. The pattern of ventilation during sleep is irregular more often in the elderly than in young adults. Repetitive periodic apneas occur in 35% to 40% of the elderly, predominantly in males during sleep stages 1 and 2.[8]

Clinical Manifestations

Signs
Pulmonary Function Tests. Total lung capacity and airway resistance are usually unchanged. The RV is increased, and the VC is decreased by approximately 25% by age 70.[12] Flow rates are de-

AGING

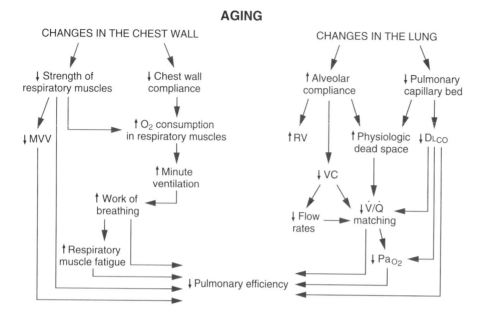

Figure 5–5. Respiratory changes with aging. MVV, Maximum voluntary ventilation; O_2, oxygen; RV, residual volume; VC, vital capacity; V/Q, ventilation-perfusion; Pa_{O_2}, arterial partial pressure of oxygen; DL_{CO}, diffusing capacity of the lungs for carbon monoxide.

creased. **Maximum voluntary ventilation** (MVV) is decreased by about 30%[11]; DL_{CO} is also decreased.

Chest Radiograph. The chest film can show a variety of changes in the bony thorax (e.g., decalcification of ribs, barrel chest, kyphosis) and in the lung parenchyma (e.g., larger air spaces, altered vascular markings).

Arterial Blood Gases. The Pa_{O_2} normally is decreased to about 75 mm Hg at age 70.[11] Usually the Pa_{CO_2} is normal or slightly elevated.

Breath Sounds. Auscultation often reveals slightly diminished breath sounds.

Cardiovascular Findings. With increased age maximum heart rate, stroke volume, and cardiac output usually decrease. Often systolic blood pressure increases.

Symptoms. The pulmonary reserve is so great that individuals usually do not consciously note any changes until the seventh or eighth decade. But even before changes in the pulmonary system are recognized, an individual has often made changes in activity patterns and recreational pursuits because of normal aging processes taking place in other body systems.

Treatment

Aging is normal—no treatment is required. The elderly should be encouraged to remain active and

fit. Although even with regular activity about 0.45 mL/kg/min of oxygen consumption is lost each year, the fit elderly person has a greater maximum oxygen consumption than the sedentary person. In fact, a sedentary elderly person beginning regular exercise can improve maximum oxygen consumption by 5% to 25% and can regain the exercise capability that was present as much as 5 to 10 years earlier.[11]

PULMONARY CAUSES OF RESTRICTIVE LUNG DYSFUNCTION

Idiopathic Pulmonary Fibrosis

Idiopathic pulmonary fibrosis (IPF) is an inflammatory process involving all of the components of the alveolar wall that progresses to gross distortion of lung architecture. The components of the alveolar wall include the epithelial cells, the endothelial cells, the cellular and noncellular components of the interstitium, and the capillary network. These components are supported by the connective tissue framework made up of collagen and elastic fibers and containing a milieu of ground substance. Other synonyms used for IPF are **cryp-**

togenic fibrosing alveolitis, interstitial pneumonitis, and **Hamman-Rich syndrome.**[13, 14]

Etiology

By definition, IPF is of unknown origin. It may be due to viral, genetic, or immune system disorders or a combination of these disorders.[15] IPF seems to be an immunologically mediated disease set in motion by an initial acute injury or infection.[16]

Pathophysiology

The lung involvement in IPF often shows patchy focal lesions scattered throughout both lungs. These lesions first show inflammatory changes and then scar and become fibrotic, distorting the alveolar septa and the capillary network. The alveolar spaces become irregular in size and shape. There can be significant progressive destruction of the capillary bed. These changes combine to cause decreased lung compliance; decreased lung volumes; increased ventilation-perfusion mismatching; decreased surface area for gas exchange; decreased diffusing capacity; increased pulmonary arterial pressure, which increases the work of the right ventricle; increased work of breathing; increased caloric requirements; and decreased functional capacity.[13, 15]

The two major pathologic components of IPF are (1) an inflammatory process in the alveolar wall (sometimes called an *alveolitis*), and (2) a scarring or fibrotic process that is thought to be secondary to the active inflammation. Both of these pathologic processes occur simultaneously within the lung.[13] There is also an increased incidence of lung cancer in IPF patients, as much as sixfold in women and 14-fold in men.[10, 16]

Clinical Manifestations

Signs

Pulmonary Function Tests. Patients with IPF typically show decreases in TLC, VC, FRC, and RV. These patients have normal flow rate values or slightly decreased flow rates owing to the decrease in lung volumes. The DL_{CO} is also decreased. As the disease progresses, the V_T is decreased and the respiratory rate increased.

Chest Radiograph. The chest films usually show a diffuse **reticulonodular pattern** throughout both lungs (Fig. 5–6). Some patients have a predominance of abnormal markings in the lower lung fields.[10] Interestingly, some IPF patients with symptoms of the disease have normal chest radiographs.[16] High-resolution computed tomography (HRCT) of the chest shows that areas of inflammation and cellularity have a ground-glass appearance, and areas with fibrosis and cystic changes have a reticular pattern.[16]

Arterial Blood Gases. The Pa_{O_2} is often decreased, but the Pa_{CO_2} is usually within normal limits. Patients are hypoxemic first with exercise; as the disease progresses, they are hypoxemic at rest.

Breath Sounds. Auscultation reveals bibasilar end-inspiratory dry rales and possibly decreased breath sounds.[10]

Cardiovascular Findings. As the pulmonary capillary bed is destroyed, about one third of IPF patients develop pulmonary hypertension.[10] This change from a low-pressure system to a high-pressure system puts a strain on the right ventricle and can cause cor pulmonale. Late in the course of IPF, patients may be cyanotic, and 40% to 75% of IPF patients have clubbing of the digits.[13]

Symptoms. Patients with IPF usually complain of an insidious onset of dyspnea on exertion, which progresses until the patient may feel short of breath even at rest. Many patients also complain of a repetitive, nonproductive cough, although some patients may have mucus hypersecretion and expectoration.[16] Patients also usually report weight loss and decrease in appetite as well as complain of fatigue. Another symptom of IPF reported by some patients is sleep disturbances with a loss of rapid eye movement sleep.[13, 15]

Treatment

Corticosteroids (usually prednisone) continue to be the mainstay in the treatment of IPF. However, cytotoxic drugs such as cyclophosphamide and azathioprine have also been used in patients who do not seem to be responsive to corticosteroids. In fact, there is now some evidence that initial treatment with steroids and cyclophosphamide or cyclophosphamide alone may be preferable.[9, 16] It is the active alveolitis that seems to have some positive response to these drugs. The progressive fibrosis is

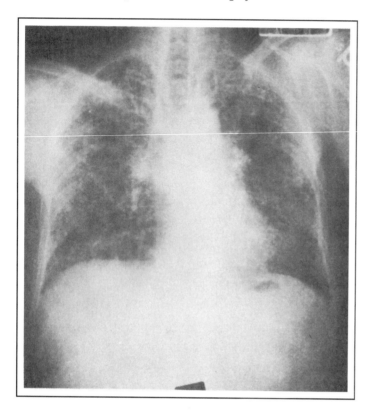

Figure 5-6. Chest radiograph of a patient with idiopathic pulmonary fibrosis, showing a diffuse reticulonodular pattern and elevated diaphragms. (From Mitchell RS. Synopsis of Clinical Pulmonary Disease. 2nd ed. St. Louis, CV Mosby, 1978, p 244.)

nonreversible, and these drugs have no effect on lung tissue that is already fibrotic.

The remaining treatment measures are supportive. They include smoking cessation, maintaining adequate oxygenation and ventilation, good nutrition, and aggressive treatment of infection.[16]

The final therapeutic intervention that can be offered to IPF patients is **lung transplantation.** Orthotopic single lung transplantation (SLT) is a viable therapeutic option for selected IPF patients.[15] In 1983 the Toronto Group reported the first long-term survival of an IPF patient with an SLT.[16] IPF is now one of the four primary diagnoses (IPF, emphysema, cystic fibrosis, pulmonary hypertension) for which lung transplantation is performed.[17] However, this surgical therapeutic intervention is not without risks (see Chapter 12), including the risk of restrictive lung dysfunction, namely obliterative bronchiolitis.

Coal Workers' Pneumoconiosis

Coal workers' pneumoconiosis (CWP) is an interstitial lung disease, an occupational **pneumoconiosis,** caused by the inhalation of coal dust. This

disease is most commonly divided into simple CWP and complicated CWP.[18]

Etiology

Coal workers' pneumoconiosis is caused by repeated inhalation of coal dust over a long period of time; usually 10 to 12 years of underground work exposure is necessary for the development of simple CWP.[19] Complicated CWP, sometimes called *progressive massive fibrosis,* usually occurs only after even longer exposure to coal dust. Anthracite coal is more hazardous than bituminous in the development of this disease.[20]

Coal workers' pneumoconiosis is not the most common respiratory disease found in this occupational group. Chronic bronchitis is even more common, usually occurs earlier, and often coexists with CWP in coal miners.

Pathophysiology

The pathologic hallmark of CWP is the coal macule, which is a focal collection of coal dust with little tissue reaction either in terms of cellular infiltration or fibrosis. These coal macules are often located at the division of respiratory bronchioles and are often associated with focal emphysema.[19] Lymph nodes are enlarged and homogeneously pigmented and are firm but not fibrotic. The pleural surface appears black owing to the deposits of coal dust. Simple CWP is a benign disease if complications do not develop. Less than 5% of cases progress to complicated CWP.[21]

The mechanism for the progression of simple CWP to complicated CWP is unknown. It has been suggested that simple CWP may progress when it is combined with infection, or silicosis, or tuberculosis, or altered immunologic mechanisms. Complicated CWP results in large confluent zones of dense fibrosis that are usually present in apical segments in one or both lungs. These zones are made up of dense, acellular, collagenous, black-pigmented tissue. The normal lung parenchyma can be completely replaced, and the blood vessels in the area then show an obliterative arteritis. These fibrous zones can completely replace the entire upper lobe.[19]

Common complications associated with complicated CWP include emphysema, chronic bronchitis, tuberculosis, cor pulmonale, and pulmonary **thromboembolism.**

Clinical Manifestations

Signs
Pulmonary Function Tests. In simple CWP, spirometric tests may be normal or may show a slight decrease in VC with a small increase in RV. There may also be a small reduction in DL_{CO}. In complicated CWP, a marked reduction occurs in TLC, VC, and FRC. Lung compliance is decreased. The diffusing capacity is also decreased. Respiratory rate is often increased.

Chest Radiograph. The chest radiograph in simple CWP shows small, discrete densities more nodular than linear. They may appear throughout both lung fields but usually are predominantly in the upper regions. In complicated CWP, the chest radiograph shows **coalescent opacities** of black fibrous tissue, usually in the posterior segments of the upper lobes or the superior segments of the lower lobes. Cavities also may be evident that are due to superimposed tuberculosis or are secondary to ischemic necrosis.

Arterial Blood Gases. The Pa_{O_2} is decreased.

Breath Sounds. With simple CWP, breath sounds may be slightly diminished, with rhonchi heard owing to the concomitant chronic bronchitis. In complicated CWP, breath sounds vary: they are markedly decreased over areas of fibrotic tissue; abnormal bronchial breath sounds are present over compressed or atelectatic lung areas; and rhonchi and rales are heard with chronic bronchitis and excess secretions.

Cardiovascular Findings. In complicated CWP, fibrotic pulmonary hypertension and cor pulmonale are common when significant portions of the lungs and pulmonary capillary beds are involved.

Symptoms. The major symptoms include severe dyspnea and cough, usually with the appearance of moderate to copious amounts of black sputum. Patients are often barrel chested and wasted in appearance. Progressive weight loss is common.

Treatment

Complicated CWP with pulmonary fibrosis is nonreversible; there is no cure for it. Supportive treatment includes cessation of exposure to coal dust, good nutrition, interventions to ensure adequate oxygenation and ventilation, and progressive exercise training to maximize the remaining lung function.

Silicosis

Silicosis, one of the occupational pneumoconioses, is a fibrotic lung disease caused by the inhalation of the inorganic dust known as free or **crystalline silicon dioxide.**[18]

Etiology

The disease as mentioned is caused by the repeated inhalation of free or crystalline silicon dioxide, which is very common and widely distributed in the earth's crust in a variety of forms including quartz, flint, cristobalite, and tridymite.[19] Industries in which silicon dioxide exposure can occur include mining, tunneling through rock, quarrying, grinding and polishing rock, sandblasting, ship building, and foundry work.[21]

Pathophysiology

Inhaled silica causes macrophages to enter the area to ingest these particles. But the macrophages are destroyed by the cytotoxic effects of the silica. This process releases lysosomal enzymes that then induce progressive formation of collagen, which eventually becomes fibrotic. Another characteristic of silicosis is the formation of acellular nodules composed of connective tissue called *silicotic nodules.* Initially these nodules are small and discrete, but as the disease progresses they become larger and coalesce. Silicosis normally affects the upper lobes of the lung more than the lower lobes. Silicosis also seems to predispose the patient to secondary infections by mycobacteria including ***Mycobacterium tuberculosis.*** Complicated silicosis follows a steadily deteriorating course that leads to respiratory failure (Fig. 5–7).[2, 21]

Clinical Manifestations

Signs

Pulmonary Function Tests. As would be expected, TLC and VC are decreased. Pulmonary compliance is decreased, and FEV_1 is diminished.

Chest Radiograph. The chest films may show small rounded opacities or nodules (simple silicosis), which can become larger over time and coalesce (complicated silicosis). The pathologic findings are seen more in the upper lung fields. The hilar lymph nodes may be enlarged and calcified.

Arterial Blood Gases. The Pa_{O_2} is decreased with exercise.

Breath Sounds. Breath sounds are decreased, particularly over the upper lobes. Rhonchi may or may not be present.

Cardiovascular Findings. There are no specific findings.

Symptoms. The major symptom is shortness of breath. Cough is also very common, and it may be productive or nonproductive.

Treatment

There is no treatment except to avoid further exposure to silica. Supportive therapy is used to counteract the patient's symptoms and includes measures to provide adequate oxygenation, ventilation, and nutrition. Annual TB screening using PPD skin testing is also recommended.[16]

Asbestosis

Asbestosis is a diffuse interstitial pulmonary fibrotic disease caused by asbestos exposure.[20]

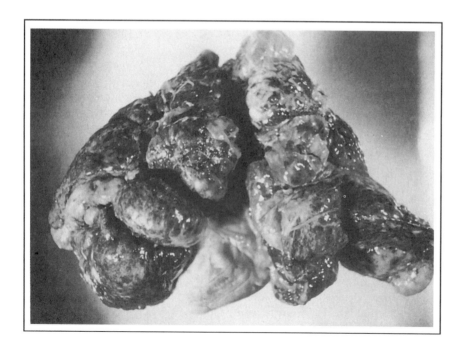

Figure 5–7. Lungs with widespread silicosis showing scarring and honeycombing. (From Fishman AP. Pulmonary Diseases and Disorders. 2nd ed. New York, McGraw-Hill, 1988, p 2238.)

Occupational asbestos exposure is also associated with an increased incidence of primary cancer of the larynx, oropharynx, esophagus, stomach, and colon.[19]

Etiology

The term *asbestos* is used generically to name a specific group of naturally occurring fibrous silicates. There are four types of commercially significant asbestos. *Chrysolite* accounts for more than 70% of the asbestos used in the United States and is primarily mined in Canada and the Commonwealth of Independent States. *Crocidolite* and *amosite* are mined primarily in South Africa. *Anthophyllite* comes from Finland.[20]

Asbestos is valued because of its resistance to fire; it has been used widely since the 1930s. Those at most risk for asbestosis are asbestos miners and millers, construction workers, shipbuilders, insulation workers, pipefitters, steamfitters, sheet metal workers, welders, workers who remove old asbestos insulation, workers employed in building renovation or demolition, and auto mechanics who work on brake linings.

Pathophysiology

How asbestos causes a fibrotic reaction is not understood. There seems to be a considerable latency period after an initial exposure, which can extend to 15 to 20 years. It is hypothesized that the asbestos fiber causes an alveolitis in the area of the respiratory bronchioles, which then progresses to peribronchiolar fibrosis owing to the release of chemical mediators. Plaques, which are localized fibrous thickenings of the parietal pleura, are common and are usually seen posteriorly, laterally, or on the pleural surface of the diaphragm. Pleural effusions may also occur with asbestosis. Also "asbestos bodies" or ferruginous bodies appear in the lungs and sputum of these patients. These rod-shaped bodies with clubbed ends seem to be an asbestos fiber coated by macrophages with an iron-protein complex.[2, 7, 19, 20]

Studies have shown conclusively that cigarette smoking has a multiplicative effect in the development of primary lung cancer in persons who have been exposed to asbestos. In addition several studies have shown a dose-response relationship between the amount of cigarette smoking and the degree of fibrotic response to inhaled asbestos.[19] Complications of asbestosis include **bronchiectasis,** pleural **mesothelioma,** and **bronchogenic carcinoma.**[7]

Clinical Manifestations

Signs
Pulmonary Function Tests. Lung compliance and therefore lung volumes are decreased. Specifically the TLC and the VC are decreased with a lesser decrease usually seen in the RV. The FEV_1, which is a measure of flow rate, is often decreased also. The DL_{CO} is decreased.

Chest Radiograph. The chest films show irregular or linear opacities distributed throughout the lung fields that are more prominent in the lower zones. Often a loss of distinct heart and diaphragmatic borders occurs owing to pleural involvement. These usually clear borders take on a "shaggy" appearance. There also may be radiographic evidence of diaphragmatic or pericardial calcification. Late in the course of the disease, the chest radiograph may show cyst formation, and the lungs may take on a honeycomb appearance.

Arterial Blood Gases. The Pa_{O_2} is decreased with exercise and, as the disease progresses, may be decreased at rest. Hypercapnia is not a usual manifestation of asbestosis, so the Pa_{CO_2} is commonly within normal limits.

Breath Sounds. Auscultation usually reveals bibasilar rales with decreased breath sounds due to the pleural thickening. Percussion is often dull at the bases.

Cardiovascular Findings. As the pulmonary capillary bed is destroyed, pulmonary hypertension develops and increases the work of the right ventricle. This can progress to cor pulmonale and cyanosis. Clubbing is more common in asbestosis than in silicosis or coal workers' pneumoconiosis.

Symptoms. The major patient complaints with asbestosis are dyspnea on exertion that progresses to shortness of breath even at rest, recurrent pulmonary infections, and chronic cough with or without sputum production. In addition, patients often report weight loss with decreased appetite and exercise tolerance.

Treatment

There is no curative treatment for asbestosis, and the disease progresses even though exposure to asbestos has ceased. Symptomatic support includes cessation of smoking, good nutrition, exercise conditioning to maximize lung function, and prompt treatment of recurrent pulmonary infections.

Bronchopulmonary Dysplasia

Bronchopulmonary dysplasia is a chronic pulmonary syndrome in neonates that occurs in some survivors of RDS who have been ventilated mechanically and have received high concentrations of oxygen over a prolonged period of time. Other names used for this syndrome are **pulmonary fibroplasia** and ventilator lung.[7, 8]

Etiology

The incidence of BPD following RDS varies from 2% to 68% in different studies.[8] The incidence increases in neonates who had low birth weights (less than 1000 g); required mechanical ventilation, particularly using continuous positive pressure; received inspired oxygen concentrations (FI_{O_2}) at 60% or higher; or received supplemental oxygen for more than 50 hours.[7, 8] In fact, BPD almost invariably develops in neonates who received oxygen at an FI_{O_2} of 60% or higher for 123 hours or more.[7] See Chapter 6 for more details on BPD.

Bronchiolitis Obliterans

Bronchiolitis obliterans is a fibrotic lung disease that affects the smaller airways. It can produce restrictive and obstructive lung dysfunction. This syndrome has been known and discussed under a variety of names including bronchiolitis, bronchiolitis obliterans with organizing pneumonia (BOOP), bronchiolitis fibrosa obliterans, follicular bronchiolitis, and bronchiolitis obliterans with diffuse interstitial pneumonia.[13]

Etiology

Bronchiolitis obliterans was first recognized in children, usually those under the age of 2 years. Pediatric bronchiolitis obliterans is often caused by a viral infection, most commonly by the *respiratory syncytial virus, parainfluenza virus, influenza virus,* or *adenovirus.*[20] An adult form of the disease has now been recognized that can occur in persons from 20 to 80 years of age and has a wider variety of causes. In the adult, bronchiolitis obliterans may be caused by toxic fume inhalation (nitrogen dioxide) or by viral, bacterial, or mycobacterial infectious agents, particularly **Mycoplasma pneumoniae.** It may be associated with connective tissue diseases, such as rheumatoid arthritis; related to organ transplantation and graft versus host reactions; or allied with other diseases, such as idiopathic pulmonary fibrosis. It also may be idiopathic, with no known cause.[13]

Pathophysiology

Bronchiolitis obliterans is characterized by necrosis of the respiratory epithelium in the affected bronchioles. This necrosis allows fluid and debris to enter the bronchioles and alveoli, causing alveolar pulmonary edema and partial or complete obstruction of these small airways. With complete obstruction, the trapped air is absorbed gradually, and the alveoli then collapse, causing areas of atelectasis. When the destruction of the respiratory epithelium is severe or widespread, it may be followed by a significant inflammatory response. This causes fibrotic changes in the adjacent peribronchial space, the alveolar walls, and the air spaces. The fibrotic changes are patchy and usually occur primarily within the bronchial tree and alveoli rather than in the interstitial lung tissue, as happens in IPF. All these changes combine to increase ventilation-perfusion mismatching; decrease lung compliance; impair gas transport; and, in some patients, cause demonstrable airway obstruction.[13]

Clinical Manifestations

Signs
Pulmonary Function Tests. The DL_{CO} is usually reduced. Lung volumes may be normal or decreased. Respiratory rate is increased. Flow rates are more frequently within normal limits but may be decreased.

Chest Radiograph. The chest radiographic findings are variable depending on the causative factor and the extent of involvement. In pediatric bronchiolitis obliterans, the chest radiograph may show hyperinflation with increased bronchial markings or subsegmental consolidation and collapse. Some children have patchy alveolar infiltrates, and others have a diffuse nodular or reticulonodular pattern consistent with interstitial inflammation and scarring. In adults the chest radiograph may first show pulmonary edema; bilateral patchy alveolar infiltrates may also be seen. Later in the clinical course, a nodular pattern consistent with fibrotic changes within the bronchial tree and alveoli may be seen.

Arterial Blood Gases. Hypoxemia is present in almost all patients; the Pa_{O_2} is therefore reduced. Carbon dioxide may be retained, resulting in respiratory acidosis, or the Pa_{CO_2} may be within normal limits.

Breath Sounds. Rales and often expiratory wheezing are heard on auscultation. Areas of decreased breath sounds are also common.

Cardiovascular Findings. Tachycardia is common.

Symptoms. Patients are often **dyspneic,** with an increased respiratory rate and a hacking, nonproductive cough. In infants chest wall retractions are often evident. Patients may be **cyanotic.** If the cause of the bronchiolitis obliterans is infectious, fever and malaise are common.

Treatment

In children treatment is supportive, usually consisting of hydration and supplemental oxygen. If the child is unable to clear secretions, postural drainage and suctioning are employed. Mechanical ventilation is rarely needed. If respiratory syncytial virus is the causative pathogen, then the antiviral agent ribavirin may be administered via aerosol.[20] Corticosteroids, antibiotics, and bronchodilators are not recommended in the treatment of pediatric bronchiolitis obliterans. In adults supplemental oxygen and proper fluid balance are also very important. Corticosteroids have proved very effective in treating adult bronchiolitis obliterans that is idiopathic, caused by toxic fume inhalation, or associated with connective tissue disease.

Pneumonia

Pneumonia is an inflammatory process of the lung parenchyma. This inflammation usually begins with an infection in the lower respiratory tract that may be caused by various microbes, including bacteria, mycoplasmas, viruses, protozoa, or a psittacosis agent. There are two categories of pneumonias: **community-acquired** pneumonias and hospital-acquired or **nosocomial** pneumonias[12, 22] (Fig. 5–8).

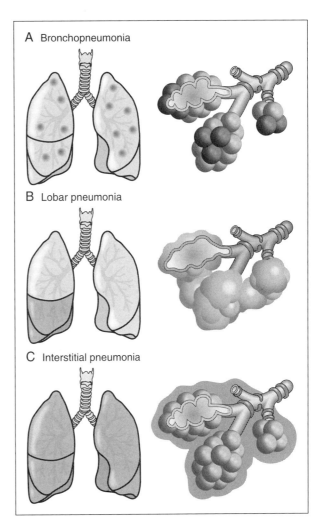

Figure 5–8. Lung infection (pneumonia) can be diffuse throughout the lung, as in bronchopneumonia (*A*) or localized, as in lobar pneumonia (*B*). Interstitial pneumonia, as found in AIDS, is often diffuse and bilateral in the interstitium (*C*). (From Damjanov, I. Pathology for the Health-Related Professions. Philadelphia, WB Saunders, 1996, Fig. 8–7, p 181.)

> ### Clinical Note: Treatment for Pneumonia
>
> Pneumonia is simply an inflammatory process of some part of the lung where gas exchange occurs that progresses beyond inflammation and develops into infection. The key to treatment of pneumonia is to first identify the microbe (virus versus gram-positive or gram-negative bacteria). Specific medical treatment (specific antibiotic) is based on identification of the microbe, although broad-spectrum medications may be initiated before identification has been made.
>
> The problem with treating pneumonia in recent years is the identification of microbes that are resistant to many forms of antibiotics. These microbes can be spread via aerosol or physical contact and can cause severe disability and even death in immunosuppressed individuals.

Etiology

Community-acquired pneumonias can be traced to the causative agent in approximately 50% of cases.[20] Although bacteria account for the majority of these pneumonias, viruses cause about one third of the pneumonias in this category.[20] More than 1 million cases of bacterial pneumonia occur each year in the United States. Approximately 50,000 people die of this disease, making it the fifth most common cause of death in the nation.[2] The most common agent causing bacterial pneumonia is *Streptococcus pneumoniae,* commonly called *pneumococcus.* Other bacterial agents that cause community-acquired pneumonias are *Legionella pneumophila, Haemophilus influenzae,* enteric gram-negative bacteria, *Staphylococcus aureus,* and anaerobic bacteria often found in the oropharynx. The mycoplasmal agent *M. pneumoniae,* the psittacosis agent *Chlamydia psittaci,* and the protozoan *Pneumocystis carinii,* can also cause community-acquired pneumonias. The viruses that are most commonly involved in community-acquired pneumonias are adenovirus, influenza virus, herpes group viruses (including cytomegalovirus), parainfluenza virus, respiratory syncytial virus, and Hantavirus that can lead to severe ARDS. Hantavirus was the cause of multiple deaths during an epidemic in the southwestern United States in 1993.[9] Although there are many infectious agents in the environment, few pneumonias develop because of the efficient de-fense mechanisms in the lung. Those who develop community-acquired pneumonias usually have been infected with an exceedingly virulent organism or a particularly large **inoculum** or have impaired or damaged lung defense mechanisms.[20]

Hospital-acquired or nosocomial pneumonias are defined as infections in the lower respiratory tract with an onset of 72 hours or more after hospitalization; they are characterized by the development of a new or progressive lung infiltrate.[20] Nosocomial pneumonias account for 10% of all nosocomial infections.[8] These opportunistic infections prey on the sickest patients in the hospital. The rate of nosocomial infections in the United States is 5.7 per 100 admissions or more than 2 million per year.[8] The most commonly identified causative agent of nosocomial pneumonias is a gram-negative bacillus, *Pseudomonas aeruginosa.*[20] Other microbes also capable of causing hospital-acquired pneumonias are *S. aureus, Klebsiella pneumoniae,* and *P. carinii.* The patients most likely to develop a nosocomial pneumonia have one or more of the following risk factors: nasogastric tube placement; intubation; **dysphagia;** tracheostomy; mechanical ventilation; thoracoabdominal surgery; lung injury; diabetes; chronic cardiopulmonary disease; intra-abdominal infection; **uremia; shock;** history of smoking; advanced age; poor nutritional status; or certain therapeutic interventions, such as the administration of broad spectrum antibiotics, corticosteroids, antacids, or high oxygen concentrations.

Pathophysiology

Bacteria and other microbes commonly enter the lower respiratory tract. It has been estimated that during sleep 45% of healthy people aspirate oropharyngeal secretions into the lower respiratory tract (Fig. 5–9).[8] However, microbial entrance into the lower respiratory tree usually does not lead to pneumonia because of the elaborate defense mechanisms within the pulmonary system. The mechanical defenses include cough, bronchoconstriction, angulation of the airways favoring impaction and subsequent transport upward, and action of the mucociliary escalator. The immune defenses include bronchus-associated lymphoid tissue, phagocytosis by polymorphonuclear cells and macrophages, immunoglobulins A and G, comple-

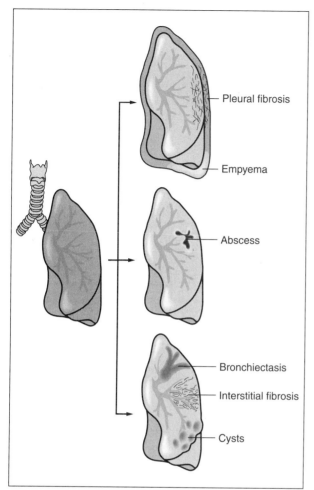

Figure 5–9. *Top,* Chronic changes in the lung can include pleural fibrosis (scarring secondary to infection or inflammation). Persistent infection in the pleural cavity is called empyema. Chronic inflammation of the pleura due to chronic irritation or infection (from occupational lung diseases, pneumonia, etc.) can cause pleural fibrosis. *Middle,* When the pneumonia is suppurative, an abscess can form. *Bottom,* Chronic infection may also lead to bronchiectasis. Chronic lung disease may also lead to interstitial fibrosis or cyst formation. (From Damjanov I. Pathology for the Health-Related Professions. 2nd ed. Philadelphia, WB Saunders, 2000, Fig. 8–9, p 183.)

ment, surfactant, and cell-mediated immunity by T lymphocytes.[20]

The most common routes for infection leading to pneumonia are inhalation and aspiration (Table 5–2). When the causative agent is bacterial, the first response to infection is an outpouring of edema fluid. This is followed rapidly by the appearance of polymorphonuclear leukocytes that are involved in active **phagocytosis** of the bacteria, and then fibrin is deposited in the inflamed area. Usually by day 5, specific antibodies are in the area fighting the bacterial infection. Clinically, bacterial pneumonia usually has an abrupt onset and is characterized by lobar **consolidation,** high fever, chills, dyspnea, tachypnea, productive cough, pleuritic pain, and leukocytosis.[1, 19, 20] When the causative agent is viral, the virus first localizes in respiratory epithelial cells and causes destruction of the cilia and mucosal surface, leading to the loss of mucociliary function. This impairment may then predispose the patient to bacterial pneumonia. If viral infection reaches the level of the alveoli, there may be edema, hemorrhage, hyaline membrane formation, and possibly the development of adult respiratory distress syndrome. Primary viral pneumonia is a serious disease with diffuse infiltrates, extensive parenchymal injury, and severe hypoxemia. Clinically, viral pneumonia usually has an insidious onset and is characterized by patchy diffuse bronchopulmonary infiltrates, moderate fever, dyspnea, tachypnea, nonproductive cough, **myalgia,** and a normal white blood cell count.[20] Usually it is impossible to identify the specific pathogen by clinical signs and symptoms or chest radiographic findings. Specific laboratory test results and other data are needed.

Clinical Manifestations

Signs
Pulmonary Function Tests. Pneumonias from any cause result in decreased lung volumes, decreased lung compliance, decreased gas exchange, increased respiratory rate, increased inspiratory pressure, and increased work of breathing. These changes are due to fluid-filled alveoli; increased ventilation-perfusion mismatching; decreased oxygen uptake; possible pulmonary capillary leakage; and pneumonia resolution, including fibrosis and scarring. For these reasons, pneumonias are usually classified as primarily restrictive in the lung dysfunction they cause.

Chest Radiograph. Bacterial pneumonia usually shows a lobar consolidation on radiographic examination. This may involve more than one lobe in one lung or may involve lobes in both lungs with confluent shadows that usually terminate at pleural surfaces. Viral pneumonia presents a different ra-

Table 5-2

Pneumonia Transmission and Treatment

PNEUMONIA TYPE	TRANSMISSION ROUTE	SUSCEPTIBLE POPULATIONS	PREFERRED DRUG
Bacterial			
Streptococcus pneumoniae	Droplet inhalation, direct contact with infected respiratory secretions, indirect contact with articles soiled by infected respiratory secretions	Infants, elderly; patients having congestive heart failure, COPD, splenectomy, alcoholism, multiple myeloma, or a predisposing viral infection	Penicillin G Tetracyclines Ampicillin
Legionella pneumophila	Inhalation of an aerosolized infected water source (drinking water, air conditioning, shower heads, lakes)	Elderly; patients having diabetes, COPD, AIDS, renal transplantation, malignancy, and alcoholism; smokers	Erythromycin
Haemophilus influenzae	Droplet inhalation, direct contact with infected respiratory secretions, indirect contact with articles soiled by infected respiratory secretions	Elderly; patients having chronic bronchitis, AIDS, alcoholism, splenectomy, chronic debilitation, or a predisposing viral infection	Ampicillin Cephalosporins
Klebsiella pneumoniae	Droplet inhalation, direct contact with infected respiratory secretions, indirect contact with articles soiled by infected respiratory secretions	Elderly in nursing homes; patients having COPD, alcoholism, diabetes, malignancy, chronic renal failure, and chronic debilitation	Aminoglycosides Cephalosporins
Pseudomonas aeruginosa	Droplet inhalation, direct contact with infected respiratory secretions, indirect contact with articles soiled by infected respiratory secretions, hematogenously, wound infection	Patients having cystic fibrosis, ARDS, or neutropenia; patients on mechanical ventilation	Carbenicillin Aztreonam Aminoglycosides
Staphylococcus aureus	Droplet inhalation, direct contact with infected respiratory secretions, indirect contact with articles soiled by infected respiratory secretions, hematogenously, aspiration	Patients having cystic fibrosis, drug addictions, splenectomy, or a predisposing viral infection	Antistaphylococcal penicillin Cephalosporins Vancomycin Clindamycin Gentamicin
Mycoplasmal			
Mycoplasma pneumoniae	Droplet inhalation, direct contact with infected respiratory secretions, indirect contact with articles soiled by infected respiratory secretions	School children; college students; patients with AIDS	Erythromycin Tetracycline Streptomycin
Viral			
Respiratory syncytial virus	Droplet inhalation, direct contact with infected respiratory secretions, indirect contact with articles soiled by infected respiratory secretions	Infants 2–5 months of age and school-aged children	Ribavirin

	Mode of Transmission	Susceptible Population	Treatment
Adenovirus	Droplet inhalation, direct contact with infected respiratory secretions or infected feces, indirect contact with articles soiled by infected respiratory secretions or feces	Children 6 months to 5 years and military recruits	None
Cytomegalovirus	Contact with infected body fluids including tears, saliva, blood, breast milk, urine, semen; can be infected in utero and by infected transplanted organs	Fetuses; patients having malignancy, AIDS, major organ transplantation, or chronic debilitation	Acyclovir analogue
Influenza virus	Droplet inhalation, direct contact with infected respiratory secretions, indirect contact with articles soiled by infected respiratory secretions	Women in the third trimester of pregnancy; elderly; patients having malignancy, heart disease, COPD, diabetes, chronic renal failure, neuromuscular disorders, or chronic debilitation	Amantadine
Fungal			
Pneumocystis carinii	Unknown, probably droplet inhalation	Premature infants, patients with AIDS, or chronic debilitation	Trimethoprim-sulfamethoxazole Pentamidine
Chlamydial			
Chlamydia psittaci	Inhalation of infected droplets, droplet nuclei, or dust from the desiccated dropping of infected birds (parrots, parakeets, turkeys, pigeons, chickens)	Persons with pet birds and workers on poultry farms and in poultry processing plants	Tetracycline Chloramphenicol

COPD, chronic obstructive pulmonary disease; AIDS, acquired immunodeficiency syndrome; ARDS, adult respiratory distress syndrome.
From Cottrell GP, Surkin HB. Pharmacology for Respiratory Care Practitioners. Philadelphia, FA Davis, 1995.

diographic picture, which is usually of a bilateral bronchopneumonia. It appears on a chest radiograph as diffuse scattered fluffy shadows, indicating patchy alveolar infiltrates, and follows the distribution of the central conducting airways. When cavities are seen in addition to the other chest radiographic findings, the pneumonia is described as a necrotizing pneumonia.

Arterial Blood Gases. Patients with pneumonia are usually hypoxemic, having a decreased Pa_{O_2}. Because most patients with pneumonia are dyspneic and tachypneic, they are blowing off an excess of carbon dioxide and so the Pa_{CO_2} may be decreased.

Breath Sounds. Auscultation findings vary depending on the amount of consolidation and the course of the particular pneumonia. Breath sounds could include any of the following: bubbling rales, rhonchi, bronchial breath sounds, decreased or absent breath sounds, a pleural friction rub, egophony, and **whispered pectoriloquy.** There is a dullness to **mediate percussion.**

Cardiovascular Findings. Patients usually have some tachycardia, particularly with high fever. Arrhythmias are uncommon.

Symptoms. Generally the symptoms of bacterial pneumonia include high fever, chills, dyspnea, tachypnea, productive cough, and pleuritic pain. A viral pneumonia produces symptoms of moderate fever, dyspnea, tachypnea, nonproductive cough, and myalgias.

Treatment

Drug therapy is the primary focus in the treatment of pneumonia, particularly antibiotics for treating bacterial pneumonia. Antibiotic therapy should be pathogen specific if the pathogen can be determined; if not, an empiric regimen of multiple antibiotics may be needed. Oxygen and temporary mechanical ventilation may be necessary in patients with refractory hypoxemia (Pa_{O_2} less than 60 mm Hg). Other supportive therapy includes postural drainage, percussion, vibration, and assisted coughing techniques for patients who are producing more than 30 mL per day of mucus or have an impaired cough mechanism.[20] Adequate hydration and nutrition are also important. Nosocomial pneumonias can also be prevented by rigorous environmental controls in hospitals. Such controls include strict guideline adherence for the prevention of contamination of ventilators and other respiratory equipment, careful aseptic patient care practices, and surveillance of infections and antibiotic susceptibility patterns in high-risk areas.

Specific Pneumonias

Bacterial Pneumonias
• **Streptococcus pneumoniae**
S. pneumoniae is more common in the elderly, in alcoholics, and in those with **asplenia,** multiple myeloma, congestive heart failure, or chronic obstructive lung disease. Seventy percent of patients report a preceding viral illness.[20] This type of pneumonia occurs more frequently during the winter and early spring. Specific signs and symptoms include rusty colored sputum, hemoptysis, bronchial breath sounds, egophony, increased tactile fremitus, pleural friction rub, severe pleuritic chest pain, pleural effusion in 25% of patients, and slight liver dysfunction.[10, 20] Complications can include **lung abscess,** atelectasis, delayed resolution in the elderly, pericarditis, **endocarditis, meningitis,** jaundice, and arthritis.[19] S. pneumoniae is treated with penicillin G, ampicillin or tetracyclines.[23] There is also a pneumococcal vaccine; this injection provides lifetime protection against 23 **serotypes** of the pneumococcus that account for 85% of all cases of pneumococcal pneumonia.[20]

Legionella pneumophila
L. pneumophila can occur in epidemic proportions because the organism is water borne and can emanate from air conditioning equipment, drinking water, lakes, river banks, water faucets, and shower heads. L. pneumophila accounts for 7% to 15% of all community-acquired pneumonias.[20] It is found commonly in patients who are on dialysis; in persons who have a malignancy, a chronic obstructive pulmonary disease (COPD), a smoking history, or are older than 50 years; and in persons who are alcoholics or diabetics. Transplant recipients, of any organ, are at the highest risk.[10] Signs and symptoms in addition to those characteristic of bacterial pneumonias include headache, myalgias, preceding diarrhea, mental confusion, **hyponatremia,** bradycardia, and liver function abnormalities. Productive coughs with purulent sputum and he-

moptysis can develop in 50% to 75% of patients.[10] However, most patients (90%) begin with a non-productive cough.[10] The chest radiograph may show **lobar** consolidation or unilateral or bilateral bronchopneumonia; rounded densities with **cavitation** may also be seen. Fifteen percent of these patients have pleural effusions. The antibiotic of choice is erythromycin. Rifampin may also be used in addition to erythromycin.[20]

Haemophilus influenzae

H. influenzae causes pneumonia particularly in children who have had their spleen removed, in patients with COPD, in alcoholics, in AIDS patients, in those with lung cancer, in patients with **hypogammaglobulinemia,** and in the elderly.[9] In addition to the expected signs and symptoms of bacterial pneumonia, *H. influenzae* often causes a sore throat. The chest radiograph may show focal lobar, lobular, multilobar, or patchy bronchopneumonia or segmental pneumonia that usually involves the lower lobes. Complications can include empyema, lung abscess, epiglottitis, otitis media, pericarditis, meningitis, and arthritis. The preferred antibiotic is ampicillin; however, 20% of patients have been shown to be resistant to ampicillin. In these cases cephalosporins, trimethoprimsulfamethoxazole, and chloramphenicol are used.[19, 20]

Klebsiella pneumoniae

K. pneumoniae may cause either a community-acquired pneumonia or a nosocomial pneumonia. The community-acquired *Klebsiella* pneumonia is seen most commonly in men over the age of 40 who are alcoholic or diabetic or who have underlying pulmonary disease. These patients may show purulent blood-streaked sputum, hemoptysis, cyanosis, and hypotension. Chest radiographic findings most frequently show right-sided involvement of the posterior segment of the upper lobe or the lower lobe segments. There may be outward bulging of a lobar fissure due to edema, and 25% to 50% of these patients have lung abscesses.[19] Complications include empyema, lung abscess, pneumothorax, chronic pneumonia, pericarditis, meningitis, and anemia. Treatment includes a two-drug therapy: an aminoglycoside and a cephalosporin. Oxygen is also used to maintain an oxygen saturation level of 80% to 85%. The mortality rate for this gram-negative pneumonia is 20%.[19]

Nosocomial *Klebsiella* pneumonia is a **fulminant** infection that causes severe lung damage and has a 50% mortality rate.[20] It affects debilitated patients in hospitals and nursing homes, middle-aged or older, who suffer from concomitant alcoholism, diabetes, malignancy, or chronic renal or cardiopulmonary disease. Their sputum is thick, purulent, and bloody or is thin and has a "currant jelly" texture. Tachycardia is common. The chest radiograph can show lobar consolidation, usually in the upper lobes, with lung abscesses, cavities, scarring, and fibrosis. A bronchopneumonia appearance may also occur. Complications are the same as those in community-acquired *Klebsiella* pneumonia. Drug therapy includes the use of aminoglycosides, cephalosporin, and antipseudomonal penicillin.[19, 20]

Pseudomonas aeruginosa

P. aeruginosa is a gram-negative bacillus and is the most common cause of nosocomial pneumonias. It causes 15% of all hospital-acquired pneumonias and affects 40% of all mechanically ventilated patients.[20] Those at most risk for this infection are patients with cystic fibrosis, bronchiectasis, **tracheostomy,** or **neutropenia** or those who are on mechanical ventilation or corticosteroid therapy. This necrotizing pneumonia causes alveolar septal necrosis, microabscesses, and vascular thrombosis and has a mortality rate of 70% in postoperative patients.[20] Signs and symptoms include confusion, bradycardia, and hemorrhagic pleural effusion. The chest radiograph shows bilateral patchy alveolar infiltrates, usually in the lower lobes with nodular infiltrates and cavitation.[20] Treatment always involves two drugs. Aminoglycosides, carbenicillin, and aztreonam are used to overcome this bacterium.[23]

Staphylococcus aureus

S. aureus causes approximately 5% of community-acquired pneumonias and can also cause nosocomial pneumonia.[20] This type of pneumonia is usually seen in infants and children under the age of 2 years, in patients with cystic fibrosis or COPD, or in patients who are recovering from influenza. The hallmark lesion seen in this pneumonia is ulcerative bronchiolitis with necrosis of the bronchiolar wall.[23] Signs and symptoms include cough with dirty salmon-pink purulent sputum, high fever, dyspnea, and pleuritic chest pain.[23] Other manifestations commonly seen in children are cyanosis, labored breathing, grunting, flaring of the nostrils, and chest wall retractions. The chest radiograph shows a diffuse bronchopneumonia, with bilateral infiltrates, cavitary lung abscesses, **pneumatoceles,** and pleural effusions. Complications include pneumothorax, lung abscess, endocarditis, and meningitis. Treatment is with antistaphylococcal penicillin, cephalosporin, vancomycin, clindamycin, and gentamicin.[19, 20, 23]

Mycoplasma Pneumonias

Mycoplasmas are the smallest free-living organisms that have yet been identified. This class of organisms is intermediate between bacteria and viruses. Unlike bacteria they have no rigid cell wall, and unlike viruses they do not require the intracellular machinery of a host cell to replicate.

Mycoplasma pneumoniae

M. pneumoniae is seen in all age groups but is more common in persons under 20 years of age. Mycoplasma pneumonias account for 20% of all community-acquired pneumonias.[20] This infection is common year round, but usually the incidence increases in the fall and winter. Mycoplasma pneumonia has also been termed *walking pneumonia* because the respiratory symptoms are often not severe enough for people to seek medical attention. The course of the disease is approximately 4 weeks, and it is very infectious; whole families may become ill once a child brings it into the home. The signs and symptoms often include many extrapulmonary manifestations that are not common in bacterial or viral pneumonias. Patients may have fever, shaking chills, dry cough, headache, **malaise,** sore throat, ear ache, arthralgias, arthritis, immune dysfunction with an **autoantibody response, meningoencephalitis,** meningitis, **transverse myelitis,** cranial nerve palsies, Guillain-Barré syndrome, myocarditis, pericarditis, gastroenteritis, pancreatitis, glomerulonephritis, hepatitis, generalized lymphadenopathy, and erythema multiforme including Stevens-Johnson syndrome.[10] The chest radiograph shows interstitial infiltrates, usually unilateral in the lower lobe; 20% of patients have a pleural effusion. Treatment is with erythromycin, tetracycline, or streptomycin.[20, 23]

Viral Pneumonias

Cytomegalovirus, varicella zoster, and **herpes simplex** cause viral pneumonias most commonly in immunocompromised hosts, such as patients who have had major organ transplants or who have AIDS or malignancy. The respiratory syncytial virus and the parainfluenza virus cause viral pneumonias in children. The adenovirus is a source of viral pneumonias in children and in military recruits. Viral pneumonias in the debilitated elderly are most commonly caused by the influenza virus. Persons at most risk for a viral pneumonia are those who have an underlying cardiopulmonary disease or who are immunosuppressed or pregnant. Complications of viral pneumonias include secondary bacterial infections, bronchial hyperreactivity and possibly asthma, chronic air flow obstruction, **tracheitis,** bronchitis, **bronchiolitis,** and **acellular hyaline membrane** formation.

Some antiviral agents are now available. **Acyclovir** is used against herpes simplex and varicella zoster. **Amantadine** is the drug of choice for influenza A. **Ribavirin** is used in children to treat the respiratory syncytial virus. Cytomegalovirus is treated with acyclovir analogue dihydroxyphenylglycol (DHPG). No drug therapy is available for all the varieties of viral agents, so treatment is often limited to supportive measures.[19, 20]

Fungal Pneumonias
Pneumocystis carinii

P. carinii, originally described as a protozoan, is now thought to be a fungal organism.[10] *Pneumocystis carinii* pneumonia (PCP) is closely associated with AIDS because nearly 75% of AIDS patients have at least one episode of PCP during their lifetime.[10] Patients with AIDS have impairment of T cell function as well as humoral immune dysfunction and thus are susceptible to infection from bacteria, viruses, fungi, and parasites. PCP is also seen in transplant patients, especially those on cyclosporine, and in patients with lymphoreticular hematologic malignancies.[9] The chest radiograph most commonly shows bilateral diffuse interstitial or alveolar infiltrates, more prominent in the perihilar regions, and a solitary pulmonary nodule.[9] PCP damages the parenchymal cells within the lung and alters the alveolar-capillary permeability. This type of pneumonia usually has a subacute course of fever, dyspnea, cough, chest pain, malaise, fatigue, weight loss, and night sweats, but the symptoms can progress to include tachypnea, reduced Pa_{O_2} and cyanosis.[9] Treatment is with trimethoprim-sulfamethoxazole. If this drug is not tolerated, then pentamidine is prescribed.[9, 12, 20]

Chlamydial Pneumonias
Chlamydia psittaci

C. psittaci causes approximately 12% of the community-acquired pneumonias in the student population and about 6% of the community-acquired pneumonias in the elderly.[20] The onset is usually insidious, with cough, sputum, hemoptysis, dyspnea, headache, myalgia, and hepatosplenomegaly.[9, 10] Complications include laryngitis, pharyngitis, encephalitis, hemolytic anemia, bradycardia, hepatitis, renal failure, and macular rash. Treatment is with tetracycline or chloramphenicol.[9, 10]

Adult Respiratory Distress Syndrome

Adult respiratory distress syndrome is a clinical syndrome caused by acute lung injury and characterized by severe hypoxemia and increased permeability of the alveolar capillary membrane. It also has been known as noncardiogenic pulmonary edema, shock lung, increased permeability pulmonary edema, and post-traumatic pulmonary insufficiency.[2, 8, 20, 22, 24]

Etiology

Adult respiratory distress syndrome can result from a variety of causes. Some of the primary causes of ARDS include

- Trauma—fat emboli, lung contusion, heart-lung transplantation, head injury
- Aspiration—drowning, gastric contents
- Drug associated—heroin, barbiturates, narcotics
- Inhaled toxins—smoke, high oxygen concentrations
- Shock—any cause
- Massive blood transfusion—sepsis
- Metabolic—acute pancreatitis, uremia
- Primary pneumonias—viral, bacterial, *P. carinii*
- Other—increased intracranial pressure, post-cardiopulmonary bypass, amniotic fluid embolism, ascent to high altitudes[2, 8, 20, 22, 24]

Approximately 150,000 cases of ARDS are diagnosed annually in the United States.[20]

> **Clinical Note: Adult Respiratory Distress Syndrome**
>
> A diagnosis of ARDS is a serious, life-threatening diagnosis, as these patients have a high in-hospital mortality rate and poor in-hospital prognosis. Fewer than 50% of the patients with this diagnosis live.

Pathophysiology

The primary pathologic change is an increase in the permeability of the microvascular pulmonary membrane. The specific cause of this change is unknown. It seems that a variety of mechanisms can be involved, depending on the specific associated etiology. Therefore, the exact mechanisms that damage the pulmonary capillary endothelial cells and the alveolar epithelial cells are still under investigation. The current theories under investigation involve the role of the neutrophils, the complement pathway, the superoxide radicals, the proteolytic enzymes, and the coagulation system.[2] When the permeability of the microvascular membrane increases, excess fluid and plasma proteins are allowed to move out of the vascular channel. This fluid leaks into the interstitial tissue and then crosses the usually tight alveolar epithelium to fill the alveoli. The change from an air-filled to a fluid-filled organ decreases markedly the compliance of the lung and all lung volumes and capacities; the work of breathing is increased. Pulmonary vascular resistance is increased; an intrapulmonary right-to-left shunt takes place; ventilation-perfusion mismatching is increased; and gas exchange is drastically reduced. In addition, surfactant production is decreased. The significant atelectasis due to edema in the interstitial spaces leads to increased pressure on the adjacent bronchioles and alveoli (Fig. 5–10).[6, 20]

Following this acute phase, ARDS may resolve completely so that the patient regains normal lung function after a period of a few months. However, some patients enter a **subacute** phase following ARDS. During this phase, alveolar fibrosis and capillary obliteration develop within the lung, which leads to chronic significant restrictive dysfunction. It is not clear why ARDS in some patients resolves completely whereas in others significant perma-

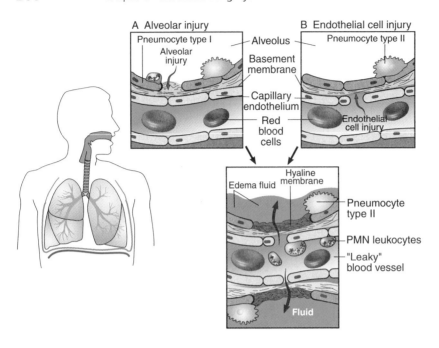

Figure 5-10. Pathogenesis of adult respiratory distress syndrome. Initial injury may be from alveolar cell injury (*A*) or systemic from endothelial cell injury (*B*). The result of injury is diffuse compromised hyaline membranes, ruptured alveolar walls, leaky blood vessels, and subsequent intra-alveolar edema fluid with polymorphonuclear (PMN) leukocyte invasion. (Adapted from Damjanov I. Pathology for the Health-Related Professions. Philadelphia, WB Saunders, 1996, Fig. 8-21, p 212.)

nent lung damage occurs. It is known that the longer the patient is on mechanical ventilation and high concentrations of oxygen, the poorer is the long-term prognosis.[20]

Clinical Manifestations

Signs

Pulmonary Function Tests. The FRC, VC, and V_T are all decreased. Owing to the decreased lung compliance, the work of breathing is increased and the respiratory rate is high. Flow rates may be normal or somewhat decreased. The DL_{CO} is usually decreased.

Chest Radiograph. Symmetric, bilateral, diffuse, fluffy infiltrates are found on the chest radiograph. These may coalesce into a diffuse haze, which essentially whites out the lung. Other findings may be present that are consistent with concomitant COPD, atelectasis, or pneumonia.

Arterial Blood Gases. The Pa_{O_2} by definition is less than 60 mm Hg in ARDS.[8] The Pa_{CO_2} is usually decreased also because of the markedly impaired gas exchange; however, if the patient has a chronic carbon dioxide–retention problem, the Pa_{CO_2} may be elevated.

Breath Sounds. Decreased breath sounds are heard over the fluid-filled areas of lung, and wet rales are a common finding. Wheezing and rhon-

chi may be heard also, depending on the precipitating cause of ARDS.

Cardiovascular Findings. Tachycardia is common with ARDS. Arrhythmias may occur also, owing to the decreased oxygenation of the myocardium and the stress placed on the heart.

Symptoms. These patients appear acutely ill. They are dyspneic even at rest, and their breathing pattern is fast and labored. They often are cyanotic. Other symptoms include headache, impaired mental status, restlessness, and increased anxiety.

Treatment

The treatment of ARDS can be divided into four areas, each with a distinct goal. The first area is treatment of the precipitating cause of the ARDS. Because of the wide variety of causes for ARDS, there is a wide variety in the treatment protocols used to address the underlying cause. The second area of treatment is aimed at supporting adequate gas exchange and tissue oxygenation until the ARDS resolves. Maintaining an adequate airway and oxygenation is usually accomplished by intubating and mechanically ventilating the patient. Most often the patient is placed on a volume-cycled ventilator with supplemental oxygen. **Positive end-expiratory pressure** (PEEP) of approximately 5 to 15 cm H_2O is often utilized.[20] The PEEP helps inflate poorly ventilated alveoli; improves gas exchange; and permits the inspired oxygen concentration to be lowered, decreasing the risk of oxygen toxicity. The third area of treatment is supportive, managing the patient's nutritional status and fluid balance. Fluid and electrolyte balance is very important in these patients. Management may mean monitoring input and output and using diuretics. Or because ARDS can be associated with multiorgan failure, it may mean the use of highly technical interventions such as **continuous arteriovenous hemofiltration** (CAVH) or dialysis in patients with chronic renal insufficiency.[8] The final focus of treatment is to prevent and treat complications of the patient's condition along with intensive care measures. Complications common in patients with ARDS are nosocomial infections, pulmonary barotrauma due to the use of PEEP, and coagulation disturbances. The prognosis in ARDS is always guarded; mortality can be as high as 50% to 70%, especially if this syndrome is associated with failure in other organ systems or is complicated by serious or repeated infections.[8, 20]

Bronchogenic Carcinoma

Bronchogenic carcinoma is a malignant growth of abnormal epithelial cells arising in a bronchus.[20] This growth or tumor may spread by infiltrating surrounding tissues or by metastasizing to other body organs, or both (Fig. 5–11). The World Health Organization has established a standard classification system that organizes bronchogenic carcinoma into four major types. They are squamous cell carcinoma, small cell carcinoma, adenocarcinoma, and large cell carcinoma.[20]

Etiology

The causes of lung cancer are many. However, it has now been well established through numerous studies that the primary causative factor is tobacco use. *Approximately 80% to 90% of lung cancers are caused by tobacco.*[10] The average cigarette smoker has 10 times the risk of developing lung cancer as the nonsmoker. The heavy cigarette smoker may have up to 25 times the risk of developing lung cancer as the nonsmoker.[10, 20] Most disturbing is

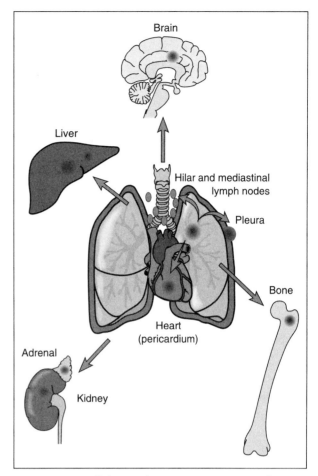

Figure 5–11. Primary lung cancer metastasizes to pleura, lymph, bone, brain, kidney, and liver. (From Damjanov I. Pathology for the Health-Related Professions. 2nd ed. Philadelphia, WB Saunders, 2000, Fig. 8–26, p 204.)

the finding that lung cancer risk is closely related and increased by starting to smoke at an early age. When children start smoking at 15 years of age or younger and continue smoking, after 50 years they have a **100-fold increased risk** of lung cancer over that of a nonsmoker.[10] Passive smoking, that is, exposure to cigarette smoke exhaled by a smoker as well as side-stream smoke, also has been proved to increase the incidence of lung cancer by approximately 20%. Like active smoking at an early age, passive smoking during childhood and adolescence may pose a significantly increased risk.[10] It is currently estimated that there are 500 to 5000 lung cancer deaths per year in the United States due to passive smoking.[9, 10]

Occupational agents have also been implicated in the development of bronchogenic carcinoma. The known carcinogens present in the workplace include radioactive material, asbestos, chromates, nickel, mustard gas, isopropyl oil, hydrocarbons, arsenic, hematite, vinyl chloride, and bischloromethyl ether.[20] Increased exposure to radon or significant air pollution also increases the incidence of lung cancer, although the relationship is very difficult to quantify. It is interesting that diets containing beta carotene (found in many green, yellow, and orange fruits and vegetables) have been shown to modestly decrease the risk for lung and other cancers.[16] In some individuals and families, a genetic predisposition for the development of lung cancer seems to be present.

Globally, it is estimated that one death occurs each minute as a result of lung cancer.[10] Currently, lung cancer accounts for 33% of all cancer deaths in men and 23% of all cancer deaths in women. Over the past 20 years the male-female ratio of lung cancer deaths has dropped from 5–7:1 to 1.4:1 as a result of the striking increase in lung cancer among women, which began about 1965.[9] It is now the leading cause of death from cancer in both men and women (surpassing breast cancer). In 1995 approximately 157,400 Americans died of lung cancer, 95,400 men and 62,000 women.[16] In the same year almost 175,000 new cases of lung cancer were diagnosed.[20] Lung cancer prognosis is bleak and unchanging. About 50% of patients die within 1 year of the diagnosis. The 5-year survival rates have not changed significantly over the past 3 decades. This means that of the 175,000 Americans diagnosed with lung cancer in 1995, fewer than 20,000 lived to see the year 2000.[16] *The majority of these people could have been spared this diagnosis, with its pain, health care costs, morbidity, and unrelenting fatal conclusion, if they had given up smoking.*

Pathophysiology

Each of the four major types of bronchogenic carcinoma is discussed separately (Fig. 5–12).

Squamous cell carcinoma accounts for 15% to 25% of all lung cancer. It arises from the bronchial mucosa after repeated inflammation or irritation caused by cancer stimuli. It is therefore the type of lung cancer most closely associated with cigarette smoking. Squamous cell carcinoma often arises in the segmental or subsegmental bronchi but can also cause a hilar tumor. It is considered a centrally located tumor and occurs in the peripheral lung only about 30% of the time. Squamous cell tumors are bulky. They cause obstructive dysfunction because they extend into the bronchial lumen, which can prevent airflow and lead to atelectasis and pneumonia. They cause restrictive dysfunction because the tumor can compress the surrounding lung tissue; cause atelectasis and pneumonia, both of which decrease the ventilation-perfusion matching; and impair gas exchange. These tumors often cavitate but do not metastasize early. When squamous cell cancer does metastasize, it most often involves the liver, adrenal gland, central nervous system, and pancreas.[20]

Small cell carcinoma, also called *oat cell carcinoma,* accounts for 20% to 25% of all lung cancer.[2] It may arise in any part of the bronchial tree; however, 75% of the time it presents as a centrally located proximal lesion.[20] It often has hilar or mediastinal lymph node involvement. This tumor usually does not extend into the bronchial lumen but spreads through the submucosa and can cause obstructive and restrictive dysfunction through compression of the surrounding lung tissue. This type of lung cancer rapidly involves the vascular channels, lymph nodes, and soft tissue. It is known to metastasize widely and early and in most patients has metastasized by the time the diagnosis is made. This tumor rarely cavitates but commonly produces hormones that can lead to a wide variety of symptoms in many different body systems not involved in direct metastasis.

A number of body organs, however, are involved in direct metastasis. Seventy-five percent of small cell carcinoma metastasizes to the central nervous system, 65% to the liver, 58% to the adrenal gland, 30% to the pancreas, 28% to bone, 20% to the genitourinary system, 10% to the thyroid, and 10% to the spleen.[20] The metastases to the central nervous system and the bone often produce clinical symptoms such as hemiplegia, epilepsy, personality changes, confusion, speech deficits, headache, bone pain, and pathologic fractures. Metastases to the liver and the adrenal glands are often clinically silent.[8] Other clinical symptoms caused by tumor hormone production that are of particular interest to the physical therapist include abnormalities in the neurologic or

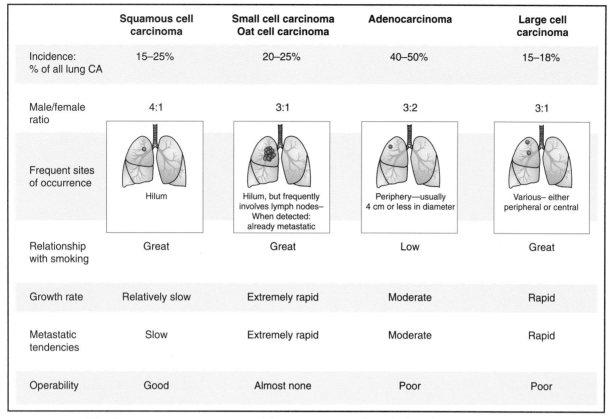

	Squamous cell carcinoma	Small cell carcinoma Oat cell carcinoma	Adenocarcinoma	Large cell carcinoma
Incidence: % of all lung CA	15–25%	20–25%	40–50%	15–18%
Male/female ratio	4:1	3:1	3:2	3:1
Frequent sites of occurrence	Hilum	Hilum, but frequently involves lymph nodes– When detected: already metastatic	Periphery—usually 4 cm or less in diameter	Various– either peripheral or central
Relationship with smoking	Great	Great	Low	Great
Growth rate	Relatively slow	Extremely rapid	Moderate	Rapid
Metastatic tendencies	Slow	Extremely rapid	Moderate	Rapid
Operability	Good	Almost none	Poor	Poor

Figure 5–12. The four most common types of lung cancer are described and compared in regard to several features, including incidence, pattern of development, growth rate, and gender representation.

muscular systems. These complications of small cell carcinoma can include progressive dementia, ataxia, vertigo, sensory neuropathy with numbness and loss of reflexes, motor neuropathy with progressive muscle weakness and wasting, atrophic paresis of the proximal limb girdle musculature, marked fatigability, osteoarthropathy, arthralgia, and peripheral edema.[20]

Adenocarcinoma includes acinar adenocarcinoma, papillary adenocarcinoma, and bronchoalveolar carcinoma and accounts for 40% to 50% of all lung cancer.[9] This is now the most common type of lung cancer in the United States.[10] The majority of these tumors are located in the periphery of the lung and may not be spatially related to the bronchial tree. These tumors may arise as a solitary nodule and may involve the pleura, causing a carcinogenic pleural effusion. Adenocarcinomas metastasize widely and often involve the central nervous system, which produces neurologic symptoms already listed under small cell carci-

noma. Approximately half of these tumors involve the hilar and mediastinal lymph nodes.[20]

Large cell carcinoma includes all tumors not categorized in the first three groups and accounts for 15% to 18% of all lung cancer.[2] These tumors are most frequently subpleural in location. Peripheral tumors are often large, lobulated, and bulky, causing compression of the normal lung tissue. They are usually sharply defined lesions, which may be necrotic or cavitate. This type of tumor spreads locally by invasion and also metastasizes widely, with more than 50% metastasizing to the brain.[20]

Prognosis for lung cancer is usually discussed in terms of 5-year survival rates according to the stage of the disease. The assigned stage number is determined by the International Cancer Staging System and is determined by the degree of lung involvement, the location of the lesion, and the metastatic spread of the disease. The 5-year survival rate for stage I is 50%, for stage II is 30%, for stage

IIIa is 17%, for stage IIIb is less than 5%, and for stage IV is 0%.[20]

Clinical Manifestations

Signs

Pulmonary Function Tests. There are no characteristic pulmonary function abnormalities associated with bronchogenic carcinoma. Some obstructive or restrictive dysfunction may be reflected in the pulmonary function test values, depending on the location and size of the lesion.

Chest Radiograph. Squamous cell carcinoma appears most often as a hilar or perihilar cavitary lesion with bronchial obstruction and atelectasis or postobstructive consolidation.[8, 20] Small cell carcinoma usually appears as a central mass, often with bulky hilar and mediastinal adenopathy.[8] Adenocarcinoma is usually seen as a peripheral tumor, often with pleural involvement and pleural effusions.[20] Large cell carcinoma is seen on a chest radiograph as a sharply defined, large, often lobulated mass in the periphery of the lung; the lesion may cavitate.[20] The chest radiograph may also show elevated diaphragms if the tumor compresses the phrenic nerve and causes paralysis of the diaphragm.

Arterial Blood Gases. Hypoxemia and hypocapnia are common as the lung cancer progresses.

Breath Sounds. Wheezing and **stridor** may be heard if the tumor is obstructing the bronchial lumen. Patients may also have breath sounds consistent with atelectasis or postobstructive pneumonia if the tumor causes these complications.

Cardiovascular Findings. Superior vena cava syndrome may be present if the tumor compresses the superior vena cava. This compression would result in neck enlargement, neck vein distention, and edema in one or both arms. Anemia is common. Recurrent or migratory **thrombophlebitis** may occur. Cardiac arrhythmias and **tamponade** may also be complications of lung cancer.

Symptoms. The symptoms and physical findings with lung cancer can be extremely variable because they result from (1) the location and growth of the primary tumor with compression of the surrounding tissue, (2) regional extension into the mediastinum, (3) metastases to other body organs, and (4) tumor-produced hormones that can affect a number of body systems.[8] The pulmonary symptoms most common to lung cancer are a cough—productive or nonproductive—and chest pain—dull or acute. Central lesions more often cause the dull, vague, persistent, but poorly localized type of chest pain.[8] Peripheral lesions usually cause a more localized, sharp, pleuritic-type chest pain.[8] If the patient's cough is productive, blood streaking of the sputum is common, but massive hemoptysis is rare. Clubbing of the digits is a common finding. Some patients develop dyspnea. Most patients have experienced an unexplained weight loss.

Treatment

The three most widely accepted forms of therapy remain surgery, radiation, and chemotherapy. Newer treatment interventions being applied to patients with lung cancer include immunotherapy, laser, brachytherapy, and nutritional therapy. Unfortunately, none of these newer treatment options has affected the overall survival rate of lung cancer patients. Surgical removal of the tumor remains the treatment of choice for all non–small cell lung carcinoma when the location of the tumor makes resection possible.[20] The more defined and smaller the lesion, the better the surgical success rate. Radiation has been used to treat all types of lung cancer. However, small cell lung carcinoma is the most radiosensitive, followed by squamous cell carcinoma and adenocarcinoma. Large cell carcinoma is the least responsive to radiation.[20] The response to radiation therapy depends on the size of the tumor and the intrathoracic spread of the cancer. Chemotherapy does not significantly benefit non–small cell lung carcinoma. The response rates are low, and the toxicity rates for the drugs used are high. Chemotherapy is the treatment of choice for small cell lung carcinoma.[20] Because small cell carcinoma metastasizes so early, surgery has little to offer patients with this type of cancer. Chemotherapy and radiation in combination with chemotherapy are often used to treat small cell carcinoma. See Chapter 7 for the effects of chemotherapy and radiation on the cardiopulmonary system.

Pleural Effusions

Pleural effusion is the accumulation of fluid within the pleural space. The fluid is a **transudate**

if it has a low-protein content and accumulates owing to changes in the hydrostatic pressure within the pleural capillaries. The fluid is an **exudate** if it has a high-protein content and accumulates because of changes in the permeability of the pleural surfaces[21] (Fig. 5–13).

Etiology

Numerous disease entities can cause pleural effusions. Transudative pleural effusions can be caused by congestive heart failure, left ventricular failure, **cirrhosis,** nephrotic syndrome, pericardial disease, myxedema, pulmonary emboli, peritoneal dialysis, or atelectasis.[10] Exudative pleural effusions can be caused by bacterial or viral pneumonias, parasitic or fungal infections, tuberculosis, mesotheliomas, bronchogenic carcinoma, **systemic lupus erythematosus** (SLE), **rheumatoid arthritis** (RA), acute **pancreatitis,** esophageal perforations, intra-abdominal abscess, asbestos exposure, uremia, sarcoidosis, or drug hypersensitivity.[16, 19, 21]

Pathophysiology

The capillaries in the parietal pleura receive blood via the high-pressure systemic arterial circulation.

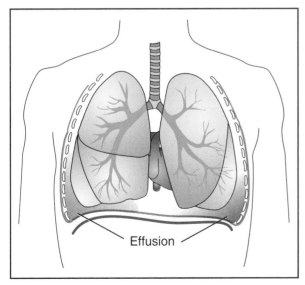

Figure 5–13. Pleural effusion is a collection of fluid in the pleural space between the thoracic cavity and the lung tissue. Pleurisy is an inflammation of the pleura. Both conditions restrict lung expansion.

> ### Clinical Note: Pleural Effusion
> The diagnosis of pleural effusion is not an indication for bronchopulmonary hygiene techniques. Instead, prevention of further pulmonary complications can be achieved with change of position, breathing exercises in different positions, and increasing activity. However, until the fluid is removed or reabsorbed, compression of the alveoli will occur, and atelectasis will be present.

The capillaries in the visceral pleura receive blood via the low-pressure pulmonary circulation. Because of this pressure gradient, fluid is constantly moving from the parietal pleural capillaries into the pleural space and is then reabsorbed into the visceral pleural capillaries. Approximately 5 to 10 liters of fluid pass through the pleural space each day using this route.[2] Additionally, each day up to one half liter of fluid and solutes can be moved out of the pleural space via the pleural lymphatics.[2, 20] Normally pleural fluid formation and pleural fluid resorption are balanced, so fluid does not accumulate in the pleural space. When this balance is disrupted by any cause and a significant amount of fluid is allowed to accumulate in the pleural space, a restrictive pulmonary impairment results.[2] The excess pleural fluid within the thorax does not allow the lungs to expand fully.

Transudative pleural effusions are associated with an elevation in the hydrostatic pressure in the pleural capillaries. This is most commonly due to left-sided heart failure, right-sided heart failure, or both. Because of the increase in the hydrostatic pressure, more fluid is moved out of the pleural capillaries and less fluid is reabsorbed. There is therefore excess fluid in the pleural space, causing a bilateral pleural effusion. Congestive heart failure is the single most common cause of transudative pleural effusions.[2]

Exudative pleural effusions are associated with an increase in the permeability of the pleural surfaces that allows protein and excess fluid to move into the pleural space. Therefore, in exudative pleural effusions the pleurae are in some way involved in the pathologic process. Most commonly, the pleurae may be involved in an inflammatory process or with neoplastic disease. Inflammatory processes such as pneumonia, tuberculosis, or pulmonary emboli with infarction can begin in the lung but extend into the visceral pleura, causing disruption of the normal pleural permeability. Cancer can also cause disruption of the normal pleural permeability, either by direct extension of a lung tumor to the pleural surface or by hematogenous dissemination of tumor cells to the pleural surface from a distant source. Tumor cells are also spread via the lymphatic system and therefore can alter the normal lymphatic clearance of the pleural space or be brought into the pleural space by the pleural lymphatics (Fig. 5–14).[2]

Clinical Manifestations

Signs

Pulmonary Function Tests. The larger the pleural effusion, the more compromised the lung volumes. Flow rates and DL_{CO} are unaffected by the pleural effusion. Pulmonary function tests may show a variety of abnormalities, depending on the underlying cause of the pleural effusion.

Chest Radiograph. Smaller pleural effusions are usually seen by noting a blunting of the costophrenic angle. Larger effusions cause a homogeneous opacity of fluid density, which may spread over the entire lung but is usually more pronounced at the bases when the patient is upright. The underlying cause of the pleural effusion if located within the thorax may also be evident on the chest radiograph.

Arterial Blood Gases. The Pa_{O_2} and the Pa_{CO_2} usually remain within normal limits. Even if the pleural effusion is large and is compressing a significant amount of lung tissue, ventilation-perfusion matching is maintained. This is accomplished by reflex vasoconstriction in the hypoventilated areas of the lung.

Breath Sounds. Bronchial breath sounds and **egophony** are usually present just above a pleural effusion. Directly over the pleural effusion, breath sounds are decreased. A pleural friction rub may also be heard if the pleural surfaces are inflamed.

Cardiovascular Findings. There are none specific to the pleural effusion. However, there may be abnormal cardiovascular findings if the pleural effusion is due to cardiovascular disease.

Symptoms. Patients may exhibit no symptoms. If the pleural effusion is large, the patient may be short of breath. If there is inflammation of the parietal pleura, the patient may have **pleuritic** chest pain. Some patients report a dry, nonproductive cough, which may result from irritation of the pleural surfaces.

Treatment

The underlying cause of the pleural effusion must be identified and treated. In many cases this treatment causes the pleural effusion to resolve secondarily.[9] Diagnostic thoracentesis is routinely used to obtain fluid and tissue samples to determine if the fluid is a transudate or exudate.[9] Thoracentesis can also be used therapeutically to remove excess pleural fluid via a large-bore needle. However, there is little evidence that patients benefit from this intervention, and it is being used less frequently.[16] A new procedure, thoroscopy, uses a rigid scope with a light source to explore the entire hemithorax. Thoroscopy can be used to biopsy the pleura, biopsy the lung, obtain pleural fluid samples, remove pleural fluid, and perform a pleurodesis, and if necessary lysis of adhesions can be accomplished.[9] Another treatment option that is used if a large infected pleural effusion (empy-

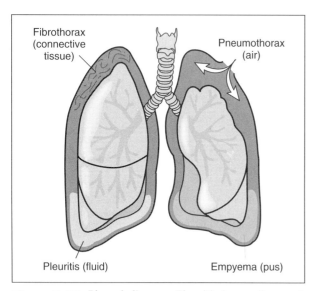

Figure 5–14. Pleural diseases. Pleuritis is usually associated with pleural effusion. Fibrothorax is an encasement of the lungs with fibrous tissue that obliterates the pleural cavity. Pneumothorax denotes the entry of air into the pleural cavity. Empyema involves pockets of pus enclosed in fibrous adhesions. (From Damjanov I. Pathology for the Health-Related Professions. 2nd ed. Philadelphia, WB Saunders, 2000, Fig. 8–28, p 205.)

ema) is present is the placement of a pleural space chest tube for drainage of this fluid.[16]

Sarcoidosis

Sarcoidosis is an enigmatic multisystem disease that is characterized by the presence of **noncaseating** epithelioid granulomas in many organs. Clinically the lung is the most involved organ[13, 14] (Fig. 5–15).

Etiology

The etiology of this disease is unknown. Infectious agents, chemicals or drugs, allergy, autoimmunity, and genetic factors have all been researched as possible causes.[10] Sarcoidosis most commonly affects young adults, with 70% of the cases diagnosed in persons 20 to 40 years of age. Sarcoidosis is more common in women than in men. The incidence is increased tenfold in black Americans when compared with whites. It is rare in Native American Indians.[21]

Pathophysiology

This disease presents with three distinctive features within the lung: **alveolitis,** formation of well-defined round or oval granulomas, and pulmonary fibrosis.[13] The alveolitis usually appears earliest and is an infiltration of the alveolar walls by inflammatory cells, especially macrophages and T lymphocytes. The core of the sarcoid granuloma contains epithelioid cells and multinucleated giant cells; there is rarely any necrosis in the core. The core is surrounded by monocytes, macrophages, lymphocytes, and fibroblasts. These granulomas may resolve without scarring, but many go on to become obliterative fibrosis, which is characterized by the accumulation of fibroblasts and collagen around the granuloma. Diffuse fibrosis of the alveolar walls is not typical in this disease, although it can occur late in the disease progression. Approximately 25% of patients with pulmonary sarcoidosis experience a permanent decrease in lung function, which over time proves fatal in 5% to 10% of patients.[13] This loss of lung function is due to restrictive lung impairment primarily, but this dis-

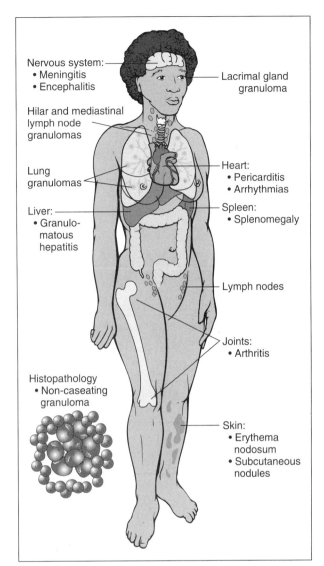

Figure 5–15. Sites that may be involved in sarcoidosis. The most common sites of granulomas are the lungs and the thoracic lymph nodes. Other extrathoracic sites are less commonly involved. The histopathologic appearance shows a noncaseating granuloma composed predominantly of epithelioid cells, macrophages, and lymphocytes. In contrast to tuberculosis, there is no central necrosis. (From Damjanov I. Pathology for the Health-Related Professions. 2nd ed. Philadelphia, WB Saunders, 2000, Fig. 8–17, p 192.)

ease also has an obstructive component. Prognosis seems to be better if the onset of pulmonary symptoms is acute. If the onset is insidious, with progressive dyspnea, then the prognosis is worse.

Sarcoidosis is a multisystem disease, and although the pulmonary system is the most commonly involved (90%), other systems are affected also. Seventeen percent of patients have ocular involvement, which can lead to blindness.[13] The most common ocular presentation is **granulomatous uveitis,** which causes redness and watering of the eyes, cloudy vision, and **photophobia.**[25] Five percent of patients have neurologic involvement, which can include **encephalopathy,** granulomatous meningitis, or involvement of the cranial nerves.[13] Other organ systems that can be involved are the liver (60% to 80%), the lymphatics (50% to 75%), the heart (30%), the skin (30%), the spleen (15%), the kidney, muscles, joints, and the immune system.[2, 7, 13, 14, 21, 25]

The progression of this disease is extremely variable. The disease can be active and resolve spontaneously, both clinically and radiographically. The disease can be inactive and stable for long periods of time with no change in clinical symptoms. The disease also can be persistent and active, with progressive loss of lung function leading to a fatal outcome.[9, 13]

Clinical Manifestations

Signs

Pulmonary Function Tests. The TLC and all lung volumes including RV are decreased. Lung compliance is decreased. The DL_{CO} is decreased primarily because of the increase in the ventilation-perfusion mismatching. Late in the disease there may be superimposed obstructive deficits, which result in decreased flow rates, especially if the patient has respiratory symptoms and/or a 20% to 30% reduction in PFT values.[16]

Chest Radiograph. Bilateral hilar **lymphadenopathy** is commonly seen on the chest radiograph. The lung parenchyma shows diffuse infiltrates with an interstitial reticulonodular pattern.

Arterial Blood Gases. Blood gas values may remain within normal limits. Late in the disease as pulmonary involvement progresses, the Pa_{O_2} falls.

Breath Sounds. The patient's respiratory rate is increased, and chest expansion is decreased. Auscultation commonly reveals bibasilar rales, decreased breath sounds in the apices due to bullae, and sometimes wheezes from bronchial obstruction.

Cardiovascular Findings. Because of the pulmonary involvement, approximately 15% of patients develop pulmonary hypertension, but this complication rarely progresses to cor pulmonale.[13] Direct effects on the heart in sarcoidosis include dysrhythmias, congestive heart failure, and papillary muscle dysfunction.

Symptoms. Approximately one third of patients with sarcoidosis experience dyspnea during the course of the disease.[21] Cough with or without sputum production is common also, and some patients complain of a vague retrosternal discomfort or fullness. Other constitutional symptoms include fever, fatigue, weight loss, and erythema nodosum.

Treatment

Treatment of this disease is difficult because it is known that some cases resolve spontaneously and others can go into long periods of remission. In treating the three pulmonary manifestations of this disease, corticosteroids are used early to suppress the alveolitis and granuloma formation, especially if the patient has respiratory symptoms and/or a 20% to 30% reduction in PFT values.[9, 16] Established granulomas with pulmonary fibrosis are relatively fixed lesions and do not respond to therapy. Corticosteroid therapy is indicated for extrapulmonary sarcoidosis involving the eyes, heart, or nervous system.[16]

CARDIOVASCULAR CAUSES OF RESTRICTIVE LUNG DYSFUNCTION

Pulmonary Edema

Pulmonary edema is an increase in the amount of fluid within the lung. Usually the pulmonary interstitium is affected first and then the alveolar spaces.[18, 20]

Etiology

Pulmonary edema has two primary causes. One is an increase in the pulmonary capillary hydrostatic pressure secondary to left ventricular failure. This is called cardiogenic pulmonary edema and is discussed in this section. Pulmonary edema can also be caused by increased alveolar capillary membrane permeability secondary to various causes.

This type of pulmonary edema is also named ARDS and was discussed under the section on Pulmonary Causes of RLD. Cardiogenic pulmonary edema is also known as high-pressure pulmonary edema, hydrostatic pulmonary edema, and hemodynamic pulmonary edema (Fig. 5–16).[8, 20]

Pathophysiology

As the left ventricle fails, its ability to contract and pump blood into the systemic circulation efficiently is diminished. This results in an increase in left atrial pressure, which is transmitted back to the pulmonary circulation. Because of this impedance to blood flow, the pressure in the microcirculation of the lung is increased, which increases the *transvascular* flow of fluid into the interstitium of the lung. The interstitial space can accommodate a small amount of excess fluid, approximately 500 mL.[20] The lymphatic drainage can be enhanced to move some excess fluid out of the tho-

rax. However, when the left atrial pressure rises above 30 mm Hg, these protective mechanisms are overcome.[20] The interstitial edema fluid disrupts the tight alveolar epithelium, floods the alveolar spaces, and moves through the visceral pleura, causing pleural effusions. The pulmonary edema fluid in cardiogenic pulmonary edema is characterized by low-protein concentrations. This finding is in contrast to that in ARDS in which the pulmonary edema fluid has elevated protein concentrations. With fluid in the alveoli and the interstitium, lung compliance is decreased; ventilation-perfusion mismatching is increased; gas exchange is disrupted; the work of breathing is increased; and there is restrictive lung dysfunction.[8, 18, 20]

Clinical Manifestations

Signs
Pulmonary Function Tests. Respiratory rate is increased and lung volumes are decreased. Flow

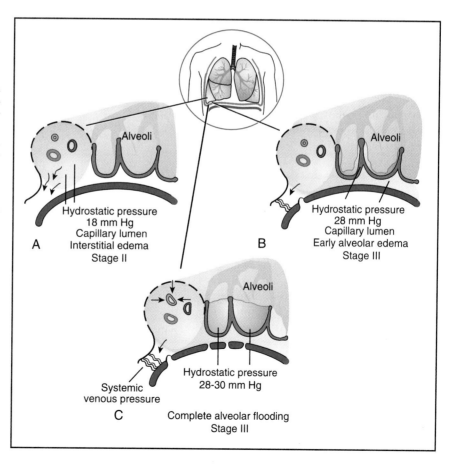

Figure 5–16. Pulmonary edema resulting from left-sided cardiac muscle failure may present in different stages. *A*, In stage II, interstitial edema results from an elevated capillary pressure (18 mm Hg), which forces fluid (plasma) into the interstitial area. *B*, Early alveolar edema occurs when the capillary hydrostatic pressure is significantly elevated (18 to 28 mm Hg), causing fluid to move from the capillary, invade the interstitium, and cross the alveolar membrane. *C*, Complete alveolar flooding occurs when the capillary hydrostatic pressure is severely elevated (>28 mm Hg), causing fluid to flood the alveoli and possibly invade the large airways.

Alveoli

Hydrostatic pressure
18 mm Hg
Capillary lumen
Interstitial edema
Stage II
A

Alveoli

Hydrostatic pressure
28 mm Hg
Capillary lumen
Early alveolar edema
Stage III
B

Alveoli

Systemic
venous pressure

Hydrostatic pressure
28-30 mm Hg

Complete alveolar flooding
Stage III
C

rates are usually normal. The DL_{CO} is normal or decreased.

Chest Radiograph. Increased vascular markings in the hilar region are characteristic of cardiogenic pulmonary edema. **Kerley B lines** are present because of prominent thickened interlobular septa. Interstitial and alveolar infiltrates can be diffuse, and pleural effusions are common.[16]

Arterial Blood Gases. The Pa_{O_2} is decreased owing to the increased ventilation-perfusion mismatching. The Pa_{CO_2} is usually decreased with the pH increased, denoting a respiratory alkalosis. Later in the clinical course, there may be carbon dioxide retention.

Breath Sounds. Wet rales with decreased breath sounds are the most common auscultatory finding. Some patients may develop marked bronchospasm and wheezing.

Cardiovascular Findings. Many patients with pulmonary edema may have a history of significant cardiac problems, including myocardial infarction, left ventricular failure, aortic or mitral valve disease, or cardiomyopathy.[16] These patients commonly have arrhythmias.

Symptoms. Patients with pulmonary edema appear in respiratory distress and may report a sense of suffocation. They are short of breath, cyanotic, and their respiratory pattern is usually fast and labored. The patient's cough is productive of pink frothy sputum. **Pallor, diaphoresis,** and restlessness are also common symptoms.

Treatment

Treatment is aimed at decreasing the cardiac preload and maintaining oxygenation of the tissues. To decrease cardiac preload, venous return to the heart is decreased, which decreases the left ventricular filling pressure. Venodilators such as morphine sulfate or sodium nitroprusside, and diuretics like furosemide are used to decrease the venous return. Other drugs, for example, dopamine, dobutamine, and digitalis may be given to improve cardiac contractility. To maintain oxygenation, supplemental oxygen is provided. Intubation with mechanical ventilation may also be necessary.[16]

Pulmonary Emboli

Pulmonary emboli are a complication of venous thrombosis, in which blood clots or thrombi travel from a systemic vein through the right side of the heart and into the pulmonary circulation, where they lodge in branches of the pulmonary artery.[2, 14]

Etiology

Pulmonary embolism is the most common acute pulmonary problem among hospitalized patients in the United States. Each year 500,000 to 1 million Americans have a pulmonary embolic event.[20] Many of these events may go unnoticed because they are clinically silent. However, approximately 10% of pulmonary embolisms result in the patient's death.[20] Thus, between 50,000 and 100,000 Americans die annually because of a pulmonary embolism, making it the third most common cause of death in the United States.[20] About one third of the deaths occur within 1 hour of the acute event. And more than half of these fatalities occur in patients in whom the diagnosis was not clinically suspect.[20]

In more than 95% of the cases, the thrombi that caused the pulmonary emboli were formed in the lower extremities.[2] In the remaining 5% of the cases, the thrombi may be formed in the pelvis, the arms, or the right side of the heart. Numerous risk factors increase the likelihood of thrombus formation in the lower extremities. These risk factors include immobilization owing to bedrest, long periods of travel, or fracture stabilization. Increased age, congestive heart failure, obesity, cancer, chronic deep venous insufficiency, trauma, cerebral vascular accident, oral contraceptives, pregnancy and the postpartum period, sickle-cell anemia, and thrombocytosis are also risk factors for pulmonary embolism. The highest risk group for thrombophlebitis is *orthopedic patients.* Studies have shown that the frequency of deep-vein thrombosis perioperatively is 80% in patients after hip or knee surgery.[16]

Pathophysiology

The pathophysiologic changes that occur following pulmonary embolism affect the pulmonary system and the cardiovascular system. The occlusion of one or more pulmonary arterial branches causes edema and hemorrhage into the surrounding lung parenchyma. This is known as *congestive atelectasis.* The lack of blood flow causes coagulative necrosis of the alveolar walls; the alveoli fill with erythrocytes, and there is an inflammatory response. Another change within the pulmonary system is the increase in the alveolar dead space because a portion of the lung is being ventilated but no longer perfused. Pneumoconstriction of the affected area occurs, with a marked decrease in alveolar carbon dioxide owing to the lack of gas exchange and the patient's respiratory pattern of hyperventilation. In addition, the alveolar surfactant decreases over a period of approximately 24 hours, which results in alveolar collapse and regional atelectasis. These changes combine to cause an acute increase in ventilation-perfusion mismatching, a decrease in lung compliance, and impaired gas exchange. If the oxygen supply is completely cut off to a portion of lung, then frank necrosis and infarction of lung tissue results. This happens in less than 10% of all pulmonary embolisms because lung tissue has three sources of oxygen: the pulmonary vascular system, the bronchial vascular system, and the alveolar gas.[20] However, infarction of lung tissue is followed by contraction of the affected tissue and scar formation.

The first cardiovascular change that occurs because of a pulmonary embolism is an increase in the pulmonary arterial resistance due to a decrease in the cross-sectional area of the pulmonary arterial bed. If this cross-sectional area is decreased by more than 50%, then the pressure needed to maintain pulmonary blood flow rises and pulmonary hypertension results.[20] This also increases the work of the right ventricle and can lead to right ventricular failure. If the pulmonary embolus is massive, right ventricular failure and cardiac arrest can occur within minutes.[8, 18, 20]

Clinical Manifestations

Signs
Pulmonary Function Tests. Lung volumes are decreased owing to the decrease in lung compliance and the congestive atelectasis. Expiratory flow rates also may be decreased owing to bronchoconstriction. Respiratory rate is increased, often markedly. These changes are transient and can resolve completely with resolution of the pulmonary embolism. If lung infarction occurs, then lung volumes remain decreased in proportion to the amount of lung tissue infarcted.

Chest Radiograph. A chest radiograph may appear normal. If changes take place, they usually occur in the lower lobes, where the blood supply is best. The chest radiograph may show a transient cone-shaped infiltrate fanning out and extending to the visceral pleura or a rounded nodular lesion. One of the pulmonary arteries may appear larger and the other smaller than normal. There may be evidence of a small pleural effusion. With unilateral pulmonary embolism and pneumoconstriction, one of the hemidiaphragms may appear elevated. These changes resolve with lysis or fragmentation of the pulmonary embolism. The only permanent change seen on chest radiograph is the scar formation secondary to lung infarction.[16]

Arterial Blood Gases. Commonly the Pa_{O_2} is decreased, and the patient is hypoxic, although if the pulmonary embolism is small, the Pa_{O_2} may be normal. The Pa_{CO_2} is decreased, and the patient's pH is elevated, denoting a respiratory alkalosis.[16]

Breath Sounds. Breath sounds are decreased in the area of pneumoconstriction; there may be some wheezing. Sometimes fine rales due to the surfactant loss and resultant atelectasis also are evident.[16]

Cardiovascular Findings. Tachycardia is almost always present. Electrocardiographic (ECG) changes are common but are usually minor and nonspecific. Arrhythmias may develop, particularly when hypoxemia develops. If the pulmonary embolism is massive, right ventricular failure and cardiac arrest can occur.[16]

Symptoms. The acute onset of dyspnea is the most common symptom; more than 90% of patients who have a pulmonary embolism complain of shortness of breath.[20] This is the only symptom for the majority of patients. The severity of the dyspnea is directly related to the amount of pulmonary vasculature involved in the embolic event. Rapid shallow breathing and tachycardia are commonly present. Apprehension and cough may be present in some patients. Syncope may be evident with a massive pulmonary embolism. Pleuritic chest pain and hemoptysis may occur with pulmonary infarction but usually do not develop for some hours following the vascular occlusion. Patients may run a low-grade fever following a pulmonary embolism.

Treatment

Treatment begins with prevention of deep-vein thrombosis. There are two methods used in preventing or minimizing deep-vein thrombosis. The mechanical approach includes ankle pumping exercises in bed, early ambulation, use of gradient compression stockings, pneumatic calf compression, and electrical stimulation of calf muscles. The pharmacologic approach includes the use of agents that decrease the hypercoagulability of the blood, such as warfarin, dextran, low-molecular-weight heparin, heparinoids, and heparin.[16] With repeated thrombus formation and embolic events, surgical placement of a transvenous device (e.g., Greenfield filter) to prevent migration of thrombi may be utilized.

Heparin therapy is most commonly used to treat pulmonary embolism. Heparin does not lyse existing clots, but prevents formation and propagation of further clots.[16] To maintain adequate tissue oxygenation, mechanical ventilation with supplemental oxygen may be required. In addition, if the patient is hypotensive or in shock, fluid therapy and vasopressors may be needed. Mild sedation and analgesia may be used to decrease anxiety and pain. Thromboembolic lysing agents (e.g., streptokinase) can be used to lyse the emboli, but this therapeutic intervention is no more effective than heparin therapy in terms of the patient's morbidity or mortality.[16] Pulmonary embolectomy is being performed less frequently owing to the increased mortality rate (50% to 94%) when compared with the mortality rate (24%) for conventional medical treatment.[16] However, this emergent surgical intervention may be indicated in patients who have large emboli and cannot receive heparin therapy or have overt right ventricular heart failure leading to cardiac arrest. The ultimate prognosis following pulmonary embolism is extremely variable. In patients who experience no shock and are treated medically, the mortality rate is 18%.[16] Patients who have pulmonary embolism and a simultaneous cardiac arrest have a 45% mortality rate. Patients who have a pulmonary embolism with extreme increases in right ventricular pressures have a 90% mortality rate.[20]

NEUROMUSCULAR CAUSES OF RESTRICTIVE LUNG DYSFUNCTION

Spinal Cord Injury

Spinal cord injury is damage to or interruption of the neurologic pathways contained within the spinal cord.[18, 26]

Etiology

A spinal cord injury can result from an acute traumatic event, often a motor vehicle accident or a diving accident, or from a pathologic process that invades the spinal cord and damages it or in some way interrupts the neurologic transmissions.

Pathophysiology

For this discussion, spinal cord injuries include cervical injuries only. A spinal cord injury in the cervical region produces paralysis or **paresis** in the arms, legs, and trunk, therefore resulting in **tetraplegia.** With this type of injury, the expiratory muscles are paralyzed or very weak, leading to an inability to cough. This ineffective cough may cause an increase in the incidence of pulmonary infections. The external intercostals are inactive, and the patient may have a functional, weak, or absent diaphragm, depending on the level of the injury (Table 5–3).[8, 26] Weakness in the inspiratory muscles results in alveolar hypoventilation, hypoxemia, and hypercapnia. Because the alveoli are not well ventilated, the patient is prone to atelectasis, particularly in the dependent lung regions, which could lead to recurrent pulmonary infections. With parts of the lung underventilated, the ventilation-perfusion matching is impaired and the diffusing capacity reduced. A cervical injury also results in the loss of the sigh reflex, which increases the incidence of atelectasis and contributes to alveolar collapse. If the patient retains use of the diaphragm, breathing dynamics are altered markedly, resulting in **paradoxical** breathing. In paradoxical

Table 5–3	
Innervation Levels of the Respiratory Muscles	
MUSCLES	LEVEL
Inspiratory	
Diaphragm	C3, C4, C5 (phrenic nerve)
External intercostals	T1–T12
Sternocleidomastoids	Cranial nerve XI (spinal accessory nerve)
Scalenes	C1, C2
Expiratory	
Internal intercostals	T1–T12
Abdominals	T7–L1

breathing the diaphragm descends on inspiration, causing the abdomen to rise and the paralyzed thoracic wall to be pulled inward. The diaphragm relaxes on exhalation, causing the abdomen to fall and the chest wall to move outward. Immediately after a cervical injury, the VC and the maximum voluntary ventilation are markedly reduced (Fig. 5–17).

Approximately 6 months after injury, the VC has improved significantly if the patient has an intact diaphragm. And although it may not be normal, the VC may have doubled since the acute postinjury period. Paradoxical breathing is also diminished or eliminated because of the developing *spasticity* in the thorax and abdomen.[8, 12, 26]

Over time pulmonary compliance is decreased owing to the shallow breathing and atelectasis within the lung, and chest wall compliance is decreased due to paralysis of the thoracic musculature and the developing thoracic spasticity. This increases the work of breathing and can lead to diaphragmatic fatigue. All these pathophysiologic alterations lead to RLD and a chronic state of hypoxemia. The patient may therefore need mechanical ventilation part time or full time or an enriched FI_{O_2} (Fig. 5–18).[2, 8, 19]

Clinical Manifestations

Signs
Pulmonary Function Tests. The TLC, VC, and inspiratory capacity (IC) are decreased. The ERV is eliminated if there are no active expiratory muscles and the RV equals the FRC. The RV is increased. Flow rates are decreased. Peak inspiratory and expiratory pressures are decreased. The respiratory rate is routinely increased and the tidal volume diminished.[26]

Chest Radiograph. The chest radiograph may be within normal limits or may show evidence of pulmonary infections and infiltrates. Over time the ribs take on a more horizontal configuration.

Arterial Blood Gases. Hypoxemia is normal in high cervical lesions of the spinal cord. The more profound the respiratory muscle weakness, the more significant the level of hypercapnia.

Breath Sounds. Usually auscultation reveals diminished breath sounds, with abnormal or adventitious breath sounds being consistent with current pulmonary infections or infiltrates.

Cardiovascular Findings. Patients with spinal cord injuries above the T7 level may have episodes of **autonomic dysreflexia (hyperreflexia).** This may result in vasoconstriction below the level of the injury, which causes hypertension. The central nervous system above the level of the injury may then try to compensate in an effort to decrease the blood pressure, causing vasodilation and bradycardia.

Symptoms. Patients with acute cervical spinal cord injuries often complain of fatigue. This fatigue is due to the inefficiency of the breathing pattern and the effort that must be made by the remaining respiratory muscles. Patients also report shortness of breath, inability to cough, inadequate voice volume, and morning headaches, this last complaint being a significant symptom of hypoxia during sleep. Patients may also be restless or irritable, both of which can be caused by hypercapnia.

Treatment

Patients with spinal cord injuries must be taught ways to strengthen and increase the endurance of any remaining ventilatory muscles via use of an

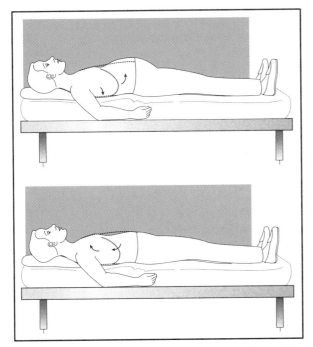

Figure 5–17. Paradoxical breathing. Note the position of the rib cage and abdomen. *Top,* Paradoxical breathing when the diaphragm is strong, but the accessory muscles are absent. *Bottom,* Paradoxical breathing during paralysis of the diaphragm.

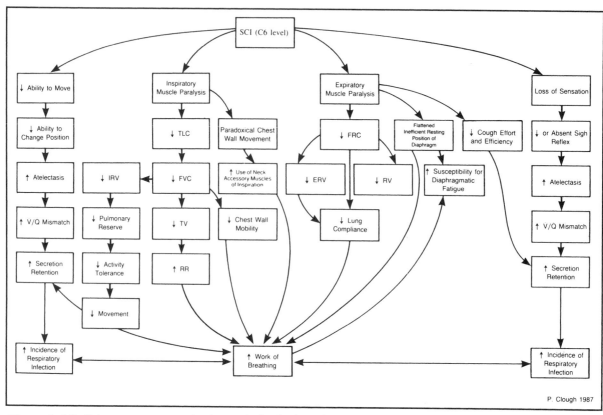

Figure 5-18. Pulmonary compromise in cervical spinal cord injury (SCI). TLC, Total lung capacity; FVC, forced vital capacity; IRV, inspiratory reserve volume; TV, tidal volume; RR, respiratory rate; FRC, functional residual capacity; ERV, expiratory reserve volume; RV, residual volume; V, ventilation; Q, perfusion; ↓, decreased; ↑, increased (From Peat M [ed]. Current Physical Therapy. Philadelphia, BC Decker, 1988, p 34.)

inspiratory muscle trainer, resistance exercises to the diaphragm, or an incentive spirometer. Patients must learn how to perform active and passive chest wall stretching, using rolling, positioning, side leaning, and air shift maneuvers. Patients, family members, or caregivers need to know how to assist the patient in clearing excess secretions with postural drainage, percussion, assisted coughing, and possibly suctioning. Learning how to perform glossopharyngeal breathing or how to operate a portable ventilator may also be necessary for selected patients.[26]

Amyotrophic Lateral Sclerosis

Amyotrophic lateral sclerosis (ALS) is a progressive degenerative disease of the nervous system that involves both upper and lower motor neurons, causing both flaccid and spastic paralysis.[1, 2]

Etiology

The cause of the disease is unknown. It occurs worldwide, and onset is usually after the age of 40. Males are affected 1.7 times as often as females.[18]

Pathophysiology

The anterior horn cells of the cervical, lower thoracic, and lumbosacral spinal segments usually are the most involved, which means that the respiratory muscles may be affected severely. Muscles innervated by the cranial nerves as well as the spinal nerves frequently are involved, causing problems with dysarthria and dysphagia. Muscle weakness and wasting are profound. Following the onset of neurologic symptoms, the average life expectancy is 3.6 years.[24] Death is often the result of acute respiratory failure.[19]

Clinical Manifestations

Signs

Pulmonary Function Tests. The TLC, IC, VC, and ERV are all decreased, and RV is usually increased, resulting in an FRC that may be within normal limits. The patient's respiratory rate usually increases as the weakness of ventilatory muscles progresses and VT is diminished. The maximum voluntary ventilation is severely reduced. Because of the profound weakness, the maximum inspiratory and expiratory pressures are also reduced.

Chest Radiograph. This parameter may be within normal limits or may show retained secretions and infiltrates that the patient is not able to clear.

Arterial Blood Gases. Owing to the compromised ventilatory pump, the Pa_{O_2} is decreased, and these patients experience marked hypoxemia. The Pa_{CO_2} is elevated because of the alveolar hypoventilation.

Breath Sounds. Auscultation usually reveals very decreased breath sounds, often with rales and rhonchi due to pulmonary infiltrates or infections.

Cardiovascular Findings. There are no specific clinical cardiovascular manifestations.

Symptoms. Patients often first notice a weakness or wasting in the muscles of the hands, although presentation of the disease can begin in the lower extremities or the trunk. This weakness may be accompanied by pain. Weakness is followed by atrophy of the muscles and muscular **fasciculations** ("snakelike" movements).[1] Patients retain normal sensation and may complain of cramping of the muscles. Patients fatigue easily, lack endurance for activities, and become dyspneic with even mild exertion.

Treatment

There is no treatment for this disease except supportive therapy to make the patient more comfortable. Physical exertion is not recommended because it tires the patient so rapidly. However, the patient should be encouraged to get out of bed and be as mobile as possible.

Poliomyelitis

Poliomyelitis (polio) is a viral disease that attacks the motor nerve cells of the spinal cord and brain stem and can result in muscular paralysis.[2]

Etiology

Polio is caused by an acute viral infection, which can reach epidemic proportions in at-risk populations. It is reported most commonly in children. This infection can now be prevented by vaccine.

Pathophysiology

The virus is **neurotropic** and has a predilection for the motor cells of the anterior horn and the brain stem. The lesions are patchy and asymmetric, and microscopically healthy and diseased cells can be seen side by side. This results in a patchy flaccid paralysis or paresis of the lower motor neuron type. Both the diaphragm and intercostal muscles may be affected, resulting in a respiratory muscle weakness that can progress to respiratory failure. There are two stages. The preparalytic stage is characterized by fever, headache, malaise, and symptoms in the gastrointestinal and upper respiratory tracts. For some patients this stage is followed by the paralytic stage, which includes tremulousness of the limbs, tenderness in the muscles, and swollen painful joints, as well as flaccid paralysis of from one to two muscles to all four limbs and the trunk.[1, 2, 19]

Clinical Manifestations (Polio with Respiratory Involvement)

Signs

Pulmonary Function Tests. The paralysis of the diaphragm, intercostals, or both results in RLD, with the lung volumes being decreased. Respiratory rate is increased and VT diminished. The maximum inspiratory and expiratory pressures are decreased. The DL_{CO} is decreased owing to the increase in ventilation-perfusion mismatching and alveolar hypoventilation.

Chest Radiograph. Films may show atelectasis or infiltrates. If the diaphragm is paralyzed, it appears elevated. Over time, if trunk musculature is paralyzed or paretic, a kyphoscoliosis may develop that would be evident on chest radiograph.

Arterial Blood Gases. The Pa_{O_2} is decreased, and the Pa_{CO_2} is elevated owing to alveolar hypoventilation and increased ventilation-perfusion mismatching.

Breath Sounds. Breath sounds are usually diminished. **Rhonchi** may be present, particularly in bulbar polio, which affects the brain stem and can result in the loss of the swallowing reflexes, thus leading to aspiration problems.

Cardiovascular Findings. There may be some transient rise in the systolic or diastolic pressures. Occasionally ECG changes may be found.

Symptoms. Patients are short of breath and anxious. Cough effort may be weak and ineffective in clearing secretions. Patients may experience any of the clinical symptoms described in the pathophysiology section.

Treatment

There is no specific treatment for poliomyelitis. Prevention through the use of oral or parenteral vaccine is very effective. Supportive therapy consisting of rest during the acute phase, with proper positioning, pain relief, good nutrition, and ventilatory support, as needed, is appropriate. Later, active range of motion exercises, strengthening exercises, bracing, and other equipment evaluation are required for patients with paralysis.

Guillain-Barré Syndrome

Guillain-Barré syndrome is a demyelinating disease of the motor neurons of the peripheral nerves.[19]

Etiology

This *idiopathic polyneuritis* is a disorder that seems to be linked to the immune system. The history of most patients with Guillain-Barré syndrome includes a viral illness followed by the ascending paralysis of this syndrome. However, the specific cause of the syndrome remains unknown.[2]

Pathophysiology

Guillain-Barré syndrome is characterized by a rapid bilateral ascending flaccid motor paralysis.

The loss of muscular strength is usually fully realized within 30 days, often within 10 to 15 days, and may leave the patient so involved that mechanical ventilation is required. Approximately 10% to 20% of all patients with Guillain-Barré syndrome develop acute respiratory failure and must be placed on a ventilator.[8] The duration of mechanical ventilation is variable but is usually between 2 weeks and 2 months.[1, 2, 8, 19]

Clinical Manifestations

Signs

Pulmonary Function Tests. Because of the profound muscular weakness seen in this syndrome, all the dynamic lung volumes are decreased. This includes the TLC, VC, IRV, ERV, and VT. The RV is usually within normal limits. Peak inspiratory and expiratory pressures are decreased. Respiratory rate is usually increased in an effort to maintain minute ventilation with a decreased VT. The DL_{CO} may also be decreased because of the increase in ventilation-perfusion mismatching and alveolar hypoventilation.

Chest Radiograph. Findings on chest films may vary widely during the course of the disease. They may include atelectasis, infiltrates, pneumonia, or neurogenic pulmonary edema.

Arterial Blood Gases. Owing to the weakness of the ventilatory pump, both hypoxia and hypercapnia are common.

Breath Sounds. Auscultation reveals diminished breath sounds that are usually most decreased at the bases. Adventitious breath sounds may also be heard during periods of pneumonia or with pulmonary infiltrates.

Cardiovascular Findings. Autonomic abnormalities can occur in Guillain-Barré syndrome, including cardiac dysrhythmias, hypertension, or postural hypotension.

Symptoms. Patients usually complain of weakness of both legs. Muscles may feel tender, and often paresthesias of the fingers and toes occur. Other sensory loss is slight.[1] When the respiratory muscles become involved, patients often report feeling dyspneic, anxious, and suffocated. Cough effort is often ineffective in clearing secretions. Patients report decreased endurance for activities and increased fatigue.

Treatment

Patients are supported throughout the syndrome's progression. Heat may be used to decrease muscular pain. Passive range of motion is begun immediately. Active exercises, including breathing exercises to assist the patient in weaning from the ventilator, should be begun as soon as the patient's condition has stabilized. Although exercise is important, patients with Guillain-Barré syndrome fatigue easily and should not be overly stressed. This polyneuropathy usually leads to complete recovery with minimal permanent sequelae. Recurrence of Guillain-Barré syndrome in the same patient is possible; in fact, patients with this syndrome are at slightly higher risk than the general public. However, even a second bout of the syndrome usually resolves.[2, 18]

Myasthenia Gravis

Myasthenia gravis is a chronic neuromuscular disease characterized by progressive muscular weakness on exertion.[1]

Etiology

Myasthenia gravis is caused by an autoimmune attack on the acetylcholine receptors at the postsynaptic neuromuscular junction. What causes the production of this antibody is unknown. This disease predominantly affects women, and its onset is usually between 20 to 40 years of age.[18]

Pathophysiology

The antibody IgG binds to the acetylcholine receptor sites, which impairs the normal transmission of impulses from the nerves to the muscles. The muscles most characteristically involved are those innervated by the cranial nerves. This causes **ptosis, diplopia, dysarthria,** dysphagia, and proximal limb weakness. The signs and symptoms of this disease may fluctuate over a period of hours or days. Severe generalized quadriparesis may develop. Approximately 10% of patients develop respiratory muscle involvement that can be life threatening.[18, 27]

Clinical Manifestations

Signs
Pulmonary Function Tests. With ventilatory pump failure, all the dynamic lung volumes and capacities are decreased. The peak inspiratory and expiratory pressures are decreased. As expected in a patient with RLD, the respiratory rate is increased and the VT decreased. The DL_{CO} is diminished owing to alveolar hypoventilation and ventilation-perfusion mismatching.

Chest Radiograph. The chest radiograph may be consistent with atelectasis or pneumonia.

Arterial Blood Gases. The patient's Pa_{O_2} is decreased, and the Pa_{CO_2} is increased because of alveolar hypoventilation and increased ventilation-perfusion mismatching.

Breath Sounds. Decreased breath sounds are common. If the patient retains secretions and cannot clear them, adventitious sounds also are heard.

Cardiovascular Findings. There are no specific clinical cardiovascular manifestations.

Symptoms. Patients with myasthenia gravis complain of weakness and fatigue of voluntary muscles, particularly those innervated by the cranial nerves. They may not be able to focus their eyes properly or to swallow. Patients are often short of breath, and their cough is weak and ineffective.

Treatment

Treatment of the disease's symptoms is with an **anticholinesterase** (pyridostigmine or neostigmine) and **plasmapheresis.** Corticosteroids, immunosuppressive drugs, and thymectomy are used in an effort to alter the disease's progression by interfering with the autoimmune abnormality.[18, 19]

Tetanus

Tetanus is a disease of the neuromuscular system caused by the neurotoxin produced by *Clostridium tetani.*[1] This anaerobic bacillus is found in the soil and the excreta of humans and animals and usually enters via a contaminated wound. The **neurotoxin** binds to the **ganglioside** membranes of the nerve synapses and blocks release of the inhibitory transmitter. This action causes severe muscle spasticity with superimposed tonic convulsions. This muscle rigidity can become so severe that the chest wall is immobilized, resulting in **asphyxia** and death. Tetanus can produce the most severe example of decreased chest wall compliance, leading to a restrictive impairment incompatible with life. The best treatment for tetanus is prevention via immunization. Prompt and careful wound debridement is also important. Once a patient has developed the disease, the tetanus antitoxin can be used to neutralize nonfixed toxin in the system. Once fixed or bound, the toxin cannot be neutralized. Supportive therapy is primarily focused on maintaining an airway and ensuring adequate ventilation.[1, 18]

Pseudohypertrophic (Duchenne's) Muscular Dystrophy

Pseudohypertrophic muscular dystrophy is a genetically determined, progressive degenerative myopathy.[18, 27]

Etiology

Pseudohypertrophic muscular dystrophy is a sex-linked (X chromosome) recessive disorder that occurs only in boys and is transmitted by female carriers. It is the most common of the *muscular dystrophies*, with a prevalence rate of 4 per 100,000 in the United States.[18, 27]

Pathophysiology

Pseudohypertrophic muscular dystrophy typically appears when boys who have this recessive gene are 3 to 7 years of age.[18] Muscle biopsy at this time shows both muscle fiber hypertrophy and necrosis with regeneration. There is also excessive infiltration of the muscle with fibrous tissue and fat. Muscle innervation is not normal in this disease, but the abnormality is due to loss of motor end plates when muscle fibers degenerate and not to neurogenic disease. The pelvic girdle is affected first, and then the shoulder girdle muscles become involved. Although the calf often shows **pseudohy-**

pertrophy, the quadriceps usually appear atrophied. The progression of the disease is steady, and most patients are confined to wheelchairs by 10 to 12 years of age. Involvement of the diaphragm occurs late in the course of this disease. However, respiratory failure and infection are the causes of death in 75% of these patients, which occurs usually by age 20.[8, 18, 27]

Clinical Manifestations

Signs
Pulmonary Function Tests. All lung volumes are decreased except the RV, which is usually increased. The TLC and VC are decreased. Because the patient is so weak, the respiratory pattern becomes inefficient with the VT decreased and the respiratory rate increased. Maximum inspiratory and expiratory pressures are also decreased.[2] The maximum voluntary ventilation is markedly decreased, often by one third of the predicted normal.[19] Chest wall compliance is decreased, and because of the microatelectasis that develops, lung compliance is also decreased. Gas diffusion is decreased owing to the increased ventilation-perfusion mismatching.

Chest Radiograph. Chest films may show atelectasis, pulmonary infection with infiltrates, or both.

Arterial Blood Gases. The Pa_{CO_2} is increased owing to alveolar hypoventilation and ventilation-perfusion mismatching. The Pa_{O_2} is often decreased, with the patient becoming hypoxic.

Breath Sounds. Breath sounds are often diminished; when a pulmonary infection and infiltrates are present, rales, rhonchi, and bronchovesicular breath sounds may be heard.

Cardiovascular Findings. The cardiac muscle is often involved, and fibrosis of the myocardium can be extensive. This change may cause abnormalities in the ECG, indicating a conduction block.

Symptoms. The usual presenting symptoms are a waddling gait, toe walking, lordosis, frequent falls, difficulty standing up from the floor, and difficulty in climbing stairs, all of which are caused by proximal pelvic girdle muscle weakness. With respiratory muscle involvement, patients first feel dyspnea on exertion and so will decrease their activity level. The dyspnea may worsen so the patient becomes dyspneic at rest and feels anxious and suffocated. Cough is weak and often ineffective in clearing secretions.

Treatment

There is no curative treatment. Supportive treatment is aimed at preserving the patient's mobility as long as possible and making the patient comfortable.

Other Muscular Dystrophies

Facioscapulohumeral Muscular Dystrophy

Facioscapulohumeral muscular dystrophy is an *autosomal dominant* disorder characterized by weakness of the facial and shoulder girdle muscles. Respiratory involvement or failure is uncommon in this type of muscular dystrophy.[8, 18]

Limb-Girdle Muscular Dystrophy

Limb-girdle muscular dystrophy is a disorder in which adults exhibit weakness of the pelvic and shoulder girdle musculature. There can be severe involvement of the diaphragm early in the course of this disease.[8, 18]

Myotonic Muscular Dystrophy

Myotonic muscular dystrophy is an autosomal dominant disorder that combines myotonia with progressive peripheral muscle weakness. Respiratory involvement and failure are common as this disease progresses.[8, 18]

MUSCULOSKELETAL CAUSES OF RESTRICTIVE LUNG DYSFUNCTION

Diaphragmatic Paralysis or Paresis

Diaphragmatic paralysis or **paresis** is the loss or impairment of motor function of the diaphragm because of a lesion in the neurologic or muscular system. The paralysis or paresis may be temporary or permanent.[19, 20]

Etiology

Unilateral paralysis or paresis of the diaphragm is most commonly caused by invasion of the phrenic nerve by bronchogenic carcinoma.[20] Another very common cause is open heart surgery. An estimated 20% of patients who undergo cardiac surgery suffer injury to the phrenic nerve owing to either cold or stretching of the nerve.[16, 20] In hemiplegic patients it is not uncommon to find paralysis of the corresponding **hemidiaphragm.** The left hemidiaphragm is involved in left hemiplegia more frequently than the right hemidiaphragm is involved in right hemiplegia.[19] Other causes of unilateral diaphragmatic dysfunction include poliomyelitis; Huntington's chorea; herpes zoster; or peripheral neuritis associated with measles, tetanus, typhoid, or diphtheria. Bilateral paralysis or paresis of the diaphragm may result from high spinal cord injury, thoracic trauma, Guillain-Barré syndrome, multiple sclerosis, muscular dystrophy, or anterior horn cell disease.[16, 19, 20]

Pathophysiology

Normally as the crural portion of the diaphragm contracts, the pleural space pressure decreases; the central tendon moves caudally; the lungs inflate; and the abdominal pressure increases, which moves the abdominal wall outward. Contraction of the costal portion of the diaphragm accomplishes these same effects and in addition causes the anterior lower ribs to expand and move in a *cephalad* direction.[8] In diaphragmatic paralysis or significant weakness, the negative pleural space pressure moves the diaphragm in a cephalad direction so that the diaphragm's resting position is elevated. During inspiration, as the pleural space pressure becomes more negative, the paralyzed diaphragm is pulled farther upward and the anterior lower ribs are pulled inward rather than being expanded.[20] These changes in ventilatory mechanics cause alveolar hypoventilation with secondary changes that are seen in the lung parenchyma. The decreased inspiratory capacity leads to microatelectasis, ventilation-perfusion mismatching, alveolar collapse, and hypoxemia. The atelectasis leads to a decrease in lung compliance and an increase in the work of breathing. These pathologic changes are heightened in the supine position.

The rib cage is elevated in the supine position, putting the rib cage musculature at a mechanical disadvantage, thereby decreasing its ability to generate an inspiratory volume.[9] Therefore, in the supine position, diaphragmatic dysfunction produces a more significant decrease in alveolar ventilation than that produced in the upright position. The changes in the ventilatory mechanics and within the lung parenchyma combine to increase the risk of pulmonary infection or pneumonia in patients with diaphragmatic dysfunction.[8, 19, 20]

Clinical Manifestations

Signs

Pulmonary Function Tests. All lung capacities and all dynamic lung volumes are decreased in proportion to the degree of diaphragmatic dysfunction. With unilateral paralysis, the TLC and VC are decreased approximately 25%.[20] With full diaphragmatic paralysis, the VC may fall below the predicted V_T, which would necessitate mechanical ventilation for the patient. Lung volumes may be further decreased when these patients change positions; the VC is decreased 30% by moving a patient with diaphragmatic paralysis from the sitting to the supine position.[19] Flow rates are also decreased in proportion to the decrease in lung volumes. The degree of weakness of the diaphragm is best measured by transdiaphragmatic pressure. The normal transdiaphragmatic pressure is higher than 98 cm H_2O.[14, 19] When the transdiaphragmatic pressure is lower than 20 cm H_2O, the patient exhibits significant respiratory distress.[19] The maximum transdiaphragmatic pressure is decreased 50%, and the maximum inspiratory pressure is decreased 40% with unilateral paralysis.[16, 20] The reduction is even more profound with bilateral involvement.

Chest Radiograph. An elevated hemidiaphragm is the classic radiographic finding. The diaphragm may show decreased, absent, or paradoxical movement on inspiration. Areas of atelectasis, especially at the bases, or pneumonia may also be evident.[16]

Arterial Blood Gases. The Pa_{O_2} is decreased with diaphragmatic dysfunction, and the decrease is more pronounced when the patient is in the supine position. The Pa_{CO_2} usually remains within normal limits with unilateral involvement. With bilateral involvement, hypercapnia results when the

patient is not able to maintain an adequate V_T and minute ventilation.

Breath Sounds. Breath sounds are usually decreased on the side of the paralysis or paresis, particularly at the base.

Cardiovascular Findings. Severe hypoxemia can cause pulmonary hypertension, which can progress to cor pulmonale.[16]

Symptoms. The patient's most common complaint is dyspnea, which is worse in the supine position. Therefore, patients often report orthopnea and use two or three pillows because they are uncomfortable and short of breath when lying flat. Patients also report difficult or labored inspiration, anxiety, insomnia, daytime somnolence, and morning headache.[16]

Treatment

Patients with unilateral diaphragmatic involvement usually do not require treatment because of the large pulmonary reserve and the other respiratory muscles that are still functional. With bilateral involvement, either full-time or part-time mechanical ventilation is often required. Diaphragmatic pacing via an intact phrenic nerve is also a possibility for some of these patients; however, the success rate with this treatment intervention is estimated at only 50%.[16, 19]

Kyphoscoliosis

Kyphoscoliosis is a combination of excessive anteroposterior and lateral curvature of the thoracic spine (Fig. 5–19).[2, 8] This bony abnormality occurs in 3% of the population. However, lung dysfunction occurs in only 3% of the population with kyphoscoliosis (Fig. 5–20).[16, 20]

Etiology

The cause of kyphoscoliosis is unknown or idiopathic in 85% of the cases. Idiopathic kyphoscoliosis is usually divided into three groups by age at onset: infantile, juvenile, and adolescent (10 to 14 years of age), with most cases appearing in the adolescent group. There is a 4:1 ratio of females to males in this group. The other 15% of the cases

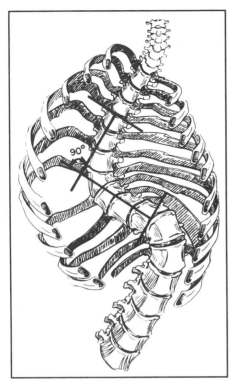

Figure 5–19. Kyphoscoliosis, showing the primary and secondary curves. The angle of curvature (90 degrees) is determined by the intersection of two lines drawn through the upper and lower limbs of the primary curve. (From Fishman AP. Pulmonary Diseases and Disorders. 2nd ed. New York, McGraw-Hill, 1988, p 2300.)

are due to known congenital causes (e.g., hemivertebrae) or develop in response to a neuromuscular disease (e.g., poliomyelitis, syringomyelia, muscular dystrophy).[16, 20]

Pathophysiology

In addition to the excessive anteroposterior and lateral curvature, the lateral displacement causes two additional structural changes. A second lateral curve develops to counterbalance the primary curve. In addition, the spine rotates on its longitudinal axis so that the ribs on the side of the convexity are displaced posteriorly and splayed, creating a *gibbous* hump, whereas the ribs on the side of the concavity are compressed. Significant spinal curvature must be present before pulmonary symptoms develop. Usually angles less than 70 degrees

do not produce pulmonary symptoms. Angles between 70 degrees and 120 degrees cause some respiratory dysfunction, and respiratory symptoms may increase with age as the angle increases and as the changes associated with aging affect the lung. Angles greater than 120 degrees are commonly associated with severe RLD and respiratory failure.[8] These skeletal abnormalities decrease the chest wall compliance, which may be as low as 25% of predicted.[8] Lung compliance is also decreased and dead space increased. The distribution of ventilation is disturbed, with more air going to the apices. Ventilation-perfusion matching is markedly impaired. These changes lead to a state of alveolar hypoventilation and a profound increase in the work of breathing—as high as 500% over normal.[8] The hypoventilation causes pulmonary hypertension, which over time causes structural changes in the vessels and thickening of the pulmonary arteriolar walls, leading to cor pulmonale. Although the respiratory muscles need to work harder to overcome the decreased pulmonary compliance, they are impaired because of the mechanical disadvantages from the thoracoabdominal deformity. When the VC is decreased to less than 40% of the predicted value, cardiorespiratory

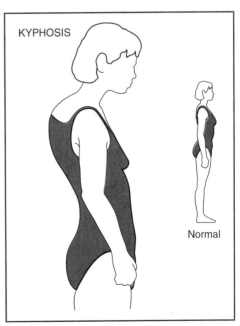

Figure 5–20. Kyphosis may cause restrictive lung defects secondary to musculoskeletal deformity and subsequent compression of the alveoli.

failure is likely to occur.[19] This usually occurs in the fourth or fifth decade of life. Sixty percent of deaths are due to respiratory failure or cor pulmonale.[19]

Clinical Manifestations

Signs

Pulmonary Function Tests. All the dynamic lung volumes and lung capacities are decreased in proportion to the degree of deformity. The RV may be normal or increased.[16] Flow rates are decreased in proportion to the decrease in the VC. Because so much energy is needed to move the chest wall, even VT is decreased, and so to try to maintain minute ventilation the respiratory rate is increased. The DL_{CO} is usually within normal limits unless the angle is 120 degrees or more, in which case it is decreased.

Chest Radiograph. The thoracic film appears grossly abnormal because of the severe deformity of the ribs and spine. The geography of the underlying lungs also is disrupted. It is not uncommon to see some lung tissue compressed with increased vascular markings, whereas other lung tissue is distended and may be emphysematous.

Arterial Blood Gases. If the angle is great enough, there is a decrease in the Pa_{O_2} and an increase in the Pa_{CO_2} owing to the chronic alveolar hypoventilation. The long-term elevation of the Pa_{CO_2} may blunt the responsiveness of the central chemoreceptors to acute changes in the Pa_{CO_2} that can put the patient at risk.

Breath Sounds. Breath sounds are usually decreased over the compressed lung.

Cardiovascular Findings. The hypoventilation causes pulmonary hypertension to develop. The arteriolar walls thicken, and cor pulmonale is common. Another complication of the chronic hypoxemia is that **polycythemia** may develop.[2, 16]

Symptoms. Patients have dyspnea on exertion, and their exercise tolerance decreases as the pulmonary restrictive impairment increases. The structural abnormality may overstretch the muscles, make them subject to spasm or overuse, or cause them to be underused and atrophied. Patients appear wasted owing to the very high caloric expenditure necessary to maintain ventilation.

Treatment

Kyphoscoliosis is treated conservatively with orthotic devices and an exercise program. Surgical intervention includes placement of Harrington's distraction strut bars. Pulmonary compromise is treated with preventive and supportive measures including immunizations, good hydration, aggressive treatment of pulmonary infections, avoidance of sedatives, supplemental oxygen, and respiratory muscle training.[9] Serious pulmonary involvement, including recurrent episodes of respiratory failure, seems to benefit from long-term nocturnal mechanical ventilation either through a chest cuirass or a positive pressure ventilator.[19, 20] Studies have shown that nasal continuous positive airway pressure (CPAP) is also beneficial, and it is now the preferred therapy.[16]

Ankylosing Spondylitis

Ankylosing spondylitis is a chronic inflammatory disease of the spine characterized by immobility of the sacroiliac and vertebral joints and by ossification of the paravertebral ligaments.[1, 12]

Etiology

Ankylosing spondylitis is an inherited arthritic condition that ultimately immobilizes the spine and results in a fixed thoracic cage.[20] It occurs predominantly in males, ages 20 to 40 years.[9]

Pathophysiology

The pulmonary impairment caused by this disease results from the markedly decreased compliance of the chest wall. With thoracic expansion so markedly decreased, ventilation becomes dependent almost entirely on diaphragmatic movement. Displacement of the abdomen during inspiration may be increased to compensate for the lack of rib expansion. Because the diaphragm is the major muscle of inspiration, the restrictive impairment involving the chest wall may result in only minimal respiratory symptoms.[8, 20] However, approximately 6% of patients with ankylosing spondylitis develop specific fibrosing lesions in the upper lobes as part of this disease process.[7] Why these lesions occur in some patients is unknown, but the immune system may be involved.[21] The pulmonary lesions may be unilateral or bilateral; they begin as small irregular opacities in the upper lobes. These lesions then increase in size, coalesce, and contract the lung parenchyma. Cavitation is frequent. The lung architecture becomes distorted, showing dense fibrosis which can lead to bronchiectasis and repeated pulmonary infections and an obstructive pulmonary deficit superimposed on the RLD.[7, 21] Apical pleural thickening is invariably present.[9]

Clinical Manifestations

Signs. The VC and IC are decreased. However, unlike many other RLD entities, the RV and the FRC are increased.[8] If upper lobe fibrosis is present, it is apparent on chest radiograph. Breath sounds are usually normal unless the upper lobes are involved, and then rhonchi consistent with bronchiectasis can be heard.

Symptoms. The major symptom is dyspnea on exertion owing to the restrictive lung impairment. Pleuritic chest pain is present in about 60% of patients.[9] With involvement of the upper lobes, symptoms may include a productive cough, progressive dyspnea, fever, and possible **hemoptysis.** Other symptoms can include low back pain, weight loss, and anorexia.[9]

Treatment

There is no curative treatment for ankylosing spondylitis. It is important to maintain good body alignment and as much thoracic mobility as possible. If there is direct lung involvement, then treatment of repeated pulmonary infections is required.

Pectus Excavatum

Pectus excavatum (funnel chest) is a congenital abnormality characterized by sternal depression and decreased anteroposterior diameter. The lower portion of the sternum is displaced posteriorly, and the anterior ribs are bowed markedly. Pulmonary function values are normal or near normal, and respiratory symptoms are uncommon. If the deformity is very severe, the patient may have decreased TLC, VC, and maximum voluntary ventilation and may complain of dyspnea on exertion, precordial pain, palpitation, and dizziness. Usually no treatment is indicated because the deformity is only cosmetic with no functional deficits.[1, 19, 20]

Pectus Carinatum

Pectus carinatum (pigeon breast) is a structural abnormality characterized by the sternum protruding anteriorly. Fifty percent of patients with **atrial** or **ventricular septal defects** have pectus carinatum. It also has been associated with severe prolonged childhood asthma. There is no pulmonary compromise associated with this structural abnormality, and no treatment is indicated.[20]

CONNECTIVE TISSUE CAUSES OF RESTRICTIVE LUNG DYSFUNCTION

Rheumatoid Arthritis

Rheumatoid arthritis is a chronic process characterized by inflammation of the peripheral joints that results in progressive destruction of articular and periarticular structures.[1, 18]

Etiology

The etiology is unknown. There is a high prevalence of RA in the United States; 4 to 6 million adults have been diagnosed with this chronic condition.[13] One third of these patients, almost 2 million people, have some pulmonary involvement as part of their disease, although it remains unclear why one or more pulmonary lesions may develop in a given patient.[21] Lung involvement with RA usually occurs between 50 to 60 years of age and is very rare in children who have RA.[13] Another distinction is that although RA is more prevalent in women, pulmonary involvement, particularly pulmonary fibrosis, is more common in men.[21]

Pathophysiology

Pulmonary involvement in RA was first recognized and reported by Ellman and Ball in 1948.[25] Rheumatoid arthritis can affect the lungs in seven different ways: pleural involvement, **pneumonitis,** interstitial fibrosis, development of pulmonary nodules, pulmonary **vasculitis,** obliterative bronchiolitis, and an increased incidence of bronchogenic cancer.[9] These different pulmonary manifestations of RA may occur individually or in combination within the lungs.[25] Pleural involvement may include pleuritis, pleural friction rub, repeated small exudative pleural effusions, and pleural thickening and fibrosis.[13, 21, 22] These pulmonary abnormalities can result in pain and some RLD. Pneumonitis causes an inflammatory reaction in the lung, including patchy infiltrates, which can resolve spontaneously or can progress to fibrotic changes. The cause of interstitial fibrosis in the patient with RA is unknown but seems to correlate with increased manifestations of **autoimmunity.**[25] Patients with a high titer of rheumatoid factor are more likely to develop interstitial fibrosis.[13]

There seems to be a temporal relationship between joint involvement and development of fibrosing alveolitis, with the joint involvement usually coming first.[13] Interstitial fibrosis can be diffuse but predominates in the lower lobes. Rheumatoid (necrobiotic) nodules usually occur subpleurally in the upper lung fields or in the interlobular septa. They may be single, multiple, unilateral, or bilateral. Spontaneous resolution of these nodules can occur. Cavitation is common.[19, 25] If a patient with RA is exposed to coal dust, pulmonary nodules known as *Caplan's syndrome* can develop. These multiple peripheral pulmonary nodules have a pigmented ring of coal dust surrounding the lesion. Rheumatoid nodules and Caplan's syndrome rarely produce significant RLD.[21, 25]

Pulmonary vasculitis often occurs adjacent to pulmonary nodules. There is intimal fibrosis in the pulmonary arterioles.[7, 25] Obliterative bronchiolitis is rare; however, the onset is usually acute and

progresses within 2 years to a fatal outcome. The bronchioles become inflamed and edematous and are then replaced with granulation tissue. The bronchial lumen is severely narrowed or obliterated.[7, 19] The increased incidence of bronchogenic cancer in RA is related to coexisting interstitial fibrosis in both smokers and nonsmokers.[9]

In addition to lung involvement with RA, chest wall compliance may be decreased significantly owing to increased rigidity of the thorax because of RA, decreased inspiratory muscle power because of rheumatoid myopathy, or decreased mobility because of pain caused by **pleurisy.** Therefore the RLD that can result in RA patients may be due to a decrease both in lung and in chest wall compliance.[13]

Clinical Manifestations

Signs
Pulmonary Function Tests. With interstitial fibrosis the VC and the volumes that make up this lung capacity decrease. The DL_{CO} also decreases, especially if there is evidence of pulmonary vasculitis. Lung compliance is reduced.

Chest Radiograph. The chest radiograph may show pleural thickening or effusion, which is unilateral in 80% of cases.[9] Rheumatoid nodules appear as rounded, homogeneous densities, most often seen in the peripheral lung fields of the upper lobes.[9] Interstitial pneumonitis may show as patchy alveolar infiltrates and increased reticulation in the lower lobes. Later, as interstitial fibrosis develops, a dense reticular or reticulonodular pattern with honeycombing appears.[9]

Arterial Blood Gases. As lung involvement becomes significant, the typical restrictive lung impairment values of a decreased Pa_{O_2} with a normal Pa_{CO_2} emerge.

Breath Sounds. Bibasilar rales are common. With fibrosis, decreased breath sounds may also occur.

Cardiovascular Findings. With pulmonary vasculitis, pulmonary hypertension occurs if enough of the pulmonary vessels are involved.

Symptoms. The common articular symptoms are warm, swollen, painful joints, with progressive destruction of the joint surfaces and impairment of the joint mechanics. The major pulmonary symptoms are progressive dyspnea with a nonproductive cough. Other symptoms can include pleuritic pain, fever, clubbing, cyanosis; hemoptysis can occur with cavitation of pulmonary nodules.[13, 19, 22] With pleural involvement only, symptoms are often minimal or may be absent in one third of patients.[9]

Treatment

Corticosteroids and immunosuppressant drugs are commonly used to treat pulmonary involvement in RA.[19, 25]

Systemic Lupus Erythematosus

Systemic lupus erythematosus (SLE) is a chronic inflammatory connective tissue disorder.[1, 18, 19]

Etiology

The etiology is unknown, although the immune system seems to be involved.[1, 19] Ninety percent of cases occur in women, and SLE is more common in black women.[8] It usually occurs between the ages of 15 and 45, most frequently in the second and third decades of life.[8] It is interesting that certain drugs (procainamide hydrochloride, phenytoin, hydralazine hydrochloride, penicillamine, isoniazid) can evoke a clinical syndrome indistinguishable from spontaneous SLE.[13]

Pathophysiology

This disorder involves the autoimmune system and is characterized by a variety of **antigen-antibody reactions.**[1] Systemic lupus erythematosus can involve the skin, joints, kidneys, lung, nervous tissue, and heart. In 50% to 90% of the cases it does involve the lungs or pleura; this incidence of pulmonary involvement is higher than that of any other connective tissue disorder.[10, 22] The most common lung involvement is pleurisy, often with the development of small bilateral exudative pleural effusions that may be recurrent, may be associated with **pericarditis,** and may lead to fibrinous pleuritis.[8, 22] Acute lupus pneumonitis is another mani-

festation of lung involvement. It usually causes hypoxemia, severe shortness of breath, cyanosis, tachypnea, and tachycardia.[8, 19, 22] There may be an accompanying pleuritis with or without pleural effusion. Acute lupus pneumonitis may resolve or may lead to chronic interstitial pneumonitis and fibrosis. Alveolar hemorrhage is a rare but life-threatening pulmonary manifestation of SLE. It can occur suddenly with no prior hemoptysis and can carry a mortality as high as 70%.[8] The reasons some patients develop recurrent pulmonary hemorrhages or have a massive intra-alveolar hemorrhage are not known. Recurrent hemorrhages can lead to interstitial fibrosis.

It has been found that diaphragmatic weakness is relatively common in SLE patients. It is now appreciated that the "shrinkage" of the lower lobes, elevated diaphragms, and bibasilar atelectasis can be attributed largely to diaphragmatic weakness. The diaphragm may show muscle atrophy and fibrosis with minimal inflammation.[8] Other ventilatory muscles may also be weak, even with no noticeable weakness in the muscles of the extremities. This muscle involvement may cause a marked restrictive ventilatory impairment in 25% of SLE patients.[9] Nephritis occurs in more than 50% of patients and is the major cause of mortality in SLE.[8]

Clinical Manifestations

Signs
Pulmonary Function Tests. With interstitial fibrosis or fibrosing alveolitis, lung volumes are decreased due to the decrease in lung compliance. Lung volumes could also be decreased owing to respiratory muscle weakness or recurrent alveolar hemorrhage. Diffusing capacity is decreased due to the increased ventilation-perfusion mismatching.[9]

Chest Radiograph. The chest radiograph can show atelectatic pneumonitis with alveolar consolidation, particularly at the bases of the lungs; elevated hemidiaphragms; the reticulonodular pattern of interstitial infiltrates; pleural effusions; or **cardiomegaly** from a pericardial effusion.[9]

Arterial Blood Gases. The Pa_{O_2} is decreased with significant restrictive impairment, and the Pa_{CO_2} is usually within normal limits.[9]

Breath Sounds. On auscultation bibasilar rales may be heard or a pleural friction rub, or both.

Cardiovascular Findings. Pericarditis is often present; pericardial effusions and pulmonary hypertension can also occur.

Symptoms. Approximately 90% of SLE patients report articular symptoms, including arthralgias and polyarthritis.[19] Pulmonary symptoms reported depend on the type of pulmonary involvement but may include dyspnea, cough without or with only scant sputum production, hemoptysis, fever, pleuritic pain, cyanosis, and clubbing. Other symptoms may include skin lesions, photosensitivity, fatigue, weight loss, **Raynaud's phenomenon,** oral or nasal septal ulcerations, and neurologic disturbances.

Treatment

Corticosteroids cause rapid improvement of acute lupus pneumonitis and, together with plasmapheresis, are also used to treat alveolar hemorrhage.[8, 22] Fibrotic changes in the lungs are irreversible, so only supportive therapy is indicated.

Scleroderma

Scleroderma (progressive systemic sclerosis) is a progressive fibrosing disorder that causes degenerative changes in the skin, small blood vessels, esophagus, intestinal tract, lung, heart, kidney, and articular structures.[1, 19]

Etiology

The etiology is unknown, and the pattern of involvement, progression, and severity of the disease varies widely. It is four times more common in women than in men and is rare in children. The majority of patients are diagnosed between 30 and 50 years of age.[22]

Pathophysiology

Within the lung, scleroderma appears as progressive diffuse interstitial fibrosis, in which collagen replaces the normal connective tissue framework of the lung. There is fibrotic replacement of the connective tissue within the alveolar walls. The pulmonary arterioles undergo obliterative changes; however, necrotizing vasculitis is rare.[19] These changes may be accompanied by parenchymal cystic sclerosis, thus increasing the restrictive impairment in the lung. At autopsy 75% to 80% of scleroderma victims show evidence of interstitial pulmonary fibrosis.[21] Pleuritis and pleural effusions are unusual, unlike in the other collagen diseases that have pulmonary involvement.[21] Carcinoma of the lung also has been reported in association with scleroderma.[19]

Esophageal dysfunction is the most frequent visceral disturbance and occurs in most patients.[22] Lung dysfunction is the second most common visceral disturbance, occurring in approximately 90% of scleroderma patients.[9, 10] The disease is often slowly progressive. However, if cardiac, pulmonary, or renal involvement is early, the prognosis is poor. Death is usually due to cardiac or renal failure.[21]

Clinical Manifestations

Signs

Pulmonary Function Tests. The TLC, VC, and all lung volumes are decreased. Lung compliance is reduced owing to the interstitial fibrosis, and chest wall compliance also may be reduced because of the scleroderma. These changes can increase markedly the work of breathing and usually result in an increased respiratory rate in an effort to maintain minute ventilation. The DL_{CO} is impaired early in this disease.

Chest Radiograph. The chest films early in the course of the disease show pulmonary infiltrates. Later the chest radiograph may show an interstitial reticular pattern with honeycombing, particularly at the bases of the lungs; pleural thickening; or aspiration pneumonia, which is common because of the decreased esophageal motility. Pericardial effusions and right-sided heart enlargement may also be seen.[9]

Arterial Blood Gases. Because of the RLD, the Pa_{O_2} is decreased, whereas the Pa_{CO_2} is usually within normal limits.

Breath Sounds. Bibasilar rales are the most common finding. Breath sounds may be diminished, and rhonchi can be present if the patient has pulmonary infiltrates or an aspiration pneumonia.[9]

Cardiovascular Findings. Pulmonary hypertension is common and can progress to cor pulmonale. Other common cardiac findings are pericarditis with pericardial effusions, arrhythmias, and conduction disturbances.

Symptoms. The most prominent symptom is exertional dyspnea, and this occurs in approximately 40% of all scleroderma patients. It is even more common in patients with Raynaud's phenomenon.[21] A nonproductive cough and clubbing of the digits are also common.

Treatment

There is no effective drug treatment for sclerodermatous pleuropulmonary disease. The interstitial fibrosis is progressive and nonreversible. There is also no drug therapy that has been shown to be effective in altering the course of scleroderma. A number of agents are used to treat specific symptoms in affected organs.[22] Lung transplantation may be an option, particularly if the scleroderma has not affected any other organ system.[9] Otherwise, only supportive treatment of pulmonary symptoms is available.

Polymyositis

Polymyositis is a systemic connective tissue disease characterized by symmetric proximal muscle weakness and pain.[18, 19, 22]

Etiology

The etiology is unknown but may involve an autoimmune reaction. The disease can occur throughout life but most commonly appears before age 15 or between 40 and 60 years of age. The disease is twice as common in women.[18, 22]

Pathophysiology

Approximately 5% to 20% of patients exhibit involvement of the lung parenchyma.[10] **Aspiration pneumonia** is the most common pulmonary abnormality and is seen in 15% to 20% of patients.[10] Other changes can include interstitial pneumonitis and fibrosis, bronchiolitis obliterans, or diffuse pulmonary infiltrates. The pleura is usually not involved. In addition to these changes, which result in a restrictive pulmonary impairment, the respiratory muscles may be weak, which increases the restrictive dysfunction. Striated muscle involvement includes inflammation, degeneration, atrophy, and necrosis. This results in profound weakness of the limb girdle muscles, the respiratory muscles, the laryngeal muscles, and the pharyngeal muscles. When the disease occurs in children, diffuse soft tissue calcification may occur also, which could decrease chest wall compliance further. Dysphagia and aspiration problems are common. Although characteristics of the disease are similar in children and adults, the onset is often more acute in children and more insidious in adults. The disease may enter long periods of remission. However, it seems to be more severe and unrelenting in patients with pulmonary or cardiac involvement.[19, 21, 22]

Clinical Manifestations

Signs. With chest wall and lung parenchymal involvement, the lung volumes are decreased and the DL_{CO} is also reduced. The chest radiograph shows peripheral lower lobe interstitial fibrosis with honeycombing.[10] Because of weakness in the ventilatory pump, alveolar hypoventilation occurs, which leads to a decrease in the Pa_{O_2}. Auscultation reveals late-inspiratory bibasilar rales.[9]

Symptoms. Patients experience progressive shortness of breath with a nonproductive cough. Neck flexors may become extremely weak so that the patient has difficulty lifting or supporting the head. Weakness of the laryngeal and pharyngeal muscles can cause dysphonia and dysphagia. As the respiratory muscles become weak, breathing becomes labored. There may also be muscle pain and tenderness and polyarthralgia. Raynaud's phenomenon is present in 9% of these patients.[19]

Treatment

Pulmonary involvement is treated with corticosteroids with good results if started early during the inflammatory phase.[19]

Dermatomyositis

Dermatomyositis is a systemic connective tissue disease characterized primarily by inflammatory and degenerative changes in the skin. The pulmonary involvement that occurs with this disease mirrors the involvement that occurs with polymyositis described earlier. The incidence of lung involvement in dermatomyositis patients is also 5% to 20%.[10, 12, 21]

IMMUNOLOGIC CAUSES OF RESTRICTIVE LUNG DYSFUNCTION

Goodpasture's Syndrome

Goodpasture's syndrome is a disease of the immune complex that is characterized by interstitial or intra-alveolar hemorrhage, glomerulonephritis, and **anemia**.[21]

Etiology

This rather rare disease is most often brought on by the presence of *antiglomerular basement membrane (anti-GBM) antibodies* that react with the vascular basement membranes of the alveolus and the glomerulus, causing pulmonary hemorrhage and glomerulonephritis. How these antibodies come to be formed is still unknown. **Prodromal** viral infections or exposure to chemical substances such as hydrocarbon solvents may be involved. Why these anti-GBM antibodies cannot be demonstrated in all patients with Goodpasture's syndrome is another mystery. This syndrome is approximately four times more prevalent in men than in women. The onset of the disease occurs between the ages of 17 and 27 in 75% of the cases.[20]

Pathophysiology

Whatever the cause of these autoantibodies, it has been shown that when they are present in the circulating blood, they crossreact with the basement membrane of the alveolar wall and deposit along the glomerular basement membrane. This results in the release of **cytotoxic** substances that damage the pulmonary and glomerular capillaries. Blood leaks from the damaged pulmonary capillaries into the interstitium and the alveolar spaces, which over time can lead to significant and widespread pulmonary fibrosis. The pulmonary hemorrhages are episodic and seem to be precipitated by nonimmunologic factors such as fluid overload, smoking, toxic exposure, or infection. Within the kidney, the damaged glomerular capillaries lead to a rapidly progressive, often necrotizing type of glomerulonephritis and renal failure.[8, 20, 21]

Clinical Manifestations

Signs
Pulmonary Function Tests. Lung volumes are decreased in proportion to the amount of pulmonary fibrosis present. The area of the lung involved and affected by the fibrosis is variable.

Chest Radiograph. The chest radiograph shows the distribution, volume, and temporal sequence of repeated pulmonary hemorrhages. Confluent densities are visible shortly after a hemorrhage into the interstitial tissue or the alveolar spaces. These diffuse, fluffy infiltrates may clear completely during remission of the disease. However, with repeated episodes of pulmonary hemorrhage, accentuated interstitial pulmonary markings persist and become visible on the radiograph. When pulmonary fibrosis develops, permanent reticulonodular infiltrates can be seen. It is also possible to see fluffy alveolar densities superimposed on a reticulonodular pattern when there is a new pulmonary hemorrhage in an already damaged and fibrotic area of lung.[9, 16]

Arterial Blood Gases. Hypoxemia is common owing to the increase in ventilation-perfusion mismatching. Pa_{CO_2} may also be decreased.

Breath Sounds. Auscultatory findings vary. With active pulmonary hemorrhage, breath sounds are decreased, and rales or rhonchi may be heard. Over areas of permanent pulmonary fibrosis, the most common findings are decreased breath sounds and dry inspiratory rales.[9]

Cardiovascular Findings. Usually the ECG is normal.

Symptoms. The most characteristic symptom is hemoptysis, which can vary from blood-tinged sputum to massive amounts of frank red blood. He-

moptysis is most often the initial symptom; it occurs at some time during the course of the disease
in virtually every case. Other pulmonary symptoms
include dyspnea, cough, and substernal chest pain.
Patients may also experience weakness, fatigue, hematuria, pallor, and fever, and 5% of these patients report arthralgias or arthritis.[9, 10]

Treatment

Treatment usually combines plasmapheresis and
immunosuppressive therapy to lower the levels of
anti-GBM antibodies circulating in the blood. Cyclophosphamide with prednisone is the regimen of
choice. Methylprednisolone may be used to treat
pulmonary hemorrhage. Dialysis is used to counteract renal failure. The overall prognosis for
Goodpasture's syndrome is poor. Until recently,
approximately 50% of the patients died within 1
year of diagnosis. One half of the deaths were due
to pulmonary hemorrhage and the other half to
renal failure.[8, 20, 21] Currently, however, it has been
recognized that there can be milder forms of the
disease and that the disease's responsiveness to
treatment can be variable. Therefore, early aggressive therapy encompassing plasmapheresis, drugs,
ventilator support, acute hemodialysis, treatment
of infection, and careful avoidance of cardiogenic
edema has been used to increase survival rates to
70% to 80%.[9]

Wegener's Granulomatosis

Wegener's granulomatosis is a multisystem disease
characterized by granulomatous vasculitis of the
upper and lower respiratory tracts, glomerulonephritis, and widespread small vessel vasculitis.[20]

Etiology

The etiology is unknown. Some studies seem to
indicate that the disease may be due to a hypersensitivity reaction to an undetermined antigen.
During the active disease process, circulating immune complexes have been identified. Immune
reactants and complexlike deposits have also been
identified in renal biopsies of patients with Wegener's granulomatosis. Although histologically the

immune system and hypersensitivity reactions seem
to be involved, the disease appears clinically as an
infectious process due to some unknown pathogen. This disease can occur at any age, but the
average age at onset is 40 years. The disease is
twice as common in males as in females.[20]

Pathophysiology

The disease often seems to start in the upper respiratory tract with necrotizing granulomas and ulceration in the nasopharynx and paranasal areas.
Inflammation with perivascular exudative infiltration and fibrin deposition in the pulmonary arteries and veins causes focal destruction. Multiple
nodular cavitary infiltrates develop in one or both
lungs. These lesions often consist of a necrotic
core surrounded by granulation tissue. Early in the
disease, the kidney shows acute focal or segmental
glomerulitis with hematuria. As the disease progresses, necrotizing glomerulonephritis leading to
kidney failure often occurs.[14, 20]

Clinical Manifestations

Signs
Pulmonary Function Tests. Lung volumes are
decreased if the lung parenchyma is significantly
involved. There may also be an obstructive component to this disease if granulomatous lesions invade and block bronchial airways. Gas diffusion
can also be impaired if the pulmonary capillary
bed has been extensively destroyed.

Chest Radiograph. The pulmonary infiltrates
seen on radiograph may be of any size or shape
and seem to have no predilection for location
within the lung. These nodular infiltrates may appear in any lobe—bilaterally or unilaterally—and
may appear hazy or with sharply defined borders.
Cavitation of these lesions is common.[14, 20] Pleural
effusions are seen in about 20% of patients.[9]

Arterial Blood Gases. A decrease in the Pa_{O_2} is
evident as more of the lung tissue and the pulmonary capillary bed are unable to participate in gas
exchange.

Breath Sounds. Auscultatory findings are variable, depending on the size and location of the
pulmonary lesions.

Cardiovascular Findings. These findings are

variable, depending on the severity of the disseminated small vessel vasculitis. Myocardial infarction can result from the vasculitis.

Symptoms. The initial symptoms often involve the upper respiratory tract and include severe **rhinorrhea;** paranasal sinusitis; nasal mucosal ulcerations; and otitis media, often with hearing loss. With pulmonary involvement, the usual symptoms include dyspnea, cough, hemoptysis, vague chest pain, or pleuritic chest pain. Other more generalized symptoms commonly noted in this disease are fever, fatigue, malaise, anorexia, weight loss, and migratory arthralgias.[9]

Treatment

The treatment of choice is with cyclophosphamide. This drug can produce marked improvement or partial remissions in 91% of patients and complete remissions in 75% of patients.[9] Without drug therapy, this disease progresses rapidly and is fatal. The mean duration between diagnosis and death is 5 months when not treated.[20] Death is most often due to renal disease progressing to kidney failure. Kidney transplantation has been used successfully in cases of renal failure.

PREGNANCY AS A CAUSE OF RESTRICTIVE LUNG DYSFUNCTION

During the third trimester of pregnancy, ventilation to the dependent regions of the lungs is impaired by the growth and position of the developing fetus. This restrictive change in ventilation is due to a decrease in chest wall compliance caused primarily by the decreased downward excursion of the diaphragm. The decreased ventilation in the bases of the lungs results in early small airway closure and increased ventilation-perfusion mismatching. The voluntary lung volumes are decreased, particularly the ERV (8% to 40%).[9] The work of breathing is increased, and the woman may feel she is unable to take a deep breath, particularly in the supine position. To counteract some of these changes and to keep the Pa_{O_2} within the normal range, the body increases the progesterone level during this trimester. The increased

level of progesterone increases the woman's ventilatory drive, which in turn increases the tidal volume and respiratory rate, thereby increasing the minute ventilation. This increase results in a decrease in Pa_{CO_2} and a rise in Pa_{O_2}, which ensures that the mother and the fetus do not become hypoxemic.[9, 12]

NUTRITIONAL AND METABOLIC CAUSES OF RESTRICTIVE LUNG DYSFUNCTION

Obesity

Obesity is defined as a condition in which the body weight is 20% or more over the ideal body weight.[18]

Etiology

Obesity is the result of an imbalance between the calories ingested and the calories expended. This imbalance may be due to overeating, inadequate exercise, a pathologic process that alters metabolism, or a psychological need or coping mechanism.

Pathophysiology

The increase in body weight represents a significant increase in body mass, and this extra tissue requires additional oxygen from the lungs and produces additional carbon dioxide, which must be eliminated by the lungs. The excess soft tissue on the chest wall decreases the compliance of the thorax and therefore increases the work of breathing. The excess soft tissue in the abdominal wall exerts pressure on the abdominal contents, forcing the diaphragm up to a higher resting position. This shift results in decreased lung expansion and early closure of the small airways and alveoli, especially at the bases or the dependent regions of the lung. These areas are hypoventilated relative to their perfusion, which can markedly increase the ventilation-perfusion mismatching and result in hypoxemia.[2, 8] In addition, some overweight individuals have demonstrated an obesity-hypoventilation syndrome, which results when there is an imbalance between the ventilatory drive and the ventilatory load.[9]

Clinical Manifestations

Signs

Pulmonary Function Tests. The ERV is especially decreased, but all lung capacities and volumes are slightly diminished. The VT may be smaller, so to maintain minute ventilation the respiratory rate is increased. However, overall the maximal voluntary ventilation is diminished.[9] In the supine position, the lung volumes are even further reduced, which can lead to alveolar hypoventilation during sleep.

Chest Radiograph. The chest film shows an increase in the adipose tissue overlying the ribs. Compression of the lung tissue in the dependent lung regions may also be evident. Over time the chest radiograph may also show an enlarged heart and small lung fields with pulmonary congestion.[9]

Arterial Blood Gases. In very obese patients, alveolar hypoventilation, increased ventilation-perfusion mismatching, oxygenation demands of the extra adipose tissue, increased work and oxygen uptake in the inspiratory muscles, and inefficient breathing patterns all combine to cause hypoxemia. The Pa_{O_2} is therefore decreased, and in some patients the Pa_{CO_2} is continually elevated, which blunts the response to acute changes in the Pa_{CO_2}.[9]

Breath Sounds. Breath sounds are diminished, particularly at the bases of the lungs.

Cardiovascular Findings. The circulatory response to obesity is an increase in the cardiac output and the circulating blood volume. This response creates more work for the heart, and both systemic and pulmonary hypertension are not uncommon, with both the right and left ventricles being stressed. Alveolar hypoventilation leads to further pulmonary hypertension. Over time, cardiac arrhythmias and congestive heart failure can result.

Symptoms. The primary symptom is dyspnea on exertion, which can become more limiting as the obesity increases. **Sleep apnea** can also occur owing to the extra soft tissue in the neck that surrounds the upper airways, causing airway obstruction during sleep.[2]

Treatment

It is becoming better recognized that obesity is a very complex disorder. It involves virtually all the body's systems via the patient's metabolism, the psychological and mental processes within the patient, and the patient's behaviors and habits. Treatment consisting of dieting and will power is usually not effective over an extended period of time. Patients who have been markedly obese over a long period usually can demonstrate expertise in dieting and remarkably significant will power. It is not unusual for these patients to have lost three or four times their body weight over their lifetime, only to regain the lost weight and more. Current treatment strategies for the obese patient combine interventions. Weight loss programs now often include extensive medical evaluation and a variety of therapeutic interventions, including diet, increased activity, behavior modification, psychological support, nutritional counseling, and family involvement. Weight loss will decrease the work of breathing, increase the vital capacity, and increase the ventilatory drive in these patients.[9] Sleep apnea is most commonly treated with weight loss, avoidance of ethanol, position therapy, dental devices, nasal CPAP, increased FI_{O_2}, and tracheostomy.[9, 10]

A great deal is still to be learned and understood about the body's metabolism: how food is broken down, stored, and eliminated; and how obesity can be reversed so that recurrence is not the norm. See Chapter 7 for more details on obesity.

Diabetes Mellitus

Diabetes mellitus is a syndrome that results from abnormal carbohydrate metabolism and is characterized by inadequate insulin secretion and **hyperglycemia**.[18]

Etiology

Diabetes mellitus has no distinct etiology but seems to result from a variable interaction of hereditary and environmental factors.[18]

Pathophysiology

The most common pathologic changes seen in diabetes mellitus result from hyperglycemia, large vessel disease, microvascular disease (particularly involving the retina and kidney), and neuropathy.[18] The effects of this metabolic disorder on the lungs have been reported, and although the incidence of pulmonary involvement does not seem to be high, it can be significant in some patients. Hyperglycemic patients have an increased incidence of pulmonary infections and tuberculosis, which is manifest more frequently in the lower lobes.[19] Diffuse alveolar hemorrhage has also been reported in diabetics and may be due to inflammation and necrosis of the pulmonary capillary endothelium. This could then be followed by fibrotic changes.[13] In a study of more than 31,000 patients with diabetes mellitus, pulmonary fibrosis was found in 0.8% of the diabetic population, which is a moderately greater incidence than that reported for the general population.[19] Juvenile diabetics have shown a decrease in elastic recoil of the lungs and in lung compliance, causing a decrease in TLC.[19, 25] These abnormalities in ventilatory mechanics are thought to be due to changes in the elastin and collagen within the lung. Another mechanism that can cause a restrictive impairment in the lung is *diabetic ketoacidosis,* which can produce a noncardiogenic pulmonary edema. The physiologic cause for this change is unclear but may be an alteration in the pulmonary capillary permeability.[19] See Chapter 7 for more details on diabetes.

TRAUMATIC CAUSES OF RESTRICTIVE LUNG DYSFUNCTION

Crush Injuries

Crush injuries to the thorax are usually caused by blunt trauma that results in pathologic damage, particularly rib fractures, flail chest, or lung contusion.[1]

Etiology

The leading cause of blunt trauma to the thorax is motor vehicle accidents. The second most com-

mon cause of thoracic crush injuries is falls, which usually occur in the home.[20]

Pathophysiology

Rib Fractures. Rib fractures most commonly involve the fifth through the ninth ribs because they are anchored anteriorly and posteriorly and are less protected than ribs 1 through 4 from the kinetic energy of a traumatic blow.[20] Even nondisplaced rib fractures can be very painful, and it is the pain on any movement of the chest wall that causes the restrictive impairment. Patients with rib fractures breathe very shallowly in an effort to keep the thoracic wall still. The muscular splinting around the fracture site also decreases chest wall excursion and lung expansion. In addition, fractured ribs may be accompanied by a **hemothorax,** which can progress to a large sanguinous effusion and empyema. This fluid in the pleural space compresses the underlying lung parenchyma and can cause fibrosis and scarring of the pleura, leading to permanent restrictive dysfunction.[8] More frequently, the pain of the rib fractures decreases significantly during the first 2 weeks after the injury, and normal lung function is restored, although coughing may cause pain for up to 6 months. Patients who have multiple rib fractures, are older than 50 years, or have underlying pulmonary or cardiovascular disease are at greater risk of developing a pneumonia following rib fracture.[4, 20]

Flail Chest. Flail chest refers to a free-floating segment of ribs due to multiple rib fractures both anteriorly and posteriorly that leave this part of the thoracic wall disconnected to the rest of the thoracic cage.[20] This segment can usually be identified by its paradoxical movement during the respiratory cycle. It moves inward during inspiration, drawn by the increase in the negative pleural space pressure. It moves outward during expiration, as the pleural space pressure approaches atmospheric pressure. Both the pain and the paradoxical movement of a part of the thoracic cage during the respiratory cycle contribute to the restrictive dysfunction. Lung volumes are decreased, and the distribution of ventilation is altered, causing an increase in ventilation-perfusion mismatching. The force of the blunt trauma that causes a flail chest is usually greater than that causing a simple rib fracture. Because the force is greater, flail chest is often associated with lung contusion.[4, 16, 20] Long-term pulmonary disability following flail chest is common; 60% of these patients have chest wall pain, chest wall deformity, dyspnea on exertion, and mild restrictive pulmonary dysfunction for months to years following the injury.[16]

Lung Contusion. Lung contusion occurs when the lung strikes directly against the chest wall. The local pulmonary microvasculature is damaged, causing red blood cells and plasma to move into the alveoli.[20] This immediately decreases the compliance of the lung, changes the distribution of inspired gases, and increases ventilation-perfusion mismatching. Although the injury due to the lung contusion may resolve in approximately 3 days, patients are at high risk for serious pulmonary complications. Approximately 50% to 70% develop a pneumonia in the contused segment, 35% develop an empyema, and some patients develop ARDS, with complete "white out" of the injured lung on chest radiograph.[4, 16, 20]

Clinical Manifestations

Signs
Pulmonary Function Tests. Crush injuries increase the respiratory rate and decrease V_T, FRC, VC, and TLC.

Chest Radiograph. The chest radiograph may appear normal if the rib fractures are not displaced. Displaced rib fractures and flail chest are easily recognized on the posteroanterior (PA) view of the chest film. A lung contusion on chest radiograph shows as focal infiltrates occurring in nonsegmental and nonlobar distribution. These infiltrates usually clear within 3 days. More diffuse infiltrates that remain more than 3 days following injury may denote a pneumonia or the development of ARDS.

Arterial Blood Gases. The Pa_{O_2} is decreased in proportion to the amount of chest wall damage and lung contusion. There is increased ventilation-perfusion mismatching.[16]

Breath Sounds. Breath sounds are diminished owing to the decrease in lung volumes and possible fluid in the pleural space. Rales may also be heard over areas of atelectasis.[16]

Cardiovascular Findings. Because the heart may be directly involved in the precipitating trauma, changes in the cardiovascular system are variable.

Symptoms. With rib fracture and flail chest,

the primary symptom is chest wall pain and tenderness to palpation. Pain is exacerbated with movement of the chest wall, particularly coughing and sneezing. Patients splint the chest wall to decrease movement during the respiratory cycle. Respiratory rate is increased, and with larger injuries patients may appear in some respiratory distress.

Treatment

Rib Fractures. Pain control is the primary treatment and can be accomplished by oral analgesics, intercostal nerve block, or epidural anesthesia depending on the extent of the injury.[20] The goal is to allow the patient to reestablish a normal breathing pattern. In patients at high risk for developing pneumonia, hospital admission may be indicated for close observation and for aggressive pulmonary hygiene in addition to pain relief.[16]

Flail Chest. Flail chest may have to be managed by mechanical ventilation when the patient's respiratory rate exceeds 40 breaths per minute, the VC progressively decreases to less than 10 to 15 mL/kg of body weight, the arterial oxygenation falls to less than 60 mm Hg with an FI_{O_2} of 50%, hypercapnia develops with the Pa_{CO_2} higher than 50 mm Hg, or other injuries sustained in the trauma necessitate its use.[20] Mechanical ventilatory support may be needed for 2 to 4 weeks. With severe chest wall injuries or marked displacement of the fracture fragments, surgical stabilization may be required. Surgery usually shortens the time the patient needs to be on mechanical ventilation, decreases the pain, and increases anatomic alignment during the healing process.[20] With less severe injuries, the flail chest may be able to be treated with excellent pain control and aggressive breathing exercises, use of an **incentive spirometer,** positioning, and coughing.

Lung Contusion. Treatment is supportive and preventive. Mechanical ventilation and supplemental oxygen may be required. Fluid monitoring to ensure against volume overload, which could lead to pulmonary edema, is important. Although corticosteroids have been used, there is no current data that show they improve the morbidity or mortality rates in these patients.[16] Deep breathing exercises, positioning, and coughing are also used to assist in clearing infiltrates and to decrease the incidence of pneumonia.[20]

Penetrating Wounds

Penetrating wounds to the thorax are usually caused by shooting or stabbing and result in pathologic damage, particularly pneumothorax, hemothorax, pulmonary laceration, tracheal or bronchial disruption, diaphragmatic injury, esophageal perforation, or cardiac laceration. Only the first three are discussed within the scope of this chapter.[1, 4]

Etiology

The leading cause of penetrating wounds to the thorax is gunshot wounds and stab wounds. Penetrating wounds to the chest are usually more specific and defined and are less likely to have the multisystem involvement more commonly seen with thoracic crush injuries.[4, 20]

Pathophysiology

Pneumothorax. Traumatic pneumothorax is defined as the entry of free air into the pleural space (Fig. 5–21). This often occurs after a penetrating wound to the thorax. A traumatic pneumothorax can be further classified as an open pneumothorax or a **tension pneumothorax.**[1]

An open pneumothorax means the air in the pleural space communicates freely with the outside environment. When air can move freely through the chest wall, into and out of the pleural space, the patient is unable to maintain a negative pleural space pressure. Because an effective negative pleural space pressure cannot be maintained in both the affected and unaffected hemithorax, the patient's ability to move air into the lungs is severely diminished. Lung volumes are decreased; lung compliance is decreased; ventilation-perfusion mismatching is increased; and gas exchange is impaired.[1]

A tension pneumothorax means air can enter the pleural space but cannot escape into the external environment. This is an acute life-threatening situation.[21] As air continues to enter and become trapped in the pleural space the intrapleural pressure rapidly increases. This causes the lung on the involved side to collapse. The mediastinal structures are pushed away from the affected side. The increased thoracic pressure causes a decrease in venous return; cardiac output falls; and systemic hypotension and shock are the result. Lung volumes are significantly reduced; lung compliance is decreased; and the alveolar-capillary surface area available for gas exchange is cut by more than 50%.[1, 4, 20]

Hemothorax. Hemothorax is the presence of blood in the pleural space. It can occur with both penetrating wounds and crush injuries to the thorax. Approximately 70% of patients with chest trauma develop a hemothorax.[16] Collection of blood in the pleural space causes compression of the underlying lung tissue and prevents lung expansion. This process usually affects the lower lobes because the blood in the pleural space is

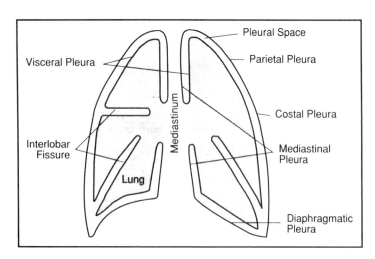

Figure 5–21. Diagram of the pleural space. (From Weinberger SE. Principles of Pulmonary Medicine. Philadelphia, WB Saunders, 1986, p 178.)

pulled by gravity to the most dependent area. Compression of the lung tissue causes an increase in ventilation-perfusion mismatching, decreases lung compliance, and promotes atelectasis. Occasionally trauma to the thorax results in a massive hemothorax, which almost always means that the heart or great vessels were injured directly.

Hemothorax can have serious sequelae if all the blood is not evacuated from the pleural space. The residual blood becomes organized into non-elastic fibrous tissue, which can form a restrictive pleural rind. This condition is known as *fibrothorax* and can limit lung expansion markedly, causing a restrictive lung dysfunction and predisposing the patient to atelectasis and pneumonic complications.[16] In addition, approximately 5% of patients with hemothorax develop an infection within the pleural space called an empyema, which can lead to further scarring of the pleural surfaces.[1, 4, 20]

Pulmonary Laceration. A laceration directly into the lung parenchyma is usually caused by a penetrating wound. It results in air and blood escaping from the lung into the pleural space and often into the environment. Therefore, a pulmonary laceration most commonly appears in combination with a pneumothorax and hemothorax. The hemothorax is usually not massive because the lung is perfused at low pressures, so the bleeding is not profuse. The restrictive impairments caused by pneumothorax and hemothorax described earlier are present, and in addition the damaged lung tissue is not participating in gas exchange.[20]

Clinical Manifestations

Signs

Pulmonary Function Tests. Respiratory rate is increased. Lung volumes are decreased; this is most marked in a tension pneumothorax. Lung volume changes are usually transient in pneumothorax and hemothorax and can return to normal. If a fibrothorax or empyema develops, lung volumes remain diminished owing to the decrease in chest wall and lung compliance.

Chest Radiograph. In pneumothorax lung collapse can readily be seen on the chest radiograph. In tension pneumothorax, the diaphragm may be flattened, the mediastinal structures shifted, the trachea deviated, and the neck veins distended, in addition to lung collapse. Hemothorax, unless massive, may be more difficult to visualize on the chest radiograph. It may appear as a subtle uniform increase in the density over the affected hemithorax.[16] Upright and decubitus films are very helpful in determining the presence of a hemothorax because the blood shifts within the pleural space with the change in position.[4, 20]

Arterial Blood Gases. Hypoxemia results from all penetrating wound injuries. The degree of hypoxemia depends on the extent of the injury and the subsequent restrictive lung dysfunction. Hypercapnia is also common.

Breath Sounds. With a pneumothorax, the patient has markedly decreased or absent breath sounds over the affected hemithorax. Breath sounds are also decreased in hemothorax, fibrothorax, and empyema.[16]

Cardiovascular Findings. Tachycardia is common in pneumothorax and decreased cardiac output, and systemic hypotension is present with a tension pneumothorax. Other cardiovascular changes are variable, depending on the involvement of the heart or great vessels in the thoracic trauma.

Symptoms. Shortness of breath is severe in pneumothorax and can also be present in hemothorax, fibrothorax, and empyema. Patients may appear in respiratory distress with an increased respiratory rate, intercostal retractions, cyanosis, and increased anxiety and agitation. Pain at the site of the chest wound is to be expected. Patients may also appear pale, cyanotic, or unconscious owing to loss of blood, systemic hypotension, hypoxemia, and shock.

Treatment

Pneumothorax. The definitive treatment of an open pneumothorax is the application of an airtight, sterile dressing over the sucking chest wound and the placement of a chest tube into the pleural space of the affected hemithorax. The chest tube is connected to suction so that the air and any fluid or blood within the pleural space can be evacuated. These measures will reexpand the collapsed lung. Mechanical ventilation and supplemental oxygen may be required until the patient can maintain tissue oxygenation independently.[16, 20]

A tension pneumothorax is treated as an emergency by inserting a needle into the pleural space to allow air to escape. This is immediately followed by placement of a chest tube connected to suction so that air can be continuously evacuated from the pleural space along with any blood or fluid.[4, 16, 20]

Hemothorax. The definitive treatment for hemothorax is to evacuate the blood from the pleural space by placement of a dependent chest tube. This chest tube is connected to suction. Autotransfusion devices are becoming more common so that the patient's own blood can be returned to the cardiovascular system to replace lost blood volume.[16] If the wound involves the lung parenchyma, the bleeding in most patients stops because of clotting and internal repair mechanisms. Only 4% of these patients require thoracotomy and surgical intervention to control the bleeding.[20] If the wound involves the heart or great vessels, then emergency surgery may be required to stop massive bleeding; this surgery takes precedence over all other treatment other than respiratory and cardiac resuscitation. Following placement of the chest tube, the patient should be monitored carefully by chest radiograph to be sure all the blood is evacuated from the pleural space. An additional chest tube may be required to accomplish this goal. If a fibrothorax does develop and impairs lung expansion, a surgical procedure known as a *decortication* may be required. A decortication removes the restrictive pleural rind, which is usually done through a minithoracotomy.[20, 21] An empyema may also develop if the hemothorax is not completely resolved. The empyema would be treated with placement of a chest tube and antibiotics.[20]

Thermal Trauma

Thermal trauma involving the pulmonary system is usually due to inhalation injuries, direct burn injuries to the thorax, or a combination of both.[12]

Etiology

Thermal trauma is usually caused by exposure to fire and smoke, particularly in an enclosed space. The effects of this exposure are dependent on what is burning, the intensity or the temperatures generated by the fire, the length of the exposure, and the amount of body surface involved.[28]

Pathophysiology

Smoke inhalation causes pulmonary dysfunction in three different ways. First is a direct injury from inhaling hot, dry air containing heated particulate matter. This injury is localized in the upper airway because most of the heat is dissipated in the nasopharynx. Nasal hairs may be scorched. There is usually edema of the laryngeal and tracheal mucosa with **laryngospasm** and **bronchospasm** almost always present. Mucus production is increased, and commonly there is damage to the mucociliary clearance mechanism. This can lead to bronchopneumonia.[12, 28]

The second cause of pulmonary dysfunction is the inhalation of carbon monoxide, a gas present in smoke. Carbon monoxide is a colorless, odorless, tasteless, nonirritating gas. Exposure to carbon monoxide can be life threatening; many suicides are committed by overexposure to carbon monoxide. This gas has more than 200 times the affinity for hemoglobin when compared with oxygen.[12] This means that when carbon monoxide is taken into the lungs it diffuses quickly into the pulmonary capillaries, enters the red blood cells, and binds with hemoglobin to form **carboxyhemoglobin.** This abnormal process decreases the available hemoglobin binding sites for oxygen and significantly decreases the oxygen-carrying capacity of the blood.[9]

The third cause of pulmonary dysfunction is the inhalation of noxious and toxic gases, the effects from which are dependent on the materials being burned. The specific pulmonary abnormalities depend on the specific gas inhaled and the length of time exposed to the gas. However, exposure to noxious gases often results in surfactant inactivation and chemical pneumonitis.[12, 24, 28] Later in the clinical course, the lungs may develop an obliterative bronchiolitis. Although this complication is uncommon, when it occurs it causes significant RLD.[9]

Direct burn injuries to the thorax cause pulmonary dysfunction in five ways.

• The pain of the burn decreases chest wall mobility.

- If the depth of the burn is third degree, involving chest wall musculature, then the effectiveness of the respiratory pump is diminished.
- Major burns involving 25% of the body surface area or more result in a massive shift of fluid from the intravascular to the interstitial spaces, causing pulmonary edema and possibly acute pulmonary insufficiency.
- With circumferential burns of the thorax, **eschar** formation may severely restrict chest wall expansion.
- Because these patients may have to be on bedrest for protracted periods of time, the pulmonary system is at risk for atelectasis and bronchopneumonia.[12, 28]

Clinical Manifestations

Signs

Pulmonary Function Tests. Constriction of the airways and edema of the airway mucosa cause marked obstructive lung dysfunction. Flow rates are decreased. Lung volumes are decreased both by decreased lung compliance due to surfactant inactivation, pulmonary edema, and atelectasis and by decreased chest wall compliance due to the direct burn injury and pain. Gas diffusion is decreased. Respiratory rate is increased in an effort to maintain minute ventilation.

Chest Radiograph. The chest radiograph often shows diffuse interstitial and intra-alveolar infiltrates owing to the shift of body fluid. Superimposed on these findings may be areas of bronchopneumonia or atelectasis.

Arterial Blood Gases. Hypoxemia is common owing to the increased ventilation-perfusion mismatching and hypoventilation. If the patient was exposed to carbon monoxide for a period of time, the Pa_{O_2} may be so low that it becomes incompatible with life.

Breath Sounds. Auscultation usually reveals decreased breath sounds; wheezing, wet rales, and rhonchi are common.

Cardiovascular Findings. Tachycardia is common. Significant thermal trauma can cause shock, cardiac arrhythmias, hypertension, hypotension, or myocardial infarction.[28]

Symptoms. Patients with thermal trauma appear dyspneic and have a repetitive, hacking, productive cough. Sputum may be **carbonaceous.**[28]

Respiratory rate is increased. Stridor and wheezing may be heard. Patients are usually very anxious and may be cyanotic.

Treatment

Treatment of the seriously burned patient is usually divided into emergency, acute, and rehabilitative care and involves monitoring and providing support and care for every body system. Treatment of the pulmonary system includes humidification, supplemental oxygen, bronchodilators, appropriate positioning, and pulmonary hygiene techniques.[28] Bronchoscopy, intubation, ventilatory support using high frequency ventilation (HFV) and PEEP, suctioning, and perhaps hyperbaric oxygen may be necessary in some patients.[9]

THERAPEUTIC CAUSES OF RESTRICTIVE LUNG DYSFUNCTION

Surgical Therapy

Surgery can be defined as a planned entry into the human body by a trained practitioner under well-controlled conditions.[1]

Etiology

The pulmonary dysfunction that results from surgical therapy is due to three primary factors: (1) the anesthetic agent, (2) the surgical incision or procedure itself, and (3) the pain caused by the incision or procedure.[1, 20]

Pathophysiology

The anesthetic agent causes a decrease in the pulmonary arterial vasoconstrictive response to hypoxia. This increases ventilation-perfusion mismatching and decreases pulmonary gas exchange. Anesthesia also depresses the respiratory control centers so that ventilatory response to hypercapnia and hypoxia is decreased.[16] Placement of an endotracheal tube increases airway resistance.[20] Placing the patient in a supine position reduces the functional residual capacity by 20%.[16] During surgery the shape and configuration of the thorax change. The anteroposterior diameter decreases, and the lateral diameter increases. The vertical diameter of the thorax also decreases, with the diaphragm moving in a cephalad direction owing to the effect of general anesthesia on central nervous system innervation of diaphragmatic tone.[16] These changes in configuration result in a further decrease in thoracic volumes; the FRC is decreased an additional 15%.[16]

If the site of surgery is in the upper abdomen or the thorax, the surgical incision causes a significant, although temporary, restrictive impairment. Following upper abdominal surgery, the VC is decreased by 55% and the FRC by 30%.[20] These decreases in lung volumes reach their greatest values 24 to 48 hours following surgery. Lung volumes then return to relatively normal values in 5 days, although full recovery may take 2 weeks.[20] Postoperative lung volume changes after upper abdominal surgery resemble changes seen in patients with unilateral diaphragmatic paralysis. In fact, diaphragmatic dysfunction has been demonstrated in some abdominal surgery patients. Diaphragmatic dysfunction also can occur following thoracic surgery, particularly if the phrenic nerve experiences hypothermic damage because of external cardiac cooling. Some studies have shown that a transverse abdominal incision results in better postoperative lung volumes and fewer postoperative pulmonary complications than the vertical midline abdominal incision. This is not a universal finding.[20] However, it is well accepted that the median sternotomy incision is better tolerated and results in fewer pulmonary complications than the posterolateral thoracotomy.[20]

The surgical procedure itself can result in a permanent restrictive impairment when lung tissue is excised. Because pulmonary reserves are significant, a *pneumonectomy* or possibly a *lobectomy* has to be performed before any measurable restrictive dysfunction results. *Thoracoplasty* is another surgical procedure that results in restrictive dysfunction. This procedure removes portions of several ribs so that the soft tissue of the chest wall can be used to collapse underlying lung parenchyma. Thoracoplasty was used to treat tuberculosis and was designed to close cavities caused by tuberculosis in the upper lobes. Currently this procedure is rarely performed, although it has been used to treat

bronchopulmonary fistulas.[1] Another surgical procedure that can result in significant restrictive lung dysfunction is **lung transplantation.** This therapeutic cause of RLD is discussed later in this section.

Surgical incisions invariably cause pain, particularly abdominal incisions and posterolateral thoracotomies. Because of the pain, the tone in the muscles of the thorax and the abdominal wall increases, thereby decreasing the chest wall compliance. This change contributes to decreased lung volumes and increased work of breathing during the postoperative period. The phenomenon of increased muscle tone in and around the incision is known as *muscular splinting of the incision* (Fig. 5–22).

Clinical Manifestations

Signs
Pulmonary Function Tests. All lung volumes are decreased; the VC is decreased by 55% and the FRC by 30% following upper abdominal surgery.[20] Flow rates are usually within normal limits but may be slightly decreased. Gas exchange is decreased temporarily because of the increase in ventilation-perfusion mismatching.

Chest Radiograph. Postoperative films often show atelectasis, which can occur at rates up to

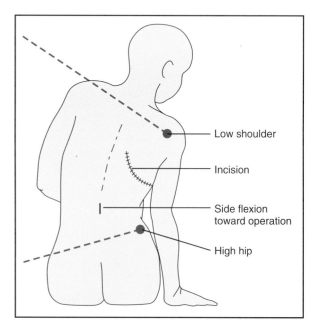

Figure 5–22. Increased muscle tone in and around the incision is known as muscular splinting of the incision.

95% of patients following abdominal or thoracic surgery.[16] The degree of atelectasis averages 4% of the thoracic cross-sectional area.[16] The chest radiograph may also show pneumonia, often involving the lower lobes, or pulmonary embolism.

Arterial Blood Gases. Hypoxia is common during the postoperative period, especially in obese or elderly patients who have cardiac or pulmonary insufficiency or in those who undergo thoracic or upper abdominal surgery. An arterial hemoglobin saturation of 90% or less was found in 35% of postoperative patients. Low oxygen saturations were associated particularly with asthma and obesity.[16] The Pa_{CO_2} may be increased, normal, or decreased, depending on the patient's breathing pattern, functioning lung tissue, and degree of pain.

Breath Sounds. The most common finding following surgery is decreased breath sounds. Rales or rhonchi also may be noted if the patient has atelectasis or pneumonia.

Cardiovascular Findings. Possible cardiovascular complications following pulmonary surgery include arrhythmias, myocardial infarction, and cardiac arrest. If a significant portion of the lung is removed, pulmonary hypertension can result.[8]

Symptoms. After surgery, patients commonly have an altered breathing pattern characterized by an increase in respiratory rate and a decrease in V_T. The cough reflex is suppressed because of the anesthesia, and voluntary coughing is difficult because of the pain. Cough is often productive of blood-streaked sputum if the patient has been intubated.

Treatment

The pulmonary status of surgical patients should be evaluated before surgery. Many patients require preoperative treatment, including deep breathing and coughing exercises and practice with an incentive spirometer. In addition, patients should abstain from smoking a minimum of 6 weeks before surgery. To prevent aspiration pneumonia, patients usually fast for 12 hours or longer before surgery. Drugs such as cimetidine or ranitidine can be used preoperatively to increase gastric pH and decrease gastric volume.[29] Postoperatively, hypoxia can be treated with inflation-hold breathing techniques, PEEP, CPAP, and occasionally with increased oxygen concentrations. Common techniques used to treat postoperative atelectasis include deep breathing exercises, early mobilization of the patient out of bed, incentive spirometry, and CPAP.[16] Nosocomial pneumonias following surgery are not uncommon following upper abdominal surgery, and 12% to 20% of patients experience this complication.[16] Nosocomial pneumonias are treated with an appropriate antibiotic and possibly with postural drainage, percussion, and vibration if the patient's secretion clearance mechanisms are impaired. Postoperative pulmonary embolism is usually treated with low-dose heparin. Prevention of venous thromboembolism may include simple leg exercises (ankle dorsi and plantar flexion), low-dose subcutaneous or adjusted-dose heparin, external pneumatic compression devices, and gradient compression stockings.[16]

Lung Transplantation

Lung transplantation can be defined as the replacement of poorly functioning lung tissue in the recipient with better functioning lung tissue (the lung tissue is never normal, there is always some preservation injury) from the donor.[30] The many aspects of this surgical therapeutic intervention are discussed in Chapter 12. Only the possible development of obliterative bronchiolitis after lung transplantation will be discussed in this section.

Etiology

Obliterative bronchiolitis (OB) is primarily a restrictive lung impairment and the major long-term complication of lung transplantation. Recent evidence suggests that chronic pulmonary rejection may be the major determinant in the cause of OB.[17] A variety of other processes may also be involved in the development of OB including viral and bacterial pneumonias, toxic inhalants, bronchial obstruction, chronic aspiration, and cytomegalovirus mismatch (seronegative recipient versus seropositive donor).[17]

Pathophysiology

Obliterative bronchiolitis clinically shows both restrictive and obstructive pulmonary function deficits and histologically shows obliteration of the terminal bronchioles.[16] This late complication of lung transplantation is seen in 20% to 40% of single lung transplant recipients.[16] It occurs most commonly between 8 and 12 months after transplant and is often preceded by an upper respiratory infection.[16] A transbronchial biopsy (TBB) is used to confirm the diagnosis (sensitivity ranging from 5% to 99%).[16, 17] In OB there is fibrotic narrowing of the bronchiolar lumen that may be irregular, regular, or totally obliterative. The smooth muscle is often destroyed and there is extension of the fibrosis into the interstitium. Early in OB there is mononuclear cell infiltration, epithelial damage, and ulceration. Later, as this complication develops and becomes more chronic, the fibrosis is more acellular, and the terminal bronchioles are completely obliterated.[30] This decreases the surface area for gas exchange. Although the patchy fibrosis seen in OB may not involve the entire transplanted lung, it does decrease lung compliance, decrease lung volumes, and increase ventilation-perfusion mismatching, all hallmarks of a restrictive lung impairment. OB is often accompanied by bronchiectasis, and recurrent respiratory infections. Death is usually due to a pneumonia from gram-negative bacteria or *Aspergillus*.[30] Infection and OB are currently the most frequent causes of post–lung transplantation death.[9]

Clinical Manifestations

Signs

Pulmonary Function Tests. IRV, ERV, and RV are all decreased. Flow rates may also be decreased and a decline in FEV_1 of more than 20% is suggestive of OB. Gas exchange is decreased due to the decreased surface area and increased ventilation-perfusion mismatching.[17]

Chest Radiograph. The chest radiograph usually remains unchanged from the early postoperative films. Films may show central bronchiectasis.[16, 30]

Arterial Blood Gases. The Pa_{O_2} is decreased, but the Pa_{CO_2} is usually within normal limits.

Breath Sounds. Auscultation can yield a variety of findings because infection and pneumonia so often occur concurrently with OB. Often there will be decreased breath sounds, and there may be rhonchi or rales.

Cardiovascular Findings. With the fibrotic changes in OB, portions of the pulmonary capillary bed are destroyed. Over time this vascular damage can lead to pulmonary hypertension. In addition, pulmonary arterioles and veins in the transplanted lung may experience chronic vascular rejection following lung transplantation. This vascular dysfunction impairs gas exchange but usually not to the degree of OB.[30]

Symptoms. The major symptom is dyspnea, which decreases exercise tolerance and progresses to shortness of breath even at rest. There is usually a cough with sputum production.[30]

Treatment

Optimal maintenance of the immunosuppressive drug regimen, prompt diagnosis and treatment of infections and episodes of acute rejection, and careful cytomegalovirus matching may all contribute to the prevention of OB.[17] Once diagnosed, OB is usually treated with high-dose methylprednisolone followed by a tapering course of oral corticosteroids. If there is no clinical response to this regimen, then azathioprine and lympholytic agents such as ALG or OKT3 may be used. Drug therapy may stabilize the pulmonary function test results but rarely is there improvement in lung function. Relapses of OB occur in 50% of these patients. Often infections complicate the intensive immunosuppression used to treat OB and frequently result in death. Because most cases of OB can only be stabilized when treated, early diagnosis and treatment are paramount in preserving lung function.[16] In the most severe cases single lung retransplantation has been used with limited success.[17]

Drug Therapy

More than 100 drugs are capable of causing RLD. Approximately 80 of these drugs adversely affect the lung parenchyma directly, causing drug-induced interstitial lung disease.[13] Other drugs affect the ventilatory pump, ventilatory drive, or chest wall compliance.[1] Most drug-induced interstitial lung disease is reversible if it is recognized early and the drug is discontinued. Drug-induced RLD contributes to the morbidity of an estimated several hundred thousand patients in the United States annually. Approximately 50% of patients treated with chemotherapeutic drugs develop some degree of interstitial pneumonitis.[13] Some patients who take chemotherapeutic drugs demonstrate pathologic alterations with no radiologic, symptomatic, or physiologic abnormalities. Therefore, probably less than 5% of all adverse drug-induced interstitial lung disease is reported or recognized.[13]

It is very difficult to predict which drugs may affect a particular person's lung adversely. The basic reason for this difficulty is insufficient knowledge. First, knowledge of the metabolites of different drugs and their effects on the lung is lacking. Second, some patients seem to have a genetic predisposition to react adversely to certain drugs but this is not well understood. Third, many patients are on multiple drugs, and the interaction of the various metabolites has not been well studied.[13]

Drug-induced interstitial lung disease probably results from a combination of mechanisms including

- Toxic effects of the drug or its metabolites
- Interference with the oxidant-antioxidant system[10]
- An indirect inflammatory reaction
- Altered immunologic processes[13]

Drugs capable of causing drug-induced interstitial lung disease are discussed by drug category.

Oxygen

High concentrations of oxygen for more than 24 hours can produce interstitial lung disease. The lung damage occurs in two phases. First is the *exudative phase*, which begins after using high oxygen concentrations for 24 to 72 hours. During this phase, perivascular, interstitial, and alveolar edema and alveolar hemorrhage and atelectasis occur. The second or *proliferative phase* is marked by **hyperplasia** of the type II pneumocytes and deposition of collagen and elastin in the interstitium, and is irreversible. Oxygen toxicity can result in significant RLD. Treatment is primarily preventive. Oxygen toxicity can be minimized by keeping the FI_{O_2} under 40% and the Pa_{O_2} under 120 mm Hg.[13]

Antibiotics

Some antibiotics used to fight infections can be neurotoxic. Drugs such as polymyxin, gentamicin, and kanamycin, when given intravenously, can cause neuromuscular blockade. This neuromuscular blockade can result in respiratory muscle paralysis, failure of the ventilatory pump, and such significant restrictive lung impairment that assisted ventilatory support may be necessary. The significance of the respiratory impairment is even greater when these drugs are used with anesthetic agents or muscle relaxants.[29]

Nitrofurantoin. This drug is an antiseptic agent used to fight specific urinary tract infections. It can cause acute or chronic interstitial pneumonitis and is responsible for more reported cases of drug-induced pulmonary disease than any other drug.[10] There seems to be no relation between the acute and chronic reactions. The acute pneumonitis is characterized by fever, dyspnea, cough, and rales; approximately 35% of patients experience pleuritic pain. The acute pneumonitis (90% of reported cases) is completely reversible if the drug is discontinued.[10] Chronic pneumonitis (10% of reported cases) mimics IPF and usually begins 6 to 12 months after initiation of the drug. Patients complain of dyspnea and a mild, nonproductive cough. There can be diffuse fibrosis with lower zone predominance. Treatment includes discontinuation of the drug, lung biopsy, and possibly corticosteroids. Therapeutic results are inconsistent and the mortality rate is 10%.[10, 13, 29]

Sulfasalazine. This drug is used to treat inflammatory bowel disease (chronic ulcerative colitis) and more recently to treat rheumatologic disorders.[10] Patients who develop lung complications complain of dyspnea and cough approximately 1 to 8 months after the initiation of the drug. Approximately half the patients also complain of fever. This can develop into interstitial pulmonary fibrosis. Treatment is to discontinue the drug. Pulmonary involvement and symptoms are reversible in most patients. Corticosteroids hasten improvement in some patients.[10] Three fatalities have been recorded as caused by sulfasalazine-induced diffuse pulmonary fibrosis.[10, 13]

Anti-Inflammatory Drugs

Gold. Gold is used in the treatment of rheumatoid arthritis, and is also being used to treat osteoarthritis and asthma, but in some patients it causes diffuse interstitial pneumonitis and fibrosis.[10]

These patients develop dyspnea and a nonproductive cough approximately 6 weeks to many months after initiation of gold therapy. Treatment is the discontinuation of the drug, which allows the reaction to regress spontaneously. Some patients with respiratory distress are given corticosteroids to speed this process.[7, 13]

Penicillamine. This drug is used to treat **Wilson's disease, cystinuria,** primary biliary cirrhosis, scleroderma, and severe rheumatoid arthritis in patients who have failed to respond to conventional therapy.[10] However, it can cause bronchiolitis obliterans, which contributes to both obstructive and restrictive lung dysfunction; Goodpasture's syndrome; or penicillamine-induced SLE. The drug is discontinued in patients who develop any of these pulmonary complications. Patients who have developed Goodpasture's syndrome are also treated with hemodialysis, immunosuppression, and plasmapheresis. Patients who have penicillamine-induced SLE may also receive corticosteroids to accelerate the resolution of this pulmonary complication.[13, 29]

Cardiovascular Drugs

Amiodarone. This antiarrhythmic drug is given for ventricular dysrhythmias that are refractory to other antiarrhythmic drugs. The pulmonary complications seem to be dose related and rarely occur if the dose is under 400 mg per day. The incidence of pulmonary complications is approximately 6%, and the pulmonary complications may be fatal in 10% to 20% of patients.[10] Patients with pulmonary involvement experience an insidious onset of dyspnea and a nonproductive cough with occasional fever and chills. Rales are heard on auscultation, and the chest radiograph shows asymmetric lesions in the lung, which appear mostly in the upper lung fields. Treatment is to discontinue the drug; the value of corticosteroids is uncertain.[10, 13]

Chemotherapeutic Drugs

These cytotoxic drugs used in cancer chemotherapy are a major cause of morbidity and mortality in the immunocompromised individual. It has been reported that the majority of these drugs can cause pulmonary fibrosis.[7] They are also responsible for causing pulmonary infiltrates, secondary neoplasms, and **non-Hodgkin's lymphoma,** all of which compromise lung function. The precise mechanism that incites the inflammatory and fibrotic response in the lung is unknown.

Dyspnea appears gradually, usually within a few weeks of the drug therapy, followed by fever and a nonproductive cough. With some drugs, symptoms may be delayed for months or years (e.g., cyclophosphamide). Early chest radiographs show asymmetric parenchymal changes in one lobe or lung; eventually these changes progress and become diffuse and uniform in distribution. Pulmonary function tests show a classic restrictive impairment. The DL_{CO} usually falls before the patient experiences the onset of any overt symptoms (except with methotrexate). Rales are heard on auscultation. Treatment consists of the discontinuation of the drug and in some cases the use of corticosteroids.[13]

Bleomycin. Bleomycin is an antibiotic used as an antineoplastic agent against squamous cell carcinomas, seminomas, and lymphomas. Ten percent of patients on this drug develop parenchymal lung disease, which proves to be fatal in 1% of the patients. The risk of lung involvement increases with higher dosages of bleomycin, if it is used with previous or concomitant thoracic radiation, if it is prescribed with current or subsequent use of high oxygen concentrations, if it is used in combination with cyclophosphamide, or if it is used in patients over the age of 70.[10, 13, 29]

Mitomycin C. Mitomycin C is an antibiotic used in conjunction with other chemotherapeutic drugs, particularly for adenocarcinoma of the esophagus, stomach, pancreas, or colon.[10] It is also used to treat breast and lung malignancies.[10] Approximately 3% to 12% of patients on this drug develop pulmonary complications. Frequency of lung involvement increases if this drug is used with radiation or with other drugs, particularly fluorouracil or the *Vinca* alkaloids.[13, 29]

Busulfan. Busulfan is an alkylating agent used to treat myeloid leukemia. Pulmonary toxicity occurs in 4% to 6% of patients. Pulmonary complications commence an average of 41 months after initiation of therapy.[10] Clinical symptoms appear insidiously; however, prognosis is poor with an estimated mortality rate of 84%.[10]

Cyclophosphamide. Cyclophosphamide is an alkylating agent used in the treatment of malignant **lymphomas,** multiple myeloma, and leuke-mias. Diffuse interstitial fibrosis can occur a few months to a few years after use of this drug; how-ever, pulmonary toxicity is uncommon (less than 1%).[10] There seems to be no age or dose correla-tion with the development of pulmonary complica-tions. The drug-induced pulmonary disease can range from one with a very long-term course to one with a rapid downhill course resulting in death.[13, 29]

Chlorambucil. Chlorambucil is an alkylating agent used to treat chronic lymphatic malignan-cies. If pulmonary complications develop, it is usu-ally 1 to 12 months before symptoms appear.[13]

Melphalan. Melphalan is an alkylating agent used in the treatment of multiple myeloma. Signif-icant RLD has been reported in only a few patients, but over half of these patients died of respiratory failure despite termination of drug therapy.[10, 13]

Azathioprine. Azathioprine is an antimetabo-lite used for treating neoplastic disease, regional enteritis, ulcerative colitis, chronic active hepatitis, rheumatoid arthritis, systemic lupus erythematosus, Wegener's granulomatosis, and rejection episodes in organ transplant patients.[10] This drug rarely causes interstitial lung disease; however, six cases have been reported in the literature.[13]

Cytarabine. Cytarabine is an antimetabolite used primarily to induce a remission in acute leu-kemia. Unlike the other drugs under discussion, cytarabine causes minimal parenchymal abnormali-ties. However, it can cause a noncardiac pulmo-nary edema, which results in RLD and has a fatal-ity rate of 69%.[10]

Methotrexate. Methotrexate is an antimetabo-lite taken for acute lymphatic leukemia and osteo-genic sarcoma in children. More recently, it is be-ing used as an anti-inflammatory agent to treat rheumatoid arthritis, psoriasis, and asthma.[10] The complication of interstitial lung disease is not dose or age related. Symptoms begin a few days to a few weeks after drug initiation, and approximately one third of patients who develop interstitial pneu-monitis have poorly formed granulomas. Treat-ment is the discontinuation of the drug; in almost all patients the lung involvement is spontaneously resolved. Corticosteroids are sometimes used.[13]

Nitrosoureas. Nitrosourea drugs (BCNU [carmustine], CCNU [lomustine], methyl-CCNU [semustine]) are used against a variety of neo-plasms, particularly intracranial neoplasm.[10] Any-where from 1% to 50% of patients on these drugs develop interstitial lung disease. Patients have a higher risk of developing pulmonary complications when higher dosages are prescribed or when these drugs are prescribed along with other agents, par-ticularly cyclophosphamide.[13] A history of cigarette smoking or pre-existing lung disease increases the risk of nitrosourea-induced lung disease.[10]

Poisons

Paraquat. Paraquat is used as a weed killer. If it is ingested, it causes acute pulmonary fibrosis. There are usually no symptoms for 24 hours after ingestion, and then the person experiences pro-gessive respiratory distress leading to death in 1 to 38 days.[7]

Other drugs can cause RLD via a variety of pathophysiologic mechanisms other than that of producing alveolar pneumonitis and fibrosis. A few of these drug categories or specific drugs are dis-cussed.

Anesthetics

Anesthetic agents such as halothane (Fluothane), methoxyflurane (Penthrane), or thiopental sodium (Pentothal) are used to provide anesthesia during surgical procedures. These agents also inhibit the respiratory centers in the medulla and therefore depress ventilation so that lung volumes are signif-icantly reduced. Assisted mechanical ventilation is usually required with the use of these drugs. The effects of these drugs and the effects of the as-sisted mechanical ventilation usually result in signif-icant but brief RLD.[1, 29]

Muscle Relaxants

Muscle relaxants such as pancuronium bromide (Pavulon), dantrolene sodium (Dantrium), diaze-pam (Valium), and cyclobenzaprine hydrochloride (Flexeril) are used to enhance surgical relaxation, overcome muscle spasm, and control shivering (with systemic hypothermia). However, because these drugs act on skeletal muscle, they also de-crease thoracic expansion, decrease chest wall compliance, and decrease pulmonary ventilation. As soon as the drug effects have worn off, the transient RLD also disappears.[1, 29]

Drug-Induced Systemic Lupus Erythematosus

Nearly 50 drugs have been reported to induce SLE, but only six regularly induce antinuclear antibodies and therefore symptomatic SLE. They are procainamide hydrochloride, hydralazine hydrochloride, practolol, penicillamine, isoniazid, and hydantoins. Patients who take one of these drugs for months or years may develop clinical SLE, and of these, 50% develop pleuropulmonary involvement, including interstitial lung disease. In the majority of patients, these changes are reversible by discontinuing the drug. Use of corticosteroids may accelerate the resolution.[13]

Illicit Drugs

Cocaine. It is estimated that there are 800,000 heroin users and over 5 million regular cocaine users in the United States.[10] Cocaine became affordable and very popular in the 1980s with the introduction of the alkaloidal form of cocaine hydrochloride known as "free base" or "crack." Crack is smoked, is usually 30% to 90% pure, and produces a rapid and intense euphoria which is extremely addictive. Lung disease is much more common among crack smokers than other cocaine users.[10] Pulmonary pathologic conditions caused by crack use include acute pulmonary hemorrhage (58%), interstitial pneumonia with or without fibrosis (38%), vascular congestion (88%), and intra-alveolar edema (77%).[10] The major symptoms of lung involvement are dyspnea (63%), cough (58%), cough with blood-stained or black sputum (34%), and chest pain (25%).[10] Fever, bronchospasm, perihilar infiltrates, hypoxemia, and respiratory failure also occur. In fact, the term "crack lung" is used to describe acute pulmonary eosinophilia or acute respiratory failure, both of which can occur after smoking free-base cocaine. These different pulmonary disorders cause acute or chronic restrictive lung dysfunction with decreased lung compliance, increased ventilation-perfusion

mismatching, decreased DL_{CO}, hypoxemia, and hypercapnia.

Treatment of acute pulmonary diseases with corticosteroids (prednisone) can result in rapid improvement. When lung tissue is repeatedly involved in hemorrhage, edema, and pneumonia, then fibrosis may result. Chronic fibrosis of the lung does not seem to respond to corticosteroids. A number of deaths have been attributed to pulmonary involvement following crack cocaine use.[10]

Heroin. An overdose of methadone hydrochloride, propoxyphene hydrochloride, or heroin can lead to a noncardiac pulmonary edema with interstitial pneumonitis. This reaction can begin within minutes of an intravenous injection or within an hour of oral ingestion. Respiration is depressed; lung compliance is decreased; hypoxemia and hypercapnia result. Treatment includes mechanically assisted ventilation and usually antibiotics to deal with the invariable aspiration pneumonia.[13]

Talc. Talc (magnesium silicate) is used as a filler in oral medications such as amphetamines, tripelennamine hydrochloride, methadone hydrochloride, meperidine, and propoxyphene hydrochloride (Darvon). When addicts inject these drugs intravenously, talc granulomatosis results. Talc granulomatosis is characterized by granulomas in the arterioles and the pulmonary interstitium. The clinical picture includes dyspnea, pulmonary hypertension, and restrictive lung impairment with a decreased DL_{CO}. Treatment is abstinence from further intravenous talc exposure. Use of corticosteroids has afforded variable results.[13]

Radiation Therapy

Radiation Pneumonitis and Fibrosis

Radiation pneumonitis or fibrosis is a primary complication of irradiation to the thorax. It usually occurs 2 to 6 months after this treatment intervention.[10, 20]

Etiology. Irradiation of the thorax is a treatment option for lymphoma (**Hodgkin's disease**), breast cancer, lung cancer, and esophageal cancer. Not all patients who receive irradiation to the thorax develop radiation pneumonitis or fibrosis. This serious pulmonary complication of irradiation seems to depend on the rate of delivery of the irradiation, the volume of lung being irradiated, the total dose, the quality of the radiation, and the concomitant chemotherapy.[2, 8, 13] Time-dose relationships are extremely important in predicting the occurrence of radiation pneumonitis or fibrosis. The number of fractions into which a dose is divided seems to be the most important factor.[8] Also important is the total dose and the span of time over which the radiation is delivered. Approximately 50% of patients undergoing irradiation of the thorax show radiologic abnormalities in the lung.[10] Only 5% to 15% of patients who receive radiation to the thorax actually develop signs and symptoms of radiation pneumonitis.[2, 10]

Currently one group of patients seems to be at higher risk for developing radiation pneumonitis or fibrosis. Bone marrow transplant patients receive whole lung irradiation; they are also on cytotoxic chemotherapeutic agents that can intensify the pneumonitis; and these patients often have a graft versus host reaction that can add to radiation damage.[8]

Pathophysiology. The pathogenesis of radiation pneumonitis or fibrosis is uncertain.[10] It is known that irradiation causes breaks in the DNA strands. When these breaks are double-stranded the cell cannot correctly repair the damage, and so the integrity of the chromosome is disrupted.[10] Chromosomal aberrations do not affect the survival or function of the cell until it tries to replicate itself. Cell death usually occurs with cell mitosis during the first or subsequent mitotic divisions. Radiation responses are seen first in cells with rapid rates of cell replication. In the lung this would include the capillary endothelial cells, the type I alveolar epithelial cells, and the type II pneumocytes. In addition to cellular death caused by molecular changes, irradiation causes an inflammatory syndrome. This inflammation may be initiated by the release of free radicals.[10]

Pulmonary injury following radiation of the thorax is usually divided into two clinical syndromes: acute radiation pneumonitis and chronic radiation fibrosis.[9] The onset of acute radiation pneumonitis is insidious, beginning 2 to 3 months after radiation. It is characterized by swelling of endothelial cells, capillary engorgement and disruption, intimal proliferation, subintimal accumulation of macrophages, and capillary occlusion and thrombosis.[9] Endothelial injury may lead to increased vascular permeability that may have a profound effect on gas exchange and ventilation-perfusion matching.

Chronic radiation fibrosis occurs 6 to 9 months after radiation and is characterized by basement membrane damage, fibroblastic proliferation, collagen deposition, capillary endothelium hyalinization and sclerosis, obliteration of alveoli, dense fibrosis, and contraction of lung volume.[8, 9, 13] There is evidence that the pneumonitis and fibrosis are two separate phases and that radiation fibrosis may not always be preceded by radiation pneumonitis.[10] It seems that the earlier the onset, the more serious and protracted the complications.[9, 21] Usually one third to one half of the volume of one lung must be irradiated for pneumonitis to develop and show any clinical symptoms.[8] Some patients have a complete resolution of the pneumonitis, but many go on to develop permanent fibrosis. Occasionally pleural effusion, spontaneous pneumothorax, bronchial obstruction, rib fractures, pericardial effusion, or tracheoesophageal fistula may further complicate the clinical picture.[9] With whole-lung irradiation, the involved fibrotic lung may contract to a remarkable degree, even causing shifts in the mediastinal structures, overexpansion of the other lung, and death. It has been reported that a late complication of radiation fibrosis may be the rapid development of adenocarcinoma of the lung. Bilateral adenocarcinoma of the lung has been described 2 years following radiation therapy for Hodgkin's disease (patient had also received chemotherapy). Malignant fibrous histiocytoma may also complicate radiation fibrosis.[10]

Clinical Manifestations

Signs

PULMONARY FUNCTION TESTS. Both lung volumes and flow rates are decreased, with the maximum impairment occurring at approximately 4 to 6 months after irradiation.[2, 13, 20] With regional irradiation, the VC and ERV are the primary volumes decreased. As more lung is irradiated, all lung volumes, the TLC, VC, IC, and RV are all decreased. The DL_{CO} is decreased because of the increased ventilation-perfusion mismatching and the decreased capillary-alveolar surface area.[9] The respiratory rate is increased and tidal volume decreased in an effort to decrease the work of breathing.[9] Lung compliance is decreased.[9] The compliance of the chest wall is usually not affected.

CHEST RADIOGRAPH. The chest radiograph shows sharply demarcated alveolar or interstitial parenchymal infiltrates limited to the radiation port.[20] Lungs may have a ground-glass or soft appearance, and the lung markings may appear hazy or indistinct. This can progress to a reticulonodular pattern that conforms in shape and location to the region of lung irradiated. Mediastinum and heart borders may become indistinct. Irradiated regions of lung may also adopt a bronchiectatic, cystic, or honeycomb appearance.[19] There are reports that some patients do develop additional changes outside the field of irradiation and even in the contralateral lung tissue.[19]

ARTERIAL BLOOD GASES. Because of the increased respiratory rate, the Pa_{CO_2} may be decreased. Hypoxemia is a common finding with respiratory distress evident even on mild exertion.

BREATH SOUNDS. During the early phase, some rales, rhonchi, or wheezes may be heard. Breath sounds are normally diminished over the involved area and this can progress to essentially absent breath sounds. Pleural rubs can occasionally be heard.

CARDIOVASCULAR FINDINGS. With the obliteration of the capillary beds, pulmonary hypertension develops, which puts an added burden on the right ventricle and can lead to cor pulmonale.[9] Thrombolytic occurrences are common. Tachycardia is extremely common in these patients.

Symptoms

The primary symptom is shortness of breath on exertion progressing to dyspnea with even minimal effort. Patients often have a repetitive, irritating cough, which may be nonproductive or may produce a white or pink sputum. Heart rate is increased. Exercise tolerance is invariably decreased. Cyanosis and clubbing of the digits may also develop. Patients may run a low-grade fever or have temperature spikes. Some patients may complain of pleuritic pain or sharp chest wall pain, which is usually due to fractured ribs caused by coughing.[13, 19]

Treatment. Asymptomatic patients with radiologic abnormalities do not require treatment.[9] Corticosteroids are used to treat acute radiation pneumonitis and may produce dramatic results. However, there are reports of a lack of response to corticosteroids, even during the acute radiation pneumonitis phase.[9] Corticosteroids offer no help in treating chronic radiation fibrosis and should not be used prophylactically because terminating corticosteroid therapy may actually precipitate radiation pneumonitis. Pneumonectomy has been reported to treat severe unilateral radiation fibrosis. Otherwise treatment is supportive and consists of oxygen therapy, cough suppression medications, analgesics, and antibiotics to treat any superimposed infection.[2, 8, 9, 19] Prophylactic antibiotics should not be used because they could predispose patients to aggressive antibiotic-resistant organisms.[9]

Prevention is the ultimate treatment, and the occurrence of radiation injury to the lung is decreasing with the refinement of radiotherapy techniques, particularly the careful tailoring of radiation fields.[7, 8]

Summary

- Restrictive lung dysfunction is not a disease; it is an abnormal reduction in pulmonary ventilation.
- Restrictive lung dysfunction can be caused by a variety of disease processes occurring in different body systems, trauma, or therapeutic measures.
- In RLD one or more of the following is abnormal: lung compliance, chest wall compliance, lung volumes, or the work of breathing.
- The classic signs of RLD include tachypnea, hypoxemia, decreased breath sounds, dry inspiratory rales, decreased lung volumes, decreased diffusing capacity, and cor pulmonale.
- The hallmark symptoms of RLD include shortness of breath, cough, and a wasted, emaciated appearance.
- Treatment interventions for RLD vary and are dependent on the cause of the restrictive impairment. Sometimes corrective measures are possible. However, once the lung has undergone fibrotic changes, the pathologic alterations are irreversible and only supportive interventions are used.
- Idiopathic pulmonary fibrosis is the pulmonary disease entity most commonly associated with RLD.
- Pneumonia is an inflammatory process within the lung which can be caused by bacteria, mycoplasmas, viruses, fungi, or chlamydial agents.

- There are four major types of lung cancer: squamous cell carcinoma, small cell carcinoma, adenocarcinoma, and large cell carcinoma. All types can cause a restrictive impairment within the lung. This restrictive impairment may be due to direct pressure from the tumor, may result from susceptibility to other disease processes in the weakened cancer patient, may be related to changes that occur as the tumor metastasizes to other body systems, or may be produced by hormones arising from the tumor, which can cause a variety of symptoms in different body systems.

- Cigarette smoking has been linked to a variety of pathologic conditions, including bronchogenic carcinoma, cancer of the mouth and larynx, esophageal cancer, kidney and urinary bladder cancer, pancreatic cancer, chronic bronchitis, emphysema, increased incidence of respiratory infection, increased frequency and severity of asthmatic attacks, coronary artery disease, myocardial infarction, peripheral vascular disease, hypertension, stroke, low birth weights in infants, increased incidence of stillbirths, impotence, burn injuries, and reduced exercise capacity.

- Neuromuscular causes of RLD include spinal cord injury, ALS, polio, Guillain-Barré syndrome, muscular dystrophy, and myasthenia gravis, and any of these disease entities can cause such a significant decrease in alveolar ventilation that a mechanical ventilator is required to maintain life.

- Crush injuries and penetrating wounds to the thorax can cause significant RLD but are almost always reversible with corrective interventions.

- More than 100 drugs have the side effect of causing restrictive lung impairment, including oxygen and the majority of drugs used in the treatment of cancer.

- Radiation fibrosis of the lung is a complication of radiation therapy and is dependent on the number of fractions into which the radiation dose is divided, the total dose of radiation, the volume of lung being irradiated, and the quality of the radiation.

References

1. Hercules PR, Lekwart FJ, Fenton MV. Pulmonary Restriction and Obstruction. Chicago, Year Book Medical Publishers, 1979.
2. Weinberger SE. Principles of Pulmonary Medicine. Philadelphia, WB Saunders, 1986.
3. Whipp BJ, Wasserman K. Exercise Pulmonary Physiology and Pathophysiology. New York, Marcel Dekker, 1991.
4. Divertie MB. The CIBA Collection of Medical Illustrations. Vol. 7: Respiratory System. 2nd ed. Summit, NJ, CIBA Pharmaceutical Company, 1980.
5. Basmajian JV. Therapeutic Exercise. 3rd ed. Baltimore, Williams & Wilkins, 1978.
6. Klusek-Hamilton H. Respiratory Disorders. Springhouse, PA, Springhouse, 1984.
7. Dunhill MS. Pulmonary Pathology. 2nd ed. New York, Churchill Livingstone, 1987.
8. Fishman AP. Pulmonary Diseases and Disorders. 2nd ed. New York, McGraw-Hill, 1988.
9. Bordow RA, Moser KM. Manual of Clinical Problems in Pulmonary Medicine. 4th ed. Boston, Little, Brown, 1996.
10. Hasleton PS. Spencer's Pathology of the Lung. 5th ed. New York, McGraw-Hill, 1996.
11. Fishman AP. Update: Pulmonary Diseases and Disorders. New York, McGraw-Hill, 1982.
12. Scully RM, Barnes MR. Physical Therapy. Philadelphia, JB Lippincott, 1989.
13. Schwarz MI, King TE Jr. Interstitial Lung Disease. Philadelphia, BC Decker, 1988.
14. Glauser FL. Signs and Symptoms in Pulmonary Medicine. Philadelphia, JB Lippincott, 1983.
15. Phan SH, Thrall RS. Pulmonary Fibrosis. New York, Marcel Dekker, 1995.
16. George RB, Light RW, Matthay MA, Matthay RA. Chest Medicine: Essentials of Pulmonary and Critical Care Medicine. 3rd ed. Baltimore, Williams & Wilkins, 1995.
17. Derenne JP, Whitelaw WA, Similowski T. Acute Respiratory Failure in Chronic Obstructive Pulmonary Disease. New York, Marcel Dekker, 1996.
18. Berkow R, Fletcher AJ. The Merck Manual of Diagnosis and Therapy. 15th ed. Rahway, NJ, Merck Sharp and Dohme Research Laboratories, 1987.
19. Baum GL, Wolinsky E. Textbook of Pulmonary Diseases. 3rd ed. Boston, Little, Brown, 1983.
20. George RB, Light RW, Matthay MA, Matthay RA. Chest Medicine: Essentials of Pulmonary and Critical Care Medicine. 2nd ed. Baltimore, Williams & Wilkins, 1990.
21. Hinshaw HC, Murray JF. Diseases of the Chest. 4th ed. Philadelphia, WB Saunders, 1980.
22. Mitchell RS. Synopsis of Clinical Pulmonary Disease. 2nd ed. St. Louis, CV Mosby, 1978.
23. Cottrell GP, Surkin HB. Pharmacology for Respiratory Care Practitioners. Philadelphia, FA Davis, 1995.
24. Boyda EK. Respiratory Problems. Oradell, NJ, Medical Economics Company, 1985.
25. Cannon GW, Zimmerman GA. The Lung in Rheumatic Diseases. New York, Marcel Dekker, 1990.
26. Peat M (ed). Current Physical Therapy. Philadelphia, BC Decker, 1988.
27. Adams JH, Corsellis JAN, Duchen LW. Greenfield's Neuropathology. 4th ed. New York, John Wiley & Sons, 1984.
28. McDonald K, Wisniewski JM. Basic Burn Seminar Notebook (unpublished). Ann Arbor, Physical Therapy Division, University of Michigan Medical Center, 1988.
29. Physicians' Desk Reference. 54th ed. Oradell, NJ, Medical Economics Company, 2000.
30. Sheppard M. Practical Pulmonary Pathology. London, Edward Arnold, 1995.

## 6

Chronic Obstructive Pulmonary Diseases

Susan L. Garritan

INTRODUCTION

Chronic obstructive pulmonary diseases (COPD) are diseases of the respiratory tract that produce an obstruction to airflow and that ultimately can affect both the mechanical function and gas exchanging capability of the lungs.

Certain physical symptoms are characteristic of obstructive lung conditions. These include chronic cough, expectoration of mucus, wheezing, and **dyspnea** on exertion. Obstructive lung conditions are diagnosed by changes in the pulmonary function test results. Important markers for COPD are a decrease in expiratory flow rates and an increase in **residual volume** (RV) (see Chapter 10).

In terms of pathologic changes, other similarities are also notable, including

- Increased mucus production (or impairment of mucus clearance)
- Inflammation of the mucosal lining of the bronchi and bronchioles
- Mucosal thickening
- Spasm of the bronchial smooth muscle

All these changes decrease the size of the bronchial lumen and increase the resistance to airflow. In addition, the loss of normal elastic recoil of lung tissue and the tendency for bronchial walls to collapse and thereby to trap air contribute to decreased airflow. Over time the entire lung may become **hyperinflated.**

Obstructive pulmonary conditions affect the efficiency and function of the lung in many ways. Respiratory muscles must work harder to overcome the resistance to airflow and to enlarge a thorax that already may be in an inflated position. **Alveolar ventilation** (gas exchange at the alveolar level) is reduced. Capillary bed surface area and alveolar wall surface area may be reduced owing to destructive changes that occur in the structure of lung tissue. This reduction results in **ventilation-perfusion mismatching** and decreased gas exchange (see Chapters 2 and 10).

Ultimately, oxygen delivery to the tissues is reduced, and carbon dioxide clearance is inadequate; decreases in Pa_{O_2} and increases in Pa_{CO_2} are noted. If **hypoxemia** (decreased Pa_{O_2}) is chronic, the patient may develop **pulmonary arterial hypertension** owing to vasoconstriction of the pulmonary artery in response to the hypoxia. **Polycythemia** (increased red blood cell count), also secondary to chronic hypoxemia, increases the **viscosity** of the blood and further increases pulmonary vascular resistance. Increased pressure in the pulmonary artery can also take place if the pulmonary capillary bed suffers a gradual loss of capillaries and area.

Cor pulmonale (right ventricular hypertrophy or dilation resulting from diseases that affect the function or structure of the lung) may ultimately develop from the resistance encountered as the right ventricle attempts to pump blood through the narrowed pulmonary artery. The development of cor pulmonale with **respiratory failure** (Pa_{O_2} less than 60 mm Hg and Pa_{CO_2} above 55 mm Hg) is frequently the cause of death in individuals with obstructive lung conditions.

Physical therapists encounter COPD as a primary or secondary diagnosis in many of the patient populations they treat. An understanding of the diseases, their responsiveness to treatment, and their general course of progression enhances our ability to provide appropriate cardiopulmonary care and complete physical therapy programs for these individuals.

UNIQUE FEATURES OF OBSTRUCTIVE LUNG CONDITIONS

Despite many similarities, important differences in etiology, pathology, and pathophysiology should be recognized in the diseases grouped under the heading of obstructive lung conditions. The dominant cause of obstruction is one important factor. The reversibility of the obstructing lesion is another important variable. In addition, the differing locations of the major sites of obstruction should be understood. By appreciating these differences, we can become more effective in designing a pulmonary care program that considers the characteristics of each disease as well as those of each patient.

Pulmonary obstructive conditions to be covered include

- **Bronchopulmonary dysplasia**
- **Cystic fibrosis**
- **Asthma**
- **Bronchiectasis**
- Chronic bronchitis
- Emphysema

Obstructive conditions may occur independently, or, frequently, they may coexist. For ease of understanding, they are presented individually, but three combinations that often develop are asthmatic bronchitis, chronic bronchitis with emphysema, and cystic fibrosis with bronchiectasis.

Over time, some obstructive conditions may result in **fibrosis** and decreased **compliance** of the lung, so that some elements of restrictive lung disease may be evident as well (see Chapter 5).

KEY CONCEPTS

Chronic airflow obstruction is defined as permanent diminution of airflow, usually assessed by testing forced expiratory airflow. There are many tests of forced expiratory airflow of which FEV_1 is just one.[1] Airflow limitation can result from two basic causes. Airflow is determined both by the pressure applied and by the resistance encountered. In the lung, pressure applied during expiratory airflow is due to the normal elastic recoil of lung tissue after it has been released from the stretched position it assumes during inspiration. Resistance encountered to airflow results from narrowing of the airways. Narrowing may be caused by inflammation, airway thickening, increased mucus, or constriction of the bronchial walls **(bronchospasm)** (Fig. 6–1).

For purposes of classifying the location of obstructive diseases, the anatomic generations of the airways are divided as follows:

- Bronchi or airways with cartilage in their walls (usually more than 2 mm in diameter)
- **Bronchioles** or airways without cartilage in their walls (usually less than 2 mm in diameter)
- Lung **parenchyma,** or alveolar units, the gas exchanging part of the lung.

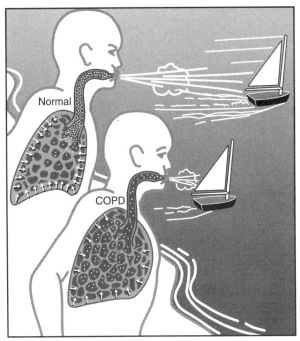

Figure 6–1. The loss of elastic recoil in lung tissue and the increased airway resistance decrease the expiratory airflow in a patient with chronic obstructive pulmonary disease as compared with the expiratory airflow in a normal subject.

Abnormalities in both the airways and the parenchyma may be present in some conditions, whereas in others one area of abnormal function may dominate.

EARLY OBSTRUCTIVE LUNG CONDITIONS

In the pediatric population, four chronic obstructive pulmonary conditions are seen:

- Bronchopulmonary dysplasia
- Cystic fibrosis
- Asthma
- Bronchiectasis

Bronchopulmonary Dysplasia

Bronchopulmonary dysplasia (BPD) is a chronic lung disease of infancy characterized by respiratory distress and oxygen dependency lasting beyond 1 month of age that follows the use of oxygen and ventilatory support to treat neonatal respiratory distress.[2] Bronchopulmonary dysplasia most commonly and more easily develops in premature infants being treated for **respiratory distress syndrome,** but it also may develop in full-term infants following **meconium aspiration,** neonatal pneumonia, **persistent fetal circulation,** or surgery when long-term ventilatory support and oxygen exposure are required.[3]

Prevalence

Bronchopulmonary dysplasia occurs in 10% to 20% of infants who require prolonged assisted ventilation and exposure to high oxygen concentrations to survive respiratory distress syndrome.[4] However, cases of BPD have been reported in infants who received only a high $F_{I_{O_2}}$ (fraction of inspired oxygen concentration) without mechanical ventilation and in infants mechanically ventilated with a low $F_{I_{O_2}}$.[5] The exact mechanism for development of BPD is unknown.

Pathology

The typical pathologic progression of BPD has four distinct phases, classified by age of occurrence (days of life).[6]

Stage I. Stage I (days 1 to 3 of life) is associated with the presence of **hyaline membrane disease,** a restrictive lung condition caused by a deficiency of pulmonary **surfactant** in immature lungs. Inadequate production of surfactant causes high **surface tension** in the alveoli and leads to the development of severe **atelectasis.** Histologic examination of autopsy results from infants has revealed complete collapse of many alveoli. In patent airways, hyaline membranes containing some **fibrin** are usually present, along with capillary congestion and edema in the **interalveolar septa** and **lymphatic spaces.**[7]

Stage II. Stage II (days 4 to 10 of life) is classified as the regeneration phase. Repair and regeneration are the most important features during this period. The medium-sized and small bronchi as well as the terminal airways become lined with **granulation** tissue. In 50% of cases, an **obliterating**

bronchitis is seen, as proliferating fibroblasts combine with cellular debris and exudates, blocking the lumina of many bronchi and terminal airways.[7] Epithelial regeneration is also sometimes excessive and reduces the lumina of some small bronchi.

Stage III. Stage III (days 10 to 20 of life) is considered the transition stage to the chronic condition of BPD. Hyaline membranes disappear, and mucus production increases.[6] The autopsy results of infants dying at this stage show that the lungs are divided into differing regions, some with **emphysematous changes** (distended terminal airways and open alveoli separated by thin septa) and some with **restrictive changes** (contracted airways, fibrous septa, and residual collapse).[7]

Stage IV. Stage IV (first month to 2 to 3 years) is defined as the chronic phase of BPD. A continuation of alternating emphysematous (with bullae formation) and atelectatic areas are present. Hypertrophy of smooth muscle and **subepithelial fibrosis** are seen in medium-sized and small bronchi. Pulmonary arterial walls are thicker, and **right ventricular hypertrophy** is also seen. The ductus arteriosus is usually patent.

Because pathologic changes caused by BPD have been documented in the autopsy results of very severe cases, milder pathologic changes may actually be present in survivors of BPD.[5]

Pathogenesis

Barotrauma (injury caused by pressure) resulting from high airway pressures utilized during ventilator management of respiratory distress syndrome plays an important role in the development of BPD.[4] Infants who are **intubated** (insertion of an endotracheal tube, necessary for mechanical ventilation) are almost five times more likely to develop BPD than infants who have only face masks or nasal prongs to provide positive airway pressure or oxygen.[8]

The use of high oxygen concentrations for prolonged periods has also been implicated in the development of BPD. The precise concentration of oxygen that is toxic depends on many factors, including maturation, nutritional status, and length of oxygen exposure. **Oxygen toxicity** increases capillary permeability, impairs **mucociliary transport,** and causes an influx of leukocytes containing proteolytic enzymes (enzymes that digest proteins in the lung's elastic fiber network).[4]

The presence of **pulmonary interstitial edema** or extra-alveolar air due to alveolar rupture from positive pressure ventilation may contribute to the development of BPD.[9] Other factors that may contribute include nutritional deficits, infectious complications, and a **patent ductus arteriosus** that increases pulmonary blood flow and interstitial fluid and further impairs pulmonary function.[4] Table 6–1 identifies contributing factors to the development of BPD.

Clinical Features

Infants with mild BPD may have only transient **tachypnea** (rapid respiratory rate) and **cyanosis** with feeding or crying. Infants with severe BPD show typical signs of acute hypoxemic respiratory distress, including tachypnea; cyanosis on room air; suprasternal, intercostal, and subcostal retractions; nasal flaring; and grunting. Infants with severe BPD may also develop pulmonary hypertension and right-sided heart failure. These infants have an increased incidence and increased severity of lower respiratory tract infections, such as **bronchiolitis** or pneumonia, and may require hospitalization for treatment. Many of their respiratory symptoms diminish with time, most likely owing to growth of parenchyma and airways.[5] Oxygen dependency and ventilator support via **tracheostomy** in some cases, however, may be necessary for 1 to 2 years.

Pathophysiology

Pulmonary Function Tests. Young children are difficult to study by pulmonary function test,

Table 6–1
Contributing Factors to the Development of Bronchopulmonary Dysplasia
Immature lungs
Barotrauma (excessive positive-pressure ventilation)
Oxygen toxicity
Endotracheal intubation
Pulmonary interstitial edema
Infection
Congestive heart failure

but use of the **partial expiratory flow volume (PEFV)** has revealed low forced expiratory rates.[10] Generally decreased lung compliance and functional residual capacity (FRC) have been reported in the early stages of BPD. An increased work of breathing has also been reported. In later tests, lung compliance continues to improve but remains below normal up to 3 years of age.[5]

Pulmonary function test results of older children with BPD have demonstrated a wide variety of responses, ranging from evidence of normality to evidence of airway obstruction and bronchial narrowing.[11]

In terms of arterial blood gases, persistent ventilation-perfusion mismatching results in hypoxemia and the need for long-term oxygen therapy and possibly ventilator support. Some infants may have long-term carbon dioxide retention.

Radiographic Findings. Initially a *ground-glass appearance* is seen on the radiograph (indicating hyaline membrane disease). This progresses to a radiograph demonstrating both atelectatic and cystic areas. Chronically, radiographs show atelectatic and fibrotic changes with some element of hyperinflation.

Medical Treatment

Medical treatment for BPD consists of the use of bronchodilators, diuretics, potassium supplements, corticosteroids, and nutritional support and in some cases prolonged oxygen support. Prompt management of lower respiratory tract infections with the appropriate antibiotic therapy is essential.

Surfactant replacement for treatment of respiratory distress syndrome is being studied in hopes of removing the need for the long-term ventilatory support that leads to the lung injury of BPD.[4]

Prognosis

The outcome for children with BPD depends on the severity of the initial disease. A small but significant number of infants die within the first year of life. In survivors, the lung grows and repairs itself, and pulmonary function may gradually improve. However, respiratory tract infections and recurrent bouts of wheezing and **pulmonary insufficiency** may develop during the first 2 years of life.[12] Infants with BPD appear to be at greater risk for growth retardation and developmental delay than infants with respiratory distress syndrome.[13]

Graded exercise stress tests and pulmonary function tests demonstrate that abnormalities persist at 10 years of age. Children with BPD continue to show evidence of airway obstruction, hyperinflation, and **airway reactivity** (bronchospasm).[14] The oldest survivors of BPD are in their early twenties, and as they mature their lung function will continue to be studied. The possibility that they may be more susceptible to progressive obstructive pulmonary disease as adults has been raised by Northway, who originally described BPD in 1967.

Cystic Fibrosis

Cystic fibrosis (CF) is a multisystem disorder involving the **exocrine glands.** Pulmonary and pancreatic problems are the most prominent clinical features, but the extent and type of involvement of different organ systems may vary in each individual.

Genetics

Cystic fibrosis is a recessively inherited genetic disorder. The incidence of the disease in whites is approximately 1 in 2500 live births, and 4% to 5% of white Americans are *heterozygous* carriers of the CF gene.[15] Although skilled medical care has resulted in increased years of survival, CF is invariably fatal. The disease is rare in orientals and blacks.

The role of genetic counseling is very important in families who have had a child, or first cousin, diagnosed with CF. The genetic defect has been localized to the long arm of chromosome 7.[15]

In 70% of individuals affected by CF worldwide, the genetic defect is caused by a deletion of three base pairs at position 508 on chromosome 7. In the remaining 30% of individuals affected by CF, 60 other mutations have been discovered. This variation in genotype explains the variability in the clinical presentation observed in CF patients.[16]

Diagnosis of CF by DNA testing has been available to families with a positive history of CF since 1985. But at this time, population screening for CF carriers is not feasible because of the large number of disease-causing mutations in the CF gene, the probability that not all the mutations have been found, and the fact that many mutations are not easily detected. Research continues the effort to discover a way to simplify the process.[16]

Pathogenesis

Although the CF gene has been localized, the basic defect causing the disease has not been identified. However, it appears that a block in the chloride permeability at the epithelial surface is a common factor in all tissues affected by CF.[15] Abnormality in ion transport explains the increased sweat chloride concentration found in the perspiration of children with CF. To explain the physiologic changes in pancreatic and lung function, however, other yet undiscovered mechanisms may also come into play.[15]

Every exocrine gland (a gland that does not secrete its product directly into the bloodstream) can be affected, although they may be affected to different degrees in individuals. Progressive obstruction of the exocrine ducts by viscous secretions seems to play a primary role in the pathogenesis of almost all manifestations of the disease. In 10% to 20% of all CF patients, the first manifestation is **meconium ileus,** or obstruction of the intestines by thick viscous meconium stool. Chronic pulmonary disease, pancreatic insufficiency, and **focal biliary cirrhosis** progress gradually throughout the course of the disease.

Pathology and Pathophysiology

Respiratory Tract. At birth the lungs of CF patients are both morphologically and functionally normal. However, soon after birth, thick secretions plug the airways and bacterial infection occurs in the lungs. Once established, the infection is difficult to eradicate despite aggressive antibiotic therapy.[15] It is unclear how the infection occurs initially, but first *Staphylococcus aureus* is found in the sputum of CF patients. Later in the disease, most patients become colonized with *Pseudomonas aeruginosa.* Less commonly found organisms include *Escherichia coli, Klebsiella,* and *Haemophilus influenzae.*[17] In later stages of CF, *Pseudomonas* is usually the predominant organism. Intensive antibiotic therapy may be partially to blame for the persist-

ence of these pathogens, but alterations in the immune system of CF patients cannot be excluded.[15]

The lung disease of CF appears to begin in the small airways with inflammation and destruction of the airway walls. Alveolar units are usually spared, but damage spreads centrally to the larger airways, and ultimately all conducting airways are inflamed. Persistent infiltration with neutrophils is the hallmark of the inflammatory process in CF.[15] There is *hyperplasia* of mucus-secreting cells, and thick secretions plug the airways. In the lungs of CF patients, the combination of hypersecretion of viscid mucus and chronic bacterial infection combine to produce an obstructive pulmonary disease that progresses eventually to severe diffuse bronchiectasis.

Repeated episodes of infection have a cumulative effect and gradually impair pulmonary function. Pulmonary function tests may be useful in tracing the natural history of the disease and also in evaluating the effectiveness of various therapeutic interventions.[17] Initially these tests reflect small airway dysfunction with reduced midexpiratory flow and increased RV (increased air trapping).[15] Later frank obstruction to airflow occurs; the FEV_1 falls; and the ratio of RV to total lung capacity (TLC) increases markedly.[15] Mild bronchoconstriction may be seen owing to slight increases in muscle tone in the airways.

Hemodynamic Changes. Early in the disease, ventilation-perfusion abnormalities widen the alveolar-arterial difference in P_{O_2} and increase the ratio of dead space to tidal volume.[17] As the disease progresses, the imbalance between ventilation and perfusion increases, and arterial hypoxemia follows. Generally pulmonary hypertension develops; cor pulmonale and right ventricular failure may follow. Late in the disease, **hypercapnia** (increased CO_2) and **respiratory acidosis** (decreased pH) are prominent features as respiratory failure develops.[17] Figure 6–2 is a diagram of the pathogenesis and progression of pulmonary disease in CF.

Clinical Features of Respiratory Involvement

Signs and Symptoms. In patients who have pulmonary involvement, increased *sputum* production and chronic cough are evident, with symp-

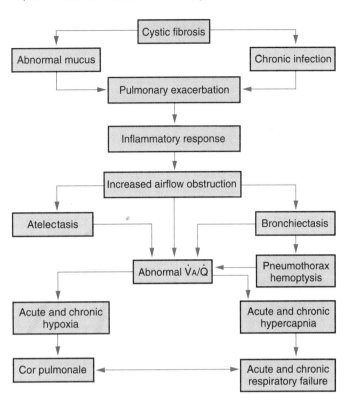

Figure 6-2. The pathogenesis and progression of pulmonary disease in cystic fibrosis. (From Fishman A. Pulmonary Diseases and Disorders. Vol. 3. 3rd ed. New York, McGraw-Hill, 1988.)

toms becoming more pronounced when a viral respiratory infection is superimposed on airways colonized with *Pseudomonas*. An increased respiratory rate and increased work of breathing may be seen with acute illness. Diffuse coarse rales, rhonchi, or wheezing may be evident, along with fever and **leukocytosis** (elevated white blood cell count). **Digital clubbing** (broadening and thickening of ends of fingers and nails seen in chronic pulmonary disease) may occur early in the course of CF.

Radiographic Findings. Radiographic findings become more abnormal as CF progresses (Fig. 6–3). Hyperinflation is frequently seen in children and may be the only abnormality initially.[15] In adults, hyperinflation is accompanied by **peribronchial** thickening due to inflammation. In advanced disease, ring shadows and **cystic lesions** may occur with areas of bronchiectasis and atelectasis also evident. The upper lobes are usually more involved than the lower lobes, and the right side is more involved than the left.[18] The pulmonary and bronchial arteries often begin to enlarge in the middle stages of disease, but the **cardiac silhouette** remains within normal limits until the disease is far advanced.

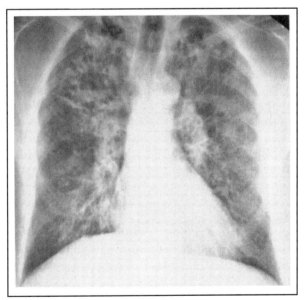

Figure 6-3. Chest radiograph of a patient with cystic fibrosis. Coarse reticulation is seen throughout the lungs with cyst formation secondary to bronchiectasis more pronounced in the upper lobes. (Courtesy of Dr. Dorothy McCauley, New York University Medical Center.)

Other Organ Involvement

Upper Airway. Sinusitis and nasal **polyps** are common in CF. Approximately 50% of adult CF patients have nasal polyps at some point.[14]

Pancreas. The pancreas is involved in 80% to 90% of CF patients. Infants with pancreatic insufficiency demonstrate failure to thrive owing to malabsorption, and older children may have **steatorrhea** (excessive fat in the feces). Pancreatic function becomes progressively more abnormal as the ducts become more obstructed by thick viscous secretions. Pancreatic enzymes that are trapped in the ducts lead to autodestruction of the pancreas. Both cystic and fibrotic changes are seen, and in advanced stages, fibrosis of the pancreas affects the **islets of Langerhans** and causes diabetes.

Liver and Biliary Tract. The liver and gallbladder are also affected by obstruction of their ducts with abnormally viscid secretions. Biliary cirrhosis may be present in infancy, and in some patients it may progress to diffuse cirrhosis and portal hypertension. **Obstructive jaundice** may also be present. **Microgallbladder** is seen in 20% to 30% of CF patients. Because of malabsorption of bile salts, gallstones are present in 13% of adults with CF.[14]

Gastrointestinal Tract. In the intestinal tract, goblet cells and hyperplasia of the mucous glands are evident. Abnormalities in intestinal mucins contribute to malabsorption of specific nutrients. Malabsorption can generally be corrected by administering pancreatic enzymes. Also, water content in the intestinal tract is reduced, probably owing to abnormalities in ion transport.[15] This reduction in liquid leaves the intestinal contents in a semisolid or solid state, in contrast to their normal, more liquid state, which can result in **fecal impaction.** Fecal impaction can also lead to **volvulus** (intestinal obstruction due to twisting of the bowel into a loop) or **intussusception** of the bowel (infolding of one segment of the intestine into an adjacent part).

Reproductive Organs. Female CF patients appear to be less fertile than other women. They demonstrate increased viscosity of cervical mucus, which fails to thin at midcycle, making sperm penetration more difficult. However, pregnancy is possible and has been carried to term in hundreds of cases.[15] In males affected with CF, the vas deferens is partially or completely obstructed, and approximately 98% of CF males are aspermatic.[17]

Laboratory Findings

A sputum culture demonstrating *P. aeruginosa* and *S. aureus,* either alone or in combination, is most common. **Sputum** cultures and sensitivities guide antibiotic therapy during treatment of exacerbations of the disease. Once present, these organisms, especially *Pseudomonas,* are rarely eradicated from the sputum.

Laboratory evaluation of malabsorption due to pancreatic insufficiency requires stool collection for 72 hours to test for residual fat content while ingestion of 100 g of fat per day is maintained. A coefficient of malabsorption of greater than 7% is considered abnormal; patients with CF often have coefficients of malabsorption of 20% to 30%.

Medical Treatment

Comprehensive and intensive medical treatment of CF patients has led to a dramatic increase in the median age of survival (age 25).[15] Individual programs must be tailored to improve or maintain function of the organs involved.

Management of Pulmonary Disease. The goals of treatment of the pulmonary disease are to prevent and treat the complications of obstruction and infection in the airways. This is done by practicing bronchial hygiene, including postural drainage with percussion and vibration, to prevent plugging of the airways (see Chapter 17) and antibiotic therapy when appropriate. Administration of aerosol, mucolytic, or bronchodilator therapies may precede the bronchial hygiene therapy.

Antibiotics. Antibiotics have been the key fac-

> **Clinical Note: Gene Therapy in CF**
>
> Since 1989, when the CF gene was isolated, gene therapy has been an area of intensive research with the goal of decreasing the clinical symptoms and disease progression associated with CF. This therapy works to correct the genetic defect and restore the chloride channel functions.

tor responsible for the increased survival of CF patients during the past few decades. When signs of pulmonary infection are evident, the appropriate antibiotic, determined by culture and sensitivity testing, is given, and bronchial hygiene therapy is increased.

Signs of Pulmonary Infection

Increased cough
Increased sputum production
Fever
Increased respiratory rate
Increased white blood cell count
New findings on auscultation or on the radiograph
Decreases in the pulmonary function test values

Antibiotics currently used to treat staphylococcal infections include dicloxacillin, cephalexin, the newer cephalosporins, and chloramphenicol.[17] Early in the pulmonary disease, *Pseudomonas* organisms may respond to tetracycline. If the *Pseudomonas* organisms are resistant to oral antibiotics, the patient must be admitted for a 2-week course of intravenous antibiotics. Usually a combination of two antibiotics is used intravenously, an aminoglycoside and a semisynthetic penicillin. The most commonly used combinations are gentamicin and carbenicillin or tobramycin and ticarcillin.[17] The combination of antibiotics is believed to work synergistically on *Pseudomonas*, and the organism is less likely to become resistant to either antibiotic.

Larger doses and more frequent administration of the aminoglycoside are prescribed to achieve higher levels of the antibiotic in the airways and the secretions. Serum concentrations of the antibiotics, renal function, and hearing are monitored to avoid toxic reactions.[17] When antibiotic therapy is required for longer than 2 weeks, use of a heparin lock or inhaled antibiotics may allow the patient to return home.

Mucolytics and Bronchodilators. Mist tents, historically used with CF patients, have been found not to be helpful in thinning secretions. However, intermittent **aerosols** are used to deliver **mucolytics** and bronchodilators. These medications should be delivered before performing **postural drainage.**

Nutrition. Management of pancreatic insufficiency is partially accomplished by ingestion of pancreatic enzyme replacements, which should be taken along with any food that contains protein, fat, or complex carbohydrates. The dose of enzymes is adjusted to attempt to maintain an adequate weight gain or an ideal weight and a relatively normal bowel pattern with a decrease in cramping and flatulence. Enzyme replacement cannot totally correct pancreatic insufficiency, so patients also require increased caloric intake. This is accomplished through the use of nutritional supplements taken orally or via nasogastric feeding. Multivitamin preparations and increased salt intake are also recommended for individuals with CF.[17]

Complications and Prognosis

The general course of CF is characterized by a gradual decrease in pulmonary function over the life span, with abrupt declines in pulmonary function when infections are present. Malnutrition may be present with severe pulmonary impairment. Certain complications, however, may occur suddenly and be life-threatening. Complications include electrolyte depletion, usually seen in hot weather, or intestinal obstruction due to an impacted fecal mass.

Pneumothorax, caused by rupture of bronchiectatic cysts or subpleural blebs, is a serious complication in CF. About 20% of patients do not survive the hospitalization during which their pneumothorax is treated.[18] Because the recurrence rate is about 50% following pneumothorax, and collapse of a lung could be fatal in CF patients, surgical treatment of pneumothorax is usually recommended.[15] **Pleurectomy, pleural abrasion,** and **oversewing** of the tear is usually effective. Atelectasis of a segment or lobe may occur, which if untreated may lead to the development of bronchiectasis in that segment. **Hemoptysis** (coughing up blood) may occur, ranging from streaking of blood in the sputum to larger quantities. When 30 to 60 mL of fresh blood is expectorated, the patient is usually hospitalized. Massive hemoptysis is uncommon in CF.[15]

With progression of the disease and during acute infections, increased hypoxia can lead to pulmonary arterial hypertension and cor pulmonale. During acute infections, oxygen and diuretics may be used to treat right heart failure. When the patient is considered to be in respiratory failure, management becomes very difficult. If the respiratory failure is due to an acute problem such as viral infection or **status asthmaticus** and prior PFTs were relatively good, mechanical ventilation is more likely to be successful. Mechanical ventilation is usually of no help when respiratory failure is due to a progressive pulmonary insufficiency despite adequate medical management.[17]

Prognosis

As mentioned earlier, the comprehensive medical treatment now available to manage patients with CF has improved median survival to 25 years of age. Thirty years ago, median survival was only a few years of age. However, most experts believe the median survival rate is now plateauing. Also because CF is such a complex clinical disorder, the variability in outcomes is wide. Some severely affected children still die at a young age, despite skillful medical management, whereas others who are more mildly affected may live into their thirties and forties. Because more than 98% of CF patients die of respiratory failure or pulmonary complications, heart-lung, bilateral single lung, and double lung transplants are being performed for end-stage CF (see Chapter 12).

Asthma

Asthma is a chronic inflammatory disease of the airways characterized by increased responsiveness of the tracheobronchial tree to a variety of stimuli. Widespread narrowing of the airways occurs when the individual comes in contact with these stimuli. Clinical manifestations of asthma include cough, dyspnea, wheezing, and an inability to expel air completely. Generally asthma is episodic in nature, with acute episodes being separated by symptom-free time periods.

Prevalence

Asthma affects both children and adults. It is estimated that approximately 4% of the population in

the United States has the disorder. Fifty percent of individuals with asthma develop the disease before age 10, and another 30% develop it before age 40.[19] Asthma that begins in childhood and is triggered by allergens is called **extrinsic asthma.** Fifty percent, or more, of these children will not "outgrow" asthma.[20] Asthma that begins after age 35 is called **intrinsic asthma** and is more severe in nature.

Pathology

Airways are dynamic structures that dilate when large amounts of air need to be moved, as during exercise, and constrict when the airways need to be protected, as during exposure to irritant gases. The ability of the airways to alter their diameter in response to both internal and external stimuli is called airway reactivity. In asthmatic individuals, airway reactivity is increased, and they develop more intense bronchoconstriction than do non-asthmatic individuals when exposed to a specific stimulus. Certain biologic functions vary during a 24-hour period, and airway reactivity appears to follow this pattern. Some asthmatics experience increased respiratory symptoms during the night and early morning. Nocturnal asthma may occur in as many as 70% to 80% of patients with asthma.[19]

Pathogenesis

Seven major types of stimuli induce acute episodes of asthma:

- Allergens
- Exercise
- Infections
- Occupational stress
- Environmental stress
- Pharmacologic stress
- Emotional stress[18]

An allergic component can be found in 35% to 55% of asthma patients. Most allergens that provoke asthma are airborne.

Initially allergens must be abundant to produce an asthmatic response, but once sensitization has occurred, only minute quantities of the substance are necessary to provoke bronchospasm. Allergens

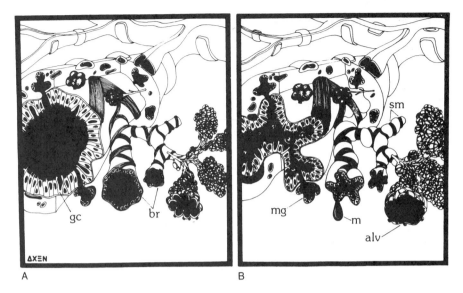

Figure 6–4. Comparison of normal (A) and asthmatic (B) airways and their surrounding tissue. gc, Goblet cell; br, bronchi; mg, mucous gland; m, mucus; sm, smooth muscle; alv, alveoli. (From Des Jardins T. Clinical Manifestations of Respiratory Disease. Chicago, Year Book Medical Publishers, 1984. Redrawn by Kenneth Axen.)

cause constriction of bronchial smooth muscle, increased secretion of mucus by bronchial glands, reduced ciliary activity, and vasodilation of blood vessels (Fig. 6–4).[19]

In a sensitized individual, inhalation of an allergen causes airflow limitation within minutes; the allergen's effect decreases in the next 30 to 60 minutes. In some individuals, the initial reaction is followed by a second wave of obstruction or what is sometimes called a *late reaction,* which may be more severe than the first and less responsive to treatment.[19]

Asthma that is exacerbated by physical exertion is identified as *exercise-induced asthma.* Attacks are characterized by cough, wheezing, and dyspnea, which resolve relatively quickly and spontaneously. The use of bronchodilators before exercise may often control attacks. The environment in which the exercise is performed may influence the development of asthma. The inhalation of cold air during exercise may precipitate an attack. Activities such as ice skating or skiing may be difficult for affected individuals. Both the lack of water content in the inspired air and the high levels of ventilation during exercise have been implicated in triggering asthmatic attacks.

Viral respiratory tract infections may also precipitate attacks. In children younger than 2 years of age, **respiratory syncytial virus** plays a major role, and with increasing age **rhinoviruses** (colds) become more important, along with influenza and

Mycoplasma infections.[19] Bacterial infections are less likely to be a cause of asthma attacks.

Certain occupations may be associated with the development of asthma. Workers in the cotton industry (those involved in the carding and spinning processes) have a higher than average incidence of asthma. Bakers exposed to cereals and flours and animal handlers also show an increased incidence of asthma. The many substances implicated in occupational asthma include metal salts; wood and vegetable dusts; pharmaceutic agents; industrial chemicals and plastics; biologic enzymes (used in detergents); and animal, bird, fish, or insect proteins.[19]

Weather changes such as increased cold or dampness may worsen asthmatic symptoms. High levels of air pollution may also trigger asthma attacks, especially when there are stagnant air masses associated with heavy pollution.

Pharmacologic agents most frequently linked with acute episodes of asthma include aspirin, drug additives such as tartrazine (yellow dye no. 5), and food preservatives such as sulfites.[19] Asthma can also be aggravated by nonselective beta-blocking drugs such as propanolol.

Emotional or psychological factors can interact with an individual's predisposition to asthma attacks. Emotions can ease or worsen the severity of the attack in approximately half of the cases.[19] However, it is unusual for psychological factors to be the cause of an attack.

Clinical Features

Signs and Symptoms. Asthma is generally episodic in nature. It is a chronic disease in which acute episodes of bronchial narrowing are interspersed with symptom-free periods. Clinical signs include intermittent wheezing and dyspnea, usually accompanied by cough. Episodes may last for a few minutes or may persist for hours or days. Young children with severe asthma or late-onset asthmatics may wheeze continuously, with variation only in severity of the wheezing.

During an attack, the patient may be in respiratory distress, using primarily the accessory muscles of respiration. The chest is often hyperinflated and hyperresonant to percussion. Auscultation reveals a prolonged expiratory phase, and diffuse wheezing may be heard on both inspiration and expiration.

Patients with a severe persistent attack of asthma that is refractory to bronchodilation medication are said to have status asthmaticus. These patients are usually in severe respiratory distress and have cyanosis (bluish discoloration of skin and mucous membranes due to lack of oxygen in the blood). They may become physically exhausted by the increased work of breathing and from sleep deprivation.[21] Auscultation during an acute attack may reveal very little air movement, with wheezing faintly heard or even absent. This is an ominous sign during a severe attack.[21] Signs of acute respiratory failure such as carbon dioxide retention, alterations in level of consciousness, and signs of cardiac failure may be evident. Patients in this type of respiratory distress require immediate attention and may require mechanical ventilation.

In asthmatics who experience only intermittent attacks, there may be no clinical signs of airway disease between attacks.

Chest Radiograph. Between attacks and during mild asthma attacks the radiograph is often entirely normal. In severe attacks, however, a radiograph may look similar to that of a patient with emphysema, and marked hyperinflation may be seen. The diaphragms may be low and flattened; the ribs are horizontal with wide interspaces and sparse vascular markings, giving a dark appearance to the lung parenchyma (Fig. 6–5).

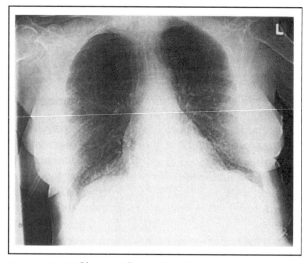

Figure 6–5. Chest radiograph of a patient during an acute attack of asthma. Note the low flattened diaphragms and horizontal ribs, indicating hyperinflation of the lungs. (Courtesy of Dr. Dorothy McCauley, New York University Medical Center.)

Pathophysiology

Obstruction to airflow, either episodic or continual with varying severity, is the predominant feature seen in the pulmonary function tests of asthmatic patients. The FEV_1 and the FEV_1 to FVC (forced vital capacity) ratio are reduced during an attack. When the FEV_1 to FVC ratio is less than 75%, obstruction to airflow is present.[21] **Maximal expiratory flow-volume** (MEFV) relationships may also be abnormal. The MEFV curve measures airflow at all lung volumes throughout the FVC maneuver, and even in asymptomatic asthma patients airflow may be reduced at lung volumes between 50% of **vital capacity** (VC) and RV.[21] This probably represents the presence of residual abnormalities in the peripheral airways. Other tests of peripheral airway function such as closing volume may also reveal abnormalities.

In performing pulmonary function tests on patients suspected of having asthma, it is very important to repeat each test after the administration (usually by aerosol) of bronchodilators. An improvement of 15% or more in the FEV_1 is considered to indicate reversibility of obstruction to airflow. Normal individuals improve 10% or less in FEV_1 measurement when their resting bronchial tone is reduced by bronchodilators.

Asthmatics often have a reduced VC and an increased FRC and RV. These signs of hyperinflation usually improve with treatment of the airways obstruction. Work of breathing may be increased when hyperinflation is present, as inspiratory muscles are at a mechanical disadvantage.

In an asthma attack, the severity of airway obstruction may be nonuniform in the lungs so that distribution of ventilation is uneven. Initially perfusion is diverted away from underventilated areas, but if obstruction becomes more widespread and severe, ventilation-perfusion mismatching worsens and arterial hypoxemia occurs. Early in the attack, minute ventilation is increased to maintain alveolar ventilation, and initially, Pa_{CO_2} is decreased (30 to 35 mm Hg). In severe attacks of obstruction, alveolar ventilation decreases and hypercapnia (Pa_{CO_2} above 45 mm Hg) results.

Laboratory Findings

A complete blood count with an absolute eosinophil count is usually ordered. Finding eosinophilia helps to identify an allergic cause of the asthma and is useful in predicting response to corticosteroids. In patients younger than 35 years of age, allergy testing (skin patch tests) may be done. Sputum should be examined for bacteria during a severe attack. If food substances are suspected allergens, the diet may need to be evaluated.

Medical Treatment

The goals of medical treatment are to relieve bronchospasm, mobilize secretions, and maintain alveolar ventilation. Drugs may be used for short-term control or long-term control with stabilization of the airway. Five categories of drugs that are used in the treatment and prevention of asthma are **sympathomimetics,** theophylline and its derivatives, anticholinergics, cromolyn, and inhaled corticosteroids (see Chapter 15).

Controlling exposure to environmental stimuli, such as smog, dust, and other irritants, may be critical in the control of asthma. Physical conditioning is believed to be beneficial in improving exercise tolerance.

Clinical Note: Changes in Asthma Treatment

Treatment for asthma has changed over the years, and recommendations now emphasize inhaled steroids (nasal and mouth) to prevent the inflammation from initiating the asthma attack, as well as decreasing the side effects the systemic medications have on the individual. Early detection of airway problems is achieved by performing daily spirometry using peak flows with a flowmeter, to assess airway patency (FEV$_1$ and FVC) changes.

Prognosis

Despite great advances in pharmacologic management, asthma-related deaths appear to be increasing. Possible explanations for this finding include complacency or lack of understanding of the disease. Overreliance on self-administered medications may be contributory also. An important goal for health care professionals working with asthmatics is to educate them and encourage them to enter the health care system earlier when experiencing symptoms of an asthma attack that are not resolving.

Bronchiectasis

Bronchiectasis is a permanent, abnormal dilation and distortion of one or more bronchi that is caused by destruction of the elastic and muscular components of the bronchial walls.

Clinical Features

Common clinical features include the following:

- Cough
- **Copious mucopurulent** sputum and **fetid breath** (having a disagreeable odor)
- Recurrent pulmonary infections
- Recurrent hemoptysis

Prevalence

The incidence of bronchiectasis is decreasing. It was common and often fatal in the preantibiotic era and is still common in developing countries. The decrease in bronchiectasis is believed to be due to greater availability of antibiotics for the treatment of respiratory tract infections and widespread use of immunization in childhood against **pertussis** (whooping cough) and measles.

Pathology

The abnormal permanent bronchial dilation involves mainly the medium-sized bronchi but extends to the more distal bronchi and bronchioles as well. Dilation of the bronchi may reach as much as four times the normal diameter. Bronchiectatic areas are often filled with purulent secretions, and the mucosal surface is swollen, inflamed, and often ulcerated. Bronchial mucous glands are dilated. Infection denudes the epithelial lining and elastic tissue; smooth muscle and surrounding cartilage are destroyed.[22] In chronic bronchiectasis, marked fibrosis occurs in and around bronchial walls, replacing muscle, mucous glands, and cartilage.

Bronchiectasis is bilateral in 30% of cases. The lower lobes are most frequently involved, with the left lower lobe involved more than three times as often as the right lower lobe. This may be because of better drainage of the wider and straighter right mainstem bronchus. Also the left mainstem bronchus is slightly compressed as the left pulmonary artery crosses it. The left lower lobe's posterior basal segment is the most frequently involved.[22]

The classification of bronchiectasis developed through a correlation between the findings of **bronchography** and the pathologic changes, both gross and microscopic, found in resected bronchiectatic lobes. Since the development of the computed tomography (CT) scan, bronchography (the instillation of a radiopaque dye into the tracheobronchial tree) is no longer used extensively in the diagnosis of bronchiectasis.

Types of Bronchiectasis

Cylindric Bronchiectasis. In **cylindric bronchiectasis,** the bronchi are tubular; the walls of the bronchi are straight and their diameter is only slightly increased. The involved bronchi come to an abrupt squared end rather than gradually ta-

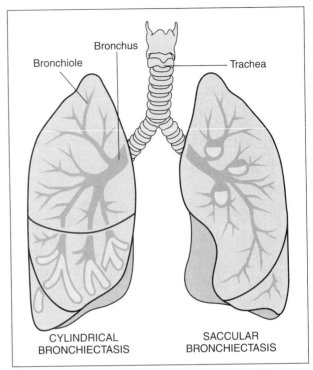

Figure 6-6. Bronchiectasis. The dilatation may be saccular or cylindrical. The lumina of the dilated bronchi contain pus and mucus. (From Damjanov I. Pathology for the Health-Related Professions. 2nd ed. Philadelphia, WB Saunders, 2000, Fig. 8–12, p 188.)

pering as do normal bronchi. The numbers of subdivisions of the bronchi appear normal by microscopic examination (see Fig. 6–6).

Varicose Bronchiectasis. In **varicose bronchiectasis,** the bronchi are generally dilated and irregular in form and size. As they extend peripherally, the bronchi terminate in a bulbous end pouch rather than tapering gradually. Irregular bulging contours are characteristic of varicose bronchiectasis. The average number of bronchial divisions is reduced to about one half of those in a normal lung on microscopic examination. In many areas the bronchial lumen is obliterated by fibrous tissue.

Saccular Bronchiectasis. In **saccular bronchiectasis,** bronchi are very dilated and ballooning in shape, especially as they progress to the periphery. The number of bronchial subdivisions is markedly reduced to one fourth or one fifth of the number normally found on microscopic examination (see Fig. 6–6).

Different classifications of bronchiectasis may coexist in the same lung, and no cause and effect relationship exists between etiology and type of bronchiectasis that develops. In general, with proper medical care bronchiectasis does not progress.

Pathogenesis

The cause of bronchiectasis is, most commonly, a **necrotizing** infection or a series of multiple infections involving the tracheobronchial walls and adjacent lung parenchyma. So-called congenital bronchiectasis is a rarer cause and is due to a variety of abnormalities in tracheobronchial structure, defects in ciliary structure or function, or alterations in the upper airway. These anatomic defects cause respiratory tract dysfunction that predisposes the child to developing bronchiectasis in early childhood. The bronchiectasis is usually not present at birth.

Before the 1950s, when extensive immunization against pertussis and measles began, pulmonary infections that developed during these childhood diseases were associated with bronchiectasis.[22] The association of measles with bronchiectasis is less prominent now in the United States, but in developing countries bronchiectasis may develop after the measles. Secondary necrotizing bacterial pneumonias that develop after pertussis can also lead to the development of bronchiectasis. Dried retained mucus and debris associated with pertussis may cause resorptive atelectasis (collapse of alveolar units caused by proximal plugging and reabsorption of distal air) and contribute to the development of bronchiectasis.

The bacterial pneumonias that predispose an individual to the development of bronchiectasis are usually necrotizing processes. These bacteria include *S. aureus, Klebsiella pneumoniae*, and *P. aeruginosa*. Tuberculosis has also been associated with subsequent bronchiectasis.

Other Causes of Bronchiectasis

Bronchial Obstruction. Bronchiectasis may develop years after an unrecognized foreign body aspiration. This type of bronchiectasis is usually localized rather than diffuse. Foreign bodies associated with aspiration include peanuts; chicken bones; or, in the pediatric population, grass (flowering head of the grass).[22] Obstructive emphysema, atelectasis, and infection usually develop behind the obstruction, setting the stage for the development of bronchiectasis.

Mucoid Impaction. Bronchiectasis may be associated with diffuse obstructive airway diseases such as asthma or chronic bronchitis. Hypersecretion of mucus may be present with these diseases, and continuing infection, mucoid impaction, blockage of peripheral bronchi, and bronchial inflammation can gradually progress to bronchiectasis.

Associated Hereditary Conditions

Immotile Cilia Syndrome. Immotile cilia syndrome is a genetic disorder in which cilia are immotile or defective owing to a molecular lesion. Symptoms of immotile cilia syndrome include sinusitis, otitis, chronic rhinitis, chronic or recurrent bronchitis, bronchiectasis, and male sterility. Cilia from these patients lack structural components called dynein arms, which are important in mucus propulsion. Consequently, in affected individuals tracheobronchial or nasal mucociliary transport is totally or nearly totally absent. The frequency of bronchiectasis associated with immotile cilia syndrome is approximately 30%. The term *ciliary dyskinesia syndrome* is used to describe those individuals whose cilia are anatomically abnormal but do display some movement, although the movement is not entirely normal.

Kartagener's Syndrome. Kartagener's syndrome is a triad of bronchiectasis, sinusitis, and situs inversus (lateral transposition of the thoracic contents; heart is located on the right). Kartagener's syndrome occurs in approximately 50% of patients with ciliary dyskinesia syndrome.

Cystic Fibrosis. Cystic fibrosis is a predisposing factor in at least half of the cases of bronchiectasis seen in persons up to the age of 20 years. Bronchiectasis is found on examination of essentially all autopsied CF victims older than 6 months of age.[22]

Clinical Features

Cough is almost always present in individuals with bronchiectasis. **Purulent** (consisting of or containing pus) sputum, which separates into three layers on standing, is characteristic of the disease: an upper layer of white or slightly greenish brown frothy secretions, a middle thin mucoid layer, and a bottom layer of thick greenish plugs. Sputum production is present in 90% of patients, and it is often greatest in the morning, after accumulating during sleep in the recumbent position. During episodes of infection, sputum increases in volume and purulence. In rare cases, sputum production is not a prominent feature, and these cases are referred to as *dry bronchiectasis.*

Patients with bronchiectasis have a tendency to develop hemoptysis. Before the widespread use of antibiotics, 40% to 70% of bronchiectatic patients developed hemoptysis.[23] Hemoptysis varies in quantity from light blood streaking to massive life-threatening bleeding.

Sinusitis is frequently associated with bronchiectasis, especially in the predisposing syndromes, such as CF and immotile cilia syndrome.

Most patients with bronchiectasis have abnormalities on auscultation of the thorax. Moist rales, or crackles, are present over the involved lobes. Rhonchi are evident during periods of mucus retention, and dullness to percussion and decreased breath sounds may be present when mucus plugging occurs. Bronchovesicular or **bronchial breath sounds** may be noted during pneumonia.

Observations of clubbing of the fingers and cyanosis were more frequent in the preantibiotic era. By the 1960s, clubbing was observed in only 7% of cases.[22] Cor pulmonale occurred in 10% to 22% of cases. Now it is a less common complication.

Radiographic Findings. Radiographic findings may be unremarkable, especially early in the disease. Later in the disease, line shadows following a bronchovascular distribution may be evident. These are caused by thickened bronchial walls, peribronchial fibrosis, and adjacent alveolar collapse.[22] If mucus plugging is significant, atelectasis or collapse of whole lobes behind the obstruction may be visible on a radiograph. With advanced saccular bronchiectasis, large cystic areas with and without fluid levels may be seen. Patchy areas of bronchopulmonary pneumonia may occur in patients with bronchiectasis.

Bronchography was done more frequently in the past to assist in diagnosis (Fig. 6–7). Currently it is done only when surgical resection of a localized bronchiectatic area is being considered. Adverse reactions to this procedure include possible allergic reactions to the dye and impairment of ventilation. Computed chest tomography (CT scan) is more frequently used for diagnostic purposes today.

Computed Tomography Scan. Cystic bronchiectasis is most easily diagnosed using a CT scan, but cylindric and varicose types may be diagnosed as well, as long as pneumonia and other causes of consolidation are eliminated. Pneumonia may look similar to bronchiectasis on a CT scan. Findings on a CT scan include dilated bronchi extending peripherally and thickened bronchial walls. Air-fluid levels may be present, and in cystic bronchiectasis clusters of cysts may be seen (Fig. 6–8).[22]

Pathophysiology

Pulmonary Function Tests. Test results in bronchiectasis depend on the extent of disease present and the coexistence of other lung diseases such as chronic bronchitis or emphysema. Patients with mild or localized bronchiectasis and no other associated diseases may have relatively normal pulmonary function test results. However, in patients with diffuse involvement, results show a pattern of airway obstruction. A reduced FVC, FEV_1, $FEV_1/$FVC, and a reduced forced expiratory flow of 25% to 75% (FEF_{25-75}) are seen as well as increased RV. In patients with associated atelectasis and fibrosis, test results show a more mixed obstructive-restrictive pattern or a largely restrictive pattern with decreased VC and decreased FRC.

Arterial Blood Gases. With extensive bronchiectasis, arterial hypoxemia may develop due to ventilation-perfusion mismatching. Carbon dioxide retention occurs only in patients with bronchiectasis associated with severe chronic bronchitis and advanced emphysema.

Hemodynamic Changes. Extensive systemic to pulmonary anastomoses occur at the precapillary level in the granulation tissue surrounding bronchiectatic segments. These anastomoses can lead to bronchial artery enlargement and left to right shunts (recirculation of oxygenated blood). In patients with severe bronchiectasis and accompanying chronic bronchitis and emphysema, hypoxia, pulmonary hypertension, and cor pulmonale may develop. The development of pulmonary hypertension and cor pulmonale is uncommon in patients with bronchiectasis alone.[22]

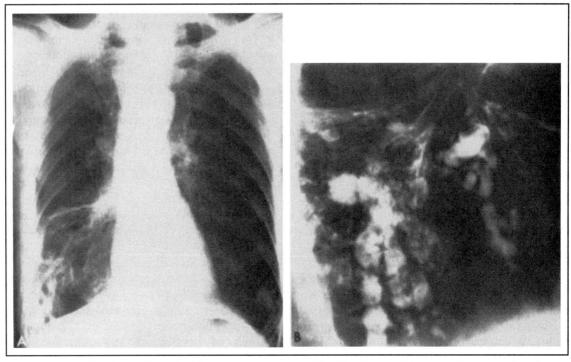

Figure 6–7. Saccullar bronchiectasis. Chest roentgenogram (*A*) of a 42-year-old man with severe chronic cough and sputum production showing increased markings extending into the right lower lobe and cystic lesions. Detail of bronchogram (*B*) confirms the presence of saccular bronchiectasis. (From Hinshaw HC, Murray JF. Diseases of the Chest. 4th ed. Philadelphia, W B Saunders, 1980, p. 597.)

Laboratory Findings

Bacteria commonly found in the sputum of bronchiectatic patients include *H. influenzae* and streptococcus pneumonia. Anaerobic bacteria may also play an important role in some cases of bronchiectasis. A Gram-stained smear of sputum shows numerous polymorphonuclear leukocytes and mixed bacterial flora, often including fusiform bacteria as well as a variety of gram-negative and gram-positive cocci. Leukocytosis is variable and may be associated with infections and active **sup-**

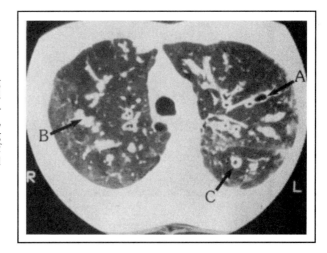

Figure 6–8. Computed tomography (CT) scan showing bronchiectasis. A, Dilated, irregularly shaped, air-filled bronchus. B, Mucoid impaction of a bronchus. The signet-ring configuration (C) is common in bronchiectasis, appearing as a dilated bronchus with its accompanying pulmonary artery, resembling a signet ring. (Courtesy of Dr. Dorothy McCauley, New York University Medical Center.)

puration. Anemia in long-standing disease is sometimes seen.[22]

Medical Treatment

The goals of treatment are to prevent the progression and to alleviate the symptoms of the disease. Control of infection and supportive measures to provide good pulmonary hygiene, including postural drainage with percussion, vibration, and shaking, are indicated. Hydration is very important to assist in thinning secretions. Eight to ten glasses of water are recommended daily. Control of bronchospasm may also be necessary.

Immunization against influenza and pneumonia is recommended for this population. Antibiotic therapy should be initiated promptly for acute infections and febrile exacerbations of bronchiectasis. The choice of antibiotic should be guided by sputum culture and sensitivity testing, which determines the most effective antibiotic for eradicating the organism. Bronchoscopy may be necessary for removal of foreign bodies if they are the cause of the bronchiectasis.

Surgical resection of a bronchiectatic segment is recommended only when symptoms of the disease are severe and interfere with the progress of a normal life. The disease must be fairly well localized. Surgery is also recommended when major hemorrhage from an eroded bronchial artery in a bronchiectatic segment cannot be controlled by bronchial arteriography and embolization.[22]

Complications and Prognosis

The complications of bronchiectasis include

- Chronic bronchial infections and episodes of **bronchopneumonia**
- Hemoptysis with possible pulmonary hemorrhage
- Obliteration of peripheral airways, with associated bronchitis and emphysema
- Chronic respiratory insufficiency
- Cor pulmonale

The greatest disability results from a combination of bronchiectasis and emphysema that produces chronic respiratory failure.[22]

Despite the use of antibiotics, the bronchiectasis could become more severe over time in already

involved segments, but its spread to previously normal areas is rare, except when a diffuse underlying process is present, such as CF or immotile cilia syndrome.[22]

In the era before antibiotics and widespread childhood immunization, bronchiectasis was considered a highly lethal disease.[23] Today mortality has improved greatly. Aside from individuals with CF and bronchiectasis, many patients with bronchiectasis live into their seventies and eighties if they receive proper treatment.[22]

ADULT OBSTRUCTIVE LUNG CONDITIONS

The prevalence of COPD is continuing to increase in the adult population. In 1990, COPD was predicted to affect as many as 30 million Americans, and it ranks as the fifth most common cause of death in the United States.[24] Although presented here separately, chronic bronchitis and emphysema are often considered together under the term COPD, because most patients have a combination of chronic bronchitis (airway disease) and emphysema (alveolar disease). The manifestation of each component may vary greatly from patient to patient. Both diseases are attributed to cigarette smoking.

Chronic Bronchitis

Chronic bronchitis is generally defined as hypersecretion of mucus sufficient to produce a productive cough on most days for 3 months during 2 consecutive years. Hypersecretion of mucus usually begins in the large airways and is not associated with airway obstruction (simple bronchitis).

> ### Clinical Note: Chronic Obstructive Pulmonary Disease
> COPD is used as a generic term for individuals with obstructive airway disease because most of these patients have a combination of chronic bronchitis and emphysema. The manifestation of the disease can vary greatly from patient to patient.

Later, hypersecretion progresses to the smaller airways, where the airway obstruction begins initially (chronic bronchitis).

Pathology

In chronic bronchitis, there is hypertrophy of the submucosal glands in the large and small bronchi and in the trachea. The ratio of gland thickness to wall thickness (Reid Index) is used as an indicator of mucous gland hypertrophy. In normal individuals this value is less than 3 to 10. In chronic bronchitis the ratio may increase to as high as 8 to 10.[25] In addition to mucous gland hypertrophy in the bronchi, there is an increase in surface epithelial secretory cells, or goblet cells, peripherally in the bronchioli, where usually they are sparse. Denudation of ciliated epithelium and **squamous metaplasia** are also seen. The degree to which the bronchioli, or small airways, are involved is the most important factor in determining disability.[25] When obstruction of the bronchioli occurs, a **bronchogram** demonstrates impairment of lung function. Peripheral filling is severely impaired, with the appearance of irregularities in the lumina of the airways and the presence of intraluminal mucus. Walls of the small airways are thickened owing to edema or inflammatory cell infiltration. The walls are also thickened by the hypertrophy of muscular and connective tissues and the increase in the height of the epithelium. Some of these changes may also be associated with infection. Deterioration of pulmonary function, however, is usually gradual and is related more to hypersecretion and the presence of mucus within the airway lumina than to infection.[25]

Pathogenesis

Chronic bronchitis is a response to chronic irritation. Cigarette smoking is the most consistently important causal factor in the development of chronic bronchitis. A persistent productive cough is highly correlated with cigarette smoking, and its severity increases with the number of cigarettes smoked. Pipe and cigar smokers have fewer symptoms than cigarette smokers.[25] Chronic bronchitis is more common in inhalers than in noninhalers and in those who extinguish and relight their ciga-

rettes.[25] It is likely that the response of airway epithelium, which is to secrete more mucus, is a nonspecific response to an irritant. The accumulation of mucus in the airways results both from epithelial hypersecretion and from defective mucociliary function.[26] Both components of mucociliary interaction are found to be impaired in smokers and in patients with chronic bronchitis.[26]

Other factors that may contribute to a lesser extent to the development of chronic bronchitis include

- Air pollution
- Second-hand smoke
- Occupational exposure to dusts, such as gold, coal, flurospar, and asbestos
- Occupational exposure to vegetable dusts, such as cotton, flax, or hemp[25]

Exposure to gases and fumes has been less well studied but may also contribute in some individuals. Heredity may also play an important role, as relatives of bronchitic patients have a higher incidence of bronchitis than the relatives of control subjects. Also bronchitics have a higher incidence of childhood respiratory infections, such as pneumonia, **pleurisy,** and acute bronchitis, than people without bronchitis.[25]

Clinical Features

The clinical presentation of chronic bronchitis is dominated by a chronic productive cough with morning expectoration and clearing of secretions accumulated during the night. Sputum is usually clear and mucoid but can become purulent during the presence of infection. Recurrent chest infections are a common feature. Bronchitic patients have a tendency to be overweight with a cyanotic cast to their lips and nailbeds. The bronchitic patient is sometimes referred to as a blue bloater or a Type B COPD patient (Fig. 6–9). These patients frequently have edema of the lower extremities because of right heart failure.

Adventitious breath sounds, such as **rhonchi** and wheezes, are frequently heard during auscultation of the chest. The expiratory phase of breathing may become prolonged as obstruction to expiration becomes more severe.

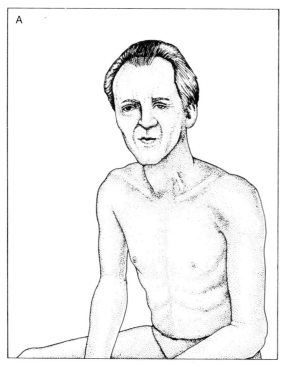
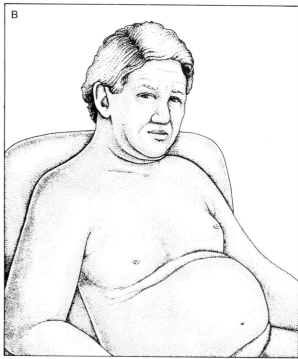

Figure 6–9. Comparison of appearance of individuals with type A dominant (*left*) and type B dominant (*right*) chronic obstructive pulmonary disease. (From Goodman CC, Snyder TEK. Differential Diagnosis in Physical Therapy. Philadelphia, WB Saunders, 1990, pp 89, 90.)

Radiographic Findings

The radiograph may be normal or may show only mild increase in peripheral markings in a bronchitic patient. Severity of disease and functional impairment cannot be estimated by the radiograph. The main use of the radiograph in this population is to help identify other possible causes of their symptoms, such as pneumonia or tumors (Fig. 6–10).

Pathophysiology

The initial lesion in the development of chronic bronchitis may be respiratory bronchiolitis, with inflammatory and obliterative changes that have been initiated by inhaled irritants (cigarette smoke) evident in the bronchioles. Early in the course of bronchitis, signs of *small airway disease* are evident. In addition to bronchiolitis and hypersecretion, other abnormalities may be seen in the small airways, such as fibrosis, ulceration, metaplasia, and increased smooth muscle mass.[25] At this point, conventional tests of airflow (FEV$_1$, FEV$_1$/FVC, maxi-

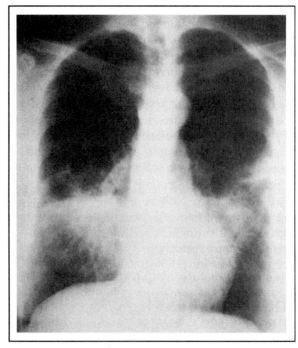

Figure 6–10. Chest radiograph showing pneumonia in a patient with bronchitis. Patchy bilateral pneumonic infiltrates affect both the right middle lobe and the lingula. (Courtesy of Dr. Dorothy McCauley, New York University Medical Center.)

mum voluntary ventilation [MVV]) may still be normal, but special tests, such as closing volume or maximal expiratory flow-volume curves (see Chapter 10), can reveal obstruction in peripheral airways.[25] Edema of the airway, intraluminal mucus, loss of elastic recoil in surrounding structures, bronchospasm, or alterations in surface tension all may contribute to the obstruction, so the cause of the functional change cannot be identified clearly. Small airway disease may not be detectable clinically, but the abnormalities are sufficient to disturb alveolar ventilation-blood flow relationships and alveolar-capillary gas exchange.[25] Pulmonary function tests and arterial blood gases may revert to normal if a person stops smoking while manifesting small airway disease.[27]

Pulmonary Function Tests. To establish the diagnosis of true chronic bronchitis, an FEV_1 of less than 65% of predicted (age, height, and sex adjusted) is considered diagnostic for chronic airflow obstruction. Also an FEV_1 to FVC ratio of less than 70% is considered diagnostic. Residual volume is increased, but VC and dynamic lung compliance are decreased.[27]

Laboratory Findings

Initially arterial blood gases reveal a Pa_{O_2} at the lower limits of normal. As the disease progresses and ventilation-perfusion mismatching increases, the Pa_{O_2} falls further and may become markedly reduced (Pa_{O_2} of 40 to 50 mm Hg); the Pa_{CO_2} may increase to 60 to 70 mm Hg or higher.

Polycythemia (increased red blood cell volume) is a commonly seen adaptation to chronic **hypoxia.** The body attempts to increase the blood's oxygen-carrying capacity by increasing the red blood cell volume. **Hematocrit** (red blood cell volume) levels may increase to 55% to 60% (normal hematocrit value is 42% to 45%). An increased hematocrit level increases blood viscosity, which increases cardiac work and decreases cardiac output.[27]

Medical Treatment

Smoking cessation is very important in the management of chronic bronchitis. Several improvements in symptoms of the disease have been noted when smoking is discontinued: (1) a decrease or resolution of signs of mucous hypersecretion, (2) a

reversal of small airways dysfunction, and (3) a slowing of the average rate of annual decline of FEV_1.[28]

Other approaches to treatment include attempts to prevent and to manage aggressively respiratory tract infections, which cause acute exacerbations of chronic bronchitis. Influenza and pneumonia vaccines are recommended.

An increased incidence of *H. influenzae* and *Streptococcus pneumoniae* bacteria has been noted in the secretions of the lower respiratory tract of patients with severe chronic bronchitis. Viruses and *Mycoplasma pneumoniae* have also been implicated as causes of acute exacerbations of chronic bronchitis.[28]

Antibiotics commonly used to manage acute exacerbations include tetracycline and erythromycin. *H. influenzae* is sensitive to tetracycline, and both *S. pneumoniae* and *M. pneumoniae* are affected by tetracycline and erythromycin. Ampicillin is also sometimes prescribed. Antiviral agents are not available for treatment.

Treatment of respiratory tract infections reduces time lost from work but does little to influence the natural history of chronic bronchitis.[29] Bronchodilators are indicated if bronchospasm is evident.

The use of low-flow oxygen (1 to 3 L/minute) may help reduce pulmonary hypertension and polycythemia and therefore improve right heart function.

Complications and Prognosis

Polycythemia, pulmonary embolism, pulmonary hypertension, respiratory failure, and cor pulmonale are the most frequent complications of chronic bronchitis. Cor pulmonale develops earlier and more frequently in COPD patients with chronic bronchitis. The predominately bronchitic patient generally has a poorer prognosis for longevity than the patient with emphysema because the former has ventilation-perfusion abnormalities that lead to respiratory failure and cor pulmonale.

Emphysema

Emphysema, an alveolar or parenchymal disease, is an abnormal and a permanent enlargement of the air spaces distal to the terminal nonrespiratory bronchioles, accompanied by destructive changes of the alveolar walls. Disturbances in lung function result from these anatomic changes, including loss of elastic recoil, excessive collapse of airways on exhalation, and chronic airflow obstruction[25] (Fig. 6–11). The diagnosis of emphysema is based on pulmonary function test findings; clinical findings, such as distant breath sounds; findings on physical examination; history; and CT scan.

Pathology

Several different types of emphysema are recognized anatomically according to the distribution of enlarged air spaces within the acinus.

Panacinar (Panlobular) Emphysema. In **panacinar emphysema,** all alveoli within the acinus are affected to the same degree; a nearly uniform destruction of most of the structures within a lobule is seen. The distinction between alveolar ducts and alveoli is lost. This type is seen in emphysema associated with **alpha$_1$-antitrypsin deficiency** and unilateral **hyperlucent lung syndrome.** The distribution is equally likely in lower and upper lobes.

Centriacinar (Centrilobular) Emphysema. In **centriacinar emphysema,** alveoli arising from the respiratory bronchiole or the proximal portion of the acinus are most affected. Alveolar ducts and alveolar sacs remain normal. Individuals with centrilobular emphysema may have no respiratory disability. Centriacinar emphysema is commonly found in the upper lobes.

Paraseptal Emphysema. In **paraseptal emphysema,** the enlarged air spaces are located at the periphery of the acinus, just under the pleura or along connective tissue septa. The enlargement is in the alveolar sacs and associated alveoli. These thin-walled, inflated areas located at the pleural surface may become bullae (subpleural air sacs of alveolar origin greater than 1 cm in diameter) and rupture, causing a spontaneous pneumothorax.

Irregular Emphysema. Irregular emphysema forms in the vicinity of scars and is related to the effects of scarring and contraction. This type is the most common and is of little clinical significance.

Pathogenesis

Cigarette smoking is the most important etiologic factor in the development of both emphysema and chronic bronchitis. Many studies suggest a rough dose-response relationship between smoking and development of emphysema. Emphysema is rare in those who have never smoked.[30] Other factors that are associated with the development of emphysema are environmental air pollution and hereditary deficiency of alpha$_1$-antitrypsin.

Emphysema is thought to result from disruption of the elastic fiber network of the lung because of an imbalance between **elastases** (proteolytic en-

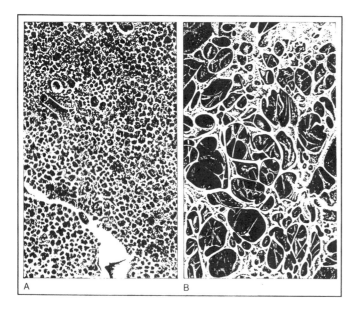

Figure 6–11. Comparison of the appearance of normal lung tissue (*A*) with the pathologic changes observable in lung tissue damaged by emphysema (*B*). (From Des Jardins T. Clinical Manifestations of Respiratory Disease. Chicago, Year Book Medical Publishers, 1984. Redrawn by Kenneth Axen.)

zymes that digest elastin) and their inhibitors.[30] The degradation of **elastin** (one component of the lung's elastic fiber network) is most important in the pathogenesis of emphysema.

Smoking produces low-level, chronic inflammation in the lungs. Increased numbers of phagocytic cells, neutrophils, and alveolar macrophages can be recovered from the lungs of smokers by bronchoalveolar lavage. Neutrophils are located mainly in alveolar walls, whereas alveolar macrophages are found in the respiratory bronchioles.[50] These cells are produced in response to the particulate matter in tobacco smoke. Both neutrophils and macrophages may release proteolytic enzymes into the lungs and be involved in the breakdown of elastin in the lungs of smokers.[30]

Smoking may also predispose an individual to emphysema through inactivation of intrapulmonary elastase inhibitors, so that elastase is unchecked in its destruction of elastin. This hypothesis has been proved in animal models but not yet in humans.[30] In addition, biosynthetic repair of pulmonary elastic tissue is reduced by smoking.[30]

A rare cause of emphysema is the inherited deficiency of alpha₁-antitrypsin, a protein that functions as a *protease* (general term for a proteolytic enzyme) inhibitor. It occurs in 1 of 6000 people in the United States, but it is more common in Sweden, where it was first detected. The concentration of alpha₁-antitrypsin in the plasma of individuals who inherit this condition is only approximately 15% of normal.[30]

The primary role of alpha₁-antitrypsin appears to be the inhibition of neutrophil elastase, because it associates with neutrophil elastase faster than with trypsin.[30] Neutrophil elastase is released during phagocytosis and helps to dispose of microorganisms, such as bacteria, by digesting them. Neutrophil elastase is active against elastin and other components of the lung's fibroelastic network, such as fibronectin and basement membrane collagen.

This unrestrained activity of elastase in the lungs, due to a deficiency of alpha₁-antitrypsin, is expected to result in the development of emphysema. From 80 to 90% of individuals with alpha₁-antitrypsin deficiency develop COPD, and their rate of deterioration of lung function (measured by annual decline in FEV₁) is nearly twice the average rate of decline for COPD patients without the deficiency.[30] When individuals with alpha₁-antitryp-

> ### Clinical Note: Alpha₁-Antitrypsin Deficiency in Emphysema
>
> Alpha₁-antitrypsin deficiency causes a rare emphysema that is found in younger individuals (50 years old and younger) who often do not have a heavy smoking history or are nonsmokers but have advanced lung dysfunction. Current medical treatment includes early identification of this deficiency and subsequent oral replacement of this protease inhibitor of human serum.

sin deficiency also smoke, symptoms appear very early, with shortness of breath evident often at age 40; nonsmokers with the condition usually become symptomatic around age 55. Panacinar emphysema, worst at the basal segments of the lung, is most often seen. Liver disease is also associated with this condition. Children are at risk for the development of **hepatitis** and **cirrhosis.** Adults have an increased incidence of chronic liver disease and **hepatoma.**[30]

Clinical Features

Patients with emphysema usually present clinically with shortness of breath and scant sputum production. They may demonstrate a barrel-shaped configuration of the chest wall, with an increased subcostal angle[31] and horizontal rather than downsloping ribs, owing to hyperinflation of the lungs. Accessory muscles of respiration may be hypertrophied, with supraclavicular retraction evident. Pursed-lip breathing may be utilized even at rest, and postures in which the upper extremities are stabilized (hand on hips in standing or forearms on knees in sitting) are commonly used for more effective utilization of the accessory muscles of breathing. Shoulders are frequently rounded because of shortening of the pectoral muscles. The respiratory rate may be rapid with a shallow depth of respiration.

The typical type A COPD patient, one with a predominately emphysematous component, is sometimes called a "pink puffer" (see Fig. 6–9). The emphysematous patient tends to be thin, sometimes **cachectic** in body build, with rosy skin tones. Distant breath sounds are frequent because of hyperinflation of the lungs; adventitious sounds are less common than in the type B patient.

Radiographic Findings

A radiograph is not considered diagnostic for emphysema. In the early stages of disease and even in some patients with advanced disease, the radiograph may be relatively normal. Centrilobular emphysema is hardest to see on a radiograph, whereas panacinar emphysema is more readily identified. When findings characteristic of emphysema are found on a chest film, the disease is very advanced. Signs of lung hyperinflation include increase in anteroposterior diameter; kyphosis; increased retrosternal air; horizontal ribs; and low, flattened diaphragms. The cardiac silhouette may be narrow and elongated because of both low diaphragms and compression from the hyperinflation of the lungs. At times bullae may also be seen. Bullae are caused by destruction of air spaces distal to the terminal bronchioles (Fig. 6–12).

Pathophysiology

The enlargement of the terminal air spaces in the lungs and the destruction of alveolar walls seen in pure emphysema cause characteristic changes in

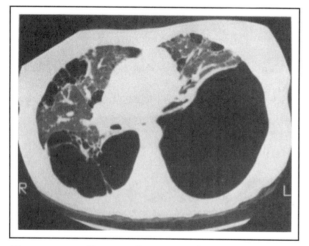

Figure 6–12. Computed tomography scan of bullous emphysema. (Courtesy of Dr. Dorothy McCauley, New York University Medical Center.)

the pulmonary function test results. In emphysema a low diffusing capacity for CO_2 is noted (using either the single-breath test or a rebreathing maneuver). However, in unaffected areas of the lung the relationship between bloodflow and ventilation is relatively well preserved so that overall Pa_{O_2} is only slightly to moderately reduced. Normally Pa_{CO_2} is slightly elevated only during acute respiratory infections.

Owing to loss of elastic recoil, some obstruction to airflow may be seen by a decrease in the FEV_1 or the FEV_1 to FVC ratio, although values are not as decreased as when chronic bronchitis is also present. Airway resistance in emphysema may be normal or slightly increased. The FRC, TLC, and RV are all markedly increased in emphysema patients.

Laboratory Findings

The hematocrit value and the pulmonary artery pressure are usually normal.

Medical Treatment

Cessation of smoking and prevention of respiratory infections are essential in the medical management of emphysema. Prophylactic immunizations against influenza and pneumonia are recommended. When emphysema coexists with bronchitis, some of the treatment methods outlined previously may be indicated.

Complications and Prognosis

Emphysema, in the absence of airway obstruction, can span 20 to 40 years of life, producing only undue breathlessness on exertion. In general, the prognosis for the patient with emphysema is much better than that for the patient with chronic bronchitis because of the preservation of ventilation and blood-flow relationships in emphysema. The emphysematous patient develops cor pulmonale only when hypoxemia is severe enough to produce pulmonary arterial hypertension.

CASE STUDIES

CASE 1—Diagnosis: Asthma

M.A. is a 31-year-old man who was diagnosed with asthma at age 7.

Past medical history: Wheezing intermittently over last 24 years. Symptoms of shortness of breath precipitated by exercise; change in temperature; and exposure to smoke, perfume, and animals. History of allergies to dogs, cats, and dust. Hospitalized once (6/87) for episode of severe bronchospasm. Pneumonia 4 times in 1988; collapsed left lower lobe 8/88.

Past surgical history: none

Smoking history: negative

Medications: Ventolin inhaler tid (three times daily), Intal inhaler tid, theophylline 200 mg bid (two times daily)

Interpretation

This case provides the opportunity for physical therapists to reinforce several important educational points regarding living with asthma which may, or may not, have been previously understood by this individual. There is evidence (history of lobar collapse and recurrent pneumonia) that mucus retention may, at times, be an issue.

Physical Therapy Evaluation

Auscultation: Expiratory wheezes in bilateral upper lobes, otherwise lungs are clear with good aeration.

Assessment with peak flow meter: Able to achieve 820 mL peak flow, but reports that he does not use it at home.

HR = 68 bpm, BP = 120/80 mm Hg.

Reported activity level: Able to jog 2 miles continuously in all seasons, except winter. Therefore, he never exercises in the winter. Always uses Ventolin inhaler prior to exercise.

Interview: Reports missing work frequently due to respiratory symptoms and coughing spasms. Reports that the pulmonologist added an inhaled steroid to his medication regimen 2 weeks ago, but he has not yet initiated its use.

Physical Therapy Treatment Goals

1. Understand the important role medications play in managing asthma.
2. Understand the importance of avoiding all asthma triggers.
3. Understand how to detect subtle changes in status of the caliber of the airways.
4. Understand how and when to perform secretion clearance techniques.
5. Understand the importance of regular aerobic exercise to overall health.
6. Understand the importance of early entry into the medical system when respiratory symptoms are worsening.

Program

1. Reinforce the importance of using prescribed medication regimens prior to any physical therapy or exercise interventions. These interventions may be ineffective and possibly harmful without proper pharmacologic support.
2. Reinforce the importance of avoidance of all animals, smoke, perfumes, and dust.
3. Encourage daily use of the peak flow meter to gain a better understanding of his normal range of values. This will make detection of changes in airway caliber easier. Ask if patient can feel the wheezing in his upper chest. If not, have him place his hands over his upper chest as he breathes to attempt to gain the ability to self-evaluate his pulmonary status.
4. Instruct in secretion clearance techniques, to be performed after the use of prescribed bronchodilator medications. Secretion clearance techniques could include conventional postural drainage with self-vibration, or preferably the active cycle of breathing technique. They should be performed if coughing spasms result in a congested sounding cough.
5. Explore an alternative form of exercise for the winter months, such as an exericse bicycle, indoor swimming, stair climbing, or use of a health club.
6. Reinforce the importance of going early to an Emergency Room or calling 911 if respiratory symptoms are unable to be controlled. Assure patient that it is better to "play it safe," and allow his doctor to decide how serious an asthma attack is or isn't. This will also relieve unnecessary worrying on the part of the patient.

Program Measures and On-going Evaluation

1. Monitor daily peak flows with peak flow meter.
2. Keep a daily exercise log.
3. Monitor absences from work.

Expected Program Outcomes

M.A. will feel confident in his ability to participate in all activities of normal living while managing his asthma effectively, with assistance, as needed, from his physician.

Pulmonary Function Test Results		Pre-Rx		Post-Rx (Bronchodilator)	
SPIROMETRY	PRED	ACTUAL	% PRED	ACTUAL	% PRED
$FEV_{0.5}$ Liters	3.10	2.33	75	2.68	86
FEV_1 Liters	4.37	3.33	76	3.77	86
$FEF_{25-75\%}$ L/sec	4.50	2.07	46	2.50	56

Case 2—Diagnosis: Bronchiectasis

R.A. is a 60-year-old woman diagnosed with bronchiectasis 9/87 following referral to a pulmonary specialist for unresolved right middle lobe and right lower lobe pneumonia.

Past medical history: 10-year history of frequent sore throats, right nasal sinus infection, and postnasal drip. Productive of moderate amounts of yellow sputum with occasional small plugs; productive 8 to 10 times daily for past 10 years. Occasional hemoptysis. Recurrent pneumonias: first in 1984, followed by pneumonia several times per year; 1987—pneumonia four times. Has experienced shortness of breath during episodes of pneumonia, as well as pleuritic pain and darker colored sputum.

Past surgical history: Hysterectomy for fibroids

Smoking history: negative

Medications: none

Diagnostic testing: Blood gas and pulmonary function test results are within normal limits.

Sputum culture (9/87): Numerous gram-negative rods; many white blood cells. Final report: *Pseudomonas aeruginosa*, moderately sensitive to tetracycline, fully sensitive to trimethoprim sulfamethoxazole (Bactrim).

CT scan (9/87): Inflammatory change within both the right middle lobe and lingula, with a suggestion of increased thickening in the region of the minor fissure and a small atelectatic area within the right middle lobe.

Interpretation

R. A. has been finally diagnosed with bronchiectasis, which she has had for some time. Secretion retention, mucus plugging, and the subsequent development of pneumonia are often seen in this condition. Bronchiectasis is sometimes overlooked, especially when sputum production is scant and hemoptysis has not occurred. It cannot be diagnosed by chest x-ray, and therefore, careful attention to the history and pattern of respiratory infections is necessary to prompt ordering a CT scan of the chest. Chest physical therapy techniques are very helpful in resolving the mucus plugging and atelectasis seen in bronchiectasis.

Physical Therapy Evaluation

Auscultation: Decreased breath sounds right midfield, posteriorly and laterally, with an occasional congested cough triggered by deep breathing.

HR = 84 bpm, BP = 110/70 mm Hg.

Musculoskeletal evaluation: Rounded shoulders with tight pectoral muscles, resulting in a slouched posture, otherwise within normal limits.

Physical Therapy Treatment Goals

1. Independence in performing secretion clearance techniques, including postural drainage, segmental expansions, manual self-treatment techniques, and the forced expiratory technique.
2. Improve aeration of right middle lobe and lingula.
3. Improve posture and spinal alignment.
4. Encourage aerobic exercise three to five times per week.

Program (to Be Performed Daily)

1. Instruct in postural drainage positions for right middle lobe and lingula; instruct in thoracic segmental expansion exercises for these areas. Instruct in self-percussion and vibration to these areas. Instruct in the forced expiratory technique. Encourage increase in fluid intake, 8 to 10 glasses of water daily.
2. Instruct in breathing maneuvers to increase collateral ventilation to the right middle lobe, such as "summed" or "stacked breathing," or use of the incentive spirometer with inhalation-hold.
3. Instruct in exercises, coordinated with breathing, to stretch the pectoral muscles and exercises to strengthen the back extensors and adductors of the scapulas.
4. Instruct in a walking, biking, swimming, or low-impact aerobic program to increase ventilation and promote cardiopulmonary fitness, along with evaluation of pulse rate.

Program Measures and On-Going Evaluation

1. Monitor sputum production and see physician if there are changes in color or consistency.
2. Monitor maximum incentive spirometry values.
3. Keep a daily exercise log.

Expected Program Outcomes

R.A. will avoid secretion retention and mucus plugging, thereby reducing her likelihood of developing pneumo-

nia. She will be able to participate in all activities of a normal active life, and will be able to reduce her coughing spasms.

Summary

- Changes seen in pulmonary function test results in obstructive pulmonary diseases are decreases in expiratory flow rates and increases in RV.
- Decreased airflow noted in COPD during expiration may be caused by loss of elastic recoil in lung tissue or resistance encountered in the airways.
- Resistance encountered in the airways in COPD may be caused by inflammation, airway thickening, mucus, or bronchospasm.
- Bronchopulmonary dysplasia is a lung disease of infancy characterized by respiratory distress and oxygen dependency lasting beyond 1 month of age following the use of oxygen and ventilatory support to treat neonatal respiratory distress.
- Cystic fibrosis is a genetic disorder resulting in abnormal function of the exocrine glands. Pulmonary and pancreatic problems are the most common clinical features.
- Asthma is a disease of the airways characterized by increased responsiveness of the tracheobronchial tree to various stimuli. Widespread narrowing of the airways occurs when these stimuli are encountered. Asthma is episodic in nature with relatively normal lung function between attacks.
- Bronchiectasis is a permanent abnormal dilation and distortion of one or more bronchi. Large amounts of mucopurulent sputum are usually produced, and recurrent pulmonary infections and hemoptysis are common.
- Chronic bronchitis (airway disease) is defined as hypersecretion of mucus sufficient to produce a productive cough on most days for 3 months during 2 consecutive years.
- Emphysema (alveolar disease) is an abnormal and permanent enlargement of the air spaces distal to the terminal nonrespiratory bronchioles accompanied by destruction of alveolar walls.
- Pulmonary diseases frequently coexist. Three common combinations are asthmatic bronchitis, chronic bronchitis with emphysema, and cystic fibrosis with bronchiectasis.
- Common signs of obstructive pulmonary disease include chronic cough, expectoration of mucus, wheezing, and dyspnea on exertion.
- Clinical signs of infection in pulmonary disease include increased cough, increased sputum production, fever, increased respiratory rate, and change in auscultatory findings.

References

1. Thurlbeck WM. Pathology of chronic airflow obstruction. Chest 97 (Suppl): 6s–10s, 1990.
2. O'Brodovich HM, Mellins RB. Bronchopulmonary dysplasia. Unresolved neonatal lung injury. Am Rev Respir Dis 132: 694–709, 1985.
3. Wedig KE, Bruce MC, Martin RJ, Fanaroff AA. Bronchopulmonary dysplasia. In: Nussbaum E, Galant S (eds). Pediatric Respiratory Disorders: Clinical Approaches. Orlando, Fla, Grune & Stratton, 1984, pp. 83–90.
4. Martin RJ, Davis PB. Relationship of neonatal and childhood lung disease to adult COPD. In: Cherniack NS (ed). Chronic Obstructive Pulmonary Disease. Philadelphia, WB Saunders, 1991, pp 286–293.
5. Katz R, McWilliams B. Bronchopulmonary dysplasia in the pediatric intensive care unit. Crit Care Clin 4:755–787, 1988.
6. Voyles JB. Bronchopulmonary dysplasia. Am J Nurs 81(3): 510–514, 1981.
7. Taghizadeh A, Reynolds EOR. Pathogenesis of bronchopulmonary dysplasia following hyaline membrane disease. Am J Pathol 82:241–256, 1976.
8. Heimler R, Hoffman RG, Starshak RJ, et al. Chronic lung disease in premature infants: A retrospective evaluation of underlying factors. Crit Care Med 16:1213–1217, 1988.
9. Watts JL, Ariagno RI, Brady JP. Chronic pulmonary disease in neonates after artificial ventilation: Distribution of ventilation and pulmonary interstitial emphysema. Pediatrics 60: 273, 1977.
10. Tepper RS, Morgan WJ, Cota K, Taussig LM. Expiratory flow limitation in infants with bronchopulmonary dysplasia. J Pediatr 109:1040–1046, 1986.
11. Smyth JA, Tabachnik E, Duncan WJ, et al. Pulmonary function and bronchial hyperactivity in long-term survivors of bronchopulmonary dysplasia. Pediatrics 68:336–340, 1981.
12. Phelan PD, Landau LI, Olinsky A. Neonatal respiratory disorders. In: Phelan PD, Landau LI, Olinsky A (eds). Respiratory Illness in Children. 3rd ed. Melbourne, Blackwell Scientific Publications, 1990, pp 17–21.
13. Meisels J, Plunkett JW, Roloff DW, et al. Growth and development of pre-term infants with respiratory distress syndrome and bronchopulmonary dysplasia. Pediatrics 77:345–352, 1986.
14. Bader D, Ramos AD, Lew CD, et al. Childhood sequelae of infant lung disease. Exercise and pulmonary function abnormalities after bronchopulmonary dysplasia. J Pediatr 110:693–699, 1987.
15. Davis PB. Cystic Fibrosis: A major cause of obstructive airways disease in the young. In: Cherniack NS (ed). Chronic Obstructive Pulmonary Disease. Philadelphia, WB Saunders, 1991, pp 297–307.
16. Iannuzzi MC, Collins FS. Genetic defect in cystic fibrosis. In: Fishman AP (ed). Update: Pulmonary Diseases and Disorders. New York, McGraw-Hill, 1992, pp 83–92.

17. Scanlin TF. Cystic fibrosis. In: Fishman AP (ed). Pulmonary Diseases and Disorders. Vol. 2. 2nd ed. New York, McGraw-Hill, 1988, pp 1273–1294.

18. Davis PB, di Sant'Agnese PA. Diagnosis and treatment of cystic fibrosis: An update. Chest 85:802–809, 1984.

19. McFadden ER Jr. Asthma: General features, pathogenesis, and pathophysiology. In: Fishman AP (ed). Pulmonary Diseases and Disorders. Vol. 2. 2nd ed. McGraw-Hill, 1988, pp 1295–1310.

20. Murray RK, Panettieri RA. Management of Asthma: The Changing Approach. In: Fishman AP (ed). Update: Pulmonary Diseases and Disorders. New York, McGraw-Hill, 1992, pp 67–82.

21. Costello JF. Asthma. In: Hinshaw HC, Murray JF (eds). Diseases of the Chest. 4th ed. Philadelphia, WB Saunders, 1980, pp 525–559.

22. Swartz MN. Bronchiectasis. In: Fishman AP (ed). Pulmonary Diseases and Disorders. Vol. 2. 2nd ed. New York, McGraw-Hill, 1988, pp 1553–1581.

23. Davis AL, Salzman SH. Bronchiectasis. In: Cherniack NS (ed). Chronic Obstructive Pulmonary Disease. Philadelphia, WB Saunders, 1991, pp 316–338.

24. Petty TL. Chronic obstructive pulmonary disease—Can we do better? Chest 97 (Suppl): 2s–5s, 1990.

25. Reid LM. Chronic obstructive pulmonary diseases. In: Fishman AP (ed). Pulmonary Diseases and Disorders. Vol. 2. 2nd ed. New York, McGraw-Hill, 1988, pp 1247–1272.

26. Wanner A. The role of mucus in chronic obstructive pulmonary disease. Chest 97 (Suppl): 11s–15s, 1990.

27. Hinshaw HC, Murray JF. Chronic bronchitis and emphysema. In: Diseases of the Chest. 4th ed. Philadelphia, WB Saunders, 1980, pp 560–590.

28. Tager IB. Chronic bronchitis. In: Fishman AP (ed). Pulmonary Diseases and Disorders. Vol. 2. 2nd ed. New York, McGraw-Hill, 1988, pp 1543–1551.

29. Higgins ITT. Epidemiology of bronchitis and emphysema. In: Fishman AP (ed). Pulmonary Diseases and Disorders. Vol. 2. 2nd ed. New York, McGraw-Hill, 1988, pp 1237–1246.

30. Senior RM, Kuhn C III. The pathogenesis of emphysema. In: Fishman AP (ed). Pulmonary Diseases and Disorders. Vol. 2. 2nd ed. New York, McGraw-Hill, 1988, pp 1209–1218.

31. Zadai CC. Rehabilitation of the patient with chronic obstructive pulmonary disease. In: Irwin S, Tecklin JS (eds). Cardiopulmonary Physical Therapy. St. Louis, CV Mosby, 1985, pp 367–381.

Cardiopulmonary Implications of Specific Diseases

Joanne Watchie

INTRODUCTION

Many diseases of body systems other than the heart and lungs also affect cardiopulmonary function. Some, like hypertension or neuromuscular diseases, have obvious associations with cardiopulmonary dysfunction; others, such as rheumatoid arthritis and the other collagen vascular diseases, are not routinely associated with cardiac and pulmonary manifestations. This chapter will present

285

the cardiopulmonary effects of a number of specific diseases and medical problems as well as their clinical implications for physical therapy intervention. The medical information presented is merely a synopsis of current knowledge and therefore is meant only as an introduction to this area. The amount of detail provided is generally proportional to the frequency with which clinicians are likely to encounter each diagnosis. The goal is to emphasize the potential for cardiopulmonary dysfunction in patients with the described diagnoses and to suggest appropriate modifications of treatment procedures. Further reading may be necessary for the physical therapist who treats a patient with one of these diagnoses.

HYPERTENSION

Hypertension (HTN) is diagnosed when diastolic blood pressure (DBP) equals or exceeds 90 mm Hg or when systolic blood pressure (SBP) is consistently higher than 140 mm Hg, with values of 130 to 139/85 to 89 mm Hg being considered high normal, as shown in Table 7–1.[1] Labile HTN refers to blood pressure (BP) that fluctuates between hypertensive and normal values. Usually individuals with HTN have elevated levels of both **systolic** and **diastolic blood pressure;** however, isolated systolic hypertension (ISH), which occurs when SBP exceeds 140 mm Hg but DBP remains within the normal range, becomes increasingly

more common in the elderly.[2, 3] Approximately 90 to 95% of individuals with HTN have no discernible cause for their disease and are said to have **primary** or **essential hypertension.** The remainder have **secondary hypertension** resulting from another identifiable medical problem, such as renovascular or endocrine disease.

Despite much research, the etiology of essential HTN continues to be unknown. Both genetic and environmental factors, such as dietary sodium excess, stress, obesity, and alcohol consumption, have been implicated. Regardless of the underlying cause(s), the result is a failure of one or more of the control mechanisms that are responsible for lowering BP when it becomes elevated.

The major determinants of arterial blood pressure are cardiac output and total peripheral resistance. If either one, or both, of these factors becomes elevated, blood pressure will rise. However, both cardiac output and total peripheral resistance are determined by a number of other factors (see Fig. 7–1). Cardiac output is the product of heart rate and stroke volume; yet, each of those factors has several determinants, as described in Chapter 2. Similarly, total peripheral resistance (TPR) is affected by several variables, including the caliber of the arteriolar bed, the viscosity of the blood, and the elasticity of the arterial walls.

Thus, there are many physiologic pathways where abnormal function can result in high blood pressure, and many of these share a number of common features, as shown in Figure 7–1. Furthermore, it is probable that the mechanisms that are responsible for initiating HTN differ from those that serve to maintain it. For example, there is evidence that many individuals with labile or early mild HTN have increased cardiac output, probably related to enhanced activity of the sympathetic nervous system and apparently normal peripheral resistance.[4, 5] However, later when HTN

Table 7–1
Blood Pressure Levels for Adults*

CATEGORY	SYSTOLIC (mm Hg)	DIASTOLIC (mm Hg)
Normal	<130	<85
High normal	130–139	85–89
Hypertension		
Stage 1 (mild)	140–159	90–99
Stage 2 (moderate)	160–179	100–109
Stage 3 (severe)	≥180	≥110

*These values are for adults aged 18 years and older who are not taking antihypertensive medications and are not acutely ill.
Source: The Sixth Report of the Joint National Committee on the Detection, Evaluation, and Treatment of High Blood Pressure. *Arch Intern Med* 157:2413–2445, 1997.

Clinical Note: Detecting Hypertension
It is important for the clinician to keep in mind that hypertension often goes undetected for many years. Labile hypertension can be particularly difficult to identify because multiple blood pressure measurements must be made to diagnose hypertension. Mild to moderate elevations in blood pressure are usually not symptomatic.

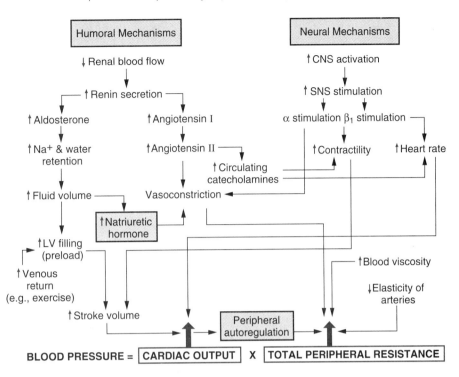

Figure 7-1. Factors contributing to elevated blood pressure. Because blood pressure is a product of cardiac output and peripheral resistance, any influence that increases either of these factors results in a rise in blood pressure. The enclosed boxes identify some of the proposed mechanisms involved in the pathogenesis of essential hypertension. Note the number of interrelationships among the different mechanisms. CNS, central nervous system; SNS, sympathetic nervous system; LV, left ventricle; ↑, increased; ↓, decreased.

becomes established, the classic findings of elevated TPR and normal or decreased cardiac output are found.[5]

The consequences of HTN are directly related to the level of BP, even within the accepted normal range. Actuarial data reveal that persons with diastolic BPs of 88 to 92 mm Hg have a 32 to 36% higher mortality rate over 20 years of follow-up than those with diastolic pressures less than 80 mm Hg.[6] Higher systolic BP levels at any given level of DBP have also been associated with an increased morbidity rate in both men and women.[3, 7–9] The most common complications of HTN include **atherosclerotic heart disease,** congestive heart failure, cerebrovascular accidents, renal failure, **dissecting aneurysm, peripheral vascular disease,** and **retinopathy.**

Hypertensive Heart Disease

Regardless of its etiology and pathophysiologic mechanisms, HTN produces a pressure overload on the left ventricle (LV), which is compensated for by left ventricular hypertrophy (LVH).[10] Initially, normal systolic LV function is maintained by the hypertrophied LV. However diastolic dysfunc-

tion with impairment of LV relaxation develops early in the course of essential HTN.[11–14] The combination of LVH and diastolic dysfunction leads to reduced LV compliance (i.e., a stiffer LV), which creates a greater load on the left atrium and resultant left atrial enlargement. In addition, LVH alters the equilibrium between the oxygen supply and demand of the myocardium. Coronary reserve is reduced in patients with HTN and LVH, even in the absence of any coronary artery stenosis.[12, 15] Thus, there is a predisposition toward myocardial ischemia and ventricular dysrhythmias. Superimposed is the role of HTN as a major risk factor for atherosclerotic heart disease (ASHD), as discussed in Chapter 3. This interaction makes it difficult to differentiate between the ischemic effects of ASHD and hypertensive heart disease.

If adequate LV filling volume is not achieved, either due to reduced filling times associated with higher heart rates or arrhythmias in which active atrial contraction is missing (e.g., atrial fibrillation, nodal rhythm, frequent premature ventricular beats), stroke volume will diminish. Thus, symptoms of inadequate **cardiac output,** such as lightheadedness or dizziness, dyspnea, and impaired exercise tolerance, can result from diastolic dysfunction rather than impaired systolic function.[16, 17]

However, as HTN becomes more severe or prolonged, impairment of systolic function may also develop, appearing as subnormal LV functional reserve initially during exercise and later at rest.[18-21]

Although normal cardiac output may be maintained for some time at the expense of pulmonary congestion, the ultimate consequence of progressive LVH is the development of left ventricular failure, as shown in Figure 7–2. A number of factors, such as further elevation of BP, increased venous return, or impaired contractile function, may precipitate decompensation and overt LV failure.

Treatment of Hypertension

The goals of antihypertensive therapy are to normalize blood pressure both at rest and during exertion and to reverse LVH and the myocardial dysfunction it creates.[1, 22-25] Pharmacologic therapy is the most commonly prescribed intervention in the

management of HTN. However, the latest medical guidelines recommend beginning with lifestyle modifications in most patients diagnosed with HTN.[1] The most effective modifications have proved to be weight reduction, sodium restriction, moderation of alcohol intake, and regular aerobic exercise.[26, 27] Although these interventions may not eliminate the need for antihypertensive medications in most patients, they often permit a lower dosage of medications to be used, thus reducing the potential for adverse side effects. In addition, because HTN tends to cluster with other coronary risk factors, such as dyslipidemia, insulin resistance, glucose intolerance, and obesity,[3] some of the interventions, such as aerobic exercise and weight reduction, by virtue of their effect on more than one factor, may significantly reduce the risk of cardiovascular disease and death.

The medications used to treat HTN fall into the following major categories: diuretics, beta-adrenergic blockers, alpha-adrenergic blockers, vasodilators, centrally acting adrenergic antagonists, cal-

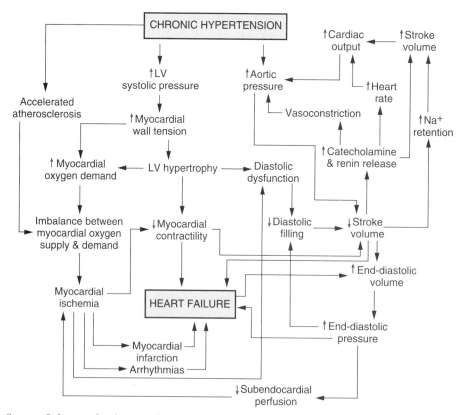

Figure 7–2. Some of the mechanisms and interrelationships in hypertension that may lead to the development of left ventricle (LV) failure. Repeating cycles tend to aggravate the problem. ↑, Increased; ↓, decreased.

cium-channel blockers, and angiotensin-converting enzyme (ACE) inhibitors. A summary of their antihypertensive effects and exercise interactions is provided in Table 7–2.[28–31] Many of these drugs have additional cardiovascular effects and side effects and may be used to treat other clinical problems. In addition, there are several new classes of antihypertensive agents, such as renin inhibitors

Table 7–2

The Antihypertensive Effects and Exercise Interactions of the Different Classes of Medications Used to Treat Hypertension

MEDICATIONS	ANTIHYPERTENSIVE ACTION	EFFECTS ON EXERCISE	SIDE EFFECTS Re EXERCISE
Beta blockers	↓ HR and contractility ↓ Renin secretion	↓ HR, ↓ SBP ↓ Ischemic ST-T changes ↓ Angina ↑ Ex. capacity in pts with angina ↓ Or ↔ ex. capacity if no angina ⊕ Training responses ? ↓ Arrhythmias May be ↑ BP during isometric ex.	Bronchospasm May mask S&S of hypoglycemia in DM ↑ Claudication Muscle fatigue and cramps ↑ K+ (hyperkalemia) Beta-blocker withdrawal
Diuretics Thiazides, loop diuretics	↓ Peripheral resistance ↓ Plasma volume	↔ Or moderate ↓ BP response ↔ HR ↔ Ex. capacity ↔ ECG	Hypokalemia → ST depression, ↑ ventricular ectopy, muscle fatigue and cramps, weakness Hypomagnesemia → PVCs Excessive diuresis → ↑ ex.-induced tachycardia, ↑ postural hypotension
K+-sparing diuretics	Same	Same	Hyperkalemia → ↑ arrhythmias
Alpha-adrenergic blockers Alpha1 Alpha2	↓ Peripheral resistance Same + ↓ CO	↓ SBP and DBP ↔ HR ↔ Ex. capacity Same	Orthostatic hypotension Post-ex. hypotension Same + Reflex tachycardia
Centrally acting alpha-adrenergic agonists	↓ Central and/or peripheral outflow of catecholamines → ↓ Plasma norepinephrine	↓ Plasma norepinephrine ↓ Or ↔ HR ↓ BP ↔ Ex. capacity ↓ Or ↔ BP response to isometric ex.	Rebound HTN on withdrawal of drug Post-ex. hypotension, dizziness, syncope
Ca2+-channel blockers	Vasodilatation	↓ BP ↓ HR (× nifedipine ↑ HR) ↓ Ischemic ST-T changes ↑ Ex. tolerance in pts with angina ↔ Ex. tolerance if no angina	Orthostatic hypotension
ACE inhibitors	Inhibits formation of angiotensin II → ↓ vasoconstriction	↓ BP ↔ Ex. tolerance	

HR = heart rate, BP = blood pressure, CO = cardiac output, SBP = systolic blood pressure, DBP = diastolic blood pressure, ex. = exercise, pts = patients, S&S = signs and symptoms, DM = diabetes mellitus, HTN = hypertension, ACE = angiotensin-converting enzyme, → = resulting in, ↑ = increased, ↓ = decreased, ↔ = little or no change, ⊕ = positive.

and angiotensin II antagonists, which are currently under investigation.[32] For more complete information on these drugs, refer to Chapter 14.

Hypertension and Exercise

Research involving hypertensive individuals has revealed that exercise capacity is reduced by 15 to 30%, even in those who are asymptomatic, when compared with age- and fitness-matched control subjects.[19, 33, 34] Stroke volume increases subnormally and peak heart rate is lower; therefore, cardiac output is decreased. There is some evidence that these changes may be due to diastolic dysfunction and impaired coronary flow reserve.[15, 19] In addition, exercise time and anaerobic threshold are also reduced.

BP measurements during exertion provide an indication of the balance between cardiac output and total peripheral resistance. The normal BP response to dynamic exercise is a rise in SBP that is proportional to the workload (approximately 7 to 10 mm Hg per MET) and little or no change in DBP ($\pm$ 10 mm Hg).[35] These responses are due to increasing cardiac output and a drop in TPR. However, once activity reaches an intensity that is predominantly anaerobic, the pressor response becomes more marked. Isometric exercise or exercise involving a small muscle mass (i.e., one arm) typically elicits minimal incremental changes in SBP and greater increases in DBP because of minimal rise in cardiac output and higher TPR.[36]

Persons with HTN frequently display abnormal BP responses to exertion.[34, 37, 38] Some individuals with normal or borderline BP values at rest develop excessive increases in systolic or diastolic BP during activity, indicating a failure to adequately reduce TPR during dynamic exercise or an excessive increase in TPR during isometric exercise. This is particularly true for emergency response team members, such as police officers and firefighters, who produce large bursts of sympathetic nervous system activity in response to an alarm. After a period of time, this physiologic response may become generalized to any stressful situation, including physical exertion, and hypertensive BP responses, especially diastolic, are frequently observed during exercise. Those with moderate HTN typically exhibit exaggerated BP responses to isometric exercise and often to isotonic exercise owing to a blunted decrease in TPR during exercise

compared to normotensive individuals.[34, 38] Additionally, they may have an impaired ability to increase cardiac output appropriately with greater demands.[18, 39] Finally, individuals with more severe HTN may display further impairment of cardiac output during exercise and more marked increases in TPR[18, 40] The net effect of these two opposing factors on BP will determine whether SBP becomes excessively increased or appears as a more normal response; DBP responses may be hypertensive.

Treatment of HTN with medications may modify the physiologic responses to exercise. Antihypertensive medications lower resting BP, but many do not maintain the same degree of effectiveness during exertion, especially with isometric activities.[18, 38, 41, 42] Thus, patients on antihypertensive medications may have acceptable BP levels at rest but display exaggerated responses to exercise. Furthermore, some of the drugs have side effects that are affected by or have an effect upon exercise, as shown in Table 7–2. Of particular concern is the **hypokalemia** that can be induced by diuretic therapy using the thiazides and loop diuretics. When combined with the systemic demands of exercise, hypokalemia can precipitate dangerous arrhythmias, skeletal muscle fatigue and cramps, weakness, and occasionally other problems. The potassium-sparing diuretics and beta blockers are associated with a greater risk of **hyperkalemia,** which can also cause arrhythmias.

A great deal of research has been directed at assessing the efficacy of exercise training for the treatment of HTN. Although the data are not consistent, the general consensus is that reductions of approximately 10 mm Hg in both systolic and diastolic BP can be achieved through exercise training in the hypertensive population. These reductions are significant enough to allow some patients to avoid or discontinue drug treatment and many others to reduce their drug dosages.[38, 43–47] In addition, exercise training has been demonstrated to

---

Clinical Note: Compliance with Exercise

The problem with exercise training as a treatment for hypertension is the high percentage of dropouts from exercise programs, or noncompliance. The effects of exercise training on blood pressure are maintained only as long as the individual remains compliant with the exercise program.

cause a significant regression of left ventricular hypertrophy.[48]

Implications for Physical Therapy Intervention

According to some estimates, approximately 40 to 50 million Americans, including nearly a third of all black adults and more than half of all adults over age 60, have high blood pressure, and a third of this population does not even know they have it.[49, 50] The prevalence of HTN increases with age. Therefore, the percentage of patients referred to physical therapy (PT) who may have recognized or unrecognized HTN is very high. Patients with any of the following diagnoses are particularly likely to have HTN: stroke, diabetes, coronary artery disease, aortic aneurysm, peripheral vascular disease, obesity, renal failure, and alcoholism. In addition, patients with chronic pain syndromes and those in high stress occupations, such as air traffic controllers, fire fighters, and middle-level and upper-level managers, may be at higher risk for HTN.

With the growing trend toward independent practice, PT may represent the mode of entry into the medical care system for a number of adults. This fact, combined with the prevalence of HTN, supports the need for inclusion of BP monitoring during the PT evaluation and treatment of all adults over the age of 35. In addition to the valuable information this might provide for both the client and the physician, the positive professional image created could improve acceptance by the medical community of the PT position as an independent health care provider. Furthermore, when a client with diagnosed HTN is seen for PT, the clinician should question the client about prescribed treatments, determine the level of compliance, and reinforce the importance of strict adherence. If the client complains of unpleasant side effects of a particular medication, he or she should be encouraged to discuss them with the physician so that a different medication can be prescribed. With so many antihypertensive agents available, most patients can receive comfortable and effective treatment.

Because BP values vary considerably during the day, it is beneficial to include monitoring during two to three different treatment sessions. Also, inasmuch as BP can be normal or borderline at rest

but become excessively elevated during exertion, it is important to monitor BP during exercise as well as at rest. The techniques for proper monitoring of BP are described in Chapter 16, but a few points that are particularly relevant to the detection and monitoring of HTN deserve emphasis here. First, proper cuff size is essential to accuracy: a cuff that is too narrow will produce a reading that is falsely elevated and one that is too wide will yield a reading that is erroneously low. Second, because there may be an **"auscultatory gap"** of up to 40 mm Hg after the first audible sounds, it is especially important to palpate for the disappearance of the radial pulse as the cuff is inflated and then continue inflation for another 30 mm Hg; otherwise, the SBP may be significantly underestimated. Third, the arm should be relaxed and supported at the level of the heart. If the arm is lower than the heart or if the arm muscles are not relaxed, the BP readings, both systolic and diastolic, will be erroneously high. When the arms are so large or misshapen that a conventional cuff does not fit properly, BP measurements will not be accurate; as an alternative, a standard BP cuff can be placed on the forearm and auscultation or palpation performed over the radial artery at the wrist.[51] Finally, a word of caution regarding the use of automated BP measurement devices during exertion: they are often both inaccurate and unreliable, tending to overestimate SBP and underestimate DBP during exercise with standard errors two to three times that of the manual method.[52–55]

If the resting BP is excessively high (SBP over 200 mm Hg or DBP above 105 to 110 mm Hg), physician clearance should be obtained before continuing with the PT evaluation or treatment. Furthermore, any evidence of target organ damage secondary to HTN, such as retinopathy, renal disease, or LVH, necessitates that BP be controlled both at rest and during exercise prior to PT intervention. Exercise should be terminated if BP becomes excessively high (SBP over 250 mm Hg or DBP over 110 mm Hg.)[28] The risk of myocardial ischemia during exercise is enhanced in individuals with HTN, especially those with evidence of LVH, and **angina** may occur. Furthermore, if LV function is impaired, **LV end-diastolic volume** and **pressure,** and therefore intrapulmonary pressures, will rise during exercise, resulting in shortness of breath.

As mentioned previously, the diastolic dysfunction that commonly occurs in HTN may impair LV filling, which becomes more clinically significant with advancing age and at higher heart rates. Many elderly patients with HTN may develop symptoms of inadequate cardiac output due to poor filling of their stiff hearts rather than impaired pump function. Some atrial and nodal arrhythmias and frequent premature ventricular complexes also reduce LV filling. Patients tolerate exercise better if their arrhythmias are controlled and if exercise intensity and heart rate (HR) responses are appropriately modulated.

Physical therapists must also consider the side effects of antihypertensive medications when designing and implementing treatment programs. The most common side effect of medications used to treat hypertension is hypotension, especially orthostatic hypotension. Caution is advised during PT treatments that result in vasodilatation, and especially during heat modalities such as the whirlpool or Hubbard tank. Moderate to vigorous exercise of large muscle groups can produce significant vasodilatation and can result in hypotension, particularly following exercise when venous return diminishes as exercise is abruptly ceased. Likewise, stationary standing, as in performing many activities of daily living, can result in venous pooling and hypotension. Finally, it is important to exercise caution when making sudden changes of position and so avoid loss of balance and falls. For patients who frequently experience orthostatic hypotension, offering encouragement to repeatedly dorsiflex the feet before standing can ameliorate symptoms by promoting greater venous return to the heart, increasing ventricular filling and stroke volume, and raising the BP.

Avoidance of breath holding and the **Valsalva maneuver,** which frequently occur during isokinetic exercise and stabilization activities, especially the "hands-and-knees" position, is particularly important in patients with HTN. The abrupt increase in BP that is associated with the Valsalva maneuver may be dangerous in these patients. As in any well-rounded exercise program, strength training is valuable for those with HTN; however, low resistances and high repetitions should be prescribed to avoid excessive BP responses.[56] Resistance training should not serve as the sole exercise training modality for persons with HTN, because it has not been shown consistently to lower BP.

Endurance training should be prescribed as part of a comprehensive PT treatment program to improve both functional capacity and hypertensive control. Aerobic exercise training can produce significant decreases (about 10 to 20 mm Hg) in both systolic and diastolic resting BP. The rise in SBP that occurs during exercise is attenuated with training. Endurance training should consist of aerobic activities, such as brisk walking, jogging, swimming, and cycling, performed at least 4 days per week for 30 to 45 minutes per session. As with other populations, typical training intensities of 60 to 85% of maximum HR may be used, but there is some evidence that lower intensities may elicit greater reductions in BP than higher intensities.[44, 57, 58] When lower training intensities are used (40 to 60%), the duration or the frequency of exercise should probably be increased so that exercise is performed for 45 to 60 minutes five or six times a week leaving at least one day of rest.

In designing an exercise prescription for clients with HTN, the standard HR formulas can be utilized when the HR response to exercise is not altered by medications (e.g., beta blockers).[57] Alternatively, a **rate of perceived exertion** (RPE) **scale** (see Chapter 16) can be used with patients, especially those who take medications that affect HR, as an indicator of exercise intensity.[59, 60] The results of an exercise stress test, if available, can be very helpful if the patient was evaluated while taking current medications. Finally, per the recommendations for physical activity issued by the Centers for Disease Control and Prevention and the American College of Sports Medicine,[61] clients should be encouraged to increase their general level of physical activity, including household chores and social, recreational, and occupational activities. Research has shown that any increase in physical activity, even in short bouts, can have health benefits. The goal is to accumulate 30 minutes or more of moderate-intensity physical activity on most days of the week.[56]

Clinical Note: Orthostatic Hypotension

Orthostatic hypotension is defined as a drop in systolic (and often diastolic) blood pressure when assuming an upright position, which often renders the individual symptomatic (dizzy, lightheaded, and sometimes passing out). It is *not* the same as a hypotensive blood pressure response to activity.

DIABETES MELLITUS

Diabetes mellitus (DM) is a chronic metabolic disorder characterized by **hyperglycemia** and caused by inadequate insulin production or ineffective insulin action. Abnormalities in the metabolism of carbohydrates, fats and proteins result. In addition, there are vascular and neuropathic components to DM, which result in abnormalities in both large vessels (macroangiopathy) and small vessels (microangiopathy) and in the **peripheral** and **autonomic nervous systems.**

There are two types of DM: type I or **insulin-dependent DM** (IDDM) and type II or **non–insulin-dependent DM** (NIDDM), which differ in etiology, clinical presentation, and pathophysiology.[62, 63] Additionally, a number of disorders are associated with secondary DM, such as pancreatic diseases (e.g., **hemochromatosis, pancreatitis, cystic fibrosis**), hormonal syndromes (e.g., **acromegaly, Cushing's syndrome, pheochromocytoma**), and drug-induced DM (e.g., Dilantin, glucocorticoids, estrogens).

Type I DM usually develops before early adulthood as a result of autoimmune destruction of the insulin-producing pancreatic beta cells.[64] The result is little or no **endogenous** insulin production. These patients develop extreme hyperglycemia, **ketosis** (the presence of ketone bodies in the blood), and the associated symptomatology, making their survival dependent upon insulin therapy.

Type II DM is considered a heterogeneous disorder which usually presents later in life (rarely before the age of 40) and is associated with obesity (70 to 90% of patients), lack of exercise, and familial tendency. Although endogenous insulin production is relatively preserved and may even be excessive in NIDDM, the great majority of patients are insulin-resistant at the cellular level because of receptor or postreceptor defects. Hyperglycemia results from an increased rate of hepatic glucose production as a consequence of hepatic insulin resistance. Ketosis is extremely rare in this group owing to the presence of at least some effective insulin.

Insulin and Glucose Physiology

The major actions of insulin are the inhibition of glucose production by the liver and the promotion of glucose transport across the cell membrane and its subsequent metabolism within the cell. Insulin also plays a role in the synthesis of glycogen, fat, and protein. Insulin deficiency results in an inability to utilize glucose as fuel, impaired protein metabolism, and increased fat mobilization with increased levels of **free fatty acids** (FFA) in the blood. When the FFAs are metabolized in the liver, ketone bodies are formed and **ketoacidosis** may develop.

A number of anti-insulin or counterregulatory hormones also participate in the regulation of glucose metabolism: **glucagon, growth hormone, cortisol,** and **catecholamines.** Of these, glucagon plays the most important role in terms of DM, in which its levels are absolutely or relatively increased. Glucagon release is stimulated by hypoglycemia, amino acids, neural influences, and stress. In the liver, it promotes the conversion of glycogen to glucose (**glycogenolysis**), the formation of glucose or glycogen from proteins and fats (**gluconeogenesis**), and the production of ketone bodies (**ketogenesis**).

Normally, physical activity induces a reduction in insulin secretion and enhanced secretion of the counterregulatory hormones, which result in stimulation of hepatic glucose production and enhanced mobilization of muscle glycogen and FFAs. Reduced insulin secretion is compensated for by a heightened sensitivity and responsiveness of the peripheral tissues to insulin. Hepatic glucose production intensifies according to glucose requirements so that blood glucose levels remain nearly constant despite large increases in glucose uptake. In diabetes, particularly IDDM, the metabolic responses to exercise are altered, as will be discussed later in this chapter.

Treatment of Diabetes

The major goal of treatment for DM is to control hyperglycemia. Achieving good control of blood glucose levels prevents acute metabolic derangements and is associated with lower morbidity and mortality rates in this disease.[65–67] Treatment is individualized and varies according to the type of DM; it may include education, diet changes, insulin therapy, oral hypoglycemic agents, and exercise. In addition, pancreas and islet cell transplantation are currently under investigation for patients with IDDM.[68]

Table 7–3

Insulin Preparations—Basic Types and Their Properties

CLASS	TYPE	ONSET	PEAK EFFECT (hr)	DURATION (hr)
Rapid acting	Regular, crystalline (CZI)	30–60 min	2–4	6–8
	Semilente	60–90 min	2–6	6–8
Intermediate acting	Neutral protamine (NPH), isophane	60–90 min	6–12	18–24
	Lente	60–90 min	6–12	18–24
Long acting	Protamine zinc (PZI)	4–8 hr	14–24	36
	Ultralente	4–8 hr	18–24	36

For patients with type I DM, insulin therapy is necessary and can be provided in a variety of forms. The most common insulin therapy consists of daily injections of insulin preparations, which are listed in Table 7–3. Usually some combination of short-, intermediate-, or long-acting insulin is used in an attempt to mimic a normal physiologic insulin profile with maintenance of basal insulin levels between meals and at night and sharp peaks at mealtimes (see Figs. 7–3 and 7–4).[69, 70] When compared to the normal insulin profile, it can be seen that patients using insulin injections often oscillate between states of insulin excess and insulin deficiency.

Intensive insulin therapy can be undertaken using multiple daily injections or **continuous subcutaneous insulin infusion** (CSII), which involves the use of an open loop insulin pump to provide a constant basal level of insulin along with preprandial boluses, in order to achieve more normal glycemic control. Both of these forms of treatment require frequent self-monitoring of blood glucose

levels (at least prior to each meal and at bedtime) so that the dosage of insulin can be adjusted according to pattern of need, size of impending meal, and anticipated exercise or activity level. The CSII pumps have come into vogue and are being used increasingly for treatment during elite sports participation. Finally, implantable insulin pumps have become available but are limited by complications, such a blockages of the intraperitoneal catheter, which require a significant number of repeat surgical procedures.[71, 72]

Hypoglycemia is the major problem associated with insulin therapy, because the level of available insulin can exceed the individual's need at times, especially during the hour or so immediately prior to mealtime. The risk of hypoglycemia increases when a meal is delayed or skipped or during strenuous or unexpected physical activity. In addition, unexpected episodes of hypoglycemia may occur because of variability in insulin activity due to the presence of insulin antibodies, which can cause insulin binding and resistance, as well as allergic reactions.[68]

During the 1990s, pancreas and islet cell transplantation have assumed a greater role in the treatment of type I DM.[73–77] Because of the need for long-term immunosuppression, with its increased risk of infection, malignancy such as lymphoma, and specific drug toxicity, pancreas transplantation is offered mainly to patients who also require immunosuppression for renal transplantation. Although there are increased surgical morbidity and mortality rates when the pancreas is also transplanted, reductions in some diabetic microvascular complications and dramatic improvements in quality of life due to complete insulin independence are significant benefits of this treatment. The net effects of pancreas/islet cell transplantation on long-term diabetic complications

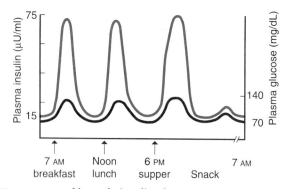

Figure 7–3. Normal insulin-glucose interrelationships throughout the day. Top line (color), plasma insulin level; bottom line (black), plasma glucose level. (From Kozak GP. Clinical Diabetes Mellitus. Philadelphia, WB Saunders, 1982, p 77.)

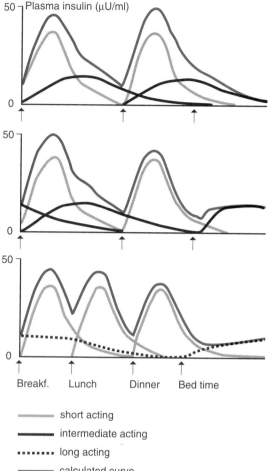

Insulin therapy regimens

short acting
intermediate acting
long acting
calculated curve

Figure 7–4. Some common insulin therapy regimens and the insulin levels they produce. The calculated curve is the sum of the plasma insulin levels derived from the combined insulin dosages. (From Krall LP [ed]. World Book of Diabetes in Practice, Vol. 3. Amsterdam, Elsevier Science Publishers BV, 1988, p 157.)

have yet to be determined. Investigations of islet cell transplantation have revealed a number of difficulties, particularly obtaining sufficient numbers of viable human islet cells (approximately 250,000 islet cells are needed to restore normoglycemia), complications related to the immunosuppressive drugs, and greater susceptibility to rejection compared with total pancreas transplantation. Research efforts are being directed at modifying the immunogenicity of islet and pancreas grafts to increase the success rates of these treatments.

The treatment of type II DM consists of diet, exercise, oral hypoglycemic agents, and sometimes insulin.[78-80] The cornerstones of treatment are diet and exercise, especially for the control of obesity. Oral hypoglycemic agents are reserved for patients who fail to control their hyperglycemia through diet and exercise (see Table 7–4). Some individuals who are not able to achieve adequate glycemic control with diet, exercise, and oral hypoglycemic agents benefit from treatment with injectable insulin, though usually only one or two doses of intermediate-acting insulin are required each day. Insulin may also be necessary during acute illness or stress situations, such as infection, myocardial infarction, trauma, and anesthesia.

The measurement of **glycosylated hemoglobin** (Hb-A_{1c}) is considered the "gold standard" as an indicator of the degree of glycemic control achieved by a diabetic over the preceding 60-day period. The test does not rely on the patient's ability to monitor or accurately record blood glucose levels, and it is not influenced by acute changes in blood glucose or by the interval since the last meal. During hyperglycemia, hemoglobin molecules become glycosylated (bound with glucose), which is a relatively irreversible process. Therefore, the level of Hb-A_{1c} within the red blood cells reflects the average level of glucose that the cell has been exposed to during its life cycle (about 120 days). Several assay methods have been developed that vary in their precision, so clinicians must become familiar with the method used at their facilities when evaluating the level of glycemic control in specific patients.

Diabetes and Exercise

Because of altered glucose and fat metabolism in individuals with DM, especially type I DM, their metabolic responses to exercise differ from those of nondiabetics. A number of important variables affect the metabolic responses to exercise in patients with IDDM: the exercise intensity, type, and duration; the type of insulin used; the injection site; the time between insulin injection and onset of exercise; and the time between exercise and the last meal. Furthermore, the metabolic responses to exercise are influenced by the level of insulin at the onset of exercise.[81-83] Commonly, there is an excess of insulin that inhibits hepatic glucose production and thus promotes the development of

Table 7-4

Oral Hypoglycemic Agents and Their Properties

MEDICATION	DURATION OF ACTION (hr)	DAILY DOSE (mg)	COMMON SIDE EFFECTS	RARE SIDE EFFECTS
Sulfonylureas			Hypoglycemia	Gastrointestinal, skin rash, liver abnormalities
Glipizide (Glucotrol)	10–30	2.5–40		
Glipizide XL (Glucotrol XL)		5–20		
Glyburide (Micronase, DiaBeta)	10–30	1.25–20		
Glyburide (micronized) (Glynase)	12–24	1.5–12		
Glymepride (Amaryl)		1–8		
Tolbutamide (Orinase, Oramide)	6–12	500–3000		
Chlorpropamide (Diabinese)	24–72	100–750		
Biguanide				
Metformin (Glucophage)	8–12	500–2500	Anorexia, nausea, abdominal discomfort, diarrhea	Lactic acidosis, pernicious anemia
Alpha-glucosidase inhibitor				
Acarbose (Precose)		75–300	Flatulence, diarrhea, abdominal cramps	

hypoglycemia. Factors associated with exercise-induced hypoglycemia include inadequate food intake preceding exercise, the rapid absorption of depot insulin from an injection site near exercising muscle, and exercising at the time of peak insulin effect. When there is an insulin deficiency with marked hyperglycemia (over 300 mg/dL) at the onset of exercise, glucose uptake by the exercising muscles will be impaired, and the additional glucose being produced by the liver will exceed peripheral utilization, resulting in even more marked hyperglycemia. The excessive mobilization of FFAs may lead to accelerated ketogenesis and ketoacidosis, which can cause coma and death.

Because patients with type I DM often have excessively high glucose levels following meals, and because exercise enhances glucose utilization by peripheral tissues, scheduling exercise to occur after meals seems practical. Although this timing works well for some patients, research has revealed that the glycemic responses to postprandial exercise are quite variable[84]; therefore, appropriate self-monitoring of blood glucose levels is indicated. There may be an increased risk of delayed hypoglycemia developing most commonly at 5 to 15 hours, but sometimes up to 24 or more hours

after the completion of exercise, especially following vigorous or prolonged exercise that is not done regularly.[85] These hypoglycemic episodes tend to occur at night, which may disturb sleep patterns and interfere with recovery, leading to significantly increased risk of morbidity/mortality versus complications, and including death, during physical activity the following day.[81]

Treatment with CSII appears to provide much more normal metabolic responses to exercise than standard insulin therapy. Because of the constant infusion of basal insulin, patients maintain steady-state plasma glucose levels throughout exercise as a result of appropriate muscle glucose uptake and hepatic glucose production. Thus, patients are even able to exercise before breakfast with minimal risk of hypoglycemia.[86] Studies have shown that reducing the action of the pump by 50% before exercise, similar to multiple injection regimens, prevents hypoglycemia.[81] The major disadvantages of CSII are the high incidence of catheter blockage and the vulnerability of the subcutaneous infusion site to trauma or disruption. Interuption of pump function for more than 2 hours can result in the relatively rapid development of insulin deficiency with hyperglycemia and ketosis.

Exercise plays a central role in the management of patients with type II DM due to its beneficial effects on glycemic control and weight loss. Research has documented a significant decrease in plasma glucose levels in patients with NIDDM following 45 minutes of moderate exercise, which may last as long as 12 to 16 hours following exercise.[87-89] For patients taking oral hypoglycemic drugs, especially the sulfonylureas, therefore, there may be some increased risk of hypoglycemia during or following prolonged exercise.[68, 78]

A number of studies have evaluated the effect of exercise training on the long-term metabolic control in both type I and type II DM. Most researchers have documented increased insulin sensitivity and favorable alterations in lipoprotein concentrations in both types of DM with exercise training.[90-95] Although improved glucose tolerance has been demonstrated in NIDDM patients following exercise training, the findings have not been consistent and the magnitude of improvement has been small and often only temporary.[90, 91, 94, 95] In patients with IDDM improved blood glucose control as measured by glycosylated hemoglobin has not been demonstrated.[96-98] However, the benefits of improved fitness level and modification of cardiovascular risk factors are sufficient reasons in and of themselves to encourage exercise training in patients with DM.

Cardiovascular and Pulmonary Complications of Diabetes

The organs most affected by DM are the eyes, kidneys, heart, and peripheral nerves. Complications develop in these organs as a result of microangiopathy with thickening or damage to the capillary basement membrane (e.g., retinopathy, nephropathy), macroangiopathy by atherosclerosis (e.g., coronary artery, cerebrovascular, and peripheral vascular disease), which tends to occur at an earlier age and with greater severity, and neuropathies involving the peripheral and autonomic nerves.[62, 68] The combination of peripheral neuropathy and arterial insufficiency leads to the frequent complications of tissue necrosis and infection, and sometimes lower extremity amputation. Because of the prevalence of

microangiopathy combined with macroangiopathy, vascular disease may be diffuse and not amenable to surgical intervention. However, there is strong evidence that good glycemic control can delay and possibly prevent the onset of retinopathy, nephropathy, and neuropathy.[63, 65, 67, 99, 100]

Cardiovascular disease is the major cause of complications and death in patients with both types of DM.[101, 102] Cardiovascular abnormalities that are more prevalent in diabetic patients include atherosclerotic heart disease, hypertension, defects in impulse conduction through the heart, congestive heart failure (CHF), autonomic neuropathy, cerebrovascular disease, and peripheral vascular disease.

Coronary artery disease (CAD), which probably results from both macro- and microangiopathy, is often diffuse and may present as angina pectoris, myocardial infarction, sudden death, and occasionally as unexplained left ventricular failure. Symptoms associated with myocardial ischemia and infarction are frequently atypical in DM: both may present "silently," that is, with little or no discomfort, or angina may appear as fatigue or dyspnea in the absence of pulmonary disease, which comes on with exertion and resolves within minutes with rest. The mortality rate associated with acute myocardial infarction (MI) is approximately two (in males) to three (in females) times that of nondiabetics.[102-104] The majority of deaths result from pump failure or arrhythmias and conduction disturbances and frequently occur up to 1 to 2 months after acute MI. Diabetics appear to have twice the risk of ventricular fibrillation, which often occurs after transfer from the cardiac care unit and is nearly always fatal.

Hypertension is approximately twice as prevalent in diabetics as in nondiabetics.[105] This finding is particularly significant because HTN accelerates both the microvascular and macrovascular complications of DM and causes irreversible myocardial damage.[106] Aggressive treatment of even borderline HTN is indicated in diabetics. However, effective treatment can be difficult to achieve in diabetics because many antihypertensive medications worsen glucose tolerance, increase lipids, or cause other severe side effects.

The incidence of congestive heart failure (CHF) is markedly increased in the diabetic population. CHF most commonly results from ASHD and hypertensive heart disease. In addition, CHF can occur in some diabetics who do not have significant coronary disease or HTN. This "diabetic cardiomyopathy" is associated with interstitial fibrosis and arteriolar hyalinization, and the degree of dysfunction is inversely related to the degree of metabolic control.[106, 107]

Autonomic defects are also very common in those with long-standing diabetes but individuals with autonomic dysfunction are often asymptomatic. Individuals who present with symptoms usually complain of postural hypotension. Autonomic dysfunction can involve predominantly the parasympathetic nervous system (PNS) or both the parasympathetic and sympathetic nervous systems.[108] The presence of autonomic neuropathy can be determined by observing the resting heart rate; the heart rate responses to the Valsalva maneuver, deep breathing, and standing; and the BP responses to standing and sustained handgrip. In patients with mainly PNS dysfunction, heart rate is elevated at rest and during the early phase of exercise, but as effort progresses, the normal activation of the sympathetic nervous system allows virtually normal HR and BP responses. However, in patients with combined defects, there is minimal HR response to stimuli, such as the Valsalva maneuver, standing up, and deep breathing, a fall in BP during standing, and blunted HR and BP responses to all phases of exercise. Techniques for assessing autonomic function are presented in the next section.

Other cardiovascular abnormalities are also observed in patients with DM. Sinus node dysfunction and AV conduction abnormalities are more common in diabetics. Also, patients with and without autonomic dysfunction demonstrate subnormal increases in oxygen consumption with work, most likely because of an impaired ability to increase cardiac output.[108, 109] Patients with DM have significantly higher incidence of peripheral and cerebrovascular disease due to the micro- and macroangiopathies associated with their diabetes.

A number of pulmonary disorders are also associated with DM. Hyperglycemic patients have a higher incidence of pulmonary infections than nondiabetics, and those with autonomic neuropathy have more sleep-related breathing problems. Pulmonary function testing often shows mild abnormalities in lung elastic recoil, diffusion capacity, and pulmonary capillary blood volume, which

are directly related to the duration of DM.[110] Diabetic ketoacidosis is related to a number of pulmonary problems including hyperventilation, pneumomediastinum, and mucus plugs in the major airways.

Implications for Physical Therapy Intervention

The abnormal metabolic responses of diabetics to exercise and the frequency of cardiovascular complications require caution in providing physical therapy to the diabetic population. Several factors need to be considered, including the necessity of pretreatment medical screening; the importance of HR, BP, and blood glucose monitoring; the potential for exercise-induced hypoglycemia; attention to the timing of exercise; and the intensity, mode, and duration of exercise.

Because of the increased incidence of asymptomatic myocardial ischemia and infarction, all patients should have a thorough medical evaluation, including graded exercise testing whenever possible, prior to starting any kind of exercise program. Ideally, adequate metabolic control should also be established before an exercise program is initiated. In the acute care setting, these precautions are frequently ignored, especially when the admitting diagnosis is not cardiac in nature. In any event, because so many patients with DM exhibit abnormal hemodynamic responses to activity, HR and BP monitoring should be included in all PT evaluations and may be indicated during treatment sessions as well. Patients with DM who do not have autonomic dysfunction frequently have hypertensive responses to exercise, as well as postexercise hypotension (thus reemphasizing the need for BP monitoring). As described earlier, patients with autonomic dysfunction also show abnormal responses to exercise (see earlier description).

Self-monitoring of blood glucose levels is essential. Monitoring just prior to exercise is extremely helpful in predicting a patient's metabolic response to treatment and should also be performed at frequent intervals following exercise initially, so the patient's need for alterations in diet or insulin dosage can be determined. Diabetics should avoid vigorous or prolonged exercise if blood glucose values are 250 to 300 mg/dL and should not exercise at all if blood glucose exceeds 300 mg/dL or if there is any ketosis.[111-113] Likewise, exercise is contraindicated if blood glucose is 80 to 100 mg/dL because of the greater risk of hypoglycemia; instead, the individual should eat a carbohydrate snack and wait until the blood glucose level has risen before initiating exercise. For those working with athletes with IDDM, more intense glucose monitoring and education are usually required because of a higher incidence of hypoglycemia during and after exercise and a greater risk of hyperglycemia during times of poor control.[112, 114, 115] In addition, athletes with IDDM may require a longer, more gradual progression to a higher level of training than is generally the case.

Exercise produces heightened sensitivity to insulin and so increases the risk of hypoglycemia, which may occur up to 24 or more hours after exercise. Therefore, patients will require a lower dose of insulin or increased carbohydrate intake prior to, during, or after exercise. Clinicians must be aware of the signs and symptoms of hypoglycemia, as described in Table 7–5. Carbohydrate snacks, such as fruit juice or soft drinks, should be readily available, with 5 to 10 g being provided for each 30 to 45 minutes of prolonged exercise, depending on intensity. Notably, drinks containing 5 to 10% carbohydrate are absorbed best, so fruit juices and most soft drinks, which contain about 12% carbohydrate, should be diluted. To minimize

the risk of hypoglycemia, patients should avoid exercising at the time of peak insulin effect or eat a carbohydrate snack a half an hour before exercise; start with moderate workloads and increase intensity gradually; use a consistent pattern of exercise (time, duration, and intensity); use exercise that can be easily quantitated if possible (which can be difficult in many PT programs); and avoid injecting insulin into tissue near the exercising muscles if patient will be exercising soon thereafter (within 40 minutes after regular insulin or within 90 minutes after intermediate insulin).[112]

The exercise prescription for those with DM must be individualized according to medication schedule, presence and severity of diabetic complications, and the goals and expected benefits of the exercise program. Because diabetics, especially those with IDDM, tend to engage anaerobic metabolism at lower heart rates,[116]* exercise HRs should not exceed 50 to 60% of predicted maximum heart rate unless the patient has a good level of physical fitness. Strenuous exercise should be avoided until reasonable diabetic control is achieved. If there is any evidence of retinopathy strenuous exercise is similarly avoided. Therapists should be watchful for any signs of exercise intolerance, as described in Chapter 16.

Because of the prevalence of autonomic dysfunction in diabetics and its associated risk for **silent ischemia** and impaired exercise tolerance, autonomic function testing may be included in the PT evaluation. One method is to measure the BP response to standing from the supine position. A fall in SBP of more than 30 mm Hg or DBP of more than 20 mm Hg may be indicative of autonomic dysfunction.[117, 118] A more reliable evaluation can be performed by measuring the beat-to-beat variation in HR during standing and deep breathing.[119] For the standing test, an ECG strip is recorded in the supine position and then as the individual quickly stands up. Using the shortest R-R interval, which usually occurs around beat 15 after starting to stand, and the longest R-R interval, which occurs about the time of beat 30, the so-called "30:15" ratio can be calculated. If the ratio is 1.0 or less, autonomic dysfunction is likely. To observe the response to deep breathing, an ECG strip is obtained at rest (sitting) and then during 1 minute of slow deep breathing at a rate of six breaths per minute. The longest and shortest R-R intervals during each breathing cycle are

Table 7–5
Signs and Symptoms of Hypoglycemia

ADRENERGIC*	NEUROGLUCOPENIC†
Weakness	Headache
Sweating	Hypothermia
Tachycardia	Visual disturbances
Palpitations	Mental dullness
Tremor	Confusion
Nervousness	Amnesia
Irritability	Seizures
Tingling of mouth and fingers	Coma
Hunger	
Nausea‡	
Vomiting‡	

* Caused by increased activity of the autonomic nervous system.
† Caused by decreased activity of the central nervous system.
‡ Unusual.

used to calculate the maximum and minimum heart rates, and the difference between these two values is used to determine autonomic function. Differences of less than 15 to 20 beats per minute (in older and younger individuals, respectively) indicate abnormal autonomic function.

Additionally, a few other factors should be emphasized in the care of diabetics. First, adequate fluid replacement, both during and after exercise, is very important for diabetics in order to avoid dehydration and maintain proper osmotic levels. Second, good footwear and careful foot hygiene with daily inspection are essential. Third, diabetics should *never* exercise alone and should always carry medical identification and a carbohydrate snack. Finally, patients should be alerted to the possibility of delayed exercise-induced hypoglycemia, which may occur up to 24 or more hours after exercise.

The PT management of diabetic patients with lower extremity amputation involves additional considerations.[120] Surgical healing following amputation is often delayed or complicated due to the circulatory abnormalities, impaired ability to fight infection, poor blood glucose control, and neuropathies associated with DM. Many of these same factors, along with visual impairment, may limit the diabetic amputee in achieving independence in donning a prosthesis, and muscle weakness due to motor neuropathy often interferes with proper prosthetic gait. The energy demands for prosthetic gait are higher than normal and increase the risk of cardiovascular complications during rehabilitation. Attention to wrist alignment when using assistive gait devices is important because of the higher incidence of carpal tunnel syndrome in diabetics.

OBESITY

Obesity can be defined as an increased accumulation of **adipose** tissue so that body mass index (body weight in kilograms divided by height in meters squared) is above 30 kg/m^2, body fat is above 25% for males or 30% for females, or body weight is more than 20% above the upper limit for height.[121] Approximately 26% of Americans are obese, a third of whom are extremely so.[122] Pathologically, there are two types of obesity, depending on the age of onset: juvenile-onset obesity is char-

acterized by an increased number, or **hyperplasia,** of **adipocytes,** and adult-onset obesity is usually associated with increased size, or hypertrophy, of the existing adipocytes.

Obesity is the result of a positive energy balance, which occurs when energy intake exceeds energy expenditure. Genetic, hormonal, and metabolic factors appear to play a role in the etiology of obesity. In fact, there are probably multiple factors, both physiologic and psychological, which vary among individuals, that interact to induce obesity. Although it is generally assumed that overeating is a primary cause of obesity, research indicates that obese individuals of all ages may consume the same number or fewer calories than their lean counterparts.[123-129] Researchers are now discovering that other factors shift the balance between energy intake and expenditure, and thus promote either body fat deposition or metabolism. For instance, diet composition appears to be at least as important as caloric content in the promotion or reduction of obesity: there is evidence that diets high in fat and refined sugar promote obesity,[123, 126, 130, 131] and those high in complex carbohydrates and fiber may assist in body fat reduction, despite the same total caloric intake.[126, 132-134] Furthermore, it is now recognized that severe calorie-restricted dieting elicits an energy conservation process with a reduction in metabolic rate that persists after the dieting period and facilitates rapid weight regain.[126, 135, 136] Frequently, this cycle is repeated a number of times, with progressive difficulty in losing weight and enhanced ability to regain any weight loss that is achieved.

Obesity represents a major health problem in this country because of its association with increased prevalences of HTN, cardiovascular disease, osteoarthritis, gastrointestinal problems, endometrial and breast cancers, glucose intolerance, type II DM, **obesity hypoventilation syndrome, sleep**

Clinical Note: Yo-Yo Dieting

The pattern of losing and regaining weight is known as yo-yo dieting, so named because the body weight goes up and down, like a yo-yo. Because very low calorie diets often result in a reduction of the resting metabolic rate, dieting may become less effective. Weight gain may occur more easily following each attempt at losing weight.

apnea, and pulmonary hypertension.[121, 137] In addition, it is associated with increased mortality rates, usually as a result of atherosclerotic heart disease, stroke, diabetes, digestive diseases, or cancer.[138, 139]

The increased prevalence of atherosclerotic heart disease in the obese is probably not due to a primary role in the pathogenesis of atherosclerosis, but rather is secondary to its association with sedentary lifestyle, HTN, hyperlipidemia, and glucose intolerance. However, a pattern of predominantly abdominal fat distribution, commonly identified using the ratio of waist-to-hip circumference, appears to be an independent risk factor for cardiovascular disease and death.[140–142] A cardiomyopathy of obesity, which consists of a syndrome of chronic circulatory congestion associated with diastolic and sometimes systolic left ventricular dysfunction in the absence of HTN or other cardiovascular disease, has been identified in morbidly obese individuals.[143] Blood volume, stroke volume, cardiac output, left ventricular end-diastolic volume, and end-diastolic filling pressure are increased with obesity, especially during exertion.[143] These result in left ventricular hypertrophy and dilatation, as well as left atrial hypertrophy due to the increased pulmonary blood volume and flow. If HTN is also present, LVH will be more marked and CHF may develop. About 75% of very obese individuals have pulmonary HTN at rest or during exercise.

The most specific pulmonary problems complicating obesity are obstructive sleep apnea and the obesity hypoventilation syndrome.[110, 144] Sleep apnea occurs in approximately 19% of obese individuals, particularly in moderately to extremely obese males, aged 40 to 60, and consists of periodic episodes of obstructive apnea at night and **hypersomnolence** during the day. During the apneic periods there are significant increases in systemic and pulmonary artery pressures and frequently cardiac arrhythmias, including sinus arrest, asystole up to 6 seconds, heart block, and ventricular tachycardia. The obesity hypoventilation syndrome occurs in about 5% of extremely obese individuals and includes hypoventilation, cyanosis, and somnolence. The result is chronic hypoxemia, hypercapnia, respiratory acidosis, and polycythemia. Chronic hypoxemia and hypercapnia stimulate pulmonary vasoconstriction, leading to worsening of pulmonary hypertension. **Biventricular hypertrophy** with pulmonary and systemic congestion are characteristic of this syndrome.

Exercise and Obesity

In obesity the resting metabolic rate and therefore cardiac output and minute ventilation relative to lean body mass are increased due to the greater body mass that must be provided with oxygen. During exercise the increase in oxygen consumption is even more marked because of the additional energy required to move the larger body segments. The resting hypoxemia that may be the result of peripheral atelectasis caused by chest wall obesity usually disappears during exercise, presumably because of deeper breathing. In obesity, the maximal oxygen consumption and anaerobic threshold are low when related to actual body weight but are normal when expressed as a ratio to height or lean body weight.

Because obesity is the result of a positive energy balance, it seems only logical that successful treatment of obesity would consist of reversing this energy imbalance through decreasing caloric intake, increasing energy expenditure, or a combination of both. Unfortunately, studies evaluating the efficacy of exercise, either as a single modality or combined with diet restriction for reducing weight, are very discouraging because of the rather low amount of weight loss that is achieved and the high dropout rates.[145–150] Yet there has been a great deal of variability in the research on obesity. Some reports have documented that the percentage of body fat decreases more with less loss of lean body weight when exercise is added to dieting[151, 152]; however, others have not found this to be the case.[153, 154] Individuals with **hyperplastic** (increased number of fat cells) obesity may be more resistant to attempted dietary restriction than those with hypertrophic (enlarged fat cells but normal number) obesity,[151] but again, not all data concur.[146] The disparity in published results may be due to a variety of factors: the type of obesity; the physiologic causes or sustaining factors involved in an individual's obesity; the age, gender, and body build of the subjects; variations in the frequency, intensity, and duration of exercise performed; the length of the training period (long term versus short term); the type of diet; and the motivation of the subjects.

Maintenance of weight loss is a major problem for many people who manage to lose weight, but has been more successful in those who continue to exercise.[155, 156] In addition, there are other demonstrable benefits of exercise in the obese, even if weight does not change. Physical training in obese individuals is associated with an improvement in glucose tolerance and a marked reduction in the insulin response to a **glucose tolerance test.**[157, 158] Also, there may be favorable shifts in the lipid profiles of obese subjects, particularly males, as a result of exercise training.[145, 150, 155, 158] As with other populations, exercise training improves exercise tolerance and increases efficiency so that daily activities can be performed more easily.[145, 147, 153, 154, 158] This improvement is particularly important in the obese, who tend to use more energy with exaggerated cardiovascular and respiratory stress to perform any form of physical work.

Implications for Physical Therapy Intervention

A number of specific considerations, when prescribing exercise for obese individuals, will maximize both safety and effectiveness. First, because of the increased prevalence of HTN and atherosclerotic heart disease in obese individuals, monitoring of the physiologic responses to exercise is indicated during physical therapy evaluation and initial treatment. A tendency toward exercise-induced syncope due to fluid imbalance resulting from calorie-restricted diets and exacerbated by exercise-induced fluid loss further emphasizes the need for BP monitoring. Second, an endurance training program should be prescribed for all patients in order to increase energy expenditure, lower cardiovascular risk factors, and improve functional efficiency. Intensity should be lower than the anaerobic threshold, or around 50 to 60% of functional capacity, in order to utilize predominantly free fatty acids as fuel. Duration and frequency should be prescribed so that a total of 1750 to 2000 calories are expended per week in a fairly even distribution. The goal is to perform 45 to 60 minutes of low to moderate intensity aerobic activity at least 3 to 5 days per week. The data from one research study suggested that prescribing exercise in multiple short bouts versus one continuous bout per day may enhance exercise adherence and weight loss while producing similar changes in cardiorespiratory fitness.[159] Non-weight-bearing exercise programs, such as cycling, swimming, or water aerobics, will decrease the stress on joints which often suffer from osteoarthritis.

Obese individuals should be encouraged to increase their general level of activity during their daily routines. This increase can be accomplished by walking whenever possible, including at least 2 to 5 minutes every hour at work or at home and during lunchtime, parking at the far end of the lot when shopping, and taking the stairs instead of the elevator for 1 to 3 flights. Creating or joining a social group that focuses on physical activity, such as a walking or cycling club, is also very helpful.

Because injuries are one of the primary reasons for discontinuing exercise in obese individuals, injury prevention is a major concern when prescribing exercise. Special considerations include obtaining a detailed history of previous injuries and joint problems; prescribing adequate warm-up, cooldown, and stretching; and encouraging a gradual progression of intensity and duration. Another concern when working with people who are obese is thermoregulation.[160] Exercise should be encouraged during the cooler times of day or in a neutral environment, and individuals should be advised to wear loose-fitting clothing and to drink plenty of water.

PTs can provide encouragement to clients who are attempting to lose weight. It is especially important to inform clients that cutting calories is essential to weight loss and that a weight loss of 5 to 10% can provide significant health benefits. Unfortunately, exercise may not provide much reinforcement at the scales, because participants often reduce body fat while increasing muscle mass. However, adding an exercise program can have a dramatic effect on health and will be very important to maintaining any weight loss that is achieved. PTs can also share other information they come across regarding specific dietary factors that might maximize the loss of fat and minimize the loss of muscle mass. For instance, as mentioned previously, there is evidence that diets high in fat and refined sugar promote obesity, and those with high amounts of complex carbohydrates and fiber may assist in body fat reduction, despite the same total caloric intake.

PERIPHERAL ARTERIAL DISEASE

Peripheral arterial disease (PAD), or more specifically **atherosclerotic occlusive disease** (AOD), involves atheromatous plaque obstruction of the large or medium-sized arteries supplying blood to one or more of the extremities (usually lower). AOD results from the same atherosclerotic process described in Chapter 3 and becomes symptomatic when the atheroma becomes so enlarged that it interferes with blood flow to the distal tissues, it ruptures and extrudes its contents into the bloodstream or obstructs the arterial lumen, or it encroaches on the media, causing weakness of that layer and aneurysmal dilatation of the arterial wall. The hemodynamic significance of the disease depends upon the location and number of lesions in an artery, the rapidity with which the atherosclerotic process progresses, and the presence and extent of any collateral arterial system. When blood flow is not adequate to meet the demand of the peripheral tissues (i.e., during activity), the patient may experience symptoms of ischemia, such as **intermittent claudication** of a lower extremity. As the disease progresses, the patient experiences more severe symptoms, such as rest pain and skin changes. Complete obstruction to flow will cause tissue **necrosis** and possibly loss of the limb.

Because atherosclerosis is a generalized disorder, most individuals with peripheral arterial insufficiency also have involvement of the coronary arteries, the carotids, or the aorta. One study noted that coronary atherosclerosis may be present in at least 90% of patients hospitalized for peripheral vascular disease.[161] Thus, those with lower extremity PAD should be assumed to have atherosclerotic heart disease, which is the main cause of higher morbidity and mortality rates in these individuals.[162–165] In fact, individuals with asymptomatic disease appear to have the same increased risk of cardiovascular events and death found in those with symptoms of claudication.[163]

Exercise and Peripheral Arterial Disease

Individuals with PAD are unable to produce the normal increases in peripheral blood flow essential for enhanced oxygen supply to exercising muscles. If the oxygen supply is not adequate to meet the increasing demand of the exercising muscles, ischemia develops and leads to the production of lactic acid. When excessive lactic acid accumulates in the muscle, pain is experienced; and when it reaches the central circulation, respiration is further stimulated and patients may experience shortness of breath.

Patients with intermittent claudication have moderate to severe impairment in walking ability. Their peak exercise capacity during graded treadmill exercise is severely limited, allowing for only light to very light activities.[166–168] Therefore, the energy requirements of many leisure and work-related activities usually exceed their capacity. Metabolic measurements during exercise testing reveal that maximal oxygen consumption and **anaerobic threshold** are reduced in patients with AOD.[166, 168] Yet, even though the anaerobic threshold may be so low that it cannot be detected, evidence of systemic lactic acidosis may be minimal because of the reduced muscle perfusion.

Several studies have documented the efficacy of exercise training in the management of patients with AOD. Increases in both pain-free and maximal walking tolerance on level ground and during constant-load treadmill exercise achieved during exercise testing have been reported.[169–177] Studies have even concluded that greater symptomatic relief and functional improvement in patients with mild to moderate claudication not requiring immediate therapeutic interventions is achieved through supervised exercise therapy rather than **percutaneous transluminal angioplasty.**[170, 178] Some studies have demonstrated the benefit of exercise for patients with rest pain.[179] Several mechanisms have been postulated to account for these improvements: increased walking efficiency, increased peripheral blood flow through changes in the collateral circulation, reduced blood viscosity, regression of atherosclerotic disease, raising of the pain threshold, and improvements in skeletal muscle metabolism. There is evidence that periods of brief repetitive walking can successfully increase oxygenation in the feet of limbs with more severe arterial obstruction.[180]

Implications for Physical Therapy Intervention

Because of the high prevalence of atherosclerotic heart disease in patients with peripheral vascular disease, all patients should receive HR and BP monitoring during PT evaluation and initial treatment. Such monitoring is especially needed when working with patients who have undergone amputation, which implies severe disease. Notably, patients with PAD may exhibit precipitous rises in BP during exercise owing to their atherosclerosis and diminished vascular bed.

Including a subjective gradation of pain for expressing claudication discomfort is extremely useful during exercise as described in Table 7–6.[28] Patients should exercise to levels of maximal tolerable pain, that is to grade 3 discomfort, in order to obtain optimal symptomatic benefit over time, possibly through enhanced collateral circulation or increased muscular efficiency.[28, 180, 181] Patients usually perform exercise in intervals often as short as 1 to 5 minutes, alternating with rest intervals of sufficient length to completely relieve pain, usually 2 to 10 minutes. As the patient progresses with the exercise program the duration of the exercise intervals is increased and the number of rest periods is reduced until 30 to 60 minutes of continuous activity can be sustained. Low-intensity exercise is recommended, as it maximizes the potential duration of the exercise bouts.

The most convenient and functional mode of exercise is walking. Non-weight-bearing activities, such as stationary cycling, rowing, swimming, or pool exercise, may allow longer duration and higher intensity exercise than weight-bearing exercise. Yet, even when these other modalities are used for training, progressive walking should also be included in the exercise prescription because of its functional importance. Exercise should be performed on a daily or twice daily basis. For patients with skin lesions, multiple brief walking periods throughout the day may be particularly helpful in promoting healing through increased tissue oxygenation.[182]

Some other important considerations should be noted. First, because cold weather induces peripheral vasoconstriction, patients with PAD require longer warm-up times before exercising in colder environments. Second, patients with PAD often have peripheral neuropathies, especially of the sensory nerves, due to chronic ischemia; and the severity of neuropathy cannot be estimated by the degree of functional impairment.[183] Sensory evaluation should be an important component of the PT evaluation, and good footwear and careful foot hygiene with daily inspection are crucial. Last, as functional status improves, other cardiovascular and orthopedic problems may become evident. Symptoms to be on the alert for include exertional angina, dyspnea, fatigue, lightheadedness or dizziness, and leg pain not of vascular origin.

RENAL FAILURE

The kidneys are complex organs whose major functions include the control of extracellular fluid volume, the regulation of serum **osmolality,** electrolyte and acid-base balances, and the secretion of hormones such as **renin** and **erythropoietin.** Thus, when renal function becomes impaired, the resultant metabolic disturbances affect virtually every other body system. Yet, **renal failure** is usually an insidious process that often presents with symptoms of only vague general **malaise** and ill health until late in its progression. Only when renal failure becomes marked, with the accumulation of water, crystalloid solutes and waste products in the blood, are the symptoms of **uremia** manifested: altered electrolyte homeostasis and acid-base imbalance, gastrointestinal distress, severe anemia, and multiple other abnormalities involving the skin, respiratory, cardiovascular, neurologic, musculoskeletal, endocrine, genitourinary, and immune systems. Chronic renal failure (CRF) results in a number of major complications: hypertension, pericarditis with pericardial effusion and sometimes **cardiac tamponade,** accelerated atherosclerosis, anemia, bleeding disorders, renal **osteodystrophy** (bone changes resembling osteomalacia and rickets occurring in patients with chronic renal failure), proximal **myopathy** (wasting and weakness of the proximal skeletal muscles), peripheral neuropathy, **peptic ulceration,** and **immunosuppression** leading to intercurrent infections.[184, 185] Al-

Table 7–6	
Subjective Gradation of Claudication Discomfort	
I	Initial discomfort (established, but minimal)
II	Moderate discomfort but attention can be diverted
III	Intense pain (attention cannot be diverted)
IV	Excruciating and unbearable pain

though most of these complications are reversible with frequent **dialysis,** patients maintained on dialysis may develop other problems, as will be described later.

Cardiovascular complications cause nearly 50% of the deaths in patients with **end-stage renal disease** (ESRD).[186-188] The majority of these deaths are due to myocardial infarction, heart failure, and cerebrovascular accidents. Hypertension is both a cause and a consequence of renal disease and greatly aggravates renal dysfunction in CRF. Accelerated atherosclerosis is related to HTN and the **hyperlipidemia** associated with CRF. Heart failure in CRF results from fluid overload, hypertension, and atherosclerotic heart disease. Uremia itself also may be associated with a cardiomyopathy.[188] In addition, patients may develop pericardial effusion from inadequate dialysis and uremia as well as dysrhythmias due to electrolyte abnormalities.

Acute or chronic renal failure also has associated pulmonary complications.[189] Pulmonary edema is the most serious problem and may be due to fluid overload as well as increased capillary permeability. Diaphragmatic weakness from a myopathic process contributes to the restrictive lung dysfunction. Other pulmonary complications that may occur include pleural effusions, pulmonary calcification, hemodialysis-induced hypoxemia and asthma, and sleep apnea.

Treatment of Chronic Renal Failure

The treatment modalities used to manage CRF include conservative management of symptoms, dialysis, and ultimately, renal transplantation. Because the clearance of toxic metabolic waste products and other substances by the kidneys remains superior to that achieved by dialysis until renal function deteriorates to 10 to 20% of normal, the conservative management of CRF is usually employed as long as possible. The primary goals of treatment are to reduce the rate of progressive deterioration in renal function and to minimize the complications of CRF. The most common interventions include control of diet, fluid balance, blood pressure, mineral metabolism, and the distressing symptoms of uremia.[184, 185] Patients with symptoms related to anemia are often treated with erythro-

poietin therapy to increase their hemoglobin concentration.[190]

When the symptoms or complications of CRF become troublesome despite conservative therapies, dialysis is indicated. Dialysis is a process that replaces the excretory functions of the kidney through the use of a semipermeable membrane and a rinsing solution (**dialysate**) to filter out toxic waste substances from the blood. In addition, dialysis allows for control of fluid and electrolyte balances. Several modes of dialysis are currently available, with hemodialysis and continuous ambulatory peritoneal dialysis being the most common. The major complications of chronic dialysis are renal osteodystrophy, anemia, vascular access infections and thromboses, **pericarditis,** and **ascites.**

Although many patients do well for more than 10 years on dialysis, success is limited by the impaired clearance of waste products and other substances and the marked impairment of the regulatory and endocrine functions normally provided by the kidneys. Therefore, renal transplantation is the treatment of choice, particularly in younger patients. It offers the best opportunity for normalization of renal function and lifestyle, but its application is dependent upon organ availability as well as immunologic matching of either living-related or cadaver kidney donors. Furthermore, transplantation can be complicated by a number of early and late immunologic, surgical, and medical events, as well as problematic side effects of the immunosuppressive medications that are required.

Exercise and Chronic Renal Failure

Most patients with CRF are extremely sedentary with poor exercise tolerance. Only 23 to 60% of patients (depending upon presence of DM or not, respectively) are able to do more than self-care,[191] and their mean exercise capacity is only 4 to 6 METs, or approximately 50% of the capacity of normal sedentary persons.[192-196] Factors that may contribute to their poor tolerance include anemia, abnormal peripheral metabolism, abnormal control of metabolic or systemic function during exercise, impaired cardiac function, and physical deconditioning. In addition, there is some evidence that skeletal muscle dysfunction is a major limiting factor for exercise capacity in these patients, because peak oxygen consumption correlates with muscle strength more closely than with hemoglobin.[197] Furthermore, leg fatigue is the most common clinical complaint limiting exercise.[198]

Hemodynamic responses to exercise are altered in patients with CRF. Heart rate responses are blunted, and blood pressure increases excessively with exercise.[192-199] Additionally, patients on hemodialysis exhibit blunted HR responses at any given relative workload, despite higher levels of **norepinephrine** compared to normal individuals, which suggests diminished **adrenergic** sensitivity.[200]

A number of studies have evaluated the responses to exercise training in selected patients with ESRD receiving hemodialysis (those without unstable angina pectoris, cardiac arrhythmias, hemodynamically significant valvular heart disease; clinically significant or symptomatic cerebrovascular, peripheral vascular, or coronary atherosclerosis; congestive heart failure; poorly controlled HTN; electrolyte imbalance; severe retinal disease; IDDM; **hypothyroidism;** or orthopedic or musculoskeletal limitations).[192-196, 201, 202] Researchers have found that exercise training sessions can be safely and successfully scheduled during dialysis,[194, 203] just prior to[192] or just following[202] dialysis, as well as on "off-dialysis" days. Most studies have documented the ability to increase maximal oxygen consumption ($VO_{2\ max}$) an average of 20 to 25% over a period of 10 weeks to 12 months of exercise training.[204] Other reported benefits of exercise training include improved lipid profiles, enhanced BP control, improved insulin sensitivity and glucose metabolism, increased red blood cell mass, increased muscle strength, and improved psychological profiles.[194, 205] Thus, some of the complications present in hemodialysis patients may be caused by their sedentary lifestyle, rather than their ESRD.

The major difficulty in implementing an exercise program for this patient population is the inability or unwillingness of the majority of patients to participate in the program. Compliance is improved if the sessions are scheduled on the days of dialysis and is highest when they are performed during dialysis. In addition, subjective reports from patients who participated in their exercise program during dialysis indicated that they found it enjoyable, were more active at home and had better endurance, experienced less muscle cramping

while on dialysis, and had fewer hypotensive responses to hemodialysis.[194]

Exercise training for selected patients after renal transplantation has also been shown to be feasible and beneficial and to increase aerobic capacity.[194, 206, 207] In addition, exercise training offers other benefits in this population: modification of coronary risk factors, prevention of corticosteroid-related myopathy, and stress reduction.

Implications for Physical Therapy Intervention

As discussed, patients with CRF are often very debilitated and have poor tolerance for activity. However, exercise training has been shown to offer a number of benefits for selected patients. Yet, the patients referred to physical therapy often have a number of the complex medical problems that excluded patients from previous research studies; for instance, a patient receiving neurologic rehabilitation for a stroke may also have diabetes, HTN, CHF, peripheral vascular disease, and renal failure.

If safe treatment is to be offered, cardiovascular monitoring is essential, and appropriate adjustments should be made to accommodate potential complications, including volume overload and electrolyte imbalances (particularly hyperkalemia), that may develop from one day to the next. Ideally, patients should be on a stable regimen of dialysis, diet, and medications; however, this is not always the case in the acute care setting, in which case additional caution must be exercised. In measuring BP in dialysis patients, care must be taken to avoid using the arm with an arteriovenous fistula. Blood pressure monitoring is also important for patients who have undergone renal transplantation because of the prevalence of hypertensive exercise responses resulting from cyclosporine therapy.[194, 208]

Exercise training programs for these patients should be low intensity initially with 2- to 5-minute exercise intervals alternating with brief (1- to 2-minute) rest periods. The exercise intervals should increase gradually with an eventual goal of 30 to 45 minutes of continuous exercise. Aerobic activities, especially those which are non-weight-bearing, are recommended. Intensity is best monitored using a rating of perceived exertion (RPE) scale[60] because calculated HRs are not tolerated by most patients. A RPE range of 12 to 13 ("somewhat hard") has been shown to be a more consistent guide than HR levels during dialysis.[195, 209] Although benefits are observed using three sessions per week, four to six sessions per week are usually recommended.[38, 194] The 6-minute walk test has been demonstrated to be an effective means of assessing functional capacity and documenting progress in this patient group.[210] Finally, because limitations may be related to muscle weakness, strength training should also be included as an important component of the exercise program. Because of the possibility of spontaneous tendon rupture in patients who have been on dialysis for more than 5 years, low resistance with high repetitions is recommended.[209]

OTHER SPECIFIC DISEASES AND DISORDERS

A wide variety of other specific diseases may be associated with cardiopulmonary complications. The presence of cardiac or pulmonary complications may affect patient tolerance for physical activity including many PT interventions. Tables 7–7 to 7–10 summarize the cardiac and pulmonary manifestations of a number of specific diseases and disorders.

Rheumatoid Arthritis and Collagen Vascular Diseases

The **collagen vascular diseases** are a diverse group of systemic diseases that are characterized by diffuse and variable abnormalities of the vasculature and inflammatory lesions involving the joints, muscles, and connective tissues, including the pericardium and pleura. Involvement of the kidneys, brain, and heart is associated with the highest morbidity and mortality rates. Pericarditis and cardiomyopathy can occur in most of these conditions, but some have very characteristic cardiovascular lesions associated with them. Collagen vascular diseases affect all of the elements of the respiratory system, either separately or in combination: the respiratory muscles, the pleura, the small airways, the interstitium, and the pulmonary vessels. Not infrequently, the pulmonary disease precedes the musculoskeletal manifestations by several months to several years.[211] The following specific collagen vascular diseases may have major cardiopulmonary involvement: rheumatoid arthritis, systemic lupus erythematosus, polyarteritis nodosa, ankylosing spondylitis, and progressive systemic sclerosis, as shown in Table 7–7. In addition, other collagen vascular diseases, such as polymyositis, dermatomyositis, and Reiter's disease are occasionally associated with cardiovascular or pulmonary dysfunction, but will not be presented here.

Table 7–7
Most Common Cardiac and Pulmonary Manifestations of the Collagen Vascular and Connective Tissue Diseases

DISEASE	CARDIAC MANIFESTATIONS						PULMONARY MANIFESTATIONS				
	P	M	E/V	CA	ECG	OTHER	Pl.	I	Pn.	Vasc.	Mm.
Systemic lupus erythematosus	++	+/−	++	+	+/−	HTN, CHF	++	+	+	+/−	+
Polyarteritis nodosa	+	++	−	++	+	HTN, CHF	−	−	−	+/−	−
Rheumatoid arthritis	++	+	+	+	+	Rare intrapulm. nodules	++	+	+	+/−	−
Ankylosing spondylitis	−	+/−	++	−	+	Ankylosis of thorax	−	+/−	+	−	−
Progressive systemic sclerosis	+	++	−	++	+	HTN, CHF, pulm. HTN	++	+	+	++	−
Marfan's syndrome	−	−	++	+	−	Aortic dissection	−	−	−	−	−
Osteogenesis imperfecta	−	−	++	−	+	AR, MVP, MR	−	−	−	−	−

P = pericardial, M = myocardial, E/V = endocardial/valvular, CA = coronary arteries, ECG = ECG changes, arrhythmias and conduction disturbances, Pl. = pleural, I = interstitial, Pn. = pneumonitis, Vasc. = vascular, Mm. = respiratory muscle weakness, + = convincing association, ++ = very common, +/− = possible association, − = no association reported for specific disease.

Table 7–8

Cardiac and Pulmonary Manifestations of Some Neurological and Neuromuscular Diseases

DISEASE/DISORDER	CARDIAC MANIFESTATIONS		OTHER MANIFESTATIONS	PULMONARY MANIFESTATIONS		
	Myocardial	CA		Mm.	Obst.	Rest.
Hemiplegia	+/−	++	HTN, CAD if vascular pathology	+	−	+
Paraplegia	−	−	Depends on level of lesion	++	−	++
Parkinson's disease	−	−	Dyskinetic respiration	+	−	+
Amyotrophic lateral sclerosis	−	−	Respiratory failure	++	−	++
Landry-Guillain-Barré syndrome	−	−	Respiratory failure	++	−	++
Myasthenia gravis	+	−	Arrhythmias, rare CHF Respiratory failure	+	−	++
Progressive muscular dystrophy	++	−	Arrhythmias Pulmonary infections	++	−	++
X-linked muscular dystrophy	+	−	Sinus arrest, atrial paralysis AV blocks	+/−	−	+/−
Limb-girdle syndromes	+	−	Abnormal ECG	+/−	−	+/−
Myotonic dystrophy	−	−	Heart blocks, ventricular tachycardia	++	−	+
Friedreich's ataxia	++	+	Arrhythmias, CHF Scoliosis, chest deformity	+/−	−	+/−

CA = coronary arteries, Mm. = respiratory muscle weakness, Obst. = obstructive lung disease, Rest. = restrictive lung disease, HTN = hypertension, CAD = coronary artery disease, CHF = congestive heart failure, AV = atrioventricular, ECG = electrocardiogram, + = convincing association, ++ = very common, +/− = possible association, − = no association reported for specific disease/disorder.

Rheumatoid arthritis (RA) is a chronic inflammatory disease that predominantly involves the joints but may affect other systems particularly when the disease is severe and long-standing. Although evidence of cardiovascular involvement, especially of the pericardium, is commonly seen during echocardiography and at autopsy, it is seldom a clinical problem.[212] Pericarditis occurs in 11 to 50% of patients. Chest pain, peripheral edema, and orthopnea are the chief complaints in these patients. Rarely patients develop constrictive pericarditis or tamponade. Other lesions sometimes seen in RA include myocarditis (up to 20% of patients with RA), arteritis of the coronary arteries (up to 20% but only rarely results in angina pectoris or myocardial infarction), varying degrees of heart block (10%), granulomatous lesions involving the heart valves (3 to 5% of patients), and aortitis (5% of patients).[212]

Pulmonary involvement with RA tends to be asymptomatic but occasionally causes major problems and is seen most often in middle-aged males, even though RA is much more common in females.[211, 213] Rheumatoid pleural disease is found at autopsy in 40 to 50% of patients with RA but is clinically apparent in about 20%. Interstitial lung disease, sometimes called rheumatoid lung, is reported in 5 to 40% of patients, depending on the methods of detection. Cough and dyspnea are common symptoms, with digital clubbing found in up to 70 to 75% of patients. The most common histologic finding is diffuse interstitial pneumonitis and fibrosis, and restrictive lung dysfunction is noted on PFTs. Upper airway involvement in RA is usually related to rheumatoid involvement of the cricoarytenoid joint, causing difficulty with inspiration in 25 to 35% of patients and occasionally resulting in stridor. Nearly one third of patients with RA exhibit obstructive lung dysfunction, usually due to bronchiolitis obliterans, which carries a poor prognosis. Some patients respond to treatment with a combination of corticosteroids and cyclophosphamide, but the majority of cases progress to hypercapnic respiratory failure. In rare cases, individuals develop intrapulmonary rheumatoid nodules (less than 1% of patients), which may become infected, cause bronchial obstruction, cavitate, or rupture into the pleural space, causing pneumothorax. Finally, there have been reports of other pulmonary problems in patients with RA, including therapeutic drug-related pulmonary dysfunction (e.g., gold, methotrexate, and cyclophos-

Table 7-9

Cardiac and Pulmonary Dysfunction Associated with Cancer Treatment

TREATMENT	CARDIAC MANIFESTATIONS				COMMENTS	PULMONARY MANIFESTATIONS		
	Ar/ECG	P	Isch.	CM		Pneum.	Fib.	Other
Radiation Therapy to Chest	+	++	+	+	Varies with Rx techniques	+	+	−
Chemotherapy Agents								
Amsacrine (AMSA)	+	−	+/−	+		−	−	−
Azathioprine	+/−	−	−	−	Atrial fibrillation	−	−	−
Bleomycin	−	+/−	−	−	Dose-dependent, O_2 sensitive	+	+	+
Busulfan	−	−	−	−	Poor prognosis	+	+	+
Carmustine (BCNU)	−	−	−	−		+	+	−
Chlorambucil	−	−	−	−	50% mortality rate	+/−	+/−	−
Chlorozotocin (DCNU)	−	−	−	−		+	+	−
Cyclophosphamide	−	+	−	+	Acute pericarditis-myocarditis	+	+	+
Cytosine arabinoside/Cytarabine	−	+/−	−	−	Unexplained pulm. edema	−	−	+
Dactinomycin	−	−	−	−		+	−	−
Daunorubicin (Daunomycin)	+	+	+	+	Dose-dependent	−	−	−
Doxorubicin (Adriamycin)	+	+	+	+	Dose-dependent	−	−	−
Etoposide	−	−	+/−	−		−	−	−
Fluorouracil (5-FU)	−	−	+	−		−	−	−
Interleukin-2	−	−	+	−		−	−	−
Lomustine (CCNU)	−	−	−	−		+	+	−
Mechlorethamine	+/−	−	−	−	PACs and tachycardia	−	−	−
Melphalan	−	−	−	−		+/−	+/−	−
Mercaptopurine	−	−	−	−	Very rare	−	−	+/−
Methotrexate	+/−	−	−	−	? Hypersensitivity	+	+/−	+
Mitomycin	−	−	−	−	Almost 50% mortality rate	+	+	+
Procarbazine	−	−	−	−	Allergic interstitial infiltrates	+	+/−	+
Semustine (methyl-CCNU)	−	−	−	−		+	+	−
Vinblastine/vincristine/vindesine	−	−	+	−	Accelerated CAD, coronary spasm	+	+	+
Bone Marrow Transplantation	++	−	−	+/−	Pulmonary edema, COPD, graft-versus-host disease	++	++	+

ar/ECG = arrhythmias/ECG changes, P = pericardial, Isch. = myocardial ischemia/infarction, CM = chronic cardiomyopathy, Pneum. = pneumonitis, Fib. = fibrosis, CAD = coronary artery disease, PAC = premature atrial complex, + = convincing association, ++ = very common, +/− = possible association, − = no reported association.

phamide), pulmonary vascular disease, and rarely a follicular bronchiolitis.

Systemic lupus erythematosus (SLE) is a multisystem autoimmune disease characterized by the production of autoantibodies and immune complexes with diffuse and widespread inflammation involving the skin, joints, brain, kidney, heart, and virtually all serous membranes. Clinical evidence of cardiac involvement is present in 18 to 56% of patients, although histologic evidence at autopsy is found in up to 90% of patients.[212, 214–219] Inflammation of the cardiac structures can result in peri-

Table 7–10

Cardiac and Pulmonary Manifestations of Some Specific Diseases

DISEASE	CARDIAC MANIFESTATIONS			OTHER MANIFESTATIONS	PULMONARY MANIFESTATIONS			
	P	M	CA		Pl.	I	Pn.	Vasc.
Sickle cell disease	−	++	+	Cardiomegaly, ↓ Exercise capacity	−	−	++	+
AIDS	+	−	−	Metastasis of Kaposi's sarcoma to heart and lungs, non-Hodgkin's lymphoma, opportunistic infections	−	+	+	−
Hepatic disease	−	+	−	Alcoholic cardiomyopathy, HTN, arrhythmias, chest pain, ascites → ↓ vital capacity, pulmonary shunting and HTN	+	−	−	−
Anorexia nervosa	−	++	−	Arrhythmias, sudden death	−	−	−	−
Bulimia	−	+/−	−	Arrhythmias Aspiration pneumonia	−	−	−	−

P = pericardial, M = myocardial, E/V = endocardial/valvular, CA = coronary arteries, Pl. = pleural, I = interstitial, Pn. = pneumonitis, Vasc. = vascular, AIDS = acquired immunodeficiency syndrome, HTN = hypertension, + = convincing association, ++ = very common, +/− = possible association, − = no association reported for specific disease.

carditis, which is usually asymptomatic but on rare occasions can cause pericardial constriction or tamponade; endocarditis with lesions most commonly on the aortic and mitral valves; myocarditis which is only rarely symptomatic; and sometimes a pancarditis in which all structures are involved. Occasionally, widespread **vasculitis** may affect the smaller coronary arteries, resulting in myocardial necrosis and fibrosis, cardiomyopathy, and sometimes rhythm and conduction disturbances. In addition, patients have an increased incidence of coronary atherosclerosis, which is related to long-term glucocorticosteroid treatment.[215, 219] Hypertension is common in patients with SLE and is the major cause of cardiac enlargement and heart failure.

Pulmonary involvement, which occurs in 35 to 75% of patients with SLE, most commonly affects the pleura.[211, 213, 220–222] Pleuritic chest pain is more common than chest x-ray evidence of pleural effusions, though massive effusions can occur. Acute pneumonitis develops in some patients; it is often infectious but can also result from the disease directly (acute lupus pneumonitis) or diffuse alveolar hemorrhage, which can be fatal. Chronic interstitial lung disease is occasionally seen and is characterized by dyspnea on exertion and bibasilar rales. Approximately 50% of patients with SLE

have decreased diffusion capacity and changes consistent with restrictive lung disease, which may be related to respiratory muscle weakness or interstitial lung disease. Diaphragmatic weakness has recently been recognized to be relatively common in SLE and is manifested as dyspnea, especially when recumbent. Patients can have mild to severe hypoxemia, Finally, pulmonary hypertension occurs in a small number of patients.

Progressive systemic sclerosis (PSS), or **scleroderma,** is an uncommon autoimmune disorder of the small arteries, microvessels, and connective tissue characterized by slowly progressive fibrosis and vascular obliteration of the skin, subcutaneous tissues, and often the visceral organs, including the gastrointestinal tract (especially the esophagus), heart, lungs, and kidneys. Cardiovascular disease, which is found in over 90% of patients with diffuse PSS, results from either primary involvement of the heart by the disease or secondary to disease of the kidneys or lungs.[223–226] Cardiomyopathy due to myocardial necrosis and fibrosis, which may result from **Raynaud's phenomenon** of the coronary arteries, is found in 50 to 80% of patients at autopsy.[212, 218] Individuals with PSS may also have CHF, heart block due to fibrosis of conducting tissue, pericarditis, and valvular abnormalities. HTN secondary to renal involvement is common in these individuals. The primary cause of death due to PSS is the combined effect of multiple pulmonary abnormalities.[227, 228] Lung abnormalities are found in 70 to 100% of patients with PSS at autopsy.[213, 229] The most frequent pathologic finding is that of interstitial fibrosis with distortion of smaller airways and bronchiolectasis. Other pulmonary complications include pleural effusions, which are usually asymptomatic, and diffuse pleural thickening. Pulmonary HTN, which occurs in 5 to 35% of patients, can develop as a primary pulmonary vasculopathy or secondary to interstitial lung disease or cardiac involvement and has an extremely poor prognosis.[230, 231] Dyspnea is the most frequent symptom, occurring in over 60% of patients, particularly those with vascular disease. Greater than 50% of asymptomatic patients have abnormal PFTs, including isolated reduction in diffusing capacity, restrictive ventilatory defects, and obstructive airway disease.[232–234] However, a sedentary lifestyle due to skin and joint restrictions often masks the symptoms of shortness of breath or dyspnea on exertion until late in the disease process. Furthermore, exercise testing reveals subclinical pulmonary abnormalities not detected during routine PFTs.[226]

Polyarteritis nodosa is a systemic disease characterized by segmental necrotizing inflammation of the medium-sized to small arteries with resultant dysfunction of multiple organ systems, including the skin, kidneys, gastrointestinal tract, spleen, lymph nodes, central nervous and musculoskeletal systems, and heart. Approximately 78% of patients exhibit signs of cardiovascular involvement, particularly hypertension and congestive heart failure.[235] Polyarteritis of the coronary arteries and their branches occurs in almost 70% of patients and can lead to myocardial infarction, which is often undiagnosed but found at autopsy.[236] The myocardial necrosis and subsequent replacement fibrosis tend to be focal and patchy throughout the left ventricular wall.[218] Chest pain, heart murmurs, pericardial friction rubs, cardiac enlargement, and electrocardiographic (ECG) abnormalities are fairly common. Heart failure caused by a combination of infarction and renal failure is a frequent cause of death in patients with polyarteritis nodosa. Although the pulmonary arteries can be involved in classic polyarteritis, clinical manifestations of pulmonary disease do not occur unless there is **allergic angiitis** and **granulomatosis** involving the pulmonary arteries and parenchyma. In addition, there may be intractable asthma and transient or progressive episodes of pneumonia. Pulmonary lesions account for approximately 50% of the deaths in patients with allergic angiitis and granulomatosis.[236]

Ankylosing spondylitis is a form of arthritis involving mainly the spine and sacroiliac joints, resulting in chronic back pain, deforming dorsal kyphosis, and possibly fusion of the costovertebral and sacroiliac joints. Cardiac involvement takes the form of a sclerosing inflammatory lesion involving the aortic root area, both immediately above and below the aortic valve, resulting in aortic insufficiency in up to 5 to 10% of patients with long-standing disease.[212, 218, 237] The inflammatory process can also involve the mitral valve, causing mitral regurgitation. Conduction disturbances through the bundle of His and its branches occur in up to one third of patients due to distortion by fibrous tissue and may be intermittent, be asymptomatic, and resolve spontaneously. Patients with severe disease may develop chronic infiltrative and fibrotic changes in upper lung fields that mimic tuberculosis, but these occur only late in the course of the disease.[211, 238, 239] Ankylosis of the costovertebral joints results in a stiff, fixated thorax, which is revealed as mild to moderate restrictive changes during pulmonary function testing. Progressive dyspnea and cough are the usual symptoms, though cyst formation and subsequent *Aspergillus* infection may cause hemoptysis. Finally, ankylosing hyperostosis of the cervical spine can cause dysphagia, foreign-body sensation, and aspiration.

Connective Tissue Diseases

Abnormalities of connective tissue of the great arteries, cardiac valves, skeletal system and skin are characteristic of a number of diseases, including **Marfan's syndrome, Ehlers-Danlos syndrome, osteogenesis imperfecta,** and **homocystinuria.** These diseases may cause minimal cardiovascular dysfunction, such as mitral valve prolapse or mild aortic root dilatation, or severe problems, such as severe aortic or mitral insufficiency, or aortic dissection and aneurysm. These manifestations probably reflect the response of abnormal connective tissue to prolonged hemodynamic stresses. Pulmonary problems may also develop in these patients.

Neuromuscular Diseases and Neurologic Disorders

A number of disorders affecting the neurologic or neuromuscular systems are associated with cardiac and pulmonary dysfunction (see Table 7–8). The incidence and severity of dysfunction in all the disorders varies widely. Cardiac abnormalities include cardiomyopathy and disorders of impulse formation and conduction. Abnormalities of pulmonary function are usually related to respiratory muscle weakness causing hypoventilation and weakness of cough, bulbar muscle weakness resulting in aspiration pneumonia, or cardiomyopathy with resultant pulmonary edema. Respiratory muscle fatigue is probably the final event responsible for respiratory failure in the neuromuscular disorders and is often precipitated by acute respiratory infection. Nocturnal mechanical ventilation in the form of cuirass ventilators, the rocking bed, and the pneumobelt or nasal positive pressure ventilation can be used to provide relief from chronic respiratory muscle fatigue and reverse microatelectasis. Thus, the incidence and severity of pulmonary hypertension and cor pulmonale can be reduced and the onset of respiratory failure can be delayed in some patients.[240, 241] Some of the more commonly encountered disorders are presented here.

Hemiplegia can result from a number of events, including cerebrovascular accidents due to thrombosis, embolism, or hemorrhage, surgical excision of a brain tumor, and trauma. Regardless of cause,

Clinical Note: Signs of Respiratory Involvement

It is important to realize that respiratory symptoms often do not correlate well with the degree of respiratory dysfunction in slowly progressive disorders. Measures of maximal inspiratory and expiratory pressures can be used to detect and monitor respiratory muscle weakness and are more sensitive than spirometric measures of lung volume. Patients with neuromuscular and myopathic disorders involving the respiratory muscles are particularly prone to desaturation during sleep. Therefore, clinicians should be attentive to the development of symptoms such as disordered sleep, morning headache, and excessive daytime somnolence and alert the patient's physician if they are noted.

weakness or spastic paralysis of the affected side of the body can include the diaphragm and intercostal muscles. Left diaphragmatic dysfunction is more common than right. Pulmonary function testing reveals decreased volumes and flows to about 60 to 70% predicted normal values.[242–244] Obviously, these abnormalities take on additional clinical significance in the presence of preexisting pulmonary disease. Respiratory failure can develop in patients whose vital capacity decreases to 25% of predicted normal values, and mechanical ventilation will be required. The usual lack of clinical symptoms in hemiplegic patients is probably due to their low level of physical exertion; however, strenuous exertion or PT activities may elicit dyspnea, especially when lying flat. There is also some evidence that both hemorrhagic and ischemic strokes are associated with nonischemic cardiac damage, most likely related to increased sympathoadrenal tone.[245] In addition, hemiplegia due to vascular pathologies may also be associated with other cardiovascular abnormalities, particularly hypertension and atherosclerotic heart disease, which are commonly found, though frequently not diagnosed, in these patients. The majority of deaths following transient ischemic attacks, stroke, and **carotid endarterectomy** are due to cardiac disease; yet only 25 to 48% of patients presenting with cerebrovascular disease have a history of coronary artery disease (CAD).[246] One angiographic study designed to define the frequency of asymptomatic CAD in patients with cerebrovascular disease found that 40% had severe CAD (defined by greater than 70% stenosis of at least one coronary artery), 46% had mild to moderate disease, and only 14% had normal coronary arteries.[247] Other studies have also documented a high prevalence of asymptomatic CAD in patients with cerebrovascular disease.[246, 248, 249] Needless to say, these data have direct implications for PT evaluation and treatment of patients with strokes (see final discussion).

Spinal cord injury (SCI) also causes pulmonary dysfunction, with the degree of dysfunction related to the severity and level of injury.[242, 244, 250] Lesions above C4 result in paralysis of the diaphragm and accessory muscles as well as the intercostal muscles and almost always necessitate ventilatory assistance. Lesions below this level will have corresponding intercostal muscle involvement and therefore some restrictive changes, but because diaphragmatic and accessory muscle function is preserved, hypoventilation does not usually occur. However, the work done by the diaphragm is many times normal in lower cervical and high thoracic injuries, and dyspnea on exertion is common. The distribution of muscle paralysis also has a profound effect on the performance of forced expiratory maneuvers, the most important of which is the cough. A discussion of this topic is beyond the scope of this chapter but can be found in Chapter 5.[250]

SCI is also associated with cardiovascular abnormalities, mostly related to interruption of autonomic nervous system signals. Acute injury to the cervical spine is frequently accompanied by cardiac arrhythmias and occasionally by sudden death. Patients with spinal cord injuries at or above the T6 level often experience serious disturbances of blood pressure. Orthostatic hypotension is common in the early phase of recovery but usually resolves over time. **Autonomic dysreflexia (hyperreflexia)** can produce elevated blood pressure when noxious visceral or cutaneous stimuli, such as a full bladder, are sensed below the level of the lesion. Finally, autonomic denervation interferes with temperature regulation so that body temperature tends to fluctuate according to the ambient temperature, especially in higher lesions; therefore, hypo- and hyperthermia can develop.

Parkinson's disease is a common dyskinetic disorder of the extrapyramidal system, which is characterized by resting muscle tremors, rigidity, slowness and poverty of motion, gait impairment, postural instability, and masklike facial expressions. Secondary parkinsonism is known to develop following some cases of encephalitis, as a result of drug abuse, and in some boxers. Although rarely recognized clinically, impaired ventilatory function occurs in 50 to 87% of patients and tends to be proportional to the severity of the skeletal muscle disease and improves with effective treatment.[251-256] Erratic, or chaotic, breathing due to the rigidity and weakness of the respiratory muscles, as well as abnormal control of ventilation, is common and may produce restrictive lung dysfunction on PFTs. Upper airway obstruction is found in 5 to 62% of patients, most likely due to involvement of the upper airway muscles.[253, 254, 256] In addition, there may be an obstructive pulmonary disease associated with Parkinson's disease.[254, 256] Finally, the medications used to treat Parkinson's disease are also associated with respiratory disease: L-dopa may

produce dyskinetic breathing and abnormal central control of ventilation, and the ergot-derived dopamine agonists can cause pleural and pulmonary fibrosis.[252] There are no specific cardiac complications associated with Parkinson's disease; however, patients often have the same cardiovascular problems (HTN, ASHD, etc.) that commonly occur in their same-aged peer group.

Amyotrophic lateral sclerosis (ALS, or Lou Gehrig's disease) is the most common motor neuron disease in the United States and is characterized by progressive neurologic deterioration without remission due to loss and degeneration of both upper and lower motor neurons. The result is a combination of spasticity and hyperreflexia and muscle wasting, weakness, and fasciculations. The average life expectancy after the onset of symptoms is 3.6 years.[257] Irreversible hypoventilation due to weakness of the intercostal muscles and diaphragm, leading to mechanical ventilator dependence and fatal respiratory failure, is common in the later stages of the disease. Also, bulbar paralysis occurs in 25% of patients, which contributes to the frequent complication of **aspiration pneumonia.** Furthermore, repetitive episodes of aspiration and airway obstruction may be responsible for the increased incidence of obstructive lung disease in patients with ALS.[258]

Landry-Guillain-Barré syndrome, or acute polyneuritis, is a **demyelinating disease** of motor neurons that is manifested by symmetric ascending paralysis. A third to a half of these patients develop complications due to respiratory muscle weakness, including weakness of the diaphragm.[244, 259-261] There is a poor correlation between peripheral muscle strength and the presence or absence of respiratory muscle weakness.[242] In addition, denervation of the bulbar muscles can occur, leading to the inability to swallow and aspiration. Approximately 25 to 30% of patients require mechanical ventilatory support during the course of their disease. The majority of deaths result from cardiopulmonary complications.[244]

Multiple sclerosis (MS) is an inflammatory demyelinating disorder of the central nervous system (CNS) of unknown etiology and is characterized clinically by periods of remissions and relapses of symptoms, although on occasion its course can be chronic and progressive. MS is the most common neurologic disease affecting young adults. Its classic clinical symptoms include paresthesias, motor weakness, blurred and double vision, dysarthria, bladder incontinence, and ataxia. Because MS can cause focal lesions anywhere in the CNS, different patterns of respiratory impairment can occur but are relatively rare. The three most common respiratory manifestations are respiratory muscle weakness, bulbar dysfunction, and abnormalities of respiratory control.[242, 244, 262-264] Pulmonary dysfunction correlates with the severity of the disease, so that quadriplegic patients with bulbar involvement are at highest risk for developing respiratory failure. Even with severe disability and impaired respiratory muscle strength, patients with MS seldom complain of dyspnea, most likely due to their low activity level and greater expiratory than inspiratory muscle dysfunction. Clinical signs that may be helpful in predicting respiratory muscle impairment are weak cough and inability to clear secretions, limited ability to count to 10 on a single breath, and upper extremity involvement. There are no specific cardiovascular abnormalities associated with MS.

Myasthenia gravis is an acquired autoimmune disorder associated with **acetylcholine** receptor deficiency at the motor end-plates affecting either the external ocular muscles selectively or the general voluntary muscle system. Abnormal fatiguability is characteristic of the disease though symptoms may fluctuate from hour to hour, day to day, or over longer periods. Cardiac involvement occurs in 10 to 40% of patients, especially those with thymoma, and may be due to heart muscle antibodies.[265-268] Focal myocarditis is the usual pathologic finding. Clinical symptoms include tachycardia and other arrhythmias, dyspnea, and rarely heart failure. Notably, drugs used to treat cardiovascular problems, such as quinidine, procainamide, lidocaine, and morphine, may adversely affect myasthenia gravis. Respiratory muscle weakness occurs in about 10% of these patients, and the resultant respiratory failure may necessitate prolonged ventilatory assistance.[269] The risk of respiratory failure may be increased by surgery, infection, and the administration of corticosteroids or antimicrobial drugs. Patients may have severe respiratory muscle involvement despite mild peripheral muscle weakness.[244] However, most patients with moderate, generalized myasthenia gravis exhibit mild to moderate reductions in forced vital capacity and both maximal inspiratory and expiratory mouth pressures.[242]

Progressive (Duchenne's) muscular dystrophy (DMD) is a lethal, X-linked recessive disorder of childhood, though approximately one third of cases arise from spontaneous mutation. It is characterized by early onset of progressive, generalized muscle weakness and pseudohypertrophy of certain muscle groups, especially the calves, resulting in the inability to ambulate by the age of 10 and death by the age of 20. Up to 90% of patients develop cardiac manifestations, with ECG abnormalities and dilated cardiomyopathy being the most typical.[270-272] Dystrophic myocardial changes occur most prominently in the posterobasal and adjacent lateral left ventricle. They consist of vacuolar degeneration and fibrous replacement of the muscle fibers as well as fatty infiltration of the heart muscle and peripheral circulatory system.[270-274] Arrhythmias and conduction disturbances also occur frequently. Involvement of the posteromedial papillary muscle sometimes causes mitral valve prolapse and mitral regurgitation. CHF usually develops in the preterminal stage of the disease. The most common cause of death is respiratory failure, which is usually precipitated by pulmonary infection. Chronic alveolar hypoventilation and poor cough due to weakness of the respiratory muscles is common by the age of 10.[242, 244, 275] Progressive kyphoscoliosis resulting from severe muscle weakness contributes to the respiratory decline. Finally, loss of the diaphragm late in the disease leads to hypercapnia and rapid deterioration.

Becker's muscular dystrophy is a milder allelic variant of DMD with more variable clinical manifestations. It presents later in life and is slower in progression, so that 50% of patients survive to age 40 and some have a near-normal life expectancy. Cardiac involvement, which is also more variable and unrelated to the extent of the musculoskeletal disease, is often more severe than in DMD. Dilated cardiomyopathy, bundle branch block, complete heart block, or tachyarrhythmias may develop.[270-272, 276] About 30% of patients develop dilated cardiomyopathy and CHF, and some patients have received heart transplants.[276, 277] Respiratory impairment develops similar to DMD, though its onset is later and its course is more slowly progressive.

Myotonic dystrophy (Steinert's disease), an autosomal dominant multisystem disease, is the most common adult form of muscular dystrophy. Symptoms usually present during adolescence or early adulthood, with premature death usually resulting from cardiopulmonary complications. It is associated with cardiac involvement, especially ECG abnormalities and arrhythmias, in at least two thirds of patients; high-grade heart block or ventricular tachycardia may cause sudden death.[278, 279] Occasionally, there is acute left ventricular failure or CHF. Respiratory muscle weakness is common in patients with myotonic dystrophy and can be severe, despite mild limb weakness. Myotonia of the respiratory muscles produces a chaotic breathing pattern, increased work of breathing, and often hypercapnia.[242, 244, 275, 280] Bulbar dysfunction and sleep-related breathing disturbances also occur. These patients are particularly susceptible to respiratory failure with general anesthesia and sedatives. Respiratory failure can also result from chronic respiratory muscle weakness, altered central control of breathing, and pneumonia.

Other types of muscular dystrophy are also associated with cardiopulmonary dysfunction.[270-272, 275, 276] Cardiomyopathy may occur in **fascioscapulohumeral (FSH) dystrophy** and **the limb-girdle syndromes,** but they are usually less prominent and heart failure is unusual. There may be cardiac gallop sounds, cardiac enlargement, and ECG abnormalities. Atrial abnormalities are present in all patients with **X-linked scapuloperoneal myopathy (Emery-Dreifuss dystrophy)** and result in sinus arrest, atrial arrhythmias, varying atrioventricular block, and permanent atrial paralysis with junctional bradycardia. Because sudden death is common in young adults, permanent pacing is recommended for ventricular rates below 50, regardless of atrial activity. FSH dystrophy and the **scapuloperoneal syndromes** have also been associated with atrial paralysis. Pulmonary function has not been studied in much detail in most of the other muscular dystrophies. FSH dystrophy affects the pelvic girdle and trunk muscles in approximately 20% of patients, and this involvement may be associated with respiratory insufficiency. Facial muscle weakness makes spirometric measures unreliable. Limb girdle dystrophy may be accompanied by chronic hypoventilation but rarely requires assisted ventilation. Finally, **oculopharyngeal muscular dystrophy** is associated with swallowing dysfunction, complicated by repeated aspiration, which may improve after cricopharyngeal myotomy.

Friedreich's ataxia is a hereditary disease characterized by progressive spinocerebellar degeneration beginning during adolescence. Progressive weakness and ataxia of the upper and lower extremities gradually develop, resulting in difficulty walking, unsteadiness of the arms and hands, and problems with writing and using eating utensils. Cardiac involvement occurs in 50 to 100% of patients and is characterized by cardiomyopathy with decreased ventricular compliance and varying degrees of hypertrophy and occasionally obstruction to ventricular outflow.[270-272, 281, 282] Cardiac problems often present as the initial manifestation of the disease, though most patients are asymptomatic, except for dyspnea, which could be explained on the basis of their neurologic disability. When other symptoms are noted, they usually consist of palpitations and angina. Arrhythmias are common, especially premature atrial contractions, atrial flutter/fibrillation, and premature ventricular contractions. Progression of the neuromuscular disease usually results in the development of respiratory failure. Death is usually caused by CHF or intercurrent infections and usually occurs within 20 to 30 years after onset of symptoms.[244, 270, 271]

Cardiopulmonary Toxicity of Cancer Treatment

The development of aggressive treatment for a number of cancers has yielded increasing survival rates and periods but has also been associated with increasing frequency of cardiac and pulmonary toxicity. There is often a synergistic effect of irradiation and some of the chemotherapeutic agents. Some of the drugs when used in combination also have a synergistic effect, which increases their degree of cardiac or pulmonary toxicity. This effect has been documented in both early and late toxicity.[283-290]

Therapeutic radiation to the chest (for the treatment of **Hodgkin's disease, non-Hodgkin's lymphoma,** or lung, esophageal, or breast cancer) necessarily exposes the heart and lungs to varying degrees and dosages of radiation, depending upon the extent of disease. The pericardium is the most commonly affected structure; pericarditis is usually mild to moderate and responsive to anti-inflammatory drugs, but can occasionally be severe and necessitate **pericardiocentesis** or **pericardiectomy** for relief of tamponade or constrictive pericarditis, respectively. Other cardiac manifestations of radiation toxicity include acute myocardial ischemia and infarction due to radiation-induced vascular injury and accelerated atherosclerosis; restrictive cardiomyopathy and ECG changes, including varying degrees of heart block, due to endocardial fibrosis; mitral regurgitation resulting from papillary muscle dysfunction; and valvular regurgitation as a consequence of endocardial valvular thickening.[291, 292] Radiation effects on cardiac tissue may occur early, even before the completion of radiotherapy, or they can appear years later, as in patients treated for Hodgkin's disease.[285, 292] Fortunately, more refined treatment techniques have resulted in dramatic decreases in the incidence of these sequelae to less than 2.5%.[293]

Chest irradiation can also produce lung injury.[290, 294-296] Acute radiation pneumonitis occurs in approximately 3 to 15% of patients who receive irradiation to the chest but in approximately 20% of patients with lung carcinoma and up to 35% of patients with Hodgkin's disease with massive mediastinal involvement (more than one third the chest diameter).[296-298] Factors that can increase the risk of developing radiation pneumonitis include concomitant chemotherapy, previous irradiation, and withdrawal of steroids. Radiation pneumonitis usually develops 2 to 3 months following completion of treatment, requires no treatment, and resolves within days to months; however, some patients (less than 5%) develop severe pneumonitis requiring hospitalization and aggressive supportive care.[298] Although frequently asymptomatic, patients often complain of dyspnea, cough, and fever. Over the next 6 to 24 months, most patients then develop gradual progressive fibrosis, which commonly stabilizes after 2 years and is usually asymptomatic. Some patients with no history suggestive of radiation pneumonitis go on to develop late pulmonary fibrosis. It is characterized primarily as a restricted lung disease, as described in Chapter 5, with varying degrees of dyspnea, depending on the amount of fibrotic lung tissue. In cases of persistent fibrosis of a large volume of lung tissue, late radiation fibrosis can be severe, with cor pulmonale and respiratory failure. The major variables associated with radiation injury to the lungs are total radiation dose (above 4000 rads), dose rate (rads/minute) and **fractionation** (rads/treatment), and volume of lung within the high-dose

region. Patients undergoing total body irradiation (TBI) in preparation for bone marrow transplantation and as systemic adjuvant treatment for pediatric and adolescent tumors, such as **neuroblastoma, rhabdomyosarcoma,** and **Ewing's sarcoma,** are also high-risk groups. Some of these patients will develop bronchiolitis obliterans, an obstructive pulmonary disease characterized by a chronic inflammatory cell infiltrate, which progresses to fibrosis and granulation and eventually COPD. Current research trials are examining agents that might modulate the fibrotic process, such as pentoxifylline, ACE inhibitors, and transforming growth factor beta antagonists.

Likewise the treatment of cancer using chemotherapeutic agents and biologic response modifiers is associated with both cardiac and pulmonary toxicity. **Cardiotoxicity** most frequently results from the use of the **anthracycline** antibiotics, doxorubicin (Adriamycin), and daunorubicin (Daunomycin). The newer analogues of doxorubicin (epirubicin, idarubicin, and pirarubicin) and another related compound (mitoxantrone) have similar, though less frequent, cardiotoxic effects.[284, 285, 299, 300] Anthracycline cardiotoxicity can develop as an acute or subacute injury, as a chronic cardiomyopathy, or as late-onset ventricular dysfunction years to decades after completing treatment. Arrhythmias and conduction disturbances are the most common manifestations of acute toxicity; more rarely, subacute left ventricular dysfunction and acute congestive heart failure can develop, as well as myocarditis, sudden death, and myocardial ischemia and infarction. Chronic cardiomyopathy presents within a year of treatment and is the most common form of damage. Late cardiotoxicity appears as a chronic cardiomyopathy appearing after a prolonged asymptomatic period in 38 to 60% of patients treated with doxorubicin, though it is clinically apparent in less than 15% of patients.[301-305] Notably, the incidence of severe cardiac abnormalities increases with the duration of follow-up.

The risk factors associated with the development of a cardiomyopathy include increasing cumulative doses (especially above 500 mg/m² for doxorubicin and above 750 mg/m² for daunorubicin); extremes of age (younger than 18 or older than 70 years); preexisting heart disease, hypertension, and diabetes; previous mediastinal radiation; rapid infusion rates; and cotreatment with other antineoplastic drugs, such as cyclophosphamide and mitomycin C. Young females may be at particular increased risk for late cardiac dysfunction, which is a major concern because doxorubicin is frequently used to treat breast cancer.[306] The prognosis with clinically apparent doxorubicin cardiomyopathy (both early and late onset) is generally poor, with the mortality rate as high as 48% in patients who present in the first month following therapy, although most patients respond to treatment and appear to stabilize.[307, 308] Fortunately, modification of treatment schedules to 48- to 96-hour infusion has greatly reduced the incidence of early cardiomyopathy.[285] Recent research has led to the development of dexrazoxane, a specific cardioprotectant agent, which dramatically decreases the cardiotoxic effects of the anthracyclines by inhibiting fee radical formation and permits the use of higher drug doses.[302, 309, 310]

Other chemotherapeutic agents have also been associated with cardiotoxicity.[284, 299, 300] Amsacrine, azathioprine, cisplatin, methotrexate, mechlorethamine, nitrogen mustard, and paclitaxel (Taxol) have been associated with arrhythmias. Cyclophosphamide in high doses has been reported to cause a rare hemorrhagic myocarditis and occasionally a cardiomyopathy. High-dose cyclophosphamide, amsacrine, and ifosfamide have been associated with impaired ventricular function and cardiomyopathies. Pericarditis is a rare complication seen in patients treated with bleomycin and dactinomycin. Finally, 5-fluorouracil (5-FU), vinblastine, vincristine, bleomycin, cisplatin, and paclitaxel have been linked to myocardial ischemia and infarction in a small percentage of patients. Recombinant technology has resulted in the development of biologic response modifiers, including the interferons, interleukins, and tumor necrosis factor, which also have some adverse cardiovascular effects. Hypotension and tachycardia are the most common problems, though there have also been reports of myocardial ischemia and infarction. These adverse effects appear to be caused by significant alterations in fluid balance rather than any native dysrhythmic or cardiotoxic properties of the drugs. Fortunately, many of the cardiac complications associated with chemotherapeutic agents and biologic response modifiers are transient and reversible.

The lungs are also a common site of chemotherapy-related toxicity, which is being recognized more frequently and associated with an increasing number of drugs (see Table 7–9).[287, 289, 311–314] Interstitial pneumonitis is the most frequently encountered manifestation of pulmonary toxicity, which presents clinically as dyspnea with or without a nonproductive cough and fever. Bleomycin has the highest incidence of interstitial pneumonitis at 3 to 50%, which is related to total dose (especially if greater than 450 to 500 mg/m², but can occur with less than 100 mg/m²).[312, 315] Other drugs that commonly cause interstitial pneumonitis include busulfan, carmustine (BCNU), mitomycin, methotrexate, neocarzinostatin, peplomycin, procarbazine, and tallysomycin S₁₀b. The most common abnormalities seen on pulmonary function testing are a decreased diffusion capacity for carbon dioxide and decreased lung volumes indicative of restrictive lung disease. There may also be arterial hypoxemia, especially with exercise. Some drugs are associated with other forms of pulmonary toxicity; the most notable is cytosine arabinoside, which causes unexplained pulmonary edema in up to 38% of patients.[316] Cyclophosphamide, chlorambucil, ara-C, fludarabine monophosphate, ifosfamide, azathioprine, dihydro-5-azacytidine, ET-18-OCH, and the biologic response modifiers are less commonly associated with pulmonary toxicity. Cyclophosphamide, bleomycin, actinomycin D, and doxorubicin may potentiate damaging effects of radiation on the lungs, whereas pulmonary toxicity from the vinca alkaloids is usually only seen in patients receiving mitomycin as well.[287, 312]

Bone marrow transplantation (BMT) involves the intravenous infusion of hematopoietic progenitor cells to reestablish marrow function in patients with bone marrow failure states, to replace diseased marrow, or as "rescue" to reconstitute marrow following high-dose chemoradiotherapy to eradicate malignancies. BMT is used in the treatment of acute and chronic leukemias, aplastic anemia, and congenital immunologic defects, as well as a variety of solid tumors. BMT can be achieved using bone marrow from an HLA-matched donor (allogeneic), an identical twin (syngeneic), or by reinfusing an individual's own bone marrow, obtained during remission or prior to high dose chemotherapy (autologous). Alternatively, peripheral-blood stem cells can be used instead of autologous BMT. Pulmonary conditions are a major cause of complications and death following BMT and may occur early or late (see Table 7–9). Pulmonary edema is common during the first 2 to 4 weeks after BMT and may result from fluid overload, myocardial injury, cyclosporin toxicity, and transfusion reactions.

The most dangerous complications of BMT are pneumonia and interstitial pneumonitis, which occur in 20 to 50% of transplant recipients and have a mortality rate of 20 to 75%.[317–324] These diseases are most commonly due to *Aspergillus* or other fungi and cytomegalovirus (CMV) infection. Interstitial pneumonitis can also result from the combined effects of the chemotherapy and total body irradiation used as treatment for the original disease or in the conditioning program immediately preceding BMT. Fortunately, the use of CMV-negative marrow and blood products, surveillance bronchoscopies, and prophylactic use of antivirals have significantly reduced the incidence of CMV pneumonia in recent years. Other pulmonary complications which may develop are pulmonary hemorrhage, bronchiolitis obliterans, pulmonary veno-occlusive disease, fat embolism, and, in allogeneic transplants, graft-versus-host disease involving the lungs.[318, 322, 325–331]

Hematologic Disorders

Anemia, or a reduced circulating red blood cell mass relative to the sex and age of an individual, results from excessive destruction of red blood cells, loss by hemorrhage, impaired red blood cell production, or a combination of these factors. The signs and symptoms associated with anemia depend upon the cause of the anemia, its extent, the rapidity of onset, and the presence of any other problems that compromise the individual's health. Anemia commonly produces fatigue, headache, and exertional dyspnea. In addition, patients with coronary disease may have increased episodes of angina with even mild anemia. A number of compensatory mechanisms are available to preserve tissue oxygenation: reduced hemoglobin-oxygen affinity, increased cardiac output, reduced peripheral vascular resistance and blood viscosity, decreased circulatory time, increased oxygen extraction, and redistribution of blood flow. Elevated cardiac output, which develops when hemoglobin values fall below 9 g/dL, appears to be due primarily to the reduction in left ventricular afterload

and an increased stroke volume, rather than an increase in heart rate, at least until the anemia is marked. Congestive heart failure can develop in severe anemia, even in the absence of cardiac disease, but usually results from the increased workload imposed on an unhealthy heart.[332]

Sickle cell disease is a genetic disease found most commonly in blacks and is characterized by hemoglobin that becomes structurally abnormal when deoxygenated so that the red blood cell is "sickle-shaped," less pliable, and "sticky." These alterations result in hemolytic anemia, which is due to the trapping and destruction of the abnormal red blood cells in the spleen; acute painful veno-occlusive crises with tissue ischemia and infarction, particularly in the spleen, central nervous system, bones, liver, kidney, and lungs; and chronic, progressive tissue and organ damage. Cardiopulmonary problems are common in sickle cell disease, as shown in Table 7–10, since both the cardiac output and oxygen extraction by the tissues are increased and the reduced oxygen content of the red blood cells leads to further sickling. Cardiomegaly is a frequent finding and is usually associated with exertional dyspnea and systolic murmurs. Exercise capacity is reduced primarily because of the diminished oxygen-carrying capacity of the blood and may be associated with an exercise-induced drop in cardiac output or myocardial ischemia.[333–336] Specific cardiac manifestations may include biventricular hypertrophy and dilatation, arteritis with proliferation and thrombosis, and myocardial degeneration, necrosis, and fibrosis.[337] Congestive heart failure is a late occurrence. The major pulmonary manifestations of sickle cell disease are recurrent pneumonias, which are a major cause of illness and death in children, and pulmonary vascular occlusion, **capillary stasis,** thrombus formation, and infarction.[338, 339] Any pulmonary disorder that causes alveolar hypoventilation or hypoxia of blood in the lungs of persons with sickle cell disease favors sickling and thrombosis. Thus, areas of pneumonia are particularly prone to in situ pulmonary thrombosis and possible infarction. Rarely, occlusive disease is sufficiently extensive to cause pulmonary hypertension and cor pulmonale. Most patients have abnormal pulmonary function tests, with decreased diffusion capacity, reduced vital capacity, arterial oxygen desaturation, and a widened alveolar-arterial oxygen tension difference.[339]

Chapter 7   Cardiopulmonary Implications of Specific Diseases   ■   319

Acquired Immunodeficiency Syndrome

Acquired immunodeficiency syndrome (AIDS) is characterized by severe immunodeficiency caused by infection of CD4$^+$ (T$_4$) lymphocytes with the human immunodeficiency virus (HIV). Pulmonary involvement is the major cause of complications and death in patients with AIDS (see Table 7–10).[340–343] Opportunistic pulmonary infections with *Pneumocystis carinii* (PCP), tuberculosis, cytomegalovirus (CMV), *Mycobacterium avium-intracellulare* (MAI), or a number of other pathogens are very common. The spectrum of HIV-associated lung diseases varies with geographic location, as well as with severity of immune compromise and the demographic make-up of the HIV-infected population in any given medical center or geographic area. Acute bronchitis and bacterial pneumonia are relatively more common among persons with higher CD4$^+$ lymphocyte counts. In addition, intravenous drug users have higher rates of bacterial pneumonia and tuberculosis than persons in other transmission categories. Other pulmonary abnormalities include diffuse interstitial pneumonitis, either idiopathic or lymphocytic; the AIDS-related pulmonary malignancies, Kaposi's sarcoma, and non-Hodgkin's lymphoma; bronchiolitis obliterans organizing pneumonia; and occasionally pulmonary hypertension.

Cardiac complications can also develop in patients with AIDS, although their prevalence is variable. In 15 autopsy series, the incidence of cardiac involvement ranges from none to 70%, depending on whether or not lymphocytic infiltration with or without myocardial necrosis is included.[344] However, the presence of clinically significant cardiac involvement occurs in about 5 to 20% of patients and only rarely is cardiac disease listed as the cause of death. The most frequent cardiac manifestation of AIDS is pericardial effusion, which is found on echocardiogram in 20 to 40% of patients and is small and asymptomatic in up to 80% of them.[345–347] In patients with AIDS, pericardial effusion can be associated with HIV infection directly, neoplastic heart disease, particularly **Kaposi's sarcoma** or lymphoma, or opportunistic infection, such as tuberculosis, MAI, or CMV.[344] Notably, the survival of patients who develop pericardial effusion is significantly shorter than those who do not,

which suggests that the development of pericardial effusion in the setting of HIV infection probably indicates end-stage disease.[348, 349] Another form of cardiac involvement, which is becoming increasingly more common with longer survival times for HIV-infected patients, is left ventricular dysfunction and dilated cardiomyopathy.[344, 350–352] The most likely etiology appears to be viral myocarditis, although myocardial involvement with lymphoma has also been documented. Other more rare cardiac complications include congestive heart failure, serious arrhythmias, and myocardial atrophy seen in patients with AIDS-associated wasting.

Hepatic Diseases

Several diseases of the liver, including **cirrhosis** and **hepatitis,** produce or are associated with multiple cardiac and pulmonary problems, as shown in Table 7–10. Approximately 15 to 45% of patients with cirrhosis, the most prevalent type of chronic liver disease in the United States, exhibit pulmonary abnormalities, especially arterial hypoxemia in conjunction with hemoglobin desaturation, hyperventilation, and pleural effusions.[353, 354] The mild to moderate hypoxemia that is found in 30 to 70% of patients with cirrhosis is attributable to "anatomic" venous admixture, which results from both high cardiac output and dilation of the pulmonary precapillaries and capillaries so that there is rapid passage of unoxygenated blood past the alveolar-capillary membranes of the lungs. The presence of ascites further compromises pulmonary function due to diaphragmatic elevation and reduced lung volumes. Additionally, patients may develop **portal-pulmonary shunting** and pulmonary hypertension. Primary biliary cirrhosis is associated with diffuse interstitial lung disease, which seems to be related to disease severity.

Chronic alcohol consumption increases the risk of developing pulmonary tuberculosis, chronic bronchitis, aspiration pneumonitis, lung abscess, and pulmonary problems from alcoholic cardiomyopathy.[354] The cardiovascular system can also be affected by chronic alcohol consumption in a variety of ways, including hypertension, cardiac arrhythmias, chest pain, and heart failure. The major cardiac abnormality specific to hepatic disease is **alcoholic cardiomyopathy,** which is responsible for up to one third of the cases of congestive cardiomyopathy (see Chapter 4).[355] In addition, up to 50% of asymptomatic alcoholics demonstrate subclinical abnormalities, including left ventricular hypertrophy, LV dilatation, and diminished contractility.[356] In addition, patients with both alcoholic and nonalcoholic cirrhosis exhibit significantly impaired cardiovascular responses to exercise, particularly marked chronotropic incompetence, failure to increase left ventricular ejection fraction, and subnormal increment in cardiac output.[357]

Eating Disorders

The two most common eating disorders are anorexia nervosa and bulimia. Both disorders occur predominantly in young, previously healthy females and have specific behavioral and psychological features as well as physiologic abnormalities, including those involving the heart and lungs, as summarized in Table 7–10.

Anorexia nervosa is characterized behaviorally by severe self-induced weight loss (at least 15% below ideal body weight) through extreme restriction of food intake and sometimes ritualized exercise. The major psychological manifestations are a distorted body image and an unreasonable concern about being "too fat," as well as denial of hunger, fatigue, and emaciation. A number of medical problems besides the characteristic amenorrhea have been reported in anorexia nervosa: salivary gland enlargement, pancreatitis, pancreatic insufficiency, liver dysfunction, thiamine deficiency, coagulopathies, electrolyte imbalance, decreased gastric emptying and intestinal mobility, hypophosphatemia, bilateral peroneal nerve palsies, hypoglycemia, osteoporosis, hypothalamic dysfunction, and cardiac abnormalities.

In addition to the considerable medical problems caused by anorexia nervosa, there is a significant mortality rate, with rates of approximately 6% over a 5-year period and 15 to 20% at 15 years.[358] Cardiac complications account for most of the deaths. Nutritional depletion results in decreased myocardial muscle mass, diminished glycogen stores, and evidence of myofibrillar destruction.[359] Both systolic and diastolic ventricular dysfunction may occur.[360–362] Mitral valve prolapse is a frequent finding. Clinically, bradycardia, relative hypotension, and abnormal exercise performance with reduced exercise tolerance (approximately 50% of

predicted normal) and blunted heart rate and blood pressure responses are common.[362–364] Multiple ECG abnormalities have been documented, and some of them, including hypokalemic-induced arrhythmias, may be responsible for episodes of sudden death. Finally, there have been reports of congestive heart failure, especially during refeeding.

Bulimia nervosa is a much more common disorder, which is characterized behaviorally by binge-eating counterposed with dieting or purging by self-induced vomiting, laxative abuse, or diuretic abuse. Psychologically, there is an awareness that the eating pattern is abnormal, a fear that eating cannot be controlled, and feelings of depression following binge eating. Because severe weight loss is not a problem for the majority of patients, many of the physiologic abnormalities seen in anorexia nervosa do not occur in most bulimic patients. However, there are major complications associated with bulimia including tooth decay, aspiration pneumonia, esophageal or gastric rupture, pneumomediastinum, pancreatitis, and neurologic abnormalities. The most significant cardiac disorders consist of cardiac arrhythmias (due to hypokalemia from vomiting and laxative abuse), which can be fatal, and occasionally ipecac-induced cardiomyopathy[363] (see Table 7–10).

CLINICAL IMPLICATIONS FOR PHYSICAL THERAPY

The most obvious implication of all the information presented in this chapter is that many patients with many different primary diagnoses may have cardiopulmonary dysfunction. Yet, the symptoms of dysfunction are often nonspecific, such as shortness of breath, lightheadedness, and fatigue, or there may not be any symptoms at all, as in HTN. The only way to determine if a patient is responding to exercise appropriately is to evaluate his/her physiologic responses by monitoring HR, BP, and other signs and symptoms during every PT evaluation. Only in this way can PTs design treatment programs that are both safe and effective.

Another important implication is that PTs must address the needs of the whole patient, not just the primary diagnosis, if the goal is truly to promote "optimal human health and function." Endurance training should be a component of the PT program for every patient who is not already performing regular aerobic exercise, except in those who are acutely ill or have debilitating neuromuscular diseases that are adversely affected by exercise. Endurance exercise facilitates the other components of almost every PT program and offers a number of additional health benefits, as discussed throughout this chapter.

Many specific guidelines have been presented in the sections on the most commonly encountered diagnoses seen by PTs, but many of them can also be applied to patients with the diagnoses presented in this last section. To summarize and reduce to the basics for practical application, the following recommendations are offered:

Guidelines for Physical Therapy Intervention

1. HR, BP, and signs and symptoms should be monitored during every PT evaluation.
2. If the patient's responses are normal, it is safe to proceed with typical treatment planning (including endurance training).
3. If the responses are abnormal, caution is indicated. They may be so abnormal that physician consultation is warranted, or they may signal that the patient's tolerance is compromised and that he or she will require frequent rests during more strenuous activities and careful attention to maintain coordinated breathing during exertion.
4. Patients with moderate to severe cardiopulmonary dysfunction will usually display symptoms of dyspnea, fatigue, and possibly lightheadedness or dizziness during activity, which should be associated with the physiologic responses detected during monitoring and then used during future treatment sessions as indicators of patient tolerance.
5. A few patients will require continued monitoring of HR, O_2 saturation, or BP during treatment sessions.
6. Some patients may benefit more from two shorter treatment sessions per day rather than one intense or prolonged session.

Guidelines for Endurance Training

Regarding endurance training, the following guidelines are suggested:

1. Patients should start slowly and increase their activity gradually.
2. The mode can consist of any form of aerobic exercise, including walking, jogging, cycling, swimming, cross-country skiing, aerobics classes, and can vary during the week.
3. Intensity may be most easily monitored by using a rating of perceived exertion (RPE) scale. A good starting place is "somewhat hard" (13 on the Borg scale of 6 to 20).[60] See Chapter 16.
4. Duration starts with the length of time a patient can exercise until fatigue begins to occur and increases about a minute or 2 per day.
5. Short rest periods (1 to 2 minutes) can be alternated with the exercise intervals if a patient has very limited endurance.
6. Patients will benefit most from twice-daily exercise periods until the duration increases to at least 20 minutes of continuous peak activity.
7. Once a patient can perform the peak aerobic portion of the program for at least 30 minutes continuously, the frequency can be reduced to 3 to 5 days per week, depending on the intensity and the goals of the patient (for control of HTN or reduction of body weight, lower intensity, longer duration exercise programs are more successful).
8. Any amount of activity is better than no activity. If a patient has a hectic day and cannot fit the entire workout in, a partial workout or multiple short bouts are preferable to skipping the workout.
9. Exercise time or distance can be recorded on a calendar in order to keep track of progress and provide motivation. Include totals for each week and month.
10. Finally, exercise should be fun! Identify activities patients enjoy or create a social aspect to their exercise program so it won't seem like a chore.

CASE STUDIES

Case 1

JF is a 76-year-old woman admitted 2 days ago because of confusion, incoherent speech, and lethargy. CT scan revealed a large parietal lobe infarct on the left. Her past medical history is significant for hypertension for 30 years, treated with hydrochlorothiazide 75 mg qd and captopril 50 mg qd. She has had type II diabetes for 15 years, treated with glyburide 5 mg every morning. Positive smoking history: 90 pack/years. The PT assessment reveals a lethargic-appearing 76-year-old woman with obvious right facial paresis, severe dysarthria, flaccid right upper extremity, decreasing tone right lower extremity though positive clonus of right ankle. She requires moderate assistance to roll supine, right side, maximal assistance to roll to left, and maximal assistance of 1 to come to sitting at edge of bed. Sitting balance is poor, with trunk lean to right.

Discussion

Admitting diagnosis of CVA indicates carotid or cerebrovascular disease
Comorbidities: diabetes (treated with oral insulin), hypertension (treated with medication)
Other risk factors for CAD and CVA: Smoking history (90 pack/years, may also have underlying COPD)

Current medical problem of CVA with hemiparesis and functional limitations implies increased work required to perform activities, probable speech and swallowing dysfunction, which increases the risk for aspiration pneumonia.

This patient, who presents with CVA and also has multiple risk factors for CAD should be monitored closely for signs and symptoms of CAD and cardiac pump dysfunction, as well as abnormal responses to exercise. Patient may also benefit from diabetic education. Patients with long-standing smoking history may have underlying COPD and may need to have oxygen saturation monitored, ABGs, and CXR.

Case 2

HS is an obese 67-year-old man admitted to the hospital with chest pain, nausea and vomiting, and positive ECG changes. His hospital course is complicated by complex ventricular dysrhythmias and CHF. He has a past medical history of HTN for 15 years for which he refuses to take any medications, hypercholesterolemia, chronic renal failure for 2 years requiring hemodialysis 3 days per week, peripheral vascular disease, and a 50 pack/year smoking history. During his PT evaluation he repeatedly asks for a cigarette.

Discussion

The patient has an admitting diagnosis of acute complicated MI and has multiple risk factors for CAD, including hypertension, obesity, hypercholesteremia, and smoking. Patient also has diagnoses of PVD and chronic renal failure requiring dialysis, which limits his activity.

The patient's constant requests for cigarettes indicate he is not ready to quit, or may not know the impact of smoking on disease.

The patient would benefit from multiple risk factor reduction, including smoking cessation, cholesterol-lowering intervention, exercise, and diet for weight loss. However, many of these risk factors are also affected by poor renal performance. Patient does not appear to be knowledgeable of the impact of the many risk factors for heart disease on all the other organs and may benefit from a comprehensive education program. Because of the multiple organ involvement patient may be a candidate for kidney transplant, the only other treatment for renal failure other than dialysis. His compliance to treatment interventions has to improve dramatically for him to be considered a candidate, however.

Case 3

MT is a 72-year-old woman admitted 6 days ago because of an intertrochanteric fracture of her right hip, S/p ORIF on day 1, and CHF.

She has a h/o HTN for 20 years and atrial fibrillation for 10 years; 1 week PTA she noted symptoms of an upper respiratory infection, then 2 days PTA noted increased shortness of breath (SOB) and 2-pillow orthopnea, then last night she had SOB at rest and had to sleep sitting up in chair. She fell getting up to go to the bathroom.

Evaluation

PMH: HTN, chronic atrial fibrillation, smoked 1 ppd for 60 years
Social: She is widowed, lives in an apartment in a retirement community, and has no children.
Meds: Digoxin 0.125 mg qd, Vasotec 10 mg bid, Catapres 0.2 mg q hs, Isordil 20 mg bid.
Review of systems: VS: P 116 bpm, BP 170/100 mm Hg, RR 26, T 38.0, Wt 77 kg
Appearance: Mildly obese, in marked distress
Neck: JVD to angle of jaw at 45 degrees
Lungs: Diffusely decreased BS, inspiratory crackles two thirds up both lungs, dull to percussion in right distal base
Cardiac: irreg-irreg rhythm, positive left parasternal lift, increased P_2, grade II/VI systolic murmur; at apex and left sternal border, positive S_3 heart sound
Abdomen: Liver palpable 3 cm below costal margins
Extremities: +2 bilateral pitting edema, skin cool and pale

Diagnostic Tests

ECG: Atrial fibrillation, ventricular rate approximately 110. LAE, LVH with strain pattern, poor R-wave progression
CXR: Marked cardiomegaly, small right pleural effusion, moderate pulmonary congestion
Right hip: Intertrochanteric fracture
Laboratory values: WNL except glucose 302 (nl 70-118), K^+ 5.7 (nl 3.3-4.6), uric acid 10.2 (nl 3.0-7.3), LDH 428 (nl 114-223), dig level 2.7 (nl 0.5-2.5)
Echocardiography: LA 60 mm Hg (nl 15-35), LV 80/70 mm Hg (D/S) (nl 40-50/25-35), Ao root 40 mm Hg (nl 20-35), IVS 14 mm Hg (nl 8-12), LV free wall 16 mm Hg (nl 8-12), RV 32 mm Hg (nl 10-26), all valves normal except mild MR, EF 28% with severe global hypokinesis
MUGA: EF 22% at rest
Hospital course: Treated with IV Lasix and diuresed to 72.2 kg. S/p ORIF right femur on day 4 and tolerated surgery well. Minimal pulmonary congestion seen on postoperative CXR. On day 5 (postoperative day 1), her BUN increased to 55 due to dehydration. She was gently rehydrated to 74 kg and her BUN dropped to 22. On postoperative day 3 she was referred to PT for GT, NWB on R. Current medications include Digoxin 0.125

mg qd, Lasix 40 mg qd, Vasotec 10 mg bid, Isordil 20 mg tid, and Aldomet 500 mg tid.

Discussion

The multiple complications involved in this case include: orthopedic dysfunction and subsequent inactivity, CHF, assumed renal dysfunction (as determined by BUN and half strength digoxin level), pulmonary involvement, irregular heart rhythm.

Summary

- Hypertension (HTN) is diagnosed when diastolic blood pressure (DBP) equals or exceeds 90 mm Hg or when systolic blood pressure (SBP) is consistently higher than 140 mm Hg, with values of 130 to 139/85 to 89 mm Hg being considered high normal.
- The consequences of HTN are directly related to the level of BP, even within the accepted normal range.
- HTN produces a pressure overload on the left ventricle (LV), which is compensated for by left ventricular hypertrophy (LVH). Initially, normal systolic LV function is maintained by the hypertrophied LV. However, diastolic dysfunction with impairment of LV relaxation develops early in the course of essential HTN. The combination of LVH and diastolic dysfunction leads to reduced LV compliance (i.e., a stiffer LV), which creates a greater load on the left atrium with resultant left atrial enlargement. In addition, LVH alters the equilibrium between the oxygen supply and demand of the myocardium.
- The latest guidelines recommend beginning with lifestyle modifications in most patients diagnosed with HTN. The most effective modifications have proved to be weight reduction, sodium restriction, moderation of alcohol intake, and regular aerobic exercise.
- Research involving hypertensive individuals has revealed that exercise capacity is reduced by 15 to 30%, even in those who are asymptomatic, when compared with age- and fitness-matched control subjects. Stroke volume increases subnormally, and peak heart rate is lower; therefore, cardiac output is decreased.
- Although the data are not consistent, the general consensus is that reductions of approximately 10 mm Hg in both systolic and diastolic BP can be achieved through exercise training. These reductions are significant enough to allow some patients to avoid or discontinue drug treatment and many others to reduce their drug dosages.
- Because BP values vary considerably during the day, it is beneficial to include monitoring during two to three different treatment sessions. Also, inasmuch as BP can be normal or borderline at rest but become excessively elevated during exertion, it is important to monitor BP during exercise as well as at rest.
- Diabetes mellitus (DM) is a chronic metabolic disorder characterized by hyperglycemia and caused by inadequate insulin production or ineffective insulin action. Abnormalities in the metabolism of carbohydrates, fats, and proteins result. In addition, vascular and neuropathic components to DM result in abnormalities in both large vessels (macroangiopathy) and small vessels (microangiopathy) and in the peripheral and autonomic nervous systems.
- Hypoglycemia is the major problem associated with insulin therapy, because the level of available insulin can exceed the individual's need at times, especially during the hour or so immediately prior to mealtime.
- A number of important variables affect the metabolic responses to exercise in patients with IDDM: the exercise intensity, type, and duration; the type of insulin used; the injection site; the time between insulin injection and onset of exercise; and the time between exercise and the last meal.
- Cardiovascular disease is the major cause of complications and death in patients with both types of DM. Cardiovascular abnormalities that are more prevalent in diabetics include atherosclerotic heart disease, hypertension, defects in impulse conduction through the heart, congestive heart failure (CHF), autonomic neuropathy, cerebrovascular disease, and peripheral vascular disease.
- Autonomic defects are also very common in patients with long-standing diabetes but are often asymptomatic; when symptoms are noted, they are usually associated with postural hypotension. Autonomic dysfunction can involve predominantly the parasympathetic nervous system (PNS) or both the parasympathetic and sympathetic nervous systems.

- Hyperglycemic diabetic patients have a higher incidence of pulmonary infections than nondiabetic individuals, and those with autonomic neuropathy have more sleep-related breathing problems. Pulmonary function testing often shows mild abnormalities in lung elastic recoil, diffusion capacity, and pulmonary capillary blood volume, which are directly related to the duration of DM.
- Because of the increased incidence of asymptomatic myocardial ischemia and infarction, all patients should have a thorough medical evaluation, including graded exercise testing whenever possible, prior to starting any kind of exercise program.
- Because of the prevalence of autonomic dysfunction in diabetics and its associated risk for silent ischemia and impaired exercise tolerance, autonomic function testing may be included in the PT evaluation. One method is to measure the BP response to standing from the supine position.
- Obesity can be defined as an increased accumulation of adipose tissue so that body mass index (body weight in kilograms divided by height in meters squared) is more than 30 kg/m², body fat is above 25% for males or above 30% for females, or body weight is more than 20% above the upper limit based on height.
- Obesity represents a major health problem in this country because of its association with increased prevalences of HTN, cardiovascular disease, osteoarthritis, gastrointestinal problems, endometrial and breast cancers, glucose intolerance, type II DM, obesity hypoventilation syndrome, sleep apnea, and pulmonary hypertension.
- Peripheral arterial disease (PAD), or more specifically atherosclerotic occlusive disease (AOD), involves obstruction of the large or medium-sized arteries supplying blood to one or more of the extremities (usually lower) by atheromatous plaques.
- Because atherosclerosis is a generalized disorder, most individuals with peripheral arterial insufficiency also have involvement of the coronary arteries, the carotid arteries, or the aorta.
- Patients with intermittent claudication have moderate to severe impairment in walking ability. Their peak exercise capacity during graded treadmill exercise is severely limited, allowing only very light to light activities.

- Because of the high prevalence of atherosclerotic heart disease in patients with peripheral vascular disease, all patients should receive HR and BP monitoring during PT evaluation and initial treatment.
- Because cold weather induces peripheral vasoconstriction, patients with PAD require longer warm-up times before exercising in colder environments.
- The kidneys are complex organs whose major functions include the control of extracellular fluid volume; the regulation of serum osmolality, electrolyte, and acid-base balances; and the secretion of hormones, such as renin and erythropoietin. Thus, when renal function becomes impaired, the resultant metabolic disturbances affect virtually every other body system.
- Chronic renal failure (CRF) results in a number of major complications: hypertension, pericarditis with pericardial effusion and sometimes cardiac tamponade, accelerated atherosclerosis, anemia, bleeding disorders, renal osteodystrophy (bone changes resembling osteomalacia and rickets), proximal myopathy (wasting and weakness of the proximal skeletal muscles), peripheral neuropathy, peptic ulceration, and immunosuppression leading to intercurrent infections.
- Acute and chronic renal failure also have associated pulmonary complications. Pulmonary edema is the most serious problem and may be due to fluid overload as well as increased capillary permeability.
- Although many patients do well for more than 10 years on dialysis, success is limited by the impaired clearance of waste products and other substances and the marked impairment of the regulatory and endocrine functions normally provided by the kidneys.
- Most patients with CRF are extremely sedentary with poor exercise tolerance: only 23 to 60% of patients (depending upon presence of DM or not, respectively) are able to do more than self-care, and their mean exercise capacity is only 4 to 6 METs, or approximately 50% of that of sedentary normal values.
- Collagen vascular disease affects all the elements of the respiratory system, either separately or in combination: the respiratory muscles, the pleura, the small airways, the interstitium, and the pulmonary vessels. Not infrequently, the pulmonary

disease precedes the musculoskeletal manifestations by several months to several years.

- Abnormalities of connective tissue of the great arteries, cardiac valves, skeletal system, and skin are characteristic of a number of diseases, including **Marfan's syndrome, Ehlers-Danlos syndrome, osteogenesis imperfecta,** and *homocystinuria*. These diseases may cause minimal cardiovascular dysfunction, such as mitral valve prolapse or mild aortic root dilatation, or severe problems, such as severe aortic or mitral insufficiency, or aortic dissection and aneurysm.

- There is often a synergistic effect of irradiation and some of the chemotherapeutic agents, and also some of the drugs when used in combination, which increases their degree of cardiac or pulmonary toxicity.

- Approximately 15 to 45% of patients with cirrhosis, the most prevalent type of chronic liver disease in the United States, exhibit pulmonary abnormalities, especially arterial hypoxemia in conjunction with hemoglobin desaturation, hyperventilation, and pleural effusions.

- The only way to determine if a patient is responding to exercise appropriately is to evaluate his or her physiologic responses. This is achieved by monitoring HR, BP, and other signs and symptoms during every PT evaluation.

- Endurance training should be a component of the PT program for every patient who is not already performing regular aerobic exercise, except those who are acutely ill or have debilitating neuromuscular diseases, which are adversely affected by exercise.

References

1. Joint National Committee on Prevention DEaToHBP. The sixth report of the Joint National Committee on prevention, detection, evaluation, and treatment of high blood pressure. Arch Intern Med 157:2413–2446, 1997 [published erratum appears in Arch Intern Med 1998 Mar 23; 158(6):573, Mar 23, 1998].
2. Cushman WC. The clinical significance of systolic hypertension. Am J Hypertens 11:182S–185S, 1998.
3. Kannel WB. Blood pressure as a cardiovascular risk factor: Prevention and treatment. JAMA 275:1571–1576, 1996.
4. Cohn JN, Limas CJ, Guiha NH. Hypertension and the heart. Arch Intern Med 133:969–979, 1974.
5. Frohlich ED. The heart in hypertension. In: Genest J, Kuchel O, Hamet P, et al (eds). Hypertension—Physiopathology and Treatment. New York, McGraw-Hill, 1983, pp 791–810.
6. Society of Actuaries & Association of Life Insurance Medical Directors of America. Blood Pressure Study 1979. Chicago, Society of Actuaries & Association of Life Insurance Medical Directors of America, 1980.
7. Kannel WB. Framingham study insights into hypertensive risk of cardiovascular disease. Hypertens Res 18:181–196, 1995.
8. Kannel WB, Wolf PA, Verter J, McNamara PM. Epidemiologic assessment of the role of blood pressure in stroke: The Framingham Study, 1970. JAMA 276:1269–1278, 1996.
9. Rutan GH, Kuller LH, Neaton JD, et al. Mortality associated with diastolic hypertension and isolated systolic hypertension among men screened for the Multiple Risk Factor Intervention Trial. Circulation 77:504–514, 1988.
10. Strauer BE. Left ventricular wall stress and hypertrophy. In: Messerli FH (ed). The Heart and Hypertension. New York, Yorke Medical Books, 1987, pp 153–165.
11. Graettinger WF, Bryg RJ. Left-ventricular diastolic function and hypertension. Cardiol Clin 13:559–567, 1995.
12. Lopez Sendon J. Regional myocardial ischaemia and diastolic dysfunction in hypertensive heart disease. Eur Heart J 14 (suppl J):110–113, 1993.
13. Smith V-E, Katz AM. Left ventricular relaxation in hypertension. In: Messerli FH (ed). The Heart and Hypertension. New York, Yorke Medical Books, 1987, pp 143–151.
14. Wikstrand J. Diastolic function of the hypertrophied left ventricle. In: Messerli FH (ed). The Heart and Hypertension. New York, Yorke Medical Books, 1987, pp 131–142.
15. Kozakova M, Palombo C, Pratali L, et al. Mechanisms of coronary flow reserve impairment in human hypertension. An integrated approach by transthoracic and transesophageal echocardiography. Hypertension 29:551–559, 1997.
16. Iriarte M, Murga N, Sagastagoitia D, et al. Congestive heart failure from left ventricular diastolic dysfunction in systemic hypertension. Am J Cardiol 71:308–312, 1993.
17. Johnson DB, Dell'Italia LJ. Cardiac hypertrophy and failure in hypertension. Curr Opin Nephrol Hypertens 5:186–191, 1996.
18. Borer JS, Jason M, Devereux RB, et al. Function of the hypertrophied left ventricle at rest and during exercise. Hypertension and aortic stenosis. Am J Med 75:34–39, 1983.
19. Lim PO, MacFadyen RJ, Clarkson PB, MacDonald TM. Impaired exercise tolerance in hypertensive patients. Ann Intern Med 124:41–55, 1996.
20. Manolas J, Kyriakidis M, Anastasakis A, et al. Usefulness of noninvasive detection of left ventricular diastolic abnormalities during isometric stress in hypertrophic cardiomyopathy and in athletes. Am J Cardiol 81:306–313, 1998.
21. Tarazi RC. Cardiovascular hypertrophy in hypertension. Arthur C. Corcoran Memorial Lecture. Hypertension 8: II187–II190, 1986.
22. Devereux RD, Agabiti-Rosei E, Dahlof B, et al. Regression of left ventricular hypertrophy as a surrogate end-point for morbid events in hypertension treatment trials. J Hypertens Suppl 14:S95–101, 1996 [published erratum appears in J Hypertens 15(1):103, Jan 1997].
23. Muiesan ML, Salvetti M, Rizzoni D, et al. Association of change in left ventricular mass with prognosis during long-term antihypertensive treatment. J Hypertens 13:1091–1095, 1995.
24. Schulman DS, Flores AR, Tugoen J, et al. Antihypertensive treatment in hypertensive patients with normal left ventricular mass is associated with left ventricular remodeling and improved diastolic function. Am J Cardiol 78:56–60, 1996.
25. Sytkowski PA, D'Agostino RB, Belanger AJ, Kannel WB.

Secular trends in long-term sustained hypertension, long-term treatment, and cardiovascular mortality. The Framingham Heart Study 1950 to 1990. Circulation 93:697–703, 1996.

26. Kaplan NM. Long-term effectiveness of nonpharmacological treatment of hypertension. Hypertension 18:I153–I160, 1991.

27. Kaplan NM. Treatment of hypertension: Insights from the JNC-VI report. Am Fam Physician 58:1323–1330, 1998.

28. American College of Sports Medicine. Guidelines for Exercise Testing and Prescription. 5th ed. Baltimore, Williams & Wilkins, 1995.

29. Fagard R, Staessen J, Thijs L, Amery A. Influence of antihypertensive drugs on exercise capacity. Drugs 46(suppl 2):32–36, 1993.

30. Head A. Exercise metabolism and beta-blocker therapy. An update. Sports Med 27:81–96, 1999.

31. Kendrick ZV, Cristal N, Lowenthal DT. Cardiovascular drugs and exercise interactions. Cardiol Clin 5:227–244, 1987.

32. Oparil S. Arterial hypertension. In: Bennett JC, Plum F (eds). Cecil Textbook of Medicine. 20th ed. Philadelphia, WB Saunders, 1996, pp 256–271.

33. Fagard R, Staessen J, Amery A. Maximal aerobic power in essential hypertension. J Hypertens 6:859–865, 1988.

34. Goodman JM, McLaughlin PR, Plyley MJ, et al. Impaired cardiopulmonary response to exercise in moderate hypertension. Can J Cardiol 8:363–371, 1992.

35. American Heart Association (The Committee on Exercise). Exercise Testing and Training of Individuals with Heart Disease or at High Risk for its Development: A Handbook for Physicians. New York, American Heart Association, 1975.

36. Blomqvist CG, Lewis SF, Taylor WF, Graham RM. Similarity of the hemodynamic responses to static and dynamic exercise of small muscle groups. Circ Res 48:I87–I92, 1981.

37. Rosenberg E, Froom P, Lewis BS, et al. Blood pressure response to exercise in normotensive and hypertensive young men. Aviat Space Environ Med 61:433–435, 1990.

38. Skinner JS. Exercise Testing and Exercise Prescription for Special Cases—Theoretical Basis and Clinical Application. Philadelphia, Lea & Febiger, 1993.

39. Pickering TG. Exercise and hypertension. Cardiol Clin 5: 311–318, 1987.

40. Balogun MO, Ajayi AA, Ladipo GO. Spectrum of treadmill exercise responses in Africans with normotension, essential hypertension and hypertensive heart failure. Int J Cardiol 21:293–300, 1988.

41. Franz IW. Blood pressure response to exercise in normotensives and hypertensives. Can J Sport Sci 16:296–301, 1991.

42. Nyberg G. Blood pressure and heart rate response to isometric exercise and mental arithmetic in normotensive and hypertensive subjects. Clin Sci Mol Med Suppl 3:681s–685s, 1976.

43. Hagberg JM, Seals DR. Exercise training and hypertension. Acta Med Scand Suppl 711:131–136, 1986.

44. Hagberg JM, Montain SJ, Martin WH, Ehsani AA. Effect of exercise training in 60- to 69-year-old persons with essential hypertension. Am J Cardiol 64:348–353, 1989.

45. Hagberg JM, Brown MD. Does exercise training play a role in the treatment of essential hypertension? J Cardiovasc Risk 2:296–302, 1995.

46. Papademetriou V, Kokkinos PF. The role of exercise in the control of hypertension and cardiovascular risk. Curr Opin Nephrol Hypertens 5:459–462, 1996.

47. Petrella RJ. How effective is exercise training for the treatment of hypertension? Clin J Sport Med 8:224–231, 1998.

48. Kokkinos PF, Narayan P, Colleran JA, et al. Effects of regular exercise on blood pressure and left ventricular hypertrophy in African-American men with severe hypertension. N Engl J Med 333:1462–1467, 1995.

49. Burt VL, Whelton P, Roccella EJ, et al. Prevalence of hypertension in the US adult population. Results from the Third National Health and Nutrition Examination Survey, 1988–1991. Hypertension 25:305–313, 1995.

50. Izzo JL, Black HR. Hypertension Primer. Dallas, American Heart Association, 1993.

51. Perloff D, Grim C, Flack J, et al. Human blood pressure determination by sphygmomanometry. Circulation 88: 2460–2470, 1993.

52. Bond VJ, Bassett DRJ, Howley ET, et al. Evaluation of the Colin STBP-680 at rest and during exercise: An automated blood pressure monitor using R-wave gating. Br J Sports Med 27:107–109, 1993.

53. Garcia-Gregory JA, Jackson AS, Studeville J, et al. Comparison of exercise blood pressure measured by technician and an automated system. Clin Cardiol 7:315–321, 1984.

54. Lightfoot JT, Tankersley C, Rowe SA, et al. Automated blood pressure measurements during exercise. Med Sci Sports Exerc 21:698–707, 1989.

55. Modesti PA, Carrabba N, Gensini GF, et al. Automated blood pressure determination during exercise test. Clinical evaluation of a new automated device. Angiology 43:980–987, 1992.

56. Gordon NF. Hypertension. In: American College of Sports Medicine. ACSM's Exercise Management for Persons with Chronic Diseases and Disabilities. Champaign, IL, Human Kinetics Books, 1997.

57. Gordon NF, Scott CB, Wilkinson WJ, et al. Exercise and mild essential hypertension. Recommendations for adults. Sports Med 10:390–404, 1990.

58. Matsusaki M, Ikeda M, Tashiro E, et al. Influence of workload on the antihypertensive effect of exercise. Clin Exp Pharmacol Physiol 19:471–479, 1992.

59. Borg G, Hassmen P, Lagerstrom M. Perceived exertion related to heart rate and blood lactate during arm and leg exercise. Eur J Appl Physiol 56:679–685, 1987.

60. Borg GA. Psychophysical bases of perceived exertion. Med Sci Sports Exerc 14:377–381, 1982.

61. Pate RR, Pratt M, Blair SN, et al. Physical activity and public health. A recommendation from the Centers for Disease Control and Prevention and the American College of Sports Medicine. JAMA 273:402–407, 1995.

62. Kahn CR, Weir GC. Joslin's Diabetes Mellitus. 13th ed. Philadelphia, Lea & Febiger, 1994.

63. Davidson MB. Diabetes Mellitus Diagnosis and Treatment. 3rd ed. New York, Churchill Livingstone, 1991.

64. Atkinson MA, Maclaren NK. The pathogenesis of insulin-dependent diabetes mellitus. N Engl J Med 331:1428–1436, 1994.

65. Chase HP, Jackson WE, Hoops SL, et al. Glucose control and the renal and retinal complications of insulin-dependent diabetes. JAMA 261:1155–1160, 1989.

66. Crofford OB. Diabetes control and complications. Annu Rev Med 46:267–279, 1995.

67. Hanssen KF, Dahl-Jorgensen K, Lauritzen T, et al. Diabetic control and microvascular complications: The near-normoglycaemic experience. Diabetologia 29:677–684, 1986 [published erratum appears in Diabetologia 29(12):901, Dec 1986].

68. Sherwin RS. Diabetes mellitus. In: Bennett JC, Plum F (eds.) Cecil Textbook of Medicine. 20th ed. Philadelphia WB Saunders, 1996, pp 1258–1277.

69. Heine RJ. The insulin dilemma: Which one to use? In: Krall LP (ed). World Book of Diabetes in Practice. New York, Elsevier Science Publishers BV, 1988.

70. Robertson RP, Klein DJ. Treatment of diabetes mellitus. Diabetologia 35(suppl 2):S8–17, 1992.
71. Renard E, Bringer J, Jaeques-Apostol D, et al. Complications of the pump pocket may represent a significant cause of incidents with implanted systems for intraperitoneal insulin delivery. Diabetes Care 17:1064–1066, 1994.
72. Saudek CD. Implantable pumps. In: Alberti KGMM, Zimmet P, DeFronzo RA (eds). International Textbook of Diabetes Mellitus. 2nd ed. New York, John Wiley, 1997, pp 939–943.
73. Gray DWR, Morris PJ. Islet transplantation. In: Alberti KGMM, Zimmet P, DeFronzo RA (eds). International Textbook of Diabetes Mellitus. 2nd ed. New York, John Wiley, 1997, pp 965–980.
74. Gray H, O'Rahilly S. Toward improved glycemic control in diabetes. What's on the horizon? Arch Intern Med 155: 1137–1142, 1995.
75. Larsen JL, Stratta RJ. Pancreas transplantation: A treatment option for insulin-dependent diabetes mellitus. Diabetes Metab 22:139–146, 1996.
76. Stratta RJ, Larsen JL, Cushing K. Pancreas transplantation for diabetes mellitus. Annu Rev Med 46:281–298, 1995.
77. Stratta RJ, Weide LG, Sindhi R, et al. Solitary pancreas transplantation. Experience with 62 consecutive cases. Diabetes Care 20:362–368, 1997.
78. Baliga BS, Fonseca VA. Recent advances in the treatment of type II diabetes mellitus [see comments]. Am Fam Physician 55:817–824, 1997.
79. Emilien G, Maloteaux JM, Ponchon M. Pharmacological management of diabetes: Recent progress and future perspective in daily drug treatment. Pharmacol Ther 81:37–51, 1999.
80. Koivisto VA. Insulin therapy in type II diabetes. Diabetes Care 16(suppl 3):29–39, 1993.
81. Peirce NS. Diabetes and exercise. Br J Sports Med 33:161–173, 1999.
82. Rybka J. Diabetes Mellitus and Exercise Czechoslovakia, ACTA Universitatis Carolinae Medica, Monograph CXVIII, 1987.
83. Vranic M, Wasserman D, Bukowiecki L. Metabolic implications of exercise and physical fitness in physiology and diabetes. In: Rifkin H, Porte D (eds). Ellenberg and Rifkin's Diabetes Mellitus—Theory and Practice. 4th ed. New York, Elsevier Science Publishing Co., 1990.
84. Caron D, Poussier P, Marliss EB, Zinman B. The effect of postprandial exercise on meal-related glucose intolerance in insulin-dependent diabetic individuals. Diabetes Care 5: 364–369, 1982.
85. MacDonald MN. Postexercise late-onset hypoglycemia in insulin-dependent diabetic patients. Diabetes Care 10:584–588, 1987.
86. Zinman B, Vranic M. Diabetes and exercise. Med Clin North Am 69:145–157, 1985.
87. Devlin JT, Hirshman M, Horton ED, Horton ES. Enhanced peripheral and splanchnic insulin sensitivity in NIDDM men after single bout of exercise. Diabetes 36: 434–439, 1987.
88. Minuk HL, Hanna AK, Marliss EB, et al. Metabolic response to moderate exercise in obese man during prolonged fasting. Am J Physiol 238:E322–E329, 1980.
89. Minuk HL, Vranic M, Marliss EB, et al. Glucoregulatory and metabolic response to exercise in obese noninsulin-dependent diabetes. Am J Physiol 240:E458–E464, 1981.
90. Bogardus C, Ravussin E, Robbins DC, et al. Effects of physical training and diet therapy on carbohydrate metabolism in patients with glucose intolerance and non-insulin-dependent diabetes mellitus. Diabetes 33:311–318, 1984.
91. Reitman JS, Vasquez B, Klimes I, Nagulesparan M. Improvement of glucose homeostasis after exercise training in non-insulin-dependent diabetes. Diabetes Care 7:434–441, 1984.
92. Ruderman NB, Ganda OP, Johansen K. The effect of physical training on glucose tolerance and plasma lipids in maturity-onset diabetes. Diabetes 28(suppl 1):89–92, 1979.
93. Saltin B, Lindgarde F, Houston M, et al. Physical training and glucose tolerance in middle-aged men with chemical diabetes. Diabetes 28 (suppl 1):30–32, 1979.
94. Schneider SH, Amorosa LF, Khachadurian AK, Ruderman NB. Studies on the mechanism of improved glucose control during regular exercise in type 2 (non-insulin-dependent) diabetes. Diabetologia 26:355–360, 1984.
95. Trovati M, Carta Q, Cavalot F, et al. Influence of physical training on blood glucose control, glucose tolerance, insulin secretion, and insulin action in non-insulin-dependent diabetic patients. Diabetes Care 7:416–420, 1984.
96. Wallberg-Henriksson H, Gunnarsson R, Henriksson J, et al. Increased peripheral insulin sensitivity and muscle mitochondrial enzymes but unchanged blood glucose control in type I diabetics after physical training. Diabetes 31: 1044–1050, 1982.
97. Wallberg-Henriksson H, Gunnarsson R, Rossner S, Wahren J. Long-term physical training in female type 1 (insulin-dependent) diabetic patients: Absence of significant effect on glycaemic control and lipoprotein levels. Diabetologia 29:53–57, 1986.
98. Zinman B, Zuniga-Guajardo S, Kelly D. Comparison of the acute and long-term effects of exercise on glucose control in type I diabetes. Diabetes Care 7:515–519, 1984.
99. Diabetes Control and Complications Trial Research Group. The effect of intensive treatment of diabetes on the development and progression of long-term complications in insulin-dependent diabetes mellitus. N Engl J Med 329:977–986, 1993.
100. Turner R, Cull C, Holman R. United Kingdom Prospective Diabetes Study 17: A 9-year update of a randomized, controlled trial on the effect of improved metabolic control on complications in non-insulin-dependent diabetes mellitus. Ann Intern Med 124:136–145, 1996.
101. Kannel WB. Lipids, diabetes, and coronary heart disease: Insights from the Framingham Study. Am Heart J 110: 1110–1107, 1985.
102. Raman M, Nesto RW. Heart disease in diabetes mellitus. Endocrinol Metab Clin North Am 25:425–438, 1996.
103. Harrower AD, Clarke BF. Experience of coronary care in diabetes. Br Med J 1:126–128, 1976.
104. Jacoby RM, Nesto RW. Acute myocardial infarction in the diabetic patient: pathophysiology, clinical course and prognosis. J Am Coll Cardiol 20:736–744, 1992.
105. Kannel WB, McGee DL. Diabetes and cardiovascular disease. The Framingham study. JAMA 241:2035–2038, 1979.
106. Sutherland CG, Fisher BM, Frier BM, et al. Endomyocardial biopsy pathology in insulin-dependent diabetic patients with abnormal ventricular function. Histopathology 14:593–602, 1989.
107. Hausdorf G, Rieger U, Koepp P. Cardiomyopathy in childhood diabetes mellitus: Incidence, time of onset, and relation to metabolic control. Int J Cardiol 19:225–236, 1988.
108. Bottini P, Tantucci C, Scionti L, et al. Cardiovascular response to exercise in diabetic patients: influence of autonomic neuropathy of different severity. Diabetologia 38: 244–250, 1995.
109. Regensteiner JG, Sippel J, McFarling ET, et al. Effects of non-insulin-dependent diabetes on oxygen consumption during treadmill exercise. Med Sci Sports Exerc 27:661–667, 1995 [corrected and republished in Med Sci Sports Exerc 1995 Jun;27(6):875–881].

110. Prakash UBS. Endocrine and metabolic diseases. In: Baum GL, Wolinsky E (eds). Textbook of Pulmonary Diseases. 5th ed. Boston, Little, Brown, 1994.

111. Franz MJ. Exercise and diabetes. In: Haire-Joshu D, ed. Management of Diabetes Mellitus—Perspectives of Care Across the Life Span. St. Louis, Mosby–Year Book, 1996, pp 162–201.

112. Fujita Y, Kawaji K, Kanamori A, et al. Relationship between age-adjusted heart rate and anaerobic threshold in estimating exercise intensity in diabetics. Diabetes Res Clin Pract 8:69–74, 1990.

113. Pollock ML, Wilmore JH. Exercise in Health and Disease. 2nd ed. Philadelphia, WB Saunders, 1990, pp 587–593.

114. Albright AL. Diabetes. In: American College of Sports Medicine. ACSM's Exercise Management for Persons with Chronic Diseases and Disabilities. Champaign, IL, Human Kinetics, 1997, pp 94–100.

115. Ebeling P, Tuominen JA, Bourey R, et al. Athletes with IDDM exhibit impaired metabolic control and increased lipid utilization with no increase in insulin sensitivity. Diabetes 44:471–477, 1995.

116. Fahey PJ, Stallkamp ET, Kwatra S. The athlete with type I diabetes: Managing insulin, diet and exercise. Am Fam Physician 53:1611–1624, 1996.

117. Clements RSJ, Bell DS. Diabetic neuropathy: Peripheral and autonomic syndromes. Postgrad Med 71:50–15, 60, 1982.

118. Clements RSJ, Bell DS. Complications of diabetes. Prevalence, detection, current treatment, and prognosis. Am J Med 79:2–7, 1985.

119. Ewing DJ. Cardiac autonomic neuropathy. In: Jarrett RL (ed). Diabetes and Heart Disease. New York, Elsevier Science, 1984.

120. Prettyman MG. Avoiding complications in people with diabetes and amputation. Adv Physical Ther 8:22–23, 1997.

121. Schteingart DE. Obesity. In: Kelley WN, et al. (eds). Textbook of Internal Medicine. 3rd ed. Philadelphia, JB Lippincott, 1997.

122. Pi-Sunyer FX. Obesity. In: Bennett JC, Plum F (eds). Cecil Textbook of Medicine. 20th ed. Philadelphia, WB Saunders, 1996, pp 1161–1167.

123. Astrup A. Dietary composition, substrate balances and body fat in subjects with a predisposition to obesity. Int J Obes Relat Metab Disord 17 (suppl 3) S32–S36, S41, 1993.

124. Bellisle F, Rolland-Cachera MF, Deheeger M, Guilloud-Bataille M. Obesity and food intake in children: Evidence for a role of metabolic and/or behavioral daily rhythms. Appetite 11:111–118, 1988.

125. Braitman LE, Adlin EV, Stanton JLJ. Obesity and caloric intake: The National Health and Nutrition Examination Survey of 1971–1975 (HANES I). J Chronic Dis 38:727–732, 1985.

126. Miller WC, Lindeman AK, Wallace J, Niederpruem M. Diet composition, energy intake, and exercise in relation to body fat in men and women. Am J Clin Nutr 52:426–430, 1990.

127. Miller WC, Niederpruem MG, Wallace JP, Lindeman AK. Dietary fat, sugar, and fiber predict body fat content. J Am Diet Assoc 94:612–615, 1994.

128. Rolland-Cachera MF, Deheeger M, Bellisle F. Nutrient balance and body composition. Reprod Nutr Dev 37:727–734, 1997.

129. Vobecky JS, Vobecky J, Shapcott D, Demers PP. Nutrient intake patterns and nutritional status with regard to relative weight in early infancy. Am J Clin Nutr 38:730–738, 1983.

130. Golay A, Bobbioni E. The role of dietary fat in obesity. Int J Obes Relat Metab Disord 21(suppl 3):S2–11, 1997.

131. Reimer L. Role of dietary fat in obesity. Fat is fattening. J Fla Med Assoc 79:382–384, 1992.

132. Fordyce-Baum MK, Langer LM, Mantero-Atienza E, et al. Use of an expanded-whole-wheat product in the reduction of body weight and serum lipids in obese females. Am J Clin Nutr 50:30–36, 1989.

133. Raben A, Jensen ND, Marckmann P, et al. Spontaneous weight loss during 11 weeks' ad libitum intake of a low fat/high fiber diet in young, normal weight subjects. Int J Obes Relat Metab Disord 19:916–923, 1995.

134. Rossner S, von Zweigbergk D, Ohlin A, Ryttig K. Weight reduction with dietary fibre supplements. Results of two double-blind randomized studies. Acta Med Scand 222:83–88, 1987.

135. Bjorntorp P, Yang MU. Refeeding after fasting in the rat: effects on body composition and food efficiency. Am J Clin Nutr 36:444–449, 1982.

136. Blackburn GL, Wilson GT, Kanders BS, et al. Weight cycling: the experience of human dieters. Am J Clin Nutr 49:1105–1109, 1989.

137. NIH. Health implications of obesity. National Institutes of Health Consensus Development Conference Statement. Ann Intern Med 103:147–151, 1985.

138. Kannel WB, D'Agostino RB, Cobb JL. Effect of weight on cardiovascular disease. Am J Clin Nutr 63:419S–422S, 1996.

139. Van Itallie TB. Health implications of overweight and obesity in the United States. Ann Intern Med 103:983–988, 1985.

140. Bjorntorp P. Abdominal fat distribution and disease: an overview of epidemiological data. Ann Med 24:15–18, 1992.

141. Casassus P, Fontbonne A, Thibult N, et al. Upper-body fat distribution: A hyperinsulinemia-independent predictor of coronary heart disease mortality. The Paris Prospective Study. Arterioscler Thromb 12:1387–1392, 1992.

142. Pouliot MC, Despres JP, Lemieux S, et al. Waist circumference and abdominal sagittal diameter: Best simple anthropometric indexes of abdominal visceral adipose tissue accumulation and related cardiovascular risk in men and women. Am J Cardiol 73:460–468, 1994.

143. Alexander JK. The cardiomyopathy of obesity. Prog Cardiovasc Dis 27:325–334, 1985.

144. Alexander JK. Obesity and the heart. Heart Dis Stroke 2:317–321, 1993.

145. Franklin B, Buskirk E, Hodgson J, et al. Effects of physical conditioning on cardiorespiratory function, body composition and serum lipids in relatively normal-weight and obese middle-aged women. Int J Obes 3:97–109, 1979.

146. Gwinup G. Effect of exercise alone on the weight of obese women. Arch Intern Med 135:676–680, 1975.

147. Kukkonen K, Rauramaa R, Siitonen O, Hanninen O. Physical training of obese middle-aged persons. Ann Clin Res 14 (suppl 34):80–85, 1982.

148. Wadden TA, Vogt RA, Andersen RE, et al. Exercise in the treatment of obesity: Effects of four interventions on body composition, resting energy expenditure, appetite, and mood. J Consult Clin Psychol 65:269–277, 1997.

149. Warwick PM, Garrow JS. The effect of addition of exercise to a regime of dietary restriction on weight loss, nitrogen balance, resting metabolic rate and spontaneous physical activity in three obese women in a metabolic ward. Int J Obes 5:25–32, 1981.

150. Weltman A, Matter S, Stamford BA. Caloric restriction and/or mild exercise: effects on serum lipids and body composition. Am J Clin Nutr 33:1002–1009, 1980.

151. Hill JO, Sparling PB, Shields TW, Heller PA. Effects of exercise and food restriction on body composition and

metabolic rate in obese women. Am J Clin Nutr 46:622–630, 1987.

152. Oscai LB, Holloszy JO. Effects of weight changes produced by exercise, food restriction, or overeating on body composition. J Clin Invest 48:2124–2128, 1969.

153. Hammer RL, Barrier CA, Roundy ES, et al. Calorie-restricted low-fat diet and exercise in obese women. Am J Clin Nutr 49:77–85, 1989.

154. Pavlou KN, Steffee WP, Lerman RH, Burrows BA. Effects of dieting and exercise on lean body mass, oxygen uptake, and strength. Med Sci Sports Exerc 17:466–471, 1985.

155. Blair SN. Evidence for success of exercise in weight loss and control. Ann Intern Med 119:702–706, 1993.

156. Pavlou KN, Krey S, Steffee WP. Exercise as an adjunct to weight loss and maintenance in moderately obese subjects. Am J Clin Nutr 49:1115–1123, 1989.

157. Bray GA. Exercise and obesity. In: Bouchard C, Shephard RJ (eds). Exercise, Fitness, and Health. Champaign, IL, Human Kinetics Books, 1990, pp 497–510.

158. Leon AS, Conrad J, Hunninghake DB, Serfass R. Effects of a vigorous walking program on body composition, and carbohydrate and lipid metabolism of obese young men. Am J Clin Nutr 32:1776–1787, 1979.

159. Jakicic JM, Wing RR, Butler BA, Robertson RJ. Prescribing exercise in multiple short bouts versus one continuous bout: Effects on adherence, cardiorespiratory fitness, and weight loss in overweight women. Int J Obes Relat Metab Disord 19:893–901, 1995.

160. Wallace JP. Obesity. In: American College of Sports Medicine ACSM's Exercise Management for Persons with Chronic Diseases and Disabilities. Champaign, IL, Human Kinetics, 1997, pp 106–111.

161. Hertzer NR, Beven EG, Young JR, et al. Coronary artery disease in peripheral vascular patients. A classification of 1000 coronary angiograms and results of surgical management. Ann Surg 199:223–233, 1984.

162. Kallero KS. Mortality and morbidity in patients with intermittent claudication as defined by venous occlusion plethysmography. A ten-year follow-up study. J Chronic Dis 34:455–462, 1981.

163. Leng GC, Lee AJ, Fowkes FG, et al. Incidence, natural history and cardiovascular events in symptomatic and asymptomatic peripheral arterial disease in the general population. Int J Epidemiol 25:1172–1181, 1996.

164. Matsubara J, Ohta T, Sakurai T, Yamada I. Natural history of intermittent claudication in the Japanese. Jpn J Surg 16:42–45, 1986.

165. Simonsick EM, Guralnik JM, Hennekens CH, et al. Intermittent claudication and subsequent cardiovascular disease in the elderly. J Gerontol A Biol Sci Med Sci 50A:M17–M22, 1995.

166. Bauer TA, Regensteiner JG, Brass EP, Hiatt WR. Oxygen uptake kinetics during exercise are slowed in patient with peripheral arterial disease. J Appl Physiol 87:809–816, 1999.

167. Eldridge JE, Hossack KF. Patterns of oxygen consumption during exercise testing in peripheral vascular disease. Cardiology 74:236–240, 1987.

168. Hansen JE, Sue DY, Oren A, Wasserman K. Relation of oxygen uptake to work rate in normal men and men with circulatory disorders. Am J Cardiol 59:669–674, 1987.

169. Boyd CE, Bird PJ, Teates CD, et al. Pain free physical training in intermittent claudication. J Sports Med Phys Fitness 24:112–122, 1984.

170. Creasy TS, McMillan PJ, Fletcher EW, et al. Is percutaneous transluminal angioplasty better than exercise for claudication? Preliminary results from a prospective randomised trial. Eur J Vasc Surg 4:135–140, 1990.

171. Dahllof AG, Holm J, Schersten T. Exercise training of patients with intermittent claudication. Scand J Rehabil Med Suppl 9:20–26, 1983.

172. Ernst EE, Matrai A. Intermittent claudication, exercise, and blood rheology. Circulation 76:1110–1114, 1987.

173. Hiatt WR, Regensteiner JG, Hargarten ME, et al. Benefit of exercise conditioning for patients with peripheral arterial disease. Circulation 81:602–609, 1990.

174. Hiatt WR, Wolfel EE, Meier RH, Regensteiner JG. Superiority of treadmill walking exercise versus strength training for patients with peripheral arterial disease. Implications for the mechanism of the training response. Circulation 90:1866–1874, 1994.

175. Jonason T, Ringqvist I, Oman-Rydberg A. Home-training of patients with intermittent claudication. Scand J Rehabil Med 13:137–141, 1981.

176. Mannarino E, Pasqualini L, Menna M, et al. Effects of physical training on peripheral vascular disease: A controlled study. Angiology 40:5–10, 1989.

177. Ruell PA, Imperial ES, Bonar FJ, et al. Intermittent claudication. The effect of physical training on walking tolerance and venous lactate concentration. Eur J Appl Physiol 52:420–425, 1984.

178. Perkins JM, Collin J, Creasy TS, et al. Exercise training versus angioplasty for stable claudication. Long and medium term results of a prospective, randomised trial. Eur J Vasc Endovasc Surg 11:409–413, 1996.

179. Larsen OA, Lassen NA. Effect of daily muscular exercise in patients with intermittent claudication. Lancet 2:1093–1096, 1966.

180. Gardner AW. Peripheral arterial disease. In: American College of Sports Medicine. ACSM's Exercise Management for Persons with Chronic Diseases and Disabilities. Champaign, IL, Human Kinetics, 1997, pp 64–68.

181. Smith RB, Perdue GD. Diseases of the peripheral arteries and veins. In: Alexander RW, Schlant RC, et al (eds). Hurst's The Heart, Arteries and Veins. 9th ed. New York, McGraw-Hill 1998.

182. Carter SA. Effects of ambulation on foot oxygen tension in limbs with peripheral atherosclerosis. Clin Physiol 16:199–208, 1996.

183. Laghi Pasini F, Pastorelli M, Beermann U, et al. Peripheral neuropathy associated with ischemic vascular disease of the lower limbs. Angiology 47:569–577, 1996.

184. Sweny P, Farrington K, Moorhead JF. The Kidney and Its Disorders. Oxford, Blackwell Scientific Publications, 1989.

185. Warnock DG. Chronic renal failure. In: Bennett JC, Plum F (eds). Cecil Textbook of Medicine. 20th ed. Philadelphia, WB Saunders, 1996, pp 556–563.

186. Leier CV, Boudoulas H. Renal disorders and heart disease. In: Braunwald E (ed). Heart Disease—A Textbook of Cardiovascular Medicine. 5th ed. Philadelphia, WB Saunders, 1997, pp 1914–1938.

187. O'Rourke RA, Brenner BM, Stein JH. The Heart and Renal Disease. New York, Churchill Livingstone, 1984.

188. Pastan SO, Mitch WE. The heart and kidney disease. In: Alexander RW, Schlant RC, et al (eds). Hurst's The Heart, Arteries and Veins. 9th ed. New York, McGraw-Hill, 1998, pp 2413–2423.

189. Prakash UBS. Renal diseases. In: Baum GL, Wolinsky E (eds). Textbook of Pulmonary Diseases. 5th ed. Boston, Little, Brown, 1994.

190. Dunn CJ, Markham A. Epoetin beta. A review of its pharmacological properties and clinical use in the management of anaemia associated with chronic renal failure. Drugs, 51:299–318, 1996 [published erratum appears in Drugs 51(5):894, May 1996.]

191. Gutman RA, Stead WW, Robinson RR. Physical activity and

employment status of patients on maintenance dialysis. N Engl J Med 304:309–313, 1981.

192. Goldberg AP, Geltman EM, Gavin JR, et al. Exercise training reduces coronary risk and effectively rehabilitates hemodialysis patients. Nephron 42:311–316, 1986.

193. Harter HR, Goldberg AP. Endurance exercise training. An effective therapeutic modality for hemodialysis patients. Med Clin North Am 69:159–175, 1985.

194. Painter PL, Nelson-Worel JN, Hill MM, et al. Effects of exercise training during hemodialysis. Nephron 43:87–92, 1986.

195. Shalom R, Blumenthal JA, Williams RS, et al. Feasibility and benefits of exercise training in patients on maintenance dialysis. Kidney Int 25:958–963, 1984.

196. Zabetakis PM, Gleim GW, Pasternack FL, et al. Long-duration submaximal exercise conditioning in hemodialysis patients. Clin Nephrol 18:17–22, 1982.

197. Diesel W, Noakes TD, Swanepoel C, Lambert M. Isokinetic muscle strength predicts maximum exercise tolerance in renal patients on chronic hemodialysis. Am J Kidney Dis 16:109–114, 1990.

198. Painter PL. Renal failure. In: American College of Sports Medicine. ACSM's Exercise Management for Persons with Chronic Diseases and Disabilities. Champaign, IL, Human Kinetics, 1997, pp 89–93.

199. Hanson P, Ward A, Painter P. Exercise training for special populations. J Cardiopulmonary Rehabil 6:104–112, 1986.

200. Kettner A, Goldberg A, Hagberg J, et al. Cardiovascular and metabolic responses to submaximal exercise in hemodialysis patients. Kidney Int 26:66–71, 1984.

201. Goldberg AP, Geltman EM, Hagberg JM, et al. Therapeutic benefits of exercise training for hemodialysis patients. Kidney Int Suppl 16:S303–S309, 1983.

202. Ross DL, Grabeau GM, Smith S, et al. Efficacy of exercise for end-stage renal disease patients immediately following high-efficiency hemodialysis: A pilot study. Am J Nephrol 9:376–383, 1989.

203. Burke E, Germaine MJ, Hartzog R, et al. Physiological responses to submaximal exercise in chronic renal failure, on and off hemodialysis. Med Sci Sports Exerc 15:157 [abstract], 1983.

204. Painter P, Messer-Rehak D, Hanson P, et al. Exercise capacity in hemodialysis, CAPD, and renal transplant patients. Nephron 42:47–51, 1986.

205. Painter P, Zimmerman SW. Exercise in end-stage renal disease. Am J Kidney Dis 7:386–394, 1986.

206. Kempeneers G, Noakes TD, van Zyl-Smit R, et al. Skeletal muscle limits the exercise tolerance of renal transplant recipients: Effects of a graded exercise training program. Am J Kidney Dis 16:57–65, 1990.

207. Miller TD, Squires RW, Gau GT, et al. Graded exercise testing and training after renal transplantation: a preliminary study. Mayo Clin Proc 62:773–777, 1987.

208. Scott JP, Hay IF, Higenbottam TW, et al. Hypertensive exercise responses in cyclosporin-treated normotensive renal transplant recipients. Nephron 56:143–147, 1990.

209. Painter P. End-stage renal disease. In: Skinner JS (ed). Exercise Testing and Exercise Prescription for Special Cases. 2nd ed. Philadelphia, Lea & Febiger, 1993, pp 351–362.

210. Fitts SS, Guthrie MR. Six-minute walk by people with chronic renal failure. Assessment of effort by perceived exertion. Am J Phys Med Rehabil 74:54–58, 1995.

211. Schwartz MI. Pulmonary manifestations of the collagen vascular diseases. In: Fishman AP, Elias JA, et al. (eds). Fishman's Pulmonary Diseases and Disorders. 3rd ed. New York, McGraw-Hill, 1998, pp 1115–1132.

212. Coblyn JS, Weinblatt ME. Rheumatic diseases and the heart. In: Braunwald E (ed). Heart Disease—A Textbook

of Cardiovascular Medicine. Philadelphia, WB Saunders, 1997.

213. Prakash UBS. Rheumatologic diseases. In: Baum GL, Wolinsky E (eds). Textbook of Pulmonary Diseases. 5th ed. Boston: Little, Brown, 1994, pp 1471–1496.

214. Doherty NE, Siegel RJ. Cardiovascular manifestations of systemic lupus erythematosus. Am Heart J 110:1257–1265, 1985.

215. Hoffman BI. Cardiac manifestations. In: Katz WA (ed). Diagnosis and Management of Rheumatic Diseases. 2nd ed. Philadelphia, JB Lippincott, 1988, pp 198–203.

216. Leung WH, Wong KL, Lau CP, et al. Cardiac abnormalities in systemic lupus erythematosus: A prospective M-mode, cross-sectional and Doppler echocardiographic study. Int J Cardiol 27:367–375, 1990.

217. Ong ML, Veerapen K, Chambers JB, et al. Cardiac abnormalities in systemic lupus erythematosus: Prevalence and relationship to disease activity. Int J Cardiol 34:69–74, 1992.

218. Schlant RC, Gonzales EB, Roberts WC. The connective tissue diseases. In: Alexander RW, Schlant RC, et al. (eds). The Heart, Arteries, and Veins. 9th ed. New York, McGraw-Hill Information Services 1998, pp 2271–2294.

219. Sturfelt G, Eskilsson J, Nived O, et al. Cardiovascular disease in systemic lupus erythematosus. A study of 75 patients form a defined population. Medicine (Baltimore) 71:216–223, 1992.

220. Bankier AA, Kiener HP, Wiesmayr MN, et al. Discrete lung involvement in systemic lupus erythematosus: CT assessment. Radiology 196:835–840, 1995.

221. Sant SM, Doran M, Fenelon HM, Breatnach ES. Pleuropulmonary abnormalities in patients with systemic lupus erythematosus: Assessment with high resolution computed tomography, chest radiography and pulmonary function tests. Clin Exp Rheumatol 15:507–513, 1997.

222. Scoggin CH. Pulmonary manifestations. In: Katz WA (ed). Diagnosis and Management of Rheumatic Diseases. 2nd ed. Philadelphia JB Lippincott, 1988, pp 204–210.

223. Anvari A, Graninger W, Schneider B, et al. Cardiac involvement in systemic sclerosis. Arthritis Rheum 35:1356–1361, 1992.

224. Botstein GR, LeRoy EC. Primary heart disease in systemic sclerosis (scleroderma): Advances in clinical and pathologic features, pathogenesis, and new therapeutic approaches. Am Heart J 102:913–919, 1981.

225. Goldman AP, Kotler MN. Heart disease in scleroderma. Am Heart J 110:1043–1046, 1985.

226. Schwaiblmair M, Behr J, Fruhmann G. Cardiorespiratory responses to incremental exercise in patients with systemic sclerosis. Chest 110:1520–1525, 1996.

227. LeRoy EC. Systemic sclerosis (scleroderma). In: Bennett JC, Plum F (ed). Cecil Textbook of Medicine. 20th ed. Philadelphia, WB Saunders, 1996, pp 1483–1488.

228. Remy-Jardin M, Remy J, Wallaert B, et al. Pulmonary involvement in progressive systemic sclerosis: Sequential evaluation with CT, pulmonary function tests, and bronchoalveolar lavage. Radiology 188:499–506, 1993.

229. Owens GR, Follansbee WP. Cardiopulmonary manifestations of systemic sclerosis. Chest 91:118–127, 1987.

230. Battle RW, Davitt MA, Cooper SM, et al. Prevalence of pulmonary hypertension in limited and diffuse scleroderma. Chest 110:1515–1519, 1996.

231. Koh ET, Lee P, Gladman DD, Abu-Shakra M. Pulmonary hypertension in systemic sclerosis: an analysis of 17 patients. Br J Rheumatol 35:989–993, 1996.

232. Diot E, Boissinot E, Asquier E, et al. Relationship between abnormalities on high-resolution CT and pulmonary function in systemic sclerosis. Chest 114:1623–1629, 1998.

233. Greenwald GI, Tashkin DP, Gong H, et al. Longitudinal changes in lung function and respiratory symptoms in progressive systemic sclerosis. Prospective study. Am J Med 83: 83–92, 1987.

234. Jacobsen S, Halberg P, Ullman S, et al. A longitudinal study of pulmonary function in Danish patients with systemic sclerosis. Clin Rheumatol 16:384–390, 1997.

235. Gray IR. Cardiovascular manifestations of collagen-vascular diseases. In: Julian DG (ed). Diseases of the Heart. Toronto, Baillière Tindall, 1989, pp 1397–1403.

236. Wolff SM. Polyarteritis nodosa group. In: Wyngaarden JB, Smith LH, Jr. (eds). Cecil Textbook of Medicine. 19th ed. Philadelphia, WB Saunders, 1992, pp 1539–1541.

237. Crowley JJ, Donnelly SM, Tobin M, et al. Doppler echocardiographic evidence of left ventricular diastolic dysfunction in ankylosing spondylitis. Am J Cardiol 71:1337–1340, 1993.

238. Tanoue LT. Pulmonary involvement in collagen vascular disease: A review of the pulmonary manifestations of the Marfan syndrome, ankylosing spondylitis, Sjogren's syndrome, and relapsing polychondritis. J Thorac Imaging 7: 62–77, 1992.

239. Wiedemann HP, Matthay RA. Pulmonary manifestations of the collagen vascular diseases. Clin Chest Med 10:677–722, 1989.

240. Celli BR, Rassulo J, Corral R. Ventilatory muscle dysfunction in patients with bilateral idiopathic diaphragmatic paralysis: Reversal by intermittent external negative pressure ventilation. Am Rev Respir Dis 136:1276–1278, 1987.

241. Carrey Z, Gottfried SB, Levy RD. Ventilatory muscle support in respiratory failure with nasal positive pressure ventilation. Chest 97:150–158, 1990.

242. Criner GJ, Kelsen SG. Effects of neuromuscular diseases on ventilation. In: Fishman AP, Elias JA, et al. (eds). Fishman's Pulmonary Diseases and Disorders. 3rd ed. New York, McGraw-Hill, 1998, pp 1561–1585.

243. Oppenheimer S, Hachinski V. Complications of acute stroke. Lancet 339:721–724, 1992.

244. Prakash UBS. Neurologic diseases. In: Baum GL, Wolinsky E (eds). Textbook of Pulmonary Diseases. 5th ed. Boston, Little, Brown, 1994, pp 1663–1690.

245. Oppenheimer SM, Hachinski VC. The cardiac consequences of stroke. Neurol Clin 10:167–176, 1992.

246. Chimowitz MI, Mancini GB. Asymptomatic coronary artery disease in patients with stroke. Prevalence, prognosis, diagnosis, and treatment. Stroke 23:433–436, 1992.

247. Hertzer NR, Young JR, Beven EG, et al. Coronary angiography in 506 patients with extracranial cerebrovascular disease. Arch Intern Med 145:849–852, 1985.

248. Di Pasquale G, Andreoli A, Pinelli G, et al. Cerebral ischemia and asymptomatic coronary artery disease: A prospective study of 83 patients. Stroke 17:1098–1101, 1986.

249. Love BB, Grover-McKay M, Biller J, et al. Coronary artery disease and cardiac events with asymptomatic and symptomatic cerebrovascular disease. Stroke 23:939–945, 1992.

250. Massery M. The patient with neuromuscular or musculoskeletal dysfunction. In: Frownfelter D, Dean E (eds). Principles and Practice of Cardiopulmonary Physical Therapy. 3rd ed. St. Louis, Mosby, 1996, pp 679–702.

251. Bateman DN, Cooper RG, Gibson GJ, et al. Levodopa dosage and ventilatory function in Parkinson's disease. Br Med J (Clin Res Ed) 283:190–191, 1981.

252. Brown LK. Respiratory dysfunction in Parkinson's disease. Clin Chest Med 15:715–727, 1994.

253. Hovestadt A, Bogaard JM, Meerwaldt JD, et al. Pulmonary function in Parkinson's disease. J Neurol Neurosurg Psychiatry 52:329–333, 1989.

254. Izquierdo-Alonso JL, Jimenez-Jimenez FJ, Cabrera-Valdivia F, Mansilla-Lesmes M. Airway dysfunction in patients with Parkinson's disease. Lung 172:47–55, 1994.

255. Mehta AD, Wright WB, Kirby BJ. Ventilatory function in Parkinson's disease. Br Med J 1:1456–1457, 1978.

256. Sabate M, Gonzalez I, Ruperez F, Rodriguez M. Obstructive and restrictive pulmonary dysfunctions in Parkinson's disease. J Neurol Sci 138:114–119, 1996.

257. Nakano KK, Bass H, Tyler HR, Carmel RJ. Amyotrophic lateral sclerosis: A study of pulmonary function. Dis Nerv Syst 37:32–35, 1976.

258. Fallat RJ, Jewitt B, Bass M, et al. Spirometry in amyotrophic lateral sclerosis. Arch Neurol 36:74–80, 1979.

259. Gracey DR, McMichan JC, Divertie MB, Howard FMJ. Respiratory failure in Guillain-Barré syndrome: A 6-year experience. Mayo Clin Proc 57:742–746, 1982.

260. Ng KK, Howard RS, Fish DR, et al. Management and outcome of severe Guillain-Barré syndrome. QJM 88:243–250, 1995.

261. Teitelbaum JS, Borel CO. Respiratory dysfunction in Guillain-Barré syndrome. Clin Chest Med 15:705–714, 1994.

262. Buyse B, Demedts M, Meekers J, et al. Respiratory dysfunction in multiple sclerosis: A prospective analysis of 60 patients. Eur Respir J 10:139–145, 1997.

263. Carter JL, Noseworthy JH. Ventilatory dysfunction in multiple sclerosis. Clin Chest Med 15:693–703, 1994.

264. Foglio K, Clini E, Facchetti D, et al. Respiratory muscle function and exercise capacity in multiple sclerosis. Eur Respir J 7:23–28, 1994.

265. Gibson TC. The heart in myasthenia gravis. Am Heart J 90:389–396, 1975.

266. Ashok PP, Ahuja GK, Manchanda SC, Jalal S. Cardiac involvement in myasthenia gravis. Acta Neurol Scand 68: 113–120, 1983.

267. Hofstad H, Ohm OJ, Mork SJ, Aarli JA. Heart disease in myasthenia gravis. Acta Neurol Scand 70:176–184, 1984.

268. Mygland A, Aarli JA, Hofstad H, Gilhus NE. Heart muscle antibodies in myasthenia gravis. Autoimmunity 10:263–267, 1991.

269. Kelly BJ, Luce JM. The diagnosis and management of neuromuscular diseases causing respiratory failure. Chest 99: 1485–1494, 1991.

270. Perloff JK. Neurological disorders and heart disease. In: Braunwald E (ed). Heart Disease—A Textbook of Cardiovascular Medicine. 5th ed. Philadelphia, WB Saunders, 1997, pp 1865–1886.

271. Swash M, Schwartz MS. Neuromuscular Diseases—A Practical Approach to Diagnosis and Management. 3rd ed. New York, Springer, 1997, pp 433–440.

272. Towbin JA, Roberts R. Cardiovascular diseases due to genetic abnormalities. In: Alexander RW, Schlant RC, et al. (eds). Hurst's The Heart, Arteries and Veins. 9th ed. New York, McGraw-Hill, 1998, pp 1877–1923.

273. Perloff JK, de Leon ACJ, O'Doherty D. The cardiomyopathy of progressive muscular dystrophy. Circulation 33:625–648, 1966.

274. Perloff JK, Henze E, Schelbert HR. Alterations in regional myocardial metabolism, perfusion, and wall motion in Duchenne muscular dystrophy studied by radionuclide imaging. Circulation 69:33–42, 1984.

275. Lynn DJ, Woda RP, Mendell JR. Respiratory dysfunction in muscular dystrophy and other myopathies. Clin Chest Med 15:661–674, 1994.

276. Steare SE, Dubowitz V, Benatar A. Subclinical cardiomyopathy in Becker muscular dystrophy. Br Heart J 68:304–308, 1992.

277. Quinlivan RM, Dubowitz V. Cardiac transplantation in Becker muscular dystrophy. Neuromuscul Disord 2:165–167, 1992.

278. Moorman JR, Coleman RE, Packer DL, et al. Cardiac involvement in myotonic muscular dystrophy. Medicine (Baltimore) 64:371–387, 1985.

279. Perloff JK, Stevenson WG, Roberts NK, et al. Cardiac involvement in myotonic muscular dystrophy (Steinert's disease): A prospective study of 25 patients. Am J Cardiol 54:1074–1081, 1984.

280. Begin P, Mathieu J, Almirall J, Grassino A. Relationship between chronic hypercapnia and inspiratory-muscle weakness in myotonic dystrophy. Am J Respir Crit Care Med 156:133–139, 1997.

281. Alboliras ET, Shub C, Gomez MR, et al. Spectrum of cardiac involvement in Friedreich's ataxia: Clinical, electrocardiographic and echocardiographic observations. Am J Cardiol 58:518–524, 1986.

282. Harding AE, Hewer RL. The heart disease of Friedreich's ataxia: A clinical and electrocardiographic study of 115 patients, with an analysis of serial electrocardiographic changes in 30 cases. Q J Med 52:489–502, 1983.

283. Alberts WM. Pulmonary complications of cancer treatment. Curr Opin Oncol 9:161–169, 1997.

284. Allen A. The cardiotoxicity of chemotherapeutic drugs. Semin Oncol 19:529–542, 1992.

285. Ewer MS, Benjamin RS. Cardiac complications. In: Holland JF, Blast RC, Jr. (eds). Cancer Medicine. 4th ed. Baltimore, Williams & Wilkins, 1997.

286. Jones RB. Respiratory complications. In: Holland JF, Blast RC, Jr. (eds). Cancer Medicine. 4th ed. Baltimore: Williams & Wilkins, 1997.

287. McDonald S, Rubin P, Phillips TL, Marks LB. Injury to the lung from cancer therapy: Clinical syndromes, measurable endpoints, and potential scoring systems. Int J Radiat Oncol Biol Phys 31:1187–1203, 1995.

288. Speyer JL, Freedberg R. Cardiac complications. In: Abeloff MD, Armitage JO (eds). Clinical Oncology. New York, Churchill Livingstone, 1995.

289. Stover DE, Kaner RJ. Pulmonary toxicity. In: DeVita VT Jr, Hellman S (eds). Cancer—Principles & Practice of Oncology. Philadelphia, Lippincott-Raven, 1997.

290. Wesselius LJ. Pulmonary complications of cancer therapy. Compr Ther 18:17–20, 1992.

291. Brosius FC, Waller BF, Roberts WC. Radiation heart disease. Analysis of 16 young (aged 15 to 33 years) necropsy patients who received over 3,500 rads to the heart. Am J Med 70:519–530, 1981.

292. Gustavsson A, Eskilsson J, Landberg T, et al. Late cardiac effects after mantle radiotherapy in patients with Hodgkin's disease. Ann Oncol 1:355–363, 1990.

293. Carmel RJ, Kaplan HS. Mantle irradiation in Hodgkin's disease. An analysis of technique, tumor eradication, and complications. Cancer 37:2813–2825, 1976.

294. Gross NJ. Pulmonary effects of radiation therapy. Ann Intern Med 86:81–92, 1977.

295. Lingos TI, Recht A, Vicini F, et al. Radiation pneumonitis in breast cancer patients treated with conservative surgery and radiation therapy. Int J Radiat Oncol Biol Phys 21:355–360, 1991.

296. Monson JM, Stark P, Reilly JJ, et al. Clinical radiation pneumonitis and radiographic changes after thoracic radiation therapy for lung carcinoma. Cancer 82:842–850, 1998.

297. Marks LB. The pulmonary effects of thoracic irradiation. Oncology (Huntingt) 8:89–106, 1994.

298. Tarbell NJ, Thompson L, Mauch P. Thoracic irradiation in Hodgkin's disease: Disease control and long-term complications. Int J Radiat Oncol Biol Phys 18:275–281, 1990.

299. Hochster H, Wasserheit C, Speyer J. Cardiotoxicity and cardioprotection during chemotherapy. Curr Opin Oncol 7:304–309, 1995.

300. Shan K, Lincoff AM, Young JB. Anthracycline-induced cardiotoxicity. Ann Intern Med 125:47–58, 1996.

301. Lipshultz SE, Colan SD, Gelber RD, et al. Late cardiac effects of doxorubicin therapy for acute lymphoblastic leukemia in childhood. N Engl J Med 324:808–815, 1991.

302. Mott MG. Anthracycline cardiotoxicity and its prevention. Ann NY Acad Sci 824:221–228, 1997.

303. Postma A, Bink-Boelkens MT, Beaufort-Krol GC, et al. Late cardiotoxicity after treatment for a malignant bone tumor. Med Pediatr Oncol 26:230–237, 1996.

304. Praga C, Beretta G, Vigo PL, et al. Adriamycin cardiotoxicity: A survey of 1273 patients. Cancer Treat Rep 63:827–834, 1979.

305. Steinherz LJ, Steinherz PG, Tan CT, et al. Cardiac toxicity 4 to 20 years after completing anthracycline therapy. JAMA, 266:1672–1677, 1991.

306. Lipshultz SE, Lipsitz SR, Mone SM, et al. Female sex and drug dose as risk factors for late cardiotoxic effects of doxorubicin therapy for childhood cancer. N Engl J Med 332:1738–1743, 1995.

307. Pratt CB, Ransom JL, Evans WE. Age-related adriamycin cardiotoxicity in children. Cancer Treat Rep 62:1381–1385, 1978.

308. Schwartz RG, McKenzie WB, Alexander J, et al. Congestive heart failure and left ventricular dysfunction complicating doxorubicin therapy. Seven-year experience using serial radionuclide angiocardiography. Am J Med. 82:1109–1118, 1987.

309. Bu'Lock FA, Gabriel HM, Oakhill A, et al. Cardioprotection by ICRF187 against high dose anthracycline toxicity in children with malignant disease. Br Heart J 70:185–188, 1993.

310. Speyer JL, Green MD, Zeleniuch-Jacquotte A, et al. ICRF-187 permits longer treatment with doxorubicin in women with breast cancer. J Clin Oncol 10:117–127, 1992 [published erratum appears in J Clin Oncol 10(5):867, May 1992]

311. Hoekman K, Vermorken JB. Incidence and prevention of nonhaematological toxicity of high-dose chemotherapy. Ann Med 28:175–182, 1996.

312. Kreisman H, Wolkove N. Pulmonary toxicity of antineoplastic therapy. Semin Oncol 19:508–520, 1992.

313. Lehne G, Lote K. Pulmonary toxicity of cytotoxic and immunosuppressive agents. A review. Acta Oncol 29:113–124, 1990.

314. Twohig KJ, Matthay RA. Pulmonary effects of cytotoxic agents other than bleomycin. Clin Chest Med 11:31–54, 1990.

315. Jules-Elysee K, White DA. Bleomycin-induced pulmonary toxicity. Clin Chest Med 11:1–20, 1990.

316. Haupt HM, Hutchins GM, Moore GW. Ara-C lung: Noncardiogenic pulmonary edema complicating cytosine arabinoside therapy of leukemia. Am J Med 70:256–261, 1981.

317. Cardozo BL, Zoetelief H, van Bekkum DW, et al. Lung damage following bone marrow transplantation: I. The contribution of irradiation. Int J Radiat Oncol Biol Phys 11:907–914, 1985.

318. Chan CK, Hyland RH, Hutcheon MA. Pulmonary complications following bone marrow transplantation. Clin Chest Med 11:323–332, 1990.

319. Cunningham I. Pulmonary infections after bone marrow transplant. Semin Respir Infect 7:132–138, 1992.

320. Fanfulla F, Locatelli F, Zoia MC, et al. Pulmonary complications and respiratory function changes after bone marrow transplantation in children. Eur Respir J 10:2301–2306, 1997.

321. Floreani AA, Sison JH Gurney J, et al. Thoracic complications related to bone marrow transplantation. Chest Surg Clin North Am 9:139–165, 1999.

322. Jules-Elysee K, Stover DE, Yahalom J, et al. Pulmonary complications in lymphoma patients treated with high-dose therapy autologous bone marrow transplantation. Am Rev Respir Dis 146:485–491 1992.

323. Schwarer AP, Hughes JM, Trotman-Dickenson B, et al. A chronic pulmonary syndrome associated with graft-versus-host disease after allogeneic marrow transplantation. Transplantation 54:1002–1008, 1992.

324. Soubani AO, Miller KB, Hassoun PM. Pulmonary complications of bone marrow transplantation. Chest 109:1066–1077, 1996.

325. Breuer R, Lossos IS, Berkman N, Or R. Pulmonary complications of bone marrow transplantation. Respir Med 87:571–579, 1993.

326. Graham NJ, Muller NL, Miller RR, Shepherd JD. Intrathoracic complications following allogeneic bone marrow transplantation: CT findings. Radiology 181:153–156, 1991.

327. Palmas A, Tefferi A, Myers JL, et al. Late-onset noninfectious pulmonary complications after allogeneic bone marrow transplantation. Br J Haematol 100:680–687, 1998.

328. Schmidt-Wolf I, Schwerdtfeger R, Schwella N, et al. Diffuse pulmonary alveolar hemorrhage after allogeneic bone marrow transplantation. Ann Hematol 67:139–141, 1993.

329. Uchiyama H, Uchiyama M, Shishikura A, et al. Bronchiolitis obliterans after bone marrow transplantation: Evaluation with lung scintigraphy. Int. J Hematol 68:213–220, 1998.

330. Witte RJ, Gurney JW, Robbins RA, et al. Diffuse pulmonary alveolar hemorrhage after bone marrow transplantation: Radiographic findings in 39 patients. AJR 157:461–464, 1991.

331. Worthy SA, Flint JD, Muller NL. Pulmonary complications after bone marrow transplantation: High-resolution CT and pathologic findings. Radiographics 17:1359–1371, 1997.

332. Shulman LN, Braunwald E, Rosenthal DS. Hematological-oncological disorders and heart disease. In: Braunwald E (ed). Heart Disease—A Textbook of Cardiovascular Medicine. 5th ed. Philadelphia, WB Saunders, 1977, pp 1786–1808.

333. Braden DS, Covitz W, Milner PF. Cardiovascular function during rest and exercise in patients with sickle-cell anemia and coexisting alpha thalassemia-2. Am J Hematol 52:96–102, 1996.

334. Covitz W, Eubig C, Balfour IC, et al. Exercise-induced cardiac dysfunction in sickle cell anemia. A radionuclide study. Am J Cardiol 51:570–575, 1983.

335. Covitz W, Espeland M, Gallagher D, et al. The heart in sickle cell anemia. The Cooperative Study of Sickle Cell Disease (CSSCD). Chest 108:1214–1219, 1995.

336. Pianosi P, D'Souza SJ, Charge TD, et al. Cardiac output and oxygen delivery during exercise in sickle cell anemia. Am Rev Respir Dis 143:231–235, 1991.

337. Wenger NK, Abelmann WH, Roberts WC. Cardiomyopathy and specific heart muscle disease. In: Hurst JW, Alexander RW, Schlant RC (eds). Hurst's The Heart, Arteries and Veins. 9th ed. New York, McGraw-Hill Information Services, 1998, pp 1278–1347.

338. Palevsky HI, Kelley MA, Fishman AP. Pulmonary thromboembolic disease. In: Fishman AP, Elias JA, et al (eds). Fishman's Pulmonary Diseases and Disorders. 3rd ed. New York, McGraw-Hill, 1998.

339. Prakash UBS. Hematologic diseases. In: Baum GL, Wolinsky E (eds). Textbook of Pulmonary Diseases. 5th ed. Boston, Little, Brown, 1994, pp 1553–1589.

340. Prakash UBS. Immunodeficiency diseases. In: Baum GL, Wolinsky E (eds). Textbook of Pulmonary Diseases. 5th ed. Boston, Little, Brown, 1994, pp 1519–1551.

341. Hopewell PC. Pulmonary manivestations of HIV infection. In: Bennett JC, Plum F (eds). Cecil Textbook of Medicine. 20th ed. Philadelphia, WB Saunders, 1996, pp 1858–1865.

342. Murray JF, Felton CP, Garay SM, et al. Pulmonary complications of the acquired immunodeficiency syndrome. Report of a National Heart, Lung, and Blood Institute workshop. N Engl J Med 310:1682–1688, 1984.

343. Murray JF, Garay SM, Hopewell PC, et al. NHLBI workshop summary. Pulmonary complications of the acquired immunodeficiency syndrome: An update. Report of the Second National Heart, Lung and Blood Institute workshop. Am Rev Respir Dis 135:504–509, 1987.

344. Cheitlin MD. AIDS and the cardiovascular system. In: Alexander RW, Schlant RC et al (eds). Hurst's The Heart, Arteries and Veins. 9th ed. New York, McGraw-Hill, 1998, pp 2143–2152.

345. Corallo S, Mutinelli MR, Moroni M, et al. Echocardiography detects myocardial damage in AIDS: Prospective study in 102 patients. Eur Heart J 9:887–892, 1988.

346. Hecht SR, Berger M, Van Tosh A, Croxson S. Unsuspected cardiac abnormalities in the acquired immune deficiency syndrome. An echocardiographic study. Chest 96:805–808, 1989.

347. Monsuez JJ, Kinney EL, Vittecoq D, et al. Comparison among acquired immune deficiency syndrome patients with and without clinical evidence of cardiac disease. Am J Cardiol 62:1311–1313, 1988.

348. Flum DR, McGinn JTJ, Tyras DH. The role of the 'pericardial window' in AIDS. Chest 107:1522–1525, 1995.

349. Heidenreich PA, Eisenberg MJ, Kee LL, et al. Pericardial effusion in AIDS. Incidence and survival. Circulation 92:3229–3234, 1995.

350. De Castro S, d'Amati G, Gallo P, et al. Frequency of development of acute global left ventricular dysfunction in human immunodeficiency virus infection. J Am Coll Cardiol 24:1018–1024, 1994.

351. Herskowitz A, Willoughby SB, Vlahov D, et al. Dilated heart muscle disease associated with HIV infection. Eur Heart J 16 (Suppl O):50–55, 1995.

352. Reilly JM, Cunnion RE, Anderson DW, et al. Frequency of myocarditis, left ventricular dysfunction and ventricular tachycardia in the acquired immune deficiency syndrome. Am J Cardiol 62:789–793, 1988.

353. Fishman AP. Pulmonary-systemic interactions. In: Fishman AP, Elias JA, et al (eds). Fishman's Pulmonary Diseases and Disorders. 3rd ed. New York, McGraw-Hill, 1998, pp 417–427.

354. Prakash UBS. Gastroenterologic diseases. In: Baum GL, Crapo JD (eds). Textbook of Pulmonary Diseases. 6th ed. Philadelphia, Lippincott-Raven, 1998, pp 1133–1157.

355. Regan TJ. Alcohol and nutritional disease. In: Schlant RC, Hurst JW, Alexander RW (eds). The Heart, Arteries and Veins. 8th ed. New York, McGraw-Hill, 1994, pp 1943–1948.

356. Mathews ECJ, Gardin JM, Henry WL, et al. Echocardiographic abnormalities in chronic alcoholics with and without overt congestive heart failure. Am J Cardiol 47:570–578, 1981.

357. Grose RD, Nolan J, Dillon JF, et al. Exercise-induced left ventricular dysfunction in alcoholic and non-alcoholic cirrhosis. J Hepatol 22:326–332, 1995.

358. Schwartz DM, Thompson MG. Do anorectics get well? Current research and future needs. Am J Psychiatry 138:319–323, 1981.

359. Moodie DS. Anorexia and the heart. Results of studies to assess effects. Postgrad Med 81:46–55, 1987.

360. Cooke RA, Chambers JB. Anorexia nervosa and the heart. Br J Hosp Med 54:313–317, 1995.

361. de Simone G, Scalfi L, Galderisi M, et al. Cardiac abnormalities in young women with anorexia nervosa. Br Heart J 71:287–292, 1994.
362. Schocken DD, Holloway JD, Powers PS. Weight loss and the heart. Effects of anorexia nervosa and starvation. Arch Intern Med 149:877–881, 1989.
363. Casper RC. The pathophysiology of anorexia nervosa and bulimia nervosa. Annu Rev Nutr 6:299–316, 1986.
364. Nudel DB, Gootman N, Nussbaum MP, Shenker IR. Altered exercise performance and abnormal sympathetic responses to exercise in patients with anorexia nervosa. J Pediatr 105:34–37, 1984.

3

Diagnostic Tests and Procedures

8

Cardiovascular Diagnostic Tests and Procedures

Ellen A. Hillegass

INTRODUCTION

Objective information on the patient's cardiovascular system is derived from data obtained from laboratory studies and from diagnostic tests and procedures. Physical therapists must be able to identify and interpret the results of these medical tests and procedures in order to assess the status of their patients' cardiovascular systems. This chapter provides the basis for an understanding of the importance and impact of medical tests that may be ordered to determine key disease states and impairments. In addition, these tests facilitate the achievement of a correct diagnosis, aid in the prevention of complications, develop information to determine a prognosis, identify subclinical disease states, and assist in the monitoring of the progress of treatments.

The tests and procedures that are discussed in this chapter include clinical laboratory studies (e.g., for cardiac enzymes and markers, cholesterol and triglycerides, and complete blood cell count), **Holter monitoring, echocardiography, contrast echocardiography, positron emission tomography (PET), computed tomography (CT), single-photon emission computed tomography (SPECT), electron beam computed tomography (EBCT), multigated acquisition or angiogram (MUGA) imaging, magnetic resonance imaging (MRI),** perfusion imaging, exercise testing, coronary angiography and ventriculography, **digital subtraction angiography, ergonovine stimulation, heart rate variability,** and **endocardial biopsy.** Table 8–1 provides an overview of all tests and their indications found in this chapter. Electrocardiography is a separate diagnostic evaluation that is covered in Chapter 9.

CLINICAL LABORATORY STUDIES

Laboratory studies provide important information regarding the clinical status of the patient. The laboratory tests that are specific to the patient with cardiac dysfunction measure the serum enzymes, blood lipids (triglycerides and cholesterol), complete blood cell count, **coagulation** profile (prothrombin time), electrolyte levels, **blood urea nitrogen** (BUN), creatinine levels, and serum glucose levels. Table 8–2 provides the laboratory studies and the normative values.

Table 8–1
Cardiovascular Diagnostic Tests and Procedures and Their Indications

TESTS FOR RHYTHM ABNORMALITIES

Holter monitor
12-Lead ECG
Exercise ECG
Electrophysiologic studies (EPS mapping)

TESTS FOR ISCHEMIA

Resting ECG (if ischemia's occurring at time of ECG)
Exercise ECG
Pharmacologic stress testing
Single-photon emission computed tomography (SPECT)
Positron emission tomography (PET)
Ergonovine challenges
Contrast echocardiography
Cardiac catheterization
Cardiac magnetic resonance imaging (MRI)

TEST FOR VALVE INTEGRITY

Echocardiography
Contrast echocardiography
Cardiac catheterization

TESTS FOR VENTRICULAR SIZE AND EJECTION FRACTION

Chest x-ray
Multigated acquisition or angiogram (MUGA) imaging
Echocardiography

TESTS FOR CARDIAC MUSCLE PUMP FUNCTIONING

MUGA
Echocardiography
Ventriculography
Digital

TESTS FOR ACUTE MYOCARDIAL INFARCTION

Cardiac enzymes and markers
Resting ECG

VASCULAR DIAGNOSTIC TESTING

Ankle brachial index
Segmental limb pressures
Pulse volume recordings
Arterial duplex ultrasonography
Exercise studies

Table 8–2
Clinical Laboratory Studies with Normative Values

MEASUREMENT	NORMATIVE VALUES
SERUM ENZYMES AND MARKERS	
Creatine phosphokinase (CPK)	5–75 mU/mL
CPK-MB isoenzyme	0–3%
Lactic dehydrogenase (LDH)	100–225 mU/mL
Aspartate aminotransferase (AST)	10–40 mU/dL
Troponin	<0.2 μg/mL
Myoglobin	<100 ng/mL
Carbonic anhydrase III	Myo/CAIII <3.2*
BLOOD LIPIDS	
Total cholesterol	<200 mg/dL
High-density lipoproteins (HDL)	
Males	>33 mg/dL
Females	>43 mg/dL
Low-density lipoproteins (LDL)	<100 mg/dL
Triglycerides	<140 mg/dL
OTHER RISK FACTORS FOR CAD	
Homocysteine	<16.2 μmol/L
C-reactive protein (CRP)	>5 mg/L
COMPLETE BLOOD CELL COUNT	
Red blood cells	
Males	4.6–6.2 × 10^6/μL
Females	4.2–5.4 × 10^4/μL
Hemoglobin	
Males	13.5–18 g/dL
Females	12–16 g/dL
Hematocrit	
Males	40–54%
Females	38–47%
White blood cells	4500–11,000/μL of whole blood
Platelets	300,000/μL
COAGULATION PROFILE	
Protime	11.6–13.0 sec
PTT	21.5–34.1 sec
ELECTROLYTES, OTHERS	
Na$^+$	136–143 mEq/L
K$^+$	3.8–5.0 mEq/L
BUN	8–18 mg/dL
Creatinine	0.6–1.2 mg/dL
Glucose	70–110 mg/dL
Albumin	>2.5 g

*Myo/CAIII = myoglobin value/carbonic anhydrase III.

Serum Enzymes and Markers

Evaluation of specific serum enzyme levels and cardiac protein markers contributes to a definitive diagnosis of myocardial necrosis and in some cases to an assessment of the degree of myocardial damage or the effectiveness of **reperfusion.** When damage has occurred to the myocardial tissue, cellular integrity is lost and intracellular cardiac enzymes are released into the circulation. These enzymes are released at a variable rate and are cleared by the kidney and other organs. Their presence can be measured by serum blood tests. However, owing to their variable release and clearing rate, their absence does not rule out the possibility of injury.

The markers that are diagnostic of cardiac injury include

- Creatine phosphokinase (CPK-MB isoenzyme)
- **Troponin**
- **Myoglobin**
- Carbonic anhydrase III
- Cardiac myosin light chains
- Lactic dehydrogenase (LDH isoenzyme 1)
- Aspartate aminotransferase (AST)

More specifically, **isoenzymes,** which are different chemical forms of the same enzyme, have been found to be most conclusive of specific muscle cell necrosis. CPK (also CK) has three isoenzymes (MB, MM, BB), which are differentiated by their tissue distribution. The CPK-MB fraction is most conclusive for myocardial injury. MM is most conclusive for skeletal muscle damage and BB for brain tissue injury. CPK-MB is considered abnormal if its serum level is greater than 3%; MB is found in healthy skeletal muscle up to 3%. CPK-MB has been used as a cardiac marker for over 35 years; however, it has been shown to be elevated after cardiac surgery and cardiopulmonary resuscitation (especially if the person was **defibrillated**) and has been shown to be abnormally elevated in patients undergoing thrombolysis with streptokinase or **tissue plasminogen activator.**[1] Chapter 14 discusses specific cardiac medications.

More recently, blood levels of the troponins have been assessed to determine myocardial damage. Elevated levels of troponin occur earlier[2] and may last for up to 5 to 7 days in plasma (normal range = 0 to 3.0 mg/mL).[3] The troponins are a group of structurally related proteins found in striated muscle cells and are bound to the actin filament. The troponins include the TnC, which binds calcium; TnI, which inhibits the interaction between actin and myosin; and TnT, which links the troponin complex to tropomyosin. With cell necrosis there is a release of the troponins into the circulation. The cardiac isoforms of cTnI and cTnT are expressed only in cardiac muscle and therefore are the two troponins tested during severe ischemia and infarction.

Current research has demonstrated an increase in the cardiac troponins with heart failure and renal insufficiency; therefore, the troponins alone may not indicate specificity of myocardial infarction.[4] Several studies have shown an increased short-term mortality rate (30 to 40 days) in individuals with elevations in cTnI and cTnT.[5–9]

Myoglobin is a heme protein found in all muscle tissue and has recently come under study as a potentially powerful diagnostic tool for acute myocardial infarction (MI). Myoglobin can be detected as early as 2 hours after injury and peaks approximately 3 to 15 hours after injury.[10] The presence of myoglobin requires ruling out possible skeletal muscle injury versus cardiac muscle injury.

Carbonic anhydrase III is a cytoplasmic protein that is present in skeletal muscle, but not in cardiac muscle. In situations of skeletal muscle injury, both the myoglobin and the carbonic anhydrase III are elevated, but the ratio is constant, whereas in acute MI the ratio is not constant, and changes within 2 to 15 hours after injury. This finding, although only recent, may prove to be more beneficial to emergency room monitoring of patients in the future than CPK and the troponins.

Skeletal and cardiac muscle contain two heavy chains and two light chains in the myosin molecule. Cardiac myosin light chains (CMLCs) have been shown to be released after myocardial infarction[11] and may have a role in identification of cardiac injury in unstable angina pectoris.[12, 13] Cardiac myosin light chains are currently difficult to separate from skeletal muscle chains and difficult to detect due to the lack of a reliable immunoassay; however, once a means of detection becomes available, this diagnostic test might prove to be the most sensitive and specific for cardiac injury.

Lactic dehydrogenase has five isoenzymes, of which LDH-1 is the most conclusive for myocardial injury. Normally LDH-2 exceeds LDH-1 activity, but after myocardial infarction LDH-1 activity exceeds LDH-2.[14] More specifically, a ratio of LDH-1 to LDH-2 greater than 1.0 is strongly suggestive of myocardial infarction. The other LDH isoenzymes are increased in the presence of heart failure, renal failure, and the like.

Enzyme and isoenzyme levels increase within the first 36 hours after myocardial injury, reaching their individual peaks at different rates (Table 8–3).[15] Marked elevation in CPK enzyme levels occurs whenever thrombolytic medications (streptokinase and tPA) are used to lyse clots. Clinically, an early or secondary peak in CPK levels followed by a more rapid decline in the CPK-MB levels is strongly suggestive of reperfusion after thrombolytic therapy.[16]

Blood Lipids

Elevation in blood lipid levels (hyperlipidemia) is considered a major risk factor contributing to cor-

Table 8–3
Cardiac Enzymes

	NORMAL SERUM LEVEL VALUES (IU)*	ONSET OF RISE (hr)	TIME OF PEAK RISE (hr)	RETURN TO NORMAL (days)
CPK	55–71†	3–4	33	3
LDH	127‡	12–24	72	5–14
SGOT	24	12	24	4

*1 IU is the amount of enzyme that will catalyze the formation of 1 μmol of substrate per minute under the conditions of the test.
†CPK-MB, 0%–3%
‡LDH-1, 14%–26%
Source: Smith AM, Theirer JA, Huang SH. Serum enzymes in myocardial infarction. Am J Nurs 73(2):277, 1973. Used with permission. All rights reserved. Copyright © 1973 The American Journal of Nursing Company.

Clinical Note: Troponin

Troponin assessment is one of the newest laboratory tests used to identify myocardial injury, and may not yet be available in smaller hospitals. When troponin information is unavailable, the therapist should depend on CPK-MB information.

Table 8–4

Total Cholesterol to High-Density Lipoprotein (HDL) Ratio as a Predictor of Heart Disease

TOTAL CHOLESTEROL/HDL RATIO	RISK OF HEART DISEASE
Men	
3.43	½ Average
4.97	Average
9.55	2× Average
23.39	3× Average
Women	
3.27	½ Average
4.44	Average
7.05	2× Average
11.04	3× Average

Source: Gordon T, Castelli WP, Hjortland MC, et al. Diabetes, blood lipids, and the role of obesity in coronary heart disease risk for women. Ann Intern Med 87: 393, 1977.

onary artery disease (CAD).[17] The concentrations of serum cholesterol and triglycerides are the blood lipids of concern. The American Heart Association defines elevated blood cholesterol levels as being higher than 200 mg/100 mL; however, the more stringent recommendations suggested by Castelli define 180 mg/100 mL as the upper end of normal.[18] Elevated cholesterol levels are associated with ingestion of excess amounts of saturated fat and cholesterol as well as with hereditary influences. Elevated triglyceride levels are defined as being higher than 150 mg/100 mL. Elevated triglyceride levels are associated with increased carbohydrate ingestion and often preclude diabetes mellitus. Caution should be taken if measurements of cholesterol and triglyceride levels are taken at the time of acute injury, as research has shown these values to be inaccurate.[19] Such measurements are most accurate when obtained before a myocardial injury or a minimum of 6 weeks after an acute injury.[19]

The usefulness of clinical laboratory reports is improved by giving a breakdown of the component parts of the total cholesterol. Current information now lists the **high-density lipoprotein (HDL)** and **low-density lipoprotein (LDL)** levels as well as the ratio of total cholesterol to HDL. Research has shown that the absolute values of total cholesterol or HDL cholesterol are of less importance than the ratio of total cholesterol to HDL cholesterol in establishing an individual's relative risk for developing CAD (Table 8–4). An increased ratio of total cholesterol to HDL cholesterol identifies a person at an increased risk for development of CAD.[20] High levels of LDL (higher than 130 mg/100 mL) also increase a person's relative risk for developing CAD. Lowering total cholesterol and especially LDL cholesterol has shown to result in a 25 to 35% reduction in cardiovascular events.[21]

Recently, several new markers have been identified that are considered to be probable new risk factors, including **lipoprotein a (Lpa),** LDL subclasses, oxidized LDL, **homocysteine,** hematologic factors (primarily fibrinogen, factor VII, and tPA), inflammatory markers such as **C-reactive protein (CRP),** and infective agents such as *Chlamydia pneumoniae* **(CPN).**[22] Elevated serum levels of a lipid particle called Lpa have been strongly associated with atherosclerosis and also identified as an independent risk factor for CAD.[21] Lpa appears to have an atherogenic and **prothrombic** effect that interferes with plasminogen and tPA binding to fibrin. Lpa levels are thought to be genetic in origin, and were found in 50% of the offspring of patients with CAD in the Framingham study.[21] Increased Lpa levels are associated with a threefold increase in the risk of a primary CAD event.[21] Response to standard treatment to lower LDL in individuals with elevated Lpa were not successful except with LDL apheresis.[21]

In addition to Lpa, the presence of an elevated amount of small dense LDL particle subtype (phenotype B) is also associated with an elevated risk for CAD (threefold increased risk).[21, 22] **Small dense LDL** is also associated with elevated triglyceride levels. Apparently small LDL particles can be moved into the vessel wall 50% faster than the large LDL particles. Treatment for presence of elevated small dense LDL particle subtype consists of low-fat diet, exercise, pharmacologic therapy with resins, niacin, and hormone replacement in women.[21]

Individuals with diabetes often have abnormal lipid levels. The most common pattern of lipid abnormalities in type 2 diabetic patients is elevated triglycerides and decreased LDL levels.[23] However, type 2 diabetic patients have a preponderance of smaller denser LDL particles, although their LDL cholesterol concentration is usually not significantly different than nondiabetics. Therefore, elevated triglyceride levels may be a better predictor of coronary heart disease in type 2 diabetics than elevated LDL levels because of the correlation with insulin resistance and small dense LDL.

Other Potential Clinical Laboratory Risk Factors for CAD

Recently elevated blood levels of homocysteine have been identified as an independent risk factor for the development of coronary heart disease.[24, 25] Low levels of folate and vitamin B_6 are related to elevated circulating homocysteine blood levels, and therefore sufficient folate intake may be an important factor in the prevention of coronary heart disease.[24, 26] The odds ratio for CAD of a 5-μmol/L homocysteine increase was discovered to be 1.6 for males and 1.9 for females.[26]

Hematologic factor, such as fibrinogen, and elevated WBC counts have been associated with increased risk of CAD. Individuals with elevated fibrinogen levels in the highest quartile demonstrated a double risk of CAD, whereas the Multiple Risk Factor Intervention Trial found that an elevated WBC count is associated with increased risk.[22, 27]

Inflammatory markers and infection markers have shown some relationship to CAD. Inflammatory markers such as CRP, an acute-phase reactant to inflammation have recently been related to increased risk for CAD. Males with CRP levels in the highest quartile may have a fivefold increase in risk of developing an MI.[22] Infection markers, including C. pneumoniae, have shown a twofold increase in risk of CAD. Systemic infection may act directly on the arterial wall, or may work by local or systemic inflammation.[22]

Because these are new risk factors with insufficient evidence to support regular screening for them, they should be measured only in families with unexplained CAD or premature CAD. Future studies documenting their efficacy in identifying CAD will be necessary prior to routine screening.

Complete Blood Cell Count

The physical therapist should evaluate the complete blood cell count for three components: hemoglobin, hematocrit values, and WBC count. Hemoglobin plays a major role in the transport of oxygen throughout the body, and the hematocrit (the amount of the blood that is cells) is a significant indicator of the viscosity of the blood. Hemoglobin values are reported as a concentration in the blood (in grams per 100 mL of blood). The normal range of hemoglobin for females is 12 to 16 g/100 mL, and for males it is 14 to 18 g/100 mL.[14]

Low levels of hemoglobin or a diagnosis of anemia will increase the work on the myocardium because of a lack of oxygen-carrying capacity and subsequently low levels of oxygen available to the tissues. In order to transport adequate oxygen to the tissues (even when the body is at rest) the heart rate is elevated and subsequently the cardiac output increase, therefore increasing the work on the myocardium. In addition, the **mean corpuscular volume (MCV)** test measures red blood cells (RBCs) in terms of individual volume. This test is used to classify anemias as microcytic (RBC size smaller than normal), normocytic, or macrocytic (larger than normal). **Microcytic anemias** are found in iron deficiency, chronic infections, chronic renal disease, and malignancies. **Normocytic anemia** (hypochromic) is found in chronic infections, lead poisoning, chronic renal disease and malignancies, whereas normochromic anemia is found in hemorrhage, hemolytic anemia, bone marrow hypoplasia, and splenomegaly. **Macrocytic anemia** is found in pernicious anemia, folic acid deficiency, hypothyroidism, and hepatocellular disease. Defining the MCV therefore assists in treatment of the cause of the anemia.[28-30]

The lower limit value for hematocrit is 37 g/100 mL for females and 42 g/100 mL for males.[14] Decreased levels of hemoglobin and hematocrit are often found in post-coronary artery bypass graft surgery patients. Elevated hematocrit levels suggest that the flow of blood to the tissues may

> ### Clinical Note: Assessment of Complete Blood Cell Count
>
> *After surgery, particularly after coronary artery by-pass graft surgery, patients will demonstrate decreased hematocrit and hemoglobin values (and usually normocytic and normochromic MCV) and may be more symptomatic with activity because of low oxygen-carrying capacity.*

be impeded because of an increase in the viscosity of the blood. Elevated hematocrit levels are often seen in individuals with chronic obstructive pulmonary disease (a response to chronic low PO_2).

White blood cells are monitored for the body's response to infectious diseases. Elevated levels of WBCs (leukocytosis) are found in response to leukemia, bacterial infection, or polycythemia (secondary to bone marrow stimulation). Some studies have identified a possible association between elevated WBC counts and increased risk of CAD.[27] Decreased WBC count (**leukopenia**) is found with bone marrow depression, acute viral infection, alcohol ingestion, and agranulocytosis. Disease processes may result in a change within individual leukocyte groups by altering morphology, function, or total numbers. Therefore, the differential WBC count is important to assess to determine possible causes of the abnormal WBC count.

Coagulation Profiles

Coagulation profiles have become an important component of the patient's medical record because of the use of thrombolytic agents to dissolve clots in the early stages of myocardial infarction. **Prothrombin time** (PT) and **partial thromboplastin time** (PTT) measure the coagulation of the blood. Streptokinase or tissue plasminogen activator

> ### Clinical Note: Cautions for Anticoagulant Therapy
>
> *If a patient has been on thrombolytics or heparin, the therapist should take extreme precautions against bumping extremities with all movement as the individual will be at a greater risk of bruising and bleeding.*

(tPA) infusion is a means of dissolving critical clots that are blocking a coronary artery and creating a potential infarction and subsequent necrosis. These thrombolytic agents are most commonly administered intravenously but can also be injected directly into the coronary arteries. After the initial infusion of thrombolytics is begun, an intravenous infusion of heparin is started. As a result, PT and PTT must be monitored closely to determine the therapeutic ranges of anticoagulation.[14] PTT will often be elevated following any thrombolytic or heparin infusion. An elevated PTT indicates an increased time to form a clot, therefore, the chance of bleeding when bruised or cut is increased and caution should be taken.

Electrolytes

All electrolyte levels should be observed when evaluating the laboratory results because disturbances in the electrolytes may affect the patient's performance. The electrolytes involved in maintaining cell membrane potential—sodium (Na^+), potassium (K^+), and carbon dioxide (CO_2)—are the most important electrolytes to monitor. Hydration state, medications, and disease can affect these values. Patients receiving diuretics (e.g., for hypertension or heart failure) should have their sodium and potassium levels monitored carefully, because some diuretics act on the kidney. The action of these medications on the kidney is on the renal tubules and collecting ducts, where these electrolytes are allowed to diffuse out or are reabsorbed from the bloodstream. Dangerously low levels of potassium (below 3.5 mEq/L) can cause serious, life-threatening arrhythmias. Dangerously high levels of potassium (above 5.0 mEq/L) can affect the contractility of the myocardium. Low levels of CO_2 can cause an **alkalotic** state, muscle weakness, and dizziness.[14]

Blood Urea Nitrogen and Creatinine

The BUN and creatinine values can be found on the same laboratory form as that reporting the electrolytes and cholesterol. The normal range for the BUN is 8 to 23 mg/dL; an elevated BUN can

> ### Clinical Note: Laboratory Values in Heart Failure
>
> Abnormal laboratory values found in heart failure include increased BUN, increased LDH, normal CPK-MB, and possible increased creatinine levels due to renal dysfunction.

be an indication of heart failure or renal failure. Elevated BUN values also indicate uremia or a retention of urea in the blood. Decreased BUN values may indicate starvation, dehydration, or even other organ dysfunction such as liver disease.

The BUN value is unsuitable as a single measure of renal function, and therefore the creatinine value should also be noted. Normal serum creatinine levels are lower than 1.5 mg/dL. Endogenous creatinine is fully filtered in the glomerulus and is not reabsorbed in the tubules in the presence of normal renal function. Therefore, the clearance of creatinine is a measure of renal efficiency. As the glomerular filtration rate declines, the creatinine level rises and the renal function is assessed as inefficient. Severely elevated creatinine levels above 4.0 mg/dL indicates severe renal insufficiency or failure. The interpretation of the BUN and creatinine concentrations is an indication of the severity of the uremia.

Serum Glucose

Serum glucose level is measured when a typical laboratory sample of blood is collected. The normal value for serum glucose is 80 to 110 mg/100 mL of blood, measured in the fasting state. The concentration is maintained within a reasonably narrow range. An elevated blood glucose level (mild hyperglycemia is 120 to 130 mg/100 mL) indicates a surplus of glucose in the blood. An elevated serum glucose value is suggestive of a **prediabetic** state and warrants testing for diabetes, such as administration of a glucose tolerance test (performed in the fasting individual following the ingestion of 100 g of glucose). Severe hyperglycemia (above 300 mg/100 mL) denotes a crisis situation that requires immediate insulin because cells lack the energy source to function, resulting in severe fatigue and subsequently inadequate meta-

bolic activity. Patients should not be exercised when blood glucose measures in the severe range.

An elevated serum glucose value may also be found in a patient with diabetes who is not well controlled on oral or injectable insulin. Testing the hemoglobin A1C (HbA1C is normally 4.8 to 6.0%) measures a diabetic's insulin control over the past 90 days, which is the life of the red blood cells that carry the hemoglobin.[14] See Chapter 7 for more information on diabetes.

Other Laboratory Values

Other laboratory values may be abnormal but not usually indicative of cardiac dysfunction and instead may be related to other comorbidities. Abnormal laboratory values should be investigated to assess for comorbidity and any effect on the cardiac system. For example, albumin, a small blood protein, is the first protein detected in the urine when there is renal damage (burns, shock, low cardiac output). Elevations in albumin are rare, but low levels of albumin may be found in chronic liver disease, protein malnutrition, chronic infection, and acute stress. Elevated bilirubin may be present when there is hemorrhage or hepatic dysfunction, whereas elevations in lipase indicate pancreatic dysfunction or pancreatitis.

OTHER NONINVASIVE DIAGNOSTIC TESTS

Holter Monitoring

Holter monitoring consists of continuous 24-hour, electrocardiographic monitoring of a patient's heart rhythm, providing information that is essential to the diagnosis and management of episodes of cardiac arrhythmias and corresponding symptoms. Holter monitoring tracings must be reliable to capture, recognize, and reproduce any abnormality in heart rhythm, particularly those that threaten life or cardiac hemodynamics.

Indications for use of the Holter monitor include identifying symptoms possibly caused by arrhythmias (e.g., dizziness, **syncope,** shortness of breath at rest as well as with activity), describing the arrhythmias noted with activity (frequency and severity), and evaluating antiarrhythmia therapy and pacemaker functioning. A common practice is to perform Holter monitoring routinely before discharging any patient who has had a myocardial infarction, because arrhythmias are commonly associated with coronary disease, ischemia, and injury.

The patient's heart rhythm is monitored by means of a transcutaneous tape recorder applied to the patient's chest wall via multiple leads and electrodes (Fig. 8–1). The patient wears the Holter monitor for 24 hours while performing normal activities (except bathing). All the patient's activities as well as any symptoms that may be felt during the 24 hours are documented by the patient. Once the recorder is removed from the patient, the tape is processed by reproducing the recording on computer or paper for visual inspection.

The physician then interprets the results and plans the treatment accordingly. Repeat Holter monitoring may be necessary once treatment has been initiated to evaluate the effectiveness of the treatment.

It is the responsibility of the physical therapist working with a patient who is wearing or has worn a Holter monitor to obtain the interpretation of the results of the Holter monitor to determine if modifications are needed in the patient's activities. For example, patients with life-threatening arrhythmias recorded by the Holter monitor should not begin physical therapy activity until treatment for the arrhythmia is initiated or modified. Increasing frequency of arrhythmias or more serious (life-threatening) arrhythmias developing with activity also require further evaluation by the physician.[31]

Patients with abnormal Holter monitor results may be referred for treadmill exercise testing to assess arrhythmias during an assessment of increased work on the heart or may be referred for echocardiography to assess valve functioning.

Patients demonstrating life-threatening arrhythmias on the Holter monitor may be referred to **electrophysiologic mapping studies (EPS),** particularly if they demonstrated sustained or nonsustained ventricular tachycardia. These individuals have a high risk of sudden death. EPS is performed to identify the specific area that may be initiating the arrhythmia by inducing the arrhythmia and subsequently attempting to restore normal rhythm with one or more antiarrhythmic medications. If the arrhythmia is induced and unable to be treated successfully by the antiarrhythmic medication, the patient may be referred for an **ablation procedure** (cauterization of the area inducing the arrhythmia) or pacing techniques, or the patient may be provided an **implantable cardiac defibrillator (ICD)** for rhythm control. Current prospective clinical trials are being conducted to determine if individuals diagnosed with coronary disease, myocardial infarctions, or congestive heart failure and those who demonstrate frequent ventricular premature beats may have improved morbidity and mortality outcomes if treated *initially* with ICD implantation rather than antiarrhythmia medications.[32, 33] Individuals with recurrent uncontrolled atrial fibrillation may be referred for similar procedures, including an implantable atrial defibrillator, or an ablation procedure.

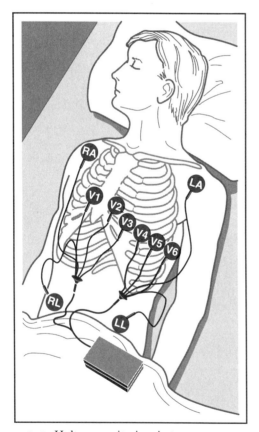

Figure 8–1. Holter monitoring is transcutaneous, with multiple leads to record heart rhythm for 24 hours.

Echocardiography

Echocardiography is a noninvasive procedure that uses pulses of reflected ultrasound to evaluate the functioning heart. A transducer that houses a special crystal emits high-frequency sound waves and receives their echoes when placed on the chest wall of the patient. The returning echoes, reflected from a variety of intracardiac surfaces, are displayed on the ultrasonographic equipment.

Echocardiography has an advantage over other cardiac diagnostic tests because the technique is completely noninvasive and gives real-time images of the beating heart. The transducer is placed on the chest wall in the third to fifth intercostal space near the left sternal border. The transducer is then tilted at various angles so that the sound waves can scan the segments of the heart. M-mode echo and two-dimensional echo (Fig. 8–2A and B) are common techniques of echocardiography, whereas Doppler echocardiography is a newer procedure. Doppler echocardiography gives information about the blood flow velocities of the heart.

Important information can be obtained from the echocardiogram, including the size of the ventricular cavity, the thickness and integrity of the interatrial and intraventricular septa, the functioning of the valves, and the motions of individual segments of the ventricular wall. Assessment of the performance of the heart muscle itself, especially the regional functioning of the left ventricle, is a valuable application of echocardiography. The degree of normal thickening of a portion of the myocardium can be assessed and is an indirect assessment of ischemia, because ischemic cardiac muscle does not thicken. Echocardiography can quantify volumes of the left ventricle, estimate stroke volume and therefore ejection fraction, and analyze motion of the valves and the heart muscle. Numerous specific problems that can be evaluated with the echocardiogram:

- **Pericardial effusion**
- **Cardiac tamponade**
- **Idiopathic congestive cardiomyopathy**
- Hypertrophic cardiomyopathy
- Mitral valve regurgitation
- Mitral valve prolapse
- Aortic regurgitation
- Aortic stenosis
- Vegetation on the valves
- Intracardiac masses
- Ischemic heart muscle
- Left ventricular aneurysm
- Ventricular thrombi
- Proximal coronary disease
- Congenital heart disease
- Interventricular thickness
- Pericarditis
- Aortic dissection
- Patency of internal mammary coronary artery bypass graft (determined with Doppler technique)

Problems exist with the image quality of standard echocardiograms owing to such confounding factors as pulmonary disease, obesity, and chest deformities. **Transesophageal echocardiography (TEE)** has solved these problems and allows an improved view of the heart and mediastinum. TEE allows for improved visualization of cardiac structures and function and is valuable in the intraoperative and perioperative monitoring of left ventricular performance as well as the evaluation of surgical results.[34–37] In addition, TEE has become established as the imaging modality of choice for the evaluation of known or suspected cardioembolic stroke.[38] TEE may also be useful in detection of those at risk for an embolic stroke and those individuals with nonvalvular atrial fibrillation.[39]

Two-dimensional echocardiographic studies during exercise, immediately after exercise, or at both times (also known as **stress echocardiography**) are currently used to evaluate ischemia-induced wall motion abnormalities noninvasively. In addition to treadmill or bicycle exercise, atrial pacing or the use of pharmacologic agents provides an "artificial exercise" situation from which two-dimensional echocardiographic studies can identify the presence and location of ischemia-induced abnormalities in the ventricular wall.[40] Stress echocardiography is especially useful for the evaluation of atypical symptoms such as dyspnea and fatigue[41] as well as for the evaluation of patients with nondiagnostic ECGs with exercise or who have atypical chest pain syndromes.[42]

The development and use of three-dimensional echocardiography, the newest form of echocardiography, provide enhanced images displaying intracardiac anatomy.[43] Three-dimensional echocardiography provides accurate quantified data previously assessed by computer analysis.[43]

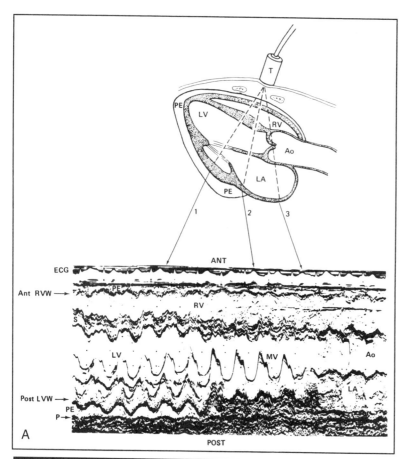

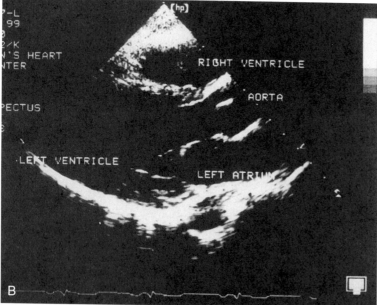

Figure 8–2. Echocardiography is a noninvasive diagnostic tool in which the transducer is placed directly over the heart. *A,* The scan through the heart is depicted in at the top. The echocardiographic movement patterns that arise from the corresponding anatomic structures are illustrated across the bottom. LV, Left ventricle; PE, pericardial effusion; T, transducer; RV, right ventricle; Ao, aorta; LA, left atrium; ANT, anterior; ECG, electrocardiogram; Ant RVW, anterior right ventricular wall; MV, mitral valve; Post LVW, posterior left ventricular wall; POST, posterior; P, pericardium. (Adapted from Sokolow M, McIlroy M, Cheitlin M, et al. Clinical Cardiology. 5th ed. East Norwalk, CT, Appleton & Lange, 1990, p 96.) *B,* Two-dimensional echocardiography (still picture from video) shows aortic valve open, with left atrium, left ventricle, and right ventricle also displayed.

Contrast Echocardiography

Using an intravenously injected contrast agent with the echocardiogram has improved the diagnostic accuracy of echocardiography in assessing myocardial perfusion and ventricular chambers.[44] The contrast agent used consists of a suspension of air-filled microspheres that act as an ultrasound tracer. Contrast echocardiography enhances the visualization of intracardiac and intrapulmonary shunts, endocardial wall motion, and ventricular wall thickness and improves the calculation of ejection fraction. In addition, contrast echocardiography appears to have potential for quantifying coronary flow and assessing myocardial viability.[45] It is a method for noninvasively assessing areas of the myocardium at risk for damage, presence or absence of coronary collateral flow, and revascularization of occluded arteries after coronary angioplasty. The use of contrast material also improves the visualization of endocardial borders, in order to discriminate between the myocardial tissue and the blood pool.[46-48] The FDA curently has approved octafluoropropane (Optison) as a contrast agent for echo imaging as it increases the endocardial border idenfication.

Contrast echocardiography has also been used with transesophageal or epicardial echocardiography (only in the operating room or in the cardiac catheterization laboratory) to assess the distribution of cardioplegia and the degree of valvular regurgitation, as well as the vascular supply of bypass grafts and bypass graft patency.[45] The future of contrast agents with echocardiography may be in the use with performance of clot lysis and for targeted gene therapy.[49]

Studies comparing contrast echocardiography with thallium-201 SPECT imaging have demonstrated similar conclusions regarding presence and amount of jeopardized myocardium, yet may involve one-half the cost of the SPECT and therefore be more cost-effective than the SPECT imaging.[44, 50]

OTHER IMAGING MODALITIES

In addition to contrast perfusion echocardiography, other imaging techniques are utilized in the diagnosis of cardiac dysfunction which may or may not utilize radioactive isotopes. Positron emission tomography (PET), computed tomography (CT), single-photon emission computed tomography (SPECT), electron beam computed tomography (EBCT), multigated acquisition imaging (MUGA), and magnetic resonance imaging (MRI) are all imaging techniques used for evaluation of coronary artery disease and cardiac dysfunction. Some of these modalities use high-speed scintillation cameras that can follow the transit of isotopes injected into the peripheral vein throught the right side of the heart, much as the dye flow that occurs with cardiac catheterization. Other methods use a camera that times the acquisition of images according to the cardiac cycle. All these tests play an important role in diagnostic evaluation of coronary artery status, each with their advantages and disadvantages, which will be discussed in the following paragraphs.

Positron Emission Tomography

Positron emission tomography is a nuclear technique that provides visualization and direct measurement of metabolic functioning, including glucose metabolism and fatty acid metabolism, as well as blood flow of the heart. PET is considered to be the gold standard for blood flow measurement and metabolic assessment of the heart, but it requires specialized technologic equipment and highly trained personnel and therefore is extremely expensive and not available at many hospitals.[51] PET has the highest resolution gain, yet given the high cost associated with PET imaging, it is unlikely it will become used routinely for cardiac imaging because there are comparable tests that are more widely available and cost less than PET imaging.[52]

PET imaging requires administration of dipyridamole to cause vasodilation of the coronary arteries while the patient is at rest, and often FD6 (18F-fluorodeoxyglucose) is administered to allow for myocardial metabolism and blood flow to be assessed in three dimensions.[53] FD6 PET imaging allows for quantification and qualification of regional myocardial tracer distribution. PET imaging demonstrates tissue viability using the metabolic tracers to detect CAD and is especially helpful in identifying the individual with severe left ventricular dysfunction who would be a candidate for re-vascularization or transplant.[53]

PET imaging has advantages over thallium imaging with exercise because it can detect jeopardized but viable myocardium[54, 55] without requiring the individual to perform an active exercise test. Patients can safely undergo PET imaging from 2 to 10 days after infarction, or when any question of impedance of flow is involved. Since the invention of thrombolytic medications to decrease infarct size, this technique has demonstrated great advantages in evaluating the effectiveness of the thrombolytic technique because the procedure can be performed so early after infarction.[56] Because of the inaccessability and cost of the procedure, other procedures have been studied and compared with the results of PET to determine equally effective diagnostic tests for myocardial blood flow. Williams determined the viable myocardium results obtained from dobutamine echocardiography was similar to the results obtained from PET imaging, and could therefore be performed when PET imaging was not an option.[57]

PET imaging has also been used as a diagnostic tool to assess brain metabolism and ischemia/injury in cerebrovascular accident and acute trauma patients.[58]

Computed Tomography

Computed tomography (CT) is used predominantly to identify masses in the cardiovascular system or to detect aortic aneurysms or pericardial thickening associated with pericarditis. Images are taken of anatomic structures; in this case, cardiac structures are viewed in slices and analyzed, and the slices are approximately 1 to 3 mm apart. Recently CT scanning has been used to assess graft patency in coronary artery bypass graft surgery patients. Because nothing is injected into the patient, this procedure is completely noninvasive and harmless, although it may not be indicated in individuals with claustrophobia.

Single-Photon Emission Computed Tomography

Single-photon emission computed tomography (SPECT) is a noninvasive method to detect and quantify myocardial perfusion defects and contractility defects and is used in conjunction with radioactive isotopes.[59] SPECT uses newer gated tomographic techniques and can be performed with the use of sestamibi (a radioactive perfusion agent) to improve the view of a myocardial perfusion study. Images are acquired with either a gamma camera, or a camera that times or "gates" the acquistion according to the cardiac cycle (via ECG). SPECT can determine contractility defects at rest by assessing both left and right ventricular ejection fraction, regional function, and ventricular volumes.[59]

SPECT imaging, although less accurate than PET imaging, is more often the diagnostic tool of choice because of the availability of these gated imaging machines and the ease of performance. Further information on SPECT is detailed in perfusion imaging with sestamibi later in this chapter.

Electron Beam Computed Tomography

Electron beam computed tomography (EBCT) is a noninvasive method to detect and quantify coronary atherosclerosis by detecting coronary calcification.[60–63] Rumberger utilized EBCT on older populations; however, recently O'Malley utilized the procedure for screening for coronary artery disease in asymptomatic active-duty U.S. Army personnel.[60, 64]

A typical EBCT scanning protocol involves a 10-minute scan involving 40 slices through the heart every 3 to 6 mm.[65] Intravenous contrast medium is not utilized, so radiation exposure is minimal (approximately one-half the radiation exposure to the average person living in the United States in 1 year).[60] EBCT detects the presence of calcium in the coronary arteries as well as the location, extent, and density of the deposits and provides a calcium scoring system. Results are given in the form of a composite score for the entire epicardial coronary system.

EBCT has been studied in individuals undergoing cardiac catheterization and has shown a sensitivity of 81 to 94% for any angiographic evidence of coronary disease and a specificity of 72 to 86%.[63, 66] EBCT currently appears to have moderate discriminating power in young, symptomatic patients with a high prevalence of obstructive disease, but its reliability with asymptomatic subjects is yet to be determined.[64]

Multigated Acquisition Imaging

Multigated acquisition (MUGA) imaging or gated pool imaging is a noninvasive technique to calculate left ventricular ejection fraction. The information gathered in this study is obtained from the electrical activity of the heart using an electrocardiograph. Multigated acquisition imaging obtains multiple individual ejection fractions knowing the heart rate and R-R intervals on the electrocardiogram and then measures the emptying curves of the heart via computer (Fig. 8–3). This technique has advantages over others in that it is noninvasive and can therefore be used on critically ill cardiac patients (e.g., those with acute cardiac failure) when other more invasive tests such as catheterization would be dangerous.[67–70]

Magnetic Resonance Imaging

Magnetic resonance imaging (MRI) is used to evaluate morphology, cardiac blood flow, and myocardial contractility.[71] However, utilization of cardiovascular MRI has been limited due to the existence of echocardiography and nuclear scintigraphy, and the familiarity with these two techniques over MRI.

MRI has similar diagnostic accuracy as PET imaging, is similarly used as a noninvasive test to assess regional blood flow problems, but is more widely available and often less expensive.[53] Nuclear magnetic resonance can produce high-resolution

tomographic pictures of the heart without using any radiation. Originally MRI was used for assessing cardiac anatomy and congenital malformations and to identify masses and thrombi. Currently MRI is being used for assessment of valvular disease, cardiac shunts, quantification of cardiac flow, and coronary artery anatomy.[72] Fayed demonstrated that the human coronary vessel wall could be noninvasively imaged in vivo with MRI, therefore providing a technique to show atherosclerotic plaque without the use of coronary angiography.[73] Future work with MRI indicates it may be the choice for detection of vulnerable plaque prior to an acute clinical event.[73, 74]

Yang et al. assessed the new cardiac MRI system, comparing it to echocardiography.[75] The new cardiac MRI (CMRI) system allows for continuous real-time dynamic acquisition and display. The CMRI was completed in less than 15 minutes and showed improved visualization of wall segments and left ventricular function as compared to the echocardiography results.[75, 76] MRI is also being used in conjunction with pharmacologic stress testing to determine significant coronary atherosclerotic plaques.[77]

Radioactive Nuclide Perfusion Imaging

As advances in cardiac medicine have evolved, assessment of coronary perfusion has been improved with the use of perfusion imaging using radioactively labeled agents. The commonly used agents include thallium-201 and **technetium-99m** (labeled sestamibi). These agents are taken up by the myocardium based on coronary blood flow. These agents can be injected following exercise or if the individual is not able to perform exercise, follow-

Figure 8–3. The R-R interval is partitioned into multiple frames. An average R-R interval is calculated by the system, and that time segment is divided into equal intervals. (From Lyons K. Cardiovascular Nuclear Medicine. East Norwalk, CT, Appleton & Lange, 1988, p. 18.)

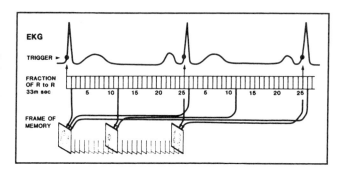

ing a pharmacologic stress test (described later in this chapter).

Thallium-201 Perfusion Imaging

Thallium-201 is an excellent perfusion tracer that is injected intravenously and used to assess acute cardiac ischemia as a result of induced physiologic stress from an exercise treadmill test, a pharmacologic induced exercise test, or when ischemia occurs spontaneously. Thallium imaging assesses blood flow and cell membrane integrity as a result of the thallium being taken up by the myocardium in proportion to the coronary blood flow in the region.[78] Cells must be both perfused and metabolically intact in order to accumulate thallium-201. Nonperfused or dead myocardium appears as "cold spots" on the scan. When exercise thallium imaging is performed, a patient is exercised to maximal exercise potential and injected with the thallium-201 1 minute prior to the end of the exercise. Immediately after the exercise test the patient is scanned using a gamma camera to assess thallium-201 uptake, and scanned again 4 hours later after the thallium has been redistributed. An area without thallium uptake (cold spot) immediately after exercise as well as 4 hours afterward is considered irreversibly damaged (scarred). An area "cold" following exercise, but reperfused 4

hours later is considered "ischemic" or "reversible" and intervention usually is indicated in such cases (Fig. 8–4).

Thallium scanning is used to predict the risk of recurrent acute myocardial infarction or death after the first acute myocardial infarction.[79–81] The use of thallium can also identify viable myocardium that could functionally improve with revascularization.[82]

As cost effectiveness of diagnostic tests is scrutinized in the current health care environment, the sensitivity and specificity of the use of thallium has been studied. Van der Wieken reported a high sensitivity (97%) and relatively high specificity (77%) for determining future events when used in individuals with acute chest pain and nondiagnostic ECGs.[83] The cost of thallium scanning increases the costs of evaluation of these patients by $500 to $800.[10] In addition, imaging equipment is available in most institutions.

The disadvantages of the use of thallium are related to the fact that it is not an ideal isotope; its low-energy photons are easily scattered and have a half-life of 73 hours. Because of the radiation exposure, the dose injected must be a low dose (approximately 2 to 4 mCi).[10] In addition, image scanning must commence within 15 to 20 minutes of the actual thallium injection, and experts in nuclear medicine must be available to perform the test and interpret the results.[10]

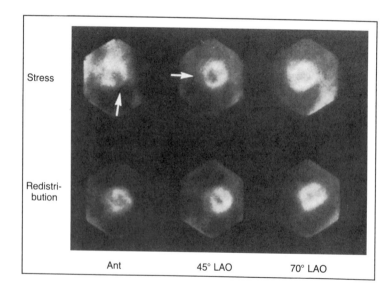

Figure 8–4. Stress-redistribution thallium scintigram of a patient with reversible apical and distal inferior perfusion defect on the anterior view and a partially reversible septal defect on the 45-degree LAO view and increased pulmonary thallium uptake on the anterior view. (From Lyons, K. Cardiovascular Nuclear Medicine. East Norwalk, CT, Appleton & Lange, 1988, p 121. Photograph by Steven A. Reisman, M.D.)

Sestamibi

Technetium-99m or sestamibi (^{99m}Tc-sestamibi), sometimes abbreviated as MIBI, has become an alternative perfusion agent to thallium-201.[79, 80, 84, 85] Like thallium-201, sestamibi is used to assess acute cardiac ischemia or infarction, and like thallium, it is taken up by the myocardium in proportion to regional blood flow.[10] The tracer can then be imaged under the gamma camera.

Whereas thallium washes out of the myocardium in proportion to blood flow, ^{99m}Tc-sestamibi remains stable, and therefore images of blood flow can be scanned immediately after administration or up to several hours later.[80, 86] Sestamibi accumulates in irreversibly damaged myocardial cells and might not demonstrate uptake in an infarction that is only a few hours old. Sestamibi is a marker of cell membrane and mitochondrial integrity as it requires active processes to occur at the level of the sarcolemma and mitochondrial membrane.[87, 88] Therefore, sestamibi is not retained in acute or chronic myocardial infarctions.

Sestamibi has demonstrated to be a more practical radioactive isotope because of its stability and has shown sensitivity and specificity for predicting any event to be 94% and 83%, respectively.[89] For predicting an acute myocardial infarction the sensitivity and specificity are 100% and 83%, respectively.[89]

One of the problems with sestamibi is that its accuracy is dependent on the skill of the operator and the knowledge and experience of the interpreter. The use of the isotope is slightly more expensive than the use of thallium-201, but it has demonstrated cost effectiveness in use with patients with nondiagnostic ECGs presenting to the emergency room.[90, 91]

Pharmacologic vasodilation with intravenous dipyridamole has been used in conjunction with the use of sestamibi for diagnostic purposes.[59] This procedure can be done while the patient is resting or in conjunction with exercise.

Sestamibi is often used in nonacute cardiac ischemic patients to assess myocardial contractility by assessing both left and right ventricular ejection fraction, regional function, and ventricular volumes.[59] Single-photon emission computed tomography (SPECT), using newer gated tomographic techniques, can be performed with sestamibi to improve the perfusion study.

PHARMACOLOGIC STRESS TESTING

When an individual is unable to perform upright exercise on a treadmill or stationary bicycle owing to severity of disease or heart failure, a neuromuscular insult (such as following a cerebrovascular accident), or a musculoskeletal disability (e.g., following recent hip or knee surgery, back pain) or is unable to achieve at least 85% of their predicted maximal heart rate on an exercise test, physiologic stress can be induced while the patient remains in a resting position by injection of a pharmacologic agent. The most common agents that are used in pharmacologic stress testing are dipyridamole, dobutamine, or adenosine.[59] Both dipyridamole and adenosine induce coronary vasodilation, a physiologic phenomenon that is difficult to occur in diseased coronary arteries, thereby affecting the perfusion image. Dobutamine acts as a stimulant (adrenergic), similar to exercise, and results in an increase in myocardial oxygen demand with the purpose of assessing myocardial oxygen supply. Another medication, **arbutamine,** has been studied in the canine model, showing promise as an additional catecholamine agent for pharmacologic stress testing.[92] Arbutamine was shown to be capable of increasing the cardiac contractility and rate incrementally.[92]

Safety of stress testing with pharmacologic agents is equivalent to the safety found in exercise testing. Safety in testing has been demonstrated in all populations including diabetics, as long as similar pretest and monitoring procedures are followed as in exercise testing.[93] In addition, pharmacologic stress testing has been shown to be safe in patients who have undergone thrombolysis following acute myocardial infarction as soon as 2 to 5 days after initiation of thrombolysis.[94]

EXERCISE TESTING

Exercise testing continues to be the single most important noninvasive procedure used in the diagnosis and management of patients with coronary artery disease, although exercise testing alone is less sensitive and specific for women versus men.

Originally exercise testing was used to measure functional capacity or to evaluate abnormalities of coronary circulation. Currently exercise testing is used for a variety of patient management problems, including

• Evaluation of chest pain suggestive of coronary disease
• Evaluation of **atypical chest pain**
• Determination of prognosis and severity of coronary artery disease
• Evaluation of the effects of medical or surgical therapy or intervention
• Evaluation of arrhythmias
• Evaluation of hypertension with activity
• Assessment of **functional capacity**
• Screening to provide an exercise prescription
• Providing motivation for a lifestyle change to reduce the risk of developing coronary artery disease

Exercise testing involves systematically and progressively increasing the oxygen demand and evaluating the responses to the increased demand. The technique varies with different modes of exercise chosen and different protocols used by the examiner. Formal exercise testing involves the following modes of exercise:

• Walking up and down steps
• Exercising on a stationary bicycle
• Using arm or wheelchair ergometry
• Walking or jogging on a treadmill at variable speeds and inclines
• Walking a specified distance as in the 6-minute walk test

Informal testing is performed to screen for exercise programs, sometimes on a group basis, and includes such tests as the 12-minute walk, Cooper's 12-minute run, the pulse recovery test, or the 1.5-mile run (Fig. 8–5).[95–97]

Safety in Exercise Testing

The physical therapist must have a clear understanding of the rationale for terminating a *low-level* exercise test. The specific criteria for termination vary from one institution to another, but the general criteria include

• An oxygen consumption level of 17.5 mL of oxygen per kg (6 METs) achieved
• 70 to 75% of age-predicted maximal heart rate achieved
• Fatigue or dyspnea
• Maximal heart rate of 120 to 130 beats per minute
• Frequent (nine or more per minute) unifocal or **multifocal** premature ventricular contractions, paired premature ventricular contractions, or ventricular tachycardia
• ST-segment depression of 1.0 to 2.0 mm
• Claudication pain
• Dizziness
• Decrease in systolic blood pressure of 10 to 15 mm Hg below peak value
• Hypertensive blood pressure (systolic over 200 mm Hg, diastolic over 110 mm Hg)
• Level 1 (out of 4) angina

Both the patient and the discharging physician benefit when a predischarge exercise test is conducted.[98] The test can facilitate the distinction between chest wall and angina pain. In addition, im-

12-Minute Walking/Running Test (distance (miles) covered in 12 minutes)							
Fitness Category				**Age (years)**			
		13–19	20–29	30–39	40–49	50–59	60+
I. Very poor	(men)	<1.30*	<1.22	<1.18	<1.14	<1.03	<.87
	(women)	<1.0	<0.96	<0.94	<0.88	<0.84	<.78
II. Poor	(men)	1.30–1.37	1.22–1.31	1.18–1.30	1.14–1.24	1.03–1.16	0.87–1.02
	(women)	1.00–1.18	0.96–1.11	0.95–1.05	0.88–0.98	0.84–0.93	0.78–0.86
III. Fair	(men)	1.38–1.56	1.32–1.49	1.31–1.45	1.25–1.39	1.17–1.30	1.03–1.20
	(women)	1.19–1.29	1.12–1.22	1.06–1.18	.99–1.11	0.94–1.05	0.87–0.98
IV. Good	(men)	1.57–1.72	1.50–1.64	1.46–1.56	1.40–1.53	1.31–1.44	1.21–1.32
	(women)	1.30–1.43	1.23–1.34	1.19–1.29	1.12–1.24	1.06–1.18	0.99–1.09
V. Excellent	(men)	1.73–1.86	1.65–1.76	1.57–1.69	1.54–1.65	1.45–1.58	1.33–1.55
	(women)	1.44–1.51	1.35–1.45	1.30–1.39	1.25–1.34	1.19–1.30	1.10–1.18
VI. Superior	(men)	>1.87	>1.77	>1.70	>1.66	>1.59	>1.56
	(women)	>1.52	>1.46	>1.40	>1.35	>1.31	>1.19

Figure 8–5. The 12-minute walk/run test, which identifies fitness category for the distance covered in 12 minutes. (From Cooper K. The Aerobic Ways. New York, Bantam Books, 1981.)

provement in exercise performance following a myocardial infarction has been related to improvement in the patient's self-confidence following a successful, uneventful predischarge exercise test.

Maximal exercise testing and testing of *high-risk* patients or post–myocardial injury patients should be done in a setting in which emergencies can be managed expertly and efficiently. Appropriate equipment, which includes emergency medications and intravenous, intubation, and suctioning materials, should be present and updated when necessary. A direct current defibrillator should be available and functioning properly. Persons performing the testing should be certified in **Advanced Cardiac Life Support,** taught by the American Heart Association, and well trained in emergency cardiac response techniques such as **defibrillation.** Written protocols describing emergency procedures to be followed should be available to all testing personnel. These can be adopted from the American Heart Association's guidelines for advanced cardiac life support.[99]

Safety is a key consideration in exercise testing, and among the most important determinants of safety are the knowledge and experience of the examiner conducting the test. The American College of Sports Medicine has published guidelines that document the knowledge and skills required for exercise testing, including a description of situations in which the involvement or presence of a physician during testing may be necessary.[100] Ellestad and Stuart published a survey of more than 500,000 exercise tests, which suggested an overall mortality rate of 0.5 per 10,000 tests and a morbidity rate of 9 per 10,000.[101]

Exercise testing by nonphysician health care professionals has been performed for more than 30 years, although the American Heart Association Committee on Stress Testing did not endorse the idea of "experienced paramedical personnel" as able to perform the tests until 1979.[102] In 1987 Cahalin published a report on the safety of testing as performed by physical therapists with advanced clinical competence (see Table 8–5).[103] In 10,577 tests performed, the mortality rate was 0.9 per 10,000 and the morbidity rate was 3.8 per 10,000. In addition, Squires reported on the safety of exercise testing of 289 cardiac outpatients with left ventricular dysfunction (ejection fraction over 35%) by paramedical personnel with physician available on call.[104] Only one serious event occurred in 289 tests, and the outcome was a successful resuscitation. In addition, Olivotto demonstrated exercise testing was safe in a community-based population of patients with hypertrophic cardiomyopathy and provides useful information on functional capacity, blood pressure responses to exercise, and presence or absence of inducible ischemia.[105]

Factors that enhance the safety of exercise testing include the use of an informed consent to be signed by the patient (Fig. 8–6), the knowledge of when to exclude a patient from proceeding with an exercise test, the knowledge of when to terminate an exercise test, the knowledge and skills to react to an abnormal response or situation, and the availability of appropriate equipment and supplies to manage an emergency (e.g., **defibrillator,** emergency medications, **intubation,** suctioning equipment).

Physical therapists wishing to conduct exercise tests on individuals older than 40 years or on persons who are at moderate to high risk of developing CAD should expect to obtain the required knowledge and skills in advanced training or in clinically supervised postprofessional education. However, all physical therapists should understand the procedures involved in exercise testing and interpretation of the test results because one of the major purposes of these tests is the development of exercise prescriptions. Exercise prescriptions are based on the results of the exercise test and other pertinent information (see Table 8–5).

Exercise Testing Equipment

Clinical monitoring tools used during exercise testing traditionally include continuous ECG monitoring, periodic measurement of blood pressure and heart rate (this can be extracted from the ECG recording; see Chapter 9), patient reported or demonstrated symptoms, and heart and lung sounds. In some testing laboratories expired gas analysis permits the assessment of oxygen uptake during the test (Fig. 8–7). Multiple-lead ECG monitoring is used to depict the electrical activity of the heart. Detection of both arrhythmias and ischemia can be made from the ECG. A detailed discussion of the interpretation of ECG data and a description of arrhythmias are presented in Chapter 9.

Table 8–5

Performance Evaluation for Independent Exercise Testing

	POINTS	SCORE		POINTS	SCORE
I. PRETEST PREPARATION AND ASSESSMENT OF PATIENT			E. Makes correct decision regarding need for post-test follow-up of patient	10	—
A. Adequate preparation in terms of having necessary materials and information (knowledge of testing protocols/guidelines)	5	—	F. Adequate supervision and instruction of electrocardiograph technician during the test	5	—
B. Consistently obtains *all* necessary information from patient's medical record	5	—	**III. TEST INTERPRETATION**		
C. Seeks additional information directly from referring physician when necessary	5	—	A. Demonstrates consistent accuracy in interpretation, assessment of physical work capacity/functional aerobic impairment, and summary remarks/recommendations	55	—
D. Consistently completes a thorough patient interview and physical examination	5	—			
E. Accurately assesses the medical database and results from the patient interview and physical examination	21	—	B. Completes test interpretation within allotted time and adequately supervises electrocardiograph technicians to ensure compliance with testing schedule	5	—
F. Checks for proper calibration of testing instrumentation and correct functioning of emergency equipment	5	—			
			TOTAL	176	
II. TEST PERFORMANCE	10	—	**IV. ABILITY TO RESPOND TO LIFE-THREATENING SITUATIONS**		
A. Consistently makes correct judgments regarding the conducting of the test			To test independently, the therapist must have:		
B. Consistently obtains accurate data before, during, and after the test	30	—	A. Clearance from the medical director of the exercise testing laboratory to take definitive action in event of an emergency		—
C. Accurately uses above information to determine test end points	10	—			
D. Accurately uses above information to determine point at which postexercise monitoring can be discontinued	5	—	B. Current American Heart Association certification in Advanced Cardiac Life Support		—

Source: Irwin SI, Techlin JS. Cardiopulmonary Physical Therapy. 2nd ed. St. Louis, CV Mosby, 1990, p 141.

Protocols for Exercise Testing

Most institutions adopt a standard protocol to facilitate comparisons of the test subject's responses from test to test session as well as for comparisons

---

Informed Consent for an Exercise Test (Sample)

1. Explanation of the Exercise Test

You will perform an exercise test on a cycle ergometer or a motor-driven treadmill. The exercise intensity will begin at a level you can easily accomplish and will be advanced in stages, depending on your fitness level. We may stop the test at any time because of signs of fatigue or you may stop when you wish because of personal feelings of fatigue or discomfort.

2. Risks and Discomforts

There exists the possibility of certain changes occurring during the test. They include abnormal blood pressure, fainting, disorder of heart beat, and in rare instances, heart attack or death. Every effort will be made to minimize these through the preliminary examination and by observations during testing. Emergency equipment and trained personnel are available to deal with unusual situations which may arise.

3. Benefits to be Expected

The results obtained from the exercise test may assist in the diagnosis of your illness or in evaluating what type of physical activities you might engage with no or low hazards.

4. Inquiries

Any questions about the procedures used in the exercise test or in the estimation of functional capacity are encouraged. If you have any doubts or questions, please ask us for further explanations.

5. Freedom of Consent

Your permission to perform this exercise test is voluntary. You are free to deny consent if you so desire.

I have read this form and I understand the test procedures that I will perform. I consent to participate in this test.

_____
Signature of Patient

_____   _____
Date   Witness

Questions: _____
_____

Response: _____
_____

Physician signature: optional.

Figure 8–6. Signing an informed consent form is one of the safety precautions taken with exercise testing. (From American College of Sports Medicine. Guidelines for Exercise Testing and Prescription. 3rd ed. Philadelphia, Lea & Febiger, 1988. Used with permission.)

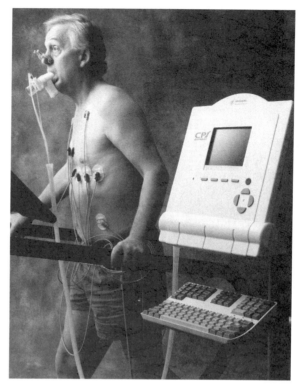

Figure 8–7. Oxygen uptake being measured directly during the exercise test. (Courtesy of Medical Graphics Corp., St. Paul, Minnesota.)

among other subjects. Standard testing procedures require a 12-lead ECG to be obtained before any test to rule out any acute ischemia or injury before testing. The patient's ECG is continuously monitored during the test. Standard procedure is to monitor a minimum of three leads during the test. Other pretest procedures include assessment of the patient's risk factor history for CAD (see Chapter 3); assessment of the patient's symptom history; and assessment of the patient's resting blood pressure, heart rate, and heart and lung auscultation.

When exercise is initiated, the workload is increased in accordance with a specific protocol. The patient's heart rate and blood pressure (and in some tests, the expired gases) are periodically monitored throughout the test and during the recovery period. Most tests are symptom limited and, as such, are terminated at the request of the patient or on the identification of an abnormality in one or more of the parameters being measured. The patient is monitored continuously during the recovery period until the pretest values are achieved. A written report documenting and interpreting the results is prepared following the test.

Testing Protocols

The most commonly used protocols in testing involve the use of either the stationary bicycle or the treadmill. Blood pressure is easier to auscultate on the stationary bicycle than on the treadmill. The bicycle also takes up less room, requires less coordination to operate, and is less expensive than the treadmill. The greatest disadvantage of the stationary bicycle, however, is that bicycling is not a daily functional activity for most persons. Therefore, patients develop muscular fatigue faster because they are using muscle groups that are not as "trained" as the muscles used for walking. Such patients do not achieve their best results, because the maximal heart rate may be well below what is considered diagnostic (85% of predicted maximal heart rate).[106] A widely used bicycle testing protocol is displayed in Figure 8–8.[107] This protocol may be employed intermittently (meaning that rests are incorporated between each work stage) rather than continuously because of the peripheral fatigue that develops. Also, the workloads may be reduced by half for females or severely deconditioned individuals.

The treadmill is relatively large, requires a patient to have balance and coordination, and is extremely noisy, making the auscultation of blood pressure very difficult. However, because walking is a functional activity, the muscles do not fatigue as rapidly as they do with cycling, and therefore the treadmill is considered to have greater diagnostic benefits. The two most common treadmill protocols are the **Bruce exercise test protocol** and the **Balke exercise protocol.** The Bruce protocol (Table 8–6) is probably most widely used in the clinical setting of hospitals because it provides normative data in the form of a nomogram to calculate functional aerobic impairment (Fig. 8–9). Previous studies have reported limitations in the ability of the functional aerobic impairment nomogram to predict functional capacity. The preferred method of predicting functional capacity is via the maximal workload performed on the treadmill test. According to Froelicher, a true test of aerobic capacity is best limited to a total exercise time of 10 minutes because of the endurance factor, which becomes significant after 10 minutes of exercise.[108]

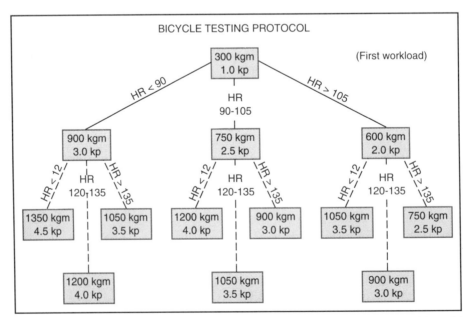

Figure 8–8. A branching bicycle testing protocol. HR, Heart rate. (Adapted from Golding LA, Myers CR, Slinning WE [eds]. The Y's Way to Physical Fitness. Rev. ed. Chicago, The YMCA of the USA, 1982, p 535, with permission of the YMCA of the USA, 101 N. Wacker Dr., Chicago IL, 60606.)

Table 8–6
Bruce Treadmill Protocol

STAGE	TIME (min)	SPEED (mph)	GRADE	MET*
I	3	1.7	10%	4–5
II	3	2.5	12%	6–7
III	3	3.4	14%	8–10
IV	3	4.2	16%	11–13
V	3	5.0	18%	14–16
VI	3	6.0	20%	17–19

*1 MET, resting metabolic rate = 3.5 mL of oxygen per kg of body weight per minute.
Source: Ellestad MH. Stress Testing Principles and Practice, 4th edition. New York, Oxford University Press, 1996.

The starting speed of the Bruce protocol is 1.7 miles per hour, which is a fairly comfortable speed for all. However, because of the rapid increases in speed and the fact the subject starts on a 10% grade, the average time a nontrained subject actually exercises during the test is between 6 and 12 minutes. In comparison, the Balke protocol (Fig. 8–10) starts at a speed of 3.3 miles per hour, which is often too fast for a deconditioned patient or an older individual, but the subject starts on a level surface and only gradually is an incline added during the protocol. The gradual workload increments allow closer attainment of a steady state at each stage and facilitate the measurement of true maximal oxygen consumption. However, the Balke protocol requires a longer time to perform owing to the gradual addition of the incline. The Balke protocol is used more widely with athletes, especially with runners, because runners typically do not train on steep inclines and because this protocol allows the athlete to attain a steady state in a shorter period of time.

Maximal and Submaximal Stress Testing

The protocols that are used are described as either maximal or submaximal; the distinction between them is the termination point of the test. **Submaxi-**

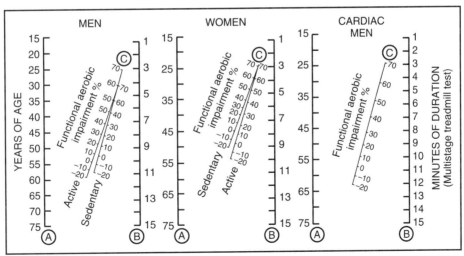

Figure 8–9. Nomograms for evaluating functional aerobic impairment (FAI) of men, women, and men with cardiac diagnosis, according to age and by duration of exercise on the Bruce protocol for sedentary and active groups. To find the FAI, identify age (in years) in the left column and identify duration of time on the Bruce treadmill protocol in the right column. With a straight edge, line up the two points and read where the straight edge intercepts the FAI nomogram for either active or sedentary. (From Bruce RL, Kusumi F, Hosmer D. Maximal oxygen intake and nomographic assessment of functional aerobic impairment in cardiovascular disease. Am Heart J 85:545–562, 1973.)

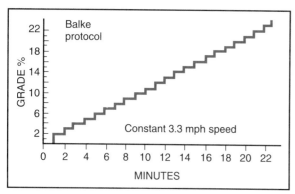

Figure 8–10. The Balke treadmill protocol.

mal tests are terminated on achievement of a predetermined end point (unless symptoms otherwise limit completion of the test). The predetermined end point may be either the achievement of a certain percentage of the patient's predicted maximal heart rate (PMHR) (e.g., 75% of PMHR) or the attainment of a certain workload (e.g., 2.5 mph, 12% grade). A special subset of submaximal testing is *low-level testing,* performed on patients during the recuperative phase after myocardial injury or coronary bypass surgery.

Maximal stress tests usually use the end point of the predicted maximal heart rate or terminate when a patient is limited by symptoms. Maximal stress testing is employed to measure functional capacity as well as to diagnose CAD. The protocol for testing involves performing a progressive workload until the patient perceives an inability to continue because of some limiting symptom such as shortness of breath, leg fatigue, or chest discomfort.

Exercise tests also may be described as intermittent or continuous. *Intermittent* testing intersperses progressive workloads with short rest periods to give the subject time to recover and decrease the effect of peripheral fatigue. *Continuous* tests utilize incrementally progressive workloads until the test is terminated because of patient symptoms or a defined end point.

Low-Level Exercise Testing

Low-level exercise testing is usually performed when patients have experienced a MI recently or have undergone coronary artery bypass graft sur-

gery. Such tests have been performed as early as 5 days after MI or surgery[109] but are more likely to be performed just before or immediately after discharge from the hospital following an acute event. Some physicians prefer to wait up to 2 weeks after the cardiac event before administering the low-level exercise test.

Low-level exercise testing may be useful in predicting the subsequent course of an MI or bypass surgery as well as for identifying the **high-risk patient.** High-risk patients exhibit an increased risk of complications or death as a result of myocardial ischemia or poor ventricular function. The high-risk patient needs more immediate intervention and should not be treated as a typical patient in a cardiac rehabilitation program. After the high-risk patient is identified, the decision on optimal medical management or surgical intervention is more easily made.

Many factors have been studied from the results of the low-level exercise test to determine the most outstanding variable for identifying high-risk patients. Exercise-induced ST-segment depression of 2.0 mm or greater on low-level exercise tests has been identified as the single most valuable indicator of prognosis after MI according to the regression analysis by Davidson and DeBusk.[110] In addition, early onset of ST-segment depression is related to increased incidence of coronary events. Starling and co-workers[111] demonstrated a significantly increased risk of death after MI when both ST-segment depression and angina were produced during low-level exercise testing in the early period after a MI. Exercise-induced angina alone was associated with subsequent coronary artery bypass surgery.[112, 113] Other variables of minor prognostic significance after MI include inappropriate blood pressure response, maximum heart rate achieved, and maximum systolic blood pressure achieved.[114, 115]

Low-level exercise testing can also provide information useful for optimal medical management after myocardial injury or surgery, including treatment for angina, arrhythmias, or hypertension. Exercise-induced arrhythmias on a low-level exercise test may be an indication for therapeutic management before hospital discharge. The incidence of sudden death has been reported to be 2.5 times higher in patients manifesting ventricular arrhythmias during low-level exercise testing.[116] Poor performance, such as limited exercise duration, has been highly correlated with increased incidence of heart failure and is associated with an increased mortality.[117]

Because of its great prognostic and therapeutic value, low-level testing is often used for screening patients who wish to participate in cardiac rehabilitation programs.[98] Activity levels for patients during rehabilitation in the home or hospital setting can be prescribed on the basis of the results of the low-level exercise test.

However, not all patients are appropriate candidates for low-level exercise testing. Safety of exercise testing early after MI has been a topic of debate because of the traditional medical belief that a recently damaged myocardium is prone to further injury, including rupture, **aneurysm,** extension of infarction, or susceptibility to serious arrhythmias.[118] However, the safety of properly conducted exercise testing was documented as early as 1973.[119] Knowledge of and adherence to contraindications for testing optimize the safety of exercise testing (Table 8–7).[106]

Institutions vary in the choice of an exercise testing protocol for low-level testing. However, a progressively increasing workload from 2 to approximately 6 METs (Metabolic Equivalent Tables, a multiple of the resting metabolic rate) is often used. Among the protocols for low-level exercise testing, the modified Naughton and modified Sheffield-Bruce protocols appear to be most widely chosen (Tables 8–8, 8–9).

Low-level exercise testing soon after MI is a safe, noninvasive method for evaluating the functional capacity for physical activity; for detecting

Table 8–8
Modified Naughton Treadmill Protocol

	TIME (min)							
	0	3	6	9	12	15	18	21
Speed (mph)	2	2	2	2	2	3	3	3
Grade (%)	3.5	7	10.5	14	17.5	12.5	15	17.5
MET	3	4	5	6	7	8	9	10

MET, resting metabolic rate.

Table 8–9
Modified Sheffield-Bruce Submaximal Protocol

STAGE	SPEED (mph)	GRADE (%)	TIME (min)
1	1.7	0	3
2	1.7	5	3
3	1.7	10	3
4	2.5	12	3

arrhythmias, angina, and hypertensive responses with exercise; for determining optimal medical management; and for predicting the risk of subsequent cardiac events.

Contraindications to Testing

Essential to safe testing is knowing who should *not* be tested. Thoroughly evaluating the patient before testing reveals any **contraindications** to testing. Absolute contraindications to maximal stress testing include the following:

- Recent MI (less than 4 to 6 weeks after the MI for a maximal, symptom-limited test) in most clinical settings
- Acute **pericarditis** or **myocarditis**
- Resting or **unstable angina**
- Serious ventricular or rapid atrial arrhythmias (e.g., ventricular tachycardia, couplets, atrial fibrillation, or atrial flutter)
- Untreated second- or third-degree heart block
- Overt congestive heart failure (pulmonary rales, third heart sound, or both)
- Any acute illness

Table 8–7
Contraindications to Low-Level Testing

Unstable angina or angina pectoris at rest
Severe heart failure (overt left ventricular failure on examination with pulmonary rales and S_3 heart sound)
Serious arrhythmias at rest
Second- or third-degree heart block
Disabling musculoskeletal abnormalities
Valvular heart disease
Blood pressure >180/105 mm Hg
Patient refuses to sign consent form

Source: Starling MR, Crawford MH, et al. Predictive value of early postmyocardial infarction modified treadmill exercise testing in multivessel coronary artery disease detection. Am Heart J 102(2):169,1981.

In addition to absolute contraindications, the general clinical status of the patient must be considered before determining whether the stress test is contraindicated. The following relative contraindications should be considered on an individual basis:

- **Aortic stenosis**
- Known left main CAD (or its equivalent)
- Severe hypertension (defined as systolic blood pressure higher than 165 mm Hg at rest, diastolic blood pressure higher than 110 mm Hg at rest, or both)
- **Idiopathic hypertrophic subaortic stenosis**
- Severe depression of the ST segment on the resting ECG
- Compensated heart failure

Terminating the Testing Session

The person administering the exercise test must observe the patient and the ECG monitor during the test continuously to decide when the test should be terminated. Guidelines for termination of the test are similar for all tests and include the following:

- Increasing frequency or pairing of premature ventricular complexes
- Development of ventricular tachycardia
- Rapid atrial arrhythmias, including atrial fibrillation or atrial flutter, with uncontrolled ventricular response rates
- Development of second- or third-degree heart block
- Increased angina pain (level 2 on a scale of 4)
- Hypotensive blood pressure response (20 mm Hg or greater decrease)
- Extreme shortness of breath
- Dizziness, mental confusion, or lack of coordination
- Severe ST-segment depression. The American College of Sports Medicine recommends termination when the ST segment is depressed 2.0 mm or more, although some testing personnel may proceed when changes of greater magnitude are demonstrated as long as there is no evidence of other abnormal responses.[100]
- Observation of the patient reveals pale and clammy skin (**pallor** and **diaphoresis**)
- Extremely elevated systolic or diastolic blood pressure, or both, which may or may not be associated with symptoms.
- On achievement of predicted maximal heart rate; it is usually safe to proceed with the test

Name _____ John Doe _____ Date _____
Age __46__ Sex __M__ Height __5'10"__ Weight __190 lb.__
Diagnosis _____ Reason for test __chest pains__
Protocol __Bruce__
Time of test __8 AM__ Time last cigarette _____ Time last meal __12__
Medications __None__ Time last dose _____
Physician _____

RESULTS

12-Lead ECG interpretation __Normal__
Minutes completed __7.05__ Limiting factor(s) __Leg fatigue__
Rest HR __84__ Rest BP __140/96__ Heart sounds __Normal__
Maximum HR __170__ Maximum BP __190/102__
BP Response __Diastolic hypertension throughout__
Chest pain __None__
Summary of ST segment changes __Negative for ischemia__
Summary of arrhythmias __Rare PAC throughout__
Physical work capacity __Poor, 30% below predicted functional aerobic impairment__
Remarks/recommendations __Patient needs an exercise program to decrease blood pressure and improve functional aerobic impairment.__

Interpreted by _____ Date _____

Figure 8–11. Worksheet for interpretation of exercise test results. (From Scully R, Barnes ML. Physical Therapy. Philadelphia, JB Lippincott, 1989, p. 537.)

beyond the predicted maximal heart rate if the patient is able and willing to continue and if other indications to terminate the test are absent.[106]
- Presence of leg fatigue or leg cramps or claudication pain
- Patient request for termination of test

Differences in criteria for termination of a low-level exercise test are listed earlier and specify different maximal heart rates, ST-segment depression, level of angina, and amount of blood pressure change allowed.

Interpretation of Results

Once the test is concluded, the results are written on a worksheet to provide data for the interpretation (Fig. 8–11). The following parameters are necessary for a thorough interpretation:

- Exercise time completed (and protocol used)
- Limiting factors (reason for termination)
- Presence or absence of chest pain at peak exercise: usually defined as positive, negative, or atypical for angina or extreme shortness of breath
- Maximal heart rate achieved
- Blood pressure response
- Arrhythmias: description of which type developed and when they occurred
- ST-segment changes: usually described as positive, negative, equivocal, or indeterminate for ischemia
  - Positive: 1.0 mm or greater horizontal or downsloping ST-segment depression (Fig. 8–12)
  - Equivocal: more than 0.5 but less than 1.0 mm horizontal or downsloping ST-segment depression or more than 1.5 mm upsloping depression
  - Negative: less than 0.5 mm horizontal or downsloping ST-segment depression[106]
  - Indeterminate: unable to measure the ST segment accurately because of the presence of any of the following: bundle branch block, medication (if patient is taking digoxin [Lanoxin]), resting ST-segment changes on the ECG, or cardiac hypertrophy
- Heart sounds: notation of pretest and post-test sounds and description of any change
- Functional aerobic impairment: can be determined from a nomogram if the Bruce treadmill

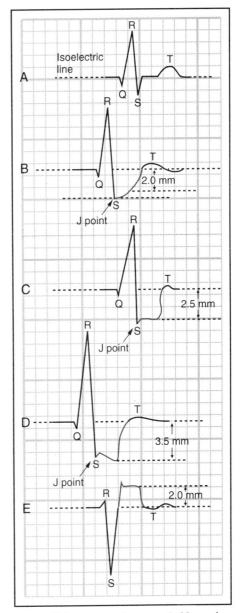

Figure 8–12. ST-segment changes. *A,* Normal segment; *B,* slowly up-sloping ST-segment depression; *C,* horizontal ST-segment depression; *D,* down-sloping ST-segment depression; *E,* horizontal ST-segment elevation.

protocol is used. This value is compared with normal values to determine impairment in functional capacity (physical work capacity).
- R wave changes: amplitude changes are considered to give additional diagnostic information in interpreting exercise test results. The normal response to exercise is a decrease in R wave ampli-

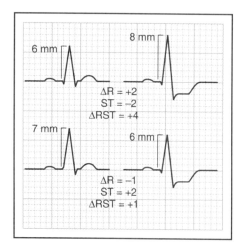

Figure 8–13. Calculation of index (RST) in two patients with ST-segment depression and R wave increased and decreased. (From Bonoris PE, et al. Evaluation of R wave amplitude changes versus ST-segment depression in stress testing. Circulation 57[5]:904–910, 1973. Reproduced by permission of the American Heart Association.)

tude. If no change or an increase in R wave amplitude occurs with exercise, the patient with CAD is considered to be at an increased risk for developing a cardiac problem in the future (Fig. 8–13).[120]

- Maximal oxygen consumption (Vo₂ max) can be calculated using formulas if not directly measured during the test (Fig. 8–14); however, this method is not very accurate.

The final summary of the exercise test should define whether the outcome of the test is normal or abnormal; if the outcome is abnormal, the summary should provide the reasons. Although the physical therapist may not actually perform the stress test, obtaining the interpretation of the re-

Treadmill:

$\dot{V}o_2$ (mL/kg/min) =
Velocity (m/min) × 1.78 (mL O₂/kg/m × (% grade + .073)

Convert mph to m/min as follows:

1609 m = 1 mile
60 min = 1 hour

1 mph = 1609 m/60 min = 26.8 m/min

Figure 8–14. Calculation of maximal oxygen consumption (VO₂max) indirectly via formula.

sults provides valuable data for developing an exercise prescription. The interpretation also provides valuable information regarding safety during exercise for the patient.

Prognostic Value of Maximal Exercise Testing

Maximal exercise testing is used as a noninvasive screening method for the detection of coronary disease. Its diagnostic accuracy in determining coronary disease is limited by the fact that it is a noninvasive test and therefore only reflects gross metabolic and electrical changes in the heart. Nonetheless, studies evaluating the specificity and sensitivity of stress testing have suggested that in appropriately chosen populations, it can be very helpful in identifying coronary disease and defining its severity.[106] **Sensitivity** is the measure of the reliability of stress testing in identifying the presence of disease. **Specificity** is the measure of the reliability of stress testing in identifying the population without disease. In general, testing demonstrates greater sensitivity and specificity in males over the age of 40 than in females. Females generally demonstrate a greater percentage of **false negative** results, but it is beyond the scope of this chapter to describe the predictive values for every potential population. However, to aid clinical judgment in predicting the risk of developing coronary artery disease, one can use Bayes' theorem to assist in predicting sensitivity and specificity of testing.[121]

The value of diagnostic stress testing is tempered by the amount of variability among examiners conducting the test. Problems with testing include amount of encouragement given to the patient, a lack of strict adherence to protocols, use of handrail support, and interpretation of ST-segment deviation and symptoms.[108]

Despite its acknowledged potential limitations, several studies have attempted to identify specific single parameters or combinations of variables that might identify a group of patients with more severe disease.[106] Ischemia, reflected by ST-segment depression, that occurs during the early stages of an exercise test has been correlated with more severe disease than ischemia that occurs at peak exercise. Goldschlager and co-workers reported an increased incidence of subsequent myocardial infarction in a group of patients who exhibited ST-segment depression at light workloads.[122] The severity of coronary disease has also been correlated with the length of recovery time (postexercise rest) for ST segment to return to normal.

Other subsets of patients have been identified who demonstrate certain signs and symptoms that suggest a greater risk for the subsequent development of a cardiac event. The signs and symptoms that have increased prognostic value include ST-segment depression, bradycardic heart rate responses, presence of angina, and maximal systolic blood pressure attained. Ellestad identified a population with more serious prognosis of disease when the magnitude of ST-segment depression was considered.[106] In addition, a subset of persons at high risk for progression of angina, MI, or death was identified by Ellestad. Persons with normal ST segments at peak effort who achieved maximal heart rates considerably below their predicted pulses (bradycardic heart rate response or **chronotropic** incompetence) demonstrated high risk of progression of angina, MI, or death. The tendency was to describe the test results as normal because the patients in Ellestad's study did not demonstrate ischemic ST-segment changes.

The presence of angina pain gives added significance when the patient demonstrates ST-segment depression during exercise. Ellestad described a subset of patients at double the risk of a subsequent coronary event when angina and ST-segment depression occurred together, as compared with patients without angina but with ST-segment depression (silent ischemia).[106]

The incidence of sudden death is increased in the following subset of patients:

- Those unable to exceed a maximal systolic blood pressure of 130 mm Hg
- Those with increased frequency and severity of arrhythmias during testing[123]

Calculating a probability score from the combination and weighing of clinical variables from the exercise test identifies the subsets of individuals at greater risk for coronary events. Many institutions are in the process of developing multiple variable analyses to increase the predictive value of exercise testing.[124] However, the use of thallium injection at peak performance also increases the information gained from the test, as well as increasing the sensitivity of the test.

Exercise Testing with Ventilatory Gas Analysis

Although exercise testing alone is diagnostic for coronary disease, exercise testing with ventilatory gas analysis using a metabolic cart can provide greater information regarding oxygen exchange, breathlessness, etc. (see Fig. 8–7). A computer is utilized in conjunction with a system that automatically samples expired air continuously, a system for measuring the volume of expired air, a system with oxygen provided electronically, and CO_2 analyzers that measure the concentration of gases that are expired. The computer is programmed to compute the oxygen consumption, caloric expenditure, and CO_2 production during rest and during any activity. The computer can provide a printout of the gas exchange and other variables every second of activity and provide information for exercise prescription as well as for diagnosis of limitation of activity. One disadvantage of utilizing the automatic computer-generated information is that the output data are accurate only if the electronic equipment and analyzers are accurate and calibrated against previously established standards.

Cardiopulmonary exercise testing with ventilatory gas analysis provides information on cardiac performance, functional limitation, and exercise limitations, particularly when the symptom limiting the individual is breathlessness or dyspnea. In assessing dyspnea, the ventilatory reserve and the dyspnea index are the most important variables. Normally 60% of an individual's maximal ventilatory reserve is utilized during activity; measurement of maximal voluntary ventilation (MVV) provides the information. Elite athletes may use the lungs' total ventilatory capacity. Dyspnea occurs when the minute ventilation VE divided by the MVV is greater than 50% (otherwise known as the dyspnea index). When the VE/MVV is greater than 70% respiratory muscle fatigue will occur within minutes. When the ratio is greater than 90% an individual cannot continue exercising more than a few seconds.[125]

Dyspnea that occurs in the presence of pulmonary disease will demonstrate early rapid and shallow breathing, with a reduction in peak ventilation and a reduction in tidal volume (VT). Both VO_{2max} and maximal volume of CO_2 production are reduced, and the peak exercise dyspnea index is 1.0.[125]

Dyspnea that occurs in the presence of heart failure produces a different outcome with exercise testing. Individuals with heart failure achieve their anaerobic threshold much earlier than healthy individuals of similar age, with a lower than normal maximal ventilation and maximal CO_2 production. The dyspnea index, however, is normal.[125]

Many advantages exist in utilizing ventilatory gas analysis with exercise testing, however, several disadvantages exist, including the fact that the equipment (a metabolic cart) is not widely available in the clinical setting. This equipment may be in hospital settings for use with resting nutritional studies, and may be loaned for exercise testing. Another disadvantage is that many patients feel claustrophobic with the mouthpiece or headpiece and may actually hyperventilate with the mouthpiece.

Exercise Testing with Imaging Modalities

Individuals may perform an exercise test to assess the myocardial oxygen supply and demand relationship (to determine if ischemia occurs during physiologic stress) and undergo additional noninvasive imaging immediately following the performance of the exercise. The use of imaging techniques such as thallium-201 or sestamibi scanning and SPECT allows for greater diagnostic accuracy and sensitivity, particularly in individuals with atypical chest pain syndromes, or in females who demonstrate low sensitivity to exercise testing alone.[89-91] Two-dimensional echocardiography is often utilized immediately after exercise testing as well. (See earlier sections on imaging and echocardiography for information.)

CARDIAC CATHETERIZATION: CORONARY ANGIOGRAPHY AND VENTRICULOGRAPHY

Cardiac catheterization is an invasive procedure that provides extremely valuable information for the diagnosis and management of patients with cardiac disease. The general goal of cardiac catheterization is to obtain objective information that can

- Establish or confirm a diagnosis of cardiac dysfunction or heart disease
- Demonstrate the severity of coronary artery disease or valvular dysfunction
- Determine guidelines for optimal management of the patient, including medical and surgical management as well as a program of exercise

The data obtained from the cardiac catheterization are as follows:

- Cardiac output
- Shunt detection
- Angiography: coronary and ventriculography
- Left and right heart pressures (hemodynamics)
  - Right atrial (normal = 0 to 4 mm Hg)
  - Right ventricle (normal = 30/2 mm Hg)
  - Pulmonary artery (normal = 30/10 mm Hg)
  - Pulmonary artery wedge (normal = 8 to 12 mm Hg)
  - Left ventricular end-diastolic (normal = 8 to 12 mm Hg)
- Ventricular ejection fraction (estimated) (normal = 65 ± 8%)

Specific determinations that can be made as a result of cardiac catheterization include

- The presence of and severity of coronary artery disease (degree of stenosis)
- The presence of left ventricular dysfunction or aneurysm or both
- The presence of valvular heart disease and the severity of the dysfunction, including aortic valve stenosis or regurgitation, mitral valve stenosis or regurgitation or prolapse, tricuspid valve dysfunction, or pulmonary valve dysfunction (amount of backward flow across valve)
- The presence of pericardial disease

Indications for Cardiac Catheterization

Because several noninvasive tests are now available that achieve sensitivities of greater than 90% and specificities above 70% for detection of ischemia and poor perfusion, cardiac catheterization is not indicated simply to diagnose angina. However, absolute indications for catheterization include the following:[59]

- Cardiac arrest or primary (not infarction-related) ventricular fibrillation
- Pulmonary edema, potentially of ischemic etiology
- Intolerance of or noncompliance with medical therapy for angina
- Job description mandate (such as commercial pilots or heavy machine operators)

In the absence of specific angina symptoms, the following are indications for catheterization:

- Significant decrease (more than 35%) in exercise duration when compared with previous exercise treadmill test or associated with significant ST-segment depression
- Progressive decline in systolic blood pressure to less than 100 mm Hg during exercise
- Evidence of symptomatic hypoperfusion during exercise such as intense diaphoresis, pallor, mental confusion, associated with decrease in blood pressure, and ST-segment depression
- Left ventricular ejection fraction below 35% with clinical evidence of ischemia
- Ventricular tachycardia emerging with exercise, especially if associated with ST-segment depression and increasing workload

Other indications for cardiac catheterization in the presence of symptoms include:

- A 25% decrease in exercise duration as compared to a previous exercise test
- Prolonged chest pain not responsive to three nitroglycerine tablets and associated with ECG changes in an individual with known CAD
- A change in angina pattern occuring with less effort, or at rest, and requiring nitroglycerine for relief
- Increasing symptoms of angina despite adjustment in medications

Procedure for Cardiac Catheterization

Cardiac catheterization involves the insertion of a catheter into the cardiovascular system to measure pressures or perform angiography (anatomic evaluation). The specific procedure includes catheterizing the right or left sides of the heart, contrast angiography, and sometimes revascularization with drugs or pacing. The procedure is invasive and is performed in a special room in the radiology department or in a special laboratory. The patient undergoing the procedure is awake but under sedation. A catheter is inserted into either the brachial artery or the femoral artery, depending on the cardiologist's expertise with an individual technique. The catheter is then passed into the great vessels and then into the great chambers under fluoroscopic control. Pressures are measured in the chambers across the valves, and cardiac output is measured to assess the competency of the valves and the function of the cardiac muscle. Finally, radiopaque contrast medium is injected into the chambers and then into the orifices of the coronary arteries (and in some cases into the aorta itself). The passage of the contrast medium is followed and filmed for closer evaluation of the integrity of the arteries and the myocardium when the procedure is completed (Fig. 8–15).

Interpreting the Test Results

On completion of the cardiac catheterization, the cardiologist reviews the films to assess the ventricular function and the severity of coronary artery stenosis. The degree of stenosis in each arterial segment is graded during the review of the film, with total occlusion graded as 100% (Fig. 8–16). One of the problems with interpreting the cardiac catheterization film is the fact that angiography is only two-dimensional. Another problem concerns reliability: the film interpretation relies either on a person's subjective judgment or on a computer to measure the degree of stenosis. However, cardiac catheterization has greater sensitivity in detecting disease than other noninvasive procedures previously presented.

Controversy exists over the indication for performing cardiac catheterization. Some critics in the medical field believe that the catheterization technique is overused and that less invasive procedures should be used before catheterization.[54, 126] Others note, however, that coronary angiography is the only test that provides information about the actual site, extent, and severity of obstruction in coronary artery disease. Cardiac catheterization has greater predictive accuracy in assessment of coronary artery disease than exercise testing. It also may be used to confirm diagnoses from other non-

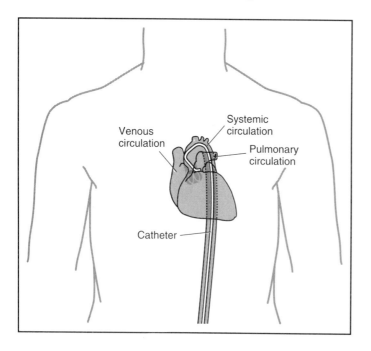

Figure 8-15. The cardiac catheterization procedure involves the passage of a catheter through the great vessels so that radiopaque contrast medium can be injected into the orifices of the coronary arteries.

invasive tests. Cardiac catheterization must be performed before any surgical intervention. Common practice demonstrates that coronary angiography and ventriculography are being performed on the majority of patients following acute myocardial infarction to assess severity of disease and amount of ventricular dysfunction resulting from the infarction. Cardiac catheterization results are very important in determining the entire clinical picture of the patient.

Digital Subtraction Angiography

Digital subtraction angiography is a technique involving the introduction of small concentrations of iodinated contrast material into a vascular bed and then analyzed by a computer to produce an angiogram without direct injection of contrast material into an artery or cardiac chamber. This procedure has shown excellent reliability with carotid circulation and bypass grafts. This procedure can also improve the quality of coronary angiograms obtained from coronary catheterization.[127]

ERGONOVINE STIMULATION

Coronary artery spasm has been demonstrated to play a role in the manifestation of ischemic heart disease. To document coronary artery spasm, one must demonstrate significant or total narrowing of

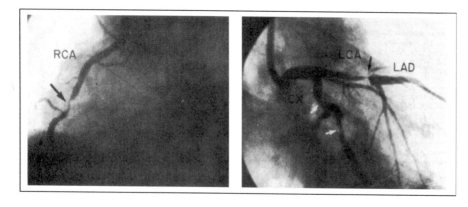

Figure 8-16. The degree of stenosis in each arterial segment is graded during review of the film, with total occlusion graded as 100%. The arrows point to areas of occlusion. LAD, Left anterior descending artery; LCA, left coronary artery; CX, circumflex artery. (From Braunwald E [ed]. Harrison's Principles of Internal Medicine. 12th ed. New York, McGraw-Hill, 1991, p. 883.)

a segment in an artery that may or may not have partial arteriosclerotic narrowing. If increased narrowing of the artery occurs and the narrowing is relieved with the administration of a vasodilator, then coronary artery spasm has been documented. Spasm is rarely documented with coronary angiography (3%).[128] Therefore, because angiography does not frequently induce the spasm, ergonovine stimulation has become an important diagnostic test for coronary spasm.

Ergonovine stimulation is used when coronary spasm is suspected, particularly in a patient with documented ECG changes during symptoms or with documented ischemic episodes and a normal coronary angiographic study. The test has a high degree of sensitivity and specificity for coronary vasospasm.[129, 130]

Ergonovine stimulation is performed in the cardiac catheterization laboratory or in the coronary care unit (if previous angiography studies have demonstrated normal coronary arteries). Either incremental doses of ergonovine are given by intravenous injections or a single bolus of ergometrine is given while a patient is monitored continuously for ECG or hemodynamic changes (particularly ST-segment elevation or major heart rate and blood pressure changes) (Fig. 8–17). The patient is monitored throughout the injections until a maximal dosage is given or until the patient experiences symptoms.

When ergonovine stimulation is performed in the cardiac catheterization laboratory, repeat angiography is performed when symptoms or changes on the ECG develop; treatment with vasodilators is initiated after spasm is documented. In the coronary care unit, the patient is treated with vasodilators when the ECG changes or when the patient complains of symptoms. When a positive response occurs to ergonovine stimulation, the patient is managed with medications that reduce or prevent the occurrence of spasm (see discussion of calcium-channel blockers in Chapter 14).

HEART RATE VARIABILITY

Studies have indicated that both the sympathetic and parasympathetic branches of the autonomic nervous system affect the frequency of sudden death and cardiovascular death after myocardial infarction.[131, 132] Methods in the past have utilized heart rate variability as measured by 24-hour Holter monitoring, looking at variability over a time period from 2 to 15 minutes.

Deep breathing has been utilized to assess variations in heart rate due to the altered vagal-cardiac activity during this activity.[133] Impairments in the vagal input can depress the variability of the heart rate during deep breathing.[134] Katz found that heart rate variability below 10 beats per minute during 6 deep respirations in 1 minute was a significant predictor of death with an odds ratio of 1.38.[133] Therefore, there may be some indication to follow heart rate variability in the asymptomatic at risk population as well as the post-MI population in the future.

ENDOCARDIAL BIOPSY

Samples of the right or left ventricular endomyocardium may be obtained at the time of catheterization to determine myocardial rejection in patients with cardiac transplant. In addition, a myocardial biopsy may be taken to diagnose hypertrophic and congenital cardiomyopathy.[127]

VASCULAR DIAGNOSTIC TESTING FOR AORTIC, PERIPHERAL, AND CAROTID DISEASE

Adequate perfusion of muscles and organs is imperative for optimal functioning and requires optimal flow through the body's vascular system. Therefore, when disease or dysfunction is suspected in any of these vessels, evaluation of the specific vascular components is performed, including physical assessment, laboratory evaluation, and diagnostic assessment.

Aortic Disease and Dysfunction and Diagnosis

The most common dysfunction identified in the aorta include aneurysms, atherosclerotic disease, aortic valve dysfunction, and arteritis. The most common diagnostic tests for aortic dysfunction include ECG, angiography, CT scan, and chest x-ray. Table 8–10 presents information on clinical, physi-

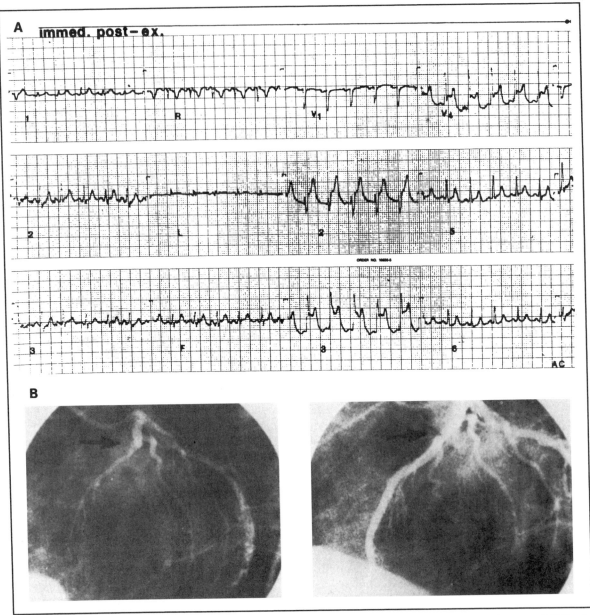

Figure 8–17. Exercise-induced ST-segment elevation in variant angina. *A,* Exercise electrocardiogram (ECG) of a 45-year-old man with exertional, rest, and nocturnal angina. The rest ECG is normal. During exercise, ST-segment elevation is present in the anterior leads, suggesting anterior wall ischemia and left anterior descending (LAD) artery obstruction. *B,* Coronary arteriogram of the same patient. The left coronary artery *(left panel)* is normal except for a 40% obstruction in the proximal LAD *(arrow).* A septal perforator is seen running behind the LAD. The patient developed spontaneous chest pain with anterior ST-segment elevation, similar to that present during exercise. Repeat angiography *(right panel)* shows the LAD totally obstructed *(arrow)* at the previous site of the minimal lesion and distal to the origin of the septal perforator, which is now seen clearly. The coronary artery spasm was relieved by sublingual nitroglycerine, and further arteriography showed that the 40% obstruction in the LAD remained unchanged. ST-segment elevation during exercise in this patient was probably caused by exercise-induced coronary artery spasm similar to that seen during spontaneous chest pain and not by a severe fixed coronary lesion. (From Dunn RF, Kell TD. Exercise-induced ST-segment elevation. Primary Cardiology Supplement to Hospital Physician 1:A79–A90, 1982. Reprinted with permission from Turner White Communications, Inc.)

Table 8-10

Aortic Aneurysms

ANEURYSM TYPE	ETIOLOGY	LOCATION	CLINICAL FEATURES	PHYSICAL FINDINGS	LABORATORY FINDINGS	TREATMENT
Arterosclerotic	Atherosclerosis	Usually abdominal (between renal arteries and aortic bifurcation)	Older males Often asymptomatic until rupture Abdominal fullness or pulsations; back or epigastric pain, worse prior to rupture	Palpable, pulsatile abdominal mass Peripheral emboli Abdominal bruit Associated peripheral vascular disease	Size measured by abdominal ultrasound Angiography less accurate at estimating size but necessary to define surgical anatomy	Rupture of >6 cm diameter: surgery <4 cm diameter
Dissecting	Hypertension Marfan's syndrome Cystic medial necrosis Aortic coarctation Trauma	Type I: proximal ascending aorta to descending aorta Type II: confined to ascending aorta Type III: begins in descending aorta and aorta and extends distally	Severe, sudden, tearing chest pain radiating to abdomen and back (occasional patient will have no pain) Aortic branch occlusions causing myocardial infarction, stroke, spinal infarction with paraplegia, renal impairment Aortic root involvement causing acute aortic insufficiency, rupture into pericardium with pericardial friction rub or tamponade	Hypertension Asymmetric pulses Signs of aortic insufficiency, neurologic involvement, or tamponade if present	ECG may show myocardial infarction Wide mediastinum on chest x-ray (not always present) CT scan usually diagnostic Angiography necessary to define surgical anatomy	Surgical indications: Ascending aortic involvement Impairment of vital organs Etiology not hypertensive Hemodynamic impairment Medical therapy may be tried in older patient with distal hypertension and lessen force of contraction (nitroprusside + beta blocker)

Source: Andreoli TE, Carpenter CC, Plum F, Smith LH: Cecil Essentials of Medicine. 2nd ed. Philadelphia, WB Saunders, 1990, p 114.

369

cal, and laboratory features for assessment of aortic aneurysms, one of the most common dysfunction secondary to atherosclerotic disease in the aorta and aortic valve dysfunction.

Peripheral Arterial Disease and Dysfunction and Diagnosis

The presence of **peripheral arterial disease (PAD)** increases with age and is most often found in the form of arteriosclerosis obliterans (or atherosclerotic narrowing) of large and medium-sized arteries supplying blood to the lower extremities, or thromboangiitis obliterans (Buerger's disease; an inflammatory process causing vessel blockage) of peripheral arteries and veins.[135, 136] Arteriovenous fistulas (abnormal communications between arteries and veins without connecting capillaries), Raynaud's phenomena (bilateral paroxysmal ischemia of fingers and toes), arterial emboli, and trauma are other peripheral arterial dysfunction that occur in the population.

The current methods to determine presence of peripheral arterial disease include history of symptoms, history of risk factors for atherosclerotic disease, physical examination of pulses, and use of noninvasive vascular tests. Table 8–11 provides general clinical, physical and laboratory features for peripheral arterial diseases.

Noninvasive vascular tests include the ankle brachial index (ABI), segmental limb pressures, pulse volume recordings (PVR), and native vessel arterial duplex ultrasonography. If invasive tests are required, arteriography with contrast or with magnetic resonance imaging.

Ankle Brachial Index

Ankle brachial index (ABI) is an noninvasive test that compares the blood pressure obtained with a Doppler in the dorsalis pedis (or posterior tibial artery) to the blood pressure in the higher of the two brachial pressures. An ABI above 0.9 is considered normal. An ABI below 0.5 is suggestive of severe arterial occlusive disease.

Research has shown that the ABI may be a marker of diffuse atherosclerosis, cardiovascular risk, and overall survival.[137] Males who had an ABI less than 0.9 demonstrated a higher relative risk of

Table 8–11

General Clinical, Physical, and Laboratory Features of Peripheral Arterial Diseases

DISEASE	PATHOLOGY	CLINICAL FEATURES	PHYSICAL FEATURES	LABORATORY/ DIAGNOSTIC
Arteriosclerosis obliterans	Atherosclerotic narrowing of large and medium-sized arteries of lower extremities	Males more than females Common in diabetics Exertional leg pain relieved with rest Cold, numb legs	Decreased or absent LE pulses Aortic, iliac, or femoral Limb ischemia, cool pale, cyanotic, shiny dry skin	Doppler and arteriography
Thromboangiitis obliterans	Intima inflammation and infiltrates, thrombi, in small to medium-sized vessels	Males more than females Occurs before age 30 Cool extremities	Cool extremities Ulcers of digits	Biopsy of artery
Arterial embolism	Emboli lodge at bifurcations, with thrombus formation	Sudden onset, painful extremity	Cold, pale extremities Absent pulses distal to embolus	Doppler
Raynaud's phenomenon	Vasospasm of digital vessels aggravated by cold, relieved by heat		White, cyanotic digits exposed to cold, hyperemic upon recirculation	None; diagnosis based on physical symptoms

death from all causes and from cardiovascular causes. In addition, in a study of men and women over 65, the lower the ABI, the greater the incidence of cardiovascular risk factors and clinical cardiovascular disease.[138]

Segmental Limb Pressures

Segmental limb pressures can aid in localizing stenoses or occlusions with the placement of pressure cuffs on the thigh, calf, ankle, and transmetarsal region of the foot and digit. The pressure is sequentially inflated in each cuff to approximately 20 to 30 mm Hg above the systolic pressure. The pressure is measured using a Doppler at each segment as the pressure in the cuff is gradually released.

Pulse Volume Recordings

The changes in the volume of blood flowing through a limb can be detected by **plethysmographic tracings.** Pressure cuffs are placed on the thigh and ankle and inflated separately to approximately 65 mm Hg while a plethysmographic tracing is recorded. The normal **pulse volume recording (PVR)** consists of a rapid systolic upstroke and rapid downstroke with a dicrotic notch. Individuals with severe arterial disease will demonstrate a more attenuated waveform with a wide downslope. Individuals with near-complete blockage will demonstrate absent waveforms.[139]

Arterial Duplex Ultrasonography

Arterial duplex ultrasonography is a more precise diagnostic test for defining arterial stenoses and occlusions. A 5.0- to 7.5-MHz transducer is used to image the supra- and infrainguinal arteries in the sagittal plane at a 60-degree Doppler angle. The five categories, ranging from normal to occluded are determined based upon the alterations in the Doppler waveform. Duplex ultrasonography is utilized to guide the interventionist when performing endovascular therapy. One limitation cited in the literature is the potential to overestimate residual stenoses following balloon angioplasty.[140]

Graft Surveillance

Graft surveillance is utilized in patients who have undergone surgical bypass graft revascularization. Stenoses have been reported in 21 to 33% of bypass cases.[141] However, once the stenosis is detected and repaired prior to thrombosis, over 80% of the grafts have been salvaged.[141] The procedure for graft surveillance is similar to arterial duplex ultrasonography. Initially the inflow artery to the bypass is imaged, followed by the proximal anastomosis; proximal, middle, and distal graft; distal anastomosis; and then the outflow artery. The peak systolic and end-diastolic velocities are determined at each segment and compared to the segment of graft proximal to the area being studied. If the peak systolic velocity to normal segment proximal to graft is greater than 2, a 50 to 75% diameter reduction is assumed. If the end-diastolic velocity is less than 100 cm/sec, then a greater than 75% stenosis is assumed to exist. Arteriography should be performed if either of these values are determined with graft surveillance.

Vein bypass grafts should be studied within 7 days of surgery, 1 month after surgery, and then every 3 months for the first year, and every 6 months after the first year.

Exercise Studies

Exercise testing provides objective documentation of functional limitation from peripheral arterial disease as well as determining the physiologic improvement following arterial stenosis intervention (andioplasty or bypass graft surgery). However, claudication often limits activity before any cardiac symptoms are evoked, and therefore, a graded exercise test may not be an effective method of evaluating cardiac disease if patients have PAD.[142] A cycle ergometer may be the choice of mode for exercise testing to reduce the effort placed on the calf muscles.[143] In the absence of a complete graded exercise test, the minimum that should be performed is an assessment of claudication during a walk on the treadmill until exercise must be ceased (sometimes referred to as the claudication time test). Ankle pressures should be assessed prior to the treadmill walk, and immediately after exercise. A postexercise drop in ankle systolic pressure confirms the diagnosis of arterial disease.[142]

Ankle pressures should be measured at 1-minute intervals until a return to the pre-exercise pressure.

Other Clinical Tests

Rubor Dependency Test. This test assesses lower extremity arterial circulation using skin color changes and positional changes. The patient begins the test supine with legs elevated 35 to 45 degrees. The legs are assessed in this position for color (pale versus normal pink), then placed in a dependent position. Normal response is to see a rapid pink flush in the feet. Arterial insufficiency will demonstrate a deep, red color (rubor) after 30 seconds in this position.

Venous Filling Time Test. This test measures the efficiency of arterial blood flow through the capillaries and into the veins. The patient is placed in the supine position and the leg or legs are elevated to drain the blood from the extremity. The leg is then placed in a dependent position and time for veins to refill is recorded. In the presence of arterial insufficiency, the time for veins to refill is greater than 15 seconds.

Peripheral Venous Disease and Diagnosis

The most common disorder involving peripheral veins is thrombosis and subsequent thrombophlebitis (inflammation of the vein secondary to thrombosis, but can occur with trauma or infection). Initial diagnosis is often made with clinical signs of red color, warmth, and swelling, but diagnostic evaluation should be performed using Doppler studies and impedance plethysmography. Occasionally venograms are performed (injected dye into the venous system rather than arterial system as in artiography).

The second most common disorder involving peripheral veins is varicose veins, which can result from thrombophlebitis, but often occur congenitally or in conditions of increased venous pressure (such as pregnancy, prolonged standing, obesity, or ascites). **Venography** is recommended to assess for severity of insufficiency and prior to any surgical or chemical treatment.

Other Clinical Venous Insufficiency Tests

Trendelenburg Test. To assess valvular competence, the patient lies supine with the leg elevated 90 degrees to empty any blood currently in the venous system. A tourniquet is placed around the thigh to occlude venous flow, and the patient assumes a standing position while the filling of the veins is assessed. Normal venous fill should occur within 30 seconds. If superficial veins fill while the tourniquet is still in place, the communicating veins are deemed incompetent. If, when the tourniquet is removed, sudden additional filling occurs, the saphenous vein valves are determined to be incompetent.

Homan's Sign. To assess for deep-vein thrombophlebitis, the patient's gastrocnemius muscle belly is squeezed while the foot is dorsiflexed with force. If the patient indicates tenderness or pain in the gastrocnemius the test is determined to be positive for thrombophlebitis, and further diagnostic testing should be performed to determine the severity of the thrombophlebitis and initiate treatment.

Carotid Artery Disease and Diagnosis

Significant internal CAD increases the risk for transient and permanent ischemic attacks to the neurologic system and represents an increased risk for coronary atherosclerosis and infarction.[144, 145]

Often, eye examination may detect ischemia; however, carotid Doppler evaluations are most widely used, especially when bruits are auscultated during the physical examination. Recently, direct visualization with duplex ultrasonography has been used and demonstrated to have excellent accuracy (duplex ultrasonography is discussed earlier).[135] Carotid duplex examination can identify plaque, stenoses, and occlusions in the internal, common, and external carotid arteries as well as the flow direction in the vertebral arteries. Research has demonstrated that the sensitivity of **carotid duplex ultrasonography** to be 85% and the specificity is 90%.[146, 147]

Graft surveillance is utilized in patients who have undergone surgical bypass graft revascularization. Stenoses have been reported in 21 to 33% of bypass cases.[141] However, once the stenosis is detected and repaired prior to thrombosis, over 80% of the grafts have been salvaged.[141]

The procedure for graft surveillance is similar to that for arterial duplex ultrasonography. Initially, the inflow artery to the bypass is imaged, followed by the proximal anastomosis; proximal, middle, and distal graft; distal anastomosis; and then the outflow artery. The peak systolic and end-diastolic velocities are determined at each segment and compared to the segment of graft proximal to the area being studied. If the peak systolic velocity to normal segment proximal to graft is above 2, a 50 to 75% diameter reduction is assumed. If the end-diastolic velocity is below 100 cm/sec, then a greater than 75% stenosis is assumed to exist. Arteriography should be performed if either of these values are determined with graft surveillance.

Vein bypass grafts should be studied within 7 days of surgery, 1 month after surgery, and then every 3 months for the first year, and every 6 months after the first year.

EXERCISE TESTING

Exercise testing provides objective documentation of functional limitation from peripheral arterial disease as well as determining the physiologic improvement following arterial stenosis intervention (angioplasty or bypass graft surgery). However, claudication often limits activity before any cardiac symptoms are evoked, and therefore, a graded exercise test may not be an effective method of evaluating cardiac disease if patients have PAD.[142] A cycle ergometer may be the choice of mode for exercise testing to reduce the effort placed on the calf muscles.[143]

In the absence of a complete graded exercise test, the minimum testing that should be performed is an assessment of claudication during a walk on the treadmill until exercise must be ceased (sometimes referred to as the claudication time test). Ankle pressures should be assessed prior to the treadmill walk, and immediately after exercise. A postexercise drop in ankle systolic pressure confirms the diagnosis of arterial disease. Ankle pressures should be measured at 1-minute intervals until a return to the pre-exercise pressure (see Fig. 8–18).

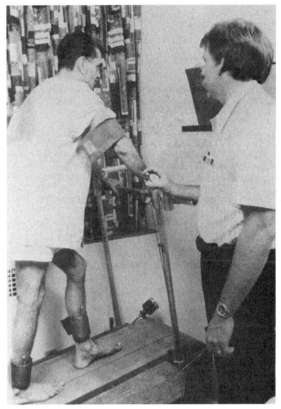

Figure 8–18. Ankle cuffs and one arm cuff are in place to facilitate postexercise pressure measurements in the treadmill stress test. (From Zwiebel WJ. Introduction to Vascular Ultrasonography. 4th ed. Philadelphia, WB Saunders, 2000, Fig. 16–9, p 240.)

CASE STUDIES

Case 1

MH is a 48-year-old woman who experienced frequent symptoms of chest pain during her aerobic workouts that were not always relieved with rest. Sometimes the symptoms would develop with emotional upset. Her past medical history included elevated cholesterol, which was to be treated with diet, and a positive family history (father with MI, CHF, and pacemaker and mother with hypertension and elevated cholesterol). MH had undergone a stress exercise test 2 months prior, experienced chest pain on the test, but there was no evidence of ischemic changes or abnormal heart rate, blood pressure, or ECG changes, so it was recommended that MH follow up with her family physician if similar symptoms persisted. Because MH continued to experience chest pain that limited her activities, MH was then referred for thallium-201 stress exercise test during which she developed chest pain after 5 minutes. The results of the thallium stress test demonstrated significant inferior perfusion defects at peak exercise that were resolved on the 3-hour postexercise scan. MH subsequently underwent single-vessel (right) percutaneous transluminal coronary angioplasty (PTCA). On the day after PTCA MH uderwent a repeat thallium stress exercise test which she performed symptom-free for 8 minutes and without any perfusion defects. MH was discharged to home and returned to her normal activities within 2 weeks.

Discussion

This case study demonstrates the inability of the standard exercise stress test to diagnose coronary artery disease in a female with significant symptoms plus significant risk factors for coronary artery disease. The thallium exercise test was definitive for coronary artery disease, intervention by PTCA was performed, and patient was symptom-free after PTCA.

Case 2

CS is a 46-year-old man who was admitted to hospital in early April from the emergency room with severe substernal chest pain of 2 hours' duration that was unrelieved with rest or antacids. On admission to the ER CS had an ECG that demonstrated acute anterior myocardial injury, and was given oxygen, morphine, nitroglycerine, and IV tPA was started. Laboratory work on admission showed an elevated troponin, and subsequent laboratory work documented elevated CPK with an elevated MB. On the admitting evaluation carotid bruits were noticed on the left. The patient was transferred to the coronary care unit.

CS had a past medical history of smoking two packs per day, family history of CAD (father died of an MI at 52), hypertension treated with Norvasc (calcium channel blocker), and was overweight, leading a sedentary lifestyle. Patient works as a CPA and experiences high stress during tax season.

CS underwent coronary catheterization and carotid angiogram within 2 hours of admission demonstrating triple-vessel disease and significant carotid occlusion (95%) on the left. CS subsequently underwent coronary artery bypass graft surgery with carotid endarterectomy.

Case 3

JH is a 35-year-old woman who went to her family physician for frequent episodes which she described as "all of a sudden my heart would race away." JH would experience shortness of breath and dizziness when these episodes occurred. JH had no significant medical history, and no significant family history of heart disease. The physician's initial evaluation revealed normal vital signs, normal resting ECG, clear lungs, but a midsystolic click on auscultation of the heart. Based upon the symptoms and the heart sounds, the physician referred JH for an echocardiogram to assess her mitral valve functioning, and a Holter monitor to assess for the racing heart symptoms. The echocardiogram identified moderate mitral valve prolapse (MVP), and the Holter monitor recorded one episode of paroxysmal atrial tachycardia that spontaneously returned to normal sinus rhythm.

JH was referred for a two-dimensional stress echo to assess exercise tolerance as JH actively took part in aerobics, tennis, and running, and was recommended to followup with physician yearly to assess mitral valve functioning. JH was also recommended to document her cardiac history whenever undergoing dental hygiene or surgical intervention as antibiotics would be recommended prophylactically because of her MVP.

Summary

- The laboratory tests that are specific to the patient with cardiac dysfunction measure the serum enzymes, blood lipids (triglycerides and cholesterol), complete blood cell count, coagulation profile (prothrombin time), electrolyte levels, BUN and creatinine levels, and serum glucose levels.
- The markers that are diagnostic of cardiac injury include creatine phosphokinase (CPK-MB isoenzyme), troponin, myoglobin, carbonic anhydrase III, cardiac myosin light chains, lactic dehydrogenase (LDH isoenzyme 1), and aspartate aminotransferase (AST).
- The enzymes that are diagnostic of cardiac injury include creatine phosphokinase, lactic dehydrogenase, and aspartate aminotransferase.
- Clinically, an early or a secondary peak in CPK levels followed by a more rapid decline in the CPK-MB levels is strongly suggestive of reperfusion following thrombolytic therapy.
- Sodium, potassium, and CO_2 are the most important electrolytes to monitor. Hydration state, medications, and disease can affect the electrolyte levels.
- Indications for use of the Holter monitor include identifying symptoms possibly caused by arrhythmias (e.g., dizziness, syncope, shortness of breath at rest as well as with activity), describing the arrhythmias noted with activity (frequency and severity), and evaluating antiarrhythmia therapy and pacemaker functioning.

- Important information can be obtained from the echocardiogram, including the size of the ventricular cavity, the thickness and integrity of the interatrial and interventricular septa, the functioning of the valves, and the motions of individual segments of the ventricular wall.
- Using an intravenously injected contrast agent with the echocardiogram has improved the diagnostic accuracy of echocardiography in assessing myocardial perfusion and ventricular chambers.
- Positron emission tomography (PET), computed tomography (CT), single photon emission computed tomography (SPECT), electron beam computed tomography (EBCT), multigated acquisition (MUGA) imaging, and magnetic resonance imaging (MRI) are all imaging techniques used for evaluation of coronary artery disease and cardiac dysfunction.
- Positron emission tomography (PET) is a nuclear assessment technique that provides visualization and direct measurement of metabolic functioning, including glucose metabolism and fatty acid metabolism as well as blood flow of the heart.
- Magnetic resonance imaging (MRI) is used to evaluate morphology, cardiac blood flow, and myocardial contractility.
- The commonly used agents include thallium-201 and technetium-99m (labeled sestamibi). These agents are taken up by the myocardium based on coronary blood flow.
- The most common agents used in pharmacologic stress testing are dipyridamole, dobutamine, and adenosine.
- Most exercise tests are symptom limited and, as such, are terminated at the request of the patient or when an abnormality is identified in one or more parameters being measured.
- Indications for uses of thallium injection with stress testing include detection of myocardial infarction and transient myocardial ischemia.
- Low-level exercise testing may be useful for predicting the subsequent course of a myocardial infarction or bypass surgery as well as for identifying the high-risk patient.
- Exercise-induced ST-segment depression of 2.0 mm or greater on low-level exercise tests has been identified as the single most valuable indicator of prognosis after myocardial infarction.
- Low-level exercise testing can also provide information useful for optimal medical management after myocardial injury or surgery, including

treatment for angina, arrhythmias, or hypertension.
- Although the physical therapist may not actually perform the stress test, obtaining the interpretation of the results provides valuable data for developing an exercise prescription.
- Sensitivity is the measure of the reliability of stress testing to identify the presence of disease. Specificity is the measure of the reliability of stress testing to identify the population without disease.
- Although exercise testing alone is diagnostic for coronary disease, exercise testing with ventilatory gas analysis using a metabolic cart can provide greater information regarding oxygen exchange, breathlessness, etc.
- Digital subtraction angiography is a technique involving the introduction of small concentrations of iodinated contrast material into a vascular bed which is then analyzed by a computer to produce an angiogram without direct injection of contrast material into an artery or cardiac chamber.
- Specific determinations that can be made as a result of cardiac catheterization include (1) severity of coronary artery disease (degree of stenosis); (2) left ventricular dysfunction or aneurysm or both; (3) valvular heart disease and the severity of the dysfunction, including aortic valve stenosis or regurgitation, mitral valve stenosis or regurgitation or prolapse, tricuspid valve dysfunction, or pulmonary valve dysfunction; (4) pericardial disease; (5) myocardial disease including cardiomyopathy; and (6) congenital heart disease.
- Ergonovine stimulation is used when coronary spasm is suspected, particularly in a patient with ECG-documented changes during symptoms or with documented ischemic episodes and a normal coronary angiographic study.
- There may be some indication to follow heart rate variability in the asymptomatic at-risk population as well as the post-MI population in the future.
- Samples of the right or left ventricular endomyocardium may be obtained at the time of catheterization to determine myocardial rejection in patients with cardiac transplant.
- PET is a nuclear assessment technique that provides visualization and direct measurement of metabolic functioning including glucose metabo-

lism, fatty acid metabolism, and blood flow of the heart without the patient performing exercise.

- Multigated acquisition imaging or gated pool imaging is a noninvasive technique to calculate left ventricular ejection fraction.

References

1. Karmazyn M. Reduction of enzyme release from reperfused ischemic hearts by steroidal and nonsteroidal prostaglandin synthesis inhibitors. Prostaglandins Leukot Med 11:299–315, 1983.
2. Adams JE, Sicard GA, Allen BT, et al. Diagnosis of perioperative myocardial infarction with measurement of cardiac troponin I. N Engl J Med 330:670–674, 1994.
3. Cummins B, Auckland ML, Cummins P. Cardiac-specific troponin-I radio-immunoassay in the diagnosis of acute myocardial infarction. Am Heart J 113:1333–1344, 1987.
4. Piano MR. Serologic markers of ischemia: Creatine kinase and the troponins. American Heart Association, 71st Scientific Sessions, November 8, 1998.
5. Katus HA, Remppis A, Neumann FJ, et al. Diagnostic efficiency of troponin T measurements in acute myocardial infarction. Circulation 83:902–912, 1991.
6. Polanczyk CA, Lee TH, Cook EF, et al: Cardiac troponin I as a a predictor of major cardiac events in emergency department patients with acute coronary care syndromes. J Am Coll Cardiol 32:8–14, 1998.
7. Heeschen C, Goldman BU, Moeller RH, et al. Analytic performance and clinical application of a new rapid bedside assay for the detection of serum cardiac troponin I. Clin Chem 44:1925–1930, 1998.
8. Christenson RH, Azzazy HM. Biochemical markers of the acute coronary syndromes. Clin Chem 44(8 Pt 2):1855–1864, 1998.
9. Ohman EM, Armstrong PW, Christenson RH, et al: Cardiac troponin T levels for risk stratification in acute myocardial ischemia. N Engl J Med 335:1333–1341, 1996.
10. National Heart Attack Alert Program Working Group. An evaluation of technologies for identifying acute cardiac ischemia in the emergency department. Ann Emerg Med 29:13–87, 1997.
11. Katus HA, Diedrich KW, Schwartz F, el al: Influence of reperfusion on serum concentrations of cytosolic creatine kinase and structural myosin light chains in acute myocardial infarction. Am J Cardiol 60:440–445, 1987.
12. Hoberg E, Katus HA, Diederich KW, et al: Myoglobin, creatine kinase-B isoenzyme, and myosin light chain release in patients with unstable angina pectoris. Eur Heart J 8:989–994, 1987.
13. Katus HA, Diedrich KW, Hoberg E, et al: Circulating cardiac myosin light chains in patients with angina at rest: Identification of a high risk subgroup. J Am Coll Cardiol 11:487–493, 1988.
14. Jacobs DS, Kasten BL, DeMott WR, Worlfson WL. Lab Test Handbook. Cleveland, Lexicomp/Mosby, 1988.
15. Smith AM, Theirer JA, Huang SH. Serum enzymes in myocardial infarction. Am J Nurs 73(2):277, 1973.
16. White HD, Cross DB, Williams BF, Norris RM. Safety and efficacy of repeat thrombolytic treatment after acute MI. Br Heart J 64(3):177–181, 1990.
17. Pollock ML, Schmidt DH. Epidemiologic Insights into Atherosclerotic Cardiovascular Disease from the Framingham Study in Heart Disease and Rehabilitation. 2nd ed. New York, John Wiley and Sons, 1986.
18. Castelli WP. Cholesterol and lipids in the risk of coronary artery disease—the Framingham Heart Study. Can J Cardiol 4(suppl A):5A–10A, 1988.
19. National Cholesterol Education Program (NCEP). Second report of the expert panel in detection, evaluation and treatment of high blood cholesterol in adults (Adult Treatment Panel II). JAMA 269:3015–3021, 1993.
20. Gordon T, Castelli WP, Hjortlan MC, et al: Diabetes, blood lipids, and the role of obesity in coronary heart disease for women. Ann Intern Med 87:393, 1977.
21. Superko HR, Fogelman A. Lipoproteins and atherosclerosis—The role of HDL cholesterol, Lp(a), and LDL particle size. Presented at the American College of Cardiology, 48th Scientific Session, March 7–10, 1999.
22. Cohen J, Wilson WF. Homocysteine, fibrinogen, Lp(a), small dense LDL, oxidative stress, and C. pneumoniae infection: How important are they? Am Coll Cardiol March 7–10, 1999.
23. American Diabetes Association, Inc. Management of dyslipidemia in adults with diabetes, position statement, January 1999. Diabetes Care 22(s1):56–59, 1999.
24. Robinson K, Arheart K, Refsum H, et al. Concentrations: Risk factors for stroke, peripheral vascular disease and coronary artery disease. European Comac Group. Circulation 97(5):437–43, 1998.
25. Glueck CJ, Shaw P, Lang JE, et al. Evidence that homocysteine is an independent risk factor for atherosclerosis in hyperlipidemic patients. Am J Cardiol 75(2):132–136, 1995.
26. Boushey CJ, Beresford SA, Omenn GS, Motulsky AG. A quantitative assessment of plasma homocysteine as a risk factor for vascular disease. JAMA 274(13a):1049–1057, 1995.
27. Evans RW, Shaten BJ, Hempel JD, et al. Homocysteine and risk of cardiovascular disease in the Multiple Risk Factor Intervention Trial. Arterioscler Thromb Vasc Biol 17(10):1947–1953, 1997.
28. Greenburg AG. Pathophysiology of anemia. Am J Med 101(2A):7S–11S, 1996.
29. Krantz SB. Pathogenesis and treatment of the anemia of chronic disease. Am J Med Sci 307(5):353–359, 1994.
30. Szaflarski NL. Physiologic effects of normovolemic anemia: Implications for clinical monitoring. AACN Clin Issues 7(2):198–211, 1996.
31. Bigger JT, Weld F, Rolnitzky L. Prevalence, characteristics and significance of ventricular tachycardia detected with ambulatory electrocardiographic recording of late hospital phase of acute myocardial infarction. Am J Cardiol 48(5):815, 1981.
32. Cappato R. Secondary prevention of sudden death: The Dutch Study, the Antiarrhythmics Versus Implantable Defibrillator Trial, the Cardiac Arrest Study Hamburg, and the Canadian Implantable Defibrillator Study. Am J Cardiol 83(5B):68D–73D, 1999.
33. Pathmanathan RK, Lau EW, Cooper J, et al. Potential impact of antiarrhythmic drugs versus implantable defibrillators on the management of ventricular arrhythmias: The Midlands trial of empirical amiodarone versus electrophysiologically guided intervention and cardioverter implant registry data. Heart 80(1):68–70, 1998.
34. Gentile R. Clinical usefulness of a new echocardiographic window: The transesophageal approach. Medicina (Firenze) 10(4):411–415, 1990.
35. Pedersen WR, Walker M, Olson JD, et al. Value of transesophageal echocardiography as an adjunct to transtho-

racic echocardiography in evaluation of native and prosthetic valve endocarditis. Chest 100(2):351–356, 1991.

36. Orihashi K, Hong YW, Chung G, et al. New applications of two dimensional transesophageal echocardiography in cardiac surgery. J Cardiothorac Vasc Anesth 5(1):33–39, 1991.

37. Font VE, Obarski TP, Klein AL, et al. Transesophageal echocardiography in the critical care unit. Cleve. Clin J Med 58:3315–3322, 1991.

38. Labovitz AJ. Embolic stroke and echocardiographic findings—What are the implications? Controversies in Clinical Echocardiography, 72nd Scientific Sessions of American Heart Association, November 9, 1999.

39. Crawford MH. Should transesophageal echocardiogram be performed in all patients with atrial fibrillation? Controversies in Clinical Echocardiography, 72nd Scientific Sessions of American Heart Association, November 9, 1999.

40. Kelly WN. Textbook of Internal Medicine. Vol. 1. Philadelphia, JB Lippincott, 1989.

41. Armstrong WF. Treadmill exercise echocardiography methodology and clinical role. Eur Heart J 18 (suppl D): D2–D8, 1997.

42. Devereux RB, Pini R, Aurigemmla GP, Roman MJ. Measurement of left ventricular mass: Methodology and expertise. J Hypertens 15(8):801–809, 1997.

43. De Castro S, Yao J, Pandian NG. Three-dimensional echocardiography: Clinical relevance and application. Am J Cardiol 81(12A):96G–102G, 1998.

44. Shaw LJ. Impact of contrast echocardiography on diagnostic algorithms: Pharmaco-economic implications. Clin Cardiol 20(10 suppl):I39–I48, 1997.

45. P'erez JE. Current role of contrast echocardiography in the diagnosis of cardiovascular diseases. Clin Cardiol 20(10 suppl):I31–I38, 1997.

46. Feinstein SB, Cheirif J, Ten Cate FJ, et al. Safety and efficacy of a new transpulmonary ultrasound contrast agent: Initial multicenter clinical results. J Am Coll Cardiol 16:316–324, 1990.

47. Crouse LJ, Cheirif J, Hanly DE. Opacification and border delineation improvement in patients with suboptimal border definition in routine echocardiography: Results of the phase III Albunex multicenter trial. J Am Coll Cardiol 22: 1494–1500, 1993.

48. Gandhok NK, Block R, Ostoic T, et al. Reduced forward output states affect the left ventricular opacificification of intravenously administered Albunex. J Am Soc Echocardiogr 10:25–30, 1997.

49. Main ML, Grayburn PA. Clinical applications of transpulmonary contrast echocardiography. Am Heart J 137(1): 144–153, 1999.

50. Cheirif J, Desir RM, Bolli R, et al. Relation of perfusion defects observed with myocardial contrast echocardiography to the severity of coronary stenosis: Correlation with thallium-201 single-photon emission tomography. J Am Coll Cardiol 19(6):1343–1349, 1992.

51. DiCarli MF, Davidson M, Little R, et al. Value of metabolic imaging with positron emission tomography for evaluating prognosis in patients with coronary artery disease and left ventricular dysfunction. Am J Cardiol 73(8):527–533, 1994.

52. Merz CN, Berman DS. Imaging techniques for coronary artery disease: Current status and future directions. Clin Cardiol 20(6):526–532, 1997.

53. Maddahi J, Blitz A, Phelps M, Laks H. The use of positron emission tomography imaging in the management of patients with ischemic cardiomyopathy. Adv Card Surg 7: 163–188, 1996.

54. Beller GA, Gibson RS: Sensitivity, specificity and prognostic significance of noninvasive testing for occult or known coronary disease. Prog Cardiovasc Dis 29:241, 1987.

55. Chan SY, Brunken RC, Buxton DB. Cardiac positron emission tomography: The foundations and clinical applications. J Thorac Imaging 5(3):9–19, 1990.

56. Berman DS, Kiat H, Van Train KF, et al. Comparison of SPECT using technetium-99m agents and thallium-201 and PET for the assessment of myocardial perfusion and viability. Am J Cardiol 66(13):72E–79E, 1990.

57. Williams MJ, Odabashian J, Lauer MS, et al. Prognostic value of dobutamine echocardiography in patients with left ventricular dysfunction. J Am Coll Cardiol 27(1):132–139, 1996.

58. Toole JF. The Willis lecture: Transient ischemic attacks, scientific method, and new realities. Stroke 22(1):99–104, 1991.

59. Graboys TB, Blatt CM. Angina Pectoris: Management Strategies and Guide to Interventions. Cado, OK, Professional Communications, Inc., 1997.

60. Rumberger JA, Sheedy PF, Breen JF, et al. Electron beam computed tomography and coronary artery disease: Scanning for coronary artery calcification. Mayo Clin Proc 71: 369–377, 1996.

61. Budoff MJ, Georgiou D, Brody A, et al. Ultrafast computed tomography as a diagnostic modality in the detection of coronary artery disease: A multicenter study. Circulation 93:898–904, 1996.

62. Kaufmann RB, Peyser PA, Sheedy PF, et al. Quantification of coronary artery calcium by electron beam computed tomography for determination of severity of angiographic disease in young patients. J Am Coll Cardiol 25:626–632, 1995.

63. Fallovollita JA, Brody AS, Bunnell IL, et al. Fast computed tomography detection of coronary calcification in the diagnosis of coronary artery disease: Comparison with angiography in patients <50 years old. Circulation 89:285–290, 1994.

64. O'Malley PG, Taylor AJ, Gibbons RV, et al. Rationale and design of the Prospective Army Coronary Calcium (PACC) Study: Utility of electron beam computed tomography as a screening test for coronary artery disease and as an intervention for risk factor modification among young, asymptomatic, active-duty United States Army personnel. Am Heart J 137(5):932–941, 1999.

65. Wang S, Detrano RC, Secci A, et al. Detection of coronary calcification with electron beam computed tomography: Evaluation of interexamination reproducibility and comparison of 3 image acquisition protocols. Am Heart J 132: 550–558, 1996.

66. Breen JF, Sheedy PF, Shwartz RS, et al. Coronary artery calcification detected with ultrafast CT as an indication of coronary artery disease. Radiology 185:435–439, 1992.

67. Ben-David Y, Shefer A, Weiss AT, et al. Early postoperative assessment of coronary artery bypass surgery using nuclear left ventriculography and atrial pacing. Thorac Cardiovasc Surg 31(6):377–381, 1983.

68. Gunnar WP, Martin M, Smith RF, et al. The utility of cardiac evaluation in the hemodynamically stable patient with suspected myocardial contusion. Am Surg 57(6):373, 1991.

69. Yang DC, Jain CU, Patel D, et al. Use of i.v. radionuclide total body arteriography to evaluate arterial bypass shunts—a new method—a review of several cases. Angiology 41(9[pt.1]):745–752, 1990.

70. Gottlieb SO, Gottlieb SH, Achuff SC, et al. Silent ischemia on Holter monitoring predicts mortality in high risk post infarction patients. JAMA 259:1030, 1988.

71. Carrol CL, Higgins CB, Caputo GR. Magnetic resonance

imaging of acquired cardiac disease. Texas Heart Inst J 23(2):144–154, 1996.

72. Colletti PM, Term MR. Magnetic resonance imaging applications to cardiac diagnosis. Biomed Instrum Technol 30(4):354–358, 1996.

73. Fayad ZA, Fuster V, Fallon JT, et al. Human coronary atherosclerotic wall imaging using in vivo high resolution MR. Presented at the American Heart Association 72nd Scientific Sessions, Atlanta, GA. November 7–10, 1999. Abstract 2742, November 9.

74. Kramer CM. Integrated approach to ischemic heart disease. The one-stop shop. Cardiol Clin 16(2):267–276, 1998.

75. Yang PC, Kerr AB, Liu AC, et al. New real-time interactive cardiac magnetic resonance imaging system complements echocardiography. J Am Coll Cardiol 32(7):2049–2056, 1998.

76. Sakuma H, Takeda K, Higgins CB. Fast magnetic resonance imaging of the heart. Eur J Radiol 29(2):101–113, 1999.

77. De Roos A, Niezen RA, Lamb HJ, et al. MR of the heart under pharmacologic stress. Cardiol Clin 16(2):247–265, 1998.

78. Bonow RO. The hibernating myocardium: Implications for management of congestive heart failure. Am J Cardiol 75(3):17A–25A, 1995.

79. Zaret BL, Wackers FJ. Nuclear cardiology. N Engl J Med 329:775–783, 855–863, 1993.

80. Ritchie JL, Bateman TM, Bonow RO, et al. Guidelines for clinical use of cardiac radionuclide imaging: A report of the American Heart Association/American College of Caardiology Task Force on Assessment of Diagnostic and Therapeutic Cardiovascular Procedures. Circulation 91: 1278–1302, 1995.

81. Cerqueira MD, Maynard C, Ritchie JL, et al. Long-term survival in 618 patient from the Western-Washington Streptokinase in Myocardial Infarction Trials. J Am Coll Cardiol 20:1452–1459, 1992.

82. Dilsizian V, Bonow RO. Current diagnostic techniques of assessing myocardial viability in hibernating and stunned myocardium. Circulation 87:1–20, 1993.

83. Van der Wieken LR, Kan G, Belfer AJ, et al. Thallium-201 scanning to decide CCU admission in patients with non-diagnostic electrocardiograms. Int J Cardiol 4:285–299, 1983.

84. Van Train KF, Garcia EV, Maddahi J, et al. Multicenter trial validation for quantitative analysis of same-day rest-stress technetium-99m-sestamibi myocardial tomograms. J Nucl Med 35:609–618, 1994.

85. Berman DS, Kiat HS, Van Train KF, et al. Myocardial perfusion imaging with technetium-99m-sestamibi: Comparative analysis of available imaging protocols. J Nucl Med 35:681–688, 1994.

86. Ritchie JL, Bateman TM, Bonow RO, et al. Guidelines for clinical use of cardiac radionuclide imaging: A report of the American Heart Association/American College of Cardiology Task Force on Assessment of Diagnostic and Therapeutic Cardiovascular Procedures. Circulation 91:1278–1302, 1995.

87. Beanlands RSB, Dawood F, Wen WH, et al. Are the kinetics of technetium-99m methoxyisobutyl isonitrile affected by cell metabolism and viability? Circulation 82:1802–1814, 1990.

88. Piwnica-Worms D, Kronauge JF, Chiu ML. Uptake and retention of hexakis(2-methoxyisobutyl isonitrile) technetium in cultured myocardial cells: Mitochondrial and plasma membrane potential dependence. Circulation 82: 1826–1838, 1990.

89. Hilton TC, Thompson RC, Williams HJ, et al. Technetium-99m sestamibi myocardial perfusion imaging in the emergency room evaluation of chest pain. J Am Coll Cardiol 23:1016–1022, 1994.

90. Weissman IA, Dickinson C, Dworkin H, et al. Emergency center myocardial perfusion SPECT: Long-term follow-up: cost-effective imaging providing diagnostic and prognostic information [abstract]. J Nucl Med 36:P88, 1995.

91. Radensky PW, Stowers S, Hilton TC, et al: Cost effectiveness of acute myocardial perfusion imaging with Tc99m sestamibi for risk stratification of emergency room patients with acute chest pain. Circulation 90:1–528, 1994.

92. Nagarajan R, Abou-Mohamed G, Myers T, Caldwell RW. A novel catecholamine, arbutamine, for a pharmacological cardiac stress agent. Cardiovasc Drugs Thera 10(1):31–38, 1996.

93. Ellhendy A, van Domburg RT, Poldermans D, et al. Safety and feasibility of dobutamine-atropine stress echocardiography for the diagnosis of coronary artery disease in diabetic patients unable to perform an exercise stress test. Diabetes Care 21(11):1797–1802, 1998.

94. Bouvier F, Hojer J, Hulting J, et al. Myocardial perfusion scintigraphy (SPECT) during adenosine stress can be performed safely early on after thrombolytic therapy in acute myocardial infarction. Clin Physiol 18(2):97–101, 1998.

95. Cooper KH. The Aerobics Way. New York, Bantam Books, 1981.

96. McGavin CR, Gupta SP, McHardy GJR. Twelve minute walking tests for assessing disability in chronic bronchitis. Br Med J 1:822–823, 1976.

97. Jones NL, Cambell EJ. Clinical Exercise Testing. 2nd ed. Philadelphia, WB Saunders, 1982.

98. Ibsen H, Kjoller E, Styperck J, et al. Routine exercise ECG three weeks after acute myocardial infarction. Acta Med Scand 198:463, 1975.

99. McIntyre KM, Lewis AJ. Textbook of Advanced Cardiac Life Support. Dallas, American Heart Association, 1983.

100. American College of Sports Medicine. Guidelines for Exercise Testing and Prescription. 4th ed. Philadelphia, Lea & Febiger, 1990.

101. Ellestad MH, Stuart RJ. National survey of exercise stress testing facilities. Chest 77:94, 1980.

102. Ellestad MH, Wan MKC. Standards for adult exercise testing laboratories. The Exercise Standards Book. Dallas, American Heart Association, 1979.

103. Cahalin LP, Blessey R, Cummer D, Simard M. The safety of exercise testing performed independently by physical therapists. J Cardiopulm Rehab 7(6):269, 1987.

104. Squires RW, Allison TG, Johnson BD, Gau GT. Non-physician supervision of cardiopulmonary exercise testing in chronic heart failure: Safety and results of a preliminary investigation. J Cardiopulm Rehab 19(4):249–253, 1999.

105. Olivotto I, Montereggi A, Mazzuoli F, Cecchi F. Clinical utility and safety of exercise testing in patients with hypertrophic cardiomyopathy. G Ital Cardiol 29(1):11–19, 1999.

106. Ellestad MH. Stress Testing Principles and Practice. Philadelphia, FA Davis, 1986.

107. Golding LA, Myers CR, Sinning WE. Y's Way to Physical Fitness. 3rd ed. Champaign, Ill, Human Kinetics, 1989.

108. Froelicher VF. Exercise and the Heart. Clinical Concepts. 2nd ed. Chicago, Year Book Medical Publishers, 1987.

109. Blessey RL. Aerobic capacity and cardiac catheterization results in 13 patients with exercise bradycardia. Med Sci Sports Exerc 8:50, 1976 (abstract).

110. Davidson DM, DeBusk RJ. Prognostic value of a single exercise test 3 weeks after uncomplicated myocardial infarction. Circulation 61:236–242, 1980.

111. Starling MR, Crawford MH, Kennedy GT, et al. Predictive

value of early post-myocardial infarction modified exercise testing in multivessel coronary artery disease detection. Am Heart J 102(2):169, 1981.

112. Schwartz K, Turner J, Sheffield L, et al. Limited exercise testing soon after MI (correlation with early coronary and left ventricular angiography). Ann Intern Med 94(6):727, 1981.

113. Fuller C, Razner A, Verani M, et al. Early post myocardial infarction treadmill stress testing. Ann Intern Med 94:734, 1981.

114. Savnamki KI, Anderson D. Early exercise test in the assessment of long term prognosis after acute MI. Acta Med Scand 209:185, 1981.

115. Weld F, Chu K, Bigger J, Rolnitzky L. Risk stratification with low level exercise testing two weeks after acute MI. Circulation 64(2):306–314, 1981.

116. Theroux P, Waters D, Halphen C, et al. Prognostic value of exercise testing soon after myocardial infarction. N Engl J Med 301(7):341, 1979.

117. Firth BG, Lange RA. Pathophysiology and management of primary pump failure. In: Gersh BJ, Rahimtoola SH (eds). Acute Myocardial Infarction. New York, Elsevier, 1991.

118. Ross J. Hemodynamic changes in acute MI. In: The Myocardium Failure and Infarction. New York, HP Publishing, 1974, p 261.

119. Ericsson M, Granath A, Ohlsen P, et al: Arrhythmias and symptoms during treadmill testing three weeks after myocardial infarction in 100 patients. Br Heart J 35:787, 1973.

120. Poyatos ME, Lerman J, Estrada A, et al. Predictive value of changes in R-wave amplitude after exercise in coronary heart disease. Am J Cardiol 54(10):1212, 1984.

121. Diamond GA, Forrester JS. Analysis of probability as an aid in the clinical diagnosis of coronary artery disease. N Engl J Med 300:1350, 1979.

122. Goldschlager H, Selzer Z, Cohn K. Treadmill stress tests as indicators of presence and severity of coronary artery disease. Ann Intern Med 85:277, 1976.

123. Bruce RA, DeRouen T, Peterson DR, et al. Noninvasive predictors of sudden death in men with coronary heart disease. Am J Cardiol 39:833, 1977.

124. Weiner DA, Ryan TJ, McCabe GH, et al. Prognostic importance of a clinical profile and exercise test in medically treated patients with coronary artery disease. J Am Coll Cardiol 3(3):772, 1984.

125. Higginbotham MB. Cardiopulmonary exercise testing; An interpretation for the cardiologist. St. Paul, MN, Medical Graphics Corporation, 1993.

126. Ross J Jr, Fisch C. Guidelines for coronary angiography. J Am Coll Cardiol 10:935, 1987.

127. Andreoli TE, Carpenter CCJ, Plum F, Smith LH. Cecil Essentials of Medicine. Philadelphia, WB Saunders, 1996, pp 91–93.

128. Maseri A. Role of coronary artery spasm in symptomatic and silent myocardial ischemia. J Am Coll Cardiol 9:249, 1987.

129. Igarashi Y, Yamazoe M, Shibata A. Effect of direct intracoronary administration of methylergonovine in patients with and without variant angina. Am Heart J 121(4[pt. 1]):1094–1100, 1991.

130. Khoshio A, Miyakoda H, Fukuiki M. Significance of coronary artery tone assessed by coronary responses to ergonovine and nitrate. Jpn Circ J 55(1):33–40, 1991.

131. Eckberg DL. Parasympathetic cardiovascular control in human disease: A critical review of methods and results. Am J Physiol 2239:H581–H593,1980.

132. Malliani A, Schwartz PJ, Zanchetti A. Neural mechanism in life threatening arrhythmias. Am Heart J 100:705–714, 1980.

133. Katz A, Liberty IF, Porath A, et al. A simple bedside test of 1-minute heart rate variability during deep breathing as a prognostic index after myocardial infarction. Am Heart J 138(1):32–38, 1999.

134. Van Ravenswaaij-Arls CA, Kollee LA, Hopman JC, et al. Heart rate variability. Ann Intern Med 118:436–447, 1993.

135. Jaff MR. Diagnostic testing in vascular medicine: The foundation for successful intervention. J Invasive Cardiol 11(10):640–644, 1999.

136. Weitz JI, Byrne J, Clagett GP, et al. Diagnosis and treatment of arterial insufficiency of the lower extremities: a critical review. Circulation. 94:3026–3049, 1996.

137. Kornitzer M, Dramaix M, Sobolski J, et al. Ankle/arm pressure index in asymptomatic middle-aged males: An independent predictor of ten year coronary heart disease mortality. Angiology 46:211–219, 1995.

138. Newman AB, Siscovick DS, Manolio TA, et al. Ankle-arm index as a marker of atherosclerosis in the cardiovascular health study. Circulation 88:837–845, 1993.

139. MacDonald NR. Pulse volume plethysmography. J Vasc Technol 18:241–248, 1994.

140. Sacks D, Robinson ML, Marinelli DL, Perlmutter GS. Evaluation of the peripheral arteries with duplex US after angioplasty. Radiology 176:39–44, 1990.

141. Bandyk DF. Ultrasonic duplex scanning in the evaluation of arterial grafts and dilatations. Echocardiography 4:251–264, 1987.

142. American Association for Cardiovascular and Pulmonary Rehabilitation. Guidelines for cardiac rehabilitation and secondary prevention programs. Champaign, IL, Human Kinetics, 1995, pp 167–169.

143. Gardner AW, Poehlman ET: Exercise rehabilitation programs for the treatment of claudication pain. A meta-analysis. JAMA 274(12):975–980, 1995.

144. Autret A, Saudeau D, Bertrand PH, et al. Stroke risk in patients with carotid stenosis. Lancet 1:888–890, 1987.

145. O'Leary DH, Polak JF, Kronmal RA, et al. Carotid artery intima and media thickness as a risk factor for myocardial infarction and stroke in older adults. N Engl J Med 340:14–22, 1999.

146. Feussner JR, Matchar DB. When and how to study the carotid arteries. Ann Intern Med 109:805–818, 1988.

147. Kirsch JD, Wagner LR, James EM, et al. Carotid artery occlusion: Positive predictive value of duplex sonography compared with arteriography. J Vasc Surg 19:642–649, 1994.

9

Electrocardiography

Ellen A. Hillegass

INTRODUCTION

Understanding the electrocardiogram (ECG) requires a basic understanding of the electrophysiology and anatomy of the heart and conduction system (see Chapters 1 and 2), an appreciation of the ECG waveforms (both their normal and abnormal presentations in different leads), and a certain amount of practice in the systematic review of 12-lead and single-lead ECG rhythm strips. After reading this chapter the therapist should be able to determine whether an ECG tracing represents a benign or a life-threatening situation and be able to begin to make appropriate clinical decisions based on this determination. Further information regarding the ECG and more advanced arrhythmia detection should be researched in texts devoted entirely to electrocardiography.

One comment should be made about nomenclature before beginning the discussion of electrocardiography. *Dysrhythmia* is the most accurate term to describe a heart rhythm that is abnormal, because the prefix *dys* means "bad" or "difficult." However, researchers do not use this term widely but rather favor the term *arrhythmia,* which means "without rhythm" or "no rhythm." In keeping with current usage, this chapter and text use arrhythmia throughout to refer to abnormal rhythm.

BASIC ELECTROPHYSIOLOGIC PRINCIPLES

The ECG is inscribed on specially ruled paper. It represents the electrical impulses of the heart and provides valuable information regarding the heart's function. The myocardium is comprised of cells that have different functions, and the ECG is the expression of these cells and their function. The four types of monocytes that compose the muscle include the typical working myocytes, which respond to the electrical stimulus to contract and pump the blood; nodal myocytes, which have the highest rate of rhythmicity but slow impulse-conduction rates; transitional myocytes, which conduct impulses twice as fast as nodal cells; and Purkinje's cells, which have a low rate of rhythmicity yet a high rate of conductivity.

Electrical stimulation makes the cell membrane more permeable to the flow of ions. As there is a predominance of potassium (K^+) on the inside of the cell and sodium (Na^+) on the outside, the electrical stimulation makes the membrane more permeable to the sodium ions so that they flow inward, creating a change in the resting state of the cells of the cardiac muscle from a negative to a positive charge on the interior. This sodium flow is referred to as the *fast channel.* The potassium ions then start to flow outward. The potassium flow is referred to as the *slow channel.* The electrical stimulation of the specialized cells that cause contraction is called **depolarization** (Fig. 9-1). As the cell becomes positive on the interior, the myocardial cells are stimulated to contract. When the potassium ion flow outward exceeds the sodium flow inward, repolarization begins. During **repolar-**

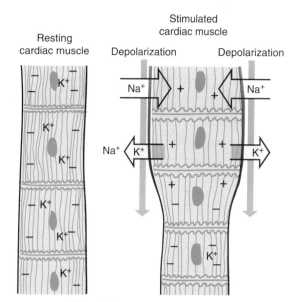

Figure 9-1. Electrical stimulation to the cardiac muscle cell membrane causes depolarization. With depolarization the membrane is more permeable to sodium ions, allowing them to flow inward and creating a positive charge on the inside.

ization, the myocardial cells return to a negative interior and a positive exterior, and muscle relaxation occurs.[1] When the wave of depolarization is moving toward a positive electrode located on the skin, the ECG records a simultaneous upward deflection (Fig. 9-2).

Cardiac muscle has three unique properties: **automaticity, rhythmicity,** and **conductivity.** Cardiac muscle cells are able to discharge an electrical stimulus without stimulation from a nerve, as is typical in all other muscle cells, demonstrating the property of automaticity. Rhythmicity is the regularity with which such pacemaking activity occurs. Cardiac muscle cells can therefore "automatically" discharge an electrical stimulus. This is particularly noticeable in the **sinoatrial (SA) node,** which is the primary pacemaker and has the most amount of automaticity of the cardiac cells.

However, other cardiac cells may discharge at any time owing to this property of automaticity, creating abnormal rates or rhythms (as in premature beats). The SA node has a normal innate automatic firing rate between 60 and 100 beats per minute. The **atrioventricular (AV) node** has an inherent firing rate of 40 to 60 beats per minute and begins to act as the pacemaker if the SA node

Stimulated
cardiac muscle

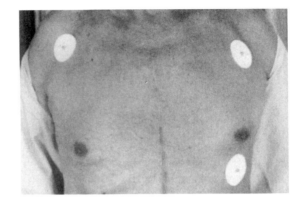

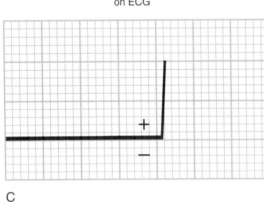

A

B

on ECG

C

Figure 9–2. When the depolarization wave (*A*) moves toward a positive electrode on the chest (*B*), the electrocardiogram (ECG) records an upward (positive) deflection (*C*).

is not functioning properly. The His-Purkinje portions of the specialized conduction system have an inherent firing rate of 30 to 40 beats per minute.

Cardiac muscle cells also have the ability to spread impulses to adjoining cells very quickly (the property of conductivity). The rapid spread can be visualized when one considers how fast the cells must depolarize and repolarize at a heart rate of 200 beats per minute. Rapid arrhythmias such as supraventricular tachycardia and slow rates due to AV blocks are examples of problems with conductivity. See Chapter 2 for further discussion of the myocytes.

THE AUTONOMIC NERVOUS SYSTEM

The autonomic nervous system has a major influence on reflex cardiac activity as a result of two counterbalancing forces: the sympathetic and the parasympathetic divisions. The effects of the two divisions determine the delicate balance between excitation and depression of cardiac activity, which can be altered in favor of one or the other by numerous physiologic and pathologic factors and in a variety of situations. The sympathetic division is equated with acceleration, and the parasympathetic division is equated with deceleration or braking.

Sympathetic Division

The sympathetic division discharges norepinephrine (noradrenalin) from its terminal nerve branches in the atria and ventricles, resulting in an excitation of the rate of impulse formation and the velocity of impulse propagation and an increase in the force of contractile fibers. The sympathetic division acts on both the SA node and the AV node as well as on the ventricles. In addition, the sympathetic division can stimulate the adrenal gland to secrete norepinephrine and epinephrine into the bloodstream. The direct action of these hormones on the heart is equal to the direct stimulation of the terminal nerve branches in the heart. Increased sympathetic activity increases the heart rate, the conduction velocity throughout the AV node, the contractility of the heart muscle, and the irritability of the heart. In addition, automaticity may increase, which can alter the normal sinus rhythm.

Parasympathetic Division

The parasympathetic division discharges acetylcholine from the terminal nerve branches. The vagus nerve is the main component of the parasympathetic division in control of the heart, and it acts primarily on the SA node as a general inhibitor on the rate of impulse formation and conduction velocity. Increased parasympathetic activity slows the heart rate and acts to slow the conduction through the AV node. Decreased parasympathetic activity increases the heart rate, the conduction through the AV node, and the irritability of the heart. Therefore, the effect of acetylcholine and the effects of vagal stimulation depress the automaticity and conductivity of the heart. See Chapter 2 for further discussion.

THE CONDUCTION SYSTEM

The conduction system is composed of myocytes arranged in a pathway that spreads the electrical

activity throughout the four chambers (two atria, two ventricles) (Fig. 9–3). The primary pacemaker that initiates the electrical impulse for the cardiac muscle is the SA node, located in the right atrium near the posterior surface and adjacent to the entry of the superior vena cava. The impulse then spreads throughout the right atrium via intra-atrial pathways and to the left atrium via **Bachmann's bundle**. The wave of atrial depolarization is represented on the ECG as the P wave. Therefore, the P wave represents atrial depolarization electrically and is normally associated with atrial contraction mechanically (Fig. 9–4). Following the spread of depolarization through the atria, the impulse then reaches the AV node, also called the junctional node, which is located near the intraventricular septum in the inferior aspect of the right atrium just superior to the tricuspid valve. The AV node delays the conduction of the electrical impulse from the atria for one tenth of a second (seen on the ECG as the isoelectric line after the P wave and before the QRS complex), allowing for the mechanical contraction of the atria to eject blood

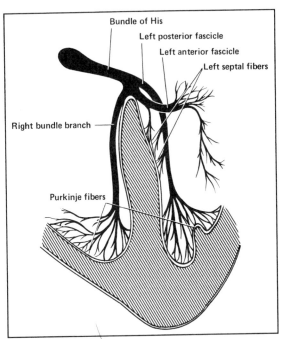

Figure 9–3. The conduction system. The pathway of electrical activity begins at the sinoatrial node and spreads to Purkinje's fibers. (From Goldman MJ. Principles of Clinical Electrocardiography. 10th ed. Los Altos, CA, Lange Medical Books, 1979.)

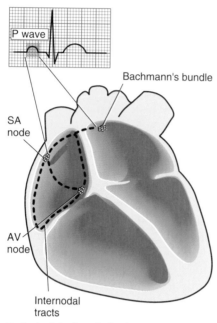

Figure 9–4. Atrial depolarization is depicted on the electrocardiographic tracing as the P wave. The impulse is spread to the left atrium via Bachmann's bundle.

into the ventricles. This is known as the **atrial kick.** The ECG depicts this delay as the P-R segment (Fig. 9–5). The P-R segment is also considered to be the isoelectric line. The impulse then passes from the AV node into the His bundle and then to the bundle branches. The bundle branches consist of a left and right division and are located in the interventricular septum (Fig. 9–6).

The right bundle branch is responsible for depolarization of the right ventricle, and the left bundle branch, which has an anterior fascicle and a posterior fascicle, is responsible for the depolarization of the left ventricle. The electrical impulses spread down the bundle branches and terminate in Purkinje's fibers, which are numerous and very small. These fibers penetrate the myocardium and stimulate muscle contraction from the apex upward toward the base of the heart in a "wringing" action. The ECG records the electrical stimulus of ventricular depolarization as the QRS complex (Fig. 9–7). The QRS complex represents ventricular depolarization and is normally followed closely by ventricular contraction. The ECG tracing may demonstrate a variety of QRS waveforms, depending on the pathologic condition or the location of the electrode, but they are generally referred to as

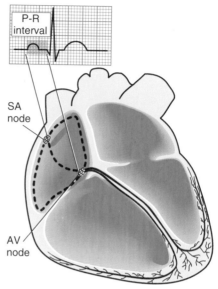

Figure 9–5. When the spread of depolarization reaches the atrioventricular node, a slight delay occurs. The electrocardiogram records this as the P-R interval.

the QRS complex regardless of the configuration. Figure 9–8 shows the various forms of QRS complexes that may be seen on an ECG.

Repolarization begins when ventricular contraction ends. Following the QRS complex, a slight pause is noted. This pause is called the ST seg-

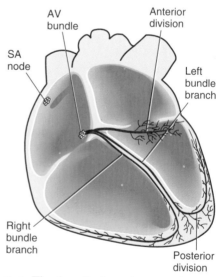

Figure 9–6. The bundle branches, consisting of a left and right division, are located within the interventricular septum. The left bundle branch has both an anterior and a posterior division.

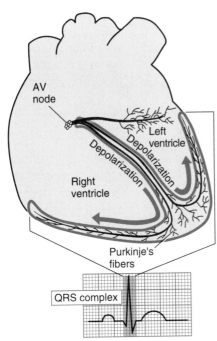

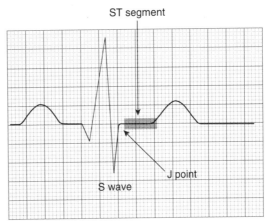

Figure 9-9. The ST segment on the electrocardiogram tracing begins at the end of the S wave and ends at the beginning of the T wave. Notice the J point, which classically is defined as the point at which the thin line of the QRS tracing turns into a thick line. The J point is also the beginning of the ST segment and is often used as the landmark when the ST segment is aberrant.

Figure 9-7. Ventricular depolarization occurs when the electric impulse reaches Purkinje's fibers. The electrocardiogram depicts ventricular depolarization in the QRS complex.

ment and is defined as the flat piece of isoelectric line that starts at the end of the QRS complex and ends at the beginning of the T wave (Fig. 9-9). The ventricle is initiating repolarization during the ST-segment phase of the ECG. This segment has very important predictive value and is discussed later.

Repolarization is complete with the ending of the T wave. The T wave represents the ventricular repolarization. Because no mechanical contraction is occurring, the T wave is strictly an electrical phenomenon that records the return of potassium inward and that of sodium outward and the change in the polarization of the cell.

THE ELECTROCARDIOGRAM RECORDING

The electrocardiogram is recorded on ruled graph paper, with the smallest divisions (or squares) being 1 mm long and 1 mm high. The height (positive deflection) or depth (negative deflection) measures the voltage as 0.1 mV/mm (Fig. 9-10). Time is represented on the graph paper by 0.04 second between each small square and 0.2 second between the large squares (Fig. 9-11) when the

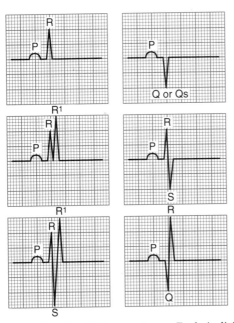

Figure 9-8. Possible QRS complexes. Each individual's electrocardiographic tracing is different.

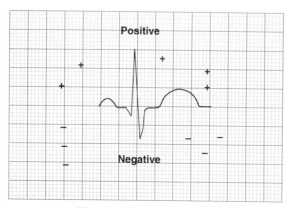

Figure 9–10. The positive or negative deflections on the electrocardiogram tracing represent voltage. Each small square is 1 mm × 1 mm.

paper speed is set at 25 mm/second. Exact time is important to note on the ECG to determine the duration of the complexes (e.g., QRS duration) and the intervals (e.g., P-R interval) as well as to identify the heart rates and arrhythmias.

The standard 12-lead ECG consists of tracings from six limb leads and six chest leads. The six limb leads are I, II, III, aVR, aVL, and aVF. Each limb lead records from a different angle, provid-

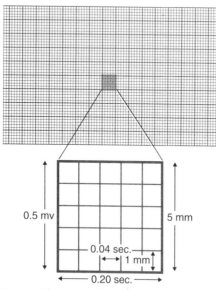

Figure 9–11. Electrocardiogram paper displays time on the horizontal axis. Each small box represents 0.04 second, and each large box represents 0.20 second. The vertical axis changes are measured in millimeters. Each small box represents 1 mm, each large box represents 5 mm.

ing a different view of the same cardiac activity. Therefore, the tracings from the various leads look different because the electrical activity is monitored from different positions. The six chest leads of the ECG are V1, V2, V3, V4, V5, and V6 and are monitored from six electrodes placed on the chest wall. The ECG tracing from the chest leads (V1 to V6) shows gradual changes in all the waves, as seen in Figure 9–12. Leads V1 and V2 are placed over the right side of the heart, and V5 and V6 are placed over the left side of the heart. Leads V3 and V4 are placed over the ventricular septum (Fig. 9–13). Figure 9–14 shows a picture of a standard 12-lead ECG with normal tracings in each of the leads, and the location of the leads on the tracing.

Four elements are specifically assessed on a 12-lead ECG tracing:

- Heart rate
- Heart rhythm
- **Hypertrophy**
- **Infarction**

A single-lead tracing, often called a *rhythm strip*, is assessed for heart rate, rhythm, and presence of arrhythmias. If hypertrophy, ischemia, or infarction is suspected, a 12-lead ECG should be obtained.

HEART RATE

The heart rate can be determined from the ECG recording by a variety of methods, including obtaining a 6-second tracing, measuring specific R waves, and counting the number of large boxes (5 mm or 0.2 second in length).

Six-Second Tracing. The investigator obtains an ECG recording that is 6 seconds in length (Fig. 9–15). The number of QRS complexes found in the 6-second recording is then multiplied by 10 to determine the heart rate per minute:

Number of QRS complexes in a 6-second recording
× 10 = heart rate per minute

R Wave Measurement. An alternative method of measuring heart rate is by identifying a specific R wave that falls on a heavy black line (large box

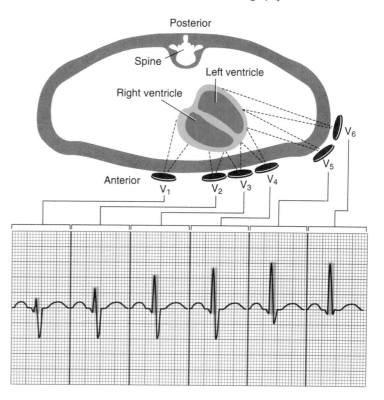

Figure 9-12. The electrocardiographic tracing from the chest leads (V1 to V6), showing the gradual changes that occur with the R and S waves.

line; Fig. 9–16). For each heavy black line that follows this R wave until the next R wave occurs the therapist counts 300, 150, 100, 75, 60, 50. Where the next R wave falls in this counting method gives the actual heart rate. To utilize this method, one must be able to memorize the specific numbers for the successive dark black lines to determine rapid heart rates from the graph paper. The one problem with R wave measurement for determining heart rate is that it cannot be used with irregular heart rhythms. For a more accurate estimate, the number of QRS complexes in a 30-

second strip must be counted and then multiplied by 2:

Number of QRS complexes in a 30-second strip
× 2 = heart rate per minute

Counting Boxes. The third method of obtaining the heart rate from the graph paper is to count the number of large boxes (5 mm or 0.2 second in length) between the first QRS complex and the next QRS complex. The number of large

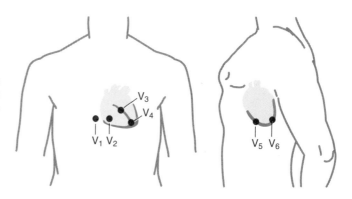

Figure 9-13. Leads V1 and V2 are placed over the right side of the heart. Leads V3 and V4 are located over the interventricular septum. Leads V5 and V6 demonstrate changes on the left side of the heart.

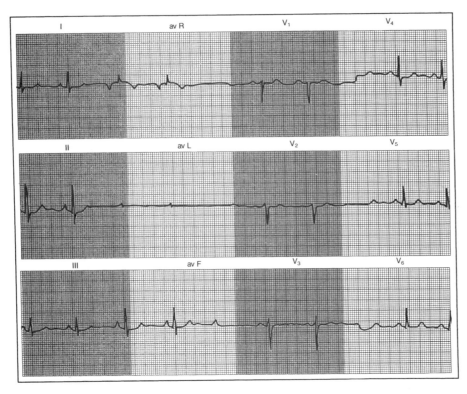

Figure 9-14. A normal 12-lead electrocardiogram tracing. Notice that aVR is the only lead in which the P wave, QRS complex, and T wave are all negative.

boxes is then divided into 300 to obtain an estimate of the heart rate:

$$300 \div \text{Number of large boxes between the first QRS complex and the next QRS complex} = \text{heart rate per minute}$$

A more accurate measurement of the heart rate can be made by counting the number of small boxes (1 mm or 0.04 second in length) between the QRS complexes and then dividing this number into 1500. This method requires much greater time to perform heart rate interpretation (Fig. 9-17).

$$\text{Number of small boxes between QRS complexes} \div 1500 = \text{heart rate per minute}$$

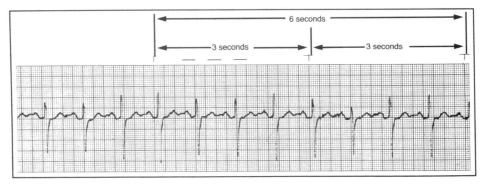

Figure 9-15. The heart rate can be determined by identifying 6 seconds on the electrocardiogram paper and counting the number of QRS complexes in the 6-second strip. The number of QRS complexes in 6 seconds multiplied by 10 gives the heart rate for 1 minute. The heart rate in this tracing is 84 bpm.

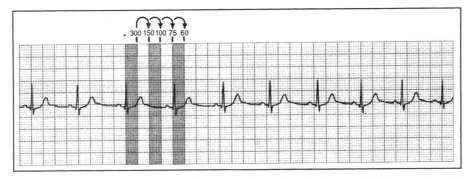

Figure 9-16. Another method of determining heart rate is to first find a specific R wave that falls on a heavy black line (see ∗). Then, count off "300, 150, 100, 75, 60, 50" for each heavy black line that follows until the next R wave falls. To find the specific heart rate, determine the difference in rate between the dark lines that encircle the R wave (for example, 300 − 150 = 150), and divide this number by 5 (the number of small boxes between the dark lines). Between 150 and 300 the distance between each small box is equivalent to 30 beats. Between 100 and 150 the distance between each small box represents 10 beats. This method assists in identifying a more accurate heart rate. The heart rate in this tracing is 72 bpm.

HEART RHYTHM

The 12-lead ECG is used primarily for determining ischemia or infarction as well as for comparing previous ECG recordings for an individual. However, for simple detection of rate or rhythm disturbances, single-lead monitoring is the appropriate choice. Single-lead monitoring via telemetry is the most common practice in stepdown intensive care units and cardiopulmonary rehabilitation programs. Single-lead monitoring is limited to detection of rate and rhythm disturbances; it *cannot* detect ischemia owing to the inability to calibrate

radiotelemetry. Hardwire systems are frequently used in the intensive care unit or cardiac care unit and should be calibrated appropriately. These systems can record **ischemia.** Twelve-lead ECG monitoring is used when ischemia is suspect or when a change in condition is noted.

Assessment Approach

To determine heart rate and rhythm from single-lead monitoring, the normal waveforms and intervals must be understood (Fig. 9–18). The wave-

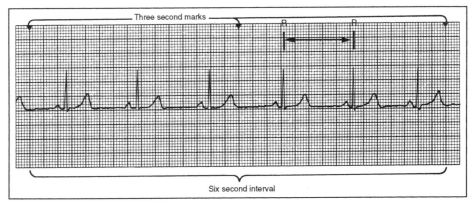

Figure 9-17. Another method of determining heart rate is to count the number of large boxes between two R waves and divide this number into 300. Or, for greater accuracy, count the number of large boxes between the R waves, multiply this number by 5 (the number of small boxes per large box), and divide this number into 1500. The heart rate in this tracing is 58 bpm. (From Wiederhold R. Electrocardiography: The Monitoring Lead. Philadelphia, WB Saunders, 1989, p 47.)

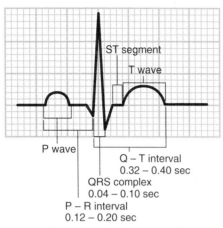

Figure 9–18. The normal electrocardiogram tracing. The P-R interval measures between 0.12 and 0.20 second. The normal duration of the QRS complex is 0.04 to 0.10 second. The normal duration of the Q-T interval is 0.32 to 0.40 second.

forms that represent depolarization of the myocardium have been labeled P, QRS, T, and U. A systematic approach to waveforms and interval measurement should be undertaken when reviewing cardiac rhythm. A systematic approach to the assessment of the cardiac cycle for rhythm and rate disturbances involves the following:

1. Evaluate the P wave. (Is it normal and upright, and is there a P wave before every QRS? Do all the P waves look alike?)
2. Evaluate the P-R interval. (Normal duration is 0.12 to 0.20 second.)
3. Evaluate the QRS complex. (Do all QRS complexes look alike?)
4. Evaluate the QRS interval. (Normal duration is 0.06 to 0.10 second.)
5. Evaluate the T wave. (Is it upright and normal in appearance?)
6. Evaluate the R-R wave interval. (Is it regular?)
7. Evaluate the heart rate (6-second strip if regular rhythm; normal rate is 60 to 100 beats per minute).
8. Observe the patient, and evaluate any symptoms. (Do the observation, symptoms, or both correlate with the arrhythmia?)

Normal Waveforms

The P wave is normally rounded, symmetric, and upright, representing atrial depolarization. A P

wave should occur before every QRS complex. The P-R interval is the interval that starts at the beginning of the P wave and ends at the beginning of the QRS complex; the portion following the P wave is also defined as the isoelectric line. The P-R interval is normally 0.12 to 0.20 second (or up to five small squares on the ECG paper). This period of time represents the atrial depolarization and the slowing of electrical conduction through the AV node.

The QRS complex follows the P-R interval and has multiple deflections and may have numerous variations, depending on the lead that is being monitored (see Fig. 9–8 for variations in the QRS complexes). The QRS complex begins at the end of the P-R interval and appears as a thin line recording from the ECG stylus, ending normally with a return to the baseline. The QRS duration reflects the time it takes for conduction to proceed to the Purkinje fibers and for the ventricles to depolarize. The normal duration is 0.04 to 0.10 second.

The ST segment follows the QRS complex, beginning where the ECG tracing transforms from a thin line to a thicker line and terminating at the beginning of the T wave. The ST segment should be represented as an isoelectric line along the same line (if measured with a ruler) as the P-R interval or the baseline. The T wave follows the ST segment and should be rounded, symmetric, and upright. The T wave represents ventricular repolarization.

The Q-T interval (from the beginning of the QRS complex until the end of the T wave) normally measures between 0.32 and 0.40 second if a normal sinus rhythm is present. The Q-T interval usually is not measured unless drug toxicity is suspected. Occasionally a U wave may follow the T wave, but its cause and clinical value are essentially unknown.

Finally, the R-R interval is reviewed throughout the rhythm strip to assess regularity of rhythm (Fig. 9–19). Normal rhythm requires a regular R-

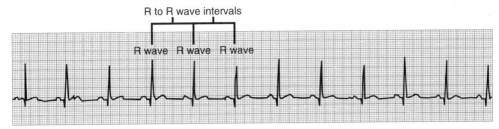

Figure 9–19. Electrocardiogram tracing demonstrating R to R intervals. R-R intervals are evaluated for regularity of rhythm. The heart rate in this tracing is 68 bpm.

R interval throughout; however, a discrepancy of up to 0.12 second between the shortest and the longest R-R interval is acceptable for normal respiratory variation. Occasionally single-lead monitoring may be affected. by artifact, such as the following:

• Muscle tremors or movement (including anything from sneezing and coughing to actual physical movement)
• Loose electrodes
• Sixty-cycle electrical interference

In most cases of artifact interference, the R-R interval is regular throughout, and the interference is seen between the R waves (Fig. 9–20).

If the R-R intervals are all regular, a 6-second strip or the counting down from 300 method can be employed to determine heart rate. Normal heart rate is between 60 and 100 beats per minute. If the R-R intervals are irregular (and greater than the acceptable range of 0.12 second for respiratory variation), a 30- to 60-second strip may be needed

to determine the heart rate and the frequency or seriousness of the arrhythmia, or both.

BASIC INTERPRETATION OF HEART RHYTHM

The key to the basic interpretation of heart rhythm in the clinical setting involves using the systematic approach as presented earlier, correlating the interpretation with the history and the signs and symptoms of the patient and then deciding if the rhythm is benign or life-threatening. If the decision is that the rhythm is truly benign, then the patient does not require ECG monitoring. If the rhythm is relatively benign, then occasional ECG monitoring may be necessary, or at least physiologic monitoring of the heart rate and blood pressure should be employed. If the arrhythmia is determined to be life-threatening, ECG monitoring as well as physiologic monitoring

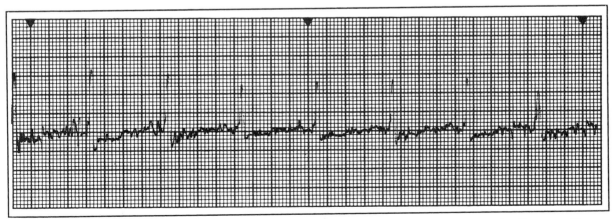

Figure 9–20. Electrocardiogram tracing of normal sinus rhythm with artifact in between the R waves. (From Wiederhold R. Electrocardiography; The Monitoring Lead. Philadelphia, WB Saunders, 1989, p 50.)

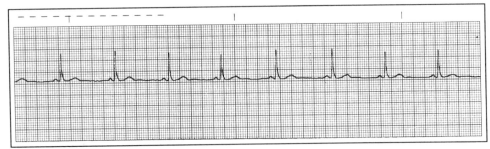

Figure 9–21. Electrocardiogram tracing of normal sinus rhythm with a heart rate of approximately 62 bpm.

should be carried out. In some cases the patient may not be a candidate for any activity or procedure until the arrhythmia is controlled.

For each of the following cardiac rhythms an ECG recording is provided along with a description of the features of each rhythm. In addition, possible etiologic factors as well as signs and symptoms that may be associated with the rhythm are explained. Treatment is discussed only so that the reader may develop an increased understanding of the whole picture of arrhythmias and their control. It should *not* be inferred that the physical therapist is responsible for the treatment of arrhythmias.

Normal Sinus Rhythm

The normal cardiac rhythm is termed *normal sinus rhythm* (NSR) and begins with an impulse originating in the SA node with conduction through the normal pathways for depolarization. Parasympathetic stimulation generally slows the rate, and sympathetic stimulation increases the rate. Figure 9–21 illustrates normal sinus rhythm. The characteristics of NSR include the following:

- All P waves are upright, normal in appearance, and identical in configuration; a P wave exists before every QRS complex.
- The P-R interval is between 0.12 and 0.20 second.
- The QRS complexes are identical.
- The QRS duration is between 0.04 and 0.10 second.
- The R-R interval is regular (or if irregular, the difference between shortest and longest intervals is less than 0.12 second).
- The heart rate is between 60 and 100 beats per minute.

Sinus Bradycardia

Sinus bradycardia differs from normal sinus rhythm only in the rate, which is less than 60 beats per minute (Fig. 9–22). The characteristics of sinus bradycardia include the following:

- All P waves are upright, normal in appearance, and identical in configuration; a P wave exists before every QRS complex.
- The P-R interval is between 0.12 and 0.20 second.
- The QRS complexes are identical.

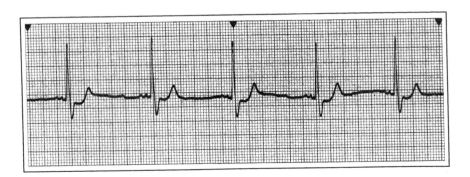

Figure 9–22. Electrocardiogram tracing illustrating sinus bradycardia with a heart rate of approximately 50 bpm. (From Wiederhold R. Electrocardiography: The Monitoring Lead. Philadelphia, WB Saunders, 1989, p 189.)

- The QRS duration is between 0.04 and 0.10 second.
- The R-R interval is regular throughout.
- The heart rate is less than 60 beats per minute.

Signs, Symptoms, and Causes

Sinus bradycardia is normal in well-trained athletes because of their enhanced stroke volume. It is also common in individuals taking beta-blocking medications. Sinus bradycardia may occur because of a decrease in the automaticity of the SA node or in a condition of increased vagal stimulation, such as suctioning or vomiting. Sinus bradycardia has been seen in patients who have traumatic brain injuries with increased intracranial pressures and in patients with brain tumors. Sinus bradycardia may also occur in the presence of second- or third-degree heart block; therefore, close evaluation of the P-R interval and the P to QRS ratio is necessary to rule out heart block.

Usually individuals with sinus bradycardia are asymptomatic unless a pathologic condition exists, at which time the individual may complain of **syncope,** dizziness, angina, or **diaphoresis.** Other arrhythmias may also develop.

Treatment

No treatment is necessary unless the patient is symptomatic. If the patient has symptoms, atropine may be used, and in some cases a temporary pacemaker may be implanted.

Sinus Tachycardia

Sinus tachycardia differs from normal sinus rhythm in rate only, which is greater than 100

> **Clinical Note: Sinus Bradycardia**
>
> Sinus bradycardia is usually non-life-threatening. The underlying cause should be sought. Some possible causes include beta-blocking medications and second- or third-degree AV block (not benign). Trained athletes with an increased resting and exercise stroke volume may also exhibit bradycardia.

beats per minute (Fig. 9–23). The characteristics of sinus tachycardia include:

- All P waves are upright, normal in appearance, and identical in configuration; a P wave exists before every QRS complex.
- The P-R interval is between 0.12 and 0.20 second.
- The QRS complexes are identical.
- The QRS duration is between 0.04 and 0.10 second.
- The R-R interval is regular.
- The heart rate is greater than 100 beats per minute.

Signs, Symptoms, and Causes

Sinus tachycardia is typically benign and is present usually in conditions in which the SA node automaticity is increased (increased sympathetic stimulation). Examples of conditions that induce sinus tachycardia include pain; fear; emotion; exertion (exercise); or any artificial stimulants such as caffeine, nicotine, amphetamines, and atropine. Sinus tachycardia is also found in situations in which the demands for oxygen are increased, including fever, congestive heart failure, infection, anemia, hemorrhage, myocardial injury, and **hyperthyroid-**

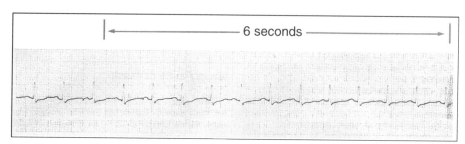

Figure 9–23. Electrocardiogram tracing illustrating sinus tachycardia (heart rate approximately 120 bpm).

ism. Usually individuals with sinus tachycardia are asymptomatic.

Treatment

Treatment for sinus tachycardia involves elimination (or treatment) of the underlying cause or, in some cases, the initiation of beta-blocker medication therapy.

Sinus Arrhythmia

Sinus arrhythmia is classified as an irregularity in rhythm in which the impulse is initiated by the SA node but with a phasic quickening and slowing of the impulse formation. The irregularity is usually caused by an alternation in vagal stimulation (Fig. 9–24). The characteristics of sinus arrhythmia include the following:

- All P waves are upright, normal in appearance, and identical in configuration; a P wave exists before every QRS complex.
- The P-R interval is between 0.12 and 0.20 second.
- The QRS complexes are identical.
- The QRS duration is between 0.04 and 0.10 second.

- The R-R interval varies throughout.
- The heart rate is between 40 to 100 beats per minute.

Signs, Symptoms, and Causes

The most common type of sinus arrhythmia is related to the respiratory cycle, with the rate increasing with inspiration and decreasing with expiration. This type of arrhythmia is usually found in the young or elderly at rest, and it disappears with activity. The other type of sinus arrhythmia is non-respiratory and therefore is not affected by the breathing cycle. Nonrespiratory sinus arrhythmia may occur in conditions of infection, medication administration (particularly toxicity associated with digoxin or morphine), and fever.[2]

Treatment

The respiratory type of sinus arrhythmia is benign and does not require any treatment. The nonrespiratory type should be evaluated for the underlying cause, and then this cause should be treated.

Sinus Pause or Block

Sinus pause or sinus block occurs when the SA node fails to initiate an impulse, usually for only one cycle (Fig. 9–25). The characteristics of sinus pause and block include the following:

- All P waves are upright, normal in appearance, and identical in configuration; a P wave exists before every QRS complex.

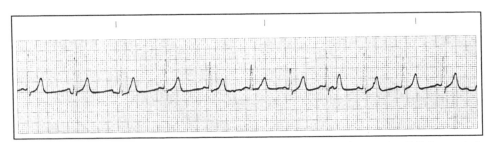

Figure 9–24. Electrocardiogram tracing showing sinus arrhythmia. Notice the varying R-R interval. In the first 3 seconds, the R-R intervals appear long, and in the second 3 seconds the intervals appear shorter.

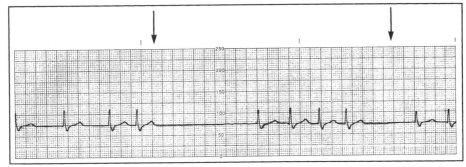

Figure 9–25. Electrocardiogram tracing of sinus pause or block (*arrows*).

- The P-R interval of the underlying rhythm is 0.12 to 0.20 second.
- The QRS complexes are identical.
- The QRS duration is between 0.04 and 0.10 second.
- The R-R interval is regular for the underlying rhythm, but occasional pauses are noted.
- The heart rate is usually 60 to 100 beats per minute.

Signs, Symptoms, and Causes

Sinus pause or block can occur for a number of reasons, including a sudden increase of parasympathetic activity, an organic disease of the SA node (sometimes referred to as sick sinus syndrome), an infection, a rheumatic disease, severe ischemia or infarction to the SA node, or a case of digoxin toxicity.[1] If the pause or block is prolonged or occurs frequently, the cardiac output is compromised, and the individual may complain of dizziness or syncope episodes.

Treatment

Treatment should be initiated when the patient is symptomatic. It involves treatment of the underlying cause, which may include reduction of digoxin, removal of vagal stimulation, and possibly treatment with atropine or implantation of a permanent pacemaker.

Wandering Atrial Pacemaker

The pacemaking activity in **wandering pacemaker** shifts from focus to focus, resulting in a rhythm that is very irregular and without a consistent pattern. Some of the impulses may arise from the AV node (Fig. 9–26). The characteristics of wandering pacemaker include the following:

- P waves are present but vary in configuration; each P wave may look different.
- A P wave exists before every QRS complex.
- The P-R intervals may vary but are usually within the normal width.

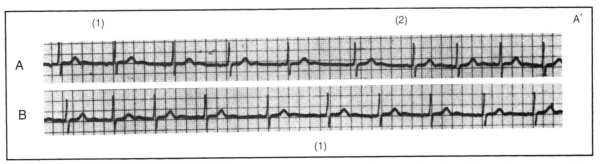

Figure 9–26. Electrocardiogram tracing illustrating a wandering atrial pacemaker. In this continuous recording B follows directly after A′. Notice that as the heart rate increases, the P waves become upright (2) and then gradually become inverted as the heart rate slows (1). (From Andreoli KG, Fowkes VH, Zipes DP, Wallace AC. Comprehensive Cardiac Care. 4th ed. St. Louis, CV Mosby, 1979.)

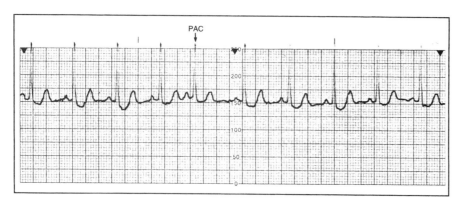

Figure 9–27. Electrocardiogram tracing showing premature atrial complex (PAC) (*arrow*).

- The QRS complexes are identical in configuration.
- The QRS duration is between 0.04 and 0.10 second.
- The R-R intervals vary.
- The heart rate is usually less than 100 beats per minute.

Signs and Symptoms

The cause is usually an irritable focus; however, the discharge of the impulse and the speed of discharge vary within the normal range. This type of arrhythmia is seen in the young and in the elderly and may be caused by ischemia or injury to the SA node, congestive heart failure, or an increase in vagal firing.[3] Usually this arrhythmia does not cause symptoms.

Treatment

This arrhythmia may lead to **atrial fibrillation,** which may require treatment; otherwise no treatment is necessary.

Atrial Arrhythmias

Premature Atrial Complexes

A **premature atrial complex** is defined as an ectopic focus in either atria that initiates an impulse before the next impulse is initiated by the SA node (Fig. 9–27). The characteristics of premature atrial complexes include the following:

- The underlying rhythm is sinus rhythm.
- Normal complexes have one P wave and one QRS wave configuration.
- The P wave of the early beat is noticeably different from the normal P waves.
- Depending on the heart rate, the P wave of the early beat may be buried in the previous T wave.
- The QRS complex involved in the early beat should look similar to the other QRS complexes.
- All P-R intervals are 0.12 to 0.20 second.
- All QRS durations are between 0.04 and 0.10 second.
- Often a pause follows the premature atrial complex, but it may not be compensatory.

Signs, Symptoms, and Causes

Causes of premature atrial complexes include emotional stress, nicotine, caffeine, alcohol, hypoxemia, infection, myocardial ischemia, rheumatic disease, and atrial damage. There may be no signs or symptoms associated with premature atrial complexes unless the pulse is palpated and the irregularity noticed.

Clinical Note: Premature Atrial Contractions

Premature atrial contractions are benign arrhythmias. They are often noticed in patients with chronic obstructive pulmonary disease.

Treatment

If the frequency of the premature atrial complexes is low, no treatment is required unless there are hemodynamic consequences. When the frequency is increased, supraventricular tachycardia or atrial fibrillation may develop.[4]

Atrial Tachycardia

The definition of **atrial tachycardia** is three or more premature atrial complexes in a row. Usually the heart rate is greater than 100 and may be as fast as 200 beats per minute (Fig. 9–28). The characteristics of atrial tachycardia include the following:

- P waves may be the same or may look different.
- P waves may not be present before every QRS complex.
- The P-R intervals vary but should be no greater than 0.20 second.
- The QRS complexes should be the same as the others that originate from the SA node.
- The QRS duration is generally between 0.04 and 0.10 second.
- The R-R intervals vary.
- The heart rate is rapid, being greater than 100 and possibly up to 200 beats per minute.

Signs, Symptoms, and Causes

The causes of atrial tachycardia include the causes of premature atrial complexes as well as those of severe pulmonary disease with hypoxemia, pulmonary hypertension, and altered pH. Atrial tachycar-dia is often found in patients with chronic obstructive pulmonary disease. Symptoms may develop owing to a compromised cardiac output if prolonged, thereby causing dizziness, fatigue, and shortness of breath.[1]

Treatment

Treatment for atrial tachycardia involves treatment of the underlying cause (if the patient is hypoxemic or if pH is altered); performance of autonomic maneuvers such as Valsalva's, breath holding, and coughing. Medications such as beta blockers, verapamil, and digoxin may be prescribed.

Paroxysmal Atrial Tachycardia

Paroxysmal atrial tachycardia (PAT) or **paroxysmal supraventricular tachycardia** (PSVT) is the sudden onset of atrial tachycardia or repetitive firing from an atrial focus. The underlying rhythm is usually normal sinus rhythm, followed by an episodic burst of atrial tachycardia that eventually returns to sinus rhythm. The episode may be extremely brief but can last for hours. The rhythm starts and stops abruptly (Fig. 9–29). The characteristics of paroxysmal atrial tachycardia include the following:

- P waves may be present but may be merged with the previous T wave.
- The P-R intervals may be difficult to determine but are less than 0.20 second.
- The QRS complexes are identical unless there is aberration.

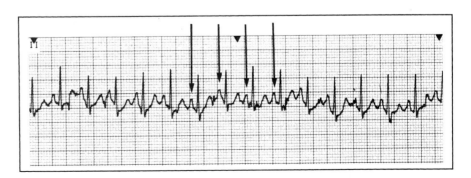

Figure 9–28. Electrocardiogram tracing showing atrial tachycardia. Note the presence of P waves (*arrows*) despite the fast heart rate (approximately 145 bpm).

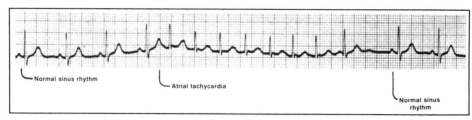

Figure 9–29. Electrocardiogram tracing illustrating paroxysmal atrial tachycardia. (From Phillips RE, Feeney MK. The Cardiac Rhythms. 3rd ed. Philadelphia, WB Saunders, 1990, p 154.)

- The QRS duration is between 0.04 and 0.10 second.
- The R-R intervals are usually regular and may show starting and stopping of the paroxysmal atrial tachycardia.
- The ST segment may be elevated or depressed, yet the magnitude of change is not diagnostically reliable.
- The heart rate is very rapid, often greater than 160 beats per minute.

Signs, Symptoms, and Causes

The causes of paroxysmal atrial tachycardia can include emotional factors; overexertion; hyperventilation; potassium depletion; caffeine, nicotine, and aspirin sensitivity; rheumatic heart disease; mitral valve dysfunction, particularly **mitral valve prolapse;** digitalis toxicity; and pulmonary embolus.[1] The clinical description of paroxysmal atrial tachycardia is a sudden racing or fluttering of the heart beat. If paroxysmal atrial tachycardia continues beyond 24 hours, it is considered to be sustained atrial tachycardia. If the rapid rate continues for a period of time, other symptoms may include dizziness, weakness, and shortness of breath (possibly even due to hyperventilation).

Treatment

Treatment includes determining the underlying cause (often in young females this would require evaluation for mitral valve prolapse); discontinuation of medications; performance of autonomic stimulation including Valsalva's maneuver, breath holding, and coughing or gagging; and, if prolonged, treatment with medications such as verapamil or beta blockers. **Carotid massage** is often performed but only in the presence of ECG monitoring.

Atrial Flutter

Atrial flutter is defined as a rapid succession of atrial depolarization caused by an ectopic focus in the atria that depolarizes at a rate of 250 to 350 times per minute. As only one ectopic focus is firing repetitively, the P waves are called flutter waves and look identical to one another, having a characteristic "sawtooth" pattern (Fig. 9–30). The characteristics of atrial flutter include the following:

- P waves are present as flutter waves having a characteristic "sawtooth" pattern.
- There is more than one P wave before every QRS complex.
- The atrial depolarization rate is 250 to 350 times per minute.
- The QRS configuration is usually normal and identical in configuration, but usually there is more than one P wave for every QRS complex.
- The QRS duration is 0.04 to 0.11 second.
- The R-R intervals may vary depending on the

> ### Clinical Note: Paroxysmal Atrial or Supraventricular Tachycardia
> Paroxysmal atrial tachycardia or paroxysmal supraventricular tachycardia is often diagnosed on ECG when a patient reports, "all of a sudden my heart was racing away." Initial treatment is to try coughing or breath-holding with a Valsalva maneuver. Treatment may require medications.

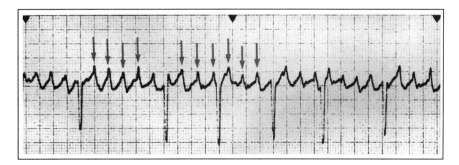

Figure 9–30. Electrocardiogram tracing of atrial flutter waves (*arrows*), with a variable block. (From Wiederhold R. Electrocardiography: The Monitoring Lead. Philadelphia, WB Saunders, 1988, p 218.)

atrial firing and number of P waves before each QRS complex. The conduction ratios may vary from 2 to 1 up to 8 to 1.

• The heart rate varies.

Signs, Symptoms, and Causes

Atrial flutter can be caused by numerous pathologic conditions, including rheumatic heart disease, mitral valve disease, coronary artery disease or infarction, stress, drugs, renal failure, hypoxemia, and pericarditis to name the most common causes.[5] As the rate of discharge from the **ectopic** focus is rapid, the critical role is played by the AV node, which blocks all the impulses from being conducted. Therefore, there may be an irregular rhythm associated with atrial flutter. This rhythm is usually not considered to be life-threatening and may even lead to atrial fibrillation. Usually no symptoms are present, and the cardiac output is not compromised unless the ventricular rate is too fast or too slow.

Treatment

Treatment for atrial flutter includes medications (digoxin, verapamil, or beta blockers are the more

> **Clinical Note: Atrial Flutter**
> Atrial flutter is relatively non-life-threatening if the heart rate is below 100 bpm at rest. Atrial flutter can be life-threatening at high heart rates. Medical treatment should be initiated if heart rate is elevated above 100 bpm at rest.

common drugs of choice) or **cardioversion** with the defibrillator paddles at 10 to 50 watts.

Atrial Fibrillation

Atrial fibrillation is defined as an erratic quivering or twitching of the atrial muscle caused by multiple ectopic foci in the atria that emit electrical impulses constantly. None of the ectopic foci actually depolarizes the atria, so no true P waves are found in atrial fibrillation. The AV node acts to control the impulses that initiate a QRS complex; therefore, a totally irregular rhythm exists. Thus, the AV node determines the ventricular response by blocking impulses or allowing them to progress forward. This ventricular response may be normal, slow, or too rapid (Fig. 9–31). The characteristics of atrial fibrillation include the following:

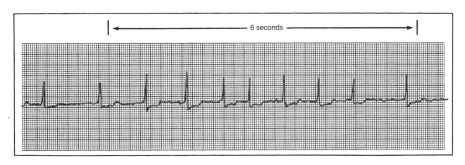

Figure 9–31. Electrocardiogram tracing of atrial fibrillation, with a ventricular response of 80 bpm. Notice the lack of P waves and the irregularly irregular rhythm.

- P waves are absent, thus leaving a flat or wavy baseline.
- The QRS duration is between 0.04 and 0.10 second.
- The R-R interval is characteristically defined as irregularly irregular.
- The rate varies but is called "ventricular response."

Signs, Symptoms, and Causes

Numerous factors may play a part in causing atrial fibrillation, including advanced age, congestive heart failure, ischemia or infarction, cardiomyopathy, digoxin toxicity, drug use, stress or pain, rheumatic heart disease, and renal failure. Atrial fibrillation presents problems for two reasons. Without atrial depolarization the atria do not contract. The contraction of the atria is also referred to as the atrial "kick." This atrial kick forces the last amount of volume to flow into the ventricles during diastole. The amount of volume that is forced into the ventricles because of atrial contraction provides up to 30% of the cardiac output. Therefore, without atrial contraction, the cardiac output is decreased up to 30%.[6]

In individuals with atrial fibrillation with heart rates (or ventricular response rates) lower than 100, the decrease in cardiac output is usually not a problem. However, as the individual exercises or if the ventricular response is greater than 100 at rest, the cardiac output may be diminished and signs of decompensation may occur. Atrial fibrillation is therefore considered relatively benign if the ventricular response is less than 100 at rest, but physiologic monitoring should be performed with exercise to assess cardiac output compensation. However, individuals who have atrial fibrillation with a ventricular response greater than 100 at rest should have physiologic monitoring during all activities, and any activity should be engaged in cautiously.

The other problem with atrial fibrillation is the potential for developing mural thrombi because of the coagulation of blood with fibrillating atria. Mural thrombi may lead to **emboli** (30% of all patients with atrial fibrillation develop emboli), so **anticoagulant** therapy is usually initiated.

> ### Clinical Note: Atrial Fibrillation
>
> Atrial fibrillation (irregular-irregular heart rhythm) is very common in the older population and is not considered life-threatening unless the heart rate is elevated at rest (above 100 is considered to be uncontrolled). Owing to a lack of "atrial kick," cardiac output is lower than normal (by 15 to 30%). Because of potential coagulation of blood with this abnormal rhythm, patients should be taking aspirin or coumadin to prevent the possibility of thrombus formation and potential cerebrovascular accident.

The classic sign of atrial fibrillation is a very irregularly irregular pulse. Symptoms occur only if the ventricular response is too rapid, which causes cardiac output decompensation.

Treatment

The treatment for atrial fibrillation usually involves pharmacologic control (e.g., digoxin, verapamil, antiarrhythmic therapy) or cardioversion. If a specific cause is identified, then treatment for that cause should be initiated. All individuals with newly diagnosed atrial fibrillation should be treated immediately with anticoagulants.

Nodal or Junctional Arrhythmias

Premature Junctional or Nodal Complexes

Premature junctional complexes are premature impulses that arise from the AV node or junctional tissue. For reasons that are not understood, the AV node becomes irritated and initiates an impulse that causes an early beat. Premature junctional complexes are very similar to premature atrial complexes except for the fact that an inverted, an absent, or a retrograde (wave that follows the QRS) P wave is present (Fig. 9–32). The characteristics of premature junctional complexes include the following:

- Inverted, absent, or retrograde P waves are present.

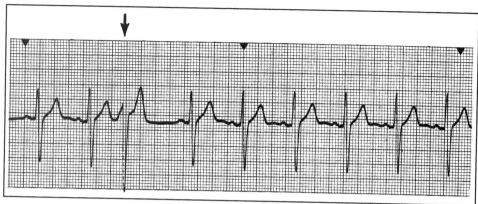

Figure 9-32. Electrocardiogram tracing of premature junctional (or nodal) complex. Note the isolated premature beat (*arrow*), which has a QRS complex of normal width. The beat comes early, however, and the P wave is absent. (From Wiederhold R. Electrocardiography: The Monitoring Lead. Philadelphia, WB Saunders, 1989, p 61.)

- The QRS configurations are usually identical.
- The QRS duration is between 0.04 and 0.10 second.
- The R-R interval is regular throughout except when the premature beats arise.
- The heart rate is usually normal (between 60 and 100 beats per minute).

Signs, Symptoms, and Causes

Some of the causes of premature junctional complexes include decreased automaticity and conductivity of the SA node or some irritability of the junctional tissue. Pathologic conditions that can cause premature junctional complexes include cardiac disease and mitral valve disease.[2] Usually no symptoms or signs are present.

Treatment

Usually no treatment is required because there are no symptoms of clinical significance.

Junctional (or Nodal) Rhythm

Junctional rhythm occurs when the AV junction takes over as the pacemaker of the heart. Junctional rhythm may be considered an escape rhythm (Fig. 9-33). The characteristics of junctional rhythm include the following:

- Absence of P waves before the QRS complex, but a retrograde P wave may be identified.
- The QRS complex has a normal configuration.
- The QRS duration is between 0.04 and 0.10 second.
- The R-R intervals are regular.
- The ventricular rate is between 40 and 60 beats per minute.

Signs, Symptoms, and Causes

Causes of junctional rhythm include a failure of the SA node to act as the pacemaker in conditions such as sinus node disease or increase in vagal tone, digoxin toxicity, and infarction or severe ischemia to the conduction system (typically right coronary artery disease). Symptoms are present only if the heart rate is too slow, which causes a compromise in the cardiac output.

Treatment

Treatment consists of identifying the cause and treating it if possible. If the rate becomes too slow (50 beats per minute or less) then the patient may develop symptoms of cardiac output decompensation, dizziness, and fatigue. In the case of symptoms and slower heart rates, the treatment involves medication to increase the rate (usually atropine or isoproterenol) or pacemaker insertion.

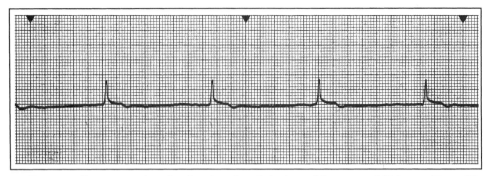

Figure 9–33. Electrocardiogram tracing showing junctional rhythm with a rate of 38 bpm. (From Wiederhold R. Electrocardiography: The Monitoring Lead. Philadelphia, WB Saunders, 1989, p 80.)

Nodal (Junctional) Tachycardia

Junctional tachycardia develops because the AV junctional tissue is acting as the pacemaker (as in junctional rhythm), but the rate of discharge is accelerated. The onset of increase in rate of discharge may be sudden, or it may be of long standing (Fig. 9–34). The characteristics of junctional tachycardia include the following:

- P waves are absent, but retrograde P wave may be present.
- The QRS configurations are identical.
- The QRS duration is between 0.04 and 0.10 second.
- The R-R interval is regular.
- The rate is usually greater than 100 beats per minute.

Signs, Symptoms, and Causes

Causes of junctional tachycardia include **hyperventilation,** coronary artery disease or infarction, post-cardiac surgery, digoxin toxicity, myocarditis, caffeine or nicotine sensitivity, overexertion, and emotional factors. When the rate is extremely rapid, the individual may experience symptoms of cardiac output decompensation.[1] Symptoms include dizziness, shortness of breath, and fatigue.

Treatment

Treatment involves identifying the cause and treating it. Digoxin is given if the underlying cause is not digoxin toxicity. Vagal stimulation may be employed or pharmacologic therapy initiated (verapamil or beta blockers).

HEART BLOCKS

First-Degree Atrioventricular Heart Block

First-degree AV block occurs when the impulse is initiated in the SA node but is delayed on the way

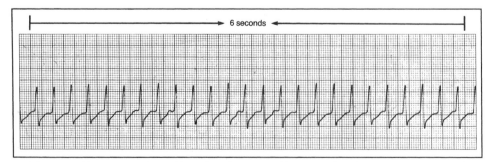

Figure 9–34. Electrocardiogram tracing of junctional tachycardia. Note the absence of P waves, illustrating atrial tachycardia.

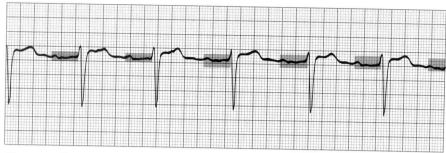

Figure 9–35. Electrocardiogram tracing of first-degree atrioventricular block (P-R interval measures approximately 0.32 second) with sinus bradycardia. (From Wiederhold R. Electrocardiography: The Monitoring Lead. Philadelphia, WB Saunders, 1989, p 87.)

to the AV node; or it may be initiated in the AV node itself, and the AV conduction time is prolonged. This results in a lengthening of the P-R interval only (Fig. 9–35).

The characteristics associated with first-degree AV block include the following:

- A P wave is present and with normal configuration before every QRS complex.
- The P-R interval is prolonged (greater than 0.20 second).
- The QRS has a normal configuration.
- The QRS duration is between 0.04 and 0.10 second.
- The R-R intervals are regular.
- The heart rate is usually within normal limits (60 to 100 beats per minute) but may be lower than 60 beats per minute.

Signs, Symptoms, and Causes

Causes of first-degree AV block include coronary artery disease, rheumatic heart disease, infarction, and reactions to medication (digoxin or beta blockers). First-degree AV block is a relatively benign arrhythmia as it exists without symptoms (unless severe bradycardia exists in conjunction with first-degree AV block); however, it should be monitored over time because it may progress to higher forms of AV block.

Treatment

Usually treatment is not warranted unless the AV block is due to reactions to medication, in which case the medication is withheld.

> **Clinical Note: First-degree AV Block**
>
> First-degree AV block is relatively benign. The only defining feature is the prolonged P-R interval (>2.0 sec).

Second-Degree Atrioventricular Block, Type I

Second-degree AV block, type I (Wenckebach's or Mobitz I heart block) is a relatively benign, transient disturbance that occurs high in the AV junction and prevents conduction of some of the impulses through the AV node. The typical appearance of **type I (Wenckebach's) second-degree block** is a progressive prolongation of the P-R interval until finally one impulse is not conducted through to the ventricles (no QRS complex following a P wave). The cycle then repeats itself (Fig. 9–36).

The characteristics of second-degree type I include the following:

- Initially a P wave precedes each QRS complex, but eventually a P wave may stand alone (conduction is blocked).
- Progressive lengthening of the P-R interval occurs in progressive order.
- As the P-R interval increases, a QRS complex will be dropped.
- This progressive lengthening of the P-R interval followed by a dropped QRS complex occurs in a repetitive cycle.

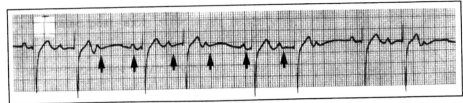

Figure 9–36. Electrocardiogram tracing showing type I second-degree heart block (Wenckebach's). The arrows identify the P waves. Notice the progressive lengthening of the P-R interval until finally a P wave exists without a QRS complex. (From Phillips RE, Feeney MK. The Cardiac Rhythms. 3rd ed. Philadelphia, WB Saunders, 1990, p 255.)

- The QRS configuration is normal, and the duration is between 0.04 and 0.10 second.
- Because of the dropping of the QRS complex, the R-R interval is irregular (regularly irregular).
- The heart rate varies.

Signs, Symptoms, and Causes

Causes of Wenckebach's heart block include right coronary artery disease or infarction, digoxin toxicity, and excessive beta adrenergic blockade; a side effect of the medication. Usually the individual with type I second-degree AV block is asymptomatic.

Treatment

Treatment is usually unnecessary because most often the individual is without symptoms and without cardiac output compromise. In rare cases, either atropine or isoproterenol have been given, or a temporary pacemaker is inserted.[7] This type of AV block rarely progresses to higher forms of AV block.

> **Clinical Note: Second-Degree AV Block (Type I)**
> Second-degree AV block or Wenckebach's heart block may be transient with severe ischemia or infarction. Treatment may include insertion of a temporary pacemaker as well as treatment for any symptoms due to slow heart rate. Rhythm may revert from this AV block with resolution of ischemia.

Second-Degree Atrioventricular Block, Type II

Second-degree AV block, **type II (Mobitz II),** is defined as nonconduction of an impulse to the ventricles without a change in the P-R interval. The site of the block is usually below the bundle of His and may be a bilateral bundle branch block (Fig. 9–37).

The characteristics of second-degree AV block type II include the following:

- A ratio of P waves to QRS complexes that is greater than 1:1 and may vary from 2 to 4 P waves for every QRS complex.

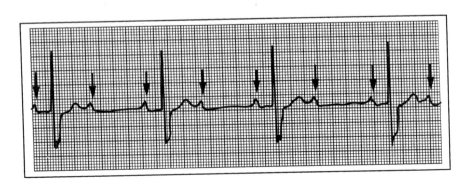

Figure 9–37. Electrocardiogram tracing of type II second-degree heart block (Mobitz II) with a heart rate of 37 bpm. Note the two P waves for every QRS complex.

- The QRS duration is between 0.04 and 0.10 second.
- The QRS configuration is normal.
- The R-R intervals may vary depending on the amount of blocking that is occurring.
- The heart rate is usually below 100 and may be below 60 beats per minute.

Signs, Symptoms, and Causes

Second-degree AV block type II occurs with myocardial infarction (especially when the left anterior descending coronary artery is involved), with ischemia or infarction of the AV node, or with digoxin toxicity. Patients may be symptomatic when the heart rate is low and when cardiac output compromise is present.[3]

Treatment

Treatment usually involves pacemaker insertion, but for immediate relief of symptoms atropine or isoproterenol may be used. The danger with type II second-degree AV block is the possibility of progression to complete heart block (third-degree AV block), which is a life-threatening condition.

Third-Degree Atrioventricular Block

In **third-degree (complete) AV block** all impulses that are initiated above the ventricle are *not* conducted to the ventricle. In complete heart block the atria fire at their own inherent rate (SA node

> ### Clinical Note: Second-Degree Type II AV Block
> Second-degree type II AV block requires temporary or permanent pacemaker insertion.

firing or ectopic foci in the atria), and a separate pacemaker in the ventricles initiates all impulses. However, there is no communication between the atria and the ventricles and thus no coordination between the firing of the atria and the firing of the ventricles, creating complete independence of the two systems (Fig. 9–38).

The characteristics of complete heart block include the following:

- P waves are present, regular, and of identical configuration.
- The P waves have no relationship to the QRS complex because the atria are firing at their own inherent rate.
- The QRS complexes are regular in that the R-R intervals are regular.
- The QRS duration may be wider than 0.10 second if the latent pacemaker is in the ventricles.
- The heart rate depends on the latent ventricular pacemaker and may range from 30 to 50 beats per minute.

Signs, Symptoms, and Causes

The causes of complete heart block usually involve acute myocardial infarction, digoxin toxicity, or degeneration of the conduction system. If a slow ventricular rate is present, then the cardiac output often is diminished, and the patient may complain

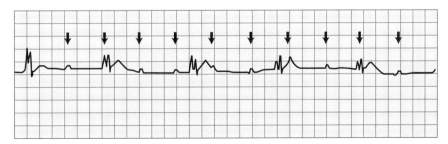

Figure 9–38. Electrocardiogram tracing showing third-degree heart block, also known as complete heart block. Notice how the P waves have their own regular rhythm (*arrows*) without interrupting the rhythm of the QRS complex. There is no communication between atrial firing and ventricular firing.

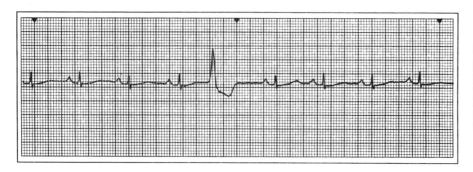

Figure 9–39. Electrocardiogram tracing of an isolated premature ventricular complex. (From Wiederhold R. Electrocardiography: The Monitoring Lead. Philadelphia, WB Saunders, 1989, p 62.)

of dizziness, shortness of breath, and possibly chest pain.

Treatment

Treatment for complete heart block involves permanent pacemaker insertion, with atropine and isoproterenol injection or infusion used in the acute situation. Complete heart block is a medical emergency.

Ventricular Arrhythmias

Premature Ventricular Complexes

Premature ventricular complexes (PVCs) occur when an ectopic focus originates an impulse from somewhere in one of the ventricles. The ventricular ectopic depolarization occurs early in the cycle before the SA node actually fires. A PVC is easily recognized on the ECG because the impulse originates in the muscle of the heart, and these myocardial cells conduct impulses very slowly compared with specialized conductive tissue. There-

fore, the QRS complex is classically described as a wide and bizarre looking QRS without a P wave and followed by a complete compensatory pause (see Fig. 9–38). Premature ventricular complexes may come in patterns (e.g., every third or fourth beat, paired together) or may be isolated. Premature ventricular beats may be identical, or they may look different. All these factors affect the seriousness of the PVCs and also affect the clinical decision-making process and treatment. See illustrations of PVCs: Unifocal (Fig. 9–39), multifocal (Fig. 9–40), frequent (bigeminy) (Fig. 9–41), R on T (Fig. 9–42), paired (Fig. 9–43), and triplet (Fig. 9–44).

The characteristics of PVCs include the following:

- An absence of P waves in the premature beat, with all other beats usually of sinus rhythm.
- The QRS complex of the premature beat is wide and bizarre and occurs earlier than the normal sinus beat would have occurred.
- The QRS duration of the early beat is greater than 0.10 second.
- The ST segment and the T wave often slope in

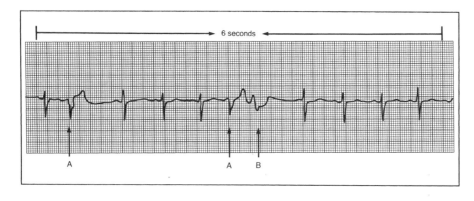

Figure 9–40. Electrocardiogram tracing of multifocal premature ventricular complexes. Note the QRS complex at A and the difference in configuration of the QRS complex at B.

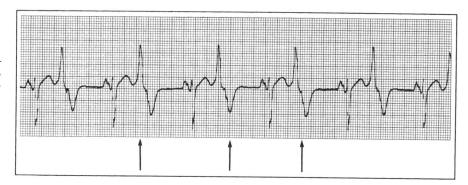

Figure 9–41. Electrocardiogram tracing showing bigeminy (premature ventricular complexes every other beat). Arrows depict premature complexes.

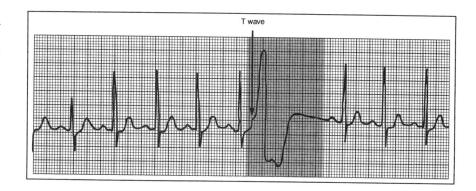

Figure 9–42. Electrocardiogram tracing of R on T premature ventricular complex (PVC). Notice the arrow depicts a PVC that begins from the top of the T wave of the preceding beat. This can be extremely dangerous, because the premature beat is firing during the refractory period and could lead to ventricular tachycardia or fibrillation.

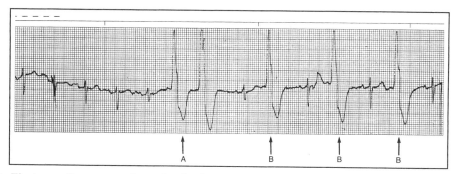

Figure 9–43. Electrocardiogram tracing of paired premature ventricular complexes (PVCs) (A). In addition, unifocal PVCs are present after paired PVCs (B).

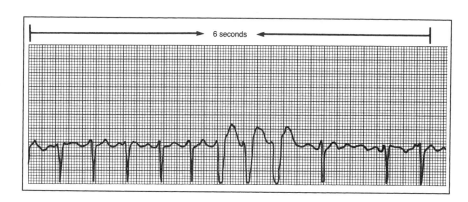

Figure 9–44. Electrocardiogram tracing of a triplet, otherwise known as a three-beat ventricular tachycardia.

the opposite direction from the normal complexes.

- The PVC is generally followed by a **compensatory pause.**
- The PVC is called bigeminy when every other beat is a PVC, trigeminy when every third beat is a PVC, and so on.
- The PVC is called unifocal if all PVCs appear identical in configuration.
- The PVCs are called **multifocal** if more than one PVC is present and the two do not appear similar in configuration.
- The PVC is paired or a couplet if two PVCs are together, a triplet or ventricular tachycardia (VTACH) if three are together in a row.
- The PVC is **interpolated** if it falls between two normal sinus beats that are separated by a normal R-R interval.

Signs, Symptoms, and Causes

The causes of PVCs are numerous. Isolated PVCs may be present owing to caffeine or nicotine sensitivity, stress, overexertion, or electrolyte imbalance (particularly **hypokalemia** or **hyperkalemia**). Premature ventricular complexes are also common in the presence of ischemia; cardiac disease; overdistention of the ventricle, as in congestive heart failure or **cardiomyopathy;** acute infarction; irritation of the myocardium or its vessels, as in cardiac catheterization; chronic lung disease and hypoxemia; and as a result of pharmacologic therapy (procan, quinidine, or digoxin toxicity).

Individuals may experience symptoms with PVCs if they are frequent or more serious in nature because they may affect the cardiac output. A skipped beat can be palpated when checking a pulse. A PVC feels like a pause or skip in the regular rhythm that usually is followed by a stronger beat. PVC cannot be diagnosed without seeing the ECG recording; therefore, the individual is placed on telemetry. The PVC may also be felt because of the decreased preload with the PVC beat, which is followed by a long compensatory pause that allows increased filling time of the ventricle and therefore an increased preload for the beat following the premature beat and subsequently an increased stroke volume. This increased stroke volume is usually what is felt in the previously asymptomatic individual and is often a con-

cern. With increased frequency of PVCs, the filling time of the ventricles decreases, which leads to a decreased preload and subsequently a decreased stroke volume. Symptoms associated with PVCs include anxiety (particularly with a new onset of arrhythmias); however, if the arrhythmias are more frequent, cardiac output may decrease, and therefore shortness of breath and dizziness may occur.

Treatment

The treatment for PVCs depends on the underlying cause, the frequency and severity of the PVCs, and the symptoms associated with them. The frequency and the type of evidence for them indicate the seriousness of the patient's condition and help to determine the clinical decision. Premature ventricular complexes are considered to be serious, or possibly life-threatening, when they

- Are paired together (see Fig. 9–43)
- Are multifocal in origin (see Fig. 9–40)
- Are more frequent than 6 per minute
- Land directly on the T wave (see Fig. 9–42)
- Are present in triplets or more (see Fig. 9–44)

Premature ventricular complexes are considered to be serious or life-threatening because they may indicate increased irritability of the ventricular muscle and may progress to **ventricular tachycardia** or **ventricular fibrillation**—two medical emergencies.

Although PVCs may be benign, a full cardiac evaluation should be performed to rule out underlying disease in the individual who demonstrates a sudden onset of PVCs.[6] If the individual has a history of arrhythmias, if the individual with arrhythmias is asymptomatic, and if the frequency or seriousness of the arrhythmias does not change, then treatment is unwarranted. If the arrhythmias

Clinical Note: Premature Ventricular Contractions

Premature ventricular contractions, when isolated, without symptoms, and fewer than 6 per minute, are usually considered benign and do not warrant treatment. When PVCs are more frequent than 6 per minute, are paired or multifocal, patients may require closer monitoring or medical treatment. Medical treatment may also cause arrhythmias and may not abate the arrhythmias.

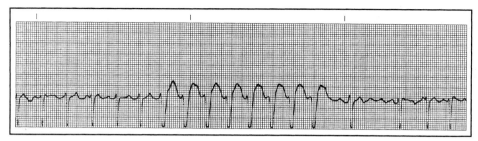

Figure 9–45. Electrocardiogram tracing showing ventricular tachycardia.

produce symptoms or appear to be more frequent either throughout the day or with increased activity, then further evaluation and possibly treatment is warranted. If an individual with chronic lung disease has a new onset of PVCs it may indicate hypoxemia, and supplemental oxygen may be necessary. Otherwise, after all the underlying causes are evaluated, antiarrhythmic medications may be warranted. Caution should be taken when an individual begins antiarrhythmic medication as antiarrhythmic medication therapy is not always effective and can even *produce* arrhythmias. See Chapter 14 for more information on the pharmacologic management of PVCs.

Ventricular Tachycardia

Ventricular tachycardia is defined as a series of three or more PVCs in a row. Ventricular tachycardia occurs because of a rapid firing by a single ventricular focus with increased automaticity (Figs. 9–44 and 9–45). The characteristics of ventricular tachycardia include the following:

- P waves are absent.
- Three or more PVCs occur in a row.
- QRS complexes of the ventricular tachycardia are wide and bizarre.
- Ventricular rate of ventricular tachycardia is between 100 and 250 beats per minute.
- Ventricular tachycardia can be the precursor to ventricular fibrillation.

Signs, Symptoms, and Causes

Causes of ventricular tachycardia include ischemia or acute infarction, coronary artery disease, hypertensive heart disease, and reaction to medications

(digoxin or quinidine toxicity). Occasionally ventricular tachycardia occurs in athletes during exercise (possibly due to electrolyte imbalance). Ventricular tachycardia indicates increased irritability as well as an emergency situation because cardiac output is greatly diminished, as is the blood pressure. Symptoms usually involve lightheadedness and sometimes syncope. A weak, thready pulse may be present. The individual may become disoriented if ventricular tachycardia is sustained. Ventricular tachycardia can progress to ventricular fibrillation and death.

Treatment

Treatment usually is an immediate pharmacologic injection (lidocaine, bretylium tosylate [bretylol], or procainamide [pronestyl]) or cardioversion or **defibrillation.** Ventricular tachycardia is considered a medical emergency.

Ventricular Tachycardia: Torsades de Pointes

Torsades de pointes is a unique configuration of ventricular tachycardia called the "twisting of the points" (Fig. 9–46). Torsades de pointes is often associated with a prolonged Q-T interval (greater than 0.5 second). The name relates to its presentation by twisting around the isoelectric line. This arrhythmia characteristically occurs at a rapid rate and terminates spontaneously.

Signs, Symptoms, and Causes

This type of ventricular tachycardia has been identified only in individuals receiving antiarrhythmic

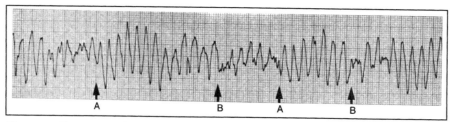

Figure 9–46. Electrocardiogram tracing showing torsades de pointes. The arrows depict the beginning (A) and ending (B) before turning of the "twisting of points." (From Phillips RE, Feeney MK. The Cardiac Rhythms. 3rd ed. Philadelphia, WB Saunders, 1990, p 393.)

therapy and for whom the medication is toxic. As cardiac output is severely diminished and as this arrhythmia often converts to ventricular fibrillation this condition is considered a medical emergency.[1] The individual who remains conscious with this arrhythmia may be extremely lightheaded or near syncope.

Treatment

Treatment is usually cardioversion.

Ventricular Fibrillation

Ventricular fibrillation is defined as an erratic quivering of the ventricular muscle resulting in no cardiac output. As in atrial fibrillation, multiple ectopic foci fire, creating asynchrony. The ECG results in a picture of grossly irregular up and down fluctuations of the baseline in an irregular zigzag pattern (Fig. 9–47).

Signs, Symptoms, and Causes

The causes of ventricular fibrillation are the same as those of ventricular tachycardia because ventricular fibrillation is usually the sequel to ventricular tachycardia.

Treatment

Treatment is defibrillation as quickly as possible followed by cardiopulmonary resuscitation, supplemental oxygen, and injection of medications. However, if the tracing appears to be ventricular fibrillation and the patient does not have a long-term history of recurrent ventricular tachycardia or ventricular fibrillation, and the patient is able to carry on a conversation, the therapist should assume this is probably only lead displacement creating artifact.

OTHER FINDINGS ON A 12-LEAD ELECTROCARDIOGRAM

Hypertrophy

Hypertrophy refers to an increase in thickness of cardiac muscle or chamber size. Signs of atrial hypertrophy can be noted by examining the P waves of the ECG for a diphasic P wave in the chest lead V1, or a voltage in excess of 3 mV. Signs of right ventricular hypertrophy are noted by changes found in lead V1 that include a large R wave and

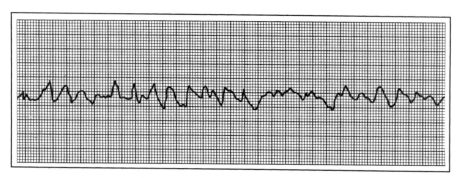

Figure 9–47. Electrocardiogram tracing showing ventricular fibrillation (coarse).

an S wave smaller than the R wave. The R wave becomes progressively smaller in the successive chest leads (V2, V3, V4, V5). Hypertrophy of the left ventricle creates enlarged QRS complexes in the chest leads in both height of the QRS (R wave) and depth of the QRS (S wave). In left ventricular hypertrophy a deep S wave occurs in V1 and a large R wave in V5. If when the depth of the S wave in V1 (in mm) is added to the height of the R wave in V5 (in mm) and the resulting number is greater than 35, then left ventricular hypertrophy is present (Fig. 9–48).

Ischemia, Infarction, or Injury

A review of an ECG to detect ischemia, infarction, or injury is performed in a variety of situations, including after any episode of chest pain that brings a patient to the physician's office or to the hospital, during hospitalization, during a follow-up examination after a cardiac event, or before conducting an exercise test. The difference between ischemia and infarction is covered in great detail in Chapter 3. In simplistic terms, ischemia literally means reduced blood and refers to a diminished blood supply to the myocardium. This can occur because of occlusion of the coronary arteries from vasospasm, atherosclerotic occlusion, thrombus, or a combination of the three. Infarction means cell death and results from a complete occlusion of a coronary artery. Injury indicates the acuteness of

the infarction. As a result of ischemia, injury, or infarction, conduction of electrical impulses is altered, and therefore depolarization of the muscle changes. As the ECG records the depolarization of the cardiac muscle, changes occur on the ECG in the presence of ischemia, infarction, or injury. The location of the ischemia, infarction, or injury is determined according to the specific leads of the ECG that demonstrate an alteration in depolarization.

Ischemia is classically demonstrated on the 12-lead ECG with T wave inversion or ST-segment depression. The T wave may vary from a flat configuration to a depressed inverted wave (Fig. 9–49). The T wave is an extremely sensitive indication of changes in repolarization activity within the ventricles.[8] Transient fluctuations in the T wave can be observed in numerous situations and must be associated with the activity and symptoms to determine if the abnormality is ischemic. For an individual who comes to a physician's office because of an episode of chest pain, T-wave inversion may be the only noticeable abnormality. If the individual took nitroglycerin while at the office and the pain disappeared before the ECG was administered, abnormalities may be absent owing to the resolution of the ischemic event.

The location of the ST segment (that portion of the ECG tracing beginning with the end of the S wave and ending with the beginning of the T wave) is another indication of ischemia or injury. Elevation of the ST segment above the baseline when following part of an R wave indicates acute

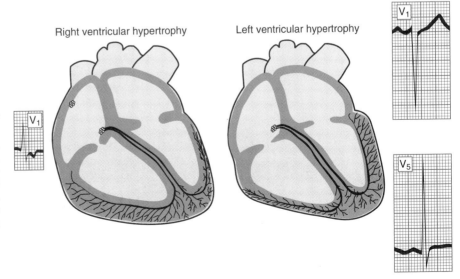

Figure 9–48. Hypertrophy is determined by looking at voltage in V1 and V5. Right ventricular hypertrophy is defined as a large R wave in V1, which gets progressively smaller in V2, V3, and V4; normally there is a very small R wave and a large S wave in V1. Left ventricular hypertrophy is defined as a large S wave in V1 and a large R wave in V5 that have a combined voltage of greater than 35 mV.

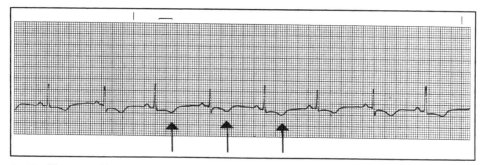

Figure 9–49. Electrocardiogram tracing showing an inverted T wave, often indicating ischemia (*arrows*).

injury (Fig. 9–50). In the presence of acute infarction, the ST segment elevates and then later returns to the level of the baseline (within 24–48 hours).[8] ST-segment elevation may also occur in the presence of a ventricular aneurysm (a ballooning out of the ventricular wall, usually following a large amount of damage to the ventricular wall). The ST-segment elevation with ventricular aneurysm never returns to the isoelectric line, and the configuration differs somewhat. The ST-segment elevation in ventricular aneurysm usually follows a large Q wave and not an R wave of the QRS complex (see Fig. 9–50). If the ECG records the presence of ST-segment elevation in the presence of acute onset of chest pain (within hours), a cardiac emergency exists and immediate treatment is indicated.

The ECG may demonstrate ST-segment depression while the patient is at rest in the presence of chest pain or of suspected coronary ischemia. The ST-segment depression in this situation represents **subendocardial infarction** and also requires immediate treatment. A subendocardial infarct is an acute injury to the myocardial wall, but it does not extend through the full thickness of the ventricular wall. Instead, the injury is only to the subendocardium (Fig. 9–51).

This ECG sign is extremely significant, because it indicates that a transmural infarction could be pending. Research has shown that an individual diagnosed with a subendocardial infarction is at extremely high risk for another infarction (this time **transmural**) within 6 weeks.[9]

Other situations may precipitate ST-segment de-

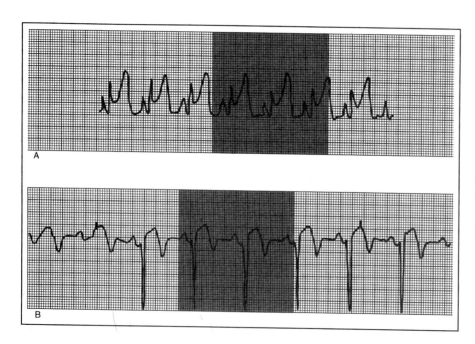

Figure 9–50. *A,* An ST-segment elevation following part of the R wave indicates acute injury. *B,* An ST-segment elevation following a large Q wave does not always indicate injury but often signals the presence of a ventricular aneurysm.

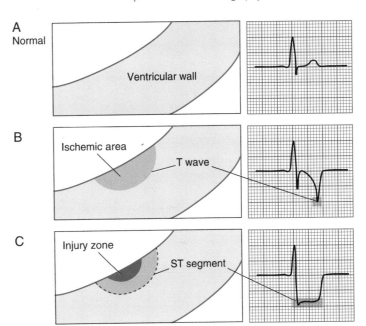

A Normal
Ventricular wall

B
Ischemic area
T wave

C
Injury zone
ST segment

Figure 9–51. An ST segment on a resting 12-lead electrocardiogram (ECG) often is indicative of subendocardial injury. *A,* Normal tracing and normal ventricular wall. *B,* Subendocardial ischemia with an ECG tracing of T wave inversion. *C,* Subendocardial injury with ST-segment depression on the ECG.

pression. ST-segment depression in the absence of suspected ischemia or angina may be caused by digitalis toxicity (see Chapter 14 for discussion of digitalis toxicity). ST-segment depression that develops during exercise, as seen during exercise testing, is defined as an ischemic response to exercise, and following rest it should return to the isoelectric line. This is an abnormal response to exercise that indicates an impaired coronary arterial supply during the exercise. This type of ischemic response should be further evaluated to determine the extent of the coronary artery involvement (see Chapter 8).

During myocardial injury, the affected area of muscle loses its ability to generate electrical impulses, and therefore alterations in the initial portion of the QRS complex occur. The cells are dead and cannot depolarize normally, which results in an inability to conduct impulses. Therefore, as ST-segment elevation or depression is diagnostic for acute infarction, the presence of a significant Q wave is also diagnostic for infarction, but the date of the infarction is not able to be determined simply by studying the ECG. The date of the infarction is determined by the patient's report of symptoms. The Q wave is the first downward part of the QRS complex (not preceded by anything else), and small Q waves may be present normally in some leads. When the Q wave is 0.04

second in duration wide (one small square on the ECG tracing) or is one third the size (height and depth included) of the QRS complex, the Q wave is considered to be *significant* and indicative of a pathologic condition (it persists as a permanent electrocardiographic "scar" from infarction [Fig. 9–52]). Therefore, any scan of the ECG should include a check for the presence of significant Q waves to identify previous infarction.

The leads that demonstrate the presence of T wave inversion, ST-segment changes, or Q waves identify the location of the ischemia, injury, or infarction. The presence of significant Q waves in the chest leads, particularly in V1, V2, V3, and V4, indicates an infarction in the anterior portion of the left ventricle. When only V1 and V2 are involved, these infarctions are often called "septal" infarctions because they primarily affect the interventricular septum. Anterior infarctions are easy to recognize if one remembers that the chest leads are placed on the anterior aspect of the left ventricle (Fig. 9–53). Referring back to Chapter 1, remember that because the left anterior descending artery primarily supplies the anterior aspect of the heart, an anterior infarction implies an occlusion somewhere in the left anterior descending artery.

An inferior infarction is identified by significant Q waves in leads II, III, and aVF (Fig. 9–54). Inferior infarctions are also referred to as *diaphrag-*

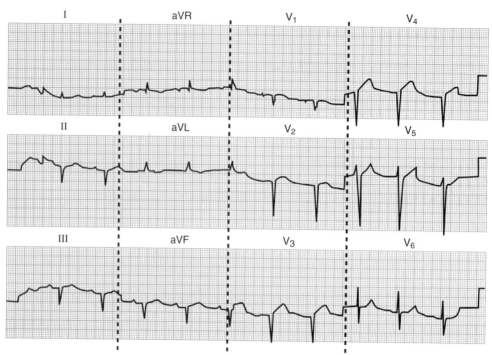

Figure 9–52. A significant Q wave is defined as a minimum of one small square wide and one third the height of the QRS. In this electrocardiogram tracing, notice the Q waves in leads II, III, and aVF and in V1, V2, V3, and V4.

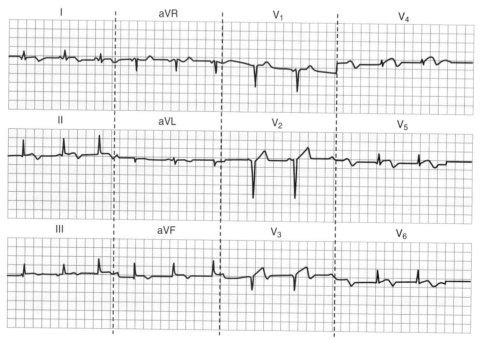

Figure 9–53. A 12-lead electrocardiogram tracing demonstrating an anterior infarction. Note the significant Q waves in V1, V2, and V3 and the inverted T waves throughout many other leads.

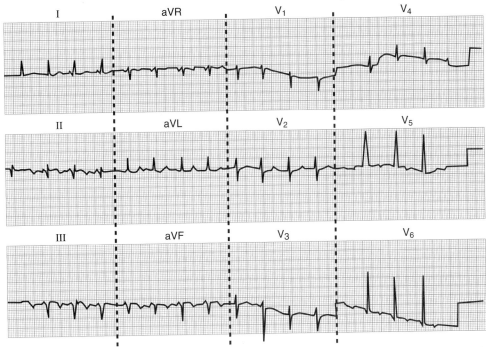

Figure 9–54. A 12-lead electrocardiogram tracing demonstrating an inferior infarction. Notice the significant Q waves in leads II, III, and aVF.

matic infarctions because the inferior wall of the heart rests on the diaphragm. Given that the right coronary artery primarily supplies the inferior aspect of the myocardium, an inferior infarction implies an occlusion somewhere in the right coronary artery. A lateral infarction demonstrates Q waves in leads I and aVL (Fig. 9–55). Because the circumflex artery supplies primarily the lateral and posterior aspects of the myocardium, an occlusion of the circumflex artery is suspected in a lateral infarction.

Probably the most difficult infarction to detect is the posterior infarction because none of the 12 leads is directly measuring the posterior aspect of the heart. Only two leads detect posterior infarcts—V1 and V2—as they measure the direct opposite wall (anterior). Therefore, the direct opposite ECG tracing of an anterior infarction in V1 and V2 should be the ECG tracing of the posterior infarction. An anterior infarction demonstrates a significant Q wave in V1 and V2 with ST-segment elevation. The mirror image of this is seen in Figure 9–56, which demonstrates a large R wave in V1 or V2 and ST-segment depression. Given that the posterior aspect of the myocardium may be

supplied by either the right coronary artery or the circumflex artery, a posterior infarction may indicate a problem in either one of these arteries. If changes in the lateral leads (e.g., I, aVL) also exist, then the circumflex artery is probably involved. However, if changes in the inferior leads exist (e.g., II, III, aVR) as well as posterior changes, then the right coronary artery is probably involved.[8]

Caution should be taken when evaluation of an ECG for an infarction is performed in the presence of left bundle branch block.[8] Identification of significant Q waves can be difficult if the conduction is delayed throughout the myocardium on the left side. Conduction may be delayed through the myocardium owing to a dysfunction in the conduction system that is secondary to genetic defect, injury, or infarction. An example of conduction delay with bundle branch block occurs when a block of the impulse occurs in the right or left bundle branch. A bundle branch block creates a delay of the electrical impulse to the side that is blocked, creating a delay in the depolarization of the myocardium that would have received the blocked impulse. When the left

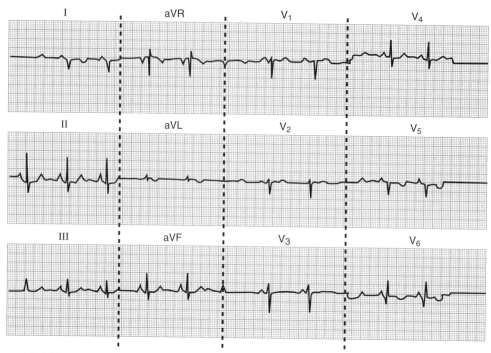

Figure 9–55. A 12-lead electrocardiogram tracing demonstrating a lateral infarction. Notice the significant Q waves in I and V5 with inverted T waves in aVL as well.

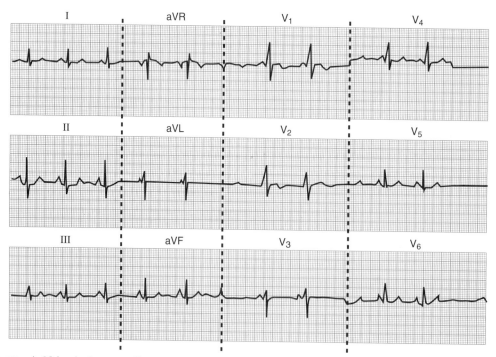

Figure 9–56. A 12-lead electrocardiogram tracing demonstrating a posterior infarction. Notice the large R waves in V1 and V2 and the inverted T waves in the same leads.

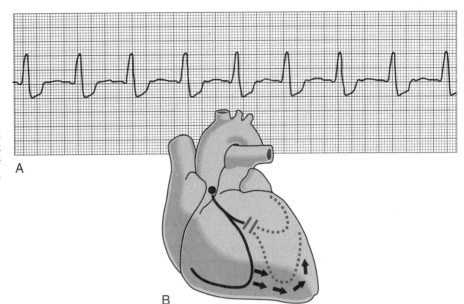

Figure 9–57. *A,* A rhythm strip demonstrating a left bundle branch block. Note the widened QRS interval. *B,* A left bundle branch block.

and right sides do not depolarize simultaneously, a widened QRS appearance is seen on the ECG tracing and sometimes two R waves. In the case of left bundle branch block, the left side of the myocardium demonstrates delayed depolarization, thereby allowing the right side of the myocardium to depolarize first and hiding any possible significant Q waves coming from the left ventricle (Fig. 9–57).

Acute **pericarditis** is a condition that causes ECG changes that differ from those caused by ischemia and infarction. These ECG changes are important to mention because they assist in the diagnosis of the condition. Acute pericarditis, defined as an inflammation of the pericardial sac, is often a complication following myocardial infarc-

tion and open heart surgery. Pericardial pain is usually intense but can closely mimic angina in location. The pain is usually aggravated or relieved by respiration and change of position. The ECG findings include ST-segment elevation, P-R interval depression, late T wave inversion, and atrial arrhythmias (often supraventricular tachycardia) (Fig. 9–58). The symptoms as well as the ECG changes are often all that is needed for diagnosis. In addition, a pericardial rub may be present during auscultation of the heart sounds.

Other abnormalities may exist on the ECG, including pacemaker functioning (Figs. 9–59 and 9–60), which is discussed in Chapter 11, and axis deviation. These abnormalities are beyond the scope of this chapter.

Figure 9–58. The 12-lead electrocardiogram illustrates acute pericarditis. Note the upward concavity of the ST segment (1) and the notching at the junction of the QRS and ST segments (2). (From Abedin Z, Conner R. 12 Lead ECG Interpretation: The Self-Assessment Approach. Philadelphia, WB Saunders, 1989, p 206.)

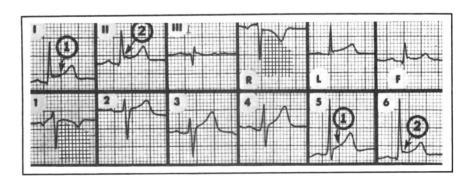

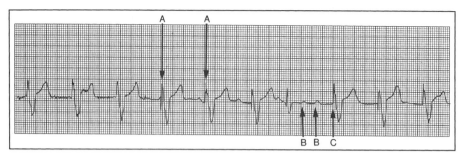

Figure 9–59. Electrocardiogram tracing showing a demand-type pacemaker set at 72 bpm. The pacemaker is firing where the arrows are pointing to straight vertical lines (A). The arrows pointing from below show the patient's own atria firing twice but without ventricular response (B). Therefore, the pacemaker initiated a beat at (C).

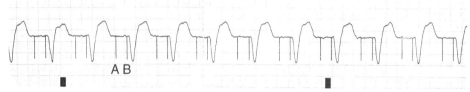

Figure 9–60. Atrioventricular sequential pacemaker rhythm. Notice the two consecutive vertical lines descending from the baseline, followed by a wide QRS complex. The first vertical line (A) initiates the depolarization of the atria, followed by the subsequent vertical line (B) which initiates the depolarization of the ventricle. *Note:* Not all QRS complexes following the firing of a pacemaker are as wide as in this rhythm strip.

CASE STUDIES

Case 1

A 68-year-old man has a history of an acute myocardial infarction that occurred 7 months ago. He subsequently underwent coronary artery bypass graft surgery exactly 1 month after the myocardial infarction. It is now 6 months since his surgery, and he is symptom-free. His goal is to return to his previously active lifestyle, so he was referred for an evaluation and exercise program.

On evaluation, his heart rate is 70, blood pressure is 124/84 mm Hg, and ECG is normal sinus rhythm. During the exercise treadmill test, he exercised at 2.5 miles per hour with 12% grade but complained of dizziness at 4.5 minutes of the exercise test. His heart rate was 110 and blood pressure was 130/78. The ECG rhythm showed a sudden onset of PVCs and a run of ventricular tachycardia. After the exercise was terminated, his rhythm slowed down to frequent PVCs and then normal sinus rhythm.

Discussion: This case demonstrates changes in the heart rhythm with increased activity. PVCs and then ventricular tachycardia occurred with increased activity, corresponding to increased irritability of the myocardium (i.e., probably secondary to ischemia). The individual was symptomatic when the arrhythmias were frequent. This patient should *not* be exercising to a HR of

110 and may need further evaluation for the abnormal response with exercise.

Case 2

A 75-year-old woman suffered a hip fracture and underwent a surgical procedure with hip pinning. Two days after the patient's operation the physical therapy order was for progressive ambulation with a walker using toe-touch gait. The patient had not been out of bed since before the fall. On evaluation, an irregular irregular heart beat was palpated. The ventricular response was approximately 100. Resting blood pressure was 110/70 mm Hg. On sitting, her blood pressure fell to 100/60 and heart rate (still irregular irregular) increased to 120. On standing, the patient complained of dizziness, and her blood pressure dropped to 90/60; her heart rate increased (still irregular irregular) to 140. The patient was returned to bed, and the physician notified. The physician left orders for the patient to spend more time sitting in a chair, so on the next visit the physical therapist brought a telemetry monitor and attached electrodes to assess the patient's rhythm. The monitor indicated that the patient had atrial fibrillation, with a ventricular response of 100 while lying supine. On sitting, heart rate again increased and blood pressure fell; the rhythm demonstrated atrial fibrillation, with a ventricular response of 120.

Discussion: This patient is experiencing uncontrolled atrial fibrillation with an HR of 100 at rest. This limits functional activity. As cardiac output is decreased when atrial fibrillation is present due to the lack of the "atrial kick," this patient may have improved performance with medication that would help the contractility of the myocardium as well as the lowering of the heart rate.

Case 3

A 21-year-old female physical therapy student was sitting in class listening to a lecture and reported that her heart was racing away and that she felt slightly lightheaded. The student had never had any real illnesses or any history of cardiac problems. When the same symptoms occurred a second time she informed one of the faculty, who happened to have an ECG monitor in her office. The student was told to wear the ECG monitor to her next class. Fortunately, the student had the same recurring symptoms, and the monitor recorded a run of paroxysmal atrial tachycardia. On auscultation of heart sounds, the student was found to have a midsystolic click. The student was referred for a full cardiac evaluation following the documented episode. The student was found to have benign mitral valve prolapse and was told to monitor episodes for frequency of occurrence and symptoms.

Discussion: Paroxysmal atrial tachycardia is a very common, usually benign, arrhythmia associated with mitral valve prolapse.

Summary

- Four cell types exist in the myocardium: working or mechanical cells, nodal cells, transitional cells, and Purkinje's cells.
- Depolarization of the cell membrane allows the influx of sodium ions into the cell and the efflux of potassium ions.
- As the cell becomes positive on the interior, the myocardial cells are stimulated to contract (called excitation coupling).
- On the ECG, the wave of depolarization is recorded as an upward deflection when moving toward a positive electrode (located on the skin).
- The cardiac muscle has three properties: automaticity, rhythmicity, and conductivity.
- The autonomic nervous system has a major influence on the cardiac system. Stimulation of the sympathetic division increases the heart rate, conduction velocity, and contractile force, and stimulation of the parasympathetic division (act-

ing primarily via the vagal nerve) slows the heart rate and the conduction through the AV node.
- The conduction system involves the spread of a stimulus via the SA node (primary pacemaker), internodal pathways, AV node, His's bundle, bundle branches, and Purkinje's fibers.
- The ECG records the electrical activity of the heart on ruled graph paper. Time is represented on the horizontal axis, and each small square is 0.04 second. Voltage is recorded on the vertical axis, and each small square is 1 mm.
- A standard 12-lead ECG consists of six limb leads and six chest leads, each recording the electrical activity from a different angle and providing a different view of the same activity in the heart.
- The ECG is reviewed to identify four areas that require interpretation: heart rate, heart rhythm, hypertrophy, and infarction.
- Numerous methods can be employed to measure heart rate from the ECG tracing, but often the 6-second strip method is the easiest if the rhythm is regular.
- Hypertrophy is detected on a 12-lead ECG by looking at the waveforms, particularly at the P wave and QRS complex for the voltage (greater than 3 mV) or configuration.
- Left ventricular hypertrophy is present if the depth of the S wave in V1 plus the height of the R wave in V5 is greater than 35 mm.
- In the presence of acute injury, the ST segment is elevated above the isoelectric line and gradually returns to the level of the isoelectric line over a period of 24 to 48 hours.
- In ventricular aneurysm, the ST segment remains elevated and does not return to the isoelectric line over time.
- ST-segment depression at rest associated with chest pain may indicate acute injury to the subendocardial wall.
- ST-segment depression that develops during exercise is an ischemic response to activity and following rest should return to the baseline.
- The presence of a significant Q wave is diagnostic for an infarction, but the date of the infarction cannot be determined from the ECG.
- A significant Q wave is 1 mm wide or one third the size of the QRS complex.
- A 12-lead ECG is used primarily for determining ischemia or infarction. Single-lead monitoring is employed for evaluating heart rate or rhythm.
- The location of the infarction is determined by

the leads on the 12-lead ECG that demonstrate changes.

- The presence of significant Q waves in V1 through V4 indicates an anterior infarction and probable involvement of the left anterior descending coronary artery.
- The presence of significant Q waves in II, III, and aVF indicates an inferior infarction and probable involvement of the right coronary artery.
- A systematic approach should be taken when evaluating the rhythm strip. All the waveform configurations should be evaluated, as well as the P-R intervals, the QRS intervals, the R-R intervals, and the rate to assess the rhythm disturbance.
- Following identification of the rhythm disturbance, an assessment of signs and symptoms should be undertaken, after which a clinical decision can be made regarding the amount of monitoring the individual will need with activity as well as the safety of activity.

References

1. Cohen M, Fuster V. Insights into the pathogenetic mechanisms of unstable angina. Haemostasis 20(suppl 1):102–112, 1990.
2. Schaper J, Schaper W. Time course of myocardial necrosis. Cardiovasc Drugs Ther 2(1):17–25, 1988.
3. Bekn Haim SA, Becker B, Edoute Y, et al. Beat to beat electrocardiographic morphology variation in healed myocardial infarction. Am J Cardiol 68(8):725–728, 1991.
4. Phillips RE, Feeney MK. The Cardiac Rhythms: A Systematic Approach to Interpretation. 3rd ed. Philadelphia, WB Saunders, 1990.
5. Scheidt S. Basic Electrocardiography: Leads, Axes, Arrhythmias. New Jersey, CIBA Clinical Symposia, 1983.
6. Berne RM, Levy MN. Cardiovascular Physiology. 6th ed. St. Louis, Mosby–Year Book, 1992.
7. Grauer K, Curry RW. Clinical Electrocardiography: A Primary Care Approach. 2nd ed. Boston, Blackwell Scientific Publishers, 1992.
8. Abedin Z, Conner RP. 12 Lead ECG Interpretation: The Self-Assessment Approach. Philadelphia, WB Saunders, 1989.
9. Valle BK, Lemberg L. Non-Q wave versus nontransmural infarction. Heart Lung 19(2):208–211, 1990.

Suggested Readings

Abedin Z, Conner RP. 12 Lead ECG Interpretation: The Self-Assessment Approach. Philadelphia, WB Saunders, 1989.
Andreoli KG, Fowkes VH, Zipes DP, Wallace AC. Comprehensive Cardiac Care. 7th ed. St. Louis, CV Mosby, 1987.
Bean DY. Introduction to ECG Interpretation. Rockville, Md, Aspen Publishers, 1987.
Cumins R. (ed). American Heart Association Advanced Cardiac Life Support. Dallas, American Heart Association, 1994.
Dubin D. Rapid ECG Interpretation. 3rd ed. Tampa, Fla, Cover Publishing, 1974.
Fenstermacher K. Dysrhythmia Recognition and Management. Philadelphia, WB Saunders, 1989.
Fisch C. Electrocardiography of Arrhythmias. Philadelphia, Lea & Febiger, 1990.
Grauer K, Curry RW. Clinical Electrocardiography: A Primary Care Approach. 2nd ed. Boston, Blackwell Scientific Publications, 1992.
Marriott HJL. Practical Electrocardiography. 8th ed. Baltimore, Williams & Wilkins, 1988.
McIntyre K, Lewis J (eds). Textbook of Advanced Cardiac Life Support. Dallas, American Heart Association, 1983.
Wiederhold R. Electrocardiography: The Monitoring Lead. Philadelphia, WB Saunders, 1988.

10

Pulmonary Diagnostic Tests and Procedures

H. Steven Sadowsky

INTRODUCTION

This chapter presents the reader with an introduction to several of the diagnostic tests and procedures commonly utilized in the assessment of patients with pulmonary disease. Although the tests and procedures described in this chapter are not necessarily performed by physical therapists, they nonetheless provide them with invaluable information. In order to apply this information to the planning, implementation, and monitoring of patient treatments, physical therapists must have a fundamental understanding of chest imaging, pulmonary function testing, bronchoscopy, arterial blood gas analysis, oximetry, and bacteriologic and cytologic tests. The incorporation of this information in the evaluative process is discussed in Chapter 17.

421

CHEST IMAGING

Largely as a result of new technologies, but also because of refinements in older techniques, there are now several imaging options in addition to the standard "plain film" radiograph. It is certainly beyond the scope of this text to present all the abnormal chest findings identifiable by these imaging techniques. Rather, this information is intended to assist in the development of a framework on which to build an understanding of these imaging techniques. A basic knowledge of how these images are produced and what they display can facilitate physician-therapist dialogue and enhance physical therapy treatment planning.

X-Rays

X-rays are produced whenever high-speed electrons undergo sudden deceleration. In an x-ray machine, electrons flowing through a wire in a vacuum-sealed cathode ray tube are focused to strike a small area on a positively charged anodal plate, resulting in the emission of x-rays. Traveling at the speed of light, x-rays have a very high frequency and a relatively short wavelength. X-rays are not reflected back like light rays; instead, they penetrate matter and are invisible. Certain phosphors become fluorescent when excited by x-rays, and these may be placed on fluorescent screens that are superimposed over photographic film to make an x-ray cassette. For a standard upright chest film, a patient is typically placed between an x-ray source and a cassette (Fig. 10–1). When the x-rays penetrate the tissues of the patient, they stimulate the fluorescent screen to emit light that exposes the film. Because scattered radiation reduces subject contrast, several different scatter reduction techniques (e.g., grids, air-gap, moving slits) are used to decrease the incidence of scattered x-rays striking the film cassette.[1–4] The radiograph thus produced is also referred to as a **roentgenogram** after Wilhelm Konrad Roentgen, who received the first Nobel Prize for Physics in 1901 for his work in defining the major properties of x-rays and the conditions necessary for their production. It was Roentgen who coined the term "x-ray."

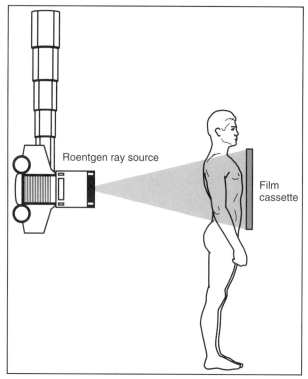

Roentgen ray source

Film cassette

Figure 10–1. For a standard posteroanterior radiograph the patient stands between the film cassette and x-ray source.

Radiographs

Despite the availability of newer methods, in most clinical settings the standard radiograph remains the predominant medium by which anatomic abnormalities resulting from pathologic processes within the chest are assessed. Consequently, a significant portion of this chapter will be devoted to the chest x-ray. The newer, more technologically advanced imaging techniques are discussed in lesser detail later in this chapter; they are generally used for the confirmatory or differential diagnostic information that they can contribute to that already obtained from a chest x-ray.

Chest radiographs provide a static view of the anatomy of the chest, and as such, they may be used to screen for abnormalities, to provide a baseline from which subsequent assessments can be made, or to monitor the progress of a disease process or treatment intervention. The principal objects shown on a chest radiograph are air, fat, water, tissue, and bone. Air in the lungs has a very low density and thus allows greater x-ray penetration, resulting in a dark image on the radiograph—**radiolucency.** At the opposite extreme is bone, which, because it is denser, allows fewer x-rays to penetrate and results in a white image on a radiograph—**radiopacity.** Depending on the densities and thicknesses of the numerous structures in the chest, the x-rays penetrating a patient are variably absorbed and create "shadows" on the x-ray film. Several other factors also affect the image depicted on a x-ray film, but are beyond the scope of this chapter. Therefore, the reader is referred to standard radiology texts for more detailed information.

The standard chest radiograph, as typically obtained in a radiology department, is routinely taken in two views: (1) a *posteroanterior* (PA) *view* with the patient in the standing position with the front of the chest facing the film cassette (Fig. 10–2) and (2) a *left lateral view* (Fig. 10–3), unless the pathologic process is known to be present on the right side of the chest (in which case, a right lateral view would be obtained). The lateral view is extremely helpful in localizing the position of an abnormality, because in the PA view the upper

and middle lobes of the lung override portions of the lower lobes. Other views that may be obtained include the following:

- *Decubitus views* are taken to confirm the presence of an air-fluid level in the lungs or a small pleural effusion. Depending upon the location of the suspected disease, the patient is placed in the supine, prone, or right or left side-lying position.
- The *lordotic view* is used to visualize the apical or middle (right middle lobe or left lingular segments) regions of the lungs, or specifically to screen for pulmonary tuberculosis, which typically manifests itself in the apical regions. The x-ray source is lowered and angled upward, and the patient may or may not be tipped slightly backward.
- *Oblique views* are taken to detect pleural thickening, to evaluate the carina, or to visualize the heart and great vessels. The patient is positioned standing diagonally (at an angle of 45 to 60 degrees to the film) with either the left or right anterior, or the left or right posterior, chest against the film cassette (anterior or posterior oblique views, respectively).

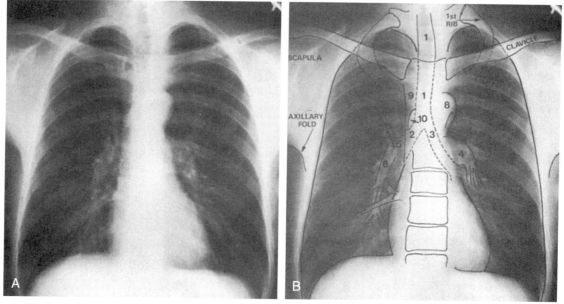

Figure 10–2. *A,* Normal chest radiograph—posteroanterior view. *B,* Same radiograph as in *A,* with the normal anatomic structures labeled or numbered: 1, trachea; 2, right mainstem bronchus; 3, left mainstem bronchus; 4, left pulmonary artery; 5, pulmonary vein to the right upper lobe; 6, right interlobular artery; 7, vein to right middle and lower lobes; 8, aortic knob; 9, superior vena cava. (From Fraser RG, Paré JAP. Diagnosis of Diseases of the Chest. Vol I. 2nd ed. Philadelphia, WB Saunders, 1977, pp 172, 173.)

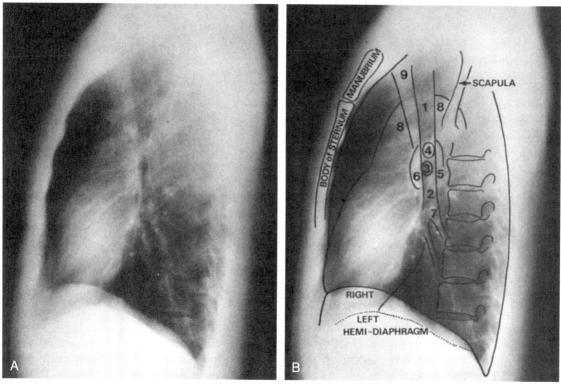

Figure 10–3. *A,* Normal chest radiograph—lateral view. *B,* Same radiograph as in *A,* with the normal anatomic structures labeled or numbered: 1, trachea; 2, right intermediate bronchus; 3, left upper lobe bronchus; 4, right upper lobe bronchus; 5, left interlobar artery; 6, right interlobar artery; 7, junction of the pulmonary veins; 8, aortic arch; 9, brachiocephalic vessels. (From Fraser RG, Paré JAP. Diagnosis of Diseases of the Chest. Vol I. 2nd ed. Philadelphia, WB Saunders, 1977, pp 174, 175.)

• The *anteroposterior (AP) view* is taken at the patient's bedside when the patient is unable to travel to the radiology department. AP radiographs are obtained with the patient either supine, semirecumbent, or sitting upright against the film cassette and facing the x-ray machine. When the film is take in the supine position, the abdominal contents tend to elevate the hemidiaphragms, the pulmonary blood flow is redistributed, and the mediastinal structures appear larger (Fig. 10–4).

The potential interpreter of radiographs is presented with several challenges, among these are the two-dimensional representation of three-dimensional objects, and the limited gray-scale "shadow" depiction of the various organs, tissues, and pathologic processes. Although it may be more likely that the clinician will have access to a radiologist's report rather than the actual radiograph, many clinical settings offer the therapist direct access to a patient's chest radiographs. Consequently, therapists should be familiar with the manner in which chest radiographs are assessed.

Examining Chest Radiographs

There is no single "best" method for examining chest radiographs, nevertheless, a systematic approach should be utilized. One approach entails starting at the center of the film and working out-

Clinical Note: Anteroposterior View

Positioning for AP views may result in a poor inspiratory effort, especially when the patient is critically ill. Clinicians observing AP films must keep this in mind when assessing the film.

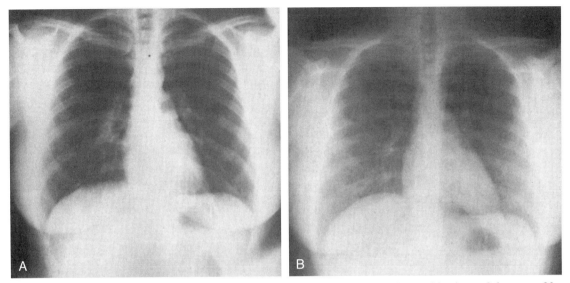

Figure 10–4. Comparison of posteroanterior (*A*) and anteroposterior (*B*) radiographic views of the same 30-year-old female. (From Kersten LD. Comprehensive Respiratory Nursing: A Decision Making Approach. Philadelphia, WB Saunders, 1989, pp 408, 409.)

ward toward the soft tissues. Another method involves starting with an examination of the bones and soft tissues, including the abdomen; the mediastinum from the larynx to the abdomen; the cardiovascular system; the hila; and finally the lung fields themselves. Independent of the method of examination, the mediastinum and hila are typically assessed for abnormal vasculature or mass lesions, the heart for changes in shape or position, and the lungs for abnormal increased density or lucency. By convention, frontal chest radiographs should be viewed as if the patient's right side was on your left side, as if you were facing each other. The left lateral chest radiograph should be viewed as if the patient's left side was facing you; the reverse is true for the right lateral view.

In the body systems approach to examining chest radiographs the overall adequacy of the image should first be addressed. The optimal radiograph should be taken with the patient holding a deep inspiration. Furthermore, the entire chest should be visible on the radiograph (see Fig. 10–2). Then, the following should be considered in turn:

• Bones and soft tissues. The size, shape, and symmetry of the bony thorax should be considered; the vertebral bodies should be faintly visible through the mediastinal shadow, and all of the other bones of the thorax should be included on the radiograph. To determine whether or not the patient is rotated to either side, the medial ends of each clavicle should be checked to see that they are equally distant from the spinous processes of the vertebral bodies (if the patient is rotated, the distances between the medial ends of the clavicles and the spinous processes will be unequal). In a PA film the clavicles often appear to be lower than in an AP film. Because of the position of the shoulders, the medial aspect of the scapulas are typically lateral to and outside the lung fields in a PA film; whereas, in an AP film, the medial borders may appear as vertical or oblique lines within the lung fields.

The various densities of the soft tissues (skin, subcutaneous fat, and muscle) normally blend together—called the **summation effect.** The width of the intercostal spaces should be considered because widened intercostal spaces may be indicative of increased thoracic volume (the best way to gain an appreciation of the normal intercostal space width is to review normal chest radiographs).

The two hemidiaphragms should appear as rounded, smooth, sharply defined shadows; the dome of the right hemidiaphragm is normally 1 to 2 cm higher than the left. The diaphragm is said to be *elevated* if, during a deep inhalation, fewer than nine ribs are visible above the level of the domes; *depressed* if more than ten ribs are visible. Where the hemidiaphragms meet the chest wall at their lateral aspects, the **costophrenic angles** are formed. The costophrenic angles are moderately deep, and they are approximately equal in size on the two sides. Opacification of the costophrenic angle is indicative of either pleural thickening (if the change has occurred over many months or years) or a pleural effusion (if the change has occurred recently). Medially, the hemidiaphragms normally form a *cardiophrenic angle* where they meet the borders of the heart.

- Mediastinum, trachea and cardiovascular system. The size of the mediastinum varies with body size, ranging from long and narrow in tall, thin persons to short and wide in short, stocky persons. Regardless, the borders of the mediastinum are generally as outlined in Figure 1–20. The trachea normally appears as a vertical translucent shadow superimposed on the mediastinal shadow in the midline, overlying the cervical vertebrae. In most cases, tracheal deviation from the midline position suggests that the patient is rotated. However, pathologic conditions can also result in tracheal deviation. For example, a large pneumothorax can push the trachea toward the contralateral side of the chest, or a massive atelectasis can pull the trachea toward the ipsilateral side of the chest. Visualization of the tracheal shadow is particularly important if the patient is intubated (has an endotracheal tube in place), because proper positioning of the endotracheal tube is determined by the proximity of its distal end to the tracheal bifurcation. The tip of a properly placed endotracheal tube should be about 2 inches above the carina when the patient's head is in the neutral position.

The heart and great vessels occupy the lower two thirds of the mediastinum, giving the mediastinum a characteristic profile. There are two distinct curves that should be noted on the right side of the cardiovascular shadow. The first, formed entirely by the right atrium, begins at the right cardiophrenic angle and proceeds superiorly. The inferior vena cava IVC) can often be seen entering the right atrium, inferiorly. The ascending aorta and the superior vena cava (SVC) form the second curve. On the left side, there are typically four curves of importance. The transverse arch and descending aorta form the first curve before the aorta passes behind the main pulmonary artery, which makes the next curve. The third curve may or may not be visible and denotes the site of the left atrial appendage. The border of the left ventricle extends downward to the diaphragm, forming the fourth curve.

- The hila. Formed by the root of the lungs (comprising the pulmonary blood vessels, the bronchi and a group of lymph nodes) the hila are at about the T4–T5 level and appear as poorly defined areas of variable density in the medial part of the central portion of the lung fields. The left hilum is partially obscured by the overlying shadow of the heart and great vessels, and it lies at a slightly higher level than the right hilum.

- The lung fields. Although the lobes of the lung cannot normally be distinguished, knowledge of lobar and segmental anatomy is crucial to an assessment of the lung fields. The left and right upper lobes and the right middle lobe lie superiorly and anteriorly within the thoracic cavity, while the lower lobes occupy the posteroinferior aspects. Although the medial segment of the right middle lobe is in contact with the right border of the heart, and the lingular segments of the left upper lobe are in contact with the left border of the heart, the lobes overlap each other considerably so that a clear localization of each lobe is not possible in the PA or AP view alone. A lateral view is essential in order to delineate accurately the lobes of the lungs and their various bronchopulmonary segments.

The *silhouette sign* (present when the normal line of demarcation between two structures is partially or completely obliterated) may be used to localize lesions within the lung fields.[5] In the critical care setting, life-support and monitoring equipment can complicate the interpretation of a chest radiograph, as demonstrated in Figure 10–5.

Clinical Note: Chronic Obstructive Pulmonary Disease

The radiograph of a patient with moderate to severe COPD will show widened intercostal spaces, flattened hemidiaphragms, squared off costophrenic angles, and rib angles that approach 90-degree angles.

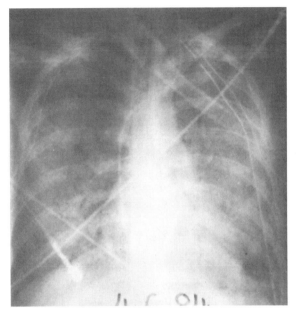

Figure 10–5. Anteroposterior radiographic view of a patient with adult respiratory distress syndrome, illustrating the additional shadows of life-support and monitoring equipment. (From Dantzker DR. Cardiopulmonary Critical Care. 2nd ed. Philadelphia, WB Saunders, 1977, p 370.)

The airways outside the mediastinum are not usually visible on a chest radiograph because of their thin walls and air-filled lumens. However, the pulmonary arteries and veins can frequently be seen as they branch and taper outward toward the periphery until they disappear in the outer third of the lung fields. By observing serial films, these *vascular markings* can be described as unchanged, increased, or decreased. Increased vascular markings are indicative of venous dilatation, while decreased vascular markings may indicate hyperinflation of the lungs.

Specific lung lesions are assessed by observing the lung fields for any abnormal density that obliterates the vascular markings or that alters the distribution of the densities within the lung fields. The lung fields should be assessed for any abnormal patterns of radiopacity. If present,

Clinical Note: Distinguishing Acute and Chronic Changes

The therapist should be able to observe the chest radiograph and distinguish between acute changes and chronic changes. Acute changes would include fluffy infiltrates or increased opacity. Chronic changes include flattened diaphragms, changes in rib angle and intercostal spaces, abnormal lung volumes, and interstitial thickening.

these abnormal patterns are typically described as either *alveolar patterns* or *interstitial patterns*, and they may be independently localized or diffuse or coexistent. Alveolar patterns are sometimes described as 'fluffy infiltrates'; they represent pathologic changes within the distal airways, e.g., pulmonary edema or alveolar pneumonia (Fig. 10–6). In contrast, interstitial patterns represent interstitial thickening, e.g., inflammation (Fig. 10–7). Interstitial disease may also assume the appearance of fine diffuse nodularity throughout the lungs. If they are of uniform size, they are called miliary nodules. The pattern of increased pulmonary vascularity often strongly resembles the interstitial pattern.

Some neonatal pulmonary diseases have unique radiographic presentations. Nevertheless, the same

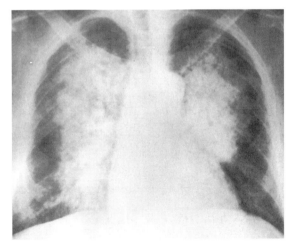

Figure 10–6. An example of the alveolar filling pattern associated with pulmonary edema in a 59-year-old male, 48 hours following a massive myocardial infarction. (From Fraser RG, Paré JAP. Diagnosis of Diseases of the Chest. Vol. II 2nd ed. Philadelphia, WB Saunders, 1977, p 1252.)

Clinical Note: Vascular Markings

Vascular markings that are increased are indicative of early left ventricular failure.

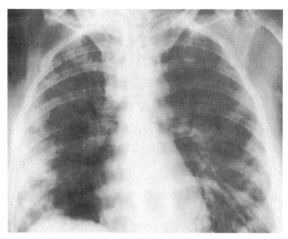

Figure 10–7. An example of the interstitial pattern associated with interstitial thickening secondary to an inflammatory process. (From Fraser RG, Paré JAP. Diagnosis of Diseases of the Chest. Vol II. 2nd ed. Philadelphia, WB Saunders, 1977, p 1289.)

Computed tomography (CT), or digital chest radiography, involves a narrow beam of x-rays moving across the field of examination in such a way as to define successive adjacent columns of tissue—a process called *translation*. Another pass is then made at a different angle—the new angle is referred to as a *rotation*. The process is repeated many times, with subsequent digitization of each analogue image into a numerical form by means of computer-based processing. Each digital image is an array (matrix) of numbers; each number representing a single element of the picture (pixel) and the value of the number defining the degree of brightness or darkness of that particular point in the image. Several digital images are then mathematically manipulated to produce a summated image for diagnostic interpretation.

general principles of radiologic assessment that are used in the assessment of older children and adults apply. To this end, the assessment must determine whether the problem is in the lungs, the heart, the mediastinum (distinct from the heart), or the thoracic wall.

Regardless of the source of the information that details the results of a radiographic chest examination, the data provided can be invaluable to the physical therapist in facilitating the choice and planning of treatment interventions and in the subsequent evaluation of treatment efficacy. Several additional chest-imaging techniques can provide the clinician with information upon which decisions regarding treatment planning or efficacy may be made. several of these techniques are briefly described here.

Tomography

Standard tomography, or sectional radiography, involves the curvilinear movement of the x-ray source and the film or screen system in opposite directions about the patient (Fig. 10–8) The shadow of the selected plane remains stationary on the moving film, while the shadows of all other planes are obliterated by their relative displacement. Standard tomography has been somewhat obviated by techniques such as computed tomography and ultrasound.[6, 7]

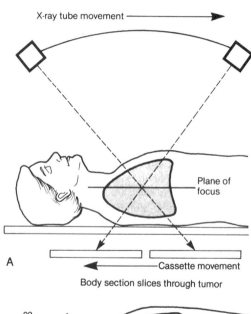

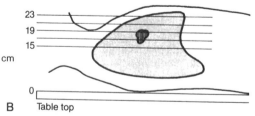

Figure 10–8. Obtaining a tomographic image of the chest. *A,* One of many focal planes that produce a tomographic image of the chest obtained as the x-ray source and the film cassette are moved. *B,* An example of several focal planes that isolate an area of pathology. (From Kersten LD. Comprehensive Respiratory Nursing: A Decision Making Approach. Philadelphia, WB Saunders, 1989, p 413.)

Magnetic Resonance Imaging

Magnetic resonance imaging (MRI) involves the interaction of stimulated hydrogen nuclei and a strong magnetic field. A MRI scanner produces a gradient magnetic field in the region of the body to be imaged. The hydrogen nuclei tend to align themselves with the magnetic field and resonate at a frequency that is proportional to the strength of the magnetic field. The gradient of nuclear resonance is proportional to the gradient of the magnetic field—magnetic resonance. The patient is then exposed to a radio signal that stimulates those nuclei whose magnetic resonance is the same as the frequency of the radio signal. These stimulated nuclei re-emit the radio signal, which is picked up by an antenna in the MRI scanner and digitally recorded by a computer, isolating a "slice of tissue" in much the same manner as that for a CT image. As soon as the re-emitted signal is recorded, a new gradient is produced in a perpendicular plane to the original slice and this new slice is stimulated and recorded. The original gradient is then restored. This excitation and retrieval process is repeated many times with the transverse gradient being applied at a slightly different angle each time.[8] The data thus obtained may be mathematically manipulated to produce a final enhanced image for interpretation, an example of which is shown in Figure 10–9. A MRI is primarily indicated for the evaluation of chest wall processes that may involve bone, muscle, fat, or pleura.

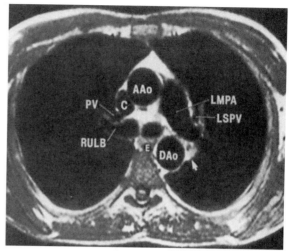

Figure 10–9. An example of a magnetic resonance image of the chest showing normal anatomy at the level of the carina. RULB, Right upper lobe bronchus; PV, right superior pulmonary vein; C, superior vena cava; AAo, ascending aorta; DAo, descending aorta; E, esophagus; LMPA, left main pulmonary artery; LSPV, left superior pulmonary vein. (From Naidich DP, Zerhouni EA, Siegelman SS. Computed Tomography and Magnetic Resonance of the Thorax. 2nd ed. New York, Raven Press, 1991, p 239.)

Clinical Note: Indications for MRI

MRIs may be indicated in individuals with abnormal chest radiographs that show a nodule or mass. An MRI could show an enhanced picture of the mass prior to surgical resection or biopsy, or may be used to enhance the pleural area to distinguish between fibrosis and the presence of nodules.

Bronchography

Bronchography is occasionally needed for the evaluation and management of some congenital pulmonary anomalies as well as some acquired diseases, usually of the tracheobronchial tree.[9] *Bronchograms* permit the study of normal and variant anatomy, and of gross pathologic changes in the bronchial wall and lumen. Contrast bronchography involves the opacification of the bronchial tree by the installation of contrast medium so that the radiographic shadows of the airways may be studied. A bronchogram demonstrating bronchiectasis of the left lower lobe bronchi is shown in Figure 10–10.

Ventilation and Perfusion Scans

Several different tests can be used to measure the gas distribution in the lungs. To measure the regional distribution of ventilation in the lungs the patient breathes xenon gas (^{133}Xe). The test is usually performed with the patient in a sitting or supine position. The patient is asked to inhale a normal tidal volume from a closed system containing a specific volume or concentration of xenon, and then to hold the breath for several seconds while photoscintigrams—ventilation scans—are made over the lung field. To determine the rate of equilibrium of the gas in the lungs, serial photoscintigrams are made over a 10- to 15-minute period with the use of a rebreathing technique.

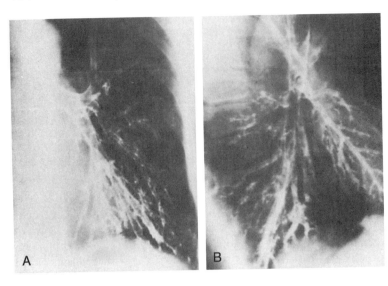

Figure 10–10. Posteroanterior (*A*) and lateral (*B*) bronchograms of the left lower lobe bronchi demonstrating the typical dilatations of bronchiectasis. (From Paré JAP, Fraser RG. Synopsis of Diseases of the Chest. Philadelphia, WB Saunders, 1983, p 561.)

Finally, to determine the washout rate of the xenon gas, the patient is returned to atmospheric breathing while serial photoscintigrams are made.

To measure the regional distribution of pulmonary blood flow in the lungs the patient is injected intravenously with radioactive iodine (^{131}I) and serial photoscintigrams—perfusion scans—are made over the lung fields as the blood perfuses the lungs.

NORMAL

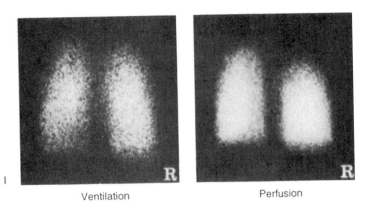

Ventilation   Perfusion

PULMONARY EMBOLISM

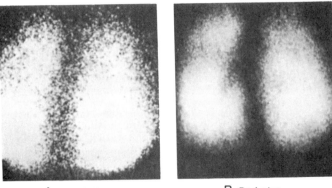

A Ventilation   B Perfusion

Figure 10–11. Examples of ventilation/perfusion scans. *Top,* Normal ventilation/perfusion scan. *Bottom,* Ventilation/perfusion scan of a patient with a pulmonary embolism showing a normal ventilation scan and an abnormal perfusion scan. (From Fraser RG, Paré JAP. Diagnosis of Diseases of the Chest. Vol I. 2nd ed. Philadelphia, WB Saunders, 1977, pp 234, 235.)

Clinical Note: Ventilation-Perfusion Scans

Ventilation-perfusion scans are usually indicated to rule out pulmonary emboli, particularly in individuals with deep-vein thrombosis.

Although they may be performed as separate tests, ventilation and perfusion scans (V/Q scans) provide the maximum amount of information when used together. Such information describes how the alveolar ventilation and pulmonary perfusion are matched in the patient. In the normal person, the V/Q scans will show greater ventilation and perfusion in the bases of the lung and less ventilation and perfusion in the apices. Normal and abnormal V/Q scans are shown in Figure 10–11.

BRONCHOSCOPY

Fiberoptic bronchoscopy has markedly decreased the necessity for contrast bronchography by permitting the direct visualization of previously inaccessible areas of the bronchial tree.[10] The typical bronchoscopic appearance of the segmental origins within each lobe is depicted in Figure 10–12.

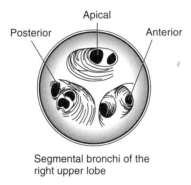

Segmental bronchi of the right upper lobe

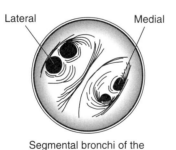

Segmental bronchi of the right middle lobe

Figure 10–12. Typical bronchoscopic appearance of the segmental bronchi of each lung.

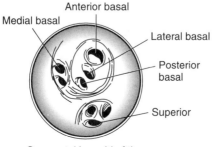

Segmental bronchi of the right lower lobe

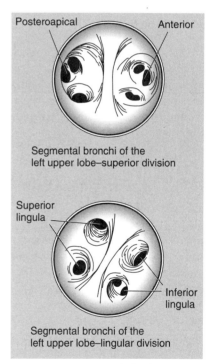

Segmental bronchi of the left upper lobe–superior division

Segmental bronchi of the left upper lobe–lingular division

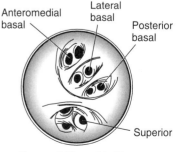

Segmental bronchi of the left lower lobe

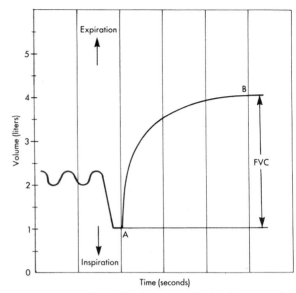

Figure 10–13. Typical spirogram obtained as a patient exhales forcefully. (From Ruppel G. Manual of Pulmonary Function Testing. St. Louis, CV Mosby, 1986, p 28.)

PULMONARY FUNCTION TESTING

Pulmonary function tests (PFTs) provide the clinician with information about the integrity of the airways, the function of the respiratory musculature, and the condition of the lung tissues themselves. A thorough evaluation of pulmonary function involves several tests that measure lung volumes and capacities, gas flow rates, gas diffusion, and gas distribution. Based on the results of PFTs, pulmonary diseases may be classified into three basic categories: obstructive, restrictive, or combined. A working knowledge of the principal test and an ability to interpret their findings are essential to the planning and implementation of effective interventions.

Tests of Lung Volume and Capacity

The basic lung volumes and capacities are defined in Chapter 2, and with the notable exception of the residual volume (RV), and therefore the functional residual capacity (FRC) and total lung capacity (TLC), lung volumes are measured by means of simple spirometry. Spirometers may be of the traditional manual waterseal type, or they may be electronic computerized devices (e.g., pneumotachometer). In either case, a graphic tracing—called a **spirogram**—of the lung volumes is typically produced to facilitate interpretation of the measurements (Fig. 10–13).

Many spirometric measurements can be accurately conducted at the bedside using relatively uncomplicated equipment (Fig. 10–14), although others necessitate the equipment found in a pulmonary function laboratory (Fig. 10–15). In either setting, the patient should be positioned in an upright sitting posture and a nose clip should be used. The patient should breathe normally into the spirometer (or other appropriate instrument) through a tight-fitting mouthpiece until a normal rhythm is established. The following is a brief description of the manner in which the spirometrically determined volumes and capacities are measured.

- Tidal volume (VT) is the total volume of air (V) moved during either inhalation or exhalation over a specific period of time (usually 1 minute) is measured, and then divided by the ventilatory rate (f): VT = V/f. The average healthy adult's VT is around 500 mL (± about 100 mL), but because there is a great deal of variability within the normal population, measurements outside the normal range (400 to 600 mL) do not necessarily indicate the presence of a disease process.
- Inspiratory reserve volume (IRV) is a component of the inspiratory capacity. The IRV has been suggested to be a valuable index of changes in resting lung hyperinflation following anticholinergic therapy in patients with chronic obstructive pulmonary disease.[11]
- Expiratory reserve volume (ERV) is assessed by having the patient to exhale maximally after a few normal breaths. The normal ERV is approximately 1000 mL, but restrictive disease processes

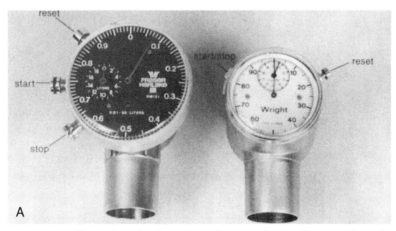
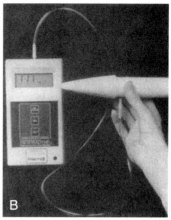

Figure 10–14. Examples of spirometers that can be used to conduct simple spirometric measurements at a patient's bedside. (From Kersten LD. Comprehensive Respiratory Nursing: A Decision Making Approach. Philadelphia, WB Saunders, 1989, Figs. 14–17, 14–18, pp 386, 387.)

(see discussion in Chapter 5) typically result in a reduced ERV.

- Vital capacity (VC) is measured by having the patient first inhale as deeply as possible, and then exhaling fully, taking as much time as is necessary to exhale completely. The normal VC ranges between 4000 to 5000 mL, representing approximately 80% of the TLC, but normal values can vary significantly, depending on age, sex, and test position. Although the VC may be normal in the early to moderate stages of obstructive lung disease, it is generally reduced in severe obstructive lung diseases. Restrictive diseases, too, may cause the VC to be decreased.
- Inspiratory capacity (IC) is measured by asking the patient to inhale maximally following a normal exhalation. The IC normally varies between 3000 and 4000 mL, but it varies widely in the normal population. The IC should represent about 75% to 80% of the vital capacity (VC) and around 55% to 60% of the TLC. Although normal values can be observed in both obstructive and restrictive lung diseases, the IC is generally reduced in both disease states. Increases in the IC usually indicate poor initial patient participation.

Residual volume (RV) is not measured directly with simple spirometry. In fact, most pulmonary function tests actually measure the FRC (by using the formula RV = FRC − ERV, the RV is then calculated).[12-14] The three most commonly used methods for determining the FRC and RV are the helium dilution method, the nitrogen washout method, and body plethysmography:

- Helium dilution method (closed-circuit method). Following a normal exhalation, the patient is connected to a closed spirometer system and breathes a known volume and concentration of helium (He) until an equilibrium is reached (carbon dioxide is eliminated through a carbon dioxide absorbent and oxygen is added at a rate equal to the oxygen consumption). Once equilibrium is reached, the FRC is calculated from the change in He concentration in the spirometer (e.g., the larger the patient's lung volume, the less the He concentration in the spirometer). It normally takes less than 5 minutes for equilibrium of the He between the patient and the spirometer to occur; however, in patients with severe obstructive disease it can take up to 30 minutes.
- Nitrogen washout method (open-circuit method). As in the He dilution test, the patient is connected to the system at the end of an exhalation. The nitrogen (N_2) concentration in the lungs is in equilibrium with the atmosphere approximately 79% so that as the patient inhales pure oxygen from the spirometer, the N_2 is "washed out" of the lungs. Because the volume of N_2 washed out of the lungs by breathing pure oxygen is proportional to the person's end-expiratory lung volume, by measuring the volume and the nitrogen percentages of the exhaled gas, the FRC is determined. The nitrogen washout

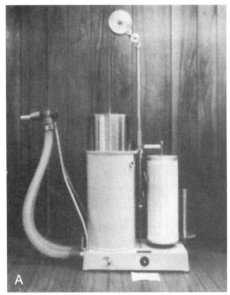

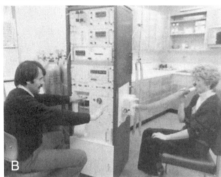

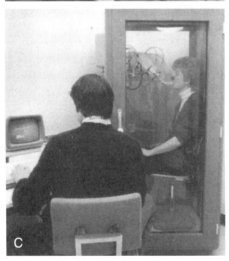

Figure 10–15. Typical pulmonary function testing equipment in a pulmonary function laboratory. *A,* Water-seal spirometer with counterweight pulley. *B,* Computerized pulmonary function system. *C,* Whole-body plethysmograph. (*A* from Ruppel G. Manual of Pulmonary Function Testing. St. Louis, CV Mosby, 1986; *B* and *C* from Kersten LD. Comprehensive Respiratory Nursing: A Decision Making Approach. Philadelphia, WB Saunders, 1989.)

method typically takes about 7 minutes to complete.

- Body plethysmography. The plethysmograph is an airtight chamber in which the patient sits; pressure transducers measure pressure both at the airway (mouthpiece) and in the chamber. The patient is placed in a plethysmograph, connected to the mouthpiece, and asked to breathe normally. At end-inspiration and end-expiration there is no airflow, and the alveolar pressure is equal to the airway pressure at that time. At a specific time (end-expiration, for example) the shutter is occluded, and the various volume and pressure values are measured. Because the body plethysmography method of FRC determination actually measures the total amount of gas in the thorax, the values obtained may be larger than those from either helium dilution or nitrogen washout techniques (any difference between the measurements is an estimate of the volume of poorly ventilated regions of the lungs).

The TLC is the sum of the VC and the RV and is the only individually diagnostic parameter in spirometry. TLC is always elevated in obstructive lung diseases and reduced in chronic restrictive lung diseases. Certain acute disorders, such as pulmonary edema, atelectasis, and consolidation, will also cause a reduction in TLC.

Tests of Gas Flow Rates

Tests that measure airflow rates during forced breathing maneuvers provide important information relating to the actual function of the lungs, the degree of impairment, and often the general location (large airways, small airways, etc.) of the problem. The basic measures of airflow rates include the following:

- Forced vital capacity (FVC) is the maximum volume of gas the patient can exhale as forcefully and as quickly as possible. FVC is measured by having the patient exhale as forcibly and as quickly as possible into a spirometer or pneumotachometer. The patient should breathe in maximally and exhale as quickly as possible. The FVC is highly dependent upon the amount of force used by the patient in early expiration at volumes near TLC. Therefore, it may be necessary to coach the patient to achieve his or her maximum expiratory effort. A normal spirographic

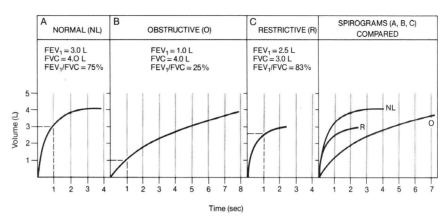

Figure 10–16. Examples and comparison of forced expiratory spirograms for normal lungs (NL), obstructive pulmonary disease (O), and restrictive pulmonary disease (R). (From Kersten LD. Comprehensive Respiratory Nursing: A Decision Making Approach. Philadelphia, WB Saunders, 1989, p 376.)

tracing of an FVC is shown in Figure 10–12. As seen in Figure 10–16, the FVC is generally reduced in both obstructive and restrictive diseases; the primary difference between the curve in the patient with restrictive disease as compared with the patient with obstructive disease is the slope of the curve. The FVC is less than the normal slow VC when airway collapse and air trapping are present. Furthermore, by analyzing the FVC with respect to the volume of air exhaled per unit time and the relationship of expiratory flow to lung volume, inferences may be made about the localization of any problem.

- Forced expiratory volume in 1 second (FEV_1) is the volume of air that is exhaled during the first second of the FVC and reflects the airflow in the large airways. The utility of the FEV_1 measurement is exemplified by the simple relationship between it and the associated degree of obstruction:
  - Little or no obstruction: FEV_1 above 2.0 L to normal
  - Mild to moderate obstruction: FEV_1 between 1.0 and 2.0 L
  - Severe obstruction: FEV_1 less than 1.0 L

This volume may also be expressed as a percentage of the FVC exhaled in 1 second ($FEV_1\%$).

Clinical Note: Reduced Forced Vital Capacity

Individuals with obstructive defects will demonstrate large lung volumes, but reduced FVC because of inability to get the air out forcefully (as in asthma or emphysema). Individuals with restrictive defects will demonstrate small lung volumes, and possibly reduced FVC because of the lack of muscle strength (as in a patient with pneumonia or severe pulmonary fibrosis).

Normally, 75% of the FVC should be exhaled within 1 second. An $FEV_1\%$ of more than 80% or 90% indicates restrictive disease, while a reduced $FEV_1\%$ indicates airway obstruction. A significant reduction in FEV_1 is associated with a higher mortality rate among both sexes, while significant declines in $FEV_1\%$ are associated with a higher all-cause mortality rate among male subjects only.[15, 16] Of course, age exerts an influence on both the FVC and the FEV_1. The average decline in FEV_1 is in the range of 40 mL per year for men and 30 mL per year for women.[17] After the late 20s to mid 30s, a progressive decline in the FEV_1 of from 20 to 50 mL per year can be expected in healthy persons, but in adults with chronic obstructive lung disease the decline is as much as 50 to 80 mL per year.

- Forced midexpiratory flow (FEF_{25-75}), previously called the maximal midexpiratory flow rate, is volume of air exhaled over the middle half of the FVC, divided by the time required to exhale it. The normal FEF_{25-75} is approximately 4 L/second (240 L/minute). Although the FEF_{25-75} has proved to be effective in detecting the presence of changes in lung function, because it depends on the FVC, it has not proved to be a particularly satisfactory parameter for use in quantifying the changes.

Numerous additional indices of lung mechanics are frequently presented on PFT reports:

- Forced expiratory flow, 200–1200 ($FEF_{200-1200}$) is the average expiratory flow during the early phase of exhalation. Specifically, it is a measure of the flow for 1 L of expired gas immediately following the first 200 mL of expired gas. The normal $FEF_{200-1200}$ is usually greater than 5 L/second (300 L/minute).

- Maximum voluntary ventilation (MVV) is the maximal volume of gas a patient can move during 1 minute (previously called the maximum breathing capacity). The patient is asked to breathe as deeply and rapidly as possible for 10, 12, or 15 seconds, the volume expired is extrapolated to yield the flow rate in L/minute. The normal value for adult males is about 160 to 180 L/minute; it is slightly lower in adult females. However, normal values can vary by as much as 25% to 30%; therefore, only major reductions in the values are clinically significant. As a rule of thumb, the MVV is typically described as being about 35 times greater than the FEV_1 value.[18]
- Peak expiratory flow (PEF) is the maximum flow that occurs at any point in time during the FVC. Normal peak flows average 9 to 10 L/second. The reliability of PEF as a clinical tool for evaluation of lung mechanics is limited because of the initial high flows that can occur even in obstructive disorders. Decreased peak flows reflect nonspecific mechanical problems of the lung, patient cooperation, and effort.
- Airway resistance (Raw) is the driving pressure necessary to move a volume of gas in a specific period of time. Mathematically, it is the ratio of the driving pressure to the flow. The most common method of measuring the airway resistance is body plethysmography. Typically, the patient is instructed to pant at V_T between 100 to 200 mL at a frequency usually greater than 100 breaths per minute. While the patient is breathing, an electronic shutter momentarily closes, creating a no-flow situation, and the alveolar pressure is determined. Normal airway resistance is between 0.5 and 2.5 cm H_2O/L/s, measured at a standardized flow of 0.5 L/second. The Raw decreases with increasing lung volumes, primarily because of the increasing airway caliber. Any factor (e.g., edema, bronchial secretions, bronchoconstriction, or vascular congestion due to inflammation) that reduces the caliber of the airway will cause an increase in airway resistance. A loss of lung elastance (increased compliance) will also cause an increase in airway resistance because of the loss of radial support in the region of the small airways. Therefore, disorders such as asthma, emphysema, and bronchitis will cause increases in airway resistance.
- Compliance (C) is the volume change in the lung per unit of pressure change; it is a measure of the distensibility of the chest or lungs. To measure the compliance of the lungs (CL), the patient is asked to swallow a balloon catheter. The catheter is positioned in the lower third of the esophagus and connected to a manometer for measurement of pressure. Pressure changes are then plotted against various lung volumes. Normal CL is approximately 0.2 L/cm H_2O. The lung-thorax compliance (CLT) is measured with body plethysmography. By serial reduction of pressures within the chambers and measurement of the resulting changes in volume, a pressure-volume curve can be plotted. Normal CLT is approximately 0.1 L/cm H_2O. From these two values, thoracic compliance (CT) can be calculated.

The various tests of breathing mechanics are measured again 5 to 20 minutes (the time depends on the specific drug and its dosage) after the administration of a bronchodilator (e.g., isoproterenol or isoetharine). In normal persons, or in persons with pure restrictive processes, there should be no difference between the before and after bronchodilator measurements. In persons with obstructive disease, bronchodilators are used primarily to measure the reversibility of the obstruction. Airway obstruction is generally said to be reversible when there is 15% or greater increase in the postbronchodilator values for at least two of the following three parameters: FVC, FEV_1, and FEF_{25-75}. However, the definition of obstruction and reversibility in clinical trials is not uniform. Moreover, at least 11 different criteria can be found in the literature to define obstruction.[19, 20]

Tests of Diffusion

The diffusing capacity of the lung (DL or DL_{CO}) is the amount of gas entering the pulmonary blood flow per unit time and is relative to the difference between the partial pressures of the gas in the alveoli and in the pulmonary blood. The DL is not so much a measure of pulmonary mechanics as it is a measure of the integrity of the functional lung unit. DL is expressed in millimeters per minute per millimeters of mercury (mL/min/mm Hg). Carbon monoxide (CO) is normally employed to measure DL because it has an affinity for hemoglobin nearly 210 times greater than that of oxygen. As long as the patient's hemoglobin is normal, all the alveolar CO should bind to hemoglobin and the partial pressure of CO in the plasma should be zero. The normal diffusing capacity of carbon monoxide is about 25 to 30 mL/min/mm Hg. Although there may be many causes for an abnormal DL_{CO} test, they can be attributed to three key factors: (1) decreased quantity of hemoglobin per unit volume of blood; (2) increased "thickness" of the alveolar-capillary membrane; and (3) decreased functional surface area available for diffusion. Loss of surface area has been identified as the primary factor. Of the two most often used tests for measuring DL_{CO}, it has been suggested that the single-breath test is of limited value because the results are influenced by unequal distribution of ventilation and diffusion, although the rebreathing method is not believed to be influenced by such inequalities.[21]

Additional Tests of Gas Exchange

Some of the gas exchange variables that may be helpful in furthering an understanding of the diagnosis of the causes of exertional dyspnea, the extent of functional impairment, or the effect of medical, surgical, or rehabilitative therapy are presented in Table 10–1. The reader is warned, however, that without an appreciation of the environmental conditions under which specific gas volumes may have been determined, dramatic errors may be made when interpreting the significance of the volumes. For example, tradition dictates that oxygen consumption ($\dot{V}O_2$) is expressed in liters per minute at standard temperature and pressure without water vapor (STPD), and expiratory minute ventilation ($\dot{V}E$) is usually expressed in liters per minute at body temperature and ambient pressure fully saturated with water vapor (BTPS). To make matters more difficult, inspiratory minute ventilation ($\dot{V}I$) is most often expressed in liters per minute at ambient temperature with ambient pressure and ambient water vapor saturation (ATPS). It may become necessary, therefore, to convert from one environmental condition to the other. The formula below demonstrates how to convert values from ATPS to BTPS:

$$(L/min\ BTPS) = (L/min,\ ATPS) \times \frac{273 + 37}{273 + T}$$
$$\times \frac{P_B - P_{H_2O}(at\ T)}{P_B - 47}$$

where 273 is the SI value (in kelvins, K) for 0°C, 37 is body temperature in °C, T is ambient temperature in °C, P_B is barometric pressure, P_{H_2O} is the partial pressure of water vapor at ambient temperature, 47 is the P_{H_2O} at 37°C. To convert values from BTPS to STPD the following formula can be used:

Table 10–1

Typical Gas Exchange Variables

VARIABLE	SYMBOL	DEFINITION
Respiratory frequency	f	Number of complete breaths per unit time
Tidal volume	V_T	Volume of air moved during either inhalation or exhalation over a specific period of time (usually 1 minute)
Minute ventilation (expiratory)	$\dot{V}E$	Volume of air exhaled per unit time
Minute ventilation (inspiratory)	$\dot{V}I$	Volume of air inhaled per unit time
Carbon dioxide output	$\dot{V}CO_2$	Volume of carbon dioxide exhaled per unit time
Oxygen uptake	$\dot{V}O_2$	Volume of oxygen consumed per unit time
Gas exchange ratio	R	Ratio of $\dot{V}CO_2$ to $\dot{V}O_2$
Ventilatory equivalent for carbon dioxide or oxygen	$\dot{V}E/\dot{V}CO_2$ or $\dot{V}E/\dot{V}O_2$	Ventilatory requirement for a given metabolic rate
Oxygen pulse	$\dot{V}O_2/HR$	Amount of oxygen consumed per heart beat

$$(\text{L/min, STPD}) = (\text{L/min, BTPS}) \times \frac{273}{273 + 37}$$

$$\times \frac{P_B - 47}{760}$$

where 760 is the value for standard barometric pressure, in mm Hg.

Flow Volume Loop

The flow volume loop or curve is not so much a pulmonary function test as a way of graphically representing the events that occur during forced inspiration and expiration. The flow volume procedure simply records flow against volume on an X-Y recorder. Following a period of normal, quiet breathing, the patient is instructed to perform a maximal inspiratory maneuver, to hold the breath for 1 to 2 seconds, to do an FVC maneuver, and then to do another maximal inspiratory maneuver. A normal flow-volume loop is shown in Figure 10–17.

The initial portion of the expiratory loop is effort-dependent, however, after the first third of the expiratory curve, the curve is effort independent and reproducible. The highest point on the expiratory curves denotes the *peak expiratory flow rate* (PEFR). The line that connects the PEFR and the end of expiration at the RV is normally straight. However, both restrictive and obstructive processes alter this effort independent portion. Values for FVC, FEV_1, peak flow, and so on, should be the same as those obtained by conventional spirometric methods.

The flow-volume loop of patients with minimal to mild small airway obstructive lung disease look essentially normal except for a slight "scooped out" appearance at the end of expiration. As the disease progresses, the PEFR becomes noticeably reduced and the scooping becomes more pronounced (Fig. 10–17). The inspiratory portion of the curve is more sensitive to central airway obstruction, whereas the expiratory portion of the curve is more sensitive to peripheral airway obstruction. The restrictive lung disease processes will show near-normal peak expiratory flow volume (FEV_t) when compared with the percentage of FVC (%FEV_t/FVC).

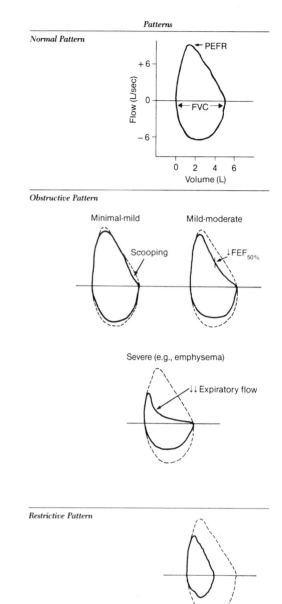

Figure 10–17. Examples of flow volume loop patterns for normal lungs, obstructive pulmonary disease, and restrictive pulmonary disease. (Adapted from Kersten LD. Comprehensive Respiratory Nursing: A Decision Making Approach. Philadelphia, WB Saunders, 1989, p 382.)

Interpretation of Basic Pulmonary Function Test Results

Pulmonary function test results are almost universally formatted to present data in columns of predicted, observed, and percentage of predicted val-

Table 10–2

Typical Effect of Obstructive and Restrictive Disease on Spirometric and Airflow Volume Measurements

MEASUREMENT	OBSTRUCTIVE	RESTRICTIVE
Tidal volume (VT)	N or $\Uparrow$	N or $\Downarrow$
Inspiratory capacity (IC)	N or $\Downarrow$	N or $\Downarrow$
Expiratory reserve volume (ERV)	N or $\Downarrow$	N or $\Downarrow$
Vital capacity (VC)	N or $\Downarrow$	$\Downarrow$
Forced vital capacity (FVC)	N or $\Downarrow$	$\Downarrow$
Residual volume (RV)	N or $\Uparrow$	N or $\Downarrow$
Functional residual capacity (FRC)	N or $\Uparrow$	N or $\Downarrow$
Total lung capacity (TLC)	N or $\Uparrow$	$\Downarrow$
Forced expiratory volume in 1 s (FEV_1)	$\Downarrow$	N
Forced expiratory flow rate between 200 and 1200 mL ($FEF_{200-1200}$)	$\Downarrow$	N or $\Downarrow$
Forced expiratory flow rate between 25% and 75% FVC (FEF_{25-75})	$\Downarrow$	N or $\Downarrow$
Maximal voluntary ventilation (MVV)	$\Downarrow$	N or $\Downarrow$
Peak expiratory flow (PEF)	N or $\Downarrow$	N or $\Downarrow$

N = normal; $\Uparrow$ = higher than normal; $\Downarrow$ = lower than normal.

ues. The predicted values (derived from a variety of nomograms) are those normally be anticipated on the basis of the patient's age (volumes decrease with age), gender (males have larger volumes than females), height (tall individuals have larger volumes than short individuals), weight, and race (American Indians, blacks, and Asians have as much as 12% to 14% lower volumes than whites).[12, 13, 22, 23] Children pose a unique challenge to prediction because their development is phasic; thus, specific nomograms are used for the pediatric population. The observed values are those actually attained by the patient. Dividing the observed value by the predicted value derives the percentage of predicted values. Generally, there should be more than 20% difference between observed and predicted values before they are considered abnormal. The generalized effects of obstructive or restrictive diseases are shown in Table 10–2.

The following points should be kept in mind when interpreting PFTs:

- Determine whether or not the results are normal.
- Determine whether the results are indicative of obstructive or restrictive disease.
- If the problem is obstructive in nature, determine its reversibility.
- Consider the history and physical examination along with serial PFTs (if available) to determine disease progression.

- Be suspicious of test results if there are signs of poor patient effort.

BLOOD GAS ANALYSIS

Blood gas analysis is crucial to the assessment of problems related to acid-base balance, ventilation, and oxygenation. Samples for blood gas analysis may be obtained from any number of sites representing different regions of the vascular bed: *arterial* samples are taken from either a needle puncture or an indwelling cannula in a peripheral artery; *venous* samples are taken from a peripheral venous puncture or catheter; *mixed venous* samples are taken from a pulmonary artery catheter. Unless otherwise specified, a blood gas sample is presumed to be arterial in origin. Arterial blood gases (ABGs) are frequently used to monitor the condition of patients in the critical care setting and to help modify respiratory interventions. A typical report of an ABG analysis contains the following measurements: arterial pH, partial pressures of carbon dioxide (Pa_{CO_2}) and oxygen (Pa_{O_2}), oxygen saturation (Sa_{O_2}), bicarbonate (HCO_3^-) concentration, and base excess (BE). Although the immediate utility of ABGs for the physical therapist may have been supplanted by the pulse oximeter, a systematic approach to a more detailed and complete interpretation of acid-base, ventilatory, or oxygenation status should not be overlooked, particularly with respect to ventilator dependent patients.

Normal Values

The laboratory "normal values" for pH and Pa_{CO_2} (7.40 and 40 mm Hg, respectively) represent the statistically determined mean values from a large representative sample population. The laboratory "normal range" may vary from institution to institution based on the particular laboratory's established normal range, which may be 1 or 2 standard deviations (SD). The narrower pH range of 7.38 to 7.42 and Pa_{CO_2} range of 38 to 42 mm Hg represents 1 SD from the normal values. The wider pH range of 7.35 to 7.45 and Pa_{CO_2} range of 35 to 45 mm Hg represents 2 SD from the normal values. For the purposes of this chapter the normal range for pH is 7.35 to 7.45; for Pa_{CO_2}, 35 to 45 mm Hg, depending on posture, age, obesity, and other factors. An even broader "clinically acceptable range" has been promoted by some clinicians.[24–27] Table 10–3 presents the normal values and normal ranges for ABG parameters.

In any systematic approach to the interpretation of ABGs, it is advantageous to focus upon three principal categories: the adequacy of alveolar ventilation, the acid-base balance, and the oxygenation status.

Adequacy of Alveolar Ventilation

The Pa_{CO_2} directly reflects the adequacy of alveolar ventilation. Given a normal Pa_{CO_2} value of 40 mm Hg, **alveolar hyperventilation** is indicated by a Pa_{CO_2} that is less than normal, and **alveolar hypoventilation** is indicated by a greater than normal Pa_{CO_2}. When a patient's Pa_{CO_2} is greater than 50 mm Hg, the condition is called **ventilatory failure.**

Ventilatory failure can only be diagnosed on the basis of the Pa_{CO_2} level, but its severity is determined from the extent of the accompanying acidemia and the rapidity of the change in pH. Sudden (acute) changes in pH hinder cellular function to a greater degree than do gradual changes, and are more often associated with a loss of alertness and coma than are gradual (chronic) pH changes. When acuity or chronicity are masked by the presence of mixed disorders, the patient's level of alertness should be used as an indicator.

The events leading to ventilatory failure can occur relatively rapidly in patients who are acutely ill, or over a period of days or weeks in patients with chronic lung disease, as they decompensate—become unable to meet the demands for the increased minute ventilation needed to maintain adequate gas exchange. Because there are no reliable means of predicting a patient's ability to avert decompensation with any certainty, monitoring of the ventilatory status is mandatory. Such monitoring consists of ongoing assessment of pH, Pa_{CO_2}, and the signs and symptoms that suggest an increased work of breathing. To determine the nature and severity of illness with accuracy, an assessment of the relationship between arterial pH and arterial CO_2 tension is necessary. Monitoring equipment is discussed in Chapters 11 and 13.

Acid-Base Balance

The assessment of blood pH provides insight to the nature and magnitude of respiratory and metabolic disorders. In general terms, the pH describes the balance between blood acids and blood bases. Specifically, it indicates the concentration of hydrogen ions (H^+) in the blood. In solution, acids give up hydrogen ions and bases, on the other hand, accept hydrogen ions.

The lungs and the kidneys regulate the two types of acids—volatile and nonvolatile—found in

Table 10–3						
Normal Ranges (± 2 SD) for Arterial Blood Gas Values						
	pH	P_{CO_2} (mm Hg)	P_{O_2} (mm Hg)	HCO_3^- (mEq/L)	BE	% SAT
Normal value	7.40	40	97	24	0	97%
Normal range	7.35–7.45	35–45	>80	22–28	±2	>95%

the body. Volatile acids readily alternate from liquid to gaseous states. The lungs regulate volatile acids, primarily represented by carbonic acid in the blood, via the excretion of CO_2. Nonvolatile acids (e.g., lactic acid or keto acid) cannot change to gases and must, therefore, be excreted by the kidneys. The principal source of nonvolatile acids is from dietary intake (organic and inorganic acids), and although the liver is where most of these nonvolatile acids are metabolized, the kidneys regulate their excretion from the body. The kidneys are also primarily responsible for regulation of the major blood base—bicarbonate (HCO_3^-). Bicarbonate is responsible for 60 to 90% of the extracellular buffering of nonvolatile acids (buffers act to prevent extreme fluctuations in hydrogen ion concentration so that cellular metabolism will not be hampered). Hemoglobin accounts for about 85% of nonbicarbonate buffering action (phosphate and serum proteins are the other nonbicarbonate buffers).

Henderson-Hasselbalch Equation

By looking at one specific component—the carbonic acid to bicarbonate ion relationship—a complete analysis of acid-base balance is possible, because the amount of hydrogen ion activity resulting from the dissociation of carbonic acid is controlled by the interrelationship of all the blood acids, bases, and buffers. The Henderson-Hasselbalch equation defines pH in terms of this relationship:

$$pH = pK + \log \frac{[HCO_3^-]}{[H_2CO_3]}$$

where pH is the negative log of hydrogen ion concentration ($-\log[H^+]$) and pK equals 6.1 (pK is a constant representing the pH at which a solute is 50% dissolved; its mathematical derivation, and that of pH, are beyond the scope of this chapter). In terms of clinically derived variables, the Henderson-Hasselbalch equation can be expressed as follows:

$$pH = pK + \log \frac{[HCO_3^-]}{s \times Pa_{CO_2}}$$

where s is the solubility coefficient for carbon dioxide, and equals 0.03. In plasma, the concentration of dissolved carbon dioxide (dCO_2) is about 1000 times greater than the concentration of carbonic acid because the catalyzing enzyme **carbonic anhydrase** does not exist in the plasma. Because it is extremely difficult to distinguish between dCO_2 and H_2CO_3, for convenience, their respective concentrations are added together and the sum is referred to as the **total** dissolved carbon dioxide in the blood. Thus, substitution of $s \times Pa_{CO_2}$ for carbonic acid is permitted because the partial pressure of carbon dioxide (P_{CO_2}) times its solubility coefficient yields the total carbon dioxide dissolved. Essentially, then, the Pa_{CO_2} can be considered to be equivalent to the plasma H_2CO_3 plus the dCO_2. Although this total dissolved carbon dioxide in the plasma is a very small portion of the total carbon dioxide content of the blood, it is extremely important because it exerts the pressure that determines the pressure gradient controlling the movement of CO_2 into or out of the blood.[24-27]

Acid-Base Terminology

Because the "normal" human blood pH is 7.4, a pH of less than 7.4 is defined as **acidemia.** The process causing the acidemia (whatever it may be) is called **acidosis.** From the Henderson-Hasselbalch equation, there are only two ways in which acidemia can occur: (1) a low HCO_3^- produces **metabolic acidosis;** and (2) a high Pa_{CO_2} is called **respiratory acidosis** (synonymous terms are alveolar hypoventilation and hypercapnia). Similarly, a pH greater than 7.4 is defined as **alkalemia,** and the process causing it is called **alkalosis.** There are also only two ways in which alkalemia can occur: (1) a high HCO_3^- is called **metabolic alkalosis;** and (2) a low Pa_{CO_2} is called **respiratory alkalosis** (alternatively called alveolar hyperventilation or hypocapnia). These four acid-base states constitute the *primary* acid-base disorders, and each elicits a *compensatory* response. For example, if some disease were to cause a decreased HCO_3^- (a *primary metabolic acidosis*), the body's response would be an attempt to decrease the Pa_{CO_2} (a *compensatory respiratory alkalosis*) to return the pH toward its normal value. In this manner, respiratory compensation for primary metabolic disorders begins in a matter of seconds by means of alveolar hyper- or hypoventilation. The kidneys compensate for primary respiratory disorders by retaining or excreting bicarbonate and hydrogen ions. However, unlike the rapidity with which respiratory compensatory activity exhibits its effect, the renal compensatory process requires 12 to 24 hours to effect significant pH change.

The relationships described in the Henderson-Hasselbalch equation permit us to "quickly" identify any of the four primary disorders based on pH and CO_2 changes. If the normal inverse relationship between pH and Pa_{CO_2} is maintained, the primary problem is most likely respiratory in nature. On the other hand, if the relationship is not maintained, the primary problem is most likely metabolic. This generalization holds true in most situations, even when combined respiratory and metabolic changes occur at the same time. However, in the face of combined disorders with large Pa_{CO_2} changes; one must keep in mind that instead of equally reflecting combined respiratory and metabolic bicarbonate changes, the Pa_{CO_2} may preferentially reflect the respiratory component. Because this makes separating metabolic and respiratory components more difficult, an additional parameter that reflects the metabolic component must be considered. The **base excess** (BE) is such parameter. The BE is a measure of the deviation of the concentration of nonvolatile acids from normal (defined as a pH of 7.40 and a Pa_{CO_2} of 40 mm Hg). As such, BE is a true nonrespiratory measurement that reflects the concentration of bicarbonate in the body. The normal range of BE is ± 2 mEq $\cdot$ L^{-1}.

The normal Pa_{O_2} is 80 to 100 mm Hg when breathing room air.[24, 27, 28] The normal newborn infant (range of 40 to 70 mm Hg) and persons over 60 years of age (in general, for every year over 60 years of age subtract 1 mm Hg from the normal minimally acceptable Pa_{O_2} of 80 mm Hg—this guideline does not apply to persons over 90 years of age) are exceptions to this rule of thumb. When the arterial oxygen tension is less than normal, a condition called **hypoxemia** is said to exist.

Interpreting Arterial Blood Gases

The reader cannot expect to interpret very unusual ABGs without a great deal of practice and clinical experience. Nonetheless, an orderly approach to the assessment of ABGs will permit the majority of blood gases to be interpreted. Interpretation of ABG data involves just a couple of basic processes:

- Assessment of ventilatory status
- Assessment of oxygenation and hypoxemic status

Assessing Ventilatory Status

There are three steps in the assessment of a patient's ventilatory status:

1. Determine whether the pH value reflects acidemia or alkalemia.
2. Classify the pathophysiologic state of the ventilatory system on the basis of the relationship between the pH and Pa_{CO_2} values. This step determines whether the blood gas values represent a primary respiratory or a primary metabolic disorder. If the normal inverse relationship between pH and Pa_{CO_2} is preserved, the primary disorder is likely to be respiratory in nature; if it is not, the primary disorder is probably metabolic.
3. Determine the adequacy of alveolar ventilation on the basis of the Pa_{CO_2} value:
   - Less than 30 mm Hg = alveolar hyperventilation
   - Between 30 and 50 mm Hg = adequate alveolar ventilation
   - Greater than 50 mm Hg = ventilatory failure

The following sample pH and Pa_{CO_2} values are offered to illustrate the preceding steps (the reader should not attempt to correlate these values with any clinical situation).

1. Sample values: pH = 7.26 and Pa_{CO_2} = 56 mm Hg. From step 1, we see that the pH value represents acidemia. From step 2, we see that the normal inverse relationship between pH and Pa_{CO_2} is maintained; thus, the values probably represent a primary respiratory acid-base disorder—respiratory acidosis. From step 3, we see that the Pa_{CO_2} represents ventilatory failure.

2. Sample values: pH = 7.56 and Pa_{CO_2} = 44 mm Hg. From step 1, we see that the pH value represents an alkalemia. From step 2, we see that the normal inverse relationship between pH and Pa_{CO_2} is not maintained; thus, the values probably represent a primary metabolic acid-base disor-

der—metabolic alkalosis. From step 3, we see that the Pa_{CO_2} indicates adequate alveolar ventilation.

The final step in the assessment of ventilatory status is the determination of the extent of the respiratory and metabolic components of the disorder. The action taken depends on whether the primary problem is respiratory or metabolic. If the primary problem is respiratory, we calculate an "expected" pH and classify the problem on the basis of acuity. To do this:

1. Determine the absolute value of the difference between the reported Pa_{CO_2} and 40.
2. Divide this number by 100.
3. Subtract half of this value from 7.40 if the reported Pa_{CO_2} is more than 40; add the entire value to 7.40 if the reported Pa_{CO_2} is less than 40.
4. Classify the problem as "acute" if the reported pH is the same as, or further from normal than the expected pH; classify the problem as "chronic" if the reported pH is closer to normal than the expected pH.

For example, in our assessment of the first set of pH and Pa_{CO_2} values we concluded that they represented a respiratory acidosis. Next, we classify the acuity of the problem in accordance with the preceding four steps:

1. $56 - 40 = 16$
2. $16 \div 100 = 0.16$
3. $7.40 - 0.08 = 7.32$ (because the reported Pa_{CO_2} is more than 40)
4. Because the reported pH is further from normal than the expected pH, we classify the problem as being acute. Thus, from our assessment of the arterial pH and P_{CO_2} values we conclude that they represent an *acute respiratory acidosis*. In fact, because the Pa_{CO_2} is greater than 50 mm Hg, we call this problem *acute ventilatory failure*.

If the primary problem is metabolic, we classify the problem on the basis of the relationship between the pH and the Pa_{CO_2}. The problem is classified as "uncompensated" if the reported pH is outside the normal range and the reported Pa_{CO_2} is within the normal range; classified as "partially compensated" if both the reported pH and Pa_{CO_2} are outside the normal range; or classified as "compensated" if the reported pH is within the normal range and the reported Pa_{CO_2} is outside the normal range. For example, in assessment of the second set of pH and Pa_{CO_2} values, we con-

cluded that they represented a metabolic alkalosis. The next step is to classify the problem on the basis the relationship between the pH and Pa_{CO_2} values. Because the pH is outside the normal range and the Pa_{CO_2} is within the normal range, we conclude that the problem is an *uncompensated metabolic alkalosis*. The extent of the metabolic problem is inferred from the base excess/deficit. To calculate the base excess/deficit:

• Calculate the expected pH
• Subtract the expected pH from the reported pH (if the value is positive, it is called base excess; if the value is negative, it is called base deficit)
• Multiply this number by 100
• Calculate the base excess/deficit by taking two thirds of this number

For example, from the second set of pH and Pa_{CO_2} values (7.56 and 44 mm Hg, respectively), we calculate the BE as follows:

• $44 - 40 = 4$
• $4 \div 100 = 0.04$
• $7.40 - 0.02 = 7.38$ (because the reported Pa_{CO_2} is more than 40)
• $7.56 - 7.38 = 0.18$ (because the number is positive, it represents a base excess)
• $0.18 \times 100 = 18$
• $18 \times \frac{2}{3} = 12$

Thus, the BE = 12 mEq/L, suggesting a fairly significant metabolic alkalosis because the normal BE is ± 2 mEq/L. Table 10–4 summarizes the classification nomenclature typically used to describe acid-base disorders.

Assessing Oxygenation and Hypoxemic Status

The oxygenation status of a patient is assessed by determining the extent to which the observed Pa_{O_2} is above or below the normal range. Generally, as

Clinical Note: Arterial Blood Gases

Arterial blood gases are assessed to determine the acuteness of the situation. For example, ABG values found in an acute respiratory illness might be pH 7.32, P_{CO_2} 52 mm Hg, and HCO_3^- 24 mEq/L. On the other hand, ABG values found in a chronic respiratory condition might be pH 7.36, P_{CO_2} 54 mm Hg, and HCO_3^- 30 mEq/L.

Table 10-4

Nomenclature for Evaluating Ventilatory and Metabolic Acid-Base Status

ACID-BASE STATUS	pH	Pa_{CO_2}
Acute alveolar hyperventilation	>7.50	<30 mm Hg
Chronic alveolar hyperventilation	7.40–7.50	<30 mm Hg
Compensated metabolic acidosis	7.30–7.40	<30 mm Hg
Partially compensated metabolic acodosis	<7.30	<30 mm Hg
Metabolic alkalosis	>7.50	35–45 mm Hg
Normal	7.35–7.45	35–45 mm Hg
Metabolic acidosis	<7.30	35–45 mm Hg
Partially compensated metabolic alkalosis	>7.50	>50 mm Hg
Chronic ventilatory failure	7.30–7.50	>50 mm Hg
Acute ventilatory failure	<7.30	>50 mm Hg

long as a patient's Pa_{O_2} is within the normal range, arterial oxygenation is considered to be acceptable. If a patient's Pa_{O_2} is between 60 and 80 mm Hg, the patient is said to be mildly hypoxemic; if it is between 40 and 60 mm Hg, moderately hypoxemic; and if it is less than 40 mm Hg, severely hypoxemic. Hypoxemia is not an absolute indicator of cellular **hypoxia**—a condition of inadequate cellular oxygenation—because other factors, such as hemoglobin level and capillary circulation, must also be considered. However, hypoxemia strongly suggests tissue hypoxia and necessitates further evaluation.

Quite frequently, patients require supplemental oxygen in the course of their medical treatment. When a patient is receiving supplemental oxygen, the adequacy of arterial oxygenation is assessed on the basis of the fraction of inspired oxygen. As a general rule, the fraction of inspired oxygen (FI_{O_2}) multiplied by 500 approximates the arterial oxygen tension expected. If that tension is not present, one may assume that the patient would be hypoxemic. For example, consider two patients, each with a Pa_{O_2} of 95 mm Hg. Patient 1 is breathing room air, so we conclude that the Pa_{O_2} represents adequate oxygenation and no hypoxemia. Patient 2, on the other hand, is receiving supplemental oxygen and has an FI_{O_2} of 0.30 (30% oxygen). If this patient were oxygenating the arterial blood normally, we would anticipate a Pa_{O_2} in the neighborhood of 150 mm Hg. Thus, we can reasonably conclude that this patient is hypoxemic.

OXIMETRY

Oximetry is a descriptive term for the various technologies available for measuring oxyhemoglobin saturation. The modern pulse oximeter involves a light-emitting diode (LED), a photodiode signal detector, and a microprocessor.[29] The LED alternately emits red and infrared light hundreds of times per second, and the microprocessor compares the signals received by the signal detector and calculates the degree of oxyhemoglobin saturation based on the intensity of transmitted light at the detector. Most units display a digital oxyhemoglobin saturation ($O_2Hb\%$) that updates every few seconds. The reader is referred to Chapter 13 for additional information regarding the clinical interpretation of oximetry values.

CYTOLOGIC AND HEMATOLOGIC TESTS

As part of the diagnostic process, many cytologic and hematologic tests are often performed on patients with pulmonary disease. These tests are helpful in the identification of disease causing organisms and in monitoring the body's responses to them.

Cytologic tests are used to identify specific microorganisms that may cause disease. Several classification schemes, often used simultaneously, describe the various microorganisms identified by cytologic testing: microorganisms are frequently described taxonomically; according to their structure (e.g., **viruses** have a simple central core of DNA or RNA encapsulated by a protein coat; **prokaryotes** have discrete cell walls, but lack nuclear membranes; **eukaryotes** have distinct cellular and nuclear membranes); with respect to their habitat (e.g., *obligate intracellular parasites* require specific cell types or cellular organelles for reproduction;

Table 10-5

Classification of Microbes

TAXONOMY	STRUCTURE	HABITAT	MORPHOLOGY
Viruses	Capsid	Obligate intracellular	Isometric, helical
Bacteria		Extracellular or facultative intracellular	
Chlamydias*	Prokaryote	Obligate intracellular	Spherical (cocci), rod-shaped (bacilli), spiral (spiro-chete)
Mycoplasmas*		Extracellular†	
Rickettsias*		Obligate intracellular	
Fungi	Eukaryote	Extracellular or facultative intracellular	
Protozoa		Extracellular, facultative or obligate intracellular	

*Sometimes classified as bacteria.
†Other habitats are possible.

facultative parasites can replicate either outside or inside cells; and extracellular parasites reproduce only outside the cell); or morphologically (e.g., spherical, rod-shaped, spiral). Bacteria are also often categorized on the basis of their staining characteristics (e.g., gram-negative, gram-positive, acid-fast) or morphology. Table 10-5 gives some examples.

Numerous microorganisms can normally be found on the skin or mucous membranes of the nasopharynx, oropharynx, and upper airway. Indigenous microbes are often referred to as normal flora (Table 10-6). The host organism is said to be colonized if the parasitic microbes cause no injury to the host's cells and is described as infected if the microbes are present below the host cells' external integument. Some parasites share a symbiotic relationship with the host (for example, vitamin B_{12} is produced by bacteria in the ileum); some are pathogenic, interfering with the host's integrity and function; and some are commensal, having no deleterious effects on a "healthy" host, but becoming opportunistically pathogenic in a compromised host. The extent to which a pathogen interferes with a host's function depends upon the virulence and number of the offending microbes: some organisms are invariably pathogenic, their identification always signifying disease; others are facultative, capable of colonization or infection, depending upon the state of the host's natural chemical and physical barriers.[30] Respiratory infections are typically divided into two groups: upper respiratory tract infection or lower respiratory tract infection. Rhinoviruses account for the majority of upper respiratory infections, although any of the commensal organisms may become pathogenic.

The tracheobronchial tree below the level of the true vocal cords is normally sterile or only minimally colonized. Lower respiratory tract infections are commonly caused by viruses, bacteria, protozoa, and fungi. Table 10-7 lists common pathogens of the lower respiratory tract. Microorganisms typically reach the lungs by inhalation, but they are occasionally transported via the blood from another infected site. Unfortunately, many medical treatments and procedures (e.g., immunosuppressive or cytotoxic therapy, intubation, catheterization, and surgical intervention) provide an opportunity for the entry of infectious agents.

Table 10-6

Common Commensal Flora of the Upper Respiratory Tract

GRAM-POSITIVE COCCI	GRAM-POSITIVE RODS	GRAM-NEGATIVE COCCI	GRAM-NEGATIVE RODS	FUNGI	PROTOZOA	VIRUSES
Streptococci Staphylococci	Actinomycetes Corynebacteria Lactobacilli	Veillonella Neisseria	Pseudomonas Haemophilus Fusobacterium Bacteroides	Candida Aspergillus	Trichomonas Selenomonas	With the exception of herpes simplex, viruses are typically pathogenic

Table 10–7

Pathogens Commonly Identified in the Lower Respiratory Tract

TYPE	PATHOGENS
Bacteria	*Streptococcus pneumoniae*
	Staphylococcus aureus
	Haemophilus influenzae
	Enterobacteriaceae
	Klebsiella pneumoniae
	Pseudomonas aeruginosa
	Legionella (all species)
	Mycoplasma pneumoniae
	Chlamydia (all species)
Fungi	*Coccidioides immitis*
	Histoplasma capsulatum
	Blastomyces dermatitidis
	Aspergillus (all species)
	Cryptococcus neoformans
	Candida (all species)
Protozoa	*Pneumocystis carinii*
Viruses	Influenza A
	Influenza B
	Adenoviruses
	Respiratory syncytial virus
	Parainfluenza viruses

Definitive diagnosis of respiratory infections depends on the isolation of specific pathogens from pulmonary secretions or the detection of pathogen-specific antibodies. Microscopic examination and culturing can proceed once appropriate specimens have been collected. Specimens are most often obtained by expectoration, but invasive techniques for specimen collection range from nasotracheal suctioning to open-lung biopsy. Expectorated sputum is the most frequently collected specimen for the diagnosis of pneumonia.[31] The utility of such specimens is controversial because the lower respiratory tract secretions are frequently contaminated by upper respiratory tract flora, making interpretation difficult. For this reason, before obtaining an expectorated specimen for culture, it is a good idea to instruct the patient to remove any dentures and to rinse the mouth with water.

Microscopic examination with various stains broadly indicates what sort of organisms are present in the specimen, but culturing is the definitive step. Culturing entails placing the specimen in a variety of cultural media in the presence and absence of oxygen and carbon dioxide, and at different temperatures for varied lengths of time. Antimicrobial therapy is not automatically initiated at the presence of a pathogen-colonization must be distinguished from infection. However, antimicrobial therapy is often initiated when the signs and symptoms of infection are recognized, even before a specific pathogen has been identified. Once a pathogen is identified, its sensitivity to various antimicrobial agents is assessed so that the antimicrobial therapy can be appropriately directed. Refer to Chapter 15 for information regarding pulmonary pharmacologic agents.

Hematologic tests also aid greatly in the assessment of cardiopulmonary disease. Typical tests include arterial blood gases (described previously), electrolyte analysis, complete blood cell (CBC) counts, and coagulation studies. The CBC count imparts information about the number of red blood cells (RBC), the hemoglobin level, the proportion of the blood that is cells (hematocrit), the number and composition of white blood cells (WBC), and the platelet count. Coagulation studies evaluate the tendency of the blood to clot.

Tables 10–8 and 10–9 present normal values for the various components of a CBC. A less than normal quantity of hemoglobin, a low RBC count, or a low hematocrit is indicative of anemia and suggests that the oxygen-carrying capacity will be decreased. Conversely, an increase in the quantity of hemoglobin, RBC count, or hematocrit is indicative of polycythemia. An increased WBC (leukocytosis) is frequently associated with a bacterial infec-

Table 10–8

Normal Values for a Complete Blood Cell Count

TEST	MALES	FEMALES
Red blood cells	4.8 to 6.0 $\times 10^6$/mm³	4.1 to 5.1 $\times 10^6$/mm³
Hemoglobin	13 to 16 g/dL or g%	12 to 14 g/dL or g%
Hematocrit	40% to 54%	37% to 47%
White blood cells	5000 to 10,000/mm³	5000 to 10,000/mm³
Platelets	200,000 to 350,000/mm³	200,000 to 350,000/mm³

Table 10-9
Differential of White Blood Cell Count

CELL TYPE	NORMAL VALUE
Neutrophils	50% to 75% Segments: 90% to 100% of total neutrophils Bands: 0% to 10% of total neutrophils
Eosinophils	2% to 4%
Basophils	Less than 0.5%
Lymphocytes	20% to 40%
Monocytes	3% to 8%

tion, whereas a decreased WBC (leukopenia) may indicate leukemia, although radiation or chemotherapy can also yield this result. An increased neutrophil count is sometimes a first indication of the body's response to inflammation or bacterial infection. An increase in the level of immature neutrophils (bands)—called a leftward shift of neutrophils—is an indication of the body's stress response (the greater the shift, the greater the stress). Eosinophilia (an increased number of eosinophils) is usually an indication of an allergic response. Viral infections often result in an increase in the number of lymphocytes. An increased number of monocytes is typical of a chronic infection. An increased number of basophils is frequently associated with some myeloproliferative disorder. Platelets are integral to a normal coagulation process; too few platelets can result in small skin hemorrhages, and too many can increase the likelihood of thrombosis.

In general, four tests are used in an evaluation of the blood's tendency to clot:

1. Bleeding time
2. Platelet count
3. Partial thromboplastin time (PTT)
4. Prothrombin time (PT)

The bleeding time measures the rate of formation of a platelet thrombus; a normal bleeding time is up to 6 minutes. The PTT measures the overall rate of both the intrinsic and common pathways (normal PTT is 32 to 70 seconds), and the PT measures the rate of the extrinsic and common pathways (normal PT is 12 to 15 seconds). Together, the PT and PTT, detect more than 95% of coagulation abnormalities. See Chapter 8 for more information on blood work.

CASE STUDY

HM was admitted to the hospital due to complaints of difficulty breathing. HM has been a cigar smoker for over 50 years, and has been diagnosed with respiratory condition of emphysema, bronchitis, and asthma. His past medical history also includes diabetes, hypertension, arthritis, and prostate cancer. On admission his vital signs included HR 106 bpm, BP 150/90 mm Hg, RR 26, temperature 100.5°F. Patient reports a change in sputum production amount and color.

ABGs: pH 7.29, P_{CO_2} 63.4 mm Hg, P_{O_2} 56 mm Hg, HCO_3^- 30 mEq/L.

During the patient's prior admission his PFTs were recorded as follows:

TLC 120% predicted
VC 115% predicted
RV 130% predicted
FEV_1 48% predicted
FEF 54% predicted

Chest x-ray showed infiltrates in right lower lobe, hyperinflation, and increased cardiac size.

Discussion

This case demonstrates the pulmonary diagnostic findings of an individual with chronic lung disease who has an acute event of pneumonia causing him to develop respiratory failure. The patient's ABGs demonstrate an acute respiratory acidosis, with partial compensation that is probably due to long-standing obstructive lung disease. His PFTs demonstrate severe obstructive airway disease, and the chest x-ray demonstrates chronic lung changes (hyperinflation) with an acute event (infiltrates in RLL).

Summary

This chapter has considered various chest imaging techniques along with a method for examining chest radiographs. Several tests of pulmonary function and their interpretation have been discussed. Finally, cytologic and hematologic tests were covered briefly. It is hoped that this information, together with that in Chapters 13 and 16, will facilitate your interpretation of evaluative findings.

• The standard radiograph is the predominant medium by which anatomic abnormalities arising from pathologic processes within the chest are assessed.
• The standard chest radiograph is typically taken in two views: posteroanterior and left lateral.
• Dark areas on a chest radiograph are termed *radiolucent;* light areas are *radiopaque.*

- In a "body systems" approach to the analysis of a chest radiograph, the examiner should examine (1) the bones and soft tissues; (2) the mediastinum, trachea, and cardiovascular system; (3) the hila; and (4) the lung fields.
- A tomogram (sectional radiograph) differs from a standard radiograph because tomography involves the curvilinear movement of the x-ray source and the imaging medium in opposite directions about the patient.
- A magnetic resonance image (MRI) is produced in much the same manner as a computed tomographic image, except that a gradient magnetic field is used to align the protons of the target tissue and then radio signals are used to stimulate them in order to create an image.
- Magnetic resonance imaging is currently limited to evaluation of chest wall (bone, muscle, fat, or pleura) processes because the expanded lungs have an insufficient density of protons for the generation of an adequate image from which to evaluate pathologic processes of the parenchyma.
- To obtain a bronchogram, the bronchial tree is opacified by the instillation of a contrast (radiopaque) medium as a radiographic or tomographic image is produced.
- Bronchograms permit the study of gross pathologic changes in the walls and lumina of the bronchial tree.
- Ventilation-perfusion scintillography (V/Q scan) is used to evaluate the regional distribution of gas and blood flow in the lungs.
- The fiberoptic bronchoscope makes the direct visualization of the bronchial tree clinically possible.
- Pulmonary function tests (PFTs) provide information about the integrity of the airways, the function of the respiratory musculature, and the condition of the lung tissues themselves. Generally, PFTs involve the assessment of lung volumes and capacities, gas flow rates, diffusion, and gas exchange.
- Pulmonary diseases are classified into three basic categories on the basis of pulmonary function testing: obstructive, restrictive, and combined.
- The three most commonly used methods for the determination of functional residual capacity (FRC) and residual volume (RV) are the helium dilution (closed-circuit) method, the nitrogen washout (open-circuit) method, and body plethysmography.

- When expressed as a percentage of the forced vital capacity, the volume of air exhaled in the first second of the maneuver ($FEV_1\%$) is one of the most useful parameters in the assessment of respiratory impairment.
- An $FEV_1\%$ of more than 80% or 90% indicates restrictive disease, while an $FEV_1\%$ of 60% or less suggests obstructive disease associated with increased morbidity and mortality rates.
- Blood gas analysis (arterial, venous, or mixed venous) allows the assessment of problems related to acid base balance, ventilation, and oxygenation. By convention, unless otherwise specified, a blood gas sample is presumed to be arterial in origin.
- The normal pH of the blood is 7.40, a pH of less than 7.40 is defined as *acidemia*, while a pH of more than 7.40 is defined as *alkalemia*. Any process that causes acidemia is called an *acidosis*, and any process that causes an alkalemia is called an *alkalosis*.
- The adequacy of alveolar ventilation is directly reflected by the Pa_{CO_2}. *Alveolar hyperventilation* is indicated by a Pa_{CO_2} that is less than normal, and *alveolar hypoventilation* is indicated by a Pa_{CO_2} that is greater than normal. When a patient's Pa_{CO_2} is greater than 50 mm Hg, the condition is called *ventilatory failure*.
- A patient's oxygenation status is assessed by determining the extent to which the observed Pa_{O_2} is above or below the normal range (generally accepted as being between 80 to 100 mm Hg, when breathing room air).
- Numerous cytologic tests are used to identify specific microorganisms that may cause disease. A cytologic sample is said to be *infected* if the parasitic microbes are present below the host cells' integument; it is *colonized* if the parasitic microbes present cause no injury to the host's cells.
- The complete blood cell (CBC) count imparts information about the number of red blood cells, the hemoglobin level, the hematocrit, the number and composition of white blood cells, and the platelet count.

References

1. Freundlich IM, Bragg DG. A Radiologic Approach to Diseases of the Chest. 2nd ed. Baltimore, Williams & Wilkins, 1997.

2. Meholic A, Ketai L, Lofgren R. Fundamentals of Chest Radiology. Philadelphia, WB Saunders, 1996.

3. Armstrong P. Imaging of Diseases of the Chest. 2nd ed. St. Louis, CV Mosby, 1995.

4. Lange S, Stark P. Radiology of Chest Diseases. New York, Thieme Medical Publishers, 1990.

5. Evans TJ. AANA Journal Course: Update for nurse anesthetists—Fundamentals of chest radiography. Techniques and interpretation for the anesthetist. AANA J 60:45–62, 1992.

6. Briggs GM. Chest imaging: Indications and interpretation. Med J Aust 166:555–560, 1997.

7. Sarinas PS, Chitkara RK, Rizk NW, et al. Imaging in lung cancer. Curropin Pulm Med 2:263–270, 1996.

8. Rinck PA, Torheim G, Lombardi M. Image postprocessing and contrast agents in clinical MR imaging—An introductory overview. Acta Radiol Suppl 412:7–19, 1997.

9. Thompson IM, Whittlesey GC, Slovis TL, et al. Evaluation of contrast media for bronchography. Pediatr Radiol 27:598–605, 1997.

10. Borchers SD, Beamis JF Jr. Flexible bronchoscopy. Chest Surg Clin North Am 6:169–192, 1996.

11. O'Donnell DE, Lam M, Webb KA. Spirometric correlates of improvement in exercise performance after anticholinergic therapy in chronic obstructive pulmonary disease. Am J Respir Crit Care Med 160:542–549, 1999.

12. Hyatt RE, Scanlon PD, Nakamura M. Interpretation of Pulmonary Function Tests: A Practical Guide. Philadelphia, Lippincott-Raven, 1997.

13. Madama VC. Pulmonary Function Testing and Cardiopulmonary Stress Testing. 2nd ed. Albany, NY, Delmar Publishers, 1998.

14. Margolis ML. PFT principles and bronchodilator testing in clinical practice: A guide for primary care physicians. Compr Ther 24:441–445, 1998.

15. Bang KM, Gergen PJ, Kramer R, Cohen B. The effect of pulmonary impairment on all-cause mortality in a national cohort. Chest 103:536–540, 1993.

16. Neas LM, Schwartz J. Pulmonary function levels as predictors of mortality in a national sample of US adults. Am J Epidemiol 147:1011–1018, 1998.

17. Ryan G, Knuiman MW, Divitini ML, et al. Decline in lung function and mortality: The Busselton Health Study. J Epidemiol Community Health 53:230–234, 1999.

18. Fulton JE, Pivarnik JM, Taylor WC, et al. Prediction of maximum voluntary ventilation (MVV) in African-American adolescent girls. Pediatr Pulmonol 20:225–233, 1995.

19. Quadrelli SA, Roncoroni AJ, Porcel G. Analysis of variability in interpretation of spirometric tests. Respiration 63:131–136, 1996.

20. Pellegrino R, Rodarte JR, Brusasco V. Assessing the reversibility of airway obstruction. Chest 114:1607–1612, 1998.

21. Jansons H, Fokkens JK, van der Tweel I, Kreukniet J. Rebreathing vs single-breath TLCO in patients with unequal ventilation and diffusion. Respir Med 92:18–24, 1998.

22. Ruppel G. Manual of Pulmonary Function Testing. 7th ed. St. Louis, Mosby, 1998.

23. Wanger J. Pulmonary Function Testing: A Practical Approach. 2nd ed. Baltimore, Williams & Wilkins; 1996.

24. Shapiro BA, Peruzzi WT, Kozelowski-Templin R. Clinical Application of Blood Gases. 5th ed. St. Louis, CV Mosby–Year Book, 1994.

25. Cornock MA. Making sense of arterial blood gases and their interpretation. Nurs Times 92:30–31, 1996.

26. Syabbalo N. Measurement and interpretation of arterial blood gases. Br J Clin Pract 51:173–176, 1997.

27. Williams AJ. ABC of oxygen: Assessing and interpreting arterial blood gases and acid-base balance. BMJ 317:1213–1216, 1998.

28. Askin DF. Interpretation of neonatal blood gases. Part II: Disorders of acid-base balance. Neonatal Netw 16:23–29, 1997.

29. Tallon RW. Oximetry: State-of-the-art. Nurs Manage 27:43–44, 1996.

30. Cotran RS, Kumar V, Collins T, Robbins SL. Robbins Pathologic Basis of Disease. 6th ed. Philadelphia, WB Saunders, 1999.

31. Burton GG, Hodgkin JE, Ward JJ. Respiratory Care: A Guide to Clinical Practice. 4th ed. Philadelphia, JB Lippincott, 1997.

4

Surgical Interventions, Monitoring, and Support

11

Cardiovascular and Thoracic Interventions

Ellen A. Hillegass

H. Steven Sadowsky

INTRODUCTION

In addition to the pathologic conditions that have already been discussed in Chapters 3 through 7, an almost unlimited number of surgical procedures and interventions can have a significant impact on the functioning of and interaction between the cardiovascular and pulmonary systems. Therefore, because an appreciation for the extent and involvement of surgical incisions is beneficial when planning and implementing therapeutic interventions for postoperative patients, the first part of this chapter introduces the reader to the most commonly used thoracic incisions. The second part of the chapter introduces interventions and devices used with patients who have cardiovascular or pulmonary disease.

CARDIOVASCULAR AND THORACIC SURGICAL PROCEDURES

Surgical Approaches

Individual surgeons develop preferences for particular surgical approaches based on their particular experiences and training. Thus, posterolateral and lateral thoracotomy incisions are most commonly used for lung resection procedures, although a median sternotomy may be employed occasionally (e.g., when lung resection is combined with a cardiac procedure).[1] Cardiac procedures are performed almost exclusively through a median sternotomy, although the great vessels sometimes are approached via a thoracotomy incision. Procedures that involve the pericardium or epicardium (e.g., pericardial biopsy, epicardial pacemaker insertion) are typically accomplished through a subxiphoid incision. Diaphragmatic procedures are commonly performed through either a lateral thoracotomy or a thoracoabdominal incision.

> ### Clinical Note: Lateral Thoracotomy
>
> Critical therapeutic interventions with individuals who undergo a lateral thoracotomy include segmental breathing to prevent or minimize atelectasis, side bending, and lateral chest wall stretching after surgery.

Posterolateral Thoracotomy

In preparation for a **posterolateral thoracotomy,** patients are generally positioned one-quarter turn from prone (operative side elevated) with the uppermost arm elevated forward, flexed at the elbow, and placed beside the head. The typical posterolateral thoracotomy incision extends downward from a point midway between the spine of the fourth thoracic vertebra and the scapula in a gently curving arch around the tip of the scapula to the fifth or sixth intercostal space at the anterior axillary line (Fig. 11–1). The serratus anterior is divided close to its muscular attachment in an effort to preserve its function and to avoid the long thoracic nerve. The pleural space is most often entered via an incision through the intercostal muscles at the fifth intercostal space, although a specific pathologic condition may dictate entry via another intercostal space.

Anterolateral Thoracotomy

Patients are positioned one-quarter turn from supine (operative side elevated) with the uppermost arm flexed at the elbow and placed beneath the back (retracting the latissimus dorsi muscle) in preparation for an **anterolateral thoracotomy.** The submammary incision curves from the fourth or fifth intercostal space at the midaxillary line to the midclavicular or parasternal region (Fig. 11–2). The pectoralis major is incised, and fibers of the serratus anterior are separated (with female patients, it is sometimes necessary for the surgeon to reflect the breast superiorly).

Lateral Thoracotomy

Patients are placed in sidelying position, operative side up, with the arm abducted, flexed at the elbow, and rotated in preparation for a **lateral thoracotomy** (excessive abduction or rotation, which might cause stretching of the brachial plexus, is avoided). There are several variations of the lateral thoracotomy incision, although it generally begins near the nipple line and extends toward the scapula (Fig. 11–3). The latissimus dorsi muscle is not incised; instead, it is retracted either anteriorly or posteriorly, and the fibers of either the serratus anterior or the intercostal muscles between the serratus interdigitations are incised to gain access

Figure 11–1. The posterolateral thoracotomy incision. This incision is often used for lung resection procedures or for procedures involving the descending thoracic aorta. (From Cooley DA. Techniques in Cardiac Surgery. 2nd ed. Philadelphia, WB Saunders, 1984, p 16.)

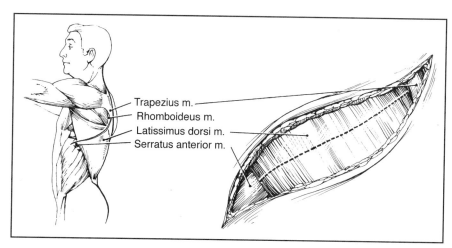

Trapezius m.
Rhomboideus m.
Latissimus dorsi m.
Serratus anterior m.

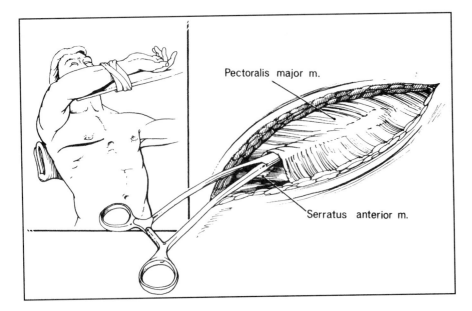

Figure 11–2. The anterolateral thoracotomy incision. This incision is not used as often as the posterolateral approach, but it is used for some cardiac procedures, pulmonary resections, and esophageal procedures. (From Cooley DA. Techniques in Cardiac Surgery. 2nd ed. Philadelphia, WB Saunders, 1984, p 14.)

to the appropriate intercostal space (most often the fourth, fifth, or sixth). Postoperative scapular winging is avoided by careful preservation of the long thoracic nerve.

Axillary Thoracotomy

An **axillary thoracotomy** is sometimes used for apical **bleb** resection or dorsal sympathectomy. Patients are placed in a sidelying position with the arm flexed at the elbow, abducted 90 degrees at

the shoulder, and rotated as for a lateral thoracotomy. From the edge of the pectoralis major, anteriorly, the incision extends posteriorly within the second intercostal space to the edge of the latissimus dorsi.

Median Sternotomy

A **median sternotomy** is probably the most frequently used incision for cardiothoracic operations.[1, 2] In preparation for a median sternotomy,

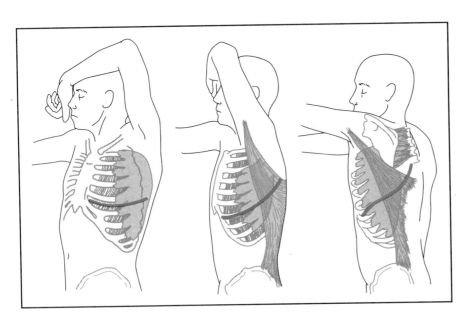

Figure 11–3. The lateral thoracotomy incision. This incision is often used because it spares the latissimus dorsi (the muscle does not have to be divided) while providing access for pneumonectomy, lobectomy, or wedge resection procedures. (Redrawn with permission from Cooper F [ed]. The Craft of Surgery, Vol. 1, Boston, Little, Brown & Co, 1964, p 197.)

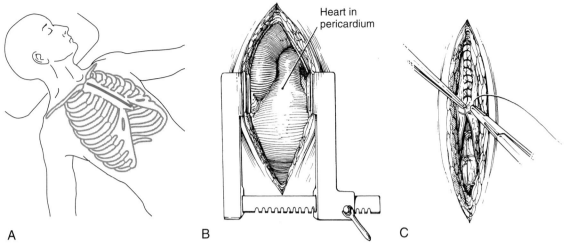

Heart in
pericardium

A   B   C

Figure 11-4. The median sternotomy incision is the most frequently used incision for cardiac procedures. *A,* The incision begins inferior to the suprasternal notch and extends below the xiphoid process. *B,* A sternal retractor maintains the incision open for access to the thoracic contents. *C,* The sternum is approximated and sutured closed with stainless steel sutures through or around the sternum; the wound is then closed in layers. (*B* and *C* from Cooley DA. Techniques in Cardiac Surgery. 2nd ed. Philadelphia, WB Saunders, 1984, pp 18, 19.)

the patient is placed in the supine position. The initial skin incision usually begins in the midline inferior to the suprasternal notch and extends below the xiphoid (Fig. 11-4*A*). The sternum is divided along its midline in a series of steps, and a sternal retractor is used to hold the incision open (Fig. 11-4*B*). At the end of the surgical procedure, the sternum is generally closed with stainless steel sutures either through or around the sternum, and the wound is closed in layers (Fig. 11-4*C*).

Thoracoabdominal Incisions

A **thoracoabdominal incision** permits procedures on the diaphragm, esophagus, biliary tract, right lobe of the liver, spleen, adrenal gland, and kidney, as well as placement of portacaval shunts. In

preparation, patients are positioned supine with the operative side rotated upward 30 to 45 degrees, the buttocks and back elevated and the arm on the operative side extended anteriorly as in a posterolateral thoracotomy. The incision usually extends from the eighth or ninth intercostal space at the posterior axillary line to the midline of the abdomen, transecting the latissimus dorsi, serratus anterior, external oblique, and rectus abdominis muscles (Fig. 11-5).

Specific Surgical Procedures

A description of all of the possible cardiovascular or thoracic surgical procedures is well beyond the scope of this chapter. However, because cardiovascular and thoracic surgical procedures are so prevalent, a few procedures deserve attention.

Percutaneous Revascularization Procedures

As discussed in Chapter 3, coronary arterial atherosclerotic disease can produce occlusive plaques that, in turn, compromise coronary arterial blood flow to such an extent that coronary arterial revascularization procedures become nec-

> **Clinical Note:**
> **Thoracoabdominal Incision**
> Individuals with a thoracoabdominal incision often have problems with coughing, deep breathing, and thoracic extension. Therefore, therapeutic interventions should be implemented early to prevent pulmonary complications, and forward flexed postures should be avoided.

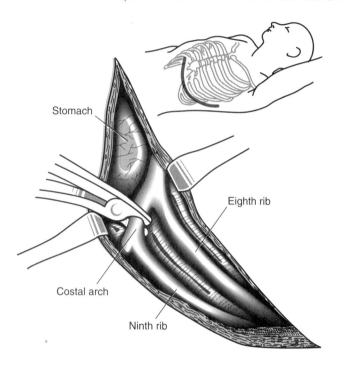

Stomach

Eighth rib

Costal arch

Ninth rib

Figure 11–5. The thoracoabdominal incision. This incision is used for procedures involving the diaphragm, the upper abdomen, or the retroperitoneal space. (Redrawn from Waldhausen JA, Pierce WS. Johnson's Surgery of the Chest. 5th ed. Chicago, Year Book Medical Publishers, 1985, p 59.)

essary to preserve myocardial integrity. Three procedures are discussed: angioplasty, arthrectomy, and stenting. Common to each of these procedures is the introduction (under fluoroscopic guidance) of a balloon-equipped catheter, via a peripheral arterial access site (e.g., femoral artery), into the coronary arterial tree to the site of the stenotic lesion. The procedure is successful if the lumen remains patent when the catheter is withdrawn and there is no ensuing angiospasm. The return of blood flow to the distribution of the previously occluded artery is immediately checked by means of an angiogram (see Chapter 8). None of the procedures is completely risk free; the arterial wall can be perforated when the lesion is penetrated, or it can rupture when the balloon is inflated.[3–6] Therefore, it is not uncommon to have a cardiac surgical suite held in reserve for the emergency remediation of any complications. Generally, however, no significant postoperative movement restrictions are associated with the procedure—patients can be ambulatory within a matter of hours following the procedure. Patients are rarely hospitalized for more than 2 to 3 days, if that long. In fact, many patients are tested, on an outpatient basis, to determine the extent of the resolution of preprocedure electrocardiographic ischemic changes and referred for outpatient cardiac rehabilitation within that time frame.

A **percutaneous transluminal coronary angioplasty (PTCA)** may be performed when a stenotic lesion is not too large, that is, when it does not completely occlude the lumen of the coronary artery. The atherosclerotic lesion is penetrated, and the balloon at the distal aspect of the catheter is inflated—compressing the central portion of the lesion outward against the wall of the artery (Fig. 11–6A). This process may be repeated with successively larger catheters to increase the lumen size as much as possible. A **directional coronary arthrectomy (DCA)** may be performed instead of, or in conjunction with, a percutaneous transluminal coronary angioplasty.[7] This procedure involves the introduction of an arthrectomy catheter through the stenotic lesion of a coronary artery. The cutter housing, which is at the distal end of the catheter through the stenotic lesion of a coronary artery,

---

Clinical Note: Percutaneous Transluminal Coronary Angioplasty

The literature reports a 70% success rate with PTCA, of which 30% undergo a repeat PTCA. Of the 30% repeat procedures, approximately 70% are successful. Less successful outcomes have been reported for women.

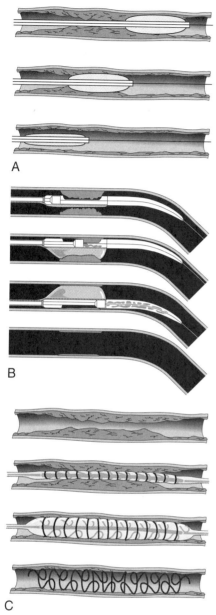

Figure 11–6. Percutaneous coronary revascularization. *A,* Percutaneous transluminal coronary angioplasty catheters are positioned at the distal end of a stenotic lesion before the balloon is inflated to compress the lesion against the arterial walls. (Redrawn from Greenhalgh RM. Vascular Surgical Techniques—An Atlas. 2nd ed. London, WB Saunders, 1989, p 315.) *B,* Atherectomy catheters are positioned so that the cutter housing is held firmly against the atheroma before the cutter is advanced. (Redrawn from Holmes DR, Garratt KN. Atherectomy. Oxford, Blackwell Scientific Publications, 1992, p 24.) *C,* Intravascular stents are positioned within a stenotic lesion before being expanded. (Redrawn from Roubin GS, King SB, Douglas JS, et al. Intracoronary stenting during percutaneous transluminal coronary angioplasty. Circulation 81[suppl IV]: IV92–IV100, 1990.)

has a longitudinal opening on one side and an inflatable balloon on the other. The opening is positioned so that it faces the atheroma, and the balloon is inflated so that the housing is fixed against the arterial wall, displacing the atheroma into the housing opening. The cutter is then activated and advanced, pushing an excised specimen into the distal part of the housing (Fig. 11–6*B*). Technologic advances have reached the point that atherectomies may now be performed using laser-tipped catheters also.

The placement of **endoluminal stents** is another means of coronary revascularization that has gained clinical acceptance.[8] Stents are tiny spring-like devices introduced into a stenotic lesion in an effort to increase the intravascular luminal diameter (Fig. 11–6*C*). Stents have been instrumental in the improvement in the safety and effectiveness of percutaneous coronary interventions. A 40% reduction has been reported in the need for repeat intervention or coronary bypass surgery over a 1-year follow-up.[9] Also, since the addition of potent antiplatelet agents such as GPIIb/IIIa (glycoprotein) inhibitors, stent placement has improved the angioplasty outcome, particularly for patients at risk for closure (diabetic and repeat stenosis patients).[10, 11]

Coronary Artery Bypass Graft

When a coronary arterial atherosclerotic lesion progresses to such an extent that the artery becomes completely occluded, or when the lesion is not amenable to percutaneous transluminal coronary angioplasty or directional coronary arthrectomy, a **coronary artery bypass graft (CABG)** may have to be performed to revascularize the myocardium. The Coronary Artery Surgery Study (CASS) concluded that surgical revascularization is the optimal choice for management of coronary artery disease when all *three* vessels are severely obstructed. A reduction in mortality rate was the clinical outcome used in the CASS study when surgical intervention was compared to medical management in patients with severe coronary artery disease and impaired left ventricular function.[12]

Vascular grafts are often procured from either or both of the saphenous veins (Fig. 11–7), but the left internal mammary artery can also be diverted for use in a coronary revascularization procedure. Following a median sternotomy, the site or

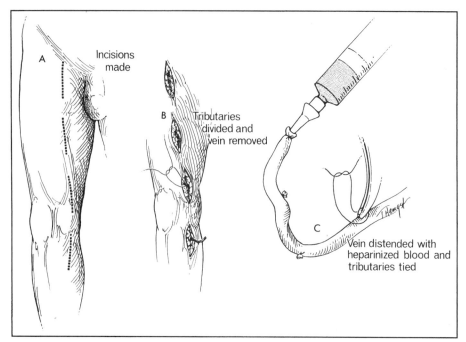

Figure 11–7. Procurement of saphenous vein grafts for use in coronary artery bypass surgery. (From Cooley DA. Techniques in Cardiac Surgery. 2nd ed. Philadelphia, WB Saunders, 1984, p 225.)

sites of coronary arterial blockage are located and isolated. When a saphenous vein graft is used, it is cut to the appropriate length and desired shape before being anastomosed above and below the occlusion (Fig. 11–8). If the internal mammary

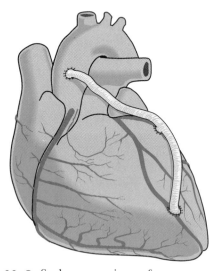

Figure 11–8. Saphenous vein grafts are anastomosed above and below the level of the occlusive lesion after they are cut to the appropriate length and desired shape.

artery is used in the revascularization procedure, it is anastomosed below the level of the occlusive lesion (Fig. 11–9). The use of internal thoracic arteries is preferable for achieving better long-term outcome, because these vessels have proved to be more resistant to graft atherosclerosis (a frequent problem with saphenous graft use).[13, 14] Once grafting is completed, the tissue layers are approximated and the wound is closed.

Recent improvements in the surgical approach include the use of smaller incisions with microinstrumentation (termed **minimally invasive direct coronary artery bypass, or MIDCAB**). MIDCAB involves a small thoracotomy and does not require the use of the heart-lung bypass machine. The procedure is limited, however, to the isolated internal mammary-LAD (left anterior descending artery) anastomosis, and therefore has not been widely adopted. Postoperative complications and recovery time are reduced, extubation is performed earlier, and patients are mobilized earlier, all potential reasons for improved surgical outcomes.

Other advances in coronary bypass grafting include the use of ultrasound guided cannulations, which have decreased the incidence of embolic

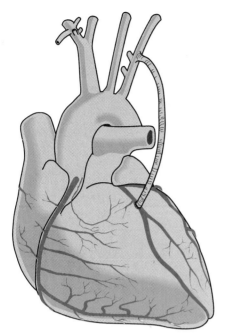

Figure 11–9. Internal mammary arterial grafts are anastomosed below the level of the occlusive lesion. (Redrawn from Waldhausen JA, Pierce WS. Johnson's Surgery of the Chest. 5th ed. Chicago, Year Book Medical Publishers, 1985, p 480.)

cerebrovascular accidents (CVAs). Again, patients do not undergo a sternotomy, but are placed on cardiopulmonary bypass by special catheters. Because the procedure is time-consuming and the technique itself is expensive, the surgical community has not adopted this procedure as a standard procedure for bypass.

A third surgical variation for coronary bypass involves a sternotomy, but no cardiopulmonary bypass, called the **off-pump coronary artery bypass (OPCAB).** The surgeon operates on a beating heart. This procedure has been more accepted than the other procedures mentioned but is not considered a standard operating procedure at the time of this publication.

Clinical Note: Coronary Artery Bypass Graft

Clinical complications observed after CABG surgery include pulmonary infection, chest wall soreness, and lower extremity discomfort or infection. Therapeutic interventions should be implemented early to prevent or minimize such complications.

Thoracic Organ Transplantation

Heart and lung transplantation is performed using a median sternotomy technique and is discussed in great detail in Chapter 12.

Surgical Interventions for Other Common Vascular Disorders

Carotid Endarterectomy

Carotid endarterectomy, although a somewhat controversial surgery from the mid-1980s to mid-1990s, has become more popular since the pub-

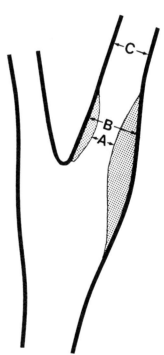

Figure 11–10. The method to measure carotid artery stenosis that was used in clinical trials demonstrating efficacy uses the narrowest part of the lumen (A) and the internal carotid size distal to the bifurcation and the atherosclerotic lesion (C). Using a theoretical bulb measurement (B) will overestimate the stenosis. This method is in agreement with the North American Symptomatic Carotid Endarterectomy Trial (NASCET) and Asymptomatic Carotid Atherosclerosis Study (ACAS) criteria for patient categorization. (From Rutherford RB. Vascular Surgery. 5th ed. Philadelphia, WB Saunders, 2000, Fig. 128–1, p 1738.)

lication of the North American Symptomatic Carotid Endarterectomy (NASCET) Trial and the Asymptomatic Carotid Atherosclerosis Study (ACAS) trial.[15, 16] Both studies provided data on appropriate patient selection, as well as data on measuring stenosis (Fig. 11–10).

Candidates for this procedure include:

- The symptomatic patient with carotid artery stenosis of 70% or greater
- The symptomatic patient with a stenosis of 50% to 69% of the carotid artery (demonstrated only modest benefit)

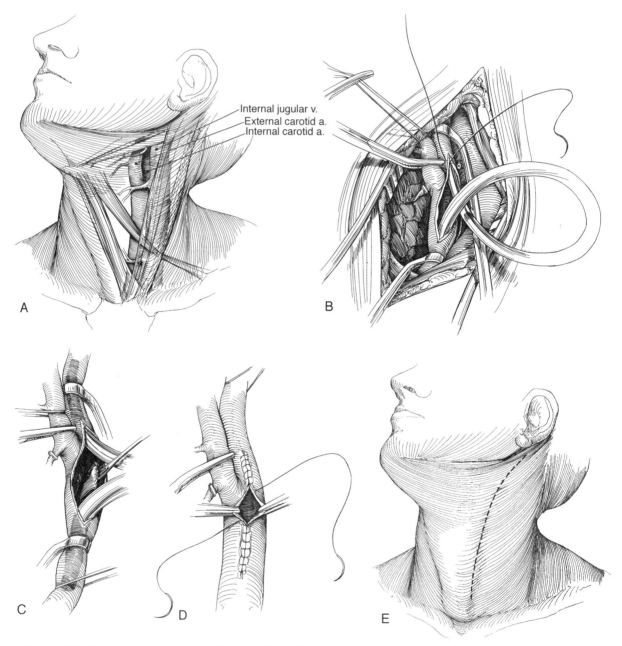

Figure 11–11. Surgical procedure for carotid endarterectomy to prevent stroke caused by atherosclerotic plaques. *A,* The anatomic position of the internal and external carotid arteries. *B,* The insertion of a temporary bypass shunt. *C,* The atherosclerotic plaque that is to be removed. *D,* The arteriotomy closure and suturing performed after the shunt is removed. *E,* The anatomic position of the closed suture (scar) present following the surgery. (From Economou SG. Atlas of Surgical Techniques. Philadelphia, WB Saunders, 1996, pp 642–647.)

- The asymptomatic patient with stenosis of 60% or greater

The procedure involves a surgical incision along the anterior border of the sternocleidomastoid muscle to allow for maximal exposure of the upper carotid artery (see Fig. 11–11A). The common and external carotid arteries are occluded with clamps, an incision is made, and a temporary bypass shunt is inserted (Fig. 11–11B). The plaque is removed (Fig. 11–11C), and the arteriotomy closed with sutures (Fig. 11–11D) while the bypass shunt is removed. The patient is left with an incision scar on the lateral aspect of the neck (Fig. 11–11E).[17]

The outcome of carotid endarterectomy, as determined from both the NASCET and ACAS trials, primarily involves a decreased risk of stroke in the vascular distribution "at risk" for many years. The risk of undergoing carotid endarterectomy was shown to increase as the severity of disease increased; therefore, those likely to benefit the most from the surgery were those who had the highest risk in undergoing the operation.[18]

The use of angioplasty in carotid artery disease is not indicated because of the risk of iatrogenic embolization; however, the use of stents may be indicated for the carotid artery.[19]

Abdominal Aortic Aneurysmectomy

Patients who undergo **abdominal aortic aneurysmectomy (AAA)** elect to have the procedure performed unless the aneurysm has ruptured (at which time the individual must have immediate surgical attention). The procedure involves a midline incision from the xiphoid to the pubis. The aorta is cross-clamped below the renal arteries and above the aneurysm, and two clamps are placed on the iliac arteries (Fig. 11–12A and B). An incision is made between the renal and iliac vessels, and the atherosclerotic material is removed (Fig.

> ### Clinical Note: Abdominal Aortic Aneurysmectomy
> Clinical techniques to assist with cough for AAA repair include splinting with pillows or towel rolls at the incisional site and forceful huffing.

11–12C). The aneurysm is then cut transversely just distal to the beginning of the aneurysm, and a graft that includes two iliac artery extensions is sutured to the aorta, and then to each iliac artery (Fig. 11–12D and E). Following completion of the suturing, the clamps are removed and circulation is evaluated prior to closing the midline incision.[17]

Because of the invasiveness of this procedure throughout the abdomen, patients undergoing this procedure are at high risk for pulmonary complications. Incisional pain and the use of the abdominal musculature in coughing discourage the patient from full inspirations as well as effective forceful huffing or coughing. Appropriate bronchial hygiene techniques are essential for decreasing the incidence of pulmonary complications, especially in patients with chronic pulmonary disease.

Peripheral Vascular Interventions

The type of intervention for peripheral vascular disease (surgical intervention versus percutaneous transluminal angioplasty and possible stenting) is determined based upon the following specific factors[18]:

- Characteristics of the lesions (location, stenosis versus occlusion, lesion length)
- Pattern of arterial occlusive disease (multilevel versus single level, runoff status)
- Patient demographics (gender, presence or absence of diabetes)
- Clinical situation (recurrent disease and indications for intervention)

> ### Clinical Note: Systemic Atherosclerosis
> The clinician should *suspect* that other vessels, besides the carotid vessels, have atherosclerosis because atherosclerosis is a systemic disease. The other vessels to suspect include the coronary arteries, peripheral vasculature, and possibly the renal vasculature.

> ### Clinical Note: Peripheral Vascular Intervention
> Weight bearing on the affected extremity is a concern with any peripheral vascular intervention; however, exercise and mobility are extremely important. Caution should always be taken to elevate the affected extremity when in the sitting position.

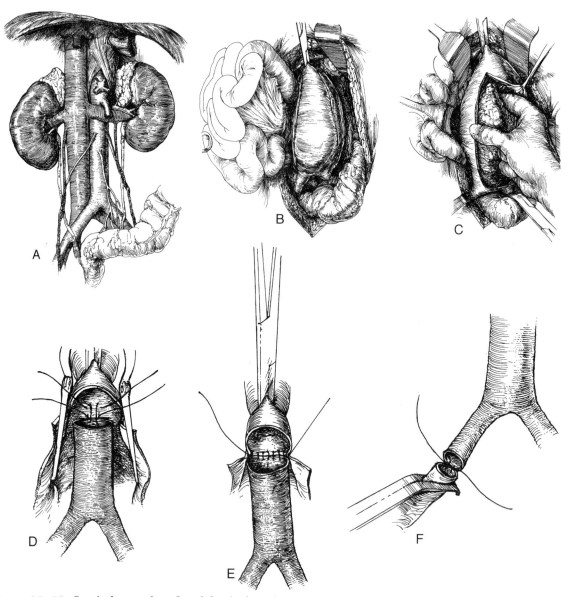

Figure 11–12. Surgical procedure for abdominal aortic aneurysmectomy to prevent spontaneous rupture of the aorta. *A,* The anatomic position of the aorta, which makes its entry into the abdominal area at the twelfth thoracic vertebra and bifurcates at the level of the iliac crest. *B,* The aortic aneurysm with the omentum and colon removed laterally to the left. *C,* The sweeping removal of the atherosclerotic material following surgical dissection. *D, E,* and *F,* suturing of the distal anastomoses. (From Economou SG. Atlas of Surgical Techniques, Philadelphia, WB Saunders, 1996, pp 648–655.)

• Intraprocedural factors (initial hemodynamic response)

In general, one of the strongest predictors of successful outcome for peripheral vascular intervention involves the clinical symptom of claudication. Patients with claudication pain have better long-term outcomes and require fewer amputations than patients with limb-threatening ischemia.[18] Angioplasty is chosen over surgery in individuals with short to moderate length stenotic disease, with mild disease in the proximal or distal arterial segments. Stents are utilized in association with angioplasty (Fig. 11–13).

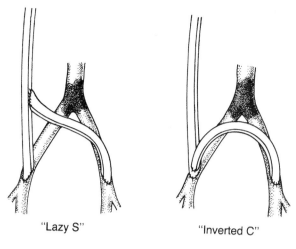

"Lazy S"   "Inverted C"

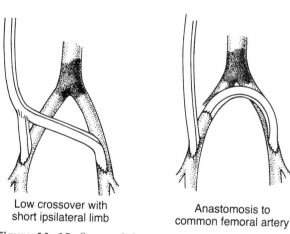

Low crossover with   Anastomosis to
short ipsilateral limb   common femoral artery

Figure 11–13. Some of the more commonly employed configurations for connecting the side limb of an axillobifemoral bypass. (From Rutherford RB. Vascular Surgery. 5th ed. Philadelphia, WB Saunders, 2000, Fig. 68–63, p 989.)

Peripheral Vascular Surgery

Surgical bypass and arterial reconstruction interventions can be performed on any vessel peripherally. Some of the more common sites include femoral-popliteal regions, aortofemoral region, infrapopliteal, and axillobifemoral (Fig. 11–14). Candidates for surgical intervention include patients with long lesions (≥0.5 cm), multiple stenoses, a very critical single stenosis in a diffusely irregular segment, or an occlusion.

Percutaneous Myocardial Revascularization: Use of Lasers. A new technique approved by the FDA for the treatment of chronic myocardial is-

chemia in those who have failed conventional bypass and angioplasty involves laser technology to create small channels in the myocardium (called **transmyocardial laser revascularization,** or **TMR**). The drilled holes do not increase the blood flow, but rather stimulate the myocardium to form small collateral vessels, and this response appears to contribute to relief of chest pain in these patients.[20, 21] Initial transmyocardial channels drilled with a CO_2 laser were used as an adjunct to coronary bypass surgery, but are now performed without surgery.[21, 22] However, CO_2 laser irradiation requires fiberoptic conduits and therefore an open thoracotomy so that the epicardial surface is exposed, placing patients at similar risk as open thoracotomy bypass surgery. To reduce the risks of open thorocotomy, the technique of percutaneous myocardial revascularization (PMR) was developed.[20] Ultraviolet or infrared laser irradiation is used in PMR and is transmitted along optical fibers without surgical intervention. The thermal effects from the laser may result in local denervation and may be the cause of the decrease in chest pain.[23]

Results have been conflicting with respect to long-term patency following TMR and PMR; however, it has been suggested that angiogenesis plays some role after these procedures. Histologic studies have demonstrated endothelialization and an increase in small capillaries in the laser-treated areas.[24–26]

Gene Therapy for the Stimulation of Angiogenesis. Recombinant human vascular endothelial growth factor (VEGF) is an agent that shows promise for stimulating the growth of new blood vessels.[27, 28] Therapeutic angiogenesis was first successfully demonstrated in humans with critical limb ischemia when gene transfer of naked DNA encoding for VEGF was used for the treatment. Improved blood flow to the ischemic limb was demonstrated on 1-year follow-up, and patients reported they were symptom-free.[27, 29]

The adult heart has been shown to have a reduced ability to produce growth factors and stimulate angiogenesis in response to ischemia. VEGF has several isoforms and is considered to be a potent angiogenic agent because it is endothelial cell specific.[29, 30] Currently experimental studies have demonstrated that both VEGF and fibroblast growth factor (FGF) can stimulate small vessel formation, as demonstrated by angiography; however, clinical benefit for patients has not been demonstrated to date (Table 11–1).[31] There is concern that stimulation of cell proliferation may cause

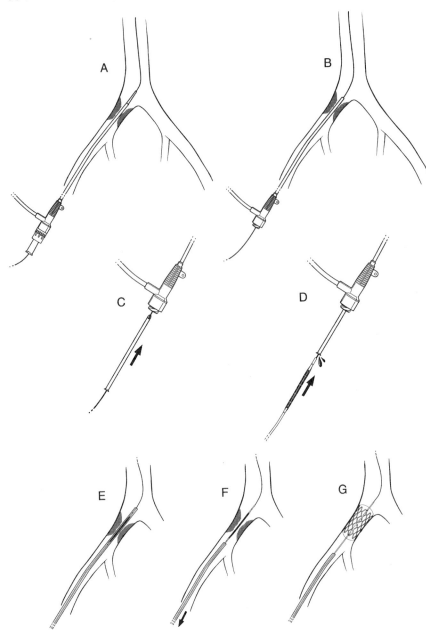

Figure 11-14. Technique of Palmaz stent placement. *A,* A long dilator and sheath are advanced across the iliac lesion. *B,* The dilator is removed, leaving the sheath across the stenosis. *C,* A metal introducer with a beveled end opens the hemostatic valve on the head of the sheath. *D,* The stent is placed at the desired location within the lesion using fluoroscopic guidance. *E* and *F,* The sheath is withdrawn to expose the mounted stent. *G,* The balloon is inflated to deploy the stent. (From Rutherford RB. Vascular Surgery. 5th ed. Philadelphia, WB Saunders, 2000, Fig. 72-7, p 1048; Schneider PA. A stent is an intravascular graft. In: Endovascular Skills. St. Louis, Quality Medical Publishing, 1998, pp 133-164.)

detrimental effects if cell proliferation occurs at the wrong site within a coronary artery (such as at an atherosclerotic plaque, therefore inducing plaque growth), or if a tumor-like hemangioma develops.[31]

Radiation

Irradiation, which is effective in treating proliferation disorders, has been investigated for the treatment of stent restenosis. When the endothelium is exposed to controlled amounts of radiation emitted from tiny seeds imbedded inside a catheter, the incidence of restenosis of the artery is reduced.[32] Early results have consistently shown a substantial benefit over standard techniques of stent alone. Treatment with radiation may also reduce the risk of restenosis in individuals who undergo angioplasty without stent placement, but again, long-term studies are needed in this area.

Table 11–1

Three Potential Mechanisms for Biorevascularization

	GENE	PROTEIN	TIME
Mechanism	Transfection ⇓ Growth factor ⇓ Angiogenesis	Growth factor ⇓ Angiogenesis	Denervation ⇓ Inflammation ⇓ Growth factors ⇓ Angiogenesis
Duration of effect	Weeks	Hours	Weeks

The natural angiogenic response initiated in chronically ischemic tissue by hypoxia-responsive growth factors is insufficient to adequately relieve ischemia. Gene transfer of growth factor genes to muscle tissue by either adenovirus, naked DNA, or several other techniques results in transcription, translation, and secretion of the growth factor locally. The growth factor then acts locally on receptors of endothelial cells to stimulate the cell cycle and promote vascular growth. Infusion of growth factor proteins is also effective, but it may require sustained or repeated infusions for maximal effect. Transmyocardial laser revascularization (TMR) uses laser technology to create small channels in the myocardium. It appears that the channels themselves do not remain patent; rather, the inflammatory reaction to the necrotic core created by the laser stimulates an angiogenic response.

Modified from Engler RL, Martin J (chairs). Joint AHA/ESC Symposium: Biorevascularization. Presented at the American Heart Association 72nd Scientific Sessions, Atlanta, GA, November 7–10, 1999. Plenary Session XI, No. 10.

Pacemaker Implantation

A cardiac pacemaker is an electronic pulse generator used to create an artificial action potential for the purpose of controlling some types of cardiac arrhythmias. Pacemakers may be used as a temporary measure to control transient arrhythmias during myocardial infarction or following cardiac surgery when vagal tone (parasympathetic stimulation) is often increased. Chronic arrhythmias (e.g., second- or third-degree heart blocks or recurrent tachyarrhythmias) may require the surgical implantation of a permanent pacemaker. The American College of Cardiology has published guidelines that discuss specific electrocardiographic indications for pacemaker implantation.[33] However, the criteria actually applied often vary from institution to institution.[34] Nevertheless, the general indications involve sinoatrial nodal disorders (e.g., bradyarrhythmias), atrioventricular nodal disorders (e.g., complete heart block, Mobitz type II arrhythmia), or tachyarrhythmias (e.g., supraventricular tachycardia, frequent ventricular ectopy) that result in hemodynamic embarrassment (signs and symptoms such as lightheadedness, fainting, blurred vision, slurred speech, confusion, or weakness) due to inadequate cardiac output. (See Chapter 9 for more information about cardiac arrhythmias and their appearance on electrocardiogram [ECG].)

Cardiac pacemakers are able to initiate myocardial depolarization by creating an electrical voltage difference between two electrodes, thus initiating an artificial depolarization spike. Figure 11–15 shows typical ECG tracings of atrially and ventricularly paced rhythms. Cardiac pacemakers employ electrical conduction configurations that are classified as being either unipolar or bipolar (Fig. 11–16). **Unipolar pacing systems** use one electrode that is in direct contact with the cardiac tissue; the second, or anodal, electrode is usually the metal housing of the pacemaker, which is located at some point distant to the myocardium. **Bipolar pacing systems** use two electrodes that are in close proximity to each other where they make contact with the myocardium. Currently, a new type of pacemaker with three leads is under study.

Rechargeable power sources for cardiac pacemakers are no longer employed, and it is highly unlikely that a pacemaker operating from a mercury zinc power source is in operation today. The vast majority of pacemakers in current clinical use operate from lithium-chemistry power sources,

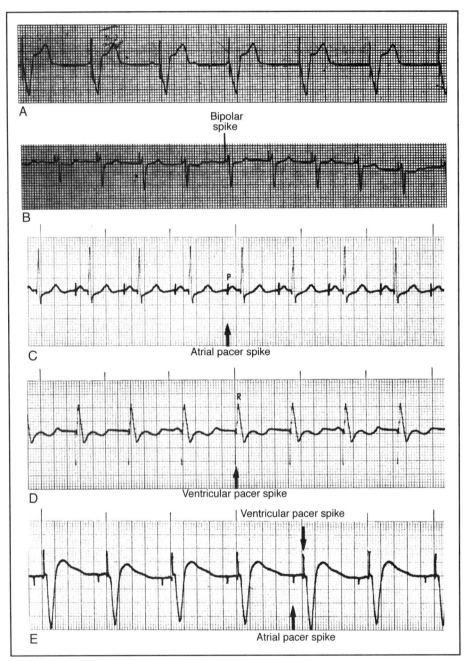

Figure 11-15. Appearance of pacemaker rhythms on electrocardiogram. *A*, Typical unipolar pacemaker spikes precede each ventricular complex. *B*, Bipolar pacemaker spikes are small (or invisible). *C*, Atrial pacemaker rhythm. *D*, Ventricular pacemaker rhythm. *E*, Sequential (atrial and ventricular) pacemaker rhythm. (*A* and *B* from Conover MB. Understanding Electrocardiography. 5th ed. St. Louis, CV Mosby, 1990, p 389. *C*, *D*, and *E* from Atwood S, Stanton C, Storey J. Introduction to Basic Cardiac Dysrhythmias. St. Louis, CV Mosby, 1990, pp 115, 116, 117.)

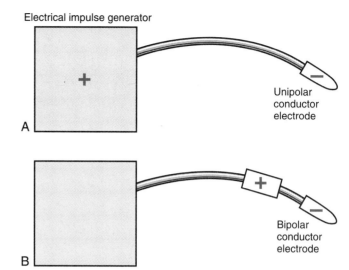

Electrical impulse generator

Unipolar conductor electrode

Bipolar conductor electrode

Figure 11-16. Pacemaker electrode configurations. *A,* Unipolar electrode. *B,* Bipolar electrode.

although "nuclear" (radioactive plutonium) **pacemakers** have been available for more than 15 years. On an actuarial basis, the 50% survival point (the battery half-life) of modern lithium–chemistry-powered pacemakers is greater than 6 years. According to Bilitch and co-workers in 1987,[35] 88% of nuclear-powered pacemakers were operational after 12 years of use.

Regardless of the electrode configuration, cardiac pacing leads are of two primary types:

• **Endocardial leads** are placed inside the right atrium, the right ventricle, or both via a transvenous route.
• **Epicardial leads** are attached directly to the surface of the right atrium or the right or left ventricle.

No matter which type of electrode is used, the pacing lead is constructed of multiple strands of conductive material so that, unlike monofilament conductors, it can withstand repeated flexure without breaking. The importance of this aspect of pacing lead construction is made abundantly clear when one considers that if a patient's heart is paced at a constant rate of 68 beats per minute, the lead flexes 35,765,280 times per year.

Endocardial lead placement can be made by means of *transvenous* (technically *pervenous* because the leads go through the vessel, not across it) insertion via the subclavian, internal jugular, or cephalic venous routes. However, the preferred route of insertion for permanent endocardial leads is via the left cephalic vein, with the impulse gen-

erator being placed in an infraclavicular pocket (Fig. 11–17).[36] The tips of these transvenous electrodes are placed in direct contact with the interior surface of either the right atrium or right ventricle, or both. A new kind of pacemaker (experimental at the time of this publication) utilizing three leads has been designed for individuals with severe heart failure. The experimental pacemaker has two leads that are attached to the right atrium and right ventricle, and the third lead is threaded inside the coronary sinus vein of the left ventricle to resynchronize the ventricles to pump more efficiently (Fig. 11–18). The two primary indications for this pacemaker are left bundle branch block and severe heart failure.

Epicardial implantation is usually accomplished during a cardiac surgical procedure. Sometimes conductive suture electrodes are sewn into the exterior myocardial wall for temporary pacing; however, in most cases electrodes are screwed, hooked, or sewn onto the myocardial surface for permanent pacing. For temporary external pacing, conductive lead wires frequently exit the chest from small subxiphoid incision. For permanent pacing,

> **Clinical Note: Cardiac Pacemakers**
> The clinician needs to know the type of pacemaker that the patient has in order to understand the ECG tracing that will be displayed, as well as whether or not there are any precautions with exercise.

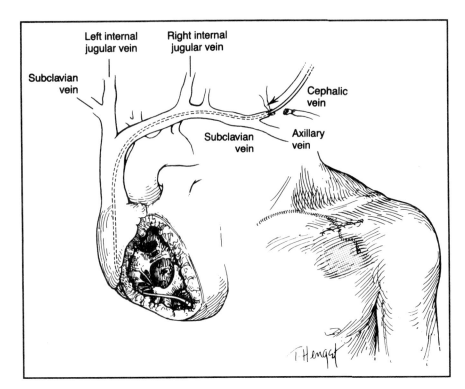

Left internal
jugular vein

Right internal
jugular vein

Subclavian
vein

Cephalic
vein

Axillary
vein

Subclavian
vein

T Henger

Figure 11–17. An endocardial electrode may be inserted transvenously (left cephalic vein depicted here) into the right atrium or ventricle and connected to a permanent pacemaker that is placed in an infraclavicular pocket. (Adapted from Cooley DA. Techniques in Cardiac Surgery. 2nd ed. Philadelphia, WB Saunders, 1984, p 79.)

Figure 11–18. The triple lead system uses two leads that are threaded into the right atrium and the right ventricle. A third lead goes inside the coronary sinus vein of the left ventricle to resynchronize the ventricles to pump more efficiently.

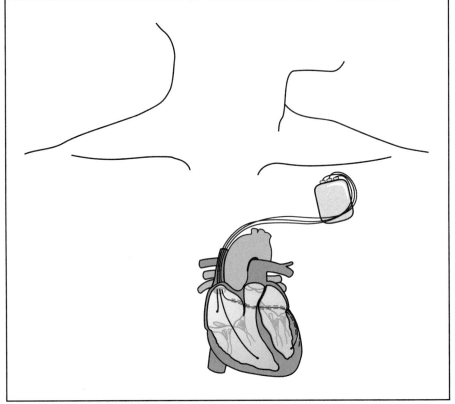

the impulse generator may be placed in a subxiphoid rectus sheath pocket (Fig. 11–19*A*). If for some reason (e.g., abdominal infection, primary thoracic entry via median sternotomy) the subxiphoid approach cannot be or is not used, a transthoracic approach may be employed (Fig. 11–19*B*).

The field of cardiac pacing has expanded explosively, creating the need for a uniform means of communicating information regarding the characteristics of a particular device. The capabilities of current pacing devices—which include telemetry; programmability; and antibradyarrhythmia, antitachyarrhythmia, and adaptive-rate pacing—far surpass those of devices from just a few years ago. In response to the need for a simple code to describe such pacing devices, the North American Society of Pacing and Electrophysiology (NASPE) and the British Pacing and Electrophysiology Group (BPEG) collaborated to devise a generic pacemaker code, the *NBG Code*.[37] The five-position NBG Code has gained widespread clinical acceptance and is summarized in Table 11–2. The first

position of the code provides a classification of the possible stimulation sites for antibradyarrhythmia pacing. The second position classifies the pacemaker's ability to "sense" either atrial or ventricular spontaneous depolarizations, or both. The third position indicates what the pacemaker does if it detects a spontaneous depolarization. The fourth position indicates the programmability or rate modulation capabilities of the pacemaker. The fifth position, if used, indicates the pacemaker's ability to prevent tachyarrhythmia. In many instances, however, only the first three positions of the NBG Code are used in clinical conversation. For example, a pacemaker that can stimulate both the atrium and the ventricle can sense spontaneous depolarizations independently in the atrium and the ventricle, can inhibit a pending stimulus in the chamber in which a spontaneous depolarization was sensed, and at the same time can trigger a ventricular stimulation (after an appropriate interval) in response to sensing a spontaneous atrial depolarization is called a DDD pacemaker. Likewise, a pacemaker that stimulates only

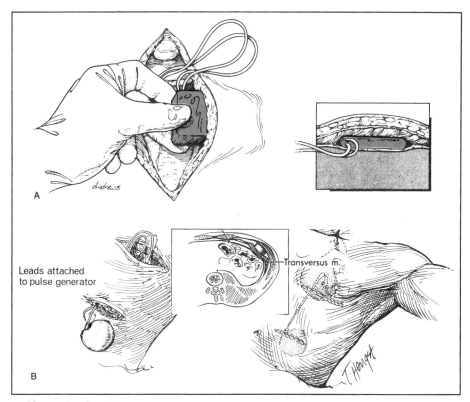

Figure 11–19. Alternative locations for pacemakers. *A,* A subxiphoid pocket, *B,* A transthoracic pocket. (From Cooley DA. Techniques in Cardiac Surgery. 2nd ed. Philadelphia, WB Saunders, 1984, pp 76, 78.)

Table 11–2

The NBG Pacemaker Code

PACING LOCATION	SENSING LOCATION	RESPONSE TO PACING	PROGRAMMABILITY/ MODULATION	ANTITACHYARRHYTHMIA FUNCTION
O = None No antibradyarrhythmia stimulation	N = None No bradyarrhythmia detecting capability	O = None No response	O = None No programmability; no rate modulation	O = None No antitachyarrhythmia capability
A = Atrium	A = Atrium Detects spontaneous atrial depolarizations	I = Inhibited Inhibits a pending stimulus when a spontaneous depolarization is detected	S = Simple programmable Capable of either or both rate and output adjustment	P = Pacing Low-energy stimulus used to interrupt tachyarrhythmia
V = Ventricle	V = Ventricle Detects spontaneous ventricular depolarizations	T = Triggered Detection produces an immediate stimulus in the same chamber	M = Multiprogrammable Can be programmed more extensively	S = Shock High-energy stimulus used to interrupt tachyarrhythmia (e.g., cardioversion or defibrillation)
D = Dual Atrium and ventricle can be stimulated to control bradyarrhythmia	D = Dual Detects spontaneous depolarizations independently in the atrium and the ventricle	D = Dual Can simultaneously inhibit and trigger a stimulus	C = Communicating Can be extensively programmed and has some "telemetry" capability	D = Dual Has both low- and high-energy capability
S = A or V Manufacturer's designation to indicate that either chamber is acceptable for pacing by a single-chamber pacemaker	S = A or V Manufacturer's designation to indicate that either chamber is acceptable for pacing by a single-chamber pacemaker		R = Rate modulation Can automatically control rate by measuring one or more other physiologic variables	

Source: Bernstein AD, Camm AJ, Fletcher RD, et al. The NASPE/BPEG generic pacemaker code for antibradyarrhythmia and adaptive-rate pacing and antitachyarrhythmia devices. PACE 10:795, 1987.

the ventricle, can sense spontaneous depolarizations only in the ventricle, and can inhibit a pending stimulus when a spontaneous depolarization is sensed is called a VVI pacemaker. Clearly, the NBG Code facilitates the exchange of a great deal of information in a very concise format. With a basic understanding of the NBG Code, the physical therapist treating a patient with a pacemaker can anticipate the patient's cardiac response capabilities for myriad situations.

Implantable Cardioverter Defibrillator

The development and continual refinement of the implantable cardioverter defibrillator (ICD, also known as automatic ICD or AICD) has been one of the most significant improvements in the treatment of life-threatening arrhythmias. An ICD is similar to a pacemaker, but is designed to correct life-threatening arrhythmias. An ICD detects and corrects all tachycardias, ventricular fibrillation, *and* bradycardia. The ICD is implanted into the patient, much like a pacemaker, and a separate programmer used to change the function of the ICD is kept at the doctor's office for follow-up care.

Patients with a left ventricular ejection fraction (LVEF) of less than 30% have a threefold to fivefold increase in incidence of sudden death. In addition to ventricular dysfunction, those individuals with frequent or complex PVCs or nonsustained ventricular tachycardia have an increased risk for sudden death. The MADIT (Multicenter Automatic Defibrillator Trial) studies patients with coronary artery disease, low left ventricular ejection fraction, and at least one episode of nonsustained ventricular tachycardia. There was close to a 50% reduction in mortality rate of those treated with ICD therapy versus pharmacologic therapy alone.[38–40] The Multicenter UnSustained Tachycardia Trial (MUSTT) provided further evidence supporting the use of the ICD in patients who have not yet had an episode of ventricular tachycardia but are at high risk for sudden death.[39, 40]

Drainage Tube Placement

Following a thoracic surgical procedure, tubes are typically placed through the chest wall to drain the affected body cavity. Although any tube penetrating the chest wall could be termed a *chest tube,* this term is generally reserved for the description of **intrapleural drainage tubes**—tubes that drain the intrapleural space—or **mediastinal drainage tubes**—tubes that drain the mediastinum. Most chest tubes are multifenestrated, and all are made of an inert material. Like endotracheal tubes, chest tubes have radiopaque markers to facilitate their localization on chest radiographs. Chest tubes and drainage collection systems permit the amount of drainage and intrathoracic blood loss to be monitored, and they provide a means by which the presence of any air leaks can be verified (Fig. 11–20).

Whenever a thoracotomy or median sternotomy is performed, the pleural cavity, mediastinum, or both are generally drained by the placement of one or more chest tubes connected to underwater seal or suction. These chest tubes drain pleural or mediastinal fluids and air with expansion of the lung. Intrapleural tubes are inserted into the second or third intercostal space (ICS) at the midclavicular line to drain air. To drain fluids, they are usually inserted at the fourth or fifth intercostal space at the anterior axillary line (sometimes as low as the eighth or ninth intercostal space at the midaxillary line). The tube's tip is advanced several inches into the pleural space; the distal end of the drainage tube may or may not be attached to a sealed drainage collection system, which may or may not be attached to suction. Posteriorly placed intrapleural tubes are not often used because they are easily kinked; they are also very uncomfortable for the patient. Mediastinal chest tubes are commonly inserted via subxiphoid incisions that are distinct from the sternotomy incision. Chest tubes normally pass obliquely through the chest wall rather than directly through at a right angle (see Fig. 11–20A). The clinician is cautioned against tipping the collection system so as not to compromise the water seal. Because disconnection of intrapleural tubes can result in collapse

> **Clinical Note: Chest Drainage Tubes and Physical Therapy**
> The presence of chest drainage tubes should not preclude the patient's participation in physical therapy activities. Mobility is encouraged unless another complication is a limiting factor.

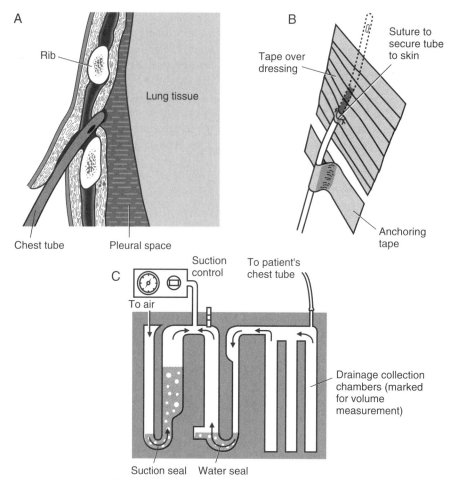

Figure 11–20. Chest drainage tubes may be placed to eliminate fluids, air, or both from the pleural or mediastinal spaces. *A,* A pleural tube being inserted into the pleural space. *B,* Once positioned, the drainage tube is sutured to the skin and covered with an occlusive dressing. *C,* Chest drainage tubes are typically connected to a collection device that may or may not be attached to suction. (*C,* redrawn from Kersten LD. Comprehensive Respiratory Nursing. Philadelphia, WB Saunders, 1989, p 776.)

of the lung, all chest tubes should be treated as if they were intrapleural drainage tubes so that proper precautions are never neglected. Nonetheless, the presence of chest drainage tubes should not preclude the patient's participation in physical therapy activities.

Much like intrapleural tubes, intra-abdominal drainage tubes are used to eliminate air or fluid from the abdominal cavity. Intra-abdominal tubes may simply drain into a collection bag by gravity or be connected to a vacuum device (e.g., Jackson-Pratt drainage tubes). Bladder drainage tubes are also common in the critical care setting. They are usually attached to "urinary catheter bags," which are also frequently used with general acute care patients as well.

CASE STUDIES

Case 1

FM is a 56-year-old man who underwent surgical removal of his right lower lobe with a lateral thoracotomy incision after the diagnosis of lung cancer. FM had a $2\frac{1}{2}$ packs per day history of smoking for the past 36 years. FM works as an automobile mechanic and requires full use of both upper extremities for his job.

Postoperatively, the patient experienced moderate to severe pain and demonstrated a moist nonproductive cough; on the second day after surgery he developed a 100.1°F temperature. Chest x-ray showed atelectasis RML and LLL and infiltrates in LLL. The patient was started on incentive spirometry and respiratory breathing treatment of a bronchodilator every 4 hours.

On the fourth postoperative day the nurse's notes documented that the patient was having difficulty feeding himself with his right arm and was using his left arm. He continued to be very inactive, and only got up to the chair with assistance. PT was ordered for mobility and ROM to right upper extremity.

Discussion: This case demonstrates the complications that can develop with a lateral thoracotomy when aggressive bronchial hygiene and ROM activities are not included early in the patient's postoperative recovery.

Case 2

ST is a 45-year-old man who underwent coronary artery bypass graft surgery for triple-vessel disease, using the left internal mammary and two saphenous vein grafts. A medical sternotomy incision was used, as well as lower leg incision for saphenous vein grafts. The patient ended up back in surgery 6 hours after entering the surgical intensive care unit because of moderate to severe amounts of blood draining in chest tubes. The patient underwent subsequent repair of postoperative bleeding. ECG after surgery showed acute inferior artery injury when compared to preoperative ECG, and both troponin and CPK-MB levels were elevated. The patient was assessed as having a perioperative inferior myocardial infarction.

ST had a past medical history of smoking, hypertension, and above normal intake of alcohol prior to surgery. Postoperatively, the patient demonstrated moist cough, was slow to respond to functional activity because of difficulty bearing weight on left lower extremity (saphenous vein graft incisions caused pain and swelling), and showed decreased ability to bilaterally raise arms over head or use arms to push himself up and out of bed. Patient was started on a ROM exercise program for upper extremities, ankle pumps for involved left lower extremity, bronchial hygiene with incentive spirometer and splinted coughing program, and gait training with a rolling walker.

Discussion: This case demonstrates the complications that may occur with coronary artery bypass surgery, including excessive postoperative bleeding (identified from the amount in the drainage tubes) and perioperative myocardial infarction.

Case 3

MB is a 74-year-old man who was seen s/p left carotid endarterectomy. MB's past medical history includes AAA 2 years prior, femoral-popliteal bypass at age 68, and CABG × 3 at 65. The patient has a long-standing history of smoking, hypertension, and elevated cholesterol. MB's nurse reports the patient has been slow to wake since surgery, was difficult to wean (just weaned) from ventilator, and seems to have difficulty using right upper extremity. Neurology consult concluded patient may have had a left cerebral embolic event since surgery and recommended stroke team to evaluate. The nurse also reports the patient seems to have difficulty

swallowing pills and coughs after attempts of swallowing pills or water. Patient has been placed on aspiration caution, and speech therapy has been asked to see patient to evaluate swallowing.

Case 4

DC is a 62-year-old man who is a plant supervisor, admitted for chest pain, emergency cardiac catheterization, and subsequently underwent CABG x 4. Patient underwent CABG × 3 eight years prior. His past medical history includes smoking (continued to smoke since initial CABG surgery), obesity, and recent history of increased family stress (wife diagnosed with stage IV breast cancer and has undergone mastectomy, bone marrow transplantation, and chemotherapy). Patient has three children living at home (ages 13, 15, and 17). Since surgery, patient has been progressing his mobility, but reports angina with ambulation of 150 ft. Patient underwent repeat cardiac catheterization after surgery, demonstrating that one vessel failed to remain open. Patient is being treated medically for angina, and is to be evaluated for functional ability and cardiac rehabilitation as an outpatient.

Discussion: Patient returned to work 4 weeks after surgery, refused to continue with cardiac rehabilitation because of scheduling conflicts, and continued to have chest pain throughout the day with low levels of activity. Patient is currently awaiting enrollment in scientific study on angiogenesis.

Summary

- The numerous surgical procedures that may be performed on the cardiovascular or pulmonary systems are generally made via one of three approaches (or modifications thereof): thoracotomy incisions are most commonly used for lung resection procedures; most cardiac procedures are performed through a median sternotomy; procedures involving the diaphragm, pericardium, or epicardium are commonly performed through a thoracoabdominal incision.
- Cardiac revascularization procedures are among the most common of cardiothoracic surgical procedures. They may be performed percutaneously (e.g., angioplasty, atherectomy, stenting) or transthoracically (e.g., bypass graft). Either approach is associated with its own postprocedure movement precautions.
- The CASS study concluded that surgical revascularization is the optimal choice for management of coronary artery disease when all *three* vessels were severely obstructed.

- The use of internal thoracic arteries is preferable for achieving improved long-term outcome.
- Recent improvements in the surgical approach include the use of smaller incisions with microinstrumentation (MIDCAB).
- Another surgical variation for coronary bypass involves a sternotomy but no cardiopulmonary bypass and is called the off-pump coronary artery bypass (OPCAB). The surgeon operates on a beating heart.
- A new technique approved by the FDA for the treatment of chronic myocardial ischemia in patients who have failed conventional bypass and angioplasty involves laser technology to create small channels in the myocardium (TMR).
- The risk of undergoing carotid endarterectomy increases as the severity of the disease increases. Those likely to benefit the most from the surgery were those who had the highest risk in undergoing the operation.
- One of the strongest predictors of successful outcome for peripheral vascular intervention involves the clinical symptom of claudication. Patients with claudication pain have better long-term outcomes and require fewer amputations than those with limb-threatening ischemia.
- If, as the result of disease or trauma, the heart is unable to generate an adequate cardiac output, cardiovascular life support equipment is frequently employed to stimulate or augment cardiac function. Pacemaker devices generate an artificial electrical stimulus to supplant or replace the heart's native rhythm of depolarization.
- Chest drainage tubes (e.g., intrapleural or mediastinal) are usually employed following cardiothoracic surgical procedures or chest trauma, or when metabolic disorders so disrupt vascular permeability and osmotic pressures that fluid collects within the thoracic cavity. Their presence should not preclude the patient's participation in physical therapy activities.

References

1. Kittle CF. Thoracic incisions. In: Baue AE (ed). Glenn's Thoracic and Cardiovascular Surgery. 5th ed. East Norwalk, Conn, Appleton & Lange, 1991.
2. Julian OC, Lopez-Belio M, Dye WS, et al. The median sternal incision in intrathoracic surgery with extracorporeal circulation: A general evaluation of its use in heart surgery. Surgery 42:753–761, 1957.
3. Dick RJ, Popma JJ, Muller DW, et al. In-hospital costs associated with new percutaneous coronary devices. Am J Cardiol 68:879–885, 1991.
4. Warner M, Chami Y, Johnson D, Cowley MJ. Directional coronary atherectomy for failed angioplasty due to occlusive coronary dissection. Catheterization Cardiovascular Diagn 24:28–31, 1991.
5. Rowe MH, Hinohara T, White NW, et al. Comparison of dissection rates and angiographic results following directional atherectomy and coronary angioplasty. Am J Cardiol 66:49–53, 1990.
6. Mansour M, Carrozza JP, Kuntz RE, et al. Frequency and outcome of chest pain after two new coronary interventions (atherectomy and stenting). Am J Cardiol 69:1379–1382, 1992.
7. Hinohara T, Selmon MR, Robertson GC, et al. Directional atherectomy. New approaches for treatment of obstructive coronary and peripheral vascular disease. Circulation 81(suppl 3):IV79–IV91, 1990.
8. Kuntz RE, Safian RD, Levine MJ, et al. Novel approach to the analysis of restenosis after the use of three new coronary devices. J Am Coll Cardiol 19:1493–1499, 1992.
9. Williams DO. Catheter-based revascularization beyond the stent. Presented at American Heart Association 72nd Scientific Sessions, Atlanta, GA, November 7, 1999. Plenary Session I: Revascularization in the 21st Century.
10. Topol EJ, Byzova TV, Plow EF. Platelet GPIIb-IIIa blockers. Lancet 353(9148):227–231, 1999.
11. Eeckhout E, Kappenberger L, Goy JL. Stents for intracoronary placement: Current status and future directions. J Am Coll Cardiol 27(4):757–765, 1996.
12. Ringzvist I, Fisher LD, Mock M, et al. Prognostic value of angiographic indices of coronary artery disease from the Coronary Artery Surgery Study (CASS). J Clin Invest 71(6): 1854–1866, 1983.
13. Lytle BW, Loop FD, Cosgrove DM, et al. Long-term (5 to 12 years) serial studies of internal mammary artery and saphenous vein coronary bypass grafts. J Thorac Cardiovasc Surg 89(2):248–258, 1985.
14. Bourassa MG, Fisher LD, Campeau L, et al. Long-term fate of bypass grafts: the Coronary Artery Surgery Study (CASS) and Montreal Heart Institute experiences. Circulation 6(1): 2, 1985.
15. North American Symptomatic Carotid Endarterectomy Trial (NASCET) Collaborators: Beneficial effect of carotid endarterectomy in symptomatic patients with high-grade stenosis. N Engl J Med 325:445–453, 1991.
16. Executive Committee for the Asymptomatic Carotid Atherosclerosis Study: Endarterectomy for asymptomatic carotid stenosis. JAMA 273:1421–1428, 1995.
17. Economou SG, Economou TS. Atlas of Surgical Techniques. Philadelphia, WB Saunders, 1996.
18. Rutherford RB. Vascular Surgery. 5th ed. Philadelphia, WB Saunders, 2000, pp 1738–1739.
19. Brown MM. Balloon angioplasty for extracranial carotid disease. In: Whittemore AD (ed). Advances in Vascular Surgery. Vol 4. St. Louis, Mosby–Year Book, 1996, pp 53–69.
20. Kim CB, Kesten R, Javier M, et al. Percutaneous method of laser transmyocardial revascularization. Catheter Cardiovasc Diagnostics 40(2):223–228, 1997.
21. Mihroseini M, Cayton MM, Shelgikar S, et al. Clinical report: Laser myocardial revascularization. Lasers Surg Med 6: 456–461, 1986.
22. Mihroseini M, Shelgikar S, Cayton MM. New concepts in revascularization of the myocardium. Ann Thoracic Surg 45:415–420, 1988.
23. Kwong KF, Kanellopoulos GK, Schuessler RB, et al. Endocardial laser treatment incompletely denervates canine myocardium. Circulation 96(suppl I):I-565, 1997.

24. Kohomoto T, Fisher PE, DeRosa C, et al. Evidence of angiogenesis in regions treated with transmyocardial laser revascularization. Circulation 94(suppl II):294, 1996.

25. Gassler N, Wintzer HO, Stubbe HM, et al. Transmyocardial laser revascularization: Histological features in human nonresponder myocardium. Circulation 95:371–375, 1997.

26. Mack CA, Magovern CJ, Hahn RT, et al. Channel patency and neovascularization following transmyocardial laser revascularization utilizing an excimer laser: Results and comparison to non-lased channels. Circulation 94(suppl I):I-294, 1996.

27. Majesky MW. A little VEGF goes a long way. Therapeutic angiogenesis by direct injection of vascular endothelial growth factor-encoding plasmid DNA. Circulation 94(12):3062–3064, 1996.

28. Takeshita S, Pu LQ, Stein LA, et al. Intramuscular administration of vascular endothelial growth factor induces dose-dependent collateral artery augmentation in a rabbit model of chronic limb ischemia. Circulation 90(5 Pt 2):II228–II234, 1994.

29. Isner JM, Pieczek A, Schainfeld R, et al. Clinical evidence of angiogenesis after arterial gene transfer of ph VEGF 165 in patients with ischemic limb. Lancet 348:370–380, 1996.

30. Isner JM, Walsh K, Symes J, et al. Arterial gene therapy for therapeutic angiogenesis in patients with peripheral artery disease. Circulation 91:2687–2692, 1995.

31. Epstein SE. Therapeutic angiogenesis. Presented at the American Heart Association 72nd Scientific Sessions, Atlanta, GA, November 7, 1999. Plenary Session I: Revascularization in the 21st Century.

32. Teirstein PS. Prevention of vascular restenosis with radiation. Texas Heart Inst J 25(1):30–33, 1998.

33. Frye RL, Collins JJ, DiSanctis RW, et al. Guidelines for permanent cardiac pacemaker implantation. J Am Coll Cardiol 4:434–442, 1984.

34. Bernstein AD. Classification of cardiac pacemakers. In: El-Sherif N, Samet P. Cardiac Pacing and Electrophysiology. 3rd ed. Philadelphia, WB Saunders, 1991, pp 494–503.

35. Bilitch M, Hauser RG, Goldman BS, et al. Performance of implantable cardiac rhythm management devices. PACE 10:389–398, 1987.

36. Reul GJ. Implantation of permanent cardiac pacemaker. In: Cooley DA. Techniques in Cardiac Surgery. 2nd ed. Philadelphia, WB Saunders, 1984, pp 75–81.

37. The NASPE/BPEG generic pacemaker code for antibradyarrhythmia and adaptive-rate pacing and antitachyarrhythmia devices. PACE 10:794–799, 1987.

38. Block M, Breithardt G. The implantable cardioverter defibrillator and primary prevention of sudden death: The Multicenter Automatic Defibrillator Implantation Trial and the Coronary Artery Bypass Graft (CABG)-Patch Trial. Am J Cardiol 83(5B):74D–78D, 1999.

39. Singh B. Sudden Cardiac Death. Presented at the American Heart Association 72nd Scientific Sessions, Atlanta, GA, November 8, 1999.

40. Connolly SJ. ICD Mortality Trials: Results and Practical Implications. Presented at the 20th Annual Scientific Sessions of the North American Society of Pacing and Electrophysiology, May 14, 1999.

## 12

Thoracic Organ Transplantation: Heart, Heart-Lung, and Lung

Tammy Versluis-Burlis
Anne Downs

INTRODUCTION

Organ transplantation has become a common procedure for managing patients with failing organs. Because of the sequelae of the transplantation procedure and alterations in patient physical performance, physical therapists have become key members of transplant teams, providing expertise in evaluation and rehabilitation of transplant recipients both before and after surgery. Although many similarities exist in the treatment of patients undergoing thoracic organ transplantation and other cardiothoracic surgeries, certain differences significantly affect physical therapy intervention and progression of activity.

In addition to a brief historical review of heart,

heart-lung, and lung transplantation, this chapter presents an overview of the surgical procedures, frequently used medications, and general complications that affect the management of transplant recipients. The physical therapy management of thoracic organ transplantation recipients, from evaluation to outpatient rehabilitation, is presented with a discussion of the similarities and differences in the treatment of heart, heart-lung, and lung transplantation recipients.

HISTORY

In the early 1900s, Carrel and Guthrie[1] first described the techniques for performing extrathoracic transplantation in animal models. Those surgical techniques were not significantly modified until 1933, when Mann[2] proposed a method for **heterotopic** (donor heart is anastomosed to the native heart without removal of the native heart) cervical cardiac transplantation. For the next 20 years, the cervical anastomosis technique was considered the most suitable method for transplantation in canines. In the 1950s, heterotopic transplantation continued to be the principal technique in the canine model, but **orthotopic** (replacement of the native heart with a donor heart) transplantation was gaining favor.

During this time, other important aspects of the heart transplantation procedure were also being explored. Marcus and colleagues[3] described the methodology for circulatory loading in a heart transplanted in the cervical position, and Webb and Howard[4] achieved organ viability for up to 8 hours in a previously refrigerated heart using an intrathoracic placement. In 1958, Goldberg and coworkers[5] reported a successful procedure for orthotopic cardiac transplantation using a cuff of the recipient's left atrium, thereby eliminating the need for separate pulmonary venous anastomoses. One year later, Cass and Brock[6] described the use of a right atrial cuff to avoid separate vena caval anastomoses.

In the 1960s, attention turned from the technical surgical aspects of the transplantation procedure toward a consideration of the damage caused to the donor organ by the recipient's intact immune system. Research by Shumway and colleagues[7, 8] led the way in studying the problem,

and in 1965 they achieved long-term survival in canine transplant recipients with the use of azathioprine and intermittent doses of steroids for **immunosuppression.**[9]

Following the increased success experienced for heart transplantation in animal models, sufficient information and experience were gained to warrant attempts in humans. The first cardiac transplantation was performed on a human in 1964, when Hardy and colleagues[10] attempted a chimpanzee-to-human heart transplant. Unfortunately, the patient survived less than an hour following the procedure. Three years later, in December of 1967, Christiaan Barnard performed the first successful human-to-human heart transplant, marking the beginning of the modern era of cardiac transplantation.[11] Even though Barnard's transplant recipient survived only 18 days before succumbing to the effects of *Pseudomonas* pneumonitis, the accomplishment led to the subsequent organization of 64 heart transplantation centers in 24 different countries by the end of 1969.[11] The initial optimism, which resulted in the performance of 101 cardiac transplantations within the first year, was tempered by postoperative immunologic difficulties, resulting in an average 1-year survival rate of 30% and a decline in the number of heart transplantation centers over the next few years.[11]

When the first human heart transplant was performed, the field of lung transplantation was experiencing a parallel development in the research laboratory. Surgeons using the canine model had been focusing on technique, immunosuppression, and effects of pulmonary denervation, prior to clinical trials in humans. In 1963, the first human lung transplant was performed by Hardy at the University of Mississippi Medical Center.[12] Although the patient died after 18 days because of renal failure, there was no evidence of immunologic rejection of the transplanted lung.[12] Hardy's operation served to demonstrate the technical feasibility of lung transplantation in humans and spurred further research in the field.

During the 1970s and early 1980s, many contributions from a team at Stanford University, directed by Norman Shumway, led to improved survival of transplant recipients by addressing the problems of postoperative care.[13–15] New surgical techniques, instrumentation for tissue sampling, a histologic grading system for tissue samples, and trials of immunosuppressive drugs all served to significantly advance the practice of thoracic transplantation. Most notably, however, the development and use of the immunosuppressant medication, **cyclosporin A** (CyA), in 1980, led to a resurgence of interest and a subsequent increase in the number of thoracic transplantation teams.[11] Cyclosporin A therapy improved the outcome of transplant recipients, resulting in fewer immunosuppressive complications compared with previous chemical agents, which were relatively nonspecific in their spectrum of action.

In the realm of heart-lung en bloc transplantation, although earlier experimental animal studies demonstrated the technical feasiblity of the procedure, difficulties with donor procurement, immunosuppression, and surgical technique remained.[16-18] In 1980, Reitz et al.[18] performed an extended study on primates that answered many questions concerning heart-lung en bloc transplantation. Instead of the previously used right thoracotomy, Reitz favored a median sternotomy and instituted cardiopulmonary bypass, which also achieved surface hypothermia of the donor organ.[18] Thus, in 1981, the first successful human heart-lung en bloc transplantation was performed by Reitz and colleagues.[16-19]

The introduction of CyA for immunosuppression and the numerous advances in the field of transplantation of other organs paved the way for the success of isolated lung transplantation in humans. In 1983, Joel Cooper and associates[20] at the University of Toronto performed the first successful single lung transplant. Immunosuppression was achieved with cyclosporine, azathioprine, and prednisone, and the patient was discharged from the hospital 6 weeks after surgery.[20] This was followed in 1986 by the first successful isolated double lung transplant, also by Dr. Cooper and the Toronto Lung Transplant Group.[21]

Both the impact of CyA and the continued advances in the field of thoracic transplantation have led to an increased number of operations and increased survival rate of recipients. The number of cardiac transplants increased from 90 in 1981 to more than 2000 performed each year since 1988, at 271 heart transplant centers.[22, 23] In 1996, the Registry of the International Society of Heart and Lung Transplantation (ISHLT) reported that through February of 1996, 34,326 heart transplantations had been performed throughout the world.[24] The actuarial 1-year survival rate for heart

transplant recipients has increased from 30% in 1969 to approximately 80% in 1996; the current 5-year survival rate is 60 to 70%, and the 10-year survival rate is 56%.[25, 26] With such impressive survival rates, cardiac transplantation is now an accepted treatment for patients with significant heart disease that can no longer be managed medically.

The number of heart-lung en bloc transplantation procedures has increased each year between 1982 and 1989.[24] Since 1989, however, the number of heart-lung en bloc transplantation procedures has declined each year.[24] The decline is likely due to the shortage of donors and the possible use of an alternative procedure, the isolated lung transplantation coupled with any needed cardiac repair. Data for 1996 indicate that 1954 heart-lung en bloc transplants were performed in 105 heart-lung transplant programs worldwide. To date, actuarial survival rate statistics for 1 year are 60%, but decrease dramatically to less than 20% at 10 years.[24]

ISHLT data for 1996 indicate that 3194 isolated single lung transplants and 1845 double lung transplants have been performed to date.[24] The current survival rate for single lung transplantation is 70% at 1 year, 62% at 2 years, 55% at 3 years, and 44% at 4 years.[24] There is an apparent reduction in the survival of recipients over the age of 60 (60%) compared to those younger than 60 years of age (70%) for a 1-year period.[24] Survival rates for bilateral (double) lung transplants are about 70% at 1 year and 55% at 4 years.

EVALUATION

Candidacy

The primary indication for heart, heart-lung, and lung transplantation is a progressive terminal cardiopulmonary disease with a limited life expectancy.[27-32] The majority of patients with end-stage disease show a marked decrease in cardiopulmonary function, require multiple medications or supplemental oxygen to carry out activities of daily living, and are no longer able to work or attend school full time. Disease processes that may lead to the need for thoracic organ transplantation are presented in Table 12–1.

The majority of heart transplants are required because of coronary artery disease, which leads to

Table 12-1

Indications for Thoracic Organ Transplantations[33-36]

Orthotopic heart
  Cardiomyopathy
  Coronary artery disease
  Congenital heart disease
  Valvular heart disease
  Cardiac tumors
  Amyloidosis
Heterotopic heart
  Patients with a high pulmonary vascular resistance
Heart-lung
  Congenital heart diseases (Eisenmenger's syndrome)
  Cystic fibrosis
  Primary pulmonary hypertension
Single lung
  Pulmonary fibrosis or other restrictive diseases
  Emphysema
  Alpha$_1$-antitrypsin deficiency
  Patients with pulmonary vascular disease
Double lung
  Patients with an infectious lung disease
  Emphysema
  Primary pulmonary hypertension
Thoracic organ repeat transplantation
  Bronchiolitis obliterans
  Graft failure
  Intractable airway problems
  Severe acute rejection
  Transplant coronary artery disease

myocardial damage and cardiomyopathy.[33] The majority of lung transplants have been performed in patients who have emphysema or cystic fibrosis.[33] The use of single organs for lung transplantation is preferable whenever feasible because such procedures double the number of candidates that can be served by available donors.

Failure of a transplanted organ is also an indication for heart, heart-lung, and lung transplantation (repeat transplantation). Hosenpud[33] reports 3% of heart and heart-lung transplants, and 4% of both single and double lung transplants, are repeat transplantation surgeries.

Criteria and Contraindications

Candidate selection criteria vary among transplant centers. Table 12–2 details the most common criteria used for placing an individual on a transplant waiting list. The criteria may be considered either absolute, meaning the criterion must be met, or relative, meaning that the criterion is important but that some centers' guidelines will not deem that it is absolutely necessary. The relative criteria identify those patients with increased chances of a successful outcome. For example, a candidate who has a good support system will be more likely to comply with the intensive regimen after transplantation.

Table 12-2

Selection Criteria for Heart and Lung Transplant Recipients[20, 23, 25-32, 126]

Absolute criteria	
NYHA class IV or III with $VO_{2\ max} < 14\ mL \cdot kg^{-1} \cdot min^{-1}$	H Tx*
Normal function or reversible dysfunction of extracardiac organ systems	H Tx, L Tx†
Transpulmonary gradient (mean PAP-mean PLWP) < 15 mm Hg without diabetic end-organ involvement	H Tx
Collagen vascular disease	H Tx
No evidence of malignancy for more than 5 years	H Tx, L Tx
Severe obstructive or restrictive lung disease or severe pulmonary hypertension	L Tx
Limited life expectancy	H Tx, L Tx
No contraindications to immunosuppression	H Tx, L Tx
Relative criteria	
Without current evidence of alcoholism, smoking, and substance abuse	H Tx, L Tx
FVC $> 50\%$ predicted and $FEV_1 > 1$ L	H Tx
Age < 60 years	H Tx, L Tx
Left ejection fraction $> 20\%$	H Tx
Sound psychological make-up and adequate social support system	H Tx, L Tx
Ability to comply with medications and follow-up regimen	H Tx, L Tx
Capable of meeting financial requirements	H Tx, L Tx
No pan-resistant organisms in sputum	L Tx
Ambulatory with rehabilitation potential	H Tx, L Tx

*H Tx = heart transplantation
†L Tx = lung transplantation.

The following are contraindications for heart, heart-lung, and lung transplantation: older than 60 years of age, pre-existing condition that would be worsened by immunosuppression, requirement for high doses of corticosteroids preoperatively, or coronary artery disease (for lung transplantation only).[28] Another contraindication is resistance to antibiotics used to treat infectious organisms.[37] Additional relative contraindications for transplantation differ from center to center, but include the presence of conditions such as previous thoracic surgeries (lung transplantation only), ventilator dependency, and the presence of certain infectious organisms (e.g., *Burkholderia cepacia*, methicillin-resistant *Staphylococcus aureus* [MRSA], vancomycin-resistant *Endococcus* [VRE]).

Medical Aspects of Evaluation

The decision to refer a patient to a transplant center for evaluation is a difficult one. The primary physician must (1) weigh the trend of the health status of the patient against the average time spent on the waiting list, and (2) find a balance between disclosing the complete spectrum of available medical treatments and offering the end-stage treatment (transplantation) before a patient is ready to fully acknowledge the gravity of the situation. If the decision is made to refer the patient to a transplant center, the patient must be evaluated by that center for acceptance into the program. The evaluation may be completed during an inpatient stay or, as is increasingly common, during outpatient visits.

The evaluation process includes a medical assessment as outlined in Table 12–3. The medical assessment provides information about the presence of any contraindications to transplantation—for example, active systemic disease and renal or hepatic insufficiency.[38] The candidate is also evaluated by members of the transplant team. Table 12–4 outlines specific information obtained by each of the team members. The screening evaluation also provides key information about social issues, patient compliance, and general health that is useful in predicting the patient's response to the transplantation process.

The transplantation candidate must be able to comply with a complicated medical regimen and have sufficient social support to endure the stres-

---

Table 12–3

Tests and Procedures for Transplant Evaluation

Laboratory tests
  Arterial blood gases
  Complete blood cell count
  Electrolytes, BUN, creatinine, liver function tests
  Chest radiograph
  Sputum culture
  Urinalysis
Pulmonary assessment
  Pulmonary function tests
  Ventilation/perfusion scan
  Computed tomography scan (when indicated)
Cardiac assessment
  12-lead electrocardiogram
  Echocardiogram
  MUGA scan
  Cardiac catheterization
  Coronary angiography
  Cardiac biopsy (when indicated)
Other
  Bone density scan (when indicated)

Key: BUN = blood urea nitrogen; MUGA = multiple uptake gated acquisition
Source: Egan TM, Kaiser LR, Cooper JD. Lung Transplantation. Curr Probl Surg 26:673–752, 1989.

Table 12–4

Evaluation by Heart, Lung, and Heart-Lung Transplant Team Members

Physicians and medical staff	Medical history
	Nature and progression of disease
	Smoking history
	Prior surgery
	Medications, including steroid usage
	Physical examination
Physical therapist	Exercise tolerance test and exercise prescription
	Musculoskeletal assessment
	Cough/mucociliary clearance
Dietitian	Ideal body weight
	Caloric intake
Social worker or pastoral care	Psychosocial assessment
Psychologist/ psychiatrist	Psychological testing

Source: Egan TM, Kaiser LR, Cooper JD. Lung Transplantation. Curr Probl Surg 26:673–752, 1989.

sors associated with both the pre- and postoperative stages of transplantation.[39, 40] The emotional reaction to the transplantation process is complex and intense. Kuhn and colleagues[41] have identified stages of emotional adjustment through which a patient progresses in dealing with his or her disease. Kuhn's stages include the pretransplant evaluation, waiting for the organ, perioperative period, in-hospital convalescence, discharge, and postdischarge adaptation. Stressors common to these stages are listed in Table 12–5.

The results of the evaluation are compiled by the transplant coordinator and provide the basis for discussion of the patient's candidacy. If accepted, the patient is placed on a waiting list; lists are maintained separately for heart, heart-lung, and lung transplantation candidates. Priority on the heart transplant list is maintained by the **United Network of Organ Sharing** (UNOS). The recipient waiting list is prioritized on the basis of severity of disease and by the date the candidate is placed on the waiting list. The highest priority (UNOS status 1) is given to potential recipients who are in the most critical state of health.[42] UNOS status 1 potential recipients are typically inpatients on mechanical circulatory support and require intravenous inotropic medications. Patients identified as status 2 are those able to be at home.

Priority on the lung transplant list is also maintained by UNOS but, unlike the heart transplant waiting list, is solely determined by the date a candidate is placed on the waiting list; no distinction is made among potential recipients based on clinical status. The only exception is a bonus of 90 days added to the time accrued on the waiting list for patients diagnosed with idiopathic pulmonary fibrosis, lessening their wait for a donor (UNOS policy No. 3.7). This reduced waiting time is necessary because of the inability of such patients to survive the typical waiting period. The median waiting time was 654 days in 1997, based on UNOS Scientific Registry data as of September 7, 1999. The average waiting time for a donor has increased because of the growing number of individuals on the waiting lists and of centers that perform transplantations.

Physical Therapy Evaluation

Physical therapy evaluation of the potential transplant candidate is similar to that of any cardiopulmonary medical or surgical patient. The physical therapist focuses on the patient's cardiac and pulmonary system limitations while assessing the candidate's musculoskeletal condition, exercise capacity, ventilatory function, and mucociliary clearance.

As with all evaluations, a focused chart review should precede the physical assessment. Past and recent history should be noted; typically, the patient will have demonstrated a decline in function over the previous 6 to 12 months. Laboratory data along with other test results, medications, and baseline vital signs will give the therapist an overall view of the patient's status. If the patient's status is critical, before proceeding with the physical therapy evaluation it is important to discuss acceptable limits of activity with the physician in charge of the patient's care.

A general evaluation for all potential transplant patients includes assessment of the following: appearance, edema, vital signs, pain, posture, range of motion, strength, bed mobility, transfers, gait, activities of daily living, and exercise tolerance.[43]

Special considerations when evaluating the heart or heart-lung transplantation candidate include an understanding of the results of specific cardiac tests, such as cardiac biopsy or ejection

---

Table 12–5

Psychosocial Stressors in Transplant Applicants and Patients

1. Coping with disabling or life-threatening illness
2. Making financial arrangements required for enrollment
   - Surgical procedure
   - Personal and family expenses
   - Postoperative medical and pharmaceutical care
3. Travel or moving to area of transplant program
4. Changes in medical management and personnel
5. Organizing an adequate support system
6. Fear of being unsuitable for transplantation
7. Onset of medical complications pre- or postoperatively
8. Guilt over the donor's life ending to save theirs

Source: Squires R. Cardiac rehabilitation issues for heart transplantation patients. J Cardiopulm Rehabil 10: 159–168, 1990, and Craven JL, Bright J, Dear CL. Psychiatric, psychosocial and rehabilitative aspects of lung transplantation. Clin Chest Med 1(2):247–257, 1990.

fraction. Ventilation and gas exchange parameters demonstrated by pulmonary function test results should be evaluated for all lung transplant candidates and selected heart and heart-lung transplant candidates, depending upon the cardiac diagnosis.

Evaluation of the patient's breathing or ventilatory function should include assessment of the breathing pattern, extent or use of accessory muscles of respiration, depth of breathing, areas of decreased chest expansion, and work of breathing. These factors should be evaluated at rest, as well as during functional activities and exercise.

In the lung transplant candidate, the efficacy of airway clearance techniques used by the patient should be evaluated by either the respiratory or physical therapist. A careful history and evaluation of sputum production patterns and preferred technique for airway clearance should be performed, noting the effectiveness and ease of techniques utilized. Auscultation of breath sounds should be included as a part of this evaluation. The foregoing components of the evaluation will assist the therapist in counseling the patient regarding (1) ways to improve current methods and (2) use of alternative techniques for airway clearance.[44]

The musculoskeletal evaluation of general strength and mobility is typical of that for other patients, but should emphasize the thoracic area. Musculoskeletal pain, posture, thoracic mobility, and muscle imbalances, wasting, or weakness are assessed by the physical therapist, so that an individualized strengthening and flexibility program may be developed.[45]

Assessment of **exercise tolerance** may be achieved in several ways. Complete cardiopulmonary exercise testing, including a maximal stress test, whereby the analysis of expired gases is evaluated, is not routinely performed at this time because exercise testing to this extreme degree is not tolerated well by transplant candidates. In the small number of studies in which such exercise testing has been reported, heart, heart-lung, and lung transplant candidates exhibit severely reduced aerobic capacities.[46, 47] In heart transplant candidates, Mancini et al[48] demonstrated that patients with a peak oxygen consumption at maximal exercise ($VO_{2\,max}$) of 14 mL/kg/min or less were at higher risk for death and should be referred for transplantation, whereas transplantation can be safely deferred in those patients with a $VO_{2\,max}$ greater than 14 mL/kg/min.

More commonly, a baseline exercise evaluation involves **submaximal treadmill** or **cycle ergometer testing.** A testing protocol with small increments in workload (Naughton, Balke-Ware) versus a testing protocol with large increments in workload (Bruce) is better suited to patients with cardiovascular or respiratory disease because it allows finer distinctions to be made with respect to what the patient is capable of achieving.[49]

A 6- or 12-minute walk has been used extensively in the evaluation of exercise tolerance in patients with pulmonary disease, and is becoming increasingly common in evaluation of patients with cardiac disease.[50–53] In the **six-minute walk test** (6MW) the patient is asked to cover as much distance as possible over a flat, measured course in 6 minutes' time. Patients with severe limitations may require one or more rest periods during the test session, whereas patients with high exercise capacity may be able to run during some or all of the time period.

During exercise testing it is necessary to monitor **oxygen saturation** levels for the heart-lung and lung transplantation candidates because they are likely to have markedly decreased values of forced expiratory volume in the first second (FEV_1) and thus are likely to exhibit oxygen desaturation during exercise.[54] It is also important to correlate the patient's oxygen saturation with hematocrit and hemoglobin levels so that a high oxygen saturation level will not be mistaken as normal in the presence of low hematocrit and hemoglobin levels.

The results of the physical therapy evaluation are used to determine whether an exercise program is indicated. Typically, exercise is contraindicated in patients with primary pulmonary hypertension (defined as an increase in normal pulmonary artery pressure, 15 to 18 mm Hg, by 5 to 10 mm Hg) because exercise aggravates the condition, causing pulmonary artery pressures to rise adversely.[55] If exercise is indicated, evaluation provides a basis for prescribing an individualized program for the patient. The physical therapy assessment also contains information that the transplant team will use in making the decision about candidacy for transplantation. For example, the therapist will note any deterrents to patient compliance with previous or current exercise or airway clearance regimen. This information could then be used to reject or defer candidacy status.

The duration of the physical therapy evaluation

period is such that it may be necessary to schedule a follow-up appointment or refer a patient elsewhere for follow-up to implement additional recommendations for exercise and to assist with airway clearance.

PREOPERATIVE REHABILITATION

Research has demonstrated that transplant candidates can achieve significant training effects from long-term rehabilitation programs.[56, 57] The training effects are achieved mainly through peripheral adaptations that provide the patient with an improved functional and exercise capacity. For example, lung transplantation centers have reported improvements of up to 39% in 6MW tests of transplant candidates participating in preoperative exercise programs.[28, 58]

Components of a preoperative rehabilitation program include the following:

1. Patient and family education regarding the surgical procedures utilized, physiologic changes that will follow surgery, and components of rehabilitation during the pre- and postoperative periods
2. Cardiovascular endurance training
3. Musculoskeletal strength and flexibility training
4. Breathing retraining

The goal of rehabilitation prior to surgery is to improve or to prevent deterioration of the candidate's physical condition. Ensuring that candidates are in the best physical condition will increase the likelihood that they will be able to endure the stresses of transplantation. Improving the status of the patients may also play a role in increasing survival of patients on the transplant waiting list, because a decline in medical status is the greatest cause of death for those patients awaiting transplantation.

Typically, the patient waiting for heart or heart-lung transplantation is encouraged to remain as active as possible within the limits of standard hemodynamic guidelines (see Chapter 18). Often the heart and heart-lung candidates' level of participation in endurance activities will be limited to minimal levels of exertion or even activities of daily living (ADLs) because of their significantly com-

promised ejection fraction and cardiac output. Pretransplant candidates may also demonstrate other unstable hemodynamic symptoms that further compromise oxygen supply to the heart and peripheral body tissues. Examples of unstable hemodynamic abnormalities include hypotension (which limits tissue perfusion), reduced lung volumes and decreased pulmonary perfusion (which may cause ventilation-perfusion mismatch), and increased pulmonary vascular resistance (which is associated with an increased respiratory rate). With increased activity these abnormalities worsen, limiting a candidate's participation in an endurance or strengthening program. If a heart or heart-lung transplant candidate is suitable for endurance training, they should be monitored closely by individuals trained to recognize inappropriate responses to exercise. The endurance training program often begins in a formal cardiac rehabilitation program and subsequently continues at home or in a community exercise program.

Other areas to be emphasized in cardiac rehabilitation focus on correct posture, mobility training, and education regarding heart and heart-lung transplant complications. The goal of rehabilitation is to maintain and potentially improve the physical condition of the patient.

Lung transplant candidates are also encouraged to begin or continue an exercise/activity program. The exercise may be done at home, in a supervised community program, or in a monitored pulmonary rehabilitation program. Some lung transplant centers require candidates to relocate close to the center in order to participate in a monitored exercise program at some point during their wait for a donor.[21, 27]

Guidelines for pulmonary rehabilitation (see Chapter 19) should be followed in the pretransplant period. Because of the variable severity of disease, lung transplant candidates will differ significantly from other participants in a pulmonary rehabilitation program. The likelihood that patients awaiting transplantation will exhibit exercise-induced hypoxemia is increased. Consequently, oxygen saturation should be monitored continuously during exercise sessions, and efforts should be made to maintain oxygen saturation at greater than 90%.[54] Although lung function may not improve, substantial increases in exercise performance have been reported in patients with end-stage pulmonary disease.[59, 60] Most patients are able to participate in 30 to 40 minutes of endurance exercise three to five times per week at 70 to 80% of predicted maximal heart rate while maintaining appropriate oxygen saturation levels.[54]

ALTERNATIVE THERAPIES TO TRANSPLANTATION

Following review by the transplantation team, patient suitability is determined. If the patient is found to be unsuitable for transplantation, this determination may be due to a number of factors, including the following: the presence of contraindications limits the potential success of the surgery, the overall benefits for the patient from the transplantation procedure are not favorable, the patient did not meet the criteria of organ system failure, or the patient opted for more conservative surgical or medical management. When any of these situations is present, the patient must be managed in other ways. For end-stage pulmonary disease, lung volume reduction surgery or biphasic positive airway pressure may be used as a replacement for lung transplantation or to improve the patient's status until a transplant is performed. Left ventricular assistive system, home pharmacologic management, or cardiac myoplasty may be used for patients with end-stage cardiac disease to improve status or to bridge the time to heart transplantation.

Alternatives To Lung Transplantation

Lung volume reduction surgery (LVRS) is a surgical procedure aimed at reducing the size of the lungs in patients with emphysema (Fig. 12–1). The surgery may be performed prior to a patient being placed on a waiting list to forestall the need for transplantation or instead of transplantation for those patients who choose not to have one. During the surgical procedure, 20 to 30% of the volume of each lung is removed. The procedure is performed via a median sternotomy incision. LVRS is performed to improve thoracic distention and chest wall mechanics. Work by Trulock and colleagues[61] demonstrates that improvement is made

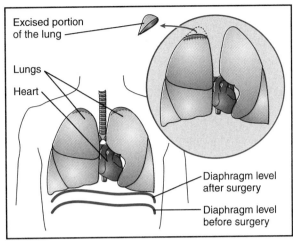

Figure 12–1. The mechanics of lung volume reduction surgery.

in both the patient's symptoms and pulmonary function by potentially improving FEV_1 by 100%. Carbon dioxide retention is decreased, and oxygen use can often be discontinued owing to the improvement in blood gas values. Other benefits documented by Sciurba[62] include clinical improvement of dyspnea, improved expiratory flow rates, improved lung volumes, and increased 6MW values. Sciurba,[63] Cooper,[64] and Trulock[62] attribute the improvements to one or more of these possibilities. The first hypothesis suggests that the surgery causes an increase in elastic recoil of the lung, creating a greater efficiency in respiratory muscle and chest wall mechanics.

The second hypothesis suggests that there may be a beneficial effect on the mechanical function of the musculoskeletal components of the respiratory system. For example, prior to surgery a patient has hyperinflated lungs and increased functional residual capacity (FRC), which presumably put the respiratory muscles at a mechanical disadvantage. Following surgery, the lung reduction decreases FRC which might allow for improved function of the respiratory muscles because they are working at a more optimal length for contraction.

The third proposed mechanism for improvement is also related to the resultant decrease in lung hyperinflation. With the reduction of lung volume, the restrictive effects caused by lung hyperinflation are ameliorated and normal cardiac filling is possible.[64] Thus, cardiac efficiency is improved and the ventilation-to-perfusion ratio is enhanced.

An ongoing multicenter trial is under way to determine the safety and effectiveness of LVRS. The objectives are to document (1) the benefits and risks over long-term follow-up (5 years), (2) the patient selection criteria that predict the best outcome, and (3) the surgical procedure (thoracoscopy versus median sternotomy) that is associated with the best outcome.[65] This effort may lead to more widespread acceptance of lung volume reduction surgery.

Progressive respiratory failure in the lung transplant candidate may necessitate the use of noninvasive **biphasic positive airway pressure** (BiPAP). BiPAP, also called **pressure release ventilation** (Fig. 12–2), utilizes a tightly fitting nasal mask to noninvasively deliver positive airway pressure during inspiration as well as on exhalation. It is indicated for patients with signs of respiratory failure despite maximal drug and oxygen therapy in an attempt to avoid intubation. Use of this device at night has resulted in a decrease in the work of breathing, headaches, and daytime fatigue, and an increase in quality of sleep and level of activity.[66, 67] BiPAP has been useful as an adjunct for patients awaiting transplantation by alleviating symptoms of respiratory failure.[67]

Alternatives to Heart Transplantation

Unfortunately, a patient with cardiac muscle dysfunction often demonstrates a deterioration in medical status quickly, not leaving adequate time for the surgical or medical procedures that could prevent the need for heart transplantation. In such instances the placement of a left or right **ventricular assistive system** or device (LVAS or LVAD) for heart transplantation candidates may be indicated to provide a bridge until a suitable donor organ becomes available and transplantation can be accomplished.

The Novacor system is a totally implantable (Fig. 12–3), electrically powered LVAS that provides permanent support of the systemic circulation in those patients for whom a suitable cardiac donor cannot yet be found.[68] It is indicated for patients with severe hemodynamic compromise for whom maximal drug therapy and other medical interventions have not proven successful. The system allows variability in pump output according to the patient's physiologic demands, allowing the patient to participate in a progressive, monitored exercise program.[69] The ability of the patient to resume activities of daily living and an exercise

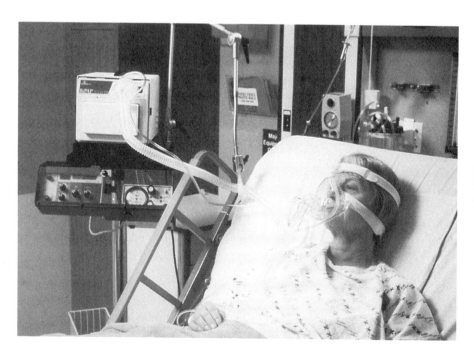

Figure 12–2. Patient on BiPAP S/T-D30. (Courtesy of Respironics, Inc., Murrysville, PA.)

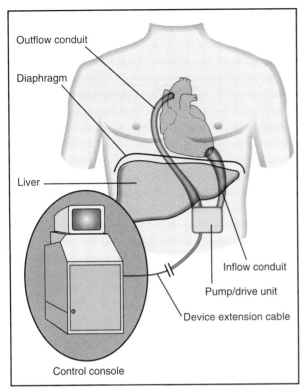

Figure 12–3. An LVAS unit can be used as a bridge until heart transplantation is available.

program leads to improved conditioning in preparation for a heart transplant. The LVAS has been used successfully as a bridge to transplant.[69]

Pharmacologic management of the patient with congestive heart failure is becoming more common as ease and portability of monitors to assess the patient's status are being developed. The major pharmacologic agents used include **angiotensin-converting enzyme inhibitors** coupled with diuretic therapy. Inotropic therapy and beta$_1$ selective antagonists may also be used as secondary agents.[70, 71] Currently, intravenous dobutamine is used in the hospital and at home to improve cardiac output. Treatment objectives associated with drug therapy include the reduction of central circulatory congestion or edema and the improvement of systemic perfusion.[70, 71] Other desirable aims include the reduction of myocardial oxygen consumption, enhancement of coronary perfusion, slowing of rapid heart rate, restoration of baroreceptor function, reversal of neurohumoral activation, restoration of cardiac size and shape, promotion of cardiac and

vascular repair, and enhancement of survival.[70, 71] If the patient with heart failure reaches a stage where they are not able to be managed at home with pharmacologic agents and they are placed on the transplant waiting list, the process of looking for a suitable donor will begin.

Cardiomyoplasty is a relatively new alternative to heart transplantation. Cardiomyoplasty is a surgical procedure in which a transformed, fatigue-resistant skeletal muscle is wrapped around the patient's heart and is stimulated electrically to contract with cardiac systole. Contraction of the skeletal muscle during systole will augment ventricular function of the failing heart.[72] It is also believed that structural reinforcement of the myocardium by the skeletal muscle prevents further dilatation of the heart and results in an increased ejection fraction.[73] The skeletal muscle typically used is the latissimus dorsi. A flap is created and a series of stimuli are applied. A burst or pulse train is delivered so that the individual muscle units will contract as a unit and be in synchrony with the cardiac beat.

DONOR SELECTION AND MATCHING CRITERIA

A suitable organ donor needs to meet the qualifications of brain death and other criteria specific to the intended transplant. These criteria are summarized in Table 12–6.

A significant shortage of suitable donor organs limits the number of transplants that can be performed, especially for lung and heart-lung transplantation. It has been estimated that only 10 to 20% of available organ donors have lungs that meet the criteria making them suitable for transplantation.[37, 74] Although all criteria should be met, centers cannot strictly adhere to the criteria because the number of ideal donors is very limited.[75]

A careful analysis is conducted to provide optimal matching of a donor and recipient based on blood work and organ size. The donor and recipient must be matched or compatible for **ABO blood group,** and an attempt is made to match **histocompatibility complexes** as closely as possible. Matching is done to decrease the chances of

Table 12-6
Criteria for Donors[17, 32, 38, 39]

Criteria for heart donors
Age less than 40
No history of cardiac disease
No present infection
No positive test for HIV or hepatitis B
No evidence of cardiac trauma
No prolonged resuscitative efforts applied prior
   to death

Criteria for lung donors
Age less than 35
Chest radiograph free of infiltrates
Arterial O_2 tension > 300 mm Hg on 100% O_2
   and 5 cm of PEEP
Clear bronchoscopy without evidence of puru-
   lent secretions or aspiration
No significant chest trauma or pulmonary contu-
   sion

Criteria for heart-lung donors
Age less than 40
No major thoracic trauma
No past history of pulmonary disease, including
   asthma
A short period of ventilation
No systemic or pulmonary infections
Normal findings on chest radiography
Normal lung compliance with a peak inspiratory
   pressure < 20 mm Hg, V_T < 15 mL/kg, and
   an RR between 10 and 14 breaths/min
Normal gas exchange
Inotropic requirement < 10 μg/kg/min dopa-
   mine or dobutamine
Normal ECG

V_T = tidal volume; RR = respiratory rate; O_2 = oxygen.

allograft rejection following surgery as well as to decrease the chances of a primary infection present in the donor from developing in the recipient.[76] For example, a cytomegalovirus (CMV)-negative recipient receiving a CMV-positive organ would develop the CMV infection.

Additional aspects of the donor organ are considered to increase compatibility with the recipient. The cardiac donor's weight should be within 20% of the recipient's unless the recipient's pulmonary vascular resistance is elevated. In this case, a larger donor is used to combat the resistance.[24, 77] Additional considerations in lung donors are compatibility with the recipient's thoracic dimensions (taken from the chest radiograph) and predicted lung volumes based on height, age, and gender.[38]

SURGICAL PROCEDURES

Cardiac Transplantation[34, 78–80]

The two methods for performing cardiac transplantation are heterotopic and orthotopic grafting. **Heterotopic transplantation,** referred to as the "piggyback" technique (Fig. 12–4), is considered to be an alternative technique and is performed less frequently than **orthotopic transplantation.** Special circumstances that may necessitate use of the heterotopic method are mismatching of size between the donor and recipient or a recipient that has an abnormally high level of pulmonary vascular resistance.[34, 81, 82] The heterotopic surgical procedure is performed without the removal of the native heart. The donor heart is connected to the patient's native heart through a median sternotomy incision in the following manner: donor right atrium to recipient right atrium and donor left atrium to recipient left atrium.[34, 42, 78–80] The four atria then function as two atria. Ascending aortas are anastomosed together, and pulmonary arteries are connected via a Dacron tube graft.[34]

Following transplantation, venous return is shared between the two hearts, and cardiac output from each heart occurs independently. This is possible as each heart is stimulated by its own electrical system. Two separate PQRST complexes are thereby seen on electrocardiogram (ECG) recordings (Fig. 12–5).[34, 81, 82]

An advantage of the heterotopic technique is the ability of the native heart to assist the donor heart with cardiac output. This assistance is especially beneficial during periods of transplant rejection and situations in which high pulmonary vascular resistance occurs. Disadvantages to heterotopic heart transplantation include the presence of **arrhythmias** and angina associated with the native heart, the need for long-term anticoagulation therapy to prevent formation of emboli due to a weak left native ventricle, the need to use a prosthetic graft for the pulmonary artery anastomosis, a higher mortality rate, and an increase in right lobe atelectasis due to the donor heart's compressing on the right lung.[32, 34, 78, 83, 84]

The more common cardiac transplant surgery uses the orthotopic technique (Fig. 12–6), which has a higher survival rate than the heterotopic method. Orthotopic heart transplantation replaces

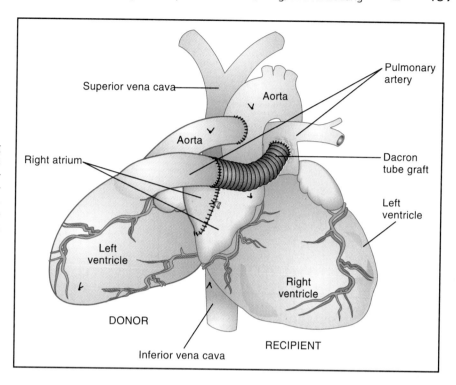

Figure 12–4. This drawing shows a completed preparation of a heterotopic heart transplant with anastomosis sites indicated by the suture lines. The donor and recipient pulmonary arteries are joined via a Dacron graft.

the recipient heart with a donor heart through a median sternotomy incision so that only one heart remains in the chest. Following the institution of cardiopulmonary bypass, the recipient heart is excised, leaving a sizable cuff of right atrium (including the sinoatrial node) and left atrium to be anastomosed with the donor's heart. The aorta and the pulmonary artery are then dissected at the valvular level. The donor heart is then prepared and connected to the recipient through the following anastomoses: left atrium to left atrial cuff, right atrium to right atrial cuff, pulmonary arterial anastomosis, and finally the aortic anastomosis. Air is aspirated out of the donor heart chambers and the patient is then taken off cardiopulmonary bypass. While the sternum remains open, pleural and mediastinal chest tubes are inserted and epicardial pacing wires are attached to the heart. Ide-

ally, the less time the heart is in transition from the donor to the recipient and the sooner surgery is completed, the better the chances for a successful recovery.[78, 83]

Currently, the technique used for orthotopic heart transplantation leaves the recipient sinoatrial (SA) node intact to avoid the need for venous anastomoses.[85] Despite a loss of blood flow, the SA node will remain functional through collateral bronchial circulation, and innervation continues to provide stimulation to the atrial remnants for contraction. Unlike the recipient atrial remnants, the donor heart's SA node is denervated and operates independently of the recipient's. Thus, two separate P waves will be seen on the ECG (Fig. 12–7). One P wave is caused by the recipient SA node and the other is from the donor SA node. The donor's P wave will continue to activate the donor

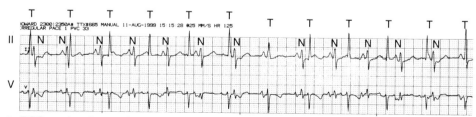

Figure 12–5. ECG tracing from a heterotopic heart transplant recipient. (T = transplanted, donor; N = native.)

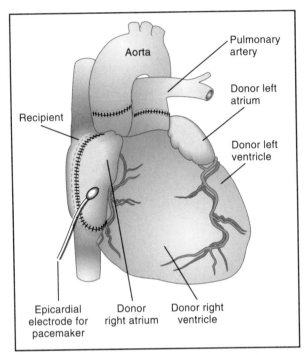

Figure 12-6. This drawing shows a completed preparation of an orthotopic heart transplant with anastomosis sites indicated by the suture lines. An atrial epicardial pacemaker electrode is in place in the donor right atrium.

heart and a resulting QRST complex will occur, providing total contraction of the donor heart to provide cardiac output.

During exercise, periods of anxiety, or other instances of sympathetic stimulation, the rate of the innervated recipient SA node will increase according to increases in the intensity of sympathetic stimulation.[85] The donor SA node rate will not respond as rapidly with sympathetic stimulation due to its state of denervation.[85]

Lung Transplantation

The lungs are harvested from the donor in this manner: the pulmonary veins are detached from the heart along with a cuff of left atrium, the pulmonary arteries are transected, and the lungs removed en bloc, divided into separate right and left lungs for implantation.[28, 86]

Initially, the technique for **double lung transplantation** was performed using a tracheal anastomosis and a double lung bloc. This technique was altered subsequently to utilize bilateral mainstem bronchial anastomoses through a median sternotomy incision.[87] Currently, the preferred procedure maintains use of mainstem bronchial anastomoses, while progressing to use of a bilateral transverse thoracosternotomy, or "clamshell incision," which provides better exposure than the median sternotomy.[88] The anastomoses for double lung transplantation, more accurately referred to as **"bilateral sequential" lung transplantation,** include the pulmonary artery anastomosis followed by the bronchial anastomoses (Figs. 12–8 and 12–9). The need for cardiopulmonary bypass has been reduced by sequential replacement of single lungs as opposed to use of a double lung bloc.[89] The airway anastomoses usually consist of end-to-end anastomoses or a "telescoping" method whereby the donor or recipient airway is inserted in the opposite airway for a distance of one cartilaginous ring.[90] The routine use of an omental pedicle wrap around the bronchial anastomoses to promote healing has been discontinued as it was not found to significantly reduce the incidence of ischemic complications.[90]

Single lung transplantation is performed similarly, using a standard posterolateral thoracotomy

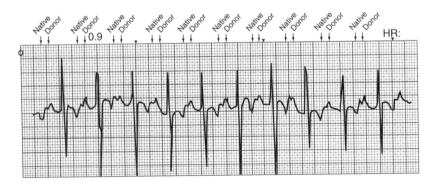

Figure 12-7. ECG tracing from an orthotopic heart transplant recipient. Note the two P waves seen prior to each QRS complex.

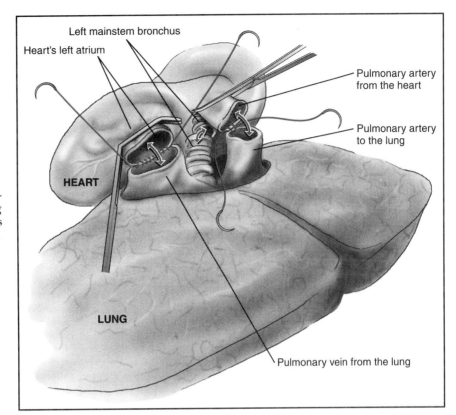

Figure 12–8. Completed preparation of a single left lung transplant with anastomosis sites designated by suture lines.

incision. The atrial anastomosis is performed first, followed by the pulmonary artery anastomosis and the bronchial anastomosis.[91] For a single lung transplantation, the side chosen is related to prior surgery, the desire to replace the worst recipient lung, and the best donor side.

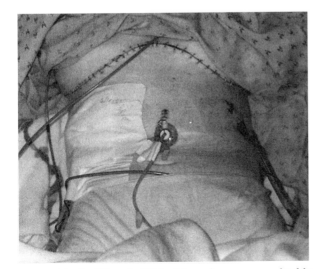

Figure 12–9. "Clamshell" incision shown on a double lung recipient. Note bilateral chest tubes, midline incision used for the omental wrap, and placement of the GI tube.

Heart-Lung Transplantation[17–19]

The operative technique for **heart-lung transplantation** begins with a median sternotomy and anterior pericardiectomy; both phrenic nerves are preserved.[92] The patient is then placed on cardiopulmonary bypass, the ascending aorta is clamped, and the heart and lungs of the patient are excised at the aorta just above the aortic valve, the atrioventricular groove of the right atrium, and across the trachea, above the level of the carina. Similar dissection is performed in the donor. The donor's heart and lungs are then flushed with a cold cardioplegic solution and cooled further with topical cold saline. Implantation occurs with anastomosis of the trachea, aorta, inferior vena cava, and superior vena cava. The heart and lungs are then resuscitated, rewarming occurs, and the thoracic cavity is closed much like what is done with the heart and lung individually.

MEDICATIONS

After surgery the transplant patient is placed on numerous medications.[93] The majority of medications are immunosuppressive agents and drugs used to combat the side effects of the immunosuppressive agents. The immunosuppressive regimen is necessary to prevent rejection of the donor organ by reducing the normal immune system's T-cell response to the foreign tissue.

Medications are initiated in the intensive care unit and continue to be part of the patient's daily regimen. Doses may be tapered to the lowest level possible to prevent rejection, but the medication is never completely stopped. Common medications are listed in Table 12–7.

Table 12–7
Commonly Used Medications for the Thoracic Organ Transplant Patient

MEDICATION	ROUTE OF ADMINISTRATION	MECHANISM OF ACTION	SIGNIFICANT ADVERSE EFFECTS
Cyclosporine (Cyclosporin A, Cy A)	IV or po	Inhibits T-lymphocyte proliferation by blocking transcription of early activation genes; inhibits macrophagic production of interleukin-1	Nephrotoxicity, hepatoxicity, HTN, HA, N&V, leukopenia & thrombocytopenia
Azathioprine (Imuran)	IV or po	Inhibit purine synthesis; powerful anti-inflammatory agent	Hepatoxicity, leukopenia, bone marrow depression resulting in thrombocytopenia, arthralgia, muscle wasting
Prednisone or Solu-Medrol	po	Inhibits cytokine synthesis; inhibits interleukin-1, -2, -6 production or synthesis by macrophages; inhibits T-cell activation; anti-inflammatory agent	CHF, HTN, edema, euphoria, insomnia, glaucoma, cataracts, ulcer formation, osteoporosis, myopathy
Orthoclone OKT3 (Muromonab-CD3)	IV	Monoclonal antibody; blocks T-cell recognition of alloantigen	N & V, chest pain, dyspnea, edema, pulmonary edema, fever, tremor, HA
Gancyclovir sodium	IV	Anti-viral agent used to treat CMV infections	Thrombocytopenia, anemia, rash, abnormal function tests
FK 506	IV or po	Similar to cyclosporin; inhibits calcium-dependent events leading to T-cell activation	HA, tremor, paresthesia, insomnia, anorexia
Additional medications: Gastric motility agents and antacids		Reduce GI upset, stimulate GI motility	
Mycostatin lozenges		Prevent yeast infections	
Bactrim (prophylactic antibiotics)		Prevent bacterial infections	

CHF = congestive heart failure, CMV = cytomegalovirus, GI = gastrointestinal, HA = headache, HTN = hypertension, IV = intravenous, po = by mouth, and N & V = nausea and vomiting.
Source: Craig CR, Stitzel RE: Modern Pharmacology. 4th ed. Boston, Little, Brown, 1994.

Table 12-8

Factors Influencing Cardiovascular Resting and Exercise Physiology After Heart Transplantation

Donor brain death
Composite atria
Surgical denervation of donor heart
Altered ventricular function
    Systolic
    Diastolic
Drug therapy
Skeletal muscle changes
    Pretransplant deconditioning
    Heart failure
Complications of transplantation
    Rejection
    Accelerated coronary sclerosis
    Hypertension
    Renal impairment
    Anemia
    Steroid side effects (e.g., myopathy)
    Donor-recipient size mismatch

Source: Banner NR, Patel N, Cox AP, et al. Altered sympathoadrenal responses to dynamic exercise in cardiac transplant recipients. Cardiovasc Res 23:965–972, 1989, and Banner NR. Exercise physiology and rehabilitation after heart transplantation. J Heart Lung Transplant 237–240, 1992.

following isolated lung transplantation.[91] The response of a denervated heart to activity differs from an innervated heart's response. In the normal heart, elevation of the heart rate from rest to 120 beats per minute (bpm) is regulated by parasympathetic withdrawal mediated by the vagus nerve. The elevation of the heart rate above 120 bpm is achieved by activation of the sympathetic system via sympathetic ganglia. At rest, the absence of parasympathetic innervation causes the donor heart rate to be elevated, often as high as 90 to 110 bpm. The higher heart rate enables the heart to achieve normal cardiac output at rest despite a lower stroke volume and left ventricular ejection fraction following transplantation.[94, 95] With exercise, the peak heart rate of a donor heart will reach only 80% of the peak rate achieved in normal subjects.[95, 96] With activity and exercise, compared with an innervated heart, a denervated heart has a delayed response in increasing its rate (Fig. 12–10).

In a normal heart, the initial response to exercise is related to the stroke volume and heart rate, providing for an increase in cardiac output, whereas in the denervated heart, the cardiac out-

POSTOPERATIVE TREATMENT

Response to Activity

Following surgery it is important for the physical therapist to note that the patient has undergone a major change in cardiovascular physiology. These changes affect the way that the transplant team cares for the patient and the way that the physical therapist works with the patient (Table 12–8). Understanding the basics of the change in cardiovascular physiology is important so that proper precautions may be taken during exercise. Typically, there are improvements in hemodynamic function allowing for an increase in aerobic endurance and activity tolerance as compared with prior hemodynamic function. This can be maximized by aerobic training following surgery.

Changes in Cardiovascular Status

Cardiac denervation occurs following heart or heart-lung transplantation and occurs infrequently

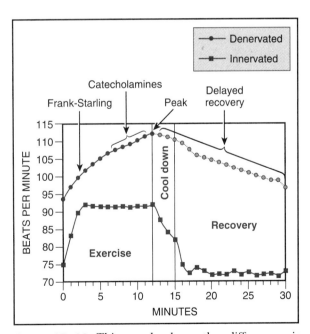

Figure 12–10. This graph shows the differences in heart rate between an innervated heart and a denervated heart. Note the higher resting heart rate of the denervated heart and its slow acceleration and recovery of heart rate with exercise and rest.

put increases, initially, due to stroke volume but heart rate does not change (**Frank-Starling mechanism**). Following the initial 5 minutes of exercise in the transplant patient, heart rate augmentation is due to increased circulating levels of catecholamines. The catecholamines cause an increase in heart rate that contributes to an increase in cardiac output. Over time, a condition known as denervation supersensitivity develops in which the organ becomes increasingly sensitive to endogenous catecholamines, such as noradrenaline.[97] Following the conclusion of exercise or activity, the heart rate may continue to increase for a few minutes before decreasing at a slower rate than normal as a result of the slow reuptake of circulating catecholamines.[43]

In a patient who has had a heterotopic heart transplant, the donor heart responds in the same manner as described for a denervated heart. Because the native heart is still innervated, it continues to respond the way it did before surgery. It is best to monitor both responses by palpation of a peripheral pulse or ECG to see how the donor denervated heart and native innervated heart respond to treatment and activity. Emphasis should be placed on the donor heart when making decisions about treatment and activity tolerance.

The delayed reaction of the denervated heart to the stimulus of activity necessitates an adequate warm-up and cool-down period in conjunction with each exercise session. This is to permit accommodation to the change in activity level.[39] Because of the decreased heart rate response to activity, heart rate monitoring will not provide an accurate measure of exercise intensity. As a substitute for measuring heart rate, a scale for rating of perceived exertion (RPE) or ventilatory response can be used as a basis for prescribing and monitoring exercise.

In the majority of recipients, resting systolic blood pressure is the same or higher than before heart transplantation.[98-100] Research has shown that the peak systolic pressure with exercise is reduced to 80% of normal.[101] At rest, diastolic BP following transplantation typically is elevated due to stiffness of the left ventricular myocardium.[101-103] Hypertension is a significant concern because the likelihood of developing ischemia with total loss of perfusion to the heart is increased.[102] Hypertensive episodes can be avoided by employing optimal patient positioning (i.e., placing the patient in upright sitting versus supine position) and by not using long periods of isometric exercise.[101-104] In the initial stages of an exercise session, the diastolic blood pressure in a healthy individual is expected to rise gradually (less than 10 mm Hg), remain the same, or drop slightly (less than 10 mm Hg). In the heart transplant recipient, blood pressure should be monitored because it may increase abnormally or may actually decline (greater than 20 mm Hg) as the result of decreased peripheral resistance and cause the patient to become hypotensive.[100, 105-107] Hypertension has been reported in lung transplant recipients, but does not occur as soon after transplantation and has a lower incidence than that reported for heart transplant recipients (66% versus 90%).[108]

Changes in Pulmonary Status

Although maximum oxygen uptake ($VO_{2\ max}$), and subsequently exercise capacity, improves significantly after heart, heart-lung, and lung transplantation, it remains well below predicted values.[109-111] The heart transplant recipient's exercise capacity is 60 to 70% of that in normal subjects, whereas recipients of heart-lung or isolated lung achieve 40 to 60% of predicted values.[46, 90, 109-111] The exercise response in single and double lung transplants, 40 to 50% and 40 to 55%, respectively, is remarkably similar, regardless of the underlying disease process.[46, 110] The anaerobic threshold has also been reported to be reduced in recipients of heart, heart-lung, and lung transplants.[43, 94, 95, 98, 101, 109] Furthermore, $VO_{2\ max}$ and anaerobic threshold do not improve 1 to 2 years after transplantation, despite a return to normal activities.[109]

Both single and double lung transplant recipients have mildly elevated respiratory rates and minute ventilation at rest. During exercise, however, the respiratory rate increases appropriately, and no ventilatory limitations are usually noted for heart-lung or lung transplant recipients.[46, 109-111]

The exercise limitation in heart-lung and lung transplant recipients may be attributable to peripheral factors, such as exercise-associated hypertension, muscle atrophy, and suboptimal nutritional status, or deconditioning, as greater attention to rehabilitation after transplantation has demonstrated improved exercise capacity with such patients.[46, 109-111]

In the heart-lung transplant recipient, there is a disruption of two major physiologic systems. Both the normal neural and vascular supplies to the heart and lungs are interrupted.[93] Revascularization occurs through collateral arteries arising from the coronary arterial circulation to feed the tracheal anastomosis, and bronchial blood flow is reestablished through retrograde flow from collateral arteries to the pulmonary arterial circulation.[112, 113] Neurogenically, denervation occurs to both afferent and efferent nerves of the heart and lungs, excluding the postganglionic efferent nerves.[113, 114]

The Acute, Postoperative Inpatient Phase

Postoperatively, patients are evaluated in the intensive care unit (ICU) by the physical therapist once they are medically stable, typically within 12 to 36 hours of surgery. Reverse isolation is observed for days to weeks depending on the transplant center and the acuteness of the transplant.[115] Transplant recipients are initially intubated and mechanically ventilated. Multiple medications are infused via intravenous lines and chest drainage tubes, and endocardial pacemaker wires, Foley catheter, and multiple monitoring devices are present. The combination of these elements confronting the physical therapist creates a challenging environment in which to perform the initial postoperative evaluation (Fig. 12–11).

Physical therapy for the transplant recipient often begins on the first day following transplantation. Intervention will continue until the patient is discharged from the hospital, at which time outpatient rehabilitation provides continuity with inpatient activities. Keeping in mind the ultimate goals of improved function and quality of life, the acute phase of rehabilitation is designed and focused on increasing functional abilities in self-care and mobility, including bed mobility, transfers, and ambulation.

Heart Transplant

In the ICU, the physical therapist's evaluation will resemble that for any patient following cardiothoracic surgery, but focuses first on impaired gas exchange, airway clearance, effects of prolonged static positioning during surgery (nerve injuries), pain, and mobility restrictions. Goals for this phase include the following: (1) optimizing pulmonary hygiene and chest wall mechanics to facilitate weaning from the ventilator and supplemental oxy-

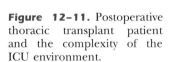

Figure 12–11. Postoperative thoracic transplant patient and the complexity of the ICU environment.

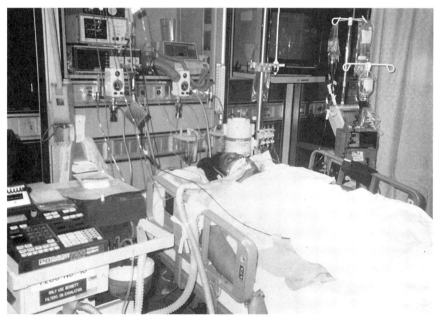

gen, (2) improving strength and range of motion in the upper extremities and thoracic area, and (3) improving exercise tolerance through ADLs and exercising at a low to moderate intensity (e.g., metabolic equivalent, or MET, level of 1 to 3).

Exercise should begin in the supine position and progress to sitting and standing (Fig. 12–12). It is essential to monitor vital signs as indicators of cardiovascular status and the patient's response to increases in activity. Although heart rate should be monitored, it should not be used as the primary indicator of the patient's response. Because the heart is denervated, blood pressure, ventilatory index, and RPE should be monitored along with signs and symptoms of fatigue (such as extreme changes in pallor, flushing, or excessive sweating) for making decisions during treatment. The physical therapist should also remember to allow time for patients to warm up adequately and adapt to changes in position before continuing with an ac-

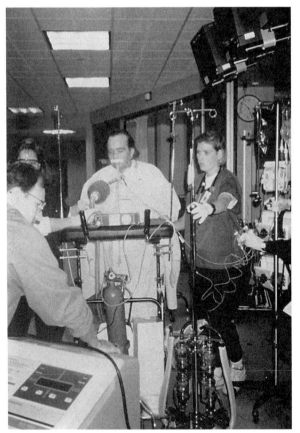

Figure 12–12. Transplant patient in the early postoperative phase, ambulating in the ICU. Note patient is being ventilated with a manual ventilation bag.

tivity.[43, 101] A proper warm-up is needed to increase stroke volume and catecholamine stimulation so that the patient's cardiac output is increased enough to meet the physical demands of the activity.

After the patient has been moved out of the ICU (typically 48 hours) or is able to increase the MET level used for activities, conventional postcardiac surgery guidelines may be followed. Table 12–9 presents examples of protocols that show a normal progression of activity used with the cardiac transplantation patient population (see also Chapter 18). Once the patient has been transferred out of the ICU, treatment focuses on achieving independence with ADLs, and increasing endurance with activities such as stationary cycling, stair climbing, and ambulation, musculoskeletal activities for posture and strengthening, and development of a home exercise program in preparation for discharge. Strengthening activities should focus on musculoskeletal deficiencies and proximal muscle groups that are more likely to be affected by the complications of steroid therapy.

Throughout the time period following transplantation, the patient needs to be educated on specific topics that are related to safety and correct performance of exercise and activity. Educational topics should include the following: proper techniques for bed mobility and transfers, sternal precautions (lifting limited to 10 lb for 6 to 8 weeks, and limitations in end range flexion and horizontal abduction), self-monitoring of HR and RPE, aerobic exercise guidelines including contraindications and progression, and signs and symptoms to serve as indicators of the development of complications. Guidelines to be used for an exercising cardiac transplant patient are provided in Table 12–10. Each patient will progress at a different rate, and complications that affect an individual patient will alter the progression of rehabilitation.

A variety of complications can affect the heart transplant recipient in the acute inpatient phase of recovery, such as bacterial infections, nonspecific **graft failure,** and **acute rejection.**[61] Within the first 30 days, the leading cause of death is nonspecific graft failure. The next most common causes of death are acute rejection and infection.[24]

Bacterial infections are common in the first 30 days, and treatment focuses on prevention through the use of barriers (masks) to reduce the incidence of opportunistic infections and insistence on good handwashing procedures for hospital staff

Table 12–9
Activity Levels for Inpatient Physical Therapy After Cardiac Transplantation

Level 1
Re-education of neuromuscular relaxation to counteract muscle tension
Re-education of thoracic and diaphragmatic breathing
Review of posture principles, body mechanics, and transfer techniques
Exercises (up to 10 repetitions, supine)
  Shoulder flexion, adduction, horizontal abduction
  Hip/knee flexion and extension
  Hip abduction
  Ankle pumps
Up in a chair 20–30 minutes
Level 2
Breathing and relaxation techniques
Exercises (up to 10 repetitions, seated)
  Shoulder exercises as before
  Shoulder circling
  Trunk rotation
  Hip/knee flexion (seated marching)
  Knee extension
  Ankle pumps
Gait: standing pregait activities (dips, weight shifting)
Up in a chair 30–60 minutes
Level 3
Exercises (up to 10 repetitions, standing)
  Head circles
  Arm circles
  Trunk rotation and lateral flexion
  Dips
  Toe raises
  Wand exercises
Gait: short walks in the room, as tolerated
Up in a chair ad lib
Level 4
Exercises (up to 10 repetitions, standing)
  Head and arm circles
  Trunk rotation and lateral flexion
  Toe raises
  Wand exercises: progress to wrist weights (1 lb)
Gait: walk in room ad lib
Level 5
Exercise and walking as per level 4 (continue through level 6)
Stationary cycle: 10 min at minimal resistance
Add cool-down stretches for quadriceps and heel cords
Level 6
Stationary cycle: 15 min at minimal resistance
Cool-down stretches as per level 5 plus hamstring stretch, continue with level 7
Level 7
Stationary cycle: 20 min at mild resistance (RPE 11–13) (include 2–3 minute slower warm-up and cool-down)

Source: Squires R. Cardiac rehabilitation issues for heart transplantation patients. J Cardiopulm Rehabil 10: 159–168, 1990.

Table 12–10
Guidelines to Use When Determining if Exercise is Appropriate for the Transplant Patient and When Progression or Termination of Exercise is Appropriate

HR > 120 bpm at rest
HR that increases > 40 bpm above the resting level with exercise
SBP > 190 mm Hg at rest
SBP increases > 40 mm Hg with exercise
SBP decreases > 10 mm Hg below the resting level with exercise
DBP > 110 mm Hg at rest
DBP increases > 15 mm Hg above the resting level with exercise
Dyspnea index > 15
RPE > 13 (somewhat hard) at rest
RPE that increases to ≥ 15 (hard) with exercise
Excessive fatigue
Vertigo
Claudication
ECG abnormalities
Mental confusion or dizziness

Source: Niset G, Hermans L, Depelchin P. Exercise and the heart transplantation: a review. Sports Med 12(6):359–379, 1992, and Kavanagh T, Yacoub MH, Mertens DJ, et al. Cardiorespiratory responses to exercise training after orthotopic cardiac transplantation. Circulation 77:162–171, 1988.

and visitors alike. In addition, antibiotics are used both prophylactically and therapeutically.

Acute rejection is characterized by either the presence of preformed antibodies or infiltrates of mononuclear cells, which lead to myocyte necrosis.[49] This invasion of mononuclear cells represents the inability of the immunosuppressive regimen to prevent activation of immune effector cells.[78] As a result of the immune system functioning properly (instead of being adequately immunosuppressed), the donor organ is not able to maintain cardiac output due to a loss in cardiac compliance and reduced coronary vasodilatation. As a result, the myocardium is at risk for ischemia because of an increased demand for oxygen with exercise and activity.[94] Acute rejection is often suspected as a complication when the patient is exhibiting signs and symptoms of exercise and activity intolerance and is then confirmed via endomyocardial biopsies. Signs and symptoms of acute rejection are found in Table 12–11. In some cases, however, rejection may not be evidenced by signs and symptoms. Reversal of the rejection process is achieved by increasing dosages of immunosuppressive medications.

Table 12-11

Signs and Symptoms of Acute Rejection

Low-grade fever
Increase in resting blood pressure
Hypotension with activity
Myalgias
Fatigue
Decreased exercise tolerance
Ventricular dysrhythmias

Progression of self-care activity and exercise may be limited by acute rejection. Rejection may be labeled as mild, moderate, or severe based on histologic classifications. If the rejection episode is mild to moderate, exercise and activity are rarely altered. If the rejection episode is moderate to severe, as demonstrated clinically by new dysrhythmias, hypotension, or fever, exercise and activity will be reduced to unresisted symptom-limited modes of activity or discontinued until the patient's status improves, as evidenced by reduction or reversal of symptoms.

Lung Transplant

Treatment of the lung transplant patient also begins when the patient is medically stable, usually on the first day following surgery. The patient remains in the ICU while intubated and mechanically ventilated. The problems and goals in this period are similar to those of the heart transplant recipient with attention given to the changes in the lungs due to pulmonary denervation. Decreased mucociliary clearance, ventilation-perfusion imbalance, and ineffective cough have been demonstrated in denervated lungs.[38, 89, 116] The initial postoperative evaluation should include the effectiveness of pulmonary hygiene, including optimal positioning, mobilization, and enhancement of cough effort.[117]

Clearance of pulmonary secretions often requires a combination of techniques, depending on the requirements for mechanical ventilation, the level of discomfort the patient is experiencing, and the airway clearance techniques with which the patient was familiar prior to surgery. Several airway clearance techniques have been shown to be effective in the mobilization of secretions including postural drainage and percussion, shaking, and manual hyperinflation, the active cycle of breathing and use of the flutter valve.[44]

The aforementioned guidelines for exercising heart transplant patients are also applicable to the lung transplant patient population. Although the HR provides an accurate measure of exercise intensity, it is helpful to use the RPE scale and respiratory rate for additional information to guide activity progression from activities in bed, to sitting up in a chair, and finally to ambulation. In the intensive care setting, mobilization of the lung transplant recipient may be accomplished by providing a wheelchair to accommodate necessary equipment such as the chest drainage tube collection boxes, portable suction unit, oxygen cylinder, and pulse oximeter. The patient then walks behind the wheelchair, using it for support, similar to a wheeled walker (Fig. 12–13).

After the patient is moved out of the intensive care setting, usually in 3 to 7 days, rehabilitation continues to focus on ventilation and airway clearance for optimal oxygen transport. Thoracic mobility exercises should be added to the rehabilitative process.[118] Breathing exercises should be incorporated into all aspects of treatment, including thoracic mobility and the cardiovascular exercise regimens, as well as coughing and airway clearance maneuvers.

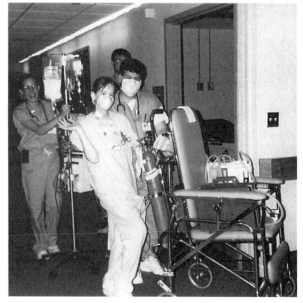

Figure 12–13. Progression of patient ambulation after leaving ICU using a wheelchair for support.

The goals for discharge from the hospital should include independence in self-care and secretion clearance if needed, increased thoracic mobility, general strength and endurance, and the ability to participate in a home exercise program. Assisted airway clearance and supplemental oxygen are usually no longer necessary at the time of discharge.

In the acute postoperative period, the most common complication in the lung transplant recipient is infection; this complication is the primary cause of death after single or double lung transplantation within the first 6 months.[119, 120] Acute rejection, determined from histologic examination of lung tissue obtained by biopsy, is also common in the lung transplant recipient, but does not appear to be a major cause of death in the acute period.[120] Treatment of rejection episodes consists of augmentation of the immunosuppressive regimen. The number of intraoperative complications as well as problems of airway dehiscence have been greatly reduced due to advances in surgical technique and increasing experience in the field of isolated lung transplantation.[119, 120]

Symptomatically, infection and rejection are both manifested by low-grade fever and leukocytosis.[119] With activity, these complications are manifested by a decrease in arterial oxygen saturation and exercise tolerance. This finding demonstrates the importance of close monitoring by the physical therapist during exercise periods.

Heart-Lung Transplant

Treatment of the heart-lung transplant patient closely resembles that of the heart and isolated lung transplant recipients. The therapist and medical staff should focus on both recipient organs and sequelae that may accompany each of them. It is important to keep in mind that the heart and lungs may exhibit signs of rejection independent of one another. Evaluation, timetables for treatment progression, and patient goals are a combination of the earlier information presented for heart and lung transplantation.

In the immediate postoperative period, the most common complications in the heart-lung transplant recipient are nonspecific graft failure and hemorrhage.[24] In the intermediate period, infection appears to be the primary cause of death,

and after 1 year, **bronchiolitis obliterans** (BO), a progressive, inflammatory lung disease, is the principal cause of death.[24]

The Postoperative Outpatient Phase

The postoperative phase begins when the patient is discharged from the hospital and continues until the patient is discharged from a formal rehabilitation program. This time frame is typically 8 to 12 weeks and is very similar to phase II cardiac rehabilitation (Fig. 12–14).[43, 118] Discharge occurs when the patient is competent with self-monitoring and independent with a home exercise program, goals are achieved, and when the patient has returned to normal daily activities, such as work or school.

If a thorough evaluation was completed as an inpatient and the patient is at the same facility, no further evaluation will be performed, excluding an exercise stress test. Depending on the previous type of exercise evaluation performed or on the level of function of the patient, the stress test may be a 6MW or a formal symptom-limited treadmill or cycle ergometer test. From the results of the stress test, the patient's exercise prescription will be determined using a combination of HR (not useful in heart transplantation recipients), RPE, MET level, and other limiting symptoms.[39, 118]

Physical therapy goals during this phase may include strengthening large proximal skeletal musculature, continued aerobic conditioning, attention to and resolution of any musculoskeletal problems, independence with a home exercise program, understanding and independence with all areas of education, and self-monitoring.[39, 118]

Frequent complications that occur as an outpatient include the following: chronic rejection, CMV infection, renal dysfunction, hypertension, **steroid myopathy,** anemia, and malignancy.[24, 39, 43, 94] Hosenpud[24] reports that late in the post-transplantation period, the three most common causes of death are cardiac allograft vasculopathy, malignancy, and acute rejection.

In heart transplant recipients, chronic rejection, also known as transplant coronary artery disease (CAD), demonstrates signs of **atherosclerosis.**[39, 94] This form of CAD is different from CAD in a native heart, as transplant CAD is diffuse and con-

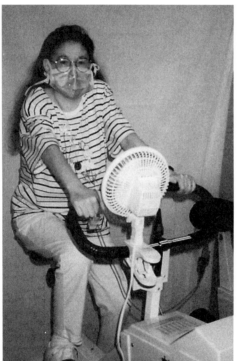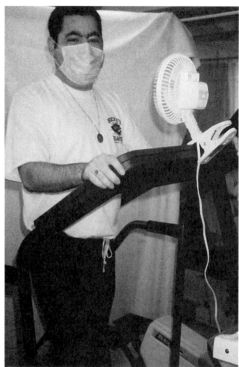

Figure 12-14. Transplant patients in the late postoperative phase, utilizing a variety of exercise modalities.

centric within the lumen.[39, 43, 93] Transplant CAD often is undetectable noninvasively, as denervation of the myocardium prevents signs of ischemia from being present. Manifestations of transplant CAD include myocardial infarction, congestive heart failure, and sudden cardiac death. The exact cause of transplant CAD is unknown; however, potential causes may include prolonged use of steroids or cyclosporine, infection, or repeated bouts of rejection.[39, 98] Treatment includes percutaneous endoluminal angioplasty, coronary artery bypass grafting, or more often than not, repeat transplantation.[39, 94] Transplant CAD is also associated with CMV infection; The infection is associated with reduced patient survival, increased episodes of rejection, and severe graft atherosclerosis.[39]

In lung transplant recipients, BO is thought to be a manifestation of chronic rejection.[119, 121-123] A persistent decline in measurements of small airway function is a predictor for the development of BO, but it must be histologically proved with specimens from a transbronchial biopsy.[121, 123-125] Prevalence of BO has been reported at 26 to 50% for isolated lung and heart-lung transplant recipients with a

reported mortality rate of 40 to 56%.[37, 121-123] As with CAD following a heart transplant, BO in lung transplant recipients has been associated with CMV infection.[121]

The current management of BO includes augmentation of immunosuppression and reinstitution of cytolytic therapy.[122, 123] Valentine[123] reported a median survival time from the diagnosis of BO in bilateral lung and heart-lung transplant recipients of nearly 3 years with minimal limitation in quality of life. However, in general, long-term survival after lung transplantation is limited primarily by BO and its complications.

The medications necessary after transplantation often produce other common complications, as seen in Table 12-7. Cyclosporine is thought to cause hypertension through alterations in the renin-angiotensin system and an increase in sympathetic neural activity.[107] Morrison[107] reports that 60 to 90% of transplant patients require medications to combat hypertension. Steroid myopathy may occur in patients who require a higher dose of steroids for adequate immunosuppression or in patients who have frequent bouts of rejection

> **Clinical Note: Steroid Myopathy**
>
> Treatment of steroid myopathy should focus on specific strengthening exercises of proximal muscle groups, especially the lower extremities necessary for weight-bearing activities. The patient should also be encouraged to continue activity and exercise at whatever level is possible.

necessitating repeated bolusing with steroids. Steroid myopathy presents with a weakness of the proximal muscles of the extremities and may be characterized by a patient's inability to climb stairs, rise from low surfaces such as a toilet seat, or increased reliance on the upper extremities when rising from a crouched or seated position. The process may be worsened by inactivity or avoidance of difficult activities.

FUTURE TRENDS IN TRANSPLANT CARE

Increases in the number and types of thoracic organ transplantations are currently constrained by the availability of donor organs.[24] As a result of the discrepancy between the number of donor organs available and the number of donor organs needed, alternative techniques and support systems must be developed to "bridge the gap" between being placed on a transplant waiting list and actually receiving a replacement organ. Other possible solutions to the donor shortage problem include perfecting the surgical technique to reduce complications and increasing the success rate of current transplantations so that recipients do not return to the list as candidates for repeat transplantation, utilizing xenograft (other species) or cadaveric organs as donors, and further investigation of the use of living related lobar transplants.

The trends demonstrate that there continues to be a need for research and monies to support the clinical application of mechanical circulatory support systems that are used to manage the patient until transplantation. The use of circulatory support systems has enabled some very critically ill patients to survive long enough to receive an organ transplantation. Now investigators are beginning to examine the feasibility of using these support systems as long-term definitive devices. If successful, the number of individuals placed on transplant waiting lists could be reduced substantially.

The number of living donor lobar transplants for patients on the lung transplant list has increased in recent years. While at Stanford University, Starnes[126] performed the first lobar transplantations from living related donors, introducing an alternative method to expand the donor pool. For this procedure, recipients are selected on the basis of deteriorating pulmonary function, hypoxia requiring mechanical ventilation, hypercapnia, or increasing antibiotic resistance. In addition to the critical status, which renders the patient unable to endure the typical waiting time on the list, the recipient's stature must be small enough to function with two donor lobes instead of entire lungs, and two family members must be identified, each of whom are willing and able to undergo a lobectomy to provide donor lobes for the recipient. Survival rate at 1 year has been reported at 71%.[126]

The use of cadaveric organ transplants is also being studied. Because respiration of lung tissue occurs directly across a gas interface, respiration at the cellular level can be accomplished in the absence of vascular perfusion. It has been hypothesized that pulmonary tissue may remain viable for a sufficient period of time post mortem to be useful for transplantation.[127] To test the feasibility of cadaver lung use, Egan et al.[127] transplanted canines with lungs of canine donors that were post mortem up to 4 hours prior to lung harvest. Recipient animals were forced to survive solely on the transplanted lung and were able to do so for up to an 8-hour observation period; the animals with the shorter postmortem donor time survived the longest. It was concluded that if the desirable period of ischemia can be increased so that reliable gas exchange function is observed for longer periods, then it may be realistic to consider eventually expanding the pulmonary donor pool using cadaver lungs as a resource.

Research is also ongoing to address the immunologic factors present in transplantation using a different species, or **xenotransplantation.** Although primate-to-human xenotransplantation has been attempted, study of the use of porcine donor organs has increased, owing to the large number of pigs available and their appropriate size and low cost.[128] Hyperacute rejection is a barrier to clinical xenotransplantation, occurring almost invariably when donor and recipient are of phylogenetically different species.[128] Lin and Platt[128] outlined new strategies for interfering with antibody-antigen interaction and the development of animals more genetically suited for transplantation, averting the occurrence of hyperacute rejection; this still leaves the recipient susceptible to more chronic forms of rejection. The recognition of the barriers to xenotransplantation at the cellular level is leading to the development and testing of therapeutic solutions in the realm of clinical xenotransplantation.[128]

Advances in medication for transplantation continue to be made. One newly approved drug is FK506 (Prograf), a second-generation immunosuppressive agent that has properties very similar to those of CyA. Actions of FK506 include selective inhibition of the transcription process that occurs in the lymphokine genes found in T lymphocytes.[129] In experimental studies, FK506 is 100 times more potent than CyA at prolonging graft survival. In addition, FK506 can be administered intermittently without loss in effectiveness, and does not produce the nephrotoxic side effects associated with CyA.[93] A second new drug, Neoral, is a form of cyclosporine that has been approved by the FDA. It is reported to be more easily absorbed than CyA, thereby potentially decreasing the amount required for adequate immunosuppression. Other medications undergoing clinical trials are polyclonal and monoclonal antibodies, developed to prevent organ rejection.

The care provided for heart, heart-lung, and lung transplant patients is also evolving at a rapid pace. Five years ago, the initial evaluation process was performed on an inpatient basis and took 5 to 7 days. Today, the majority, if not all, of the evaluation is performed on an outpatient basis and only takes 2 to 3 days. Compared to a few years ago, the patient placed on the waiting list today may be able to stay at home longer and participate in a preoperative program at a local facility on an outpatient basis instead of immediately moving to the city of the transplant facility and participating in preoperative rehabilitation at the transplant facil-

ity. Another major change in the course of care is the length of the hospital stay following transplantation. Initially, a patient was hospitalized as long as 1 to 2 months following surgery. This has been significantly shortened to an average length of stay of 2 to 3 weeks, with patients being followed as outpatients after discharge.

For the rehabilitation staff, fewer days in the hospital means that the number of physical therapy visits is decreased and the goals must be accomplished more quickly than in the past. As a result, physical therapy extenders (physical therapist assistants and aides or technicians) often participate in the transplant patient's rehabilitation treatment under the supervision of a physical therapist.

According to Hosenpud,[24] as of February 7, 1996, a total of 41,319 thoracic transplants had been performed at 500 centers worldwide. Although the number of procedures performed has plateaued in the last few years, many more candidates are waiting for a chance to be among those who have received transplants.

Thoracic organ transplantation has evolved from an experimental procedure into an accepted mode of treatment for individuals with end-stage cardiac and pulmonary disease. The twentieth century has been witness to the prolongation of survival following transplantation from a period of survival of only 18 days after the first successful heart transplant to the current 1-year survival rate of 79% for heart transplantation, 60% for heart-lung, and 75% for lung transplantation.[24] The survival rate for patients undergoing a *repeat* thoracic transplantation is much lower, with 1- and 3-year survival rates being 50 and 45% for heart transplantation, 28 and 22% for heart-lung, and 42 and 24% for lung transplantation, respectively.[24]

As increasing numbers of patients with end-stage disease are offered thoracic transplantation as a therapeutic option, the importance of keeping abreast of new developments in this evolving field cannot be overstated. Tremendous advances have been made in surgical technique, medications, and the surveillance and management of complications. As members of the health care team, physical therapists are challenged to utilize high-level skills of evaluation and treatment in order to contribute to a successful outcome for this select group of patients.

CASE STUDIES

Case 1. The Lung Transplant Patient with Cystic Fibrosis

MA is a thin 35-year-old man with end-stage cystic fibrosis, characterized by lower respiratory tract infections often requiring hospitalization, pancreatic insufficiency, airway obstruction, chest wall hyperinflation, thoracic kyphosis, digital clubbing, and oxygen desaturation with activity. Patient has thick, tenacious secretions and he is almost continuously taking antibiotics to treat his infections. Patient lives approximately 1.5 hours away from transplant center.

Evaluation

Subjective: MA has been attending a pulmonary rehabilitation program for exercise in his hometown for the past year, although inconsistently. Airway clearance (postural drainage and percussion) is performed by staff after exercise sessions, but patient admits to not doing additional airway clearance other than coughing. MA wears supplemental oxygen only during exercise. Patient's hobby is collecting rare and antique books and he reads the Bible regularly.
Pulmonary: Crackles and wheezes on auscultation, especially in upper lobes bilaterally. At rest, patient uses accessory muscles, with RR 24, SaO_2 92%, HR 89 bpm.
Activity: During a 6-minute walk test, MA walked 1932 feet without resting, required 5 L of O_2 to maintain SaO_2 at 90% or higher, with HR 110 to 142 bpm, and RPE 17.

Pretransplant Period

MA was placed on the waiting list for a double lung transplant. The patient agreed to attend pulmonary rehabilitation three times a week and to perform airway clearance at least twice daily. The patient also started coming to the transplant center every other month for an exercise re-evaluation and to attend the lung transplant support group. During this time, MA was instructed in use of the Flutter for airway clearance, reviewed exercises for chest mobility, and increased supplemental oxygen use to continuous, as his resting SaO_2 percentage was in the low 80s. The patient continued to be hospitalized at times of severe exacerbation. MA's 6-minute walk distance increased by almost 100 feet in the first year but then showed a decrease as the patient's condition worsened. The last 6-minute walk prior to transplantation was 1862 feet with 8 L of O_2 required to maintain SaO_2 at 90% or more, with HR 132 to 162 bpm, and RPE 18.

Post-Transplant Period

MA received a double lung transplant 2 years and 7 months after being placed on the list. Physical therapy treatment began within 24 hours and included turning and positioning, airway clearance maneuvers, breathing exercises, chest mobility exercises, and progressive ambulation. MA was weaned from the ventilator as well as supplemental oxygen and progressed to walking 800 feet with assistance required only for equipment such as chest tubes and IV pole. At this point, MA resumed exercise on the treadmill and bicycle ergometer while still an inpatient. His discharge from the hospital was delayed due to gastrointestinal problems, and he was discharged $2\frac{1}{2}$ weeks after transplantation.

A 6-minute walk test was performed 4 weeks after transplant: MA covered 1946 ft on room air with SaO_2 of 95 to 98%, HR 120 to 148 bpm, and RPE 14. He continued to receive outpatient pulmonary rehabilitation at the transplant center and was discharged to his hometown $3\frac{1}{2}$ months after transplant. At time of discharge, MA was walking on treadmill at 4.0 mph at a 10% grade for 30 min, and was able to use the bicycle ergometer or stepper for 30 min continuous exercise. The 6-minute walk at time of discharge was 2415 ft on room air with SaO_2 of 95 to 98%, HR 126 to 160 bpm, and RPE 16.

Case 2. The Heart Transplant Patient

JJ is a 44-year-old man with end-stage congestive heart failure (CHF) due to dilated cardiomyopathy. Cardiac risk factors include a positive family history and a 30-year history of tobacco use.

Medical Evaluation

Tests: Cardiac catheterization showed 100% blockage of RCA, 90% blockage of left main coronary artery, and ejection fraction = 7%. Complication: pericatheterization MI.
Activity: Unable to perform low-level activity without signs and symptoms of severe CHF.

Pretransplant Period

An attempt was made to manage JJ's CHF with pharmacologic support. Despite maximal pharmacologic support, JJ's CHF worsened. At this time an intra-aortic balloon pump was inserted to mechanically assist JJ's heart; the balloon pump was also unsuccessful. Following the failure of the balloon pump, a biventricular assist device (BIVAD) was implanted into JJ's chest. JJ was then referred to PT for evaluation and treatment.

Physical Therapy Evaluation

Subjective: JJ was intubated, communicating with paper and pencil, following multistep commands.
Pulmonary: Crackles present in bilateral lower lobes. RR = 20, IMV = 8, 60% oxygenation, SaO_2 = 95%
Cardiac: HR = 90 to 110 bpm. Rhythm: irregular BP = 110/70 mmHg BIVAD: pump flow 5 to 6 L/min.
Musculoskeletal: No abnormalities found in ROM, strength 2/5 UE's, 2/5 LE's, all mobility skills required

moderate to maximal assist. Impairments identified: decreased strength, decreased activity tolerance, ineffective secretion clearance.
Treatment: Bronchopulmonary hygiene and suctioning, deep breathing exercises (DBE), coughing techniques, progressive mobility skills, strengthening exercises, and endurance training (stationary cycling and gait). Treatment was initiated with low-level skills and progressed as JJ was able to tolerate higher level skills and increases in intensity and duration. He was seen twice a day with a perfusionist present initially to ensure adequate cardiac output with changes in position and exercise.

Post-Transplant Period

JJ received an orthotopic heart transplant 40 days after being placed on the transplant waiting list. Physical therapy was re-initiated 24 hours following heart transplantation. His pretransplant treatment program was again begun, and JJ was discharged to home 3 weeks later. Functional status at discharge was independent with transfers, gait, DBE, coughing techniques, and his strength had increased to 3+/5. Home health physical therapy was set up for the patient to bridge the time until he could attend a formal cardiac rehabilitation program.

Summary

- The primary indication for heart, heart-lung, and lung transplantation is a terminal cardiopulmonary disease.
- Single organ transplantation is preferred for lung transplants when possible to help decrease the donor shortage.
- Priority on transplant waiting lists is maintained by UNOS.
- Candidates for transplantation are evaluated by transplant team members and must meet certain eligibility criteria.
- The physical therapist assesses the patient's cardiac and pulmonary system limitations as well as musculoskeletal condition, exercise capacity, ventilatory function, and mucociliary clearance.
- The preoperative rehabilitation program will include patient and family education, cardiovascular endurance training, musculoskeletal strength and flexibility training, and breathing retraining.
- The goal of preoperative rehabilitation is to improve or prevent deterioration of the candidate's physical condition.
- A candidate who is better conditioned prior to transplantation has a better chance postopera-

tively of improving physical capacity and function.
- Alternatives to thoracic organ transplantation to "bridge the gap" while waiting for a suitable donor or to replace transplantation include lung volume reduction surgery, BiPAP, LVAS, cardiomyoplasty, and pharmacologic management.
- Donor organs are selected and matched to the recipient on the basis of blood type and organ size.
- Surgical procedures:

  Heart: orthotopic (performed more often) or heterotopic, heart is denervated, ECG demonstrates two separate P waves.

  Lung: single lung or double lung, lungs are denervated.

  Heart-lung: heart and lungs are denervated.
- Medications are used to prevent rejection and infection. Additional medications are used to combat the side effects of immunosuppressive medication.
- Special adherence to universal precautions needs to be followed with the transplant patient.
- When exercising a patient following heart transplantation, it is critical to have a sufficient warm-up and cool-down period to permit the denervated heart to accommodate the change in activity level and maintain cardiac output. This accommodation occurs in the warm-up by an increase in stroke volume provided by the contracting muscles and increases in catecholamine release.
- For all thoracic transplant patients, the following vital signs should be monitored: HR, BP, RR, RPE, and SaO_2. The HR of a heart transplant recipient will not increase linearly with activity progression secondary to denervation.
- The transplant patient should be assessed postoperatively within 12 to 36 hours.
- Inpatient treatment and goals focus on improving or correcting impaired gas exchange and ineffective airway clearance; patient positioning; pain reduction; and reducing mobility restrictions.
- Outpatient treatment and goals focus on strengthening large skeletal musculature, weight-bearing exercise, continued aerobic conditioning, resolution of any musculoskeletal problems, the home exercise program, education, and independence with self-monitoring.

- Frequent complications of the transplant patient include rejection, infection, CMV infection, steroid myopathy, anemia, and malignancy.
- The physical therapist needs to be alert for transplant complications, which can often manifest themselves initially in the exercise response. For example, rejection may be noted in a lung transplant patient by a decrease in SaO_2 and reduced exercise tolerance during a rehabilitation session.
- Future trends in transplant care include new operative techniques, xenograft transplants, cadaver organ transplants, living related lobar transplants, and advances in pharmacologic management.

References

1. Carrel A, Guthrie CC. The transplantation of veins and organs. Am Med 10:1101–1102, 1905.
2. Mann FC, Priestly JT, Markowitz J, Yater WM. Transplantation of the intact mammalian heart. Arch Surg 26:219–224, 1933.
3. Marcus E, Wong SNT, Luisada AA. Homologous heart grafts: Transplantation of the heart in dogs. Surg Forum 2:212–217, 1951.
4. Webb WR, Howard HS. Restoration of function of the refrigerated heart. Surg Forum 8:302, 1957.
5. Goldberg M, Berman EF, Akman LC. Homologous transplantation of the canine heart. J Int Coll Surg 30:575–586, 1958.
6. Cass MH, Brock R. Heart excision and replacement. Guy's Hosp Rep 108:285–290, 1959.
7. Lower RR, Shumway NE. Studies of orthotopic homotransplantation of the canine heart. Surg Forum 11:18–19, 1960.
8. Dong E, Hurley EJ, Lower RR, Shumway NE. Isotopic replacement of the totally excised canine heart. J Surg Res 2:90–94, 1962.
9. Lower RR, Dong E, Shumway NE. Long-term survival of cardiac homografts. Surgery 58:110–119, 1965.
10. Hardy JD, Chavez CM, Kurrus FD, et al. Heart transplantation in man. JAMA 188:1132–1140, 1964.
11. McGregor CGA. Evolution of heart transplantation. Cardiol Clin 8:3–10, 1990.
12. Hardy JD, Webb WR, Dalton ML, et al. Lung homotransplantation in man. JAMA 186:1065–1074, 1963.
13. Caves PK, Schulz WP, Dong EJ, et al. New instrument for transvenous cardiac biopsy. Am J Cardiol 33:264–267, 1974.
14. Morris RE, Dong EJ, Struthers CM, et al. Immunological detection of human cardiac rejection. Surg Forum 25:282–284, 1974.
15. Griepp RB, Stinson EB, Dong EJ, et al. Use of antithymocyte globulin in human heart transplantation. Circulation 45 (suppl 1):147–153, 1972.
16. Kirklin JK. Heart-lung transplantation (editoral). Am J Med 85:3, 1988.
17. Hutter JA, Despins P, Higenbottam T, et al. Heart-lung transplantation: better use of resources. Am J Med 85:4–21, 1988.
18. Reitz BA, Burton NA, Jamieson SW, et al. Heart and lung transplantation: autotransplantation and allotransplantation in primates with extended survival. J Thorac Cardiovasc Surg 80:360–372, 1980.
19. Reitz BA, Wallwork JL, Hunt SA, et al. Heart-lung transplantation. N Engl J Med 306:557–564, 1982.
20. The Toronto Lung Transplant Group. Unilateral lung transplantation for pulmonary fibrosis. N Engl J Med 314:1140–1145, 1986.
21. Cooper JD, Patterson GA, Grossman R, et al. Double-lung transplant for advanced chronic obstructive lung disease. Am Rev Respir Dis 139:303–307, 1989.
22. Kaye MP, Elcombe SA, O'Fallon WM. The International Heart Transplantation Registry: The 1984 report. J Heart Transplant 4:290–292, 1985.
23. Solis E, Kaye MP. The Registry of the International Society for Heart Transplantation: Third official report—June 1986. J Heart Transplant 5:2–5, 1986.
24. Hosenpud JD, Novick RJ, Bennett LE, et al. The registry of the international society for heart and lung transplantation: Thirteenth official report—1996. J Heart Lung Transplant 15:655–674, 1996.
25. Hosenpud JD, Novick RJ, Breen TJ, Daily OP. The Registry of the International Society for Heart and Lung Transplantation: Eleventh official report—1994. J Heart Lung Transplant 13:561–570, 1994.
26. Kaye MP. The Registry of the International Society for Heart and Lung Transplantation: Tenth official report—1993. J Heart Lung Transplant 12:541–548, 1993.
27. Egan TM, Detterbeck FC, Mill MR, et al. Improved results of lung transplantation for patients with cystic fibrosis. J Thorac Cardiovasc Surg 109:224–235, 1995.
28. Egan TM, Westerman JH, Lambert CJ Jr, et al. Isolated lung transplantation for end-stage lung disease: A viable therapy. Ann Thorac Surg 53:590–596, 1992.
29. Levine SM, Anzueto A, Peters JI, et al. Single lung transplantation in patients with systemic disease. Chest 105:837–841, 1994.
30. Low DE, Trulock EP, Kaiser LR, et al. Lung transplantation of ventilator-dependent patients. Chest 101:8–11, 1992.
31. Fisher JD. New York Heart Association Classification. Arch Intern Med 129:836, 1972.
32. Young JB, Naftel DC, Bourge RC, et al. Matching the heart donor and heart transplant recipient: Clues for successful expansion of the donor pool—A multivariable, multi-institutional report. The Cardiac Transplant Research Database Group. J Heart Lung Transplant 13:353–365, 1994.
33. Hosenpud JD, Novick RJ, Breen TJ, et al. The Registry of the International Society for Heart and Lung Transplantation: Twelfth official report—1995. J Heart Lung Transplant 14:805–815, 1995.
34. Novitzky D, Cooper C, Barnard C: The surgical technique of heterotopic heart transplantation. Ann Thorac Surg 36:476, 1983.
35. Michler RE, McLaughlin MJ, Chen JM, et al. Clinical experience with cardiac retransplantation. J Thorac Cardiovasc Surg 106:622–631, 1993.
36. Novick RJ, Kaye MP, Patterson GA, et al. Redo lung transplantation: A North American-European experience. J Heart Lung Transplant 12:5–16, 1995.
37. Deleted in print.
38. Egan TM, Kaiser LR, Cooper JD. Lung transplantation. Curr Probl Surg 26:673–752, 1989.
39. Squires R. Cardiac rehabilitation issues for heart transplantation patients. J Cardiopulm Rehabil 10:159–168, 1990.

40. Craven JL, Bright J, Dear CL. Psychiatric, psychosocial and rehabilitative aspects of lung transplantation. Clin Chest Med 11(2):247–257, 1990.
41. Kuhn WF, Davis MH, Lippman SB. Emotional adjustment to cardiac transplantation. Gen Hosp Psychiatry 10:108–113, 1988.
42. Bolman RM. Cardiac transplantation: The operative technique. Cardiovasc Clin 20:133–145, 1990.
43. Fick AW, Holloway V. Rehabilitation of the postsurgical cardiac patient. In: Manual of Physical Therapy. New York, Churchhill Livingston, 1989, pp 593–609.
44. Downs AM. Clinical application of airway clearance techniques. In: Frownfelter DL, Dean E (eds). Principles and Practice of Cardiopulmonary Physical Therapy, 3rd ed. St. Louis, Mosby–Year Book, 1996.
45. Biggar DG, Melen JE, Trulock EP, et al. Pulmonary rehabilitation before and after lung transplantation. In: Kasaburi R, Petty TL (eds). Principles and Practice of Pulmonary Rehabilitation. Philadelphia, WB Saunders, 1993, pp 459–467.
46. Howard DK, Iademarco EJ, Trulock EP. The role of cardiopulmonary exercise testing in lung and heart-lung transplantation. Clin Chest Med 15(2):405–420, 1994.
47. Ross DJ, Waters PF, Waxman AD, et al. Regional distribution of lung perfusion and ventilation at rest and during steady-state exercise after unilateral lung transplantation. Chest 104:130–135, 1993.
48. Mancini DM, Eisen J, Kussmaul W, et al. Value of peak exercise oxygen consumption for optimal timing of cardiac transplantation in ambulatory patients with heart failure. Circulation 83:778–786, 1991.
49. ACSM Guidelines for Exercise Testing and Prescription. 4th ed. Philadelphia, ACSM, 1995, pp 60–62, 134–165.
50. McGavin CR, Gupta SP, McHardy GJR. Twelve-minute walking test for assessing disability in chronic bronchitis. Br Med J 1:822–823, 1976.
51. Butland R. Two-, six-, and 12-minute walking tests in respiratory disease. Br Med J 284:1607–1608, 1982.
52. Guyatt GH, Sullivan MJ, Thompson PJ, et al. The 6-minute walk: A new measure of exercise capacity in patients with chronic heart failure. Can Med Assoc J 132:919–923, 1985.
53. No reference.
54. Sullivan MJ, et al. Exercise training in patients with severe left ventricular dysfunction: Hemodynamic and metabolic effects. Circulation 81:78, 1990.
55. Steele B: Timed walking tests of exercise capacity in chronic cardiopulmonary illness. J Cardiopulm Rehabil 16:25–33, 1996.
56. Malen JF, Boychuk JE. Nursing perspectives on lung transplantation. Crit Care Nurs Clin North Am 1:707–721, 1989.
57. Janicki JS, Weber KT, Likoff MJ, et al. Exercise testing to evaluate patients with pulmonary vascular disease. Am Rev Resp Dis 129:593, 1984.
58. Stevenson LW, et al. Improvement in exercise capacity of candidates awaiting heart transplant. J Am Coll Cardiol 25(1):163–170, 1995.
59. The Toronto Lung Transplantation Group. Experience with single-lung transplantation for pulmonary fibrosis. JAMA 259:2258–2262, 1988.
60. Moser KM, Bokinsky GE, Savage RT, et al. Results of a comprehensive rehabilitation program: Physiologic and functional effects on patients with chronic obstructive pulmonary disease. Arch Intern Med 140:1596–1601, 1980.
61. Holden DA, Stelmach KD, Curtis PS, et al. The impact of a rehabilitation program on functional status of patients with chronic lung disease. Respir Care 35(4):332–341, 1990.
62. Trulock EP, Cooper JD. Reduction pneumoplasty for COPD [abstract]. Chest 106:52s, 1994.
63. Sciurba FC, Rogers RM, Keenan RJ, et al. Improvement of pulmonary function and elastic recoil after lung reduction surgery for diffuse emphysematous lung. Ann Thorac Surg 57:1038–1039, 1994.
64. Cooper J. Technique to reduce air leaks after resection of emphysematous lung. Ann Thorac Surg 57:1038–1039, 1994.
64a. Benditt JO, Albert RK. Lung reduction surgery: Great expectations and a cautionary note. Chest 107:297–298, 1995.
65. MacIntyre NR (Principal Investigator), Tapson V, Davis RD, et al. Clinical Centers for Lung Volume Reduction Surgery for Emphysema: A Multicenter Assessment and Prospective Patient Registry. Proposal for NHLBI RFP-HR-97-02, August 19, 1996.
66. Padman R, Von Nesson S, Goodill J, et al. Noninvasive mechanical ventilation for cystic fibrosis patients with end stage disease. Pediatr Pulm A232:297, 1992.
67. Hill AT, Edenborough EP, Cayton RM, et el. Nasal intermittent positive pressure ventilation in cystic fibrosis: More than a bridge to transplantation? Pediatr Pulm A285:259, 1995.
68. McCarthy PM, Portner PM, Tobler HG, et al. Clinical experience with the Novacor ventricular assist system: Bridge to transplantation and the transition to permanent application. J Thorac Cardiovasc Surg 102:578–587, 1991.
69. Maddocks RM. Case study: Novacor left ventricular assist system in end-stage cardiac dysfunction. Phys Ther Practice 1(4):62–69, 1992.
70. Stevenson LW. Advanced congestive heart failure. Postgrad Med 5:97–116, 1994.
71. Armstrong PW, Moes BW. Medical advances in the treatment of congestive heart failure. Circulation 6:7941–7952, 1988.
72. Chiu RCJ. Dynamic cardiomyoplasty: An overview. PACE 14(1):577–583, 1991.
73. Chachques J, Grandjean P, Carpentier A. Patient management and clinical follow up after cardiomyoplasty. J Cardiovasc Surg 6, 1989.
74. Cooper JD, Pearson EG, Patterson GA, et al. Technique of successful lung transplantation in humans. J Thorac Cardiovasc Surg 93:173–181, 1987.
75. DiSesa VJ, Mull R, Daly ES, et al. Cardiac transplant donor heart allocation based on prospective tissue matching. Ann Thorac Surg 58:1050–1053, 1994.
76. McGregor CGA. Current state of heart transplantation. Br J Hosp Med 37:310–318, 1987.
77. Sadowsky HS. Cardiac transplantation: A review. Phys Ther 76(5):498–515, 1996.
78. Hakim MG, Gill SS. Heart transplantation: Operative techniques and postoperative management. J La State Med Soc 145:233–240, 1993.
79. Yacoub M, Mankad P, Ledingham S. Donor procurement and surgical techniques for cardiac transplantation. Semin Thorac Cardiovasc Surg 2:153–161, 1990.
80. Frazier O, Okereka O, Cooley D: Heterotopic heart transplantation in three patients at the Texas Heart Institute. Tex Heart Inst J 12:221, 1985.
81. Novitzky D, Coooper C, Rose A: The value of recipient heart assistance during severe acute rejection following heterotopic cardiac transplantation. J Cardiovasc Surg 25:287, 1984.
82. Bourge RC, Naftel DC, Costanzo-Nordin MR, et al. Pretransplantation risk factors for death after heart transplantation: A multi-institutional study—The Transplant Cardiologists Research Database Group. J Heart Lung Transplant 12:549–562, 1993.

83. Livi U, Milano A, Bortolotti U, et al. Results of heart transplantation by extending recipient selection criteria. J Cardiovasc Surg (Torino) 35:377–382, 1994.

84. Bexton R, Hellestrand K, Cory-Pearce R: Unusual atrial potentials in a cardiac transplant recipient. Possible synchronization between donor and recipient atria. J Electrocardiol 16:313, 1983.

85. Calhoon JH, Grover FL, Gibbons WJ, et al. Single lung transplantation: Alternative indications and technique. J Thorac Cardiovasc Surg 101:816–825, 1991.

86. Griffith BP, Hardesty RL, Armitage JM, et al. A decade of lung transplantation. Ann Surg 218(3):310–320, 1993.

87. Patterson GA. Double lung transplantation. Clin Chest Med 11(2):227–233, 1990.

88. Khaghani A, Tadjkarimi S, Al-Kattan K, et al. Wrapping the anastomosis with omentum or an internal mammary artery pedicle does not improve bronchial healing after single lung transplantation: Results of a randomized clinical trial. J Heart Lung Transplant 13:767–773, 1994.

89. Egan TM, Cooper JD. Surgical aspects of single lung transplantation. Clin Chest Med 11(2):195–205, 1990.

90. Craig CR, Stitzel RE: Modern Pharmacology, 4th ed. Boston, Little, Brown, 1994.

91. Schaefers JH, Frost AE, Waxman MB, et al. Cardiac innervation following double lung transplantation [abstract] Am Rev Respir Dis 137:245, 1988.

92. Augustine SM, Baumgartner WA, Stuart S, Acker MA. Heart and lung transplantation and cardiomyoplasty for end-stage cardiopulmonary disease. In: Baumgartner WA, Owens SG, Cameron DE, Reitz BA (eds). Johns Hopkins: Manual of Cardiac Surgical Care. St. Louis, Mosby–Yearbook, 1994.

93. Niset G, Hermans L, Depelchin P. Exercise and heart transplantation: A review. Sports Med 12(6):359–379, 1992.

94. Badenhop DT. The therapeutic role of exercise in patients with orthotopic heart transplant. Med Sci Sports Exerc 277:975–985, 1995.

95. Banner NR, Patel N, Cox AP, et al. Altered sympathoadrenal response to dynamic exercise in cardiac transplant recipients. Cardiovasc Res 23:965–972, 1989.

96. Banner NR. Exercise physiology and rehabilitation after heart transplantation. J Heart Lung Transplant 11(4):237–240, 1992.

97. Kavanagh T, Yacoub MH, Mertens DJ, et al. Cardiorespiratory responses to exercise training after orthotopic cardiac transplantation. Circulation 77:162–171, 1988.

98. Campeau L, Pospisil L, Grondin P, et al. Cardiac catheterization findings at rest and after exercise in patients following cardiac transplantation. Am J Cardiol 2:523–528, 1970.

99. Greenberg ML, Uretsky BF, Reddy PS, et al. Long-term hemodynamic follow-up of cardiac transplant patient treated with cyclosporine and prednisone. Circulation 71:487–494, 1985.

100. Kavanagh T, Yacoub MH. Exercise training in patients after heart transplantation. Ann Acad Med Singapore 21:372, 1992.

101. Rudas L, Pflugfelder PW, Kostuk WJ. Comparison of hemodynamic responses during dynamic exercise in the upright and supine postures after orthotopic cardiac transplant. J Am Coll Cardiol 16:1367, 1990.

102. Hausdorf G, Banner NR, Mitchell A, et al. Diastolic function after cardiac and heart-lung transplantation. Br Heart J 62:123–132, 1989.

103. Paulus WJ, et al. Deficient acceleration of left ventricular relaxation during exercise after heart transplantation. Circulation 86:1175, 1992.

104. Kao AC, Van Trigt PR, Shaeffer-McCall GS, et al. Central and peripheral limitations to upright exercise in untrained cardiac transplant recipients. Circulation 89:2605–2615, 1994.

105. Kao AC, Van Trigt PR, Shaeffer-McCall GS, et al. Allograft diastolic dysfunction and chronotropic incompetence limit cardiac output response to exercise two to six years after heart transplantation. J Heart Lung Transplant 14:11–22, 1995.

106. Griepp RB, Stinson ED, Dong E Jr, et al. Hemodynamic performance of the transplanted human heart. Surgery 70:88–96, 1971.

107. Morrison RJ, Short HD, Noon GP, et al. Hypertension after lung transplantation. J Heart Lung Transplant 12:928–931, 1993.

108. Ross DJ, Waters PF, Mohsenifar Z, et al. Hemodynamic responses to exercise after lung transplantation. Chest 103:46–53, 1993.

109. Orens JB, Becker FS, Lynch JP, et al. Cardiopulmonary exercise testing following allogeneic lung transplantation for different underlying disease states. Chest 107:144–149, 1995.

110. Levy RD, Erns P, Levine SM, et al. Exercise performance after lung transplantation. J Heart Lung Transplant 12:27–33, 1993.

111. Sadeghi AM, Guthaner DF, Wexter L, et al. Healing and revascularization of the tracheal anastomosis following heart-lung transplantation. Surg Forum 33:236–238, 1982.

112. Otulana BA, Higenbottam MD, Wallwork J. Causes of exercise limitation after heart-lung transplantation. J Heart-Lung Transplant 11:S244–251, 1992.

113. Springall DR, Polakk JM, Howard L, et al. Persistence of intrinsic neurones and possible phenotypic changes after extrinsic denervation of human respiratory tract by heart-lung transplantation. Am Rev Respir Dis 141:1538–1546, 1990.

114. McGregor CG. Cardiac transplantaton: surgical considerations and early postoperative management. Mayo Clin Proc 67:577–585, 1992.

115. Egan TM, Cooper jD. The lung following transplantation. In: Crystal RG, West JB, et al (eds). The Lung. New York, Scientific Foundations. 1991, pp 2205–2215.

116. Dolovich M, Rossman C, Chambers C, et al. Muco-ciliary function in patients following single lung or lung/heart transplantation. Am Rev Respir Dis [abstract] 135:363, 1987.

117. Downs AM. Physical therapy in lung transplantation. Phys Ther 76:626–642, 1996.

118. Butler BB. Physical therapy in heart and lung transplantation. In: Irwin S. Tecklin JS (eds). Cardiopulmonary Physical Therapy, 3rd ed. St. Louis, Mosby–Year Book, 1995.

119. Chaparro C, Maurer JR, Chamberlain D, et al. Causes of death in lung transplant recipients. J Heart Lung Transplant 13:758–766, 1994.

120. Bando K, Paradis IL, Komatsu K, et al. Analysis of time-dependent risks for infection, rejection, and death after pulmonary transplantation. J Thorac Cardiovasc Surg 109:49–59, 1995.

121. Keller CA, Cagle PT, Brown RW, et al. Bronchiolitis obliterans in recipients of single, double, and heart-lung transplantation. Chest 107:973–980, 1995.

122. Sundaresan S, Trulock EP, Mohanakumar T, et al. Prevalence and outcome of bronchiolitis obliterans syndrome after lung transplantation. Ann Thorac Surg 60:1341–1347, 1995.

123. Valentine BG, Robbins RC, Berry GJ, et al. Actuarial survival of heart-lung and bilateral sequential lung transplant

recipients with obliterative bronchiolitis. J Heart Lung Transplant 15:317–383, 1996.

124. Yousem SA, Berry GJ, Cagle PT, et al. Revision of the 1990 working formulation for the classification of pulmonary allograft rejection: Lung rejection study group. J Heart Lung Transplant 15:1–15, 1996.

125. Nathan SD, Ross DJ, Belman MJ, et al. Bronchiolitis obliterans in single lung transplant recipients. Chest 107:967–972, 1995.

126. Starnes VA, Burr ML, Schenkel FA, et al. Cardiopulmonary physiology in adult and pediatric lobar transplanta-

tion recipients: one year follow-up. J Heart Lung Transplant 15(1) [abstract], 1996.

127. Egan TM, Lambert CJ Jr, Reddick R, et al. A strategy to increase the donor pool: Use of cadaver lungs for transplantation. Ann Thorac Surg, 52:1113–1121, 1991.

128. Lin SS, Platt JL. Immunologic barriers to xenotransplantation. J Heart Lung Transplant 15:547–555, 1996.

129. Hayes DH. Immunosuppressants of today. In: Johnston C (ed). Statlander LifeTIMES Magazine. Pittsburgh, Statlander Drug Distribution Co., 1997.

## 13

Monitoring and Life-Support Equipment

H. Steven Sadowsky

INTRODUCTION

This chapter discusses equipment commonly used for monitoring and supporting the lives of patients with severe cardiovascular or pulmonary disease. Although it is true that much of the monitoring and life-support equipment is often restricted to the confines of the critical unit, this kind of equipment is making its way ever more frequently into long-term and outpatient rehabilitation, as well as home care settings.

Pressure-recording, volume-measuring, and flow-sensing instruments are frequently used for graphically and numerically displaying the variables that are felt to reflect a patient's specific physiologic status. Much of the equipment is electronic and consists of some or all of the following basic components: (1) a device to detect the physiologic event of interest, (2) an amplifier to increase the magnitude of the signal from the sensor, and (3) a recorder or meter to display the resultant signal. Although many variables must be considered in the process of clinical physiologic monitoring, with respect to subsequent life-support interventions the principal areas of concern involve hemodynamic, electrocardiographic, and ventilatory components.

509

HEMODYNAMIC MONITORING AND LIFE SUPPORT

Hemodynamic monitoring generally involves observing or calculating, and then assessing, some specific cardiovascular pressures. In addition to the stethoscope and sphygmomanometer, a pressure transducer, pressure transmission (connective) tubing, and a pressure monitor or recorder are frequently used—especially in the ICU or CCU. Currently, a typical pressure transducer is a disposable, solid-state piezoelectric device (Fig. 13–1A) that can be mounted easily on the patient, the patient's bed, or an IV pole. The piezoelectric pressure transducer is similar to a strain gauge in principle; the piezoelectric crystal creates a change in voltage when it is strained. When pressure is applied to a piezoelectric crystal its shape is dis-

torted, causing a reorientation of electrical charges within the crystal. The distortion causes a displacement of the positive and negative charges within the crystal, producing surface changes in opposite polarity on opposite sides of the crystal. The resultant voltage is amplified and converted into a graphic or numeric image on a monitor. The transducer, the connective tubing, and an indwelling catheter are typically filled with a heparinized saline solution, producing a continuous fluid column. When calibrated in relation to the standard anatomic reference level at which the catheter tip is assumed to rest (the phlebostatic point), this fluid-filled monitoring system should be accurate to within 1 mm Hg.[1, 2]

The presence of the various catheters and tubes associated with the process of hemodynamic monitoring should not be considered a contraindication to physical therapy intervention because the assessment of hemodynamic and pulmonary function at the patient's bedside has become standard

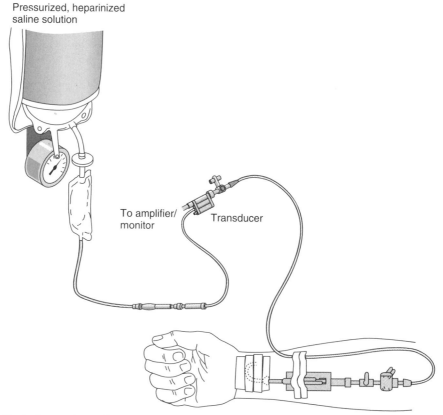

Pressurized, heparinized saline solution

To amplifier/ monitor

Transducer

Figure 13–1. Typical transducer for continuous monitoring of arterial blood pressure. For perspective on the size, consider that the actual transducer is smaller than the diameter of a U.S. quarter.

in the care of the critically ill patient. Therefore, knowledge of normal hemodynamic values, and the implications of deviations from normal, is essential to the implementation of physical therapy treatment plans. Normal values for the cardiovascular hemodynamic parameters commonly monitored are listed in Table 13–1.

ARTERIAL PRESSURES

Arterial blood pressure is the result of the rate of flow of blood (cardiac output) through and against the resistance of the circulatory system (systemic vascular resistance, or SVR). In the severely ill patient with hemodynamic compromise, a low stroke volume and excessive peripheral vasoconstriction may make **Korotkoff's sounds** (the

sounds heard over an artery when blood pressure is determined by the auscultatory method) impossible to hear. Therefore, in addition to a blood pressure cuff, an intra-arterial catheter frequently connects a monitoring device to a pressure transducer so that continuous measurement of systolic, diastolic, or mean arterial pressures can be displayed (Fig. 13–1B). In addition, an indwelling arterial catheter provides a convenient route of access for arterial blood sampling to assist in the assessment of ventilatory efficacy. A relatively recent advance in noninvasive monitoring of critically ill patients involving continuous blood pressure measurement by means of a finger cuff may eventually replace indwelling catheter placement in many instances.[3, 4]

The diastolic blood pressure is the lowest point of declining pressure resulting from the runoff of

Table 13–1
Common Hemodynamic Parameters

PARAMETER	COMMON ACRONYM	NORMAL VALUES
Arterial blood pressures	BP	
Systolic	SBP	90–140 mm Hg
Diastolic	DBP	60–80 mm Hg
Right atrial pressure	RAP	0–8 mm Hg (mean)
Right ventricular pressures		
Systolic	RVs	15–30 mm Hg *or*
End-diastolic	RVEDP	0–8 mm Hg
Pulmonary artery pressures	PAP	
Systolic	PAs	15–30 mm Hg
Diastolic	PAd	5–15 mm Hg
Pulmonary artery wedge pressure	PWP, PCWP	4–15 mm Hg (mean)
Left atrial pressure	LAP	4–12 mm Hg (mean)
Left ventricular pressures		
Systolic	LVs	100–140 mm Hg
End-diastolic	LVEDP	4–12 mm Hg
Calculated Values		
Mean arterial pressure $\dfrac{SBP + (2 \cdot DBP)}{3}$	MAP or $\overline{BP}$	70–110 mm Hg
Mean PAP $\dfrac{PAs + (2 \cdot PAd)}{3}$	$\overline{PAP}$	8–20 mm Hg
Systemic vascular resistance $\dfrac{MAP - RAP}{\dot{Q}} \cdot 80$	SVR	800–1200 dynes $\cdot$ sec^{-1} $\cdot$ cm^{-1}
Pulmonary vascular resistance $\dfrac{\overline{PAP} - PWP}{\dot{Q}} \cdot 80$	PVR	<100 dynes $\cdot$ sec^{-1} $\cdot$ cm^{-1} *or* $\frac{1}{6}$ SVR

Clinical Note: Systolic Blood Pressure Changes

The systolic blood pressure (the maximum systolic left ventricular pressure) reflects the compliance of the large arteries and the total peripheral resistance. In the normal adult, systolic pressure is usually about 120 mm Hg, ranging from 90 to 140 mm Hg, although it normally increases with age. The Joint National Committee on Prevention, Detection, Evaluation, and Treatment of High Blood Pressure[5] suggests that systolic blood pressures of nonsleeping subjects below 135 mm Hg are normal. Regardless of age, systolic blood pressure should be expected to increase with exertion in a fairly linear fashion. Typically, increases of 7 to 8 mm Hg per metabolic equivalent (MET) increase in work rate intensity are not uncommon in apparently healthy persons.[6] The blood pressure response of patients with cardiovascular disease taking vascular active medications can be quite variable. Nevertheless, it is unarguably considered unsafe if the systolic blood pressure exceeds 225 to 230 mm Hg. If the systolic blood pressure falls or fails to increase as work load increases, it may be assumed that the functional reserve capacity of the heart has been exceeded. If such situations develop, activity should be curtailed or terminated.[2, 5-7]

Clinical Note: Mean Arterial Pressure

The MAP is useful clinically because it yields one number that relates to cardiac output and the SVR.

blood from the proximal aorta to the peripheral vessels, and it reflects the velocity of the runoff and the elasticity of the arterial system. Because the duration of the diastolic period of the cardiac cycle is directly related to the heart rate, the longer the period of diastole, the more the dia-

stolic pressure falls. The diastolic blood pressure normally ranges from 60 to 80 mm Hg, although it increases somewhat with the aging process. It does not change much during repetitive, rhythmic-type activities involving the lower extremities, such as bicycling, walking, or running. However, during upper extremity exercise or isometric exercise involving any muscle group, the diastolic blood pressure normally increases. Just as there is an upper limit for systolic blood pressure, activity should be curtailed or halted if the diastolic blood pressure exceeds 130 mm Hg.[2, 5-7] A normal arterial pressure tracing is depicted in Figure 13-2.

The **mean arterial pressure (MAP)** is the average pressure tending to push blood through the circulatory system, and it reflects the tissue perfusion pressure. The MAP is closer to the diastolic than the systolic pressure because the duration of diastole is greater than that of systole. The MAP is not, therefore, a true arithmetic mean of systolic and diastolic pressures, but rather slightly less than the average of the two pressures. The normal MAP varies between 70 and 110 mm Hg; a MAP of less than 60 mm Hg indicates an inadequate tissue perfusion pressure.

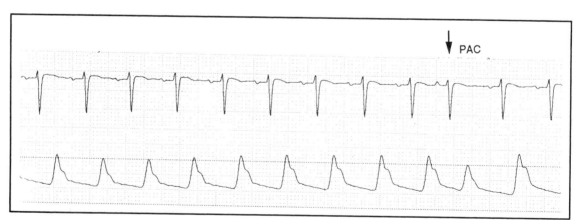

Figure 13-2. Electrocardiogram and arterial pressure tracings (sinus tachycardia at a rate between 110 and 120 beats per minute). The tenth ECG complex is a premature atrial complex (PAC); note the resultant decrease in the area of the tenth arterial pressure wave.

Right Atrial Pressure (Central Venous Pressure)

In the 1950s, the central venous pressure was estimated by measuring the vertical distance from the sternal angle to the level of the pulsating blood in one of the neck veins. In the 1960s, central venous catheters were developed, which allowed central venous pressures to be measured directly from the proximal superior vena cava by a water manometer. The term **right atrial pressure (RAP)** more correctly describes the anatomic and physiologic origins of what has traditionally been referred to as the central venous pressure. The advent of modern electronics has permitted the continuous monitoring of RAP to assess cardiac function and intravascular fluid status. Additionally, the catheter may be used as a route for medication or fluid administration, blood sampling, and emergency placement of a temporary pacemaker.

Although it was originally believed that the CVP was a reliable reflection of both right and left ventricular filling pressures, it is now recognized that there is generally a poor correlation between these two pressures as a result of the indirect temporal relationship of left ventricular dysfunction and the RAP.[8-10] Normally, the mean RAP is less than 5 mm Hg, ranging from 0 to 8 mm Hg.[2, 7] Subclavian and jugular insertion sites are most common for RAP access, and should not be an impediment to physical activity.

Pulmonary Artery Pressures

The introduction of RAP monitoring in the early 1960s was a breakthrough in direct bedside monitoring of cardiac function. However, flow and pressure abnormalities distal to the RAP catheter render meaningful evaluation of left ventricular filling pressures impossible. Thus, the development of the flow-directed, balloon-tipped pulmonary artery catheter in the 1970s permitted bedside assessment of left ventricular function. The modern pulmonary artery catheter permits direct measurement of right atrial and pulmonary arterial pressures, determination of mixed venous oxygen saturation and cardiac output, calculation of systemic and **pulmonary vascular resistance (PVR),** and pacing of the atrium and ventricles. The pulmonary artery catheter is typically introduced via a central venous access point (e.g., internal jugular or subclavian vein), passing from the vena cava into the right atrium, through the right atrioventricular (tricuspid) valve into the right ventricle, through the pulmonary valve and into the pulmonary artery (Fig. 13–3).

Because the left ventricular end-diastolic pressure (LVEDP) reflects the compliance of the left ventricle, it is the primary indicator of left ventricular performance. However, the LVEDP is difficult (even risky) to measure and is not monitored clinically—direct measurement of LVEDP is performed in the angiography laboratory as part of the coronary catheterization procedure. Fortuitously, though, the pressures in the left ventricle and in the left atrium are equal at the end of diastole because the mitral valve is still open (in the absence of mitral valve disease). Moreover, because there are no valves in the pulmonary venous system, the pressures in the pulmonary veins, the pulmonary capillaries, and the pulmonary artery are also equal at the end of diastole. Thus, the pulmonary artery end-diastolic (PAd) pressure is essentially equal to the LVEDP (normally less than 12 mm Hg) in the absence of disease.

In such situations, the pulmonary capillary wedge pressure (PWP or PCWP, normally less than 12 mm Hg) will be intermittently monitored. Note that during PWP monitoring, the distal balloon at the tip of the catheter is inflated, thus "wedging" the catheter into a branch of the pulmonary artery.

Clinical Note: Right Atrial Pressure

Elevations in RAP may result from fluid overload, right ventricular failure, tricuspid insufficiency, or chronic left ventricular failure. Low RAP may be indicative of hypovolemia and dehydration.

Clinical Note: Pulmonary Vascular Resistance

If the PVR is elevated (as might be seen with pulmonary embolism, hypoxia, chronic lung disease, or other dead-space-producing disorders), the pulmonary artery pressure will reflect the high PVR instead of the LVEDP.

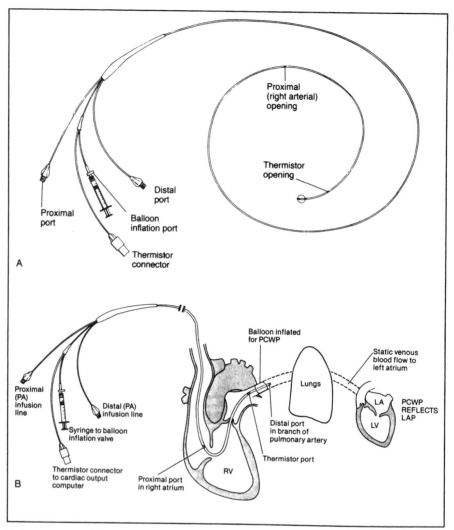

Figure 13–3. Pulmonary arterial catheter. *A,* Typical multilumen pulmonary artery catheter. *B,* The pulmonary artery catheter passes through the right atrium and ventricle to rest in the pulmonary artery. (*A* from Darovic GO. Hemodynamic Monitoring: Invasive and Noninvasive Clinical Application. Philadelphia, WB Saunders, 1987, p 140. *B* from Kersten LD. Comprehensive Respiratory Nursing. Philadelphia, WB Saunders, 1989, p 758.)

When treating patients who have pulmonary arterial lines, recognition of the "normalcy" of the potential waveforms is key to deciding whether or not it is advisable to perform physical therapy. An RAP waveform should be recognizable when right atrial pressures are being monitored; likewise, it should be possible to recognize a pulmonary arterial waveform when pulmonary artery pressures are being monitored. Normal wave configurations for right atrial, right ventricular, pulmonary artery, and pulmonary artery wedge pressures are shown in Figure 13–4.

Cardiac Output

The amount of blood ejected with each contraction of the heart is called the stroke volume (SV).

Clinical Note: Pulmonary Artery Catheterization

It is important to keep in mind that patients should not be engaged in physical therapy if the catheter is in the "wedge" position, because there is a very real possibility of rupturing the pulmonary artery.

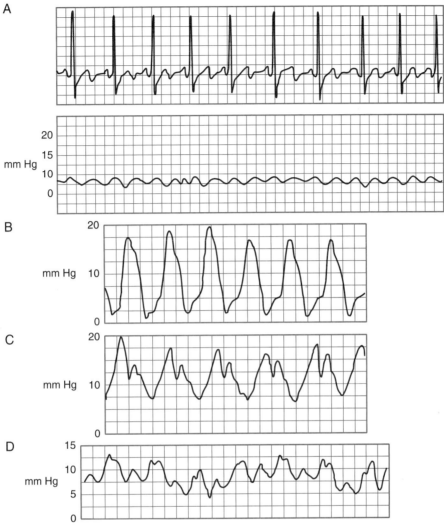

Figure 13–4. Normal pressure tracings of the right side of the heart. *A,* Electrocardiogram and concurrent right atrial pressure tracings. *B,* The right ventricular pressure waveform normally is observed only when the catheter is initially being inserted. *C,* Pulmonary arterial pressure waveform. *D,* Capillary wedge pressure waveform.

The amount of blood pumped by the heart per unit of time is termed the cardiac output ($\dot{Q}$), and unless an intracardiac shunt is present, the output of both the right and left ventricles is essentially

the same. The normal resting $\dot{Q}$ is 4 to 8 L per minute, and the normal SV ranges from 60 to 130 mL.[2, 7] Cardiac output normally increases as activity increases. However, pathologic conditions can greatly affect $\dot{Q}$ and impinge upon an individual's homeostatic tolerance.

Cardiac output is generally determined clinically by the **thermodilution method.** A cold bolus of saline is injected into the right atrium via the proximal lumen of a flow-directed, thermal-sensitive catheter (e.g., PA line); the resultant temperature change is sensed by a thermistor near the tip of the catheter located in the pulmonary artery. A temperature-time curve is constructed, and

Clinical Note: Proper Catheter Positioning

It is generally *not* normal to see a right ventricular or a "wedge" waveform when the catheter is properly positioned. If the clinician thinks that the catheter may be improperly positioned, physical therapy should be withheld until the correct catheter position is confirmed.

$\dot{Q}$ is calculated.[11] The mean SV is calculated by dividing the cardiac output by the ventricular rate over a specific period of time. Conditions such as an arteriovenous fistula, anoxia, and Paget's disease may ultimately decrease the peripheral vascular resistance and increase $\dot{Q}$ by increasing venous return to the heart. Conversely, conditions that result in decreased blood volume will reduce the venous return to the heart, decreasing $\dot{Q}$.

Unfortunately, simple $\dot{Q}$ measurements do not take into account an individual's specific needs with respect to actual body size. For this reason, the cardiac output per square meter of body surface area, the **cardiac index,** is often reported. The normal cardiac index for adults is approximately 3.0 L/min/m². A cardiac index of less than 2.2 L/min/m² is considered diagnostic of **cardiogenic shock.**[7] Cardiogenic shock is a condition in which the blood supply to the body tissues is insufficient because of inadequate $\dot{Q}$.

Mixed Venous Oxygen Saturation

The supply of oxygen to the tissues depends on $\dot{Q}$, hemogloblin level, and arterial oxygen saturation. Dissolved oxygen diffuses out of the capillaries and into the cells because of the pressure gradient that exists between them. The partial pressure of oxygen in the blood (PO_2) is normally just about 100 mm Hg at the arteriolar end of the capillary bed and about 5 mm Hg at the cell, so oxygen diffuses into the cells according to the gradient. By the time the blood reaches the venous end of the capillary bed, the Pv_{O_2} (partial pressure of venous oxygen) is about 40 mm Hg. Because the oxygen bound to the hemoglobin in the blood replenishes the dissolved oxygen that diffused out to the cells, the low Pv_{O_2} causes oxygen to dissociate from hemoglobin, as described by the oxyhemoglobin dissociation curve. Venous blood, therefore, is about 75% saturated with oxygen.[12, 13]

The amount of oxygen returning to the heart is called the venous oxygen reserve. When tissue demands for oxygen increase—as with exercise or increased metabolic rate resulting from a fever—the normal physiologic response is to increase oxygen supply and preserve the venous oxygen reserve. The oxygen supply is normally increased through an increase in $\dot{Q}$ and minute ventilation ($\dot{V}E$). Some patients (those with hypoxemia, anemia, heart failure, or pulmonary edema) cannot increase their oxygen supply in response to demand. When supply fails to meet demand, the venous oxygen reserve is affected because the tissues extract what they need as long as there is oxygen bound to the hemoglobin to replenish the dissolved oxygen taken by the cells. If the cellular demand for oxygen cannot be met, anaerobic metabolism ensues and lactic acidosis may result.

Mixed venous blood (customarily denoted by $\bar{v}$) represents the average of venous blood from all parts of the body. Venous blood is considered to be mixed when it has reached the pulmonary artery. Under normal conditions, the oxygen saturation of mixed venous blood ($S\bar{v}_{O_2}$) is in the range of 60% to 80%.

The pulmonary artery catheter permits intermittent or continuous monitoring of $S\bar{v}_{O_2}$ and may be crucial for monitoring critically ill patients during the process of weaning from mechanical ventilators because it allows for evaluation of the tissues' need for oxygen and the adequacy with which that need is being met.[14, 15]

The presence of hemodynamic monitoring lines should alert the clinician to a level of heightened awareness to the signs of intolerance of treatment that are commensurate with the level of acuity that necessitated the placement of the motoring line(s). For example, a patient requiring the placement of a pulmonary arterial line is generally less hemodynamically stable than a patient without one.

Remember that the clinical skills of observation and assessment should dictate clinical action. Attention should be paid to the trends demonstrated by hemodynamic variables, rather than to the value of any single parameter. Attention paid only to the values displayed on a bedside monitor, or comparison of observed values to norms without

> ### Clinical Note: Oxygen Saturation
>
> *Because changes in oxygen saturation are prompted by changes in the Pa_{O_2}, and because venous saturation is decreased only when oxygen supply fails to meet the demand, the $S\bar{v}_{O_2}$ can be a sensitive indicator of oxygen supply or demand status.*

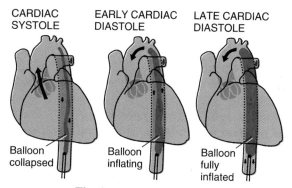

CARDIAC SYSTOLE   EARLY CARDIAC DIASTOLE   LATE CARDIAC DIASTOLE

Balloon collapsed   Balloon inflating   Balloon fully inflated

Figure 13-5. The intra-aortic balloon counterpulsation device is positioned in the descending aorta just below the orifice of the left subclavian artery. (Redrawn from Waldhausen JA, Pierce WS. Johnson's Surgery of the Chest, 5th ed. Chicago, Year Book Medical Publishers, 1985, p 273.)

Clinical Note: Effect of the Level of the Transducer

For every inch that the phlebostatic point is located above or below the level of the transducer, an error of approximately 2 mm Hg is introduced in the pressure displayed on a bedside monitor (either falsely high or low, respectively).

---

regard to the entire patient picture, contributes to an increased likelihood of inappropriate action.

As an example, consider the patient with a pulmonary artery systolic pressure (as displayed on a bedside monitor) of 22 mm Hg while he or she is in the supine position during activity. With such knowledge, a clinician might decide that the patient could tolerate more aggressive bed mobility activities. Accordingly, the clinician might proceed to sit the patient at the edge of the bed to concentrate on breathing control and balance interventions. If this hypothetical patient's right atrium were then 18 inches above the transducer because, as is customary, the transducer level was not readjusted, the pulmonary artery systolic pressure displayed on the bedside monitor would be 36 mm Hg higher than the actual value. Thus, if the clinician failed to take into account the effect of the change in the patient's position with respect to the transducer, and if the displayed pulmonary artery systolic pressure were 55 mm Hg, the clinician could misinterpret the reading as being suggestive of a significantly hypertensive response. The clinician could conclude that the patient was not tolerating the position change, and prematurely return the patient to the supine position. This error could be compounded if the clinician were to then inform the physician that the patient could not tolerate the upright sitting position because he developed a pulmonary artery systolic pressure of 55 mm Hg (instead of the actual acceptable value of 19 mm Hg). Because an error of as little as 6 mm Hg could result in significant errors in the medical therapeutic response, the clinician in such a situation should (1) move the transducer to the new level of the phlebostatic point or (2) note the value displayed with the phlebostatic point in the new position and make judgments in accordance with the new number (assuming there are no other indications of the patient's intolerance) so as to minimize the chances of misinterpretation.

Intra-aortic Balloon Counterpulsation

Sometimes, either as the result of pathologic insult or surgical intervention, patients become so hemodynamically unstable that **intra-aortic balloon counterpulsation (IABC)** is used to augment the diastolic blood pressure and to increase coronary blood flow. The balloon catheter is usually inserted into one of the femoral arteries and advanced until its tip is just below the level of the left subclavian artery orifice (Fig. 13-5; IABC is also discussed in Chapter 4). When activated, the balloon is deflated during left ventricular systole—lowering left ventricular systolic pressure—and inflated during diastole—increasing diastolic pressure and coronary blood flow. The timing for balloon inflation is based on either the R wave of the ECG or the patient's arterial pressure pulse.

Clinical Note: Movement During Intra-aortic Balloon Catheterization

As long as hip flexion for the involved limb is kept below 70 degrees, the patient can usually participate in bed mobility and range of motion activities with an IABC catheter in place. Out of bed activities are contraindicated until the IABC catheter is removed.

Electrocardiographic Monitoring

The electrocardiogram (ECG) is a graphic representation of the electrical activity of the heart. An electrocardiographic tracing demonstrates depolarization and repolarization of the atria and ventricles, although atrial repolarization is masked by ventricular depolarization. The position of the positive (recording) electrode in relation to the spread of the electrical impulse is referred to as the lead. By convention, there are 12 electrocardiographic leads: three standard limb leads, three augmented limb leads, and six precordial leads. In the critical care unit, patients are routinely monitored using only one or two of several possible leads for heart rate and rhythm. A standard 12-lead ECG is typically requested only for definitive analysis if irregularities are newly noted. Basic electrocardiographic interpretation is discussed in Chapter 9.

VENTILATORY MONITORING AND LIFE SUPPORT

Bedside Pulmonary Function Measurement

Respiratory physical therapy interventions are designed to promote bronchial hygiene, improve breathing efficiency, or promote physical reconditioning. To this end, the therapists involved may need to perform bedside pulmonary function testing or monitoring to ascertain treatment efficacy. Table 13–2 lists some of the parameters that may be measured at the bedside using relatively small and portable volume-collecting or flow-sensing devices. Additional tests may be performed at the bedside, but they require more sophisticated equipment. Nomograms have been developed specifically for certain patient populations and should be referred to before drawing conclusions regarding the normalcy of pulmonary function tests.[16] However, it is generally accepted that pulmonary function results should be within 80% and 120% of predicted values. Particularly with respect to weaning from mechanical ventilation, bedside spirometry or pulmonary function testing is indispensable. Several parameters, reflecting oxygenation status, ventilatory mechanics, respiratory muscle strength, and ventilatory demand may predict weaning success.[15, 17–23]

Oxygenation may be inferred from several clinically obtainable measurements. For example, an acceptable arterial oxygen saturation (Sa_{O_2}) and Pa_{O_2} (partial pressure of arterial oxygen) with an FI_{O_2} of 0.5 mm Hg or less is often cited as a criterion guideline preparatory to weaning attempts, as long as the Pa_{O_2}/FI_{O_2} ratio is greater than 200 mmHg.[18, 23] The literature regarding criteria for oxygenation during the weaning process

Table 13–2

Pulmonary Function Parameters Readily Obtainable at the Bedside

PARAMETER	COMMON ACRONYM	DEFINITION
Respiratory frequency	f	Number of breaths per minute
Tidal volume	V_T	Volume of air inhaled or exhaled with each normal resting breath
Minute ventilation	$\dot{V}_E$	Volume of air exhaled per minute
Vital capacity	VC Nonforced or timed	Volume of air that can be expelled from the lungs following full inspiration
Forced vital capacity	FVC	Volume of air that can be quickly and forcibly expelled from the lungs following full inspiration
Forced expiratory volume per unit time	FEV_t	Volume of air that can forcibly be exhaled per unit of time (e.g., FEV_1 = volume in 1 second)
Peak expiratory flow	PEF	Highest flow rate attained in a forced expiratory maneuver
Maximal/inspiratory force or negative inspiratory force	MIF or NIF	Greatest negative pressure achieved during an inspiratory effort

generally predates the widespread use of positive end-expiratory pressure (PEEP) and pressure support ventilation (PSV) for the treatment of adult respiratory distress syndrome; nonetheless, a PEEP of 7.5 cm H_2O or less and a PSV level of 10 cm H_2O or less is desirable prior to the initiation of the weaning process.

Although ventilatory mechanics are probably best inferred in most cases by the inspiratory capacity (IC), a tidal volume of at least 5 mL/kg and a static system compliance greater than 30 mL/cm H_2O are often considered predictive of weaning success. Likewise, a vital capacity (VC) of at least 15 mL/kg and a negative (maximal) inspiratory force (NIF or MIF) of more than 20 cm H_2O have with been suggested as suitable predictors.[20, 23, 24]

The patient's ability to meet ventilatory demand may be inferred from expiratory minute ventilation (VE), dead-space to tidal-volume ratio (VDVT), and CO_2 production (VCO_2). A VE less than 10 L/min, for a Pa_{CO_2} of 40 mm Hg, is one parameter that is highly predictive of weaning success.[20, 23, 24]

Monitoring the forces generated by the respiratory muscles is important because they are the only skeletal muscles upon which life is directly dependent. For the respiratory muscles, which work primarily in terms of elastic and resistive loads, force-length and force-velocity relationships are inferred from measurements of pressure (force developed, divided by surface area over which it acts), changes in volume (inferring changes in length), and flow rate of volume change (inferring velocity).

> ### Clinical Note: Inferring Respiratory Muscle Strength
> Respiratory muscle strength may be inferred from the MIF, IC or VC, peak flow rate, or forced expiratory volume in 1 second (FEV_1).

Airway Adjuncts

An **oral pharyngeal airway** (Fig. 13–6A) is a semirigid tube of plastic or rubber shaped to fit the

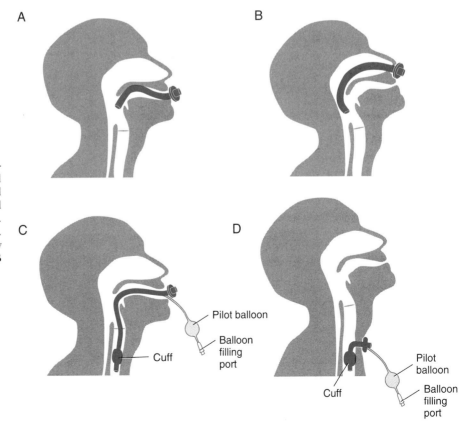

Figure 13–6. Airway adjuncts. *A*, Oral pharyngeal tube. *B*, Nasal pharyngeal tube. *C*, Oral endotracheal tube. *D*, Tracheostomy tube. (Redrawn from Kersten LD. Comprehensive Respiratory Nursing. Philadelphia, WB Saunders, 1989, p 630.)

natural curve of the soft palate and tongue. It is used to hold the tongue away from the back of the throat and maintain airway patency. The oral airway may also be used as a bite block. The **nasal pharyngeal airway** (Fig. 13–6*B*) is a soft latex or rubber tube inserted through one of the nares. It follows the wall of the naso- and oropharynx to the base of the tongue. The nasal airway is generally better tolerated because it is less likely to stimulate a gag reflex in the semiconscious or alert patient. However, the clinician is cautioned that when nasal airways are left in place for prolonged periods of time, interference with normal sinus drainage may occur. Nonetheless, when properly utilized, both the oral and the nasal airways may reduce mucosal trauma by providing a pathway for suctioning of the hypopharynx.

An endotracheal tube (Fig. 13–6*C*), an artificial airway inserted into the trachea, is made of silicone rubber or polyvinyl chloride and is generally disposable. An **oral endotracheal tube** is inserted via the mouth, and a **nasal endotracheal tube** is inserted via the nose; the specific rationale for using each type of tube may vary regionally. Regardless of the route, endotracheal intubation is usually undertaken as a last resort when other means of airway management have or are likely to fail. There are four primary reasons for employing endotracheal intubation: (1) upper airway obstruction, (2) inability to protect the lower airway from aspiration, (3) inability to clear secretions from the lower airways, or (4) need for positive pressure mechanical ventilatory assistance. A radiopaque line extending the length of the tube, or a marker at the distal end of the tube, facilitates location of the endotracheal tube by x-ray. Endotracheal tubes are beveled at their distal ends, and they are usually labeled near their proximal ends with the manufacturer's name, tube type, and internal diameter (ID) in millimeters. Unfortunately, there is no clear standard for reporting tube sizes. Instead of ID size, French size and Jackson size may be reported (for an approximate conversion of ID size to French size, multiply the ID size by 4).[25]

Modern adult endotracheal tubes typically have low-pressure, large-volume inflatable cuffs at their distal ends. Inflating the cuff stabilizes the endotracheal tube and seals the airway so that only air can move through the tube. A pilot balloon, attached to the cuff inflating tube, provides an indication of whether or not the cuff is inflated. Neo-

natal and pediatric endotracheal tubes generally do not have cuffs. A standard 15-mm adapter or universal adapter is attached at the proximal end of the endotracheal tube to facilitate connection to mechanical ventilators, manual resuscitation bags, or other respiratory modalities.

A **tracheostomy tube** (Fig. 13–6*D*) is an artificial airway inserted into the trachea, via a tracheostomy, below the level of the vocal cords. A tracheostomy may be performed for several reasons, but it is not normally an emergency procedure. In the critical care setting, a tracheostomy usually follows prolonged endotracheal intubation and is performed to minimize tracheal or vocal cord injury. The tracheostomy tube is short (2 to 6 inches long), but otherwise similar to an endotracheal tube except that it is not beveled at its distal end. An external flange near the proximal end of the tube is usually labeled with the manufacturer's name and internal or external diameter in millimeters. The flange serves to stabilize the tube in the trachea and as a base from which the tube may be secured to the patient's neck. Some tracheostomy tubes have a removable inner cannula to facilitate cleaning of the tube. There are several types of special-use tracheostomy tubes, and the clinician should be aware of the type of tube being used with the patient so that any special precautions are noted. For example, the fenestrated tube has a hole cut into the superior aspect of the outer cannula, which permits utilization of the upper airway with the tube in place if the inner cannula is removed.

Although most tracheostomy tubes are cuffed, there are many situations in which the cuff is deflated. For example, when assessing the patient's ability to protect the lower airway during swallowing, the cuff may be deflated. The reader is referred to clinical experts or specialized texts for further details regarding inflation and deflation of tracheostomy cuffs.

Clinical Note: Inflation and Deflation of Tracheostomy Cuffs

The clinician is advised to inquire whether the tracheostomy cuff should be inflated or deflated if it is ever found deflated. The cuff should not *be inflated or deflated capriciously; dire consequences for the patient may result.*

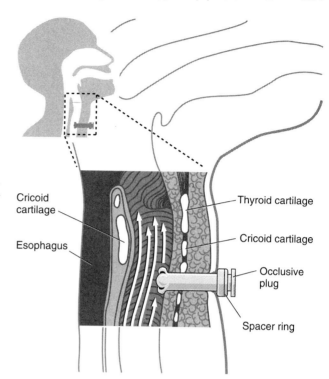

Figure 13-7. Tracheostomy button. (Adapted from Kersten LD. Comprehensive Respiratory Nursing. Philadelphia, WB Saunders, 1989, p 660.)

A **tracheostomy button** (Fig. 13–7) may be used as an intermediate step between mechanical ventilation and spontaneous breathing in the process of weaning a patient from mechanical ventilatory support. The tracheostomy button permits the upper airway to be used for spontaneous ventilation, while providing a means of maintaining the tracheostomy stoma as a direct access route to the lower airway until the patient no longer requires assistance to clear bronchial secretions.

MECHANICAL VENTILATION

Positive-Pressure Ventilators

There are two primary reasons that mechanical ventilation might be instituted for a patient—ventilatory failure and hypoxemia. Positive-pressure ventilation is used almost exclusively for mechanical ventilatory assistance. The positive pressure from the ventilator provides the force that delivers gas into the patient's lungs by increasing intrathoracic pressure to expand the chest wall. The termi-

nation of gas flow allows the chest wall to recoil to the resting position, thus exhaling the gas. Mechanical ventilators are generally classified according their cycling mechanism, that is, the method used to stop the inspiratory phase and initiate the expiratory phase. Basically, there are three types of mechanical ventilators: (1) pressure-cycled (e.g., Bird series,* Bennett series*); (2) volume-cycled (e.g., Bear series,* Bennett MA series,* Monaghan 225,* Ohio CCV-2*); and (3) time-cycled (e.g., Engstrom,* Emerson series,* Siemens Servo series,* Bourns BP200, Bird Babybird*). Of course, many of these machines can be cycled by more

---

*Manufacturers for these ventilators are as follows: Bird series, Bird Products Corporation, 3101 E. Alejo Road, Palm Springs, CA 92262; Bennett series, Puritan Bennett Corporation, 12655 Beatrice Street, Los Angeles, CA 90066; Bear series, Bourns-Bear Medical Systems, Inc., 2085 Rustin Ave., Riverside, CA 92507; Monaghan 225, Monaghan Medical Corporation, Franklyn Bldg., Rt. 9 North, P.O. Box 978, Plattsburgh, NY 12901; Ohio CCV-2, Ohmeda, 303 Ohmeda Drive, P.O. Box 7550, Madison, WI 53707; Engstrom, 600 Knight's Bridge Parkway, Lincolnshire, IL 60069; Emerson series, J.H. Emerson Co., 22 Cottage Park Ave., Cambridge, MA 02140; Siemens Servo series, Siemens-Elma Ventilator Systems, 2360 N. Palmer Drive, Schaumburg, IL 60195; Hamilton Veolar, Hamilton Medical, Inc., P.O. Box 30008, Reno, NV 89520.

than one mechanism. Newer and more sophisticated ventilators that use computer and microprocessor technology do not lend themselves to simple classification (e.g., Bear 5,* Bennett 7200,* and Hamilton Veolar*).

Knowledge of the basic components and terminology associated with the mechanical ventilator will assist the clinician in being better prepared to monitor the mechanically ventilated patient. The tubing that connects the patient to the ventilator is called the **circuit** (Fig. 13–8). The circuit generally consists of wide-bore tubing and valves that attach either to a mask or mouthpiece, or directly to an endotracheal or tracheostomy tube. In some institutions, an additional port in the terminal end of the circuit permits suctioning while maintaining the integrity of the circuit and obviates the need to disconnect the endotracheal tube from the circuit (Fig. 13–8A). During the performance of various bronchial hygiene procedures, or simply to facilitate positioning for patient comfort, the circuit may need to be disconnected from the patient. Disconnection may mean simply removing a mask or mouthpiece, as would be done with the termination of an intermittent positive-pressure breathing (IPPB) treatment, or it may involve disengaging the circuit from an endotracheal or tracheostomy tube in conjunction with hyperoxygenation. This latter effort necessitates stabilizing the endotracheal or tracheostomy tube while the circuit is removed, taking care to assure that the patient is not inadvertently extubated (endotracheal or tracheostomy tube removed), and then manually ventilating the patient with a self-inflating resuscitation bag (discussed later).

By convention, mechanical ventilation may be provided for the patient by several modes. Controlled ventilation is the provision of positive-pressure breaths at a set rate without regard for patient participation. Assist or assist-control ventilation is the provision of positive-pressure breaths at a set rate, unless the patient triggers the machine by creating a negative inspiratory force less than the preset threshold pressure of the machine. In this case, the machine delivers a positive-pressure breath at the rate established by the patient's efforts. **Intermittent mandatory ventilation (IMV)** or **synchronized intermittent mandatory ventilation (SIMV)** is the provision of a preset number of ventilator breaths in conjunction with a source of gas from which the patient may spontaneously breathe. In the IMV mode, the mandatory breath is delivered at a preset rate, regardless of the phase of the patient's spontaneous efforts. In the SIMV mode, the mandatory breath is initiated by the patient's spontaneous inspiratory effort. **Pressure support ventilation (PSV)** is the augmentation of the inspiratory phase of a patient's spontaneous ventilatory efforts with a preset amount of positive pressure. Figure 13–9 shows the pressure curves generated by various ventilatory modes and some of the airway maneuvers.

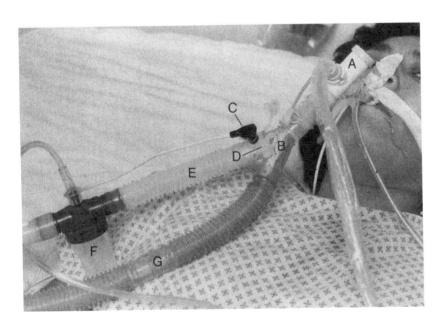

Figure 13–8. A disposable ventilator circuit with an integral endotracheal suctioning device. A, Integral, closed endotracheal suction adapter. B, Y-connector. C, Temperature probe for modulating gas temperature. D, Proximal pressure part (not in use here) for monitoring proximal airway pressure. E, Inspiratory limb of the ventilator circuit. F, In-line nebulizer for medication administration. G, Expiratory limb of the ventilator circuit. (From Kersten LD. Comprehensive Respiratory Nursing. Philadelphia, WB Saunders, 1989, p 710.)

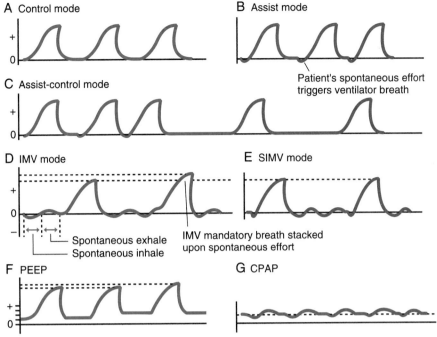

Figure 13-9. Pressure waves produced by several different modes of mechanical ventilation. *A*, Control mode. *B*, Assist mode. *C*, Assist-control mode. *D*, Intermittent mandatory ventilation (IMV) mode. *E*, Synchronized intermittent mandatory ventilation (SIMV) mode. *F*, Positive end-expiratory pressure (PEEP). *G*, Continuous positive airway pressure (CPAP) (see text for details). (Adapted from Kersten LD. Comprehensive Respiratory Nursing. Philadelphia, WB Saunders, 1989, p 712.)

Mechanical ventilation is frequently associated with a veritable alphabet soup of acronyms and terms that are used to describe various airway maneuvers that augment or modify a patient's ventilatory status. Four of these terms are noted here:

1. **Inspiratory hold** is a maneuver in which either the preset pressure or predetermined volume is reached and held for a predetermined (by the operator) period of time before exhalation is initiated.
2. **Positive end-expiratory pressure (PEEP)** is a threshold-like resistance applied after exhalation that permits the circuit pressure to drop to a set level above atmospheric pressure.
3. **Expiratory retard** is an orificial resistance applied to exhalation whereby the circuit pressure is permitted to drop slowly to atmospheric level as the expiratory gas flow ceases.
4. **Constant positive airway pressure (CPAP)** is the application of an elevated baseline pressure (greater than atmospheric) from which a patient spontaneously breathes.

Clinical Note: Artificial Ventilation

When a therapist notes that a patient is being ventilated artificially, the amount of ventilatory support must be identified. If the patient is receiving IMV 12, this means the ventilator is giving the patient 12 breaths per minute. However, if the patient is receiving IMV 2, the patient is breathing mostly on his or her own with the ventilator supplying 3 breaths per minute. When the ventilator pops off during treatment or movement, a therapist would have greater immediate concern for the patient on IMV 12 versus one on IMV 2.

Clinical Note: Constant Positive Airway Pressure

During the process of weaning the patient from the ventilator, the pressure support is often the last component to be eliminated. Therefore, prior to extubation, patients are usually given a trial of CPAP.

Negative-Pressure Ventilators

Mention should be made of a couple of negative-pressure ventilators. The **cuirass** (Fig. 13–10) is a rigid shell that encloses the patient's anterior thorax so that subatmospheric pressure can be exerted within the shell. A vacuum cleaner–like pump generates the negative pressure. The shells are usually custom-made for each patient, although prefabricated shells are available. The cuirass is probably not more widely used because (1) it tends to be noisy, (2) provision of patient care may be hampered, and (3) regulation of inspiratory/expiratory ratios is difficult. These units are useful, however, for providing augmentation to spontaneously breathing patients with weakened respiratory musculature. Additionally, ventilatory mechanics are more physiologic than they are with positive-pressure machines, and many patients do not require a tracheostomy. Patients requiring intermittent or periodic ventilatory assistance (e.g., patients with Guillain-Barré syndrome or amyotrophic lateral sclerosis) may benefit from such ventilators. Of course, the **"iron lung"** (Fig. 13–11), made famous during the poliomyelitis epidemics of the 1940s and 1950s, is still in use by some patients today. In fact, it is often used at night by patients so that they can rest sufficiently to assume the task of spontaneous ventilation during the daytime.

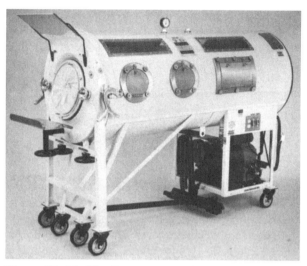

Figure 13–11. The Emerson iron lung. An iron lung is a large, relatively airtight chamber into which a patient is placed, with the head exposed. An adjustable plastic ring is used to achieve a seal around the patient's neck. The Emerson iron lung is the oldest commercially available mechanical ventilator in the United States. (From Branson RD, Hess DR, Chatburn RL. Respiratory Care Equipment. Philadelphia, JB Lippincott, 1995, p 429.)

Supplemental Oxygen-Delivery Devices

Physical therapists working with patients while they are receiving supplemental oxygen must be familiar with several types of oxygen systems. In the intensive care unit, patients' mechanical ventilators or other supplemental oxygen devices are connected to the hospital's bulk oxygen system outlets at the bedside. However, for transport or ambulation, or in the long-term or home-care settings, portable oxygen tanks or cylinders are used. This section of the chapter will consider the portable systems, such as cylinders or liquid oxygen canisters, which permit oxygen to accompany a patient away from the bedside.

The storage of compressed oxygen in tanks or cylinders is a common method of supplying oxygen for portable or out-of-hospital needs. Medical gas cylinders are made of steel, aluminum, or chrome-molybdenum. Aluminum cylinders are most useful in situations in which weight is a major concern or during some medical diagnostic procedures (for example, magnetic resonance imaging). By convention, in the United States, oxygen cylinders

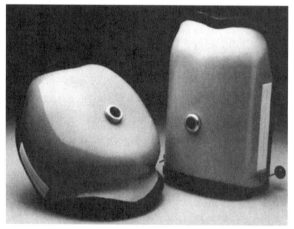

Figure 13–10. Chest cuirass. An electric pump is used to intermittently create a negative pressure within the shell when it is positioned over the patient's anterior chest. (From Branson RD, Hess DR, Chatburn RL. Respiratory Care Equipment. Philadelphia, JB Lippincott, 1995, p 428.)

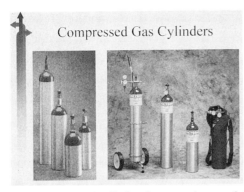

Compressed Gas Cylinders

Figure 13–12. The E-cylinder has a volume of 620 L. Although the cylinder, regulator/flow meter, and transport device have a total weight of about 17 pounds, the E-cylinder is probably still the most widely used compressed gas container for supplemental oxygen.

---

are color coded in green and are labeled "Oxygen." In other countries, the color code for oxygen cylinders is white. Nonetheless, practitioners should always check the cylinder label to identify the contents before use.

Although cylinders vary in size, the most common types are the small E-cylinder (in the hospital or outpatient setting; Fig. 13–12) and the large H-cylinder (in the home care setting). When full, an oxygen cylinder exerts about 2200 pounds per square inch (psi) of pressure. A pressure regulator reduces the high pressures from the gas in the cylinder to a lower working pressure, usually 50 psi, before the gas enters the flowmeter. The flowmeter measures and controls the flow of oxygen to the patient. When full, E-cylinders contain approximately 620 L of oxygen; H-tanks contain about 6900 L. Depending on the liter flow needed for the specific delivery device, the clinician can calculate the amount of time left at the given flow rate by using the following formula:

$$\frac{\text{psi} \times \text{k}}{\text{desired flow rate}}$$

where psi = pounds per square inch (read from the regulator dial), and k = cylinder constant (3.14 for H-tank, 0.28 for E-cylinder). The cylinder constant is a conversion factor that allows the cylinder pressure to be converted to liters of gas.

Portable liquid oxygen systems (Fig. 13–13) are in common use outside the hospital setting be-

cause of their relatively greater capacity and lighter weight. Under very high pressure, oxygen liquefies. As a liquid, oxygen occupies 1/860 the volume of gas at standard atmospheric pressure. A typical liquid oxygen system can provide oxygen for approximately 8 hours at a flow rate of 2 L/minute and will weigh about 10 lb; an E-cylinder system will last about 5 hours at a similar flow rate and weighs about 17 lb.[26] Given that 1 L of liquid oxygen weighs 2.5 lb (1.1 kg) and 1 L of liquid oxygen produces 860 L of gaseous oxygen, in order to determine the duration of flow available from a liquid oxygen container, calculate as follows:

Weight of liquid oxygen
= current container weight (lb)
− empty container weight (lb)

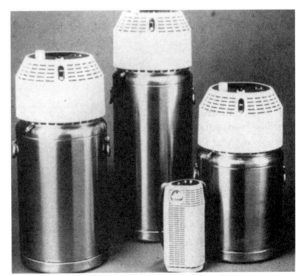

Figure 13–13. Stationary and portable liquid oxygen (LOX) units. (From Branson RD, Hess DR, Chatburn RL. Respiratory Care Equipment. Philadelphia, JB Lippincott, 1995, p 42.)

$$\text{Gas in system} = \frac{\text{weight of liquid oxygen (lb)} \times 860}{2.5 \text{ lb/L}}$$

$$\text{Duration of flow} = \frac{\text{gas remaining (L)}}{\text{flow rate (L/min)}}$$

For example, if a therapist fills a portable container with 3 lb of liquid oxygen from the stationary container and a patient requires a flow of 4 L/minute, how long will the oxygen in the portable container last?

$$\text{Gas remaining} = \frac{3 \text{ lb} \times 860}{2.5 \text{ lb/L}} = 1032 \text{ L}$$

$$\text{Duration of flow} = \frac{1032 \text{ L}}{4 \text{ L/min}} = 258 \text{ minutes}$$

$$= 4 \text{ hours, 18 minutes}$$

The gases used for therapeutic purposes are stored with all water vapor removed, that is, 100% dry. Depending on the gas flow rate, the frequency and duration of use, and the patient's state of hydration, the lack of humidity could irritate the mucosa of the pulmonary passageways. At low flow rates (less than 4 L/minute) humidification of the gases may not be necessary. At flow rates of less than 10 L/minute, simple humidifiers (Fig. 13–14) may be used to add sufficient humidity to make the gas comfortable. When the upper airway is bypassed—for example, when the patient has a tracheostomy tube in place or is intubated—the gas must be heated to increase its capacity to carry water vapor. Heated humidifiers are often used when flow rates exceed 10 L/minute or when the upper airway is bypassed. Aerosolized water is another means by which medical gases may be humidified. Nebulizers (Fig. 13–15), of which there are many types, are used to produce aerosols.

Oxygen administration devices include nasal cannulas, masks, tents, hoods, and incubators. The **nasal cannula** is the most commonly used delivery device. It is generally intended to be used with oxygen flow rates between 1 and 6 L/minute for adults, and as low as 1/16 L in neonates (Fig.

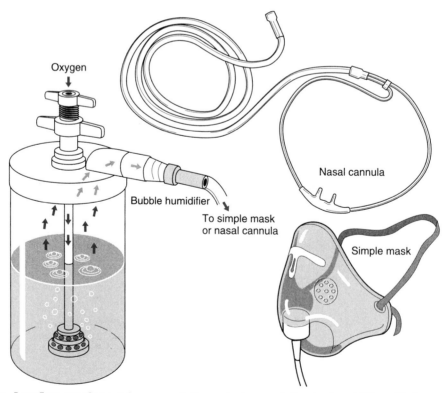

Figure 13–14. Low-flow supplemental oxygen delivery devices and flow-by humidifier. (Redrawn from Kersten LD. Comprehensive Respiratory Nursing. Philadelphia, WB Saunders, 1989, pp 608, 609.)

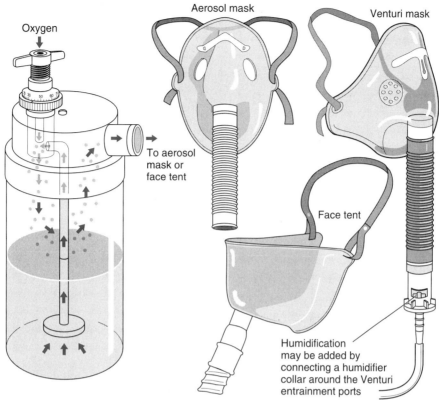

Figure 13–15. High-flow supplemental oxygen delivery devices and aerosol nebulizer. (Redrawn from Kersten LD. Comprehensive Respiratory Nursing. Philadelphia, WB Saunders, 1989, pp 581, 585.)

13–14). Whether or not a humidifier is used in conjunction with a nasal cannula may depend on individual physician preference. However, at flows exceeding 3 or 4 L/minute the nasal mucosa may become dried and irritated with sustained use of nonhumidified gas.[26, 27] An accurate fraction of inspired oxygen (FI_{O_2}) cannot be delivered with a nasal cannula because respiratory rate, tidal volume, and anatomic dead space are so variable among patients.[28] Nonetheless, as Table 13–3 shows, we assume that the approximate FI_{O_2} is increased by 4% with each 1 L/minute increase in oxygen flow rate when the patient is breathing regularly. The delivery of an accurate and consistent FI_{O_2} requires that the flow of gas be sufficient to exceed the patient's peak inspiratory flow demand, which generally requires higher flow rates than can be tolerably achieved by nasal cannula. Under such conditions, any of several different types of masks are used to deliver supplemental oxygen.[29]

The **simple mask** (Fig. 13–14) is designed to provide a flow of gas into a face piece that fits over the patient's nose and mouth. Some simple masks also include a diluter to add room air and thus increase the total gas flow as the oxygen flows into the mask. The oxygen percentage that can be delivered with a simple mask ranges from 35% to 55%, at flow rates of 5 to 10 L/minute (for adults). As is true with nasal cannulas, whether a humidifier is used in conjunction with a simple mask may depend on individual physician preference. However, at oxygen concentrations exceed-

---

Clinical Note: Oxygen Masks

Patients who are breathing through their mouths will often not receive the benefit of an increased flow rate through a nasal cannula. These patients may benefit from using a mask to improve oxygenation in the blood.

Table 13-3

Approximate FI_{O_2} Achieved with Different Oxygen Delivery Devices

DEVICE	OXYGEN FLOW RATE	FI_{O_2}
Nasal cannula (estimated FI_{O_2}, assuming normal $\dot{V}E$)		
	1 L/min	0.24
	2 L/min	0.28
	3 L/min	0.32
	4 L/min	0.36
	5 L/min	0.40
	6 L/min	0.44
Simple mask		
	5–6 L/min	0.35
	6–7 L/min	0.45
	7–10 L/min	0.55
Aerosol mask		
	10–12 L/min	0.35–1.0 (depends on setting)
Venturi mask (O_2 flow rates are minimums to be used with specific-sized orifice for desired FI_{O_2})		
	4 L/min	0.24*
	4 L/min	0.28*
	6 L/min	0.31
	8 L/min	0.35*
	8 L/min	0.40*
	10 L/min	0.50

* FI_{O_2} depends on the size of the orifice or the entrainment ports; these vary among manufacturers.

ing 30%, the nasal and oral mucosa may become dried and irritated with sustained use of nonhumidified gas.

The **aerosol mask** (Fig. 13–15) was originally designed for the administration of aerosolized medications. However, these masks are widely used for the administration of controlled percentages of oxygen at flow rates slightly greater than those for simple masks (10 to 12 L/minute), to exceed the patient's inspiratory demand. Typically, aerosol masks are used in conjunction with a nebulizer to humidify the gas. The FI_{O_2} is regulated between 35% and 100% by means of an adjustable air entrainment port on the nebulizer. Increasing the FI_{O_2} setting closes the entrainment port and decreases the dilution of the oxygen.

The **Venturi mask** (Fig. 13–15) generally provides a greater flow of gas to a patient by entraining room air through a side port. The FI_{O_2} is selected by changing either the size of the orifice

through which oxygen is delivered or the size of the entrainment ports, and adjusting the oxygen flow rate. Venturi masks operate by application of the Bernoulli principle: oxygen enters the larger flexible tubing via a narrowed orifice, creating a relative negative pressure within the tubing, which pulls room air through the entrainment ports. These masks may or may not be humidified. Table 13–3 details the oxygen flow rates and FI_{O_2} delivered by Venturi masks (different manufacturers' devices may provide different FI_{O_2} values).

In the pediatric setting, oxygen tents, hoods, or incubators are frequently used. In an **oxygen tent,** the FI_{O_2} attained depends on the incoming gas flow, the canopy volume, and the degree to which the tent is sealed. Tents generally envelop the patient's upper torso or entire body. Continuous oxygen monitoring is necessary because patient care requires entering the tent. This, therefore, alters the FI_{O_2}. Ice reservoirs are often incorporated for temperature control. An **oxygen hood,** a small plastic enclosure placed over the patient's head, permits nursing care or other treatment without hindering oxygen therapy. An **incubator** may be used for similar reasons as an oxygen tent, but it generally provides for warming instead of cooling of the environment.

Nasal continuous positive airway pressure (nCPAP) and **bilevel positive airway pressure (biPAP)** ventilators (Fig. 13–16) are being used increasingly to provide noninvasive ventilatory support in the management of obstructive sleep apnea, chronic ventilatory failure, and acute respira-

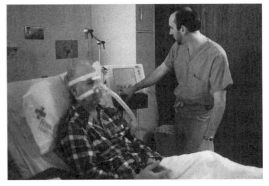

Figure 13-16. A tight-fitting nasal mask is used to convey bilevel positive airway pressure to augment the ventilation of a spontaneously breathing patient. This patient is receiving noninvasive ventilation from a BiPAP system. (Photograph of BiPAP Vision System courtesy of Respironics, Inc., Pittsburgh, PA.)

tory failure for infants, children, and adults. Nasal continuous positive airway pressure is currently the treatment of choice in cases of obstructive sleep apnea syndrome.[30] It has been suggested that biPAP improves ventilation and vital signs more rapidly than nCPAP in patients with acute pulmonary edema.[31]

Other Mechanical Devices

Additional equipment that is not readily placed in the previously discussed categories includes incentive spirometers and resistive breathing devices, mechanical percussors, and manual resuscitators. Although they might be more correctly termed adjuncts to treatment, these devices are frequently employed by physical therapists in the treatment of patients with respiratory dysfunction.

INCENTIVE SPIROMETRY AND INSPIRATORY RESISTANCE DEVICES

Approximately six to nine times an hour, the normal adult takes a deep inhalation, or sigh, that approaches the total lung capacity. In a pattern of shallow breathing, without periodic deep breaths, yawns, or sighs, a gradual alveolar collapse develops that if not corrected or reversed, can lead to gross **atelectasis** (see Chapter 5 for discussion of the pathology). Trauma, disease, and surgical procedures all contribute to such abnormal patterns of breathing. Additionally, an inadequate inspiratory capacity inhibits the patient's cough strength. For example, a patient may alter the respiratory patterns, avoiding prolonged inspiratory efforts and coughing as a result of incisional pain or muscle weakness. Therefore, breathing exercises that incorporate sustained maximal inspiratory efforts with coughing assistance techniques may be indicated.

The **incentive spirometer** is designed to provide patients with immediate visual feedback regarding achievement of preset goals while they perform sustained maximal inspiratory maneuvers. This visual input, it is hoped, encourages patients to continue to use the unit and to work toward increasing their maximal inspiratory effort. Two types of

incentive spirometers are commonly used in the clinic—flow and volume spirometers (Fig. 13–17).

Flow incentive spirometers are flow-dependent. Generally, they consist of one or more chambers containing a table tennis–like ball. Inhalation elevates the ball(s) and keeps it floating as long as the flow of air is of sufficient magnitude. Unfortunately, a very brisk flow rate will pull the ball(s) to the top of the chamber with a relatively low-volume breath. Alternately, a breath with an especially slow flow rate may achieve total lung capacity without moving the ball(s).

Volume incentive spirometers permit the selection of preset volumes that directly indicate whether the actual volume is achieved. The commonly used volume spirometers have a bellows or piston that registers the volume achieved. The clinician adjusts an indicator to the desired inspiratory goal.

Although the patient is encouraged to use either incentive spirometer independently, neither device should be placed at the patient's bedside without first providing proper instruction for its use. Several brands of incentive spirometers are commercially available.

Physical therapists are unique in their ability to assess and intervene in the rehabilitation of unused muscles. Although it is easy to see the atrophy of arm or leg muscles following the removal of a plaster cast and to appreciate that the prolonged disuse of these muscles may predispose them to weakness and rapid fatigue, too often this same association is not made with reference to the respiratory muscles following prolonged mechanical ventilatory support. A fundamental principle of exercise training is to work a muscle to the point of fatigue and then allow it to rest.

In a study on respiratory muscle strengthening and endurance training in which chronic obstructive pulmonary disease (COPD) patients utilized 3- to 5-second maximal inspiratory efforts in con-

> **Clinical Note: Incentive Spirometers**
> Incentive spirometers are great tools to use for measurement of pulmonary outcomes. Therefore, an outcome of treatment may be the amount of volume the patient can inspire using the incentive spirometer.

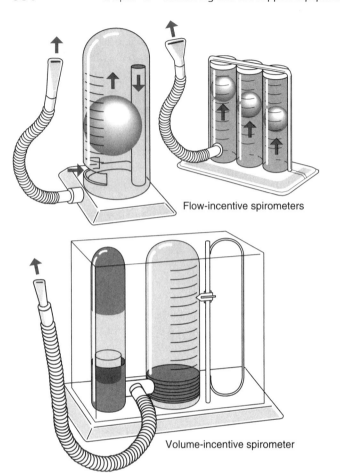

Flow-incentive spirometers

Volume-incentive spirometer

Figure 13–17. Flow- and volume-incentive spirometers. (Redrawn by permission of Sherwood Medical, St. Louis, MO.)

junction with expiratory maneuvers at 20% increments over their vital capacity ranges for strength training, and ventilation to exhaustion three to five times daily for endurance training, Leith and Bradley[32, 33] showed that strength trainers increase maximal inspiratory pressures by 55% and that endurance trainers increased their ability to sustain hyperpnea from 81% to 96% of their pretraining maximal voluntary ventilation (MVV, largest volume that can be breathed per minute with voluntary effort) while increasing their MVV by 14%. In another investigation, Gross et al.[34] reported that an 8-week regimen of 30 minutes of daily inspiratory resistance training by quadriplegic patients resulted in a 21.5% increase in mean maximal inspiratory force (MIF). Thus, resistive inspiratory training may be a beneficial treatment tool (see Chapter 19 for more details).

MECHANICAL PERCUSSORS

The modalities of percussion and vibration, as employed in the performance of a bronchial hygiene regimen, constitute a significant portion of the treatment time. Judiciously applied, these modalities have been shown to augment the mobilization and elimination of excessive secretions. Yet, as many therapists can attest, these techniques can be difficult to learn and quite fatiguing if not performed properly. Electrically or pneumatically powered mechanical percussors are commercially available to ameliorate these difficulties. However, the efficacy of these mechanical adjuncts is as highly dependent on their proper use as is the efficacy of the manual techniques. Although it may be true that these devices conserve the therapist's energy, they eliminate an often overlooked and underrated nonverbal communication system between therapist and patient—touch.

MANUAL RESUSCITATORS

Instances may exist in which the therapist must disconnect the patient from the mechanical ventilator for a prolonged period of time (e.g., transfer or ambulation training, endotracheal suctioning). In such instances, the patient will require ventilatory assistance by use of a manual resuscitator. Several manufacturers produce manual resuscitators, and the valve systems of each are unique. There are also occasions that necessitate the use of portable, battery-powered mechanical ventilators. Clinicians should become thoroughly familiar with the equipment utilized by their patients.

Manual resuscitation bags (Fig. 13–18) are self-inflating; when compressed, they deliver a volume of gas to the patient by means of one-way valves. When the bag is compressed, gas enters the valve and pushes the diaphragms against the exhalation ports. The flow of gas then opens the inhalation valve, permitting gas to flow to the patient. When flow from the bag ceases and exhalation begins, exhaled gas from the patient pushes the inhalation valve closed and opens the diaphragms, allowing gas to flow out the exhalation ports. The bag intake port may be fitted with an oxygen reservoir system to deliver oxygen-enriched breaths. Manual resuscitation bags may be used to stimulate or mimic a cough and/or to augment V_T and supplement oxygen for intubated and nonintubated patients.

Case Study

Patient is a 38-year-old woman with familial polyposis. This case progresses through 98 days of this patient's hospitalization; it represents the way that things can change rapidly in the critical care setting. Initially, the patient appears to have presented a rather straightforward case for a typical surgical revision of a continent ileostomy (Koch pouch). Unfortunately, between hospital day (HD) 4 and HD 6, her situation deteriorated as she developed adult respiratory distress syndrome (ARDS).

From HD 6 to HD 18, the patient's hemodynamic and oxygenation status continued to deteriorate, she required neuromuscular blockage (vecuronium) and a change of ventilatory support mode (volume control via synchronized intermittent mandatory ventilation, SIMV, to pressure control ventilation, PCV) in order to provide adequate minute ventilation.

A physical therapy consultation was requested when the patient was medically paralyzed. At that time, the patient could best be categorized as suffering impaired ventilation and respiration with mechanical ventilation secondary to respiratory failure (pattern 6-I in the Association APT, Guide to Physical Therapist Practice. Part 1: A description of patient/client management. Part 2: Preferred practice patterns. Phys Ther 77(11): 1997; revised July 1999). The physical therapist initiated therapeutic exercise to maintain joint range of motion and chest wall mobility until HD 40, when the patient underwent an exploratory laparotomy. The patient's ventilatory status improved marginally over that period of time.

On HD 44, physical therapy was reordered. On HD 57, the physical therapist noted decorticate posturing with PROM; neuromuscular blockage was increased. By HD 69, the patient had improved sufficiently to permit reduction of sedation and neuromuscular blockage. Bed mobility training and hemodynamic challenges (tilt table and dangling) were incorporated into the treatment regimen. By HD 83, the patient had progressed to standing activities. By HD 86, the patient was extubated. Physical therapy progressed to gait training and general strengthening exercises. The patient was finally discharged from the hospital on HD 98.

Diagnosis: familial polyposis, 15 years pta
Past medical history:
  Colectomy and ileostomy, 13 years pta
  Hepatitis C, secondary to blood transfusion, 13 years pta

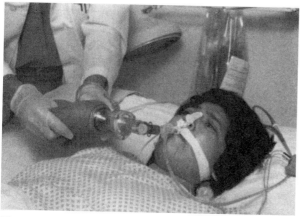

Figure 13–18. Self-inflating manual resuscitation bag being used to manually ventilate an intubated patient. (Reproduced with permission from Kersten LD. Comprehensive Respiratory Nursing. Philadelphia, WB Saunders, 1989, p 630.)

Dilatation and curettage, secondary to persistent serosanguineous vaginal drainage, 12 years pta
Hysterectomy and right oophorectomy, 12 years pta
Exploratory laparotomy and left oophorectomy, 11 years pta
Revision of ileostomy, 11 years pta
Revision of stenotic ileostomy with a Koch pouch, 10 years pta
Transabdominal revision of ileostomy, 10 years pta
Koch pouch revision, $5\frac{1}{2}$ years pta

Hospital course:

HD 1   Admit for Koch pouch revision
HD 2   Transabdominal revision of Koch pouch
HD 4   Episode of acute shortness of breath: treated with Lasix 20 mg
        1600 CXR ordered, reveals patchy bilateral perihilar infiltrates with bibasilar haziness fading superiorly, consistent with either moderate pulmonary edema, diffuse pneumonia, or early ARDS; all else is normal
        2251 Diffuse patchy opacity throughout both lung fields with confluence involving the lower lung fields bilaterally and loss of both hemidiaphragms, suggestive of worsening pulmonary edema, progressive ARDS, of diffuse pneumonia; possibility of bilateral pleural effusions can not be excluded
        2330 Unchanged from 2251
HD 6   Transferred to ICU due to persistent dyspnea, fever (38° C axillary), leukocytosis, and bilateral pulmonary infiltrates on CXR. Placed on 100% O_2 via double high flow nebulizers
        1045 ABG: pH 7.41, PCO_2 44, PO_2 171, HCO_3^- 28, SO_2 100%, Hb 9.3, RR 41
        1450 ABG: pH 7.41, PCO_2 51, PO_2 69
        Patient intubated due to ventilatory failure; right radial arterial and right internal jugular lines placed
        Mechanically ventilated: SIMV 12, VT 600, FIO_2 1.0, PEEP +5, PS +5, PIP 38, total RR 20
        Sedated with versed (2 mg prn) and fentanyl IV with 100 μg qh due to agitation and subsequent difficulty with ventilatory support (RR to 40, PIP to 50); Δ PEEP +10, FIO_2 0.5
        Started vancomycin 1 g IV q12h and imipenem 50 mg IV q6h
        TPN - D25 AA6C 60 mL qh with 250 mL 20% IV fat q24h
HD 7   Δ PEEP +12, Δ PS + 20
HD 8   Temperature 38° C (axillary)
        Abdominal CT scan − 5 × 5 × 3 cm fluid collection posterior to the bowel loops—Koch pouch(?), moderate bilateral pleural effusions
        Δ VT 700, Δ PEEP +10, Δ VT 700
        CXR—interval improvement in the intersti-

tial changes consistent with pulmonary edema
        Δ TPN to D20 AA5C @ 65 mL qh; fats same
HD 9   Temperature 38.8° C (axillary)
        Δ PEEP +8
        CXR—increasing bilateral patchy opacities with air bronchograms suggest worsening pulmonary edema
HD 10   Temperature 39° C (axillary)
        Jejunal feeding tube placed
        PIPs increased (high 40s)
        Add erythromycin, 750 mg q6h
HD 11   TPN discontinued, tube feeding begun with FS Osmolite and FS Jevity (1:1) @ 75 mL qh
        RR 38, PIP 48; Δ ventilator to AC 18, VT 600, PEEP +8, FIO_2 0.5; RR 20;
        ABG: pH 7.45, PCO_2 32, PO_2 69, HCO_3^- 26, SO_2 95%, Hb 9.5; Δ FIO_2 to 0.6
HD 12   Patient disconnected self from ventilator during bout of agitation
        2215 Questionable seizure activity; ABG; pH 7.30, PCO_2 51, PO_2 74.8; reconnected to ventilator, Δ FIO_2 to 1.0
        2250 ABG: pH 7.49, PCO_2 36, PO_2 238; Δ FIO_2 to 0.8 and weaned to 0.60; PIP in high 40s to low 50s
HD 13   Blood pressure and oxygenation labile; PIP in mid-50s, Δ AC to 20; Δ PEEP to +15
HD 14   Erythromycin discontinued
HD 15   Vancomycin and imipenem discontinued; blood cultures sent; internal jugular line clotted; sonography reveals thrombus in right internal jugular; Δ to left internal jugular line; CXR shows no change in bilateral opacities
HD 16   Oxygenation remains labile (FIO_2 0.8 to 1.0) and PIP in high 50s; hypertensive systolic pressures (200/100); sedation increased (fentanyl to 450 μg qh; Valium to 40 mg qh); vecuronium begun (2 to 4 mg prn), Δ AC to 22
HD 17   Vancomycin 1 g IV q12h; amphotericin B 15 mg IV (with Benadryl 25 mg) q24h, then 45 mg IV (with hydrocortisone 25 mg) q24h
        2100 BP 160s/90s; SpO_2 82% (FIO_2 1.0); ABG; pH 7.32, PCO_2 69, PO_2 46, SO_2 76%
        2115 CXR shows moderate left pneumothorax
        2200 Thoracostomy tube placed in left 5th ICS, midaxillary line
HD 18   Doxycycline 200 mg IV and amphotericin B 45 mg IV (with 25 mg hydrocortisone)
        Δ ventilator to PCV @ 60 with AutoPEEP +15, rate 24, FIO_2 0.9
        ABG: pH 7.35, PCO_2 70, PO_2 80 SO_2 95%
        Δ PCV to 53 and frequency to 28
        Physical therapy consultation
HD 19   Doxycycline 100 mg IV q12h
        0615 CXR shows new right apical pneumothorax

0930 Thoracostomy tube placed in right 2nd
ICS midclavicular line
1930 CXR shows new 40% left pneumothorax with left CT in situ
2145 Thoracostomy tube placed in left 3rd
ICS, midaxillary line
HD 20 Δ Amphotericin B to 25 mg IV q24h
1200 Thoracostomy tube placed in left 2nd
ICS, midclavicular line
HD 23 Because of inconsistent Vт on PCV, Δ ventilator to SIMV 25, Vт 500, PS +10, PEEP +15,
FI_{O_2} 0.65; PIPs now in 60s
ABG; pH 7.27, PCO_2 75, PO_2 86, SO_2 95%, Hb
8.5
HD 28 CXR shows increased right basal pneumo-
thorax
Thoracostomy tube placed in right 5th ICS,
anterior axillary line
HD 36 Thoracostomy tubes removed from right 5th
ICS, anterior axillary line and left 2nd ICS,
midclavicular line
HD 37 CXR shows increased right basal pneumo-
thorax
Thoracostomy tube placed in right 5th ICS,
midaxillary line; infrarenal abscess still sus-
pected
HD 40 Patient to OR, for exploratory laparotomy
No "resume physical therapy" orders among
postoperative orders
HD 44 Physical therapy reordered
SIMV 26, Vт 500, PEEP +5, FI_{O_2} 0.4
HD 51 Hypertonic posturing (decorticate) noted with
PROM, MDs notified
HD 55 SIMV 14, Sa_{O_2} 98%
HD 57 Hypertonic posturing and extreme agitation
elicited by minimal changes in tactile stimula-
tion
SIMV 18, FI_{O_2} 0.35, PIP 52
Sedation and neuromuscular blockade in-
creased
HD 59 Thoracostomy tubes removed from right 2nd
ICS, midclavicular line and left 3rd ICS,
midaxillary line
HD 63 SIMV13, PS +20
HD 69 Agitation and hypertonus progressively dimin-
ishing over last week; sedation concomitantly
reduced, SIMV 9, MDs request "more vigorous
physical therapy intervention"
HD 70 Tone reduction, ROM and maximally assisted
bed mobility activities yield modified long sit-
ting in bed
HD 72 SIMV 8, PS +10
HD 73 SIMV 7, FI_{O_2} 0.30; ABG: pH 7.33, PCO_2 46,
PO_2 96, SO_2 97%
Dangling @ EOB with maximal assistance
HD 76 Thoracostomy tubes removed from right 5th
ICS, anterior axillary line and left 5th ICS, midaxillary line
HD 83 SIMV 6, standing × 3 (<1 min each) with
maximal assist of 1

HD 84 Δ to CPAP/PS +10
HD 85 CPAP/PS +5
HD 86 Extubated; NC @ 4 L/min
HD 90 NC @ 2 L/min; transferred out of ICU, bed
mobility/transfer training
HD 91 O_2 prn via NC @ 2 L/min, gait training
HD 98 Discharged from hospital

Summary

- Airway adjuncts (e.g., oral or nasal pharyngeal airways, nasal or oral endotracheal tubes, tracheostomy tubes) are used to facilitate the removal of excess secretions from the pharynx, trachea, or large proximal airways; to prevent aspiration of oral or gastric contents into the lungs; to provide access for the administration of mechanical ventilatory support and supplemental oxygen.
- Bedside hemodynamic monitoring entails the observation and periodic recording of various vascular pressures (e.g., peripheral arterial, right atrial, pulmonary arterial) and volumes (e.g., cardiac output). Changes in the various parameters can provide insights regarding the patient's cardiovascular responses to physical therapy intervention.
- Bedside pulmonary function monitoring (e.g., simple spirometry, and arterial blood gas analysis) provides information that is helpful in the assessment of the patient's ventilatory mechanics, respiratory muscle strength, ventilatory demand, and oxygenation status. Several of these parameters may be helpful in predicting the success of weaning from mechanical ventilatory support.
- The need for mechanical ventilatory assistance does not prevent patients from participating in physical therapy. With a little creativity and preplanning on the part of the therapist, patients can participate in therapeutic exercise, balance, and ambulation interventions even while receiving mechanical or manual ventilatory assistance.

References

1. Gardner RM. Accuracy and reliability of disposable pressure transducers coupled with modern pressure monitors. Crit Care Med 24:879–882, 1996.
2. Darovic GO. Hemodynamic Monitoring: Invasive and Noninvasive Clinical Application. 2nd ed. Philadelphia, WB Saunders, 1995, p 875.

3. Voogel AJ, van Montfrans GA. Reproducibility of twenty-four-hour finger arterial blood pressure, variability and systemic hemodynamics. J Hypertens 15:1761–1765, 1997.

4. Hirschl MM, Binder M, Herkner H, et al. Accuracy and reliability of noninvasive continuous finger blood pressure measurement in critically ill patients. Crit Care Med 24:1684–1689, 1996.

5. National Heart Lung and Blood Institute. The Sixth Report of the Joint National Committee on Prevention, Detection, Evaluation and Treatment of High Blood Pressure. U.S. Department of Health and Human Services, 1999.

6. American College of Sports Medicine, Roitman JL, Kelsey M. ACSM's Resource Manual for Guidelines for Exercise Testing and Prescription. 3rd ed. Baltimore, Williams & Wilkins, 1998, p 715.

7. Daily EK, Schroeder JS. Techniques in Bedside Hemodynamic Monitoring. 5th ed. St. Louis, CV Mosby, 1994, p 450.

8. Chakko S, Woska D, Martinez H, et al. Clinical, radiographic, and hemodynamic correlations in chronic congestive heart failure: Conflicting results may lead to inappropriate care. Am J Med 90:353–359, 1991.

9. Ansley DM, Ramsay JG, Whalley DG, et al. The relationship between central venous pressure and pulmonary capillary wedge pressure during aortic surgery. Can J Anaesth 34:594–600, 1987.

10. Samii K, Conseiller C, Viars P. Central venous pressure and pulmonary wedge pressure. A comparative study in anesthetized surgical patients. Arch Surg 111:1122–1125, 1976.

11. Lehmann KG, Platt MS. Improved accuracy and precision of thermodilution cardiac output measurement using a dual thermistor catheter system. J Am Coll Cardiol 33:883–891, 1999.

12. Cathelyn JL, Samples DA. SvO_2 monitoring: Tool for evaluating patient outcomes. Dimens Crit Care Nurs 17:58–66, 1998.

13. Ahrens T. Technology utilization in the cardiac surgical patient: SvO_2 and capnography monitoring. Crit Care Nurs Q 21:24–40, 1998.

14. Ahrens T. Continuous mixed venous (SvO_2) monitoring. Too expensive or indispensible? Crit Care Nurs Clin North Am 11:33–48, 1999.

15. Jubran A, Mathru M, Dries D, Tobin MJ. Continuous recordings of mixed venous oxygen saturation during weaning from mechanical ventilation and the ramifications thereof. Am J Respir Crit Care Med 158:1763–1769, 1998.

16. Ruppel GL. Spirometry. Respir Care Clin North Am 3:155–181, 1997.

17. Brochard L. Discontinuation of mechanical ventilation. Monaldi Arch Chest Dis 53:348–349, 1998.

18. Esteban A, Alia I. Clinical management of weaning from mechanical ventilation. Intensive Care Med 24:999–1008, 1998.

19. Farias JA, Alia I, Esteban A, et al. Weaning from mechanical ventilation in pediatric intensive care patients. Intensive Care Med 24:1070–1075, 1998.

20. Mancebo J. Weaning from artificial ventilation. Monaldi Arch Chest Dis 53:350–354, 1998.

21. Nava S. Noninvasive techniques of weaning from mechanical ventilation. Monaldi Arch Chest Dis 53:355–357, 1998.

22. Ely EW, Bennett PA, Bowton DL, et al. Large scale implementation of a respiratory therapist-driven protocol for ventilator weaning. Am J Respir Crit Care Med 159:439–446, 1999.

23. Vassilakopoulos T, Roussos C, Zakynthinos S. Weaning from mechanical ventilation. J Crit Care 14:39–62, 1999.

24. Marini JJ. What derived variables should be monitored during mechanical ventilation? Respir Care 37:1097–1107, 1992.

25. Kersten LD. Comprehensive Respiratory Nursing: A Decision-Making Approach. Philadelphia, WB Saunders, 1989, p 864.

26. Branson RD, Hess D, Chatburn RL. Respiratory Care Equipment. 2nd ed. Philadelphia, JB Lippincott, 1998, p 754.

27. Campbell EJ, Baker MD, Crites-Silver P. Subjective effects of humidification of oxygen for delivery by nasal cannula. A prospective study. Chest 93:289–293, 1988.

28. Redding JS, McAfee DD, Gross CW. Oxygen concentrations received from commonly used delivery systems. South Med J 71:169–172, 1978.

29. Burkhart JE Jr, Stoller JK. Oxygen and aerosolized drug delivery: Matching the device to the patient. Cleve Clin J Med 65:200–208, 1998.

30. Resta O, Guido P, Picca V, et al. Prescription of nCPAP and nBiPAP in obstructive sleep apnoea syndrome: Italian experience in 105 subjects. A prospective two centre study. Respir Med 92:820–827, 1998.

31. Mehta S, Jay GD, Woolard RH, et al. Randomized, prospective trial of bilevel versus continuous positive airway pressure in acute pulmonary edema [see comments]. Crit Care Med 25:620–628, 1997.

32. Bradley ME, Leith DE. Ventilatory muscle training and the oxygen cost of sustained hyperpnea. J Appl Physiol 45:885–892, 1978.

33. Leith DE, Bradley M. Ventilatory muscle strength and endurance training. J Appl Physiol 41:508–516, 1976.

34. Gross D, Ladd HW, Riley EJ, et al. The effect of training on strength and endurance of the diaphragm in quadriplegia. Am J Med 68:27–35, 1980.

Pharmacology

14

Cardiovascular Medications

Kate Grimes and Meryl Cohen

INTRODUCTION

"Pharmacology can be broadly defined as the science dealing with interactions between living systems and molecules, especially chemicals introduced from outside the system. . . . A drug . . . [is] . . . any small molecule that, when introduced into the body, alters the body's function by interactions at the molecular level."[1] By strict definition, therefore, a drug may cause disease (e.g., environmental chemicals and hazardous wastes) as well as treat and prevent disease (e.g., medical pharmacology). More specific to this discussion is the role of drugs within a medical setting to prevent, treat, and identify cardiovascular disease.

Although medications have significantly broadened the management of cardiovascular dysfunction, "a drug cannot impart a new function to a cell . . . it modulates ongoing function."[2] The impact of pharmacologic management for the patient with a cardiovascular disorder cannot be underestimated. The responsibility of the physical therapist in treating any individual is to understand the effects and potential side effects of the individual's drug regimen as well as the drugs' influence on the outcome of the physical therapy intervention. This chapter presents the pharmacologic clinical management of the most common cardiovascular dysfunctions.

To appreciate the impact and complexity of drug management, a few supportive concepts should be introduced. Drugs may be prescribed by their generic or trade name. Genetic prescriptions incorporate the name of the chemical substance or substances that make up the drug; the trade name (brand name) is the name that the individual drug company assigns to its own product. In this chapter, the generic name appears first, the trade name or names follow in parentheses, for example, **verapamil** (Calan, Isoptin).

The goal of drug therapy is to prescribe the appropriate medication for the individual's needs with the expectation that the medication is delivered to the site of action in adequate strength (therapeutic level) to elicit the appropriate clinical response. The foundation of this goal rests on two broad concepts, **pharmacokinetics** and **pharmacodynamics**.[3] Pharmacokinetics addresses how the drug is absorbed, how much of the drug is available to be delivered to the target site or sites (**bioavailability**), how the drug is distributed (**distribution**), and how the drug is metabolized and excreted (**clearance**). Pharmacodynamics deals with

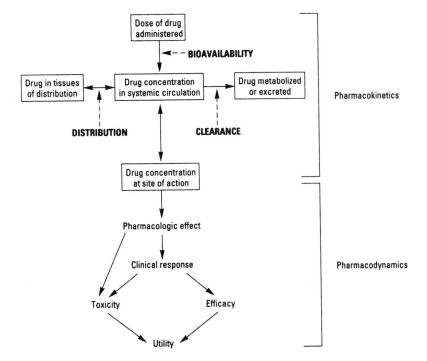

Figure 14-1. Schematic representation of the pharmacokinetic and pharmacodynamic processes. (From Katzung BG [ed]. Basic and Clinical Pharmacology. 5th ed. East Norwalk, CT, Appleton & Lange, 1992, p 29.)

the mechanism of the drug action and the relationship between the drug concentration and the clinical effect[4] (Fig. 14–1).

PHARMACOKINETICS

Pharmacokinetics is affected by many factors, not the least of which is individual metabolism. Any disease or dysfunction of the gastrointestinal system, liver, and kidneys can influence the bioavailability and clearance of the drug. Nutritional habits, use of antacids and laxatives, as well as the natural process of aging itself, may also alter an individual's response to a particular drug regimen by affecting both the bioavailability of the drug through altered metabolism and the drug clearance through the gastrointestinal and renal systems.

Drugs may be administered to the body through different access routes; the two most common are by mouth or by injection. By mouth (oral, or p.o.) is also known as **enteral,** indicating that the drug enters the gastrointestinal system before it enters the circulation. Injection is one form of **parenteral** administration, a nongastrointestinal (i.e., nonenteral) route. Parenteral routes bypass the absorption within the gastrointestinal system. See Table 14–1 for examples of drug routes.

Bioavailability

The route of administration affects the bioavailability of the drug and the length of time it takes the drug to work. Drugs taken by mouth are absorbed from the stomach and intestine and then pass through the liver (portal circulation) before reaching the systemic circulation. The active drug may be partially inactivated if it is metabolized in the liver or gastrointestinal system. This partial inactivation as a result of metabolic processes is known as the **first pass effect.** The greater the first pass effect, the less bioavailability of the drug. The liver is the principal organ of drug metabolism and therefore the principal organ for first pass effect. In order to avoid the first pass effect, critical care drugs such as **lidocaine** (Xylocaine) and **morphine** are given intravenously.

Parenteral routes by definition bypass the gas-

Table 14–1

Common Routes of Drug Administration

ROUTE	COMMENTS
Parenteral	No gastrointestinal absorption
	Fast acting
Injection	Valuable in emergencies
	May cause pain and tissue damage at injection site
intravenous (IV)	May deliver a high concentration of drug quickly
subcutaneous (SQ)	Self-administered
intramuscular (IM)	
intrathecal (spinal)	
intraperitoneal	
Buccal (sublingual)	
Inhalational	Quick delivery of drug to bronchi and alveoli for local effect
	Gaseous anesthetic
	Useful with drugs that vaporize quickly
Enteral	Absorbed through the gastrointestinal system
By mouth (p.o.)	Convenient
tablets or capsules	Most common
enteric coated	Effective absorption
sustained release	Usually most economical
chewable	
Liquid	Effective with children
oral solutions	
elixir	
Rectal	May have local or systemic effects
	Effective when gastrointestinal upset precludes use of oral
Transdermal	Slowly absorbed, prolongs blood levels

Source: Adapted from Gilman AG, Goodman LS, Rall TW, Murad F (eds). Goodman and Gilman's The Pharmacologic Basic of Therapeutics. 7th ed. New York, Macmillan, 1985, pp. 3–10; and Katzung BG (ed). Basic and Clinical Pharmacology. 4th ed. East Norwalk, Conn, Appleton & Lange, 1989.

trointestinal system, and although there may be some first pass effect through the lungs, the bioavailability is greater and the onset of action is faster than with enteral medications. Because of their fast onset of action, parenteral medications, particularly those using the intravenous and **sublingual** routes, are a key component in the management of hemodynamic stability in emergency and critical care settings. Drugs administered through sublingual routes enter the circulation through the systemic veins that drain the highly vascular oral mucosa and do not pass through the gastrointestinal system or portal circulation. **Nitroglycerin** is perhaps the most widely used sublingual medication.

Distribution

After the drug is absorbed into the bloodstream, the next phase of pharmacokinetics occurs: the distribution of the drug throughout the body by means of the circulatory system. Drug distribution may be general or restricted, depending on the ability of the drug to pass through particular cell membranes and on the permeability of the capillaries for the particular drug. Differential distribution may occur as a result of one of the following: drug binding to proteins (especially plasma protein), difficulty of drugs crossing the blood-brain barrier of the central nervous system, or storage of drugs within body tissues (particularly adipose and muscle tissues). Drugs bind to proteins both in the tissues and in the plasma; the most common plasma proteins are **albumin** and **alpha₁-acid-glycoprotein.** As a result of the protein-drug binding, the drug is unavailable to bind with its receptor sites and therefore is unable to exert its pharmacologic effect. Although protein-drug binding is a reversible and dynamic process, it may temporarily limit drug distribution.

Clearance

"Clearance of a drug is the rate of elimination by all routes relative to the concentration of drug in any biologic fluid."[3] Routes of elimination are through the renal, biliary, and pulmonary systems and through fecal matter. The kidneys serve as the most important route for overall drug elimination, whereas the lungs are the major organs for the excretion of gaseous substances. A dysfunction within any of these systems or an inadequate circulatory system to distribute the unbound drug interferes with the clearance of the drug from the

body. Drug toxicity may occur if clearance is impeded (e.g., by kidney dysfunction) because the drug level increases. Insufficient drug levels may result if the drug is cleared too rapidly, as it is with diarrhea or vomiting.

Half-life

The time it takes for the plasma concentration of the drug to be reduced by 50% is known as the **half-life.** Half-life serves as a rough indicator of the length of time the effects of the medication will last. The longer the half-life, the longer the effect of the drug.

The frequency of the administration of medication is influenced by a drug's half-life; some medications must be taken four times a day (qid) to be most effective; others may be taken only once (qd), twice (bid), or three times a day (tid). Patients should not try to manipulate the timing of their medications once a routine has been established. Medications need to be taken at regular intervals; a delay in taking the medication, for example, waiting until after a physical therapy appointment, only delays the onset and effectiveness of the medication. In some instances, once a medication schedule has been interrupted, such as a delay in taking pain medications, the prescribed dosage may be insufficient for patient comfort or desired action. An example of different half-lives can be seen with two commonly used cardiac medications, **digoxin** (Lanoxin) and **propranolol** (Inderal). The half-life of digoxin is 36 hours; that of propranolol is only 3 to 6 hours.

Dosage

In deciding the appropriate dosage of a drug, four variables must be considered:

- The amount of drug to be administered at one time
- The route of administration
- The interval between doses
- The period of time over which drug administration is to be continued[3]

Drugs may be administered by two common methods: continuous input or intermittent doses. Sustained release by mouth and infusions by intravenous or subcutaneous routes are examples of continuous input. The continuous insulin pump is an example of a subcutaneous continuous infusion; intravenous nitroglycerin given temporarily during the acute stages of myocardial ischemia is an example of an intravenous continuous infusion. Medications given at certain time intervals throughout the day by any route are examples of intermittent doses.

PHARMACODYNAMICS

Pharmacodynamics helps us to understand the critical role of drug receptors. Drugs do not have isolated effects on isolated tissues. Drug receptors are located throughout the body; therefore, the drug affects all the receptors specific to the drug's structure.

Drug receptors are cellular macromolecules that are generally, but not exclusively, cellular proteins. The best identified protein receptors are regulatory proteins that mediate the actions of neurotransmitters, hormones, and **autacoids**—a local hormone-like substance that includes histamines, polypeptides (e.g., angiotensin, bradykinin), and prostaglandins. Besides regulatory proteins, other common drug receptors are enzymes, transport proteins, and structural proteins. The drug and its receptor form a complementary relationship, likened to a lock and key. Receptors may have biochemical functions common to many cells, and, as a result, no drug produces a single effect or affects only a specific tissue. Drugs therefore have primary effects, secondary effects, and side effects. In choosing the appropriate drug, an individual's tolerance to the drug is determined not only by the primary effect but, just as important, by the impact of the secondary and side effects. An example of such a drug-receptor relationship that has generalized systemic effects is that of digitalis and the sodium-potassium pump. Digoxin not only has direct cardiac effects, such as decreased conduction through the A-V node and increased myocardial contractility, but it may also affect blood chemistry resulting in hypokalemia. Because of digitalis's widespread effects on many types of tissue, varied side effects and a low threshold for toxicity can exist for this powerful drug.

Drugs are selective regarding the type of receptor to which they are attracted but cannot be absolutely specific to a single effect or to a type of tissue. **Selectivity** means that when a certain concentration of the drug exists, the drug is preferentially attracted to one group or a subgroup of receptors. An example of selectivity can be seen within a very common group of cardiac drugs, the beta blockers. The receptors for the beta blockers (the subgroups beta$_1$ and beta$_2$) are found within the autonomic nervous system. The drug **atenolol** (Tenormin) is a selective beta blocker, affecting primarily the beta$_1$ receptors; propranolol (Inderal) is a nonselective beta blocker, affecting both beta$_1$ and beta$_2$ receptors.

Agonists and Antagonists

Drugs can be broadly classified as agonists or antagonists. An **agonist** is a drug that initiates a sequence of physiologic and biochemical changes within the cell. An **antagonist** acts as an inhibitor of agonistic activity by inactivating the receptor. A drug may be a complete or partial agonist or antagonist. Many cardiac drugs serve their function by acting as antagonists (e.g., beta-adrenergic antagonists [beta blockers] and calcium-channel antagonists [calcium-channel blockers]).

Receptors

Although drug receptors are found in many cells of the body, the most common sites for cardiac drug-receptor interactions are the autonomic nervous system (Table 14–2), the kidneys, and the vascular smooth muscle. Other sites such as the central nervous system for the management of hypertension and the blood cells for their role in clotting and lysis are also critically important for achieving cardiovascular stability.

Autonomic Nervous System

Understanding the autonomic nervous system requires a thorough review of its anatomy; please refer to Chapter 1 for more complete detail. The

Table 14-2
Autonomic Receptor Types

NAME	TYPICAL LOCATIONS
Cholinoceptors	
*Muscarinic M_1	Central nervous system neurons, sympathetic postganglionic neurons, some presynaptic sites
*Muscarinic M_2	Myocardium, smooth muscle, some presynaptic sites
Nicotinic	Autonomic ganglia, skeletal muscle neuromuscular endplate, spinal cord
Adrenoceptors	
Alpha$_1$	Postsynaptic effector cells, especially smooth muscle
Alpha$_2$	Presynaptic adrenergic nerve terminals, platelets, lipocytes, smooth muscle
Beta$_1$	Postsynaptic effector cells, especially heart; lipocytes, brain, presynaptic noradrenergic nerve terminals
Beta$_2$	Postsynaptic effector cells, especially smooth muscle
Dopamine	Brain and postsynaptic effectors, especially vascular smooth muscle of the splanchnic and renal vascular beds. Presynaptic receptors on nerve terminals, especially in the heart, vessels, and gastrointestinal system

*Assignment of muscarinic receptor subtypes is still tentative (Eglen, 1986).

Source: Katzung BG (ed). Basic and Clinical Pharmacology. 5th ed. East Norwalk, Conn, Appleton & Lange, 1992, p 75.

autonomic nervous system contains two divisions: the sympathetic and the parasympathetic nervous systems. One of the distinctions between the two is their postganglionic neurotransmitter substance: acetylcholine in the parasympathetic system and norepinephrine in the sympathetic system. As a result of their neurotransmitters, the receptors of the parasympathetic nervous system are known as **cholinergic,** and the receptors of the sympathetic are known as **adrenergic.** The two subdivisions of the adrenergic receptors are the alpha and beta adrenoceptors. Both alpha and beta receptors are responsive to the **catecholamines:** norepinephrine, released at the local level from the sympathetic postganglionic fibers, and epinephrine, released

from the adrenal medulla into the circulatory system. The sensitivity of each receptor to catecholamines differs, as do the location and action of each receptor. When alpha receptors in the vascular smooth muscle are stimulated, contraction occurs; when beta receptors are stimulated in the vascular smooth muscle, relaxation occurs. Both alpha and beta receptors are divided further into alpha$_1$ and alpha$_2$ and beta$_1$ and beta$_2$ (Table 14-3). Use of beta-adrenergic antagonists (beta blockers) has formed a cornerstone in the management of coronary artery disease over the past 30 years. Drug research is in progress regarding the new and expanding role for alpha receptors, either alone or in combination with beta receptors.

Adrenergic agonists are also known as **sympathomimetics.** The sympathomimetics are a group of drugs that mimic the activity of the endogenous chemicals of the sympathetic nervous system, particularly the catecholamines epinephrine, norepinephrine, and dopamine. Adrenergic agonists (e.g., beta blockers) are also known as **sympatholytics**—drugs that block the action of the sympathetic nervous system.

Cholinergic receptors are either **muscarinic** or **nicotinic.** The site of action for muscarinic receptors is on autonomic effector cells; within the heart these receptors are in the atria and sinoatrial and atrioventricular nodes. The site of action for nicotinic receptors is the end plates of skeletal muscle and autonomic ganglion cells. Cholinergic receptors have minimal direct clinical influence on the cardiovascular system from a pharmacologic point of view. Compared with the expansive impact of the adrenergic receptors, the pharmacologic impact of cholinergic receptors is significantly less.

Stimulation by cholinergic activating drugs (e.g., acetylcholine) through the muscarinic receptors results in decreased contractility and heart rate and a reduction in peripheral vascular resistance. Stimulation by cholinergic blocking drugs (e.g., atropine) through the muscarinic receptors results in increased heart rate. Nicotinic receptor stimulation of the autonomic ganglia has sympathetic-like effects on the cardiovascular system and may result in tachycardia and hypertension. Blocking of the nicotinic receptors' influence on the cardiovascular system decreases arteriolar and venomotor

Table 14-3
Distribution of Adrenoceptor Subtypes

TYPE	TISSUE	ACTIONS
Alpha$_1$	Most vascular smooth muscle (innervated)	Contraction
	Pupillary dilator muscle	Contraction (dilates pupil)
	Pilomotor smooth muscle	Erects hair
	Rat liver	Glycogenolysis
	Heart	Increase force of contraction
Alpha$_2$	Postsynaptic central nervous system adrenoceptors	Probably multiple
	Platelets	Aggregation
	Adrenergic and cholinergic nerve terminals	Inhibition of transmitter release
	Some vascular smooth muscle (noninnervated)	Contraction
	Fat cells	Inhibition of lipolysis
Beta$_1$	Heart	Increase force and rate of contraction
	Fat cells	Activate lipolysis
Beta$_2$	Respiratory, uterine, and vascular smooth muscle	Promote smooth muscle relaxation
	Skeletal muscle	Promote potassium uptake
	Human liver	Activate glycogenolysis

Source: Katzung BG (ed). Basic and Clinical Pharmacology. 4th ed. East Norwalk, Conn, Appleton & Lange, 1989, p 98.

tone, thereby decreasing both blood pressure and venous return. Cholinergic drugs that simulate parasympathetic activity are known as **parasympathomimetic** or cholinergic agonists; conversely, drugs that block cholinergic activity are known as **parasympatholytic** or cholinergic antagonists (Table 14–4).

Kidney

Drug receptor sites within the kidneys are found within the proximal tubule, collecting tubule and ducts, and Henle's loop. Refer to the section on antihypertension drugs and to Figure 14–7 for the site of action and the effect of specific drugs.

Vascular Smooth Muscle

Cardiac drug receptors within vascular smooth muscle are primarily adrenoceptors; they include the subtypes of alpha$_1$, beta$_2$, and alpha$_2$ adrenoceptors. Nitrates, calcium-channel blockers, and the alpha$_1$ adrenergic blockers are examples of drug classes that act at the vascular smooth muscle receptor sites (see Table 14–3).

PHARMACOLOGIC MANAGEMENT

Management of cardiac dysfunction often involves the prescription of a multifaceted drug regimen that must be dynamic in its ability to respond to an individual's needs. Long-term use of certain drugs may cause a desensitization of the receptor to that drug such that the dosage may need to be altered, the drug replaced, or an additional drug prescribed to supplement the initial drug. The cost of drugs often influences which drug (generic or trade) or class of drugs is prescribed when a choice is available. Patient compliance is also influenced by drug cost; some patients choose to decrease the frequency of their medications "to save money" or avoid taking the drug at all. Patients are often unaware of the consequences of self-

Table 14-4
Effects of Direct-Acting Cholinoceptor Stimulants

ORGAN	RESPONSE
Eye	
Sphincter muscle of iris	Contraction (miosis)
Ciliary muscle	Contraction for near vision
Heart	
Sinoatrial node	Decrease in rate (negative chronotropy)
Atria	Decrease in contractile strength (negative inotropy)
	Decrease in refractory period
Atrioventricular node	Decrease in conduction velocity (negative dromotropy)
	Increase in refractory period
Ventricles	Small decrease in contractile strength
Blood vessels	Dilation (via EDRF)
Arteries	Constriction (high dose direct effect)
Veins	Dilation (via EDRF)
	Constriction (high dose direct effect)
Lung	
Bronchial muscle	Contraction (bronchoconstriction)
Bronchial glands	Stimulation
Gastrointestinal tract	
Motility	Increase
Sphincters	Relaxation
Secretion	Stimulation
Urinary bladder	
Detrusor	Contraction
Trigone and sphincter	Relaxation
Glands	
Sweat, salivary, lacrimal, nasopharyngeal	Secretion

EDRF = endothelium releasing factor.
Source: Katzung BG (ed). Basic and Clinical Pharmacology. 5th ed. East Norwalk, Conn, Appelton & Lange, 1992, p 86.

Clinical Note: Drug Substitution

If a patient does not tolerate certain side effects of a drug, another drug in the same class may often be substituted with acceptable results.

regulation of medications; many cardiac drugs cannot be stopped abruptly without significant deleterious effects. Previously tolerated drugs may suddenly become problematic following the flu, gastrointestinal upset, or change in metabolism.

The awareness by all health care professionals that a drug cannot work effectively unless it is taken as prescribed should sensitize prescribers of drugs to the issues that contribute to noncompliance: cost of drug, difficulty in following a complicated drug regimen, poorly tolerated side effects, and undesirable interactions with other prescribed medications are just a few examples. Often a drug that is poorly tolerated may be exchanged for a similar drug that produces the same clinical effect but with less troublesome side effects to the patient.

ANTI-ISCHEMIC DRUGS

Dramatic changes have taken place during the latter part of the twentieth century in the pharmacologic management of ischemic heart disease. With the introduction of beta blockers, calcium-channel blockers, thrombolytic agents, and the critical care regimen of **vasopressors** and positive **inotropes,** hemodynamic stability has been established in many individuals who formerly might have led the lifestyle of the "cardiac cripple" at best or faced death at worst. Coronary artery disease still exists, however, holding the unfortunate distinction of being the number one cause of death in the United States. Present drug therapy focuses on the sequelae of this ravaging disease as well as risk factor prevention. Perhaps with aggressive lifestyle changes, especially in regard to nutrition, physical activity, stress management, frugal management of blood lipid levels, blood pressure, and blood glucose, the twenty-first century will render a discussion such as this obsolete.

Physiology

The heart is an oxygen-dependent organ whose energy needs are met by aerobic metabolism. Oxygen is delivered to the myocardium and conducting tissues via the coronary arteries. Adequate myocardial oxygen supply is dependent on many factors, most particularly the coronary blood flow, the oxygen-carrying capacity of blood, and the anatomy of coronary arteries (especially the lumen diameter). When myocardial oxygen demand (MVO_2) increases, such as with exercise, myocardial oxygen supply is increased by an increase in coronary blood flow.

Multiple factors influence the demand for myocardial oxygen, such as afterload, systolic wall tension, wall thickness, contractile state, preload, heart rate, and left ventricular volume and diameter. Although many factors influence myocardial oxygen demand, MVO_2 may be clinically assessed as the product of heart rate and systolic blood pressure. This clinical method for MVO_2 assessment is called the double product or **rate-pressure product** (RPP).

Demand is increased under conditions that increase heart rate, blood pressure, or both: exercise; increased systemic vascular resistance; high output states such as pregnancy, fever, and increased thyroid function; anemia; emotional stress; and anxiety are but few examples.

Pathophysiology

Unlike striated muscle, the myocardium can function without adequate oxygen for only a relatively short period of time. Coronary blood flow is the prime mechanism for supplying oxygenated blood to the myocardium. Inadequate oxygenated blood may result from either inadequate blood flow (**ischemia**) or inadequate arterial oxygenation (**hypoxemia**). When coronary blood supply is inadequate to meet the myocardial oxygen demands, the myocardium becomes **ischemic.** Clinically, the most common cause of decreased supply is coronary artery disease (CAD). The atherosclerotic plaque associated with coronary artery disease reduces the lumen size and therefore reduces blood flow. Lumen diameter may also be decreased as a result of spasm of the smooth muscle within the endothelium of the coronary artery; spasm may occur in the presence or absence of coronary artery disease.

In an acute myocardial infarction, a thrombus may form at the site of the atherosclerotic lesion and further occlude the lumen. Three steps are necessary for thrombus formation[5]:

- A conducive surface (such as damaged intravascular endothelium) on which the thrombus can form
- A sequence of platelet-mediated events: platelet adhesion, followed by platelet aggregation, followed by release of agents further stimulating platelet aggregation and vasoconstriction
- Activation of the clotting mechanism and the formation of fibrin

A clot is made up of insoluble fibrin filaments and platelets that join together to form a durable mesh. Clot formation occurs through a series of complex interactions involving platelets, tissue thromboplastin, clotting factors, prothrombin, fibrinogen, and fibrin. Fibrin comes from the protein fibrinogen that is produced in the liver and present in the plasma. Fibrinogen is a stable structure and converts to fibrin only under the influence of **thrombin.**

Thrombin comes from **prothrombin,** a normal protein constituent of plasma. The formation of thrombin from prothrombin requires a highly complex, integrated network. Adequate calcium, phospholipids, and at least seven plasma proteins (factor XI, factor XII, factor IX, factor VIII, factor X, factor V, factor XIII) are necessary for thrombin formation. Also required is the interaction of **thromboplastin** released by the injured tissue, with factor X (Fig. 14–2).[6] The role of platelets and the clotting factors necessary for the formation of thrombin are referred to as the intrinsic clotting factors; the role of tissue thromboplastin is referred to as the extrinsic clotting factors.

Once clot formation has occurred, the process of clot lysis, under normal conditions, requires many days. The plasma enzyme plasmin actively digests the fibrin, fibrinogen, and prothrombin.[6] Plasmin, however, must first be activated by its precursor, plasminogen (Fig. 14–2B).

Pharmacologic Intervention

Pharmacologic management of myocardial ischemia involves the reestablishment of a balance between myocardial oxygen supply and myocardial oxygen demand. Drugs that decrease either heart rate or systemic blood pressure decrease myocardial oxygen demand. Drugs that increase arterial

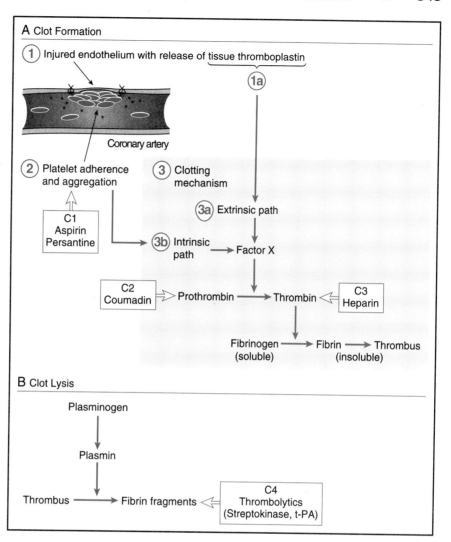

Figure 14-2. *A,* Clot formation. 1, At the site of an atherosclerotic lesion, injured endothelium releases tissue thromboplastin (1a). 2, As a result of the exposed endothelial surface, platelets begin to adhere to its surface and aggregate. 3, The clotting mechanism is very complex and is presented here in simplified form. 3a, With the release of thromboplastin, the extrinsic clotting cascade begins. 3b, The intrinsic clotting cascade begins in response to the injured endothelium and influenced by platelets. The common point for both the intrinsic and extrinsic pathways is factor X, which facilitates the eventual formation of fibrin from fibrinogen by activating thrombin from prothrombin. *B,* Clot lysis can be achieved through the antiplatelet agents aspirin and Persantine (C1), the anticoagulant Coumadin (warfarin, C2), the anticoagulant heparin (C3), or thrombolytics (e.g., streptokinase and t-PA, C4), which activate plasminogen into plasmin at the site of action of these specific drugs.

lumen size by decreasing either coronary arterial spasm or thrombus increase myocardial oxygen supply. At present, no drug exists that directly decreases a fixed atherosclerotic lesion. Reduction of risk factors for coronary artery disease and directed lipid management with or without the use of drugs have been postulated to result in a regression of coronary plaque.

Decreasing Myocardial Oxygen Demand

Current medications used to decrease MVO_2 are beta blockers, which decrease heart rate, calcium-channel blockers, which inhibit coronary vaso-

spasm, and nitrates, which decrease peripheral vascular resistance, and decrease the preload or venous return.

Beta Blockers (Table 14–5). Beta-adrenergic antagonists compete with the catecholamines epinephrine and norepinephrine for beta receptor binding sites, thereby preventing the catecholamines from binding. Beta-antagonist activity may be complete (without catecholamine stimulation) or partial (some catecholamine stimulation). Of the two beta subtypes, $beta_1$ receptors are found primarily in the myocardium and have an equal affinity for epinephrine and norepinephrine; $beta_2$ receptors are also found in the myocardium (especially the atria), but comparatively more are within the peripheral circulation and bronchi, and they

Table 14–5

Beta-Adrenergic Antagonists: Beta Blockers

CATEGORY	GENERIC (TRADE)
Nonselective	Propranolol (Inderal)
	Timolol (Blocadren)
	Nadolol (Corgard)
	Pindolol (Visken)
	Labetalol (Normodyne)
	Sotalol (Betapace)
	Carteolol (Cartrol)
Beta$_1$ selective	Metoprolol (Lopressor)
	Atenolol (Tenormin)
	Acebutolol (Sectral)
	Esmolol (Brevibloc)
	Alprenolol
Beta$_2$ selective	Butoxamine
Alpha and beta antagonists	Labetalol (Normodyne, Trandate)
	Carvedilol (Coreg)

have a higher affinity for epinephrine. Inhibition of catecholamine stimulation by beta blockers affects the cardiovascular system by decreasing heart rate, decreasing contractility, decreasing cardiac output, and decreasing blood pressure.

Drugs that block both beta$_1$ and beta$_2$ receptors are referred to as nonselective; drugs that block beta$_1$ receptors are referred to as cardioselective or beta$_1$ selective. Patients with disease processes involving the peripheral circulation and bronchi (the sites of beta$_2$ receptors) pose a challenging problem in drug management when they require beta blockers. Beta$_1$-selective drugs rather than a nonselective beta blocker are usually prescribed for patients with chronic obstructive pulmonary disease or peripheral vascular disease to avoid the vasoconstriction effects of beta$_2$ antagonists. Because no beta$_1$-selective antagonist is able to avoid completely interactions with beta$_2$ receptors, caution must be exercised in the prescription of beta blockers as with all drugs. At present, the class of beta$_2$-selective antagonists is limited to the drug butoxamine, which has little cardiovascular effect except to inhibit an increase in both heart rate and smooth muscle relaxation.

In a relatively newer class of drugs, beta blockers may combine with alpha-adrenergic blockers. This combination results in a decrease in systemic vascular resistance without a compensatory increase in heart rate. The alpha blocking component causes vasodilation and thus results in de-

creased systemic vascular resistance (SVR). A decrease in SVR would normally be accompanied by a compensatory increase in heart rate. The beta-blocking component suppresses this compensatory rise in heart rate that would be expected with alpha blockade alone and therefore also limits the increase in MVo$_2$. This class of drugs, of which **labetalol** (Normodyne, Trandate) is an example, is used primarily for hypertension control.

Side Effects of Beta Blockers. The potential side effects associated with the use of beta blockers are varied. "Three major mechanisms . . . (of side effects) . . . are through (1) central nervous penetration (dreams), (2) smooth muscle spasm (bronchospasm and cold extremities), and (3) exaggeration of the cardiac therapeutic actions (bradycardia, heart block, excess negative inotropic effect with heart failure)."[8] Beta$_1$-selective drugs such as atenolol (Tenormin) should have fewer peripheral side effects of bronchospasm, cold extremities, worsening claudication, and sexual dysfunction than nonselective drugs like propranolol (Inderal). Beta blockers also may cause fatigue, insomnia, masking of symptoms of hypoglycemia in diabetic patients, impaired glucose tolerance, **hypertriglyceridemia,** and decreased high-density lipoprotein (HDL) cholesterol. **Pindolol** (Visken) and **acebutolol** (Sectral), however, do not appear to decrease HDL cholesterol.

Clinical Considerations. The popularity of beta blockers as part of an anti-ischemic regimen cannot be disputed. Beta blockers, however, have also been used in the treatment of the following conditions: hypertension, cardiac arrhythmias; glaucoma; hyperthyroidism; mitral valve prolapse; and various neurologic disorders, such as migraine headaches, alcohol withdrawal, and anxiety. Awareness of the potential side effects of beta blockade for these patient populations is certainly clinically relevant. As with patients with peripheral vascular disease and chronic obstructive pulmonary disease, the use of beta$_1$-selective drugs may also be preferred for patients with diabetes. Beta$_2$ receptors of

Clinical Note: Beta Blockers

Beta blockers may mask the symptoms of hypoglycemia. Therefore, caution should be taken with patients with diabetes on beta blockers when initiating exercise programs, and progressing the exercise prescription.

the liver activate glycogenolysis; however, a nonselective beta blocker suppresses this action. Use of a $beta_1$-selective drug minimizes the suppression of this critical function. Poor tolerance of one beta blocker does not mean that all beta blockers will be poorly tolerated; experimentation and trial and error are credible clinical tools in assessing the compatibility of the patient-drug interaction.

Beta blockers are negative inotropes, therefore they are used cautiously in patients with impaired LV function (e.g., when ejection fraction is below 35%). Carvedilol is a relatively new beta blocker that also has alpha blocking properties; it is being used in the patient population with congestive heart failure. If a patient on a beta blocker begins to complain of dyspnea, ankle or extremity edema, orthopnea, or other signs of heart failure, the appropriate physical therapy intervention is to avoid treatment until the primary physician has been notified. Once the patient has stabilized and is medically cleared to continue with physical therapy, treatment should begin slowly and patient tolerance should be assessed on an ongoing basis.

Beta blockers decrease both resting and exercise heart rates. Before prescribing aerobic exercise for a patient on beta blockers, it is necessary to know the results of the patient's performance on an exercise tolerance test given with the same drug and dosage that the patient is presently taking. There does not appear to be a reliable relationship between heart rate and drug dosages among individual drugs. A patient who was changed from propranolol (Inderal) to metoprolol (Lopressor) has a different exercise heart rate response on each drug and may therefore need a new exercise prescription, a new exercise tolerance test, or both.

A potentially interesting relationship may exist between weight control and beta blockers. Fat cells have $beta_1$ receptors, which, when stimulated, activate **lipolysis.** With beta blockade, lipolysis is inhibited. Clinical observation has been that patients on beta blockers have a difficult time achieving weight loss. Whether this is owing to decreased metabolism, fatigue, lipocyte inhibition, or some other factor or combination of factors remains to be seen.

Calcium-Channel Blockers.
Calcium-channel blockers do not fit exclusively into either category of decreasing myocardial oxygen demand or increasing myocardial oxygen supply; they influence both. They decrease myocardial oxygen demand by decreasing arterial blood pressure and may increase supply by facilitating vascular smooth muscle relaxation. Calcium-channel blockers are discussed in detail under the section regarding increasing myocardial oxygen supply; its effects on myocardial oxygen demand as well as supply are discussed at that time.

Nitrates.
First synthesized in 1846, nitroglycerin and its analogues are perhaps one of the oldest anti-ischemic medications. This group of drugs is unusually selective; that is, the effect of nitrates is almost exclusively on smooth muscle cells, in particular on vascular smooth muscle. Nitroglycerin acts in at least three ways:

- As a venodilator, thus decreasing venous return (preload)
- As an arteriodilator, thus decreasing afterload
- As a relaxant for coronary artery smooth muscle, thus possibly increasing coronary blood supply

The possibility that nitrates may also redistribute blood flow to ischemic subendocardial tissue has been postulated.[9] The major contribution to anti-ischemia from nitroglycerin, however, comes from its decrease of myocardial demand, specifically in its ability to decrease venous return and left ventricular filling pressures. Besides their use for anti-ischemia, nitrates may also be prescribed for the management of congestive heart failure by decreasing preload and for the control of diastolic hypertension.

Many different preparations of nitrates are available. Routes of administration and duration of action vary widely among the preparations, from the immediate- and short-acting sublingual nitroglycerin to the slow-release, longer-acting transdermal patch (Table 14–6).

Clinical Considerations.
Perhaps the side effect of nitrate therapy most troublesome to patients is headache, particularly with the short-acting sublingual tablet and in the "adjustment" stage when a long-acting transdermal patch is started. Other potential side effects resulting from the vasodilator action are

- Hypotension
- Reflex tachycardia
- Flushing of the skin
- Nausea and vomiting

Table 14–6
Nitrate Preparations

GENERIC NAME	TRADE OR COMMON NAME	DURATION AND COMMENTS
Amyl nitrate inhalation	Aspirol, Vaporole	10 sec–10 min
Nitroglycerin (glyceryl trinitrate)	Nitro-Bid, Nitrostat, others	
sublingual		$1\frac{1}{2}$ min–1 hr peak: 2 min
spray		Effects apparent in 5 min: duration unknown
percutaneous ointment		3–4 hr
oral, sustained relief		8–12 hr
intravenous		During infusion and 30 min after infusion
transdermal patch	Nitrodur	Suggest wearing patch 12–14 hr: remove after 10–12 hr
	Transderm-Nitro	
	Nitrodisc	
Isosorbide dinitrate	Isordil, Sorbitrate	
sublingual		5–60 min
oral		15 min–4 hr
chewable		2 min–$2\frac{1}{2}$ hr
oral, sustained release	ISMO	reported 2–6 hr free from angina
Isosorbide mononitrate	ISMO	
Pentaerythritol tetranitrate		
sublingual	Peritrate	10–30 min
oral	Pentrinitrol	30 min–12 hr
oral	Pentafin	4–5 hr
sustained release	Vasitol	30 min–12 hr
Erythrityl tetranitrate		
oral	Tetranitrol	30 min–4 hr
oral	Erythrol tetranitrate	30 min–2–4 hr
sublingual	Cardilate	5 min–2–4 hr

Source: Adapted from Opie LH (ed). Drugs for the Heart. 2nd expanded ed. Philadelphia, WB Saunders, 1987, pp 22–23; and Hahn AB, Barkin RL, Oestrich, SJK, Pharmacology in Nursing. 15th ed. St. Louis, CV Mosby, 1982, p 595.

Because hypotension may accompany the use of nitrates, it may be recommended that patients who are taking sublingual nitroglycerin for the first time sit down. If a patient in the physical therapy clinic takes a sublingual nitroglycerin tablet either before or as a result of a physical therapy intervention, it is important to reevaluate both the intervention and the patient (e.g., heart rate, blood pressure) before making a decision to continue. Use of prophylactic sublingual nitroglycerin is sometimes recommended before exercise, but this decision must be by physician order and cannot be decided solely by the physical therapist and patient. Patients should also be told to store nitroglycerin in a dark glass jar and to keep it tightly closed; once the jar is opened the tablets begin to lose their potency. Unused sublingual nitroglycerin should be discarded within 3 months of opening unless suggested otherwise by the manufacturer. Active sublingual nitroglycerin gives a burning sensation when placed under the tongue. If the nitroglycerin does not "burn," the effect of the drug may be substantially reduced. Nitroglycerin is also available in the form of a lingual spray, which has a longer shelf life than the sublingual preparations.

Long-acting nitrates may cause a nitrate tolerance to develop, such that the drug receptors become desensitized. Use of interval dosage, with nitrate-free times (often at night), may prolong receptor site sensitivity. Patients must be informed that they are not to alter their prescribed drug schedule without consulting their health care provider. Nitrates must be given along their prescribed route; for example, taking sublingual nitroglycerin orally markedly decreases its effectiveness.

Increasing Myocardial Oxygen Supply

Pharmacologic interventions to increase myocardial oxygen supply in coronary artery disease are limited. Although calcium-channel blockers and nitrates may have secondary effects of coronary vasodilation and calcium-channel blockers can decrease coronary artery spasm, no direct way exists to increase coronary blood flow in the presence of ischemic heart disease. Over the past decade, the management of an acute myocardial infarction has broadened to include the use of thrombolytic and antiplatelet agents.

Thrombolytic Agents. The purpose of these drugs is to acutely destroy (lyse) or decrease the blood clot (thrombus) formation that occurs within the coronary artery at the time of the myocardial infarction. In doing so, some coronary blood flow within the affected area is maintained, and reduction in infarction size may be possible. Use of thrombolytic therapy is reserved for a selected group of patients. Although protocols may vary among institutions, general guidelines are that thrombolytic agents should be given within 3 to 4 hours from the onset of myocardial ischemia and with evidence of ST-segment elevation on the electrocardiogram (ECG).[10] For certain patients, thrombolytic treatment may be effective up to 6 hours after the onset of ischemic symptoms if there is persistent ST-segment elevation with symptoms yet no evidence of extensive Q wave development on the ECG.[10] The patient should have no history of bleeding abnormalities, cerebral vascular events, or uncontrolled hypertension. Even under ideal conditions, only 75% of patients are successfully *reperfused* with thrombolytic therapy, and of those that are reperfused, 10% to 20% experience early reocclusion.[10] Thrombolytic agents facilitate the conversion of plasminogen to plasmin, and therefore clot lysis can occur quickly rather than over a period of days.

Streptokinase (Kabikinase, Streptase), **urokinase** (Abbokinase), and **alteplase recombinant tPA** (Activase, t-PA) **anisoylated plasminogen streptokinase activator complex** (APSAC, Anistreplase, Eminase) are examples of thrombolytic agents presently used in the United States. Other drugs undergoing study are single-chain urokinase plasminogen activators

(SCU-PA, prourokinase). Streptokinase liberates plasmin from plasminogen. It is not fibrin-specific and therefore produces systemic lysis. In contrast, t-PA is fibrin-specific, thereby causing fewer systemic effects than streptokinase. Clinically, however, no significant difference in the risk of serious bleeding complications has been identified among the thrombolytic agents.[11]

Clinical Considerations. Care must be taken with thrombolytic agents to avoid situations of potential tissue trauma such as venipunctures, manual shaving, resistive exercises, or soft tissue injury because the patient's blood clotting ability is markedly altered during this period. Cardiac rehabilitation physical therapy, including progressive ambulation, may proceed within established acceptable guidelines.

Although thrombolytic agents may limit the amount of myocardial tissue damage, the use of these agents is not without risk. Thrombolytic agents are not absolutely tissue-specific; therefore, systemic bleeding may occur as well as lysis of the coronary thrombus. Potential undesirable side effects include

- Cerebrovascular accidents
- Genitourinary bleeding
- Gastrointestinal bleeding

Ventricular arrhythmias are common within the acute time frame following thrombolysis and are believed to be in response to tissue reperfusion and do not therefore require prolonged antiarrhythmic management.

Antiplatelet Agents. Antiplatelet agents are given prophylactically to prevent thrombus formation by decreasing the platelets' ability to adhere and aggregate at the site of the injury. Commonly used agents for this purpose are **salicylic acid** (aspirin, ASA) and **dipyridamole** (Persantine) (Fig. 14–2).

Advances in the understanding of clot formation have led to the development of two additional groups of platelet inhibitors. Glycoprotein IIb/IIIa (gp2b/3a) inhibitors block platelet receptors from binding to fibrinogen, consequently limiting platelet aggregation. Abciximab (Reapro) and eptifibatide (Integrelin) are commonly used gp2b/3a inhibitors. A second group of antiplatelet agents

Table 14-7

Common Drugs and Sites of Action*

Anticoagulants

Heparin sodium (Heparin): decreases thrombin activity, thereby preventing formation of stable clot

Warfarin sodium (Coumadin): decreases prothrombin activity

Antiplatelets

Decrease platelet aggregation

Acetylsalicylic acid (aspirin)
Dipyridamole (Persantine)
Abciximab (Reapro)
Eptifibatide (Integrilin)
Tirofiban (Aggrastat)
Clopidogrel (Plavix)
Ticlopidine (Ticlid)

Thrombolytic Agents

Facilitate the conversion of plasminogen to plasmin

Streptokinase (Streptase)
Urokinase (Abbokinase)
Alteplase recombinant tPA (Activase)
Anistreplase (Eminase)

*See Figure 14-2.

interfere with ADP activator, decreasing the available energy source for platelet aggregation processes. Clopidogrel (Plavix) and ticlopidine (Ticlid) are common drugs that act in this way.[12]

Anticoagulants. **Anticoagulants** are used prophylactically to prevent blood clot formation. These agents inhibit the formation of thrombin and therefore negate the influence of thrombin on fibrinogen. Anticoagulants may also be used when a thrombus is already formed to prevent emboli. Commonly used agents are **heparin** (Liquaemin Sodium) and **warfarin** (Coumadin). Table 14-7 summarizes common drugs and their sites of action.

Calcium-Channel Blockers. There are two sources of calcium:

• Intracellular calcium, stored within the sarcoplasmic reticulum
• Extracellular calcium, stored within the plasma

Different tissue types have an affinity for the different sources of calcium. Smooth muscle in both the coronary arteries and peripheral vascular system and in the sinoatrial and atrioventricular nodes is more dependent on extracellular calcium; striated muscle, myocardium, and coronary veins have a primary affinity for intracellular calcium.

Calcium plays a key role in muscular contraction. The process of muscular contraction requires the availability of actin, myosin, troponin, tropomyosin, and calcium. In order for actin and myosin to form crossbridges, calcium must bind with **troponin.** Troponin, when not bound to calcium, inhibits coupling of actin and myosin. In the absence of calcium, troponin is free to inhibit the actin-myosin interaction, thereby inhibiting contraction. Calcium-channel blockers block the entrance of calcium into the cell from the extracellular stores. Calcium-channel blockers therefore prevent smooth muscle contractions within the coronary artery (i.e., coronary spasm).

Calcium-channel blockers were initially used as part of an anti-ischemic regimen because of their ability to decrease vasospasm in the coronary arteries. In addition to that primary role, specific calcium-channel blockers are now also used for

• Arrhythmia control, particularly supraventricular tachycardia
• Blood pressure control
• Reducing the incidence of reinfarction in patients with non-Q wave infarcts
• Treatment of postinfarction angina (Table 14-8).

(See the following sections on drug management of hypertension and arrhythmia for further discussion.)

"Calcium channel antagonists have made a substantial contribution to the patients with ischemic heart disease. For patients with postinfarction ischemic syndromes, the addition of a calcium channel antagonist to the medical regimen can often provide salutary effects."[11] Myocardial ischemia causes an influx of calcium ions into the cell. This increase in intracellular calcium elevates the cellular metabolic rate, which, in turn, elevates myocardial oxygen demand. Ischemia increases the energy demand on tissue that already has compromised perfusion. When calcium-channel blockers are used for postinfarction ischemia, potential infarction size may be decreased.

Clinical Considerations. Although calcium-channel blockers are relatively safe drugs with few serious side effects, these medications may have negative inotropic properties at high doses; therefore

Table 14–8

Calcium-Channel Blockers

GENERIC (TRADE)	COMMON USAGE*	SIDE EFFECTS COMMON TO ALL
Nifedipine (Procardia, Adalat)	Blood pressure control	Orthostatic hypotension†
		Ankle edema
Verapamil (Isoptin, Calan)	Supraventricular arrhythmias	Flushing
Diltiazem (Cardizem)	Ischemic heart disease	Peripheral edema
		Constipation‡
		Headache
Nicardipine (Cardene)	Blood pressure control	Dizziness
Isradipine (Dyna-Circ)	Similar to nifedipine but may have less reflex tachycardia	Tachycardia
		Cough reflex¶
Amlodipine (Lotrel, Norvasc)	Blood pressure control	Tremor, dry mouth¶¶
Bepridil (Vascor)	Chronic stable angina	GI upset
Felodipine (Plendil)	Blood pressure control	Pharyngitis; do not take with grapefruit juice (specific to nisoldipine)
Nimodipine (Nimotop)		
Nisoldipine (Sultar, Solar)	Blood pressure control	

*Prevention of coronary spasm is common to all.
†Especially nifedipine and nicardipine.
‡Especially verapamil and diltiazem.
¶Especially amlodipine.
¶¶Especially bepridil.

clinical observation for heart failure is warranted. **Orthostatic hypotension** often occurs in the initiation and regulation of dosages of **nifedipine** (Procardia), so the clinician should be sensitized to watching for orthostatic signs and symptoms when initiating an increase in activity orders or when assisting the patient out of bed for the first time.

HEART FAILURE

"In the United States, an estimated 400,000 individuals develop heart failure annually: it is thus the most common inpatient diagnosis of patients older than 65 years. . . . The most common causes of congestive heart failure in the United States are as follows: (1) coronary artery disease with destruction of contractile muscle tissue, (2) systemic hypertension, (3) chronic alcoholism, (4) diabetes mellitus, (5) idiopathic dilated cardiomyopathy, (6) valvular heart disease."[13]

Heart failure may be chronic, low level, and easily managed by oral medications over a period of years. Heart failure may also be acute and life-threatening, requiring the use of parenteral medications to maintain an adequate cardiac output and tissue perfusion. The medical management of heart failure includes preload reduction with diuretics, venodilators, or angiotensin-converting enzyme (ACE) inhibitors; increased inotropy with cardiac glycosides, sympathomimetics, or bipyridines; and afterload reduction with arteriodilators, calcium-channel blockers, or ACE inhibitors.

Physiology

For a more complete review of cardiovascular physiology, please refer to Chapter 2. This discussion will serve only as a brief review of key concepts influential in the drug management of heart failure.

The heart is a pump, the function of which is to provide oxygenated blood to all parts of the body. The amount of blood that the heart is able to pump per minute is called the cardiac output. Cardiac output is directly affected by stroke volume (the amount the left ventricle pumps out with each heart beat) and the heart rate (the number of heart beats per minute). The factors that influence stroke volume are preload, afterload, and contractility. Preload—the filling pressure of the left ventricle (left ventricular end diastolic pressure)—is influenced by venous return and the distensibility of the left ventricle. Afterload—the resistance against which the left ventricle contracts—is influenced by arterial pressure and resistance across the aortic valve. Contractility (inotropy)—the ability of the myocardial muscle to contract—is dependent on adequate amounts of sodium, potassium, and calcium to facilitate cellular depolarization and actin-myosin interaction. Drugs that increase myocardial contractility are known as positive inotropes and drugs that decrease contractility as negative inotropes.

Pathophysiology

Heart failure occurs when the heart is unable (i.e., fails) to provide sufficient cardiac output safely and effectively to serve the body. Heart failure occurs, therefore, because of an inadequate heart rate, stroke volume, or both or, more specifically, because of failure of their components: rhythm, preload, afterload, or contractility. There are a variety of situations that may induce heart failure, such as

- Arrhythmias (especially if cardiac output is impaired as a result)
- Increased preload associated with fluid overload
- Increased afterload as seen with hypertension
- Significant loss of contractile tissue such as with a myocardial infarction
- Significant decrease in contractility as a result of ischemia or cardiomyopathy

The most common cause of CHF, however, is coronary artery disease (CAD), particularly in those patients who have had a previous MI. There are many degrees of heart failure, from mild, in which the symptoms of decreased cardiac output are apparent only with moderate activity, to severe, in which the heart fails to provide adequate cardiac output even at rest. Heart failure is a chronic progressive disease and therefore requires dynamic, ongoing reevaluation and aggressive pharmacologic intervention as determined by the degree of hemodynamic compromise. Heart failure, however, may also remain mild over a period of years, hemodynamically well controlled with medications.

Pharmacologic Intervention

Drug management of heart failure attempts to address the underlying contribution to the failure and to maintain an adequate cardiac output. Initial treatment of mild heart failure involves regulating fluids, decreasing preload, decreasing afterload, and improving contractility through oral medications. As the hemodynamic compromise progresses and the clinical picture worsens, medical management broadens to include parenteral medications, oxygen, and sedation (to decrease anxiety and metabolic energy) (see Table 14–15). The six categories of drugs commonly used for the management of heart failure are

- Diuretics
- Positive inotropes
- Vasodilators
- Calcium-Channel Blockers
- Angiotensin-Converting Enzyme Inhibitors
- Morphine (Table 14–9)
- Beta blockers

There are no exclusive drug categories used to treat diastolic dysfunction. Pharmacologic management requires that treatment improve the relaxation of the cardiac muscle.

Diuretics

As a first-line drug for the management of heart failure, diuretics decrease circulating blood volume, thereby decreasing preload. Diuretics encourage **diuresis** and influence water and electrolyte balance by inhibiting sodium and water reabsorption. The influence on diuresis is dependent on the site of action of the drug within the kidneys. The strongest diuretics are those that act at Henle's loop (loop diuretics); the milder diuretics are those that act on the proximal tubules and the collecting tubules and ducts. The most common diuretic for symptomatic heart failure is the loop diuretic **furosemide** (Lasix), which, besides sodium inhibition, also inhibits the movement of potassium and chloride across the plasma membrane of the ascending Henle's loop. The subsequent section on antihypertension drugs provides an expanded list of diuretics and their sites of action (see Fig. 14–7; Table 14–12).

Table 14-9

Pharmacologic Management of Heart Failure

CATEGORY	GENERIC (TRADE) NAME	SIDE EFFECTS AND COMMENTS
Diuretics		
Thiazide Thiazide-like Loop Potassium sparing Osmotic Combination	See Table 14-12	
Positive Inotropes		
Cardiac glycosides Digitalis	Digitoxin (Crystodigin) Digoxin (Lanoxin) Deslanoside (Cedilanid-DIV)	Toxicity common
Sympathomimetics Beta$_1$	Dobutamine (Dobutrex)* Prenalterol	Arrhythmias
Nonselective beta	Epinephrine (Adrenalin Chloride)* Isoproterenol (Isuprel)*	Tachycardia
Dopaminergic	Dopamine (Intropin, Dopastat)*	Myocardial ischemia similar to beta
Mixed alpha and beta	Norepinephrine (Levophed)*	May cause dangerous decrease in peripheral blood flow owing to peripheral and visceral vasoconstriction.
Bipyridines	Amrinone (Inocor)*	Nausea and vomiting Thrombocytopenia Ventricular ectopy Liver abnormalities
Vasodilators		
Venodilators Nitrates Arteriolar	See Table 14-6 Hydralazine (Apresoline) Minoxidil (Loniten) Milrinone (Primacor)* Enoximone (Perfan) (investigational)* Vesnarinone (investigational)	Hydralazine: tachycardia Palpitations, orthostatic hypotension, rebound hypotension Fluid retention Both hydralazine and minoxidil should be used with a beta blocker and diuretic. Minoxidil is useful when renal failure accompanies heart failure.
	Nifedipine (Procardia) Diazoxide (Hyperstat IV)	See Table 14-8
Combined arteriolar and venodilator	Sodium nitroprusside (Nipride)	Rapid onset of action, delivery via infusion pump May result in excess hypotension, metabolic acidosis, and arrhythmias
Angiotensin-Converting		
Enzyme inhibitors	Captopril (Capoten) Enalapril (Vasotec) Lisinopril (Prinivil, Zestril)	Hypotension Renal failure Neutropenia Skin rashes Taste disturbances
Analgesic		
	Morphine sulfate (Morphine, MS Contin)	Used in acute pulmonary edema

*Parenteral.

553

Positive Inotropes

Three categories of drugs increase contractility: cardiac glycosides, sympathomimetics, and bipyridines.

Cardiac Glycosides. One of the oldest classes of cardiac medications, cardiac glycosides is represented by the drug **digitalis.** Digitalis is available in several different preparations, the most common of which are **digitoxin** (Crystodigin) and digoxin (Lanoxin, Lanoxicaps). Digoxin appears to be the more commonly used of the two preparations, perhaps owing to its comparatively shorter half-life and therefore decreased risk of toxicity. Digitalis increases contractility by inhibiting the sodium-potassium-ATPase enzyme, which normally provides the energy for the sodium-potassium pump (NA$^+$-K$^+$ pump). The Na$^+$-K$^+$ pump expels Na$^+$, accumulated during depolarization, from the cell and brings in K$^+$ during repolarization. By binding to the enzyme, digitalis inhibits the active transport of sodium and potassium, thereby increasing intracellular sodium. An increase in intracellular sodium results in an ionic exchange of intracellular sodium for extracellular calcium (Ca^{2+}). The resultant increase in intracellular calcium stimulates large quantities of calcium to be released from the sarcoplasmic reticulum and to be available for excitation-contraction. Myocardial contractility is therefore increased as a result of increased calcium. Patients in chronic heart failure who experience limited hemodynamic compromise are commonly managed with digitalis.

Diuretics and digitalis are frequently prescribed together as successful agents for the management of chronic heart failure. In the setting of heart failure, particularly with ventricular dilation, myocardial contraction is often inefficient and results in an increase in myocardial oxygen demand. Diuretics reduce preload with resultant improvement in the ventricular length-tension relationship. This improved mechanical advantage optimizes the actin-myosin interaction, and contractility becomes more energy efficient. Myocardial oxygen demand is reduced, and heart failure improves.

Besides its positive inotropic effects, digitalis also has both negative **chronotropic** (decreased heart rate) and negative **dromotropic** (conduction delay) action, the dromotropic effect being primarily on the atrioventricular conduction system. The bradycardic and delayed atrioventricular node conduction effect of digitalis is especially useful in the treatment of atrial fibrillation (see the subsequent section on antiarrhythmic drugs).

Digitalis toxicity may occur for a variety of reasons. The more common causes are

• The interaction of digitalis with other drugs
• Decreased renal function
• Altered gastrointestinal absorption

Examples of drugs known to interact in this manner with digitalis are **quinidine** (various preparations and trade names, Duraquin, Cardioquin), **amiodarone** (Cordarone), verapamil (Calan, Isoptin), potassium-sparing diuretics, and antibiotics. Antacids, a high-fiber diet, and chemotherapeutic agents may decrease the bioavailability of digitalis. The typical patient with digitalis toxicity is usually elderly, in **atrial fibrillation,** with underlying heart disease of many years, abnormal renal function, and concomitant pulmonary disease.

Signs and symptoms of digitalis toxicity include the following:

• Gastrointestinal problems—anorexia, nausea, vomiting, diarrhea
• Neurologic problems—malaise, fatigue, vertigo, colored vision (especially green or yellow halos around lights), insomnia, depression, facial pain
• Cardiologic problems—palpitations, arrhythmias, syncope
• Hematologic problems—high digoxin levels especially with low potassium and altered blood urea nitrogen (BUN) and creatinine

Sympathomimetics. Drugs that bind to the adrenoceptors and partially or completely mimic the actions of epinephrine or norepinephrine are known as sympathomimetics. The use of sympathomimetics, given parenterally in the treatment of heart failure to optimize cardiac output, is reserved for hemodynamically compromised patients within a critical care setting (see Tables 14–9, 14–12, and 14–16).

Stimulation of beta$_1$ adrenoceptors of the myocardium results in an increased calcium influx into myocardial cells with resultant electrical and mechanical influences: increased sinus node firing, enhanced atrioventricular conduction, and increased myocardial contractility. Stimulation of beta$_2$ adrenoceptors causes dilation of smooth muscles of the bronchi and blood vessels, with myocardial effects similar to those of beta$_1$. Pharmacologic stimulation of beta$_1$ and beta$_2$ agonist receptors in a failing heart therefore increases contractility, and beta$_2$ stimulation decreases afterload by its peripheral arterial vasodilatory effect. Use of these drugs is limited to acute interventions in a critical care setting because prolonged use of beta stimulators may lead to receptor desensitization and decreased inotropy. Unwanted ventricular arrhythmias may develop in response to the increased myocardial oxygen cost from pharmacologically induced improved contractility. Increased myocardial oxygen cost may further aggravate ischemia.

Examples of beta agonist adrenoceptors are the following: selective beta$_1$: **dobutamine** (Dobutrex), **norepinephrine (Levophed),** prenalterol; nonselective beta$_1$ and beta$_2$: epinephrine (Adrenalin Chloride), **isoproterenol** (Isuprel). Relatively selective beta$_2$ agonists are used primarily in the management of respiratory dysfunction.

Another category of sympathomimetic agonists is **dopamine** (Intropin). Dopamine stimulates beta$_1$ myocardial receptors, D-1 (dopamine) vascular receptors, and alpha vascular receptors. Dopamine is used when heart failure is accompanied by systemic hypotension because it acts as both a positive inotrope (via beta$_1$ receptors) and a vasopressor (via alpha receptors). The combined beta and alpha effect increases cardiac output through increased contractility and increases blood pressure through both peripheral vascular vasoconstriction and increased cardiac output. At low doses, dopamine (via its D-1 receptors) causes selective vasodilation and therefore increased blood flow to the renal, cerebral, coronary, and mesenteric arterial beds.

Dopamine (Intropin) and dobutamine (Dobutrex) are often used together in the management of heart failure with accompanying hypotension. Although both are potent beta-adrenergic agonists, dobutamine has no alpha-adrenergic stimulation and therefore cannot increase blood pressure through vasoconstriction, whereas dopamine is able to do so. Moderate doses of both drugs, when given together, have been demonstrated to maintain arterial blood pressure, decrease pulmonary artery wedge pressure, and increase contractility.

Bipyridines. As a group, bipyridines act as positive inotropes and vasodilators. They are often recommended for the treatment of heart failure that has failed to respond to other drug management. The inotropic effect of these drugs differs from that of the previous two drugs in that bipyridines increase myocardial contractility without altering the Na$^+$-K$^+$ pumping mechanism (as does digoxin) or stimulating the adrenoceptors (as does dopamine). Bipyridines increase intracellular calcium influx by inhibition of the cyclic **nucleotide phosphodiesterase.** Amrinone (Inocor) was the first drug in this category approved for use with patients with severe CHF not responding adequately to digitalis, diuretics, or vasodilators. Amrinone is relatively specific for myocardial and vascular smooth muscle because its vasodilatory effects are balanced between preload and afterload. Overall effects of amrinone are an increase in cardiac output, reduction in preload, and decrease in afterload. In preload reduction, as measured by decreased pulmonary artery wedge pressure, amrinone is more effective than dopamine (Intropin) or dobutamine (Dobutrex); as a positive inotrope and vasodilator, it is intermediate between nitroprusside (Nipride) and dobutamine. Milrinone (Primacor) has a mechanism of action similar to that of amrinone and is approved for intravenous use. Use of oral milrinone has been shown in one long-term study to increase morbidity and mortality rates of patients with severe heart failure; the mortality rate was reported to have increased by 30%.[14]

Vasodilators

Both arterial and venous vasodilators are used in the management of heart failure as afterload and preload reducers, respectively. Arterial vasodilators are useful only when arterial hypotension is not present. Arterial vasodilators decrease afterload, which decreases left ventricular myocardial oxygen demand. Reduction in preload may also decrease myocardial oxygen demand by decreasing ventricular volume, thus improving the length-tension relationship of the myocardial fibers. The improvement allows for a greater actin-myosin interaction and more effective contractility. Myocardial oxygen demand may be reduced as the efficiency of the contraction improves.

Drugs that exhibit vasodilator properties are the following:

- Smooth muscle relaxants such as nitroglycerin, nitroprusside (Nipride), and **hydralazine** (Apresoline)
- Calcium-channel blockers
- Morphine
- ACE inhibitors
- Alpha-adrenergic antagonists (see Tables 14-9 and 14-12)

Alpha antagonists are primarily used for the management of hypertension rather than heart failure. Reflex tachycardia and a compensatory increase in blood volume with long-term use have been identified as potential detrimental side effects of alpha antagonists. **Prazosin** (Minipress) and **terazosin** (Hytrin) are examples of alpha$_1$ antagonists (see Table 14-12).

Venodilators. Nitrates reduce the preload via venodilation. Nitrates are available in many forms, including topical, sublingual, and oral. Please refer to the previous section on anti-ischemic drugs and Table 14-6 for further discussion.

Arteriodilators. Hydralazine (Apresoline) and **minoxidil** (Loniten) decrease afterload by decreasing arterial resistance. Because there is a potential increase in side effects when hydralazine is used alone, it is commonly used in combination with a diuretic and a beta blocker. Please refer to the section on antihypertension drugs and Table 14-12 for further discussion.

Combined Arteriolar and Venous Dilators. Nitroprusside (Nipride) affects both arterial resistance and venous capacitance. When it is given parenterally, it has a rapid onset of action and is effective in the treatment of severe heart failure with or without **cardiogenic shock.**

Calcium-Channel Blockers

Calcium-channel blockers work by relaxing the smooth muscle within the arterial walls, which results in a decreased afterload. Nifedipine is the most potent peripheral vasodilator of the calcium-channel blockers. Please refer to the sections on anti-ischemic and antiarrhythmic drugs and to Table 14-8 for further discussion.

Angiotensin-Converting Enzyme Inhibitors

When cardiac output is decreased, such as with symptomatic heart failure, perfusion of the renal artery is also decreased. Decreased renal perfusion stimulates the release of **renin** from the afferent arteriole of the glomerulus. Renin, along with a renin substrate, forms **angiotensin I,** which converts into **angiotensin II** (see Fig. 14-9). "This reaction is catalyzed by angiotensin converting enzyme (ACE), which is located in many organs, including the lung, the luminal membrane of vascular epithelial cells, and the **juxtaglomerular** apparatus itself."[15] Angiotensin II has two key effects: an increase in systemic vascular resistance owing to its potency as a vasoconstrictor and an increase in extracellular volume owing to renal sodium and water retention via aldosterone stimulation.[15] When the reaction of angiotensin I to angiotensin II is inhibited, the effects of angiotensin II are significantly limited.

Angiotensin-converting enzyme inhibitors are used in the management of heart failure to decrease the excess intravascular volume that occurs as a result of sodium and water retention. A decrease in volume decreases preload. A decrease in preload in a failing heart decreases myocardial oxygen demand and may improve contractility (refer to sections on diuretics and antihypertensive drugs). Commonly used ACE inhibitors for heart failure are

- **Captopril** (Capoten)
- **Enalapril** (Vasotec)
- **Lisinopril** (Zestril) (see Tables 14-9 and 14-12)

ACE inhibitors are also used in patients with suppressed LV dysfunction but without signs of overt heart failure. The findings of the SOLVD study (Studies of Left Ventricular Dysfunction) in which asymptomatic patients with ejection fractions of 35% or less were treated with enalapril, showed a significant reduction in the incidence of symptomatic heart failure and the rate of related hospitalizations.[16] Pfeffer et al.[17] reported an improvement in survival and reduced morbidity and cardiovascular mortality rates in asymptomatic patients with an ejection fraction of 40% or less who were treated with captopril following an MI. The mechanism of action of the ACE inhibitors in these cases is complex and not fully understood, but they may play a favorable role in limiting adverse ventricular remodeling and ventricular dilatation after MI.[17]

Morphine

The use of morphine in the treatment of severe heart failure has proved invaluable for both its analgesic and its hemodynamic effects. Morphine decreases preload via marked venodilation and exhibits mild arterial vasodilation. The anxiety and effort of dyspnea associated with severe heart failure appear to improve with the administration of morphine.

Beta Blockers

Carvedilol, a new beta blocker that also has alpha blocking properties is both a preload and afterload reducer. It is being used for treatment of NYHA class II and III CHF, usually with concomitant use of ACE inhibitors, digoxin, and diuretics. However, it may also be used with patients unable to tolerate ACE inhibitors. Drug dosages must be titrated very slowly and the patient must be closely monitored for adverse effects, especially for blood pressure decreases down to the vasodilatory effect and reduction in heart rate due to beta blockage.

Clinical Considerations

The importance of recognizing the side effects of all drugs has previously been stated and yet bears repetition. In the case of digoxin (Lanoxin), for example, the side effects may be perceived initially by the patient as "just not feeling well"; the correlation of those feelings to the specific drug may go unnoticed. Many patients seen by physical therapists for noncardiac reasons are taking digoxin. Any new patient complaint should be evaluated in light of its relationship to digoxin and reported to the physician. If patients are on digoxin because of atrial fibrillation, the physical therapist must recognize that they will have an irregular pulse. In addition, atrial fibrillation with a ventricular response at rest greater than 110 beats per minute warrants evaluation before continuing with an exercise program. Resting pulses should be taken for a full minute when atrial fibrillation or any other rhythm disturbance is present owing to the irregularity of the rhythm.

Signs and Symptoms

For the therapist who is seeing a patient on an outpatient basis, the signs and symptoms of impending heart failure may be subtle over a period of days; therefore, the therapist should be alerted to any complaints of dyspnea, ankle swelling, weight gain (1–2 lb in 2 days), or the presence of an S_3 heart sound or lung crackles. If these symptoms are present, the patient should not be exercised until a physician is contacted and the situation clarified or remedied. In the case of severe heart failure warranting parenterally delivered vasopressors and positive inotropes to maintain an appropriate cardiac output at rest, progressive exercise is not recommended until the patient is hemodynamically stable. As the patient becomes hemodynamically stable, appropriate treatment interventions may include the following: techniques to maintain good alveolar expansion and gas exchange, education regarding energy conservation techniques (e.g., arms supported on pillows for activities of daily living to decrease upper extremity energy requirements), and initiation of low level activity. As stroke volume decreases, heart rate compensatorily rises to prevent cardiac output from falling further. Therefore, when the patient has tachycardia at rest it is inappropriate to begin an exercise program without clear direction and mutual understanding of the treatment goals from all members of the health care team.

Patients on diuretics may also become dehydrated because of excess diuresis. Their complaints may be of lightheadedness, weakness, fatigue, or an irregular pulse. Symptoms may be more pronounced when standing as compared with sitting or lying down. Clinical signs may be resting tachycardia and postural hypotension. Patients should not participate in an exercise regimen until the situation has been stabilized and the patient has appropriately rehydrated (and replaced electrolytes if needed) under a physician's guidance.

ANTIARRHYTHMIC AGENTS

Disturbances in cardiac rhythm are known as arrhythmias. They are the result of irregularities in heart pacemaker or conduction tissue function. Arrhythmias present a broad spectrum of clinical consequences: they may be benign and remain undetected throughout life or prove fatal upon initial presentation (e.g., sudden death). Arrhythmias are recognized clinically as irregularities in the rhythm of the heartbeat on palpation, auscultation, or ECG tracing. They are labeled according to the anatomic origin of the abnormal beat (e.g., atrial, nodal, or ventricular), their frequency (e.g., tachycardia or bradycardia), and their relationship to the previous beat (e.g., premature or late).

Electrolyte imbalances, drug toxicity, excessive nicotine or caffeine ingestion, emotional stress, **hyperthyroidism,** or **mitral valve prolapse** syndrome can all produce arrhythmias. On correction of these conditions, persistent cardiac rhythm disturbances that are hemodynamically significant require drug therapy. The focus of antiarrhythmic therapy, therefore, is to maintain adequate cardiac output in the presence of pacemaker or conduction tissue disease.

Physical therapists must be alert to the etiology and presence of arrhythmias, their hemodynamic consequences, and the efficacy of the antiarrhythmic agent prescribed. Drugs suppress arrhythmias (abnormal impulse formation or conduction) by altering cell membrane permeability to specific ions, for example, sodium and calcium. Although exercise may be responsible for production of arrhythmias, electrolyte imbalances and toxic level of antiarrhythmic drugs are other nondisease states that may be arrhythmogenic.

Physiology

To understand how antiarrhythmic agents suppress rhythm disturbances, it is necessary to review the unique characteristics of normal myocardial pacemaker and conduction system functioning. See Chapter 9 for an in-depth discussion of cardiac arrhythmias. Inherent myocardial properties of automaticity, excitability, and conduction depend on the resting polarity of pacemaker (nodal) and myocardial conduction tissue (Purkinje's fibers). Refer to Chapter 2 for further information. This specialized conduction system is able to initiate, respond to, and conduct a stimulus as long as an adequate transmembrane potential exists. Resting cell polarity depends on two factors:

• The membrane permeability to sodium, calcium, potassium, and chloride ions
• The duration between action potentials (diastole)

The cardiac action potential is thought to result from an orderly and sequential change in membrane permeability to various ions. The characteristic time course has been described by phases and separated into "fast" and "slow" responses (Fig. 14–3). Whereas membrane permeability to sodium alone is felt to be responsible for the rapid upstroke of phase 0 depolarization found in normal atrial and ventricular contractile cell action potential, membrane permeability to both calcium and sodium is responsible for the slow phase 0 depolarization of sinus and atrioventricular nodal cell action potential. Repolarization via the "fast" channels can be described by three phases:

• Phase 1 is the early rapid phase and depends on membrane permeability to chloride.
• Phase 2 is the plateau phase affected by calcium and potassium movement across the membrane.
• Phase 3 is the final rapid phase of repolarization, primarily influenced by membrane permeability to potassium.

These three phases of repolarization cannot be distinguished clearly in cells with slower action potentials (see Fig. 14–3B). Phase 4 is the period of diastole and is constant in many atrial and ventricular contractile cells that rest indefinitely until stimulated. However, sinus node, atrioventricular node, and Purkinje's fibers have a unique ability to spontaneously depolarize and self-excite by achieving a threshold at which more rapid depolarization occurs.

Both myocardial contractile and conduction tissue are refractory to restimulation when the cell membrane is still depolarized. When the membrane is partially repolarized (phase 3), excitation

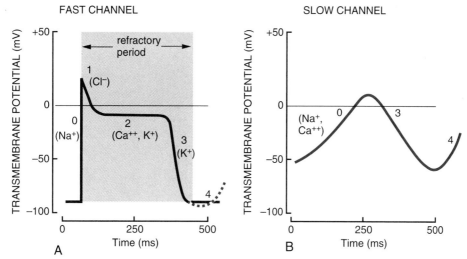

Figure 14–3. Schematic representation of phases of action potential (AP) in fast and slow depolarization. The primary ion movement responsible for AP is noted at each phase. *A,* Fast response AP (black line) begins with a relatively greater negativity and has a rapid rate of depolarization and a plateaued repolarization. This AP is found in ordinary atrial, ventricular, and Purkinje's fibers. Purkinje's fibers demonstrate a fast depolarization phase (0) but also have similar phase 4 diastole characteristics of self-excitation as in the slow channel (red dotted line). *B,* Slow response AP (red line) begins with a less negative voltage and has a slower depolarization phase (0). Repolarization lasts longer and exhibits a slow, spontaneous depolarization during phase 4 diastole. This AP is found in sinoatrial and atrioventricular nodal cells.

becomes possible but not usual, and the cell is in a "relative" refractory state (see Fig. 14–3).

Pathophysiology

The action potential and the diastolic interval between action potentials are affected by changes in the

- Maximum diastolic potential
- Slope of phase 4 depolarization
- Threshold potential required to depolarize the cell[18]

Figure 14–4*A, B,* and *C* demonstrate slowing of the heart rate by changes in any of these three action potential parameters. Numerous cardiac conditions, including cell hypoxia, ischemia, scarred tissue, and medications, can alter these parameters and can cause some cardiac cells that normally have fast action potentials to become faster or much slower, and slow action potentials to respond faster or slower than normal. When any of these alterations in the action potential occur, slow, fast, or escape rhythms may become manifest. For example, if sinoatrial node cells have

an excess of potassium (**hyperkalemia**), the resting polarity is greater than normal (more negativity). Consequently, more sodium has to enter the cell to fully depolarize the membrane, and more sodium has to leave the cell to complete repolarization. This excess of sodium and potassium creates a longer interval before the occurrence of another action potential, as illustrated in Figure 14–4*A.* Each heart beat reflects the mechanical event triggered by the electrical conduction of an action potential. Hence, a longer period between action potentials is seen clinically as a slower heart rate. Additionally, if the interval is long enough, pacemaker cells in the atrioventricular node may depolarize spontaneously, producing an "escape" action potential or a premature nodal heart beat. Similarly, if normal cell membrane integrity is disturbed and sodium permeability increases, cells may depolarize and repolarize more rapidly, causing an increase in heart rate.

In addition to the changes in the action potential, variability in the duration of the refractory period of the action potential can cause arrhythmias. In certain conditions, diseased myocardial cells repolarize and conduct slower than neighboring healthy myocardial cells, enabling "reentry" to

occur. Reentry, a common cause of rhythm disturbances, occurs when one impulse reenters and excites areas of the heart that have already been
stimulated by the original impulse (Fig. 14–5). For
reentry to occur, there must be

- Some obstacle blocking normal impulse conduction
- Another "avenue" for the impulse to be conducted through the tissue (unidirectional block)
- Sufficient time for the impulse to travel via this
alternative "avenue" (that is, long enough so that
after the impulse passes through this tissue, the

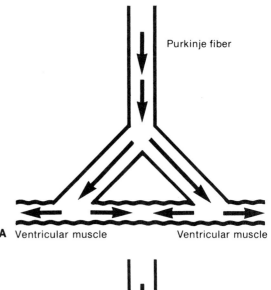

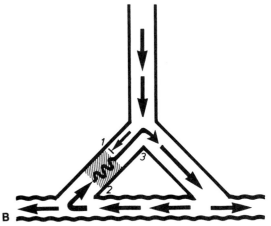

Figure 14–5. Conduction pathway. *A,* Normal conduction pathway of a depolarization wave through a Purkinje fiber to ventricular muscle. The depolarization
wave arrives simultaneously at all portions of ventricular
muscle and then extinguishes. *B,* Reentry circuit model
with unidirectional block. The depolarization wave is
blocked at the ischemic zone (1); however, it is able to
depolarize the ventricular muscle from the opposite direction (2). By the time the impulse passes through this
ischemic area, the healthy muscle is repolarized and responds to this impulse (3) before the next impulse can
be generated from the SA node. Drugs can abolish the
arrhythmia by improving forward conduction at 1 or by
preventing conduction at 2. (Modified from Tyndall A.
A nursing perspective of the invasive approach to treatment of ventricular arrhythmias. Heart Lung 12:6, 1983;
reproduced from Cohen M, Michael T. Cardiopulmonary Symptoms in Physical Therapy Practice. New York,
Churchill Livingstone, 1988, p 161.)

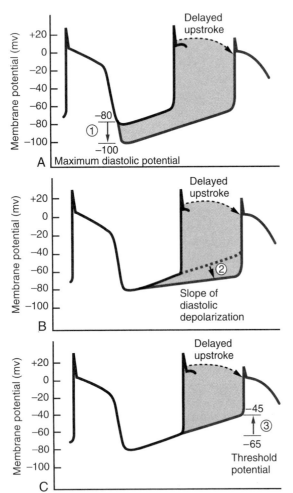

Figure 14–4. Determinants of action potential rate and
diastolic interval, as seen in Purkinje's fibers. The rate
can be slowed (and the interval lengthened; shaded
area) by three diastolic mechanisms: more negative maximum diastolic potential (*A*), reduction of the slope of
diastolic depolarization (*B*), or more positive threshold
potential (*C*). (Adapted from Katzung BG [ed]. Basic
and Clinical Pharmacology. 5th ed. East Norwalk, CT,
Appleton & Lange, 1992, p 169.)

surrounding tissue will have repolarized and will
be able to "accept" the impulse)

When these three conditions exist, the single or
repetitive conduction of a "secondary" pacemaker

occurs and is manifested clinically as a premature beat or a series of premature beats. Disease conditions such as myocardial ischemia with resultant hypoxia can cause partial depolarization and "unidirectional" block, providing the setting for reentrant rhythms. The slower repolarization rate of such disease tissue slows the reentrant impulse so that healthy surrounding tissue is no longer refractory and can respond to stimulation by this "secondary" pacemaker, subsequently making the healthy tissue refractory to the primary pacemaker.

Reentry is probably responsible for many cardiac arrhythmias, including atrial and ventricular flutter and fibrillation, supraventricular tachycardia involving accessory pathway or nodal reentry, and many ventricular tachycardias.[19] New technology enables precise identification of the origin and physiology of the reentrant rhythm. With this knowledge, physicians can plan treatment with more accuracy, including pharmacologic alteration of the action potential.

Pharmacologic Intervention

Suppression of arrhythmias by pharmacologic intervention can be complex. Although antiarrhythmic agents can reverse lethal rhythms, it is unclear that these drugs promote longevity. They can depress cardiac inotropy and may even produce arrhythmias owing to their effect on the action potential **(arrhythmogenic).** Antiarrhythmic agents act to inhibit abnormal impulse formation or conduction by altering cell membrane permeability to specific ions. The exact interaction of antiarrhythmics with various ionic channels is not well understood. As discussed in Chapter 2, current theory proposes the existence of activation and inactivation "gates," which control the flow of sodium, calcium, potassium, and chloride ions depending on stimulation. Classification of antiarrhythmic drugs according to their effects on the action potential of myocardial and pacemaker cell gates is found in Table 14–10. Significant overlapping of drug properties exists across all categories. For purposes of clarity, those classes acting primarily on the ionic channels to stabilize the membrane (classes 1 and 4) are discussed first. Beta blockers, which also appear in this classification, are discussed next (class 2), and lastly, class 3 drugs, which have properties of the previous classes, are

> ### Clinical Note: Suppression of Arrhythmias
>
> *Caution:* Some antiarrhythmic drugs may actually *induce* arrhythmias in some individuals (prorhythmic effect).

presented. Additionally, two classes of antiarrhythmics, beta blockers and calcium-channel blockers, not only are effective in the treatment of arrhythmias but also are used as anti-ischemic and antihypertensive agents (as is discussed elsewhere in this chapter).

Membrane Stabilizers

Class 1 Drugs. Class 1 drugs primarily affect the fast sodium channel and act like local anesthetics. Subclasses A, B, and C all significantly block the sodium channel of depolarized cells, but vary in the degree of sodium-channel block in normal cells. Similarly, class 1 drugs prolong the refractory period of depolarized cells but vary in their effect on normal cells. Prolongation of the refractory period of diseased tissue inhibits reentry by creating bidirectional block in these cells (see Fig. 14–5). Lidocaine (Xylocaine), a class 1B agent, facilitates propagation of the original (sinoatrial) stimulus by shortening the **refractory period** of normal cell action potentials while slowing or completely blocking the potential reentrant stimulus in diseased tissue. Lidocaine is a very effective drug for ventricular arrhythmia management in the early hours of an acute myocardial infarction when ischemic cells are in varied states of polarization. In this clinical setting, combinations of abnormal conduction and abnormal impulse formation are often responsible for many postinfarction arrhythmias.

In general, class 1 drugs are very effective in the treatment of ventricular tachycardia (VT). They may be useful in the treatment of supraventricular tachycardia (SVT), with class, 1A being the most effective. The ECG of a patient on a class 1 antiarrhythmic drug may exhibit a prolongation of the QRS duration, with a normal or prolonged P-R interval.

Class 2 Drugs. Class 2 antiarrhythmic agents —beta blockers—do not directly affect the cell

Table 14–10
Classification of Antiarrhythmic Drugs

CATEGORY	PHYSIOLOGIC EFFECT*	DRUG: GENERIC (TRADE NAME)	COMMENTS
Class 1			
Membrane depressants (sodium channel blockers)	Depolarized cells ↑ Na⁺ channel block ↑ Refractory period ↓ Pacemaker activity		
1A	Normal cell ↑ Na⁺ channel block ↑ Refractory period	Quinidine (Biquin, Cardioquin) Disopyramide (Norpace, Rythmodan) Procainamide (Pronestyl)	Gastrointestinal side effects Myocardial depressant Urinary retention effect; myocardial depressant Lupus erythematosus
1B	Normal cell No effect	Lidocaine (Xylocaine) Mexiletine (Mexitil) Tocainide (Tonocard) Phenytoin (Dilantin) Moricizine (Ethmozine)†	Signs of central nervous system abnormality (tremors, nausea) may indicate toxicity Anticonvulsant; effective with digoxin-induced arrhythmias; acts as 1C
1C	Normal cell ↑↑ Na⁺ channel block ∅, ↑ Refractory period	Flecainide (Tambocor) Propafenone (Rythmol)	Primarily for ventricular arrhythmias; effective with PVCs; arrhythmogenic during exercise; defibrillation problems
Class 2			
Beta adrenoceptor blockers	Depolarized cell ∅ Effect on Na⁺ channel ↑ Refractory period Normal cell Variable effect	See beta blocker Table 14–5 Sotalol	Effective with ventricular and supraventricular arrhythmias
Class 3			
Refractory period alterations	↑↑↑ Refractory period ↓ Pacemaker activity Sympatholytic	Amiodarone (Cordarone) Bretylium tosylate (Bretylol) Ibutilide fumarate (Corvert)	Class 1A, 2, 4 properties; useful with ventricular and supraventricular arrhythmias; may transiently increase pacemaker activity
Class 4			
Calcium-channel blockers	All cells ↑↑↑ Ca⁺⁺ channel blockade Depolarized cells ↑ Na⁺ channel block ↑ Refractory period ↓ Pacemaker activity Sympatholytic	See calcium-channel blocker Table 14–8	Verapamil (Isoptin, Calan) is most effective in this group for treatment of supraventricular tachycardia

* General effect on action potential; individual agents may differ slightly.
† Controversial classification; acts like 1C as well.
↑ slight increase
↑↑ moderate increase
↑↑↑ significant increase
↓ decrease
∅ no change

membrane. They indirectly alter the action potential by blocking sympathetic excitation of the heart to control cardiac rhythm disturbances. They are especially indicated for the treatment of supraventricular and ventricular arrhythmias that occur in the post–myocardial infarction period and arrhythmias that occur during exercise. Beta blockers are prescribed cautiously owing to their negative inotropic activity. Patients taking beta blockers may have a prolongation of the P-R interval on their ECG tracing.

Class 3 Drugs. The class 3 drugs act primarily to prolong the refractory period of cardiac tissue, thereby slowing repolarization and making it more difficult for myocardial cells to respond to stimulation. They may be effective in both SVT and VT. Amiodarone (Cordarone), one of the two drugs currently in this class, has properties of class 1A, 2, 3, and 4 agents. Amiodarone may adversely affect a variety of bodily systems, causing the following effects: exacerbation of arrhythmias, sinus bradycardia, photosensitivity, hepatotoxicity, skin pigmentation, corneal deposits, peripheral neuropathy, alveolitis, and general malaise.

Class 4 Drugs. Class 4 drugs primarily block the slow calcium channel. Like class 1 drugs, they prolong the refractory period and decrease pacemaker activity of depolarized cells. The ECG of a patient on calcium-channel blockers may show a prolonged P-R interval and no effect on the QRS complex. Verapamil (Isoptin, Calan) demonstrates the most antiarrhythmic properties in this class and is significantly more effective in the treatment of SVT than of VT.

Digitalis

Digitalis, not found in the preceding classification, is a cardiac glycoside that may also be used in arrhythmia management. In the healthy heart, it directly enhances vagal tone (parasympathetic nervous system), whereas in the failing heart, it depresses adrenergic action (sympathetic nervous system); both actions result in slowing the heart and depressing conduction through the atrioventricular node. Hence, digitalis can be used to prevent conduction of atrial arrhythmias into the ventricles. Digitalis administration, however, can predispose an individual to arrhythmias, owing to its action on the electrophysiologic properties of the heart. Commonly used in the treatment of conges-

tive heart failure, digitalis "poisons" (inhibits) the sodium-potassium pump (review previous section in this chapter). This causes excessive calcium to accumulate in the cell, along with intracellular sodium. Although this increased calcium enhances myocardial cell contraction, thereby ameliorating heart failure, the increased sodium causes a decrease in intracellular potassium. As intracellular potassium falls, maximal diastolic membrane potential decreases (less negativity), and the slope of phase 4 depolarization increases (see Fig. 14–4). The resultant increase in automaticity and ectopic activity can increase the likelihood of arrhythmias. Hence, whether prescribed for heart failure or management of rapid atrial heart rates, serum digitalis concentration and electrolyte levels should be monitored carefully.

Clinical Considerations

Pharmacologic management of arrhythmias is most successful when approached in a systematic fashion. First, adequate documentation of the arrhythmia is made by clinical evaluation, electrocardiogram, or electrophysiologic study. Assessment of hemodynamic compromise, consequences, and symptom prevalence in an emergency or long-term care setting is considered. Second, once a drug is chosen, its efficacy is evaluated by clinical and electrocardiographic observation with possible electrophysiologic study. Third, the adequacy of the dosage is measured by determination of drug concentration in the blood. Intolerance to antiarrhythmic agents and drug toxicity are common problems. Current prescription of antiarrhythmics is empirical, and several agents may need to be tried before one is found that is both effective and well tolerated by the patient. Rapid advances in electrophysiologic study and testing have helped verify the effectiveness of certain agents. Additionally, as this technology progresses, new combinations of drugs are developed (see Table 14–10).

Health professionals responsible for monitoring the exercise response of patients on antiarrhythmic agents should understand the basis of arrhythmia production and suppression. Exercise is commonly the culprit in the production of arrhythmias (Table 14–11). However, abnormal electrolyte levels or toxic levels of a drug may be responsible for cardiac rhythm disturbances. A medication prescribed to inhibit arrhythmias can in fact become

Table 14–11
Associations of Arrhythmias with Exercise

Normal cardiovascular system
Coronary artery disease
Mitral valve prolapse
Left ventricular trabeculations
Digitalis
Hypokalemia
Cardiomyopathy
Left ventricle outflow obstruction
Aortic stenosis
Hypertrophic cardiomyopathy
Long–Q-T interval syndromes
Idiopathic
Quinidine induced
Phenothiazine induced
Proarrhythmias due to antiarrhythmic drugs
   (Flecainide)
Pulmonary disease

Source: Froelicher V, Marcondes G. Manual of Exercise Testing. St. Louis, CV Mosby, 1989, p 303.

arrhythmogenic if therapeutic serum levels are exceeded. Arrhythmias, regardless of their etiology, must be interpreted by the health care provider. The hemodynamic effects and potential consequences of the arrhythmia dictate subsequent patient management and program planning.

ANTIHYPERTENSIVE THERAPY

Although surveys vary, an estimated 10% to 15% of North Americans have arterial hypertension (defined elsewhere in text).[20, 21] Of those who obtain medical treatment, most are prescribed diet or exercise or drug therapy, or a combination of these. The goal of hypertensive therapy is to prevent the negative effects of chronic blood pressure elevation. Sustained hypertension results in increased morbidity and mortality rates associated with renal failure, coronary disease, and stroke. Owing to the absence of symptoms from high blood pressure and the numerous side effects of available drug agents, noncompliance with therapy is common. Further risk of noncompliance is created by the frequent use of multiple drugs to control blood pressure.

Physiology

A number of physiologic factors combine to create normotension in the cardiovascular system. At any one moment, several mechanisms interact to maintain adequate pressure in the circulation to allow vital systems to function. Carotid baroreceptors and kidney sensors detect changes in blood pressure and trigger appropriate alterations in cardiac output and peripheral vascular resistance to maintain normotension. These alterations are regulated at three anatomic sites: the arterioles, the postcapillary venules, and the heart. A fourth site, the kidneys, acts to control blood pressure by regulating intravascular volume (cardiac preload). The sympathetic nervous system and **humoral** mechanisms, that is, renin-angiotensin-aldosterone system, continuously control the interaction of simultaneous changes at each site, influencing compensatory mechanisms between anatomic sites (Fig. 14–6).

Pathophysiology

In the majority of individuals with hypertension, the threshold of stimulation of both the **baroreceptors** and the renal blood volume-pressure control systems is "set" too high.[20, 21] This causes a delay in the initiation of central and peripheral

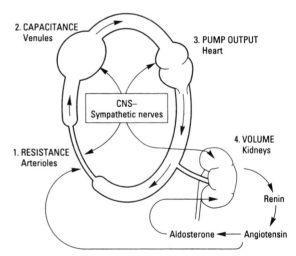

Figure 14–6. Anatomic sites of blood pressure control. (From Katzung BG [ed]. Basic and Clinical Pharmacology. 5th ed. East Norwalk, CT, Appleton & Lange, 1992, p 140.)

changes involved in the maintenance of normotension. Once baroreceptors are stimulated, the sympathetic nervous system and the kidneys usually respond normally. However, just as in normotensive individuals, if one anatomic site is "blocked" for some reason (e.g., disease, drug), other sites compensate to maintain a blood pressure level that no longer stimulates the baroreceptors. When this baseline blood pressure level is pathologically elevated, another of the remaining three anatomic sites of blood pressure regulation warrants blocking. Hence several pharmacologic agents are used to "limit" multiple normal physiologic blood pressure control mechanisms. The use of several agents also allows lower dosages of each agent and hence fewer side effects from each drug.

Pharmacologic Intervention

Classification of antihypertensive drugs is related to their primary receptor site and mode of action.

- Diuretics, which act on kidneys to reduce volume
- Those that act to limit sympathetic nervous system activity
- Vasodilators (arterial and venous)
- Those that act on the renin-angiotensin-aldosterone system at the kidney

At present, no drug has been found effective and safe in directly altering baroreceptor activity. Newer agents have been developed that act on two or more of the anatomic sites of blood pressure control. For example, a diuretic and beta blocker, or diuretic and ACE inhibitor, may be combined into one pill or tablet to facilitate patient self-management. Names of these drugs are beyond the scope of this text but can be found in any current pharmacopoeia.

Diuretics

Alterations in intravascular blood volume have a significant effect on blood pressure. Diuretics, the most commonly prescribed antihypertensive agents, act to reduce circulating volume and thereby lower blood pressure. Acting at various sites along the renal tubule or Henle's loop, diuretics will alter the reabsorption of sodium, consequently affecting the retention of water (Fig. 14–7). Furosemide

(Lasix), a **"loop" diuretic,** acts on the medullary ascending limb of Henle's loop and has the greatest diuresing effect. Carbonic anhydrase inhibitors, acting on the proximal tubules, and potassium-sparing diuretics, acting on the collecting tubules and ducts, are the most mild diuretics. The **sulfonamide diuretics** (thiazides and thiazide-like drugs) have moderate diuretic effects. These act on the cortical ascending limb of Henle's loop and the distal tubule. Thiazides are a frequently prescribed diuretic; however, they have been associated with hyperlipidemia when administered in high doses.

Clinical Considerations. The physician may choose to prescribe diuretic therapy from a long list of agents (Table 14–12). The choice of diuretic depends on the severity of the hypertension and the drug's side effects. The potency of the drug is dependent on its site of action in the **nephron** (see Fig. 14–7). Combinations of diuretics can be prescribed to treat hypertension. Caution should be used when patients taking diuretics are encouraged to participate in aerobic exercise. Volume reduction and electrolyte disturbances can predispose the exercising individual to hypotension or arrhythmias, respectively. Hypokalemia can be a serious consequence of diuretic therapy when

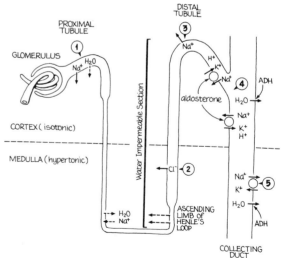

Figure 14–7. Sites of action of diuretic agents in the nephron: (1) carbonic anhydrase inhibitors; osmotic diuretics; (2) "loop" diuretics; (3) sulfonamide diuretics; (4) aldosterone antagonists; (5) potassium-sparing diuretics. (From Marquez-Julio A, Whiteside C. Diuretics. In: Kalant H, Roschlau W, Sellers M [eds]. Principles of Medical Pharmacology. 4th ed. New York, Oxford University Press, 1985.)

Table 14–12		

Antihypertensive Agents

CATEGORY	GENERIC (TRADE NAME)	COMMENTS
Diuretics		
High ceiling (loop)	Bumetanide (Bumex, Burinex) Ethacrynic acid (Edecrin) Furosemide (Lasix, Furomide, Dryptal) Frusemide (Frusetic, Frusid) Piretanide (Arlix)	Mild to severe hypokalemia may occur with diuretics, necessitating K^+ supplementation.
Sulfonamide (thiazide and thiazide-like)	Hydrochlorothiazide* (HydroDIURIL, Esidrix, Oretic, Direma) Chlorothiazide (Diuril, Saluric) Quinethazone (Hydromox, Aquamox) Bendroflumethiazide (Naturetin) Methylclothiazide (Duretic, Enduron, Aquatensen) Polythiazide (Renese) Trichlormethiazide (Naqua, Metahydrin) Metolazone (Zaroxylin, Mykrox, Diulo) Indapamide (Lozol, Natrilix) Chlorthalidone* (Hygroton) Bendrofluazide (Aprinox, Centyl, others) Benzthiazide (Aquatag, Exna, Hydrex) Cyclothiazide (Anhydron [discontinued]) Hydroflumethiazide (Diurcardin, Hydrenox, Saluron) Cyclopenthiazide (Navidrex)	
Carbonic anhydrase inhibitors	Acetazolamide (Diamox) Dichlorphanamide (Daranide) Methazolamide (Neptazane)	
Potassium-sparing	Spironolactone (Aldactone, Alatone) Triamterene (Dyrenium, Dytac) Amiloride (Midamor) Potassium canrenoate (Spiroctan-M)	Hyperkalemia may occur with K^+-sparing agents.
Osmotic combination diuretics	Mannitol (Osmitrol) Hydrochlorothiazide and: Triamterene (Dyazide, Maxzide) Spironolactone (Aldactazide) Amiloride hydrochloride (Moduretic, Moduret) Frusemide and: Amiloride (Frumil) Triamterene (Frusene)	
Sympathetic Nervous System Inhibition		
Central nervous system acting	Clonidine (Catapres) Methyldopa (Aldomet)	May have side effects of sedation, mental depression, and sleep disturbances.
Ganglion blocking	Trimethaphan (Arfonad) Mecamylamine (Inversine) Reserpine (Serpasil)	
Postganglion blocking	Guanethidine (Ismelin Sulfate) Guanadrel (Hylorel)	May cause hypotension that is increased with exercise and upright posture.

Table 14–12

Antihypertensive Agents *Continued*

CATEGORY	GENERIC (TRADE NAME)	COMMENTS
Alpha$_1$-adrenergic blocking	Prazosin (Minipress) Phenoxybenzamine (Dibenzyline) Terazosin (Hytrin) Trimazosin (Cardovar) Phentolamine† (Regitine) Doxazosin mesylate (Cardura)	Prazosin is both a venous and an arterial dilator.
Alpha$_1$- and alpha$_2$-adrenergic blocking	Phenoxybenzamine (Dibenzyline) Phentolamine (Regitine)	Useful in treating pheochromocytoma HTN; decreases peripheral vascular resistance; increases cardiac output
Beta-adrenergic blocking ***Vasodilators***	See beta blockers, Table 14–5	
Venodilators Arteriolar dilators	Nitrates (see Table 15–6) Hydralazine (Apresoline) Minoxidil (Loniten) Diazoxide (Hyperstat IV) Calcium-channel blockers (see Table 14–8)	Hydralazine and Minoxidil are used for outpatient, long-term therapy, while nitroprusside and diazoxide are parenteral agents, used in emergent conditions; Ca^{++} channel blockers are used in both acute and chronic conditions.
Combination arteriolar and venodilator ***Angiotensin-Converting Enzyme Inhibitor***	See alpha$_1$-adrenergic blockers, above Nitroprusside (Nipride)	Nitroprusside is preferred over IV alpha$_1$-adrenergic blockers.
	Captopril (Capoten) Enalapril (Vasotec) Lisinopril (Zestril, Prinivil) Quinapril HCL (Accupril) Fosinopril sodium (Monopril) Benazepril (Lotensin) Ramipril (Altace) Moexipril (Univasc)	Severe hypotension in some patients who are hypovolemic due to diuretics, salt restriction, or gastrointestinal fluid loss. Dry hacking cough in 15–20% of patients
Angiotensin II Receptor Antagonist	Losartan (Cozaar) Candesartan cilexetil (Atacand) Irbesartan (Avapro) Telmisartan (Micardis) Valsartan (Diovan)	Additive effects with hydrochlorothiazide; may be better tolerated than ACE inhibitors; side effects of dizziness, insomnia, leg cramps, GI symptoms, upper respiratory effects

*Diuretic agents most commonly used and least expensive.
†Blocks alpha$_2$ receptors also; given by intravenous infusion, it has a rapid action, lasts only minutes, and is expensive.

potent agents are prescribed. Usually potassium supplementation is prescribed to prevent a potentially unstable electrolyte environment. Hyperkalemia may occur with potassium-sparing diuretics.

Drugs Acting on the Sympathetic Nervous System

Blood pressure is influenced by sympathetic nervous system regulation of cardiac output and pe-

ripheral vascular resistance. Pharmacologic agents can be used to alter sympathetic nervous system activity to control blood pressure in the following ways (see Table 14–12):

• Centrally acting compounds reduce neural transmission from vasopressor centers in the brainstem, inhibiting vasoconstriction.
• Ganglionic blockers limit vasoconstriction that is normally mediated by norepinephrine released at autonomic ganglia. However, parasympathetic

nervous system inhibition occurs with these drugs also.

- Postganglionic blockers inhibit norepinephrine release from postganglionic adrenergic neurons in the heart and vessels, thereby reducing cardiac output and limiting vasoconstriction.
- Blocking alpha adrenoceptors in arterioles and venules prevents vasoconstriction normally induced by norepinephrine; hence, peripheral vascular resistance is reduced.
- Blocking beta adrenoceptors in heart and juxtaglomerular cells responsible for the release of renin limits cardiac output and vasoconstriction, respectively.

Clinical Considerations. A typical second drug group used to control hypertension when a mild diuretic alone is ineffective is the beta-adrenergic blocking agents (see Table 14–5). If these drugs cannot be prescribed because of their negative inotropy or chronotropy, vasomotor center-acting agents typically can be used. Potential side effects and frequency of drug administration are also considered in making decisions about the appropriate sympathetic nervous system inhibition therapy for hypertension.

Vasodilators

This group of antihypertensive drugs acts directly on vascular smooth muscle cells to reduce peripheral vascular resistance (arterial dilation) or venous return to the heart (venous dilation). Systolic hypertension can be treated effectively with arterial dilators. Hydralazine (Apresoline), minoxidil (Loniten), and diazoxide (Hyperstat IV) are examples of arterial dilators. Calcium-channel blockers reduce blood pressure by inhibiting actin and myosin coupling within vascular smooth muscle, thereby promoting smooth muscle dilation (discussed earlier in this chapter). Venodilators are especially effective in the treatment of diastolic hypertension because they reduce cardiac preload and end-diastolic pressure (see Table 14–12). Sodium nitroprusside (Nipride) is both a venous and arterial dilator. Vasodilators can be administered either orally or intravenously; the latter the route of choice for rapid treatment of malignant hypertension.

In response to vasodilation, compensatory sympathetic activation such as tachycardia, reflex vaso-

constriction, increased aldosterone, and elevated plasma renin often occurs. For these reasons, in the management of hypertension, vasodilators are usually used in combination with beta blocking or other sympathetic nervous system-inhibiting drugs. In addition, simultaneous diuretic therapy can limit fluid retention caused by the compensatory increase in aldosterone associated with the use of vasodilators.

Drugs Acting on the Renin-Angiotensin System

Three of the stimulants for renin production by the renal cortex are (1) a drop in renal artery pressure, (2) sympathetic nervous system stimulation, and (3) sodium reduction. Renin reacts to form angiotensin I, and in the presence of a converting enzyme (ACE), angiotensin I forms angiotensin II (Fig. 14–8). This latter substance is a potent vasoconstrictor that influences aldosterone production and subsequent sodium retention, all factors that result in blood pressure elevation. Unlike vasodilators, ACE inhibitors do not result in reflex sympathetic nervous system activity. Studies provide strong evidence of the efficacy of ACE inhibitors in blood pressure management in patients with depressed ejection fraction, further accounting for their escalating utilization (see Table 14–12).[11]

A new class of antihypertensive agents act as angiotensin II receptor antagonists. These agents specifically block angiotensin II receptors. As a result, vasoconstriction and aldosterone secretions are reduced. Blood pressure is lowered by decreased vascular tone and decreased water and sodium retention (see Table 14–12).[22]

PHARMACOLOGIC MANAGEMENT OF LIPID DISORDERS

In 1985 a turning point occurred in the awareness and management of lipid disorders in the United States. In that year the National Institutes of Health Consensus Conference concluded what many practitioners had believed for years: elevated blood cholesterol levels, especially low-density lipoprotein

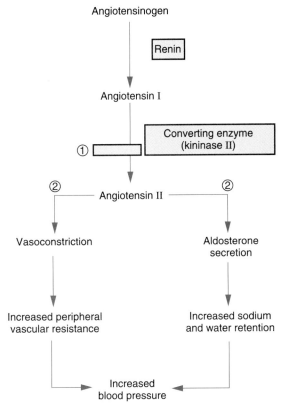

Figure 14-8. Site of action of captopril (Capoten) blockade at 1 and angiotensin II receptor blockade at 2. (Adapted from Katzung BG [ed]. Basic and Clinical Pharmacology. 5th ed. East Norwalk, CT, Appleton & Lange, 1992.)

(LDL), were associated with premature coronary heart disease and, most important for clinical practice, lowering the LDL levels decreased the risk of developing coronary heart disease. The panel recommended guidelines for treatment, including dietary and pharmacologic interventions as well as screening programs to identify persons at risk. Since that time people have become familiar with the terms *good cholesterol* (HDL) *bad cholesterol* (LDL), and *saturated fat,* not only from the medical establishment but also from the media, food corporations, and fast-food restaurants. Thus, early detection of lipid abnormalities has improved because of advances within the medical community and as a result of consumer education.

Cholesterol is a naturally occurring fatlike substance that is found within various tissues of the body: cell membranes, hormones, and plasma. Approximately 93% of all cholesterol is found in cell membranes, and the other 7% circulates within the blood plasma. A relatively small amount of the circulating cholesterol is used by the adrenals and gonads for hormone synthesis, and another small proportion is used by peripheral cells in building and maintaining membranous structures. Cholesterol is transported in the blood within a lipid molecule, which in turn is carried by *lipoproteins.* Therefore, because cholesterol is attached to the lipoproteins within the blood, assessment of cholesterol abnormalities involves lipoprotein assessment.

Three specific lipoproteins carry blood cholesterol:

- Low-density lipoproteins (LDL)
- High-density lipoproteins (HDL)
- Very low density lipoproteins (VLDL)

Triglycerides, a glycerol molecule with three fatty acid chains, makes up about 80% of VLDL with the remaining 20% being cholesterol.

Hypercholesterolemia is defined as elevated plasma cholesterol concentration greater than 240 mg/dL with normal triglycerides; HDL deficiency is identified as an HDL cholesterol level less than 35 mg/dL with normal VLDL and LDL. There are five types of lipid abnormalities that have been associated with an increased risk for atherosclerosis (Table 14–13). These types generally present as some combination of increased LDL, decreased HDL, increased triglycerides, and increased total cholesterol.

Drug therapy is recommended after at least a 6-month trial of diet in all patients without coronary artery disease (CAD) or CAD risk factors. With LDL cholesterol levels higher than 190 mg/dL the goal is to reduce LDL cholesterol levels to less than 160 mg/dL. Drug therapy is also recommended after dietary therapy in patients with 2 or more CAD risk factors and LDL cholesterol higher than 160 mg/dL with the goal of reducing the LDL level to < 130 mg/dL. In patients with known CAD or atherosclerotic vascular disease, the goal of drug and nutritional therapy is to reduce LDL to 100 mg/dL or less. The most commonly used medications for lipid reduction include anion exchange resins, niacin, fibric acid derivatives, HMG CoA reductase inhibitors, and fish oils.[23] The goal of lipid management is to decrease lipid levels by a combination of diet, exercise, and med-

Table 14–13

Lipid Abnormalities

LIPID	ABNORMALITY
Type I:	Normal total cholesterol Increased triglycerides ? Low HDL
Type II: IIa:	Increased total cholesterol Increased LDL Normal triglycerides
IIb:	Increased LDL Increased VLDL Increased total cholesterol Increased triglycerides
Type III:	Increased LDL Increased total cholesterol Increased triglycerides
Type IV:	Increased triglycerides Increased VLDL Normal total cholesterol
Type V:	Increased triglycerides Increased cholesterol Increased VLDL

HDL, high-density lipoprotein; LDL, low-density lipoprotein; VLDL, very low density lipoprotein.

ications as needed to attain acceptable levels. See Table 14–14 for drug management.

Side Effects

Some of the more common side effects include the following: gastrointestinal distress (e.g., constipation, diarrhea, nausea), liver function abnormalities, skin rashes and flushing (especially with niacin), increased bleeding time (especially with fish oils), slight increase in gallstone formation (gemfibrozil); increased blood glucose levels (niacin), and potential to worsen glucose levels in diabetics (niacin).

Lovastatin may contribute to headaches, sleep disturbances, decreased sleep duration, fatigue, and muscle cramping. **Pravastatin,** another HMG-CoA reductase inhibitor, does not cross the blood-brain barrier as does lovastatin and therefore may have less effect on the central nervous system.

Table 14–14

Classifications of Lipid-Lowering Drugs

ANION EXCHANGE RESINS/BILE ACID SEQUESTRANTS

Cholystyramine (Questran)
Colestipol (Colestid)

Primary Effect:

Decreases LDL
  (1) binds intestinal bile, causing fecal excretion of bile acids
  (2) increase LDL receptor activity

FIBRIC ACID DERIVATIVES

Clofibrate (Atromid-S)
Gemfibrozil (Lopid)
Fenofibrate (not available in U.S.)

Primary Effect:

Decreases triglycerides
  (1) reduces ability of free fatty acids to form triglycerides
  (2) increases intravascular breakdown of VLDL

Secondary Effect:

Increases activity of lipoprotein lipase

Useful in Treating:

Type IIa, type IIb

HMG–CoA REDUCTASE INHIBITOR/"STATINS"

Lovastatin (Mevacor)
Pravastatin (Pravachol)
Simvastatin (Zocor)
Fluvastatin (Lescol)
Atorvastatin (Lipitor)
Cervistatin (Baycol)

Primary Effect:

Decreases LDL
  (1) increases LDL receptor activity
  (2) inhibits cholesterol synthesis

Secondary Effect:

Increases HDL

Useful in Treating:

Type IIa, type IIb; type III; type IV; type V

NICOTINIC ACID

Niacin

Primary Effect:

Decreases LDL, decreases triglycerides
  (1) reduces hepatic synthesis of VLDL
  (2) decreases plasma levels of free fatty acids

Table 14–14
Classifications of Lipid-Lowering Drugs *Continued*

Secondary Effect:
Increases HDL

Useful in Treating:
Type IIa, type IIb; type III

FISH OILS

Omega-3 fatty acid (many over-the-counter varieties, e.g., superEPA)

Primary Effect:
Decreases triglycerides

Useful in Treating:
Type IIa, type IIb, type III, type IV; type V

LDL, low-density lipoprotein; VLDL, very low density lipoprotein; HDL, high-density lipoprotein.
Source: Adapted from Rakel R.: Conn's Current Therapy 1999. Philadelphia, WB Saunders, 1999, p 570.

Adverse side effects are more likely with combinations of drug therapy rather than single agent management; for example, HMG-CoA reductase agents (stains), when combined with niacin, increases the risk of liver toxicity; stains with gemfibrozil or niacin may provoke myosistis, muscle tenderness, and fatigue. Caution must be observed in prescribing fibric acids for patients who are on oral anticoagulants, as their anticoagulation effect may be potentiated.

Clinical Considerations

Because of the potential for worsening glucose levels, niacin and fish oils are not recommended for the diabetic patient. Liver enzyme levels should be checked within the first 6 weeks and again at 3- and 6-month intervals as needed for patients on lovastatin, niacin, and gemfibrozil. General fatigue, achiness, and abdominal discomfort may accompany elevated lipid levels. Patients who exercise and take lovastatin often complain of muscle achiness and should be evaluated for possible drug-induced side effects and exercise intolerance.

CARDIAC DRUGS USED IN CRITICAL CARE

Many pathologic conditions warrant observation and management in the critical care setting. The hemodynamic instability caused by an underlying pathologic condition often requires quick responsiveness by the medical staff. Administration of appropriate pharmacologic agents and close monitoring of their effects can significantly alter the outcome of therapy. Numerous cardiovascular conditions may be responsible for systemic compromise. Common etiologies include

- Acute myocardial ischemia or infarct
- Congestive heart failure and pulmonary edema
- Cardiac structural abnormalities
- Cardiac conduction system disease

Clinical presentations of these cardiac dysfunctions may include

- Hypoxia
- Pain
- Alterations in blood pressure (e.g., hypertension or hypotension)
- Shock
- Alterations in heart rate
- Heart rhythm abnormalities

Whenever possible, drug therapy is directed at removal of the underlying pathologic condition, for example, thrombolysis (discussed elsewhere in this chapter). In addition to providing the patient with oxygen to help reverse hypoxia, pharmacologic therapy may focus on the manipulation of the autonomic nervous system to favorably alter hemodynamics. Drug agonists and antagonists of the parasympathetic and sympathetic nervous systems are used to induce changes in vasomotor tone, cardiac inotropy, and chronotropy. Cardiac output may be further improved by the administration of antihypertensive agents (those acting independent of the autonomic nervous system) and antiarrhythmic drugs. Elimination of pain, induction of sedation, and prevention of the complications of bedrest may also be addressed with drug therapy in the critical care setting.

Pharmacologic management of the patient in the cardiac critical care setting is often guided by invasive measurement as well as by symptoms. For example, when prescribing a vasodilator, the physician must closely monitor left ventricular filling pressures **(preload)** and cardiac output. Patients with dyspnea and high-filling pressures might benefit from venodilators to reduce preload, whereas patients with fatigue and low cardiac output might benefit from arteriodilators to improve forward output.[24] Table 14–15 categorizes hemodynamic indices found in acute myocardial infarction and suggests guidelines for use of pharmacologic agents in this setting.

Oxygen

Although oxygen is not frequently thought of as a drug, it should be thought of as a drug, and it warrants a brief discussion in the context of pharmacologic considerations in cardiac critical care. Tissue hypoxia caused by disturbances in cardiac output can rarely be improved by the administration of oxygen. However, oxygen therapy is usually beneficial when concomitant hypoxemia exists.[25] Pulmonary edema, often a finding with congestive heart failure, can hinder oxygen diffusion in the lung, thereby decreasing arterial oxygen content. The administration of oxygen may help limit the severity of hypoxemia and consequent tissue hypoxia. In addition, when hemoglobin concentration is reduced, as in anemia or in conditions that cause hemoglobin to **desaturate,** the administra-

tion of oxygen is considered beneficial. Oxygen delivery systems are discussed in Chapter 10.

Agents That Affect the Autonomic Nervous System

The autonomic nervous system (ANS) exerts significant control over cardiovascular function. A complex system of feedback loops coordinates reflex responses of the sympathetic and the parasympathetic nervous systems. Transmission of impulses from the autonomic portion of the central nervous system to the effector organ to be stimulated occurs via neurotransmitter substances. As discussed in the introduction, most preganglionic fibers, and all parasympathetic nervous system postganglionic fibers, release *acetylcholine.* Most sympathetic nervous system postganglionic fibers release norepinephrine (noradrenaline). These substances can be partially or completely mimicked by pharmacologic agents (e.g., sympathomimetics, parasympathomimetics, or sympathetic or parasympathetic nervous system agonists). Similarly, receptors in the effector organ can be partially or completely blocked by pharmacologic agents (e.g., adrenoceptor or cholinoceptor blocking agents or sympathetic or parasympathetic nervous system antagonists).

Table 14–15

Suggested Therapeutic Interventions in Relation to Hemodynamic Indices Found in Acute Myocardial Infarction

HEMODYNAMIC CATEGORY	CARDIAC OUTPUT	LEFT VENTRICULAR FILLING PRESSURE	SUGGESTED THERAPY
Normal	Normal	Normal	Observation
Hypovolemia	Decreased	Decreased or normal	Volume replacement
Pulmonary congestion	Normal	Raised	Diuretics
Left ventricular failure			
Moderate	Decreased	Raised	Afterload reducing agents, with or without diuretics
Severe (cardiogenic shock)	Markedly decreased	Raised	Circulatory assist (counterpulsation) Afterload reducing agents Use of inotropic agents if other measures do not increase cardiac output*

*E.g., dopamine (Intropion, Dopastat), dobutamine (Dobutrex).
Adapted from Sokolow M, McIlroy M, Cheitlin M. Clinical Cardiology. 5th ed. East Norwalk, Conn, Appleton & Lange, 1990.

When negative alterations in mean arterial blood pressure are sensed, **adrenoceptors** and **cholinoceptors** are stimulated. Appropriate modification of peripheral vascular resistance and cardiac output are orchestrated (Fig. 14–9). In a critically ill cardiac patient, pharmacologic agents can act on the autonomic nervous system receptors to help bring about a hemodynamic stability and an effective cardiac output. By fine manipulation of the degree of vasodilation, vasoconstriction, or cardiac inotropy, an adequate mean arterial blood pressure can be established with drug therapy. Table 14–16 lists drugs that act as agonists or antagonists to the sympathetic and parasympathetic nervous systems to control blood pressure in the critical care setting. Because of the reflex nature of the feedback "loop" of the autonomic nervous system, the effects of these agents are monitored closely. Although some drugs are receptor selective, some act on multiple receptor sites. Often drugs are used in combinations in an attempt to reduce or augment certain hemodynamic responses, which further emphasizes the importance of medical observation. Epinephrine (Adrenalin Chloride), for example, is both an alpha-adrenergic agonist and a beta-adrenergic agonist; clinically, however, it usually acts only as a beta agonist.

Non-ANS Antihypertensive Agents

In addition to manipulating the autonomic nervous system with drugs to manage arterial blood pressure in critical care, physicians can also prescribe other antihypertensive agents. Sodium nitro-

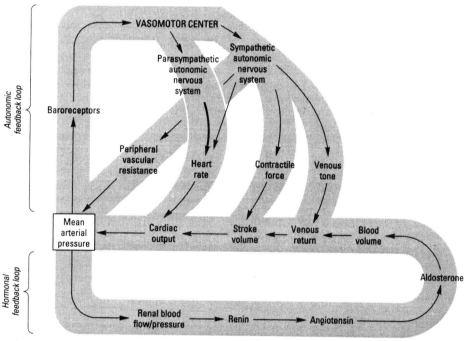

Figure 14–9. Autonomic and hormonal control of cardiovascular function. Note that at least two feedback loops are present: the autonomic nervous system loop and the hormonal loop. In addition, each major loop has several components. Thus, the sympathetic nervous system directly influences four major variables: peripheral vascular resistance, heart rate, force, and venous tone. The parasympathetic nervous system directly influences heart rate. Angiotensin II directly increases peripheral vascular resistance (not shown), and the sympathetic nervous system directly increases renin secretion (not shown). Because these control mechanisms are designed to maintain normal blood pressure, the net feedback effect of each loop is negative in that it tends to compensate for the change in arterial blood pressure that evoked the response. Thus, decreased blood pressure due to blood loss would be compensated for by increased sympathetic outflow and renin release. Conversely, elevated pressure due to the administration of a vasoconstrictor drug would cause reduced sympathetic outflow and renin release and increased parasympathetic (vagal) outflow. (From Katzung BG [ed]. Basic and Clinical Pharmacology. 5th ed. East Norwalk, CT, Appleton & Lange, 1992, p 76.)

Table 14–16

Drugs Affecting the Autonomic Nervous System: Agents Commonly Used in Critical Care

AUTONOMIC NERVOUS SYSTEM RECEPTOR	ACTION	AGONIST GENERIC (TRADE) NAME	ANTAGONIST GENERIC (TRADE) NAME
ADRENOCEPTOR Alpha$_1$	Contraction of vascular smooth muscle	Phenylephrine (Neo-Synephrine) Methoxamine (Vasoxyl)	See antihypertensives, Table 14–12 (alpha$_1$ blockers)
Alpha$_2$	Contraction of vascular smooth muscle Platelet aggregation	Clonidine (Catapres) Alpha-methyl-norepinephrine	Tolazoline (Priscoline) Yohimbine (Yohimex)
Combined alpha$_1$ and alpha$_2$		Epinephrine* (Adrenalin Chloride) Norepinephrine† (Levophed)	Phentolamine (Rogitine)
Beta$_1$	Increased force and rate of cardiac contraction	Norepinephrine† (Levophed) Dobutamine (Dobutrex) Prenalterol (investigational)	See beta blockers, Table 14–5
Beta$_2$	Relaxation of vascular, respiratory smooth muscle	Albuterol (Proventil, Ventolin) Terbutaline (Brethine) Metaproterenol (Alupent, Metaprel)	See beta blockers, Table 14–5
Combined beta$_1$ and beta$_2$		Isoproterenol‡ (Isuprel) Epinephrine* (Adrenalin Chloride)	See beta blockers, Table 14–5
Dopaminic	Vasodilation	Dopamine (Intropin)	
CHOLINOCEPTOR Muscarinic	Decreased rate and force of atrial conractoin Decreased peripheral vascular resistance	Acetylcholine (Miochol) Edrophonium§ (Tensilon)	Atropine (Isopto Atropine)

*Epinephrine is also called adrenalin; it acts primarily as a beta agonist.
†Norepinephrine is also called noradrenalin or levarterenol.
‡Isoproterenol is also called isoprenaline.
§This is not a direct-acting agonist; rather it acts indirectly by inhibiting acetylcholinesterase, thereby increasing acetylcholine.

prusside (Nipride), a potent peripheral vasodilator, and intravenous nitroglycerin are frequently used. The intravenous nitroglycerin produces a slightly greater reduction in preload and a slightly lesser reduction in afterload as compared with those of sodium nitroprusside.[26] Although both agents are effective in reducing blood pressure, the intravenous nitroglycerin is the emergency drug of choice in the treatment of congestive heart failure associated with ischemic heart disease. Sodium nitroprusside is the parenteral treatment of choice for hypertension emergencies.

As discussed earlier in this chapter, diuretics act to reduce central venous pressures by decreasing venous return. Furosemide (Lasix) is a potent, rapidly acting diuretic, often administered parenterally in the emergency treatment of pulmonary congestion in the presence of left ventricular dysfunction.

Antiarrhythmic Agents

Life-threatening arrhythmias are commonly treated in cardiac critical care units. In addition to electrical cardioversion of unstable rhythms, pharmacologic intervention is the mainstay of medical treatment. Lidocaine (Xylocaine) is the drug of choice for the suppression of ventricular ectopy in critically ill patients. It is used both **prophylactically** for patients with acute myocardial ischemia and therapeutically for patients suffering ventricular tachycardia or fibrillation. In emergencies, it is delivered as a bolus injection that is followed by a subsequent continuous intravenous infusion.

When lidocaine (Xylocaine) cannot control ventricular arrhythmias, **procainamide** (Pronestyl) can be useful. **Bretylium tosylate** (Bretylol), a class 3 antiarrhythmic, has been used in the treatment of ventricular fibrillation when lidocaine, procainamide, and electrical defibrillation fail. Verapamil (Isoptin, Calan), a calcium-channel blocker (class 4 antiarrhythmic), has been used in the management of supraventricular tachycardia not requiring **cardioversion.** Acute management of new onset paroxysmal supraventricular tachycardia (PSVT) is often treated with adenosine, a naturally occurring endogenous purine nucleoside. Adenosine (Adenocard) is very effective in terminating PSVT when a reentry pathway involving either the sinus node or AV node is involved, including the tachycardias associated with Wolff-Parkinson-White syndrome. Adenocard is given as a rapid IV bolus; its peak effect occurs within seconds.

Finally, digitalis may be used to control the ventricular response rate to atrial flutter or fibrillation. Unfortunately, it may cause significant toxicity and adverse drug interactions in critically ill patients. Although digitalis may successfully convert **paroxysmal supraventricular tachycardia** to normal sinus rhythm, it may alternatively convert atrial flutter to atrial fibrillation. Digitalis's effects on contractility are less potent than those of sympathomimetic parenteral inotropes, such as dobutamine (Dobutrex) or norepinephrine (Levophed) and therefore digitalis typically is not used for this purpose in critical care.

Other Pharmacologic Agents Used in Critical Care

Other pharmacologic agents frequently used in critical care include anticoagulants, such as heparin (Liquaemin Sodium), sedatives to reduce agitation and anxiety, and analgesics. Morphine sulfate, included in this last group, is the drug of choice for management of myocardial ischemic pain.

However, it is also very useful in the treatment of acute cardiogenic pulmonary edema. It is a potent vasodilator and acts to increase venous capacitance as well as to relieve pulmonary congestion. Electrolyte replacement is also a common occurrence in the management of the critically ill patient. Imbalances of potassium, sodium, or magnesium often occur as a result of compromised renal function and/or excess fluid administration.

As patients become hemodynamically stable, the prescription of many of the potent drugs described in this section is discontinued and replaced by oral medications. Readers interested in additional information regarding drugs used in critical care are encouraged to refer to the *Textbook of Advanced Cardiac Life Support* published by the American Heart Association.

CARDIAC PHARMACOLOGY IN THE GERIATRIC POPULATION

All drugs, not just those prescribed for cardiac problems, may have altered pharmacokinetics and pharmacodynamics in the elderly. Normal aging involves changes in body composition and function (Table 14–17). Specifically, decreases in renal function and altered blood flow (as in coronary artery disease and congestive heart failure) are responsible for adverse or suboptimal reactions to cardiac drugs. The elderly also exhibit increased sensitivity to the toxic effects of cardiac drugs such as antiarrhythmics, digitalis, or beta blockers. Other disease states such as liver or nutritional deficiencies, which often accompany aging, can alter the effectiveness of cardiac drug therapy. In addition, numerous socioeconomic and practical considerations can affect the degree of compliance by the elderly with these drug regimens.

Alteration in Pharmacokinetics

Elderly patients may have difficulty with absorption, distribution, or metabolism of cardiac drugs. Effective drug elimination is dependent on adequate renal function. The typical age-related de-

Table 14–17

Average Changes in Body Composition and Function with Age

AREA OF CHANGE	CHANGE FROM AGE 20 TO AGE 80 (%)
Body fat/total body weight	+35
Plasma volume	−8
Plasma albumin	−10
Plasma globulin	−10
Total body water	−17
Extracellular fluid (from age 20 to age 65)	−40
Conduction velocity	−20
Cardiac index	−40
Glomerular filtration rate	−50
Vital capacity	−60
Cardiac output	−30–40
Splanchnic and renal blood flow	−40

Source: Kalant H, Roschlau W, Sellers M. Principles of Medical Pharmacology. 4th ed. New York, Oxford University Press, 1985, p 68.

cline in kidney competency significantly increases the likelihood of drug accumulation and subsequent toxicity. This problem of drug accumulation is especially relevant with regard to the older patient's cardiac conduction system. The elderly are more susceptible to arrhythmias. Positive inotropes, such as digitalis, and antihypertensive agents, such as diuretics, can be particularly dangerous. These drugs alter electrolytes involved in conduction tissue depolarization. Inadequate drug elimination and consequent accumulation can cause cardiac irritability and a higher incidence of arrhythmias.

"Specific drugs" that are poorly tolerated by older persons include class Ib antiarrhythmics (see Table 14–10). These drugs tend to be associated with mental confusion in this population. The antihypertensives methyldopa, reserpine, and clonidine can decrease mental acuity and produce sedation at increased doses in geriatric individuals (see Table 14–12). In addition, propranolol, a nonselective beta-adrenergic antagonist, can cause confusion, sleep disturbance, and depression in older persons. Postural hypotension can result from certain antihypertensive drugs (e.g., Prazosin initiation) as well as ACE inhibitors used in conjunction with diuretics.[27] The combination of sensitivity to these drugs, and the blunted baroreceptor responsiveness in geriatric patients, enables postural hypotension to occur occasionally.

Therapeutic Indications

Cardiovascular drugs are used for treatment of the same conditions in the elderly as in other age groups. At this time, it appears prudent to reduce lipid levels in both primary and secondary prevention of coronary artery disease, and anticholesterolemic agents may be prescribed.

Socioeconomic Issues

As with most drugs, the effectiveness of cardiovascular agents depends on numerous practical concerns. Elderly patients often demonstrate difficulty with full compliance with drug prescriptions. In addition to financial concerns, they may have several physicians prescribing drugs and no one monitoring the effects of drug combinations. Patients may get confused and forget a dose. When elderly patients feel good, they may choose to discontinue taking the drug, or the side effects themselves may discourage patients from taking the drug. Although these issues may occur in younger age groups, the elderly are especially susceptible to these problems. Dementia or physical inability may also hamper adequate utilization of cardiovascular drugs. Seemingly simple items such as reading drug labels, removing bottle caps, or distinguishing pill color can present major obstacles to visually impaired or physically disabled elderly patients. Drug holders with the day of the week written on each compartment may improve compliance with medications.

Safe and effective use of cardiovascular agents in the geriatric population can be enhanced by knowledgeable health care providers and educated patients and family members. Drug regimens should be simplified whenever possible, with small initial doses and progressive titration until a therapeutic response is reached. Additionally, when working with the older patient, the medical team should remain alert to adverse drug reactions and interactions, taking care to avoid provoking a drug reaction that would be worse than the disease itself.

CARDIAC PHARMACOLOGY IN THE NEONATE AND PEDIATRIC POPULATIONS

Although many pharmacologic agents used to treat adult cardiac conditions are also used to treat **neonate** and pediatric patients, the younger population's response may demonstrate significant clinical differences. The immature organism can demonstrate unpredictable responses because of the unique pharmacokinetic and pharmacodynamic reactions found during each stage of development. Additionally, most cardiac drug activity has been studied in adults, and the paucity of controlled research on the immature patient causes further concern regarding optimal drug therapy in this population.

Alteration in Pharmacokinetics

Adequate plasma concentrations of a drug can be influenced by proper administration and absorption of the agent. Newborns absorb drugs more slowly than children, whereas children may have difficulty swallowing medicines. Drugs delivered intravenously bypass the absorption process; however, choosing the intravenous route increases the risks of fluid overload. The relative intolerance of infants to the volumes of fluid needed to carry a drug warrants slower rates of infusion and at times negligible concentrations if the drug is eliminated at the same rate.

As the infant develops, changes in body composition and plasma protein binding capacity affect the distribution of a drug. Total body water decreases as adipose tissue increases and fluid shifts between body compartments. Drugs are less avidly bound to plasma proteins in neonates and infants than in children and adults. Development of the liver and kidneys affects metabolism and elimination of a drug, with both organs showing decreased function at birth. However, infants and young children may metabolize drugs faster than adults.

Alteration in Pharmacodynamics

The ability of the infant or child to respond to adequate concentrations of a cardiac drug is influenced by structural concerns that are unique to the developing organism.[28, 29] Although not well studied in humans, fetal and newborn puppies and lambs exhibit (1) stiffer, less compliant ventricles; (2) smaller myocardial cells (adjusted for weight and size); and (3) a higher proportion of noncontractile to contractile tissue (e.g., mitochondria to **myofilaments**) as compared with the adult. Sympathetic nervous system innervation of the heart and periphery are decreased at birth and continue to develop during the first few months of life. Infants and young children have a higher baseline heart rate; this, in combination with a lower stroke volume, which has a limited ability to increase, means that the ways to improve cardiac output with drugs may be impaired.

Therapeutic Indications

Cardiac conditions in pediatric populations that warrant pharmacologic intervention usually include heart failure, blood pressure abnormalities, and arrhythmias. Digoxin (Lanoxin), a commonly used inotrope, is better tolerated in infants and young children than in adults, and usually achieves a satisfactory response at lower doses (normalized for weight and size). Other inotropes frequently used include isoproterenol (Isuprel), dopamine (Intropin, Dopastat), and dobutamine (Dobutrex). Because the immature heart is limited in its ability to increase stroke volume, inotropic agents may be less effective in it than in an adult heart. Therefore, increases in cardiac output may depend on drug-induced increases in heart rate.

Vasodilators such as sodium nitroprusside (Nipride) and nitroglycerin (Nitro-Bid, Nitrostat, and others) are often used in treating patients with severe congestive cardiomyopathy and post–cardiac surgery patients. They are used with special caution in newborns owing to the immature peripheral vascular resistance mechanisms of the sympathetic nervous system and the consequent enhanced risks of hypotension.

Drug therapy for pediatric patients parallels therapy for adults. The same agents are used for the same physiologic abnormalities. The immature heart, lungs, and systemic vascular structures require individualized therapeutic regimens. Understanding the progressive nature of the organism's development and the exact stage of maturity greatly influences the clinical efficacy of cardiac pharmacotherapy for this population.

PHARMACOLOGIC MANAGEMENT OF DIABETES

Pharmacologic management for the diabetic patient includes the use of either oral hypoglycemic agents or insulin (Tables 14–18 and 14–19). Patients with impaired insulin production, insulin resistance, or both are placed on oral agents; patients with chronic insulin deficiency or absence of endogenous insulin production from the beta cells of the pancreas are managed with insulin.

Clinical Considerations

One of the important components of a safe exercise program is avoidance of exercise-induced hypoglycemia. Signs and symptoms of hypoglycemia include

- Weakness
- **Diaphoresis**
- Mental confusion
- Muscle rigidity

For patients with coronary artery disease, angina or an anginal equivalent may occur. In insulin-dependent diabetics, hypoglycemia may occur during or immediately following the exercise session or hours after the session has ended as the muscles are replenishing their energy stores. Knowledge of the type of insulin that a person is taking and avoidance of exercise during its peak effect is crucial to avoid augmentation of exercise-induced hypoglycemia (see Table 14–19). During the beginning days of an exercise program, insulin-dependent patients should monitor their blood glucose both before and after exercise to understand their individualized response to exercise. Patients

Table 14–18

Oral Hypoglycemic Agents Used in Diabetic Management

CATEGORY	GENERIC NAME	TRADE NAME	ACTION
Sulfonylureas			Stimulates pancreatic insulin secretion
First generation	Tolbutamide	Orinase	
	Chlorpropamide	Diabinese	
	Tolazamide	Tolinase	
	Acetohexamide	Dymetor	
Second Generation	Glyburide	Micronase, Diabeta	
	Micronized glyburide	Glynase	
	Glipizide	Glucotrol	
	Glipizide GTS	Glucotrol XL	
	Glimepiride	Amaryl	
	Repaglinide	Prandin	
Biguanides	Metformin	Glucophage	Suppresses hepatic glucose production
Alpha-Glycosidase Inhibitors	Acarbose	Precose	Impairs carbohydrate absorption
	Miglitol		
Thiazolidinediones	Rosiglitazone	Avandia	Enhances insulin sensitivity at peripheral muscle
	Pioglitazone	Actos	

Source: Adapted from Rakel R., Conn's Current Therapy 1999. Philadelphia, WB Saunders, 1999, pp 545–546.

Table 14–19

Types of Insulin

INSULIN	ONSET* (HR)	PEAK ACTION* (HR)	DURATION OF ACTION* (HR)
Short-acting			
Regular	0.5–1.0	2–5	5–8
Semilente	1.0–1.5	3–8	8–16
Intermediate-acting			
NPH	1–1.5	6–14	18–28
Lente	1–2.5	6–14	18–28
Long-acting			
PZI	4–8	None	24–36
Ultralente	4–8	None	24–36
Very rapid acting			
Humalog	0.1–0.5	0.5–2.5	3–4

*Considerable interindividual variation for these times.
NPH, neutral protamine Hagedorn; PZI, protamine zinc insulin.
Source: Rakel R (ed). Conn's Current Therapy 1999. Philadelphia, WB Saunders, 1999, p 551.

should make certain that their blood sugar is appropriate before starting exercise and may need to take a supplemental snack within the 60 to 90 minutes before beginning (Table 14–20). Patients should be encouraged to carry a readily available carbohydrate source, for example, hard candy or jelly beans, and to meet with a nutritionist for specific diet instruction. It is prudent for any physical therapy department that treats insulin-dependent patients to have easy access to juice and sugar.

Patients whose blood sugar level is greater than 250 mg/dL should not exercise until cleared by physician who knows their metabolism because blood sugar may in fact increase in this situation. Blood sugar levels of greater than 250 mg/dL are often accompanied by the presence of **ketones** in the urine. When this occurs, exercise is absolutely contraindicated until improved glycemic control has been established.

Patients should be reminded not to inject insulin into muscle but into subcutaneous tissue. Exercise of a limb that has received an insulin injection should be avoided for at least 60 to 90 minutes or until the peak effect of the insulin has been reached. Exercising the limb sooner than that may cause the insulin effect to peak prematurely because the increased blood flow associated with exercise facilitates the entry of insulin into the blood. As with all patients, adequate fluid intake is important before, during, and after exercise beyond 30 minutes in duration.

Awareness that blisters from ill-fitting footwear may lead to prolonged healing and may develop complications is sufficient reason to instruct patients to choose footwear wisely. Within the physical therapy department, avoiding situations that may bruise the patient is very important for all patients but particularly for diabetic patients. Patients with diabetic **retinopathy** should avoid any head-down position or situation that would cause a blood pressure reading of greater than 180 mm Hg systolic. **Peripheral neuropathy** may make walking on uneven surfaces unsafe for the patient, and routine activities of daily living may be cumbersome and difficult.

Hypoglycemia may also occur in the noninsulin-dependent diabetic patient, although this is not seen as frequently as it is in insulin-dependent patients.

PHARMACOLOGY AND HEART TRANSPLANTATION

Survival after **orthotopic heart transplantation** has improved dramatically since the first procedure was performed in 1967. Advances in drug specificity have played a major role in the current 1-year survival rate, which exceeds 80%.[30] Rejection and infection have been the primary precursors of early

Table 14–20

General Guidelines for Making Food Adjustments for Exercise

TYPE OF EXERCISE AND EXAMPLES	IF BLOOD GLUCOSE IS:	INCREASE FOOD INTAKE BY:	SUGGESTIONS OF FOOD TO USE
Exercise of short duration and of low to moderate intensity (walking a half mile or leisurely bicycling for less than 30 minutes)	Less than 100 mg/dL 100 mg/dL or above	10 to 15 g of carbohydrate per hour Not necessary to increase food	1 fruit or 1 starch/bread exchange
Exercise of moderate intensity (1 hour of tennis, swimming, jogging, leisurely bicycling, golfing, etc.)	Less than 100 mg/dL 100 to 180 mg/dL 180 to 300 mg/dL 300 mg/dL or above	25 to 50 g of carbohydrate before exercise, then 10 to 15 g per hour of exercise 10 to 15 g of carbohydrate Not necessary to increase food Don't begin exercise until blood glucose is under better control	1/2 meat sandwich with a milk or fruit exchange 1 fruit or 1 starch/bread exchange
Strenuous activity or exercise (about 1 to 2 hours of football, hockey, racquetball, or basketball games; strenuous bicycling or swimming; shoveling heavy snow)	Less than 100 mg/dL 100 to 180 mg/dL 180 to 300 mg/dL 300 mg/dL or above	50 g of carbohydrate, monitor blood glucose carefully 25 to 50 g of carbohydrate, depending on intensity and duration 10 to 15 g of carbohydrate Don't begin exercise until blood glucose is under better control	1 meat sandwich (2 slices of bread) with a milk and fruit exchange 1/2 meat sandwich with a milk or fruit exchange 1 fruit or 1 starch/bread exchange

Source: Franz MJ, Norstrom RD, Norstrom J. Diabetes Actively Staying Healthy [DASH]: Your Game Plan for Diabetes and Exercise, Minneapolis, International Diabetes Center, 1990; Wayzata, Minn, DCI Publishing, pp 112–113.

death in this population. A combination of improved techniques used to monitor and detect early rejection and newer **immunosuppressive** pharmacologic agents may account for this reduction in morbidity and mortality rates. Clinical and laboratory research continues in an attempt to identify agents that act on specific components of the **immune system** while leaving other systems unaffected. Thus far, no one drug satisfies this goal. Medical centers vary considerably in their pharmacologic protocols for the heart transplant population.

Immune Mechanism

The immune system is a complex network of humoral and cellular functions that protect human beings from foreign substances (**antigens**). This system is stimulated when a heart is implanted in a patient with end-stage heart disease, because the recipient's immune system recognizes the donor heart as foreign.

Lymphocytes, mononuclear cells that circulate in the blood and lymph, interact with foreign substances to protect the body from invasion. Two types of lymphocytes, T cells and B cells, mediate cellular and humoral immunity, respectively. Current immunosuppressive therapy limits organ rejection by interfering with lymphocyte development, activation, and proliferation.

Pharmacologic Intervention

Corticosteroids

Corticosteroids were the first group of drugs to be recognized as having lympholytic properties. **Prednisone** is the most commonly used immunosuppressor in this drug class. It is **cytotoxic** to certain subsets of T cells and further suppresses **antibody, prostaglandin,** and **leukotriene** synthesis, all important components of the immune system. Lymphocyte formation may be diminished because precursor lymphoid cells (stem cells) are sensitive to prednisone. Unfortunately, long-term use of **steroids** has deleterious sequelae such as **osteoporosis** and impaired healing. The development of additional immunosuppressive agents (as discussed later) has enabled heart transplant recipients to be maintained on lower doses of steroids, thereby reducing the incidence of their negative side effects.

Cyclosporine

Before **cyclosporine** (Sandimmune) began to be used for immunosuppression of patients undergoing heart transplantation, 1-year survival rates were at best 65%.[30] Cyclosporine use, either alone or in combination with prednisone, has resulted in a lower incidence of rejection and infection in this population.[31] This agent appears to act at an early stage in stem cell differentiation to block T cell activation. It does not appear to affect already converted lymphoblasts. The lymphocytes it does affect recover their normal function after the drug is eliminated from the system.

Although cyclosporine appears to be impressive as a highly selective agent that is effective against a subpopulation of lymphocytes, it has a considerable number of side effects. Besides promoting **lymphoma,** cyclosporine causes **nephrotoxicity** and consequent hypertension. Elevated blood pressure due to cyclosporine is usually well controlled by one or two agents, such as ACE inhibitors and beta blockers.[30]

Azathioprine

Azathioprine (Imuran) interferes with the wave of lymphocyte proliferation that occurs after the antigen stimulates the immune system. It is especially effective against T cells but can also block humoral immune responses. Toxicity to azathioprine results in bone marrow depression and hepatic dysfunction. Gastrointestinal disorders may occur at higher doses.

> ### Clinical Note: Drug Interaction
> Keep in mind that all drugs have indications for use and side effects when used alone. However, with multiple drug regimens that are prescribed, there exists the chance of interaction of drugs, and possibly increased side effects—some being negative or counterproductive. When in doubt, consult the pharmacist about the interactions as well as the effect or side effects that are observed.

Antilymphocyte Antibodies

Several medical centers regularly use **antilymphocytic globulin, antithymocytic globulin,** or both for immunosuppression. Injection of an animal (e.g., horse, rabbit) with human lymphocytes provokes the animal's immune mechanism to form antibodies to human lymphocytes. The animal's antilymphocytic globulin can then be injected into the transplant recipient, which ultimately causes cytotoxic destruction of the recipient's lymphocytes. Using these agents does increase the risk of cancer, however, because of the suppression of the normal defense system against carcinogens. Another antibody, OKT3 (a monoclonal antibody), has been found effective in blocking both cytotoxic activity of human T cells and the generation of other T cell function.

CASE STUDIES

Case 1. Anti-Ischemia and Lipid Management

Mr. H is a 52-year-old business executive who underwent a routine physical examination for business insurance reasons. At the time of the physical, he stated that he was feeling fine. On further questioning, he acknowledged that his weekly tennis game was getting a bit slow; in fact he needed to switch from playing singles to playing doubles because he found himself becoming more easily winded. Mr. H attributed this to being out of shape, having slowly gained 20 lb over the last 5 years and having been unable to give up his one pack per day cigarette habit. Blood pressure on the day of the physical was 148/100 mm Hg; the patient stated that he was a little nervous. Random, nonfasting cholesterol total was 270 mg/dL; patient was instructed to have a fasting lipid profile performed within the week. It was recommended that Mr. H have a baseline exercise tolerance test (ETT), to which he agreed.

Mr. H underwent a treadmill ETT using the Bruce protocol; total duration 5 minutes 30 seconds, at which time the test was stopped because Mr. H complained of difficulty breathing and chest heaviness. Vital signs at maximum work capacity were a heart rate of 170, blood pressure of 180/100 mm Hg. The ECG was interpreted as positive for ST-segment depression at a heart rate of 160 and a blood pressure of 170/100. Mr. H was told that his ETT was positive for ischemia and that the medical recommendation at the time was to enter a supervised cardiac rehabilitation program to begin aggressive lifestyle and health habit alterations, including moderate exercise, smoking cessation, education to CAD and medications, nutritional counseling, and stress management strategies. Patient also began taking atenolol and was instructed in the use of sublingual nitroglycerin (NTG).

Mr. H was next seen 2 years later when he came to the emergency department with a chief complaint of chest heaviness unrelieved by nitroglycerin. Patient had been doing yard work when the discomfort first appeared about 2 hours earlier. Mr. H took NTG at the time of the discomfort, but he noted it didn't burn. (The bottle had been opened originally 2 years ago.) He was given one aspirin to chew while he was in the ambulance. In the emergency department, Mr. H's ECG was significant for marked ST-segment elevation in the inferior leads. Medical evaluation determined that Mr. H would be an appropriate candidate for thrombolytic therapy, and he was begun on the hospital's streptokinase protocol and, as soon as he was pain-free, was admitted to the coronary care unit.

In the coronary care unit, the patient continued to follow the streptokinase protocol, including the use of continuous infusion heparin. Patient ruled in for a small inferior myocardial infarction; ejection fraction by cardiac ultrasound was 50%. Mr. H was begun on cardiac rehabilitation by physical therapy on hospital day 2. Patient did well with activity progression and appeared to understand and agree with discharge instructions. Mr. H was discharged on atenolol and diltiazem and was given a new prescription for NTG. Predischarge ETT was negative for ischemia at a heart rate of 110 beats per minute; Mr. H was given a follow-up appointment for maximal ETT in 6 weeks.

Mr. H called his physician to state that he was having recurrent chest discomfort 4 weeks after the inferior myocardial infarction was treated with streptokinase. Chest discomfort usually occurred while Mr. H was taking his 20-minute walk, but during the previous evening the discomfort came while he was eating. All symptoms were relieved with NTG. Physician ordered an ETT (Bruce protocol) for that day. Test was stopped at $2\frac{1}{2}$ minutes when the ECG showed significant ST-segment depression in leads II, III, and aVF at a heart rate of 80 beats per minute. Patient felt his usual chest discomfort, which was relieved with NTG. Mr. H was sent for an emergency cardiac catherization, which was significant for an 80% occlusion in the right coronary artery (RCA) and 30% to 50% lesions in the circumflex artery. Patient underwent percutaneous transluminal coronary angioplasty of the RCA. Discharge medications included persantine, diltiazem, and atenolol. Predischarge blood work indicated that Mr. H's lipid profile (mg/dL) was as follows: total cholesterol 265, LDL 190, HDL 20, and triglycerides 275. Type IIb hyperlipoproteinemia was diagnosed, and Mr. H was begun on Mevacor. Mr. H admitted that he had not followed through with the recommendations for either smoking cessation or nutritional counseling in the past but was determined to do so this time.

Mr. H was seen for regularly scheduled physician visits throughout the following year. He was compliant with diet, exercise, and smoking cessation and had lost 30 lb. Resting heart rate was 54 beats per minute, blood pressure was 90/60. Physician decreased both the atenolol and diltiazem by half. A repeat lipid profile was scheduled for 3 months.

Three months later, a fasting lipid profile showed the following: total cholesterol 160, HDL 45, LDL 90, triglycerides 125. Mr. H had lost another 10 lb and was exercising for 50 minutes, four times a week within his training heart rate range; he stated that he never felt better in his life. Mr. H underwent a modified Bruce ETT; his duration was 14 minutes 20 seconds, and his maximum vital signs were heart rate 145 beats per minute and blood pressure 170/70. Test was negative for ischemia at that level.

Case 2. Antiarrhythmia

Mr. J is a 52-year-old businessman who was admitted to the coronary care unit after complaining of 2 hours of substernal chest pain, nausea, and diaphoresis. His ECG was consistent with an inferior wall myocardial infarction. Thirty minutes after his arrival in the coronary care unit he developed frequent unifocal premature ventricular contractions, bigeminy, couplets, and several short runs (5 beats) of ventricular tachycardia. A bolus of lidocaine (Xylocaine) was administered, and an intravenous drip was started. Forty-eight hours after admission, the lidocaine was discontinued. No further ventricular ectopy was noticed, and long-term antiarrhythmic therapy was not necessary.

Case 3. Antiarrhythmia

Mr. P is a 68-year-old retired dentist who began to notice occasional "flutters" in his chest accompanied by slight dizziness. He had suffered an anterolateral wall myocardial infarction 8 years earlier and had been taking Isordil, atenolol, and diltiazem. He checked his pulse when he had these episodes, and it felt "as if his heart stopped beating after every second beat." He called his physician, who ordered a 24-hour Holter monitor. A review of the Holter showed multifocal premature ventricular contractions in bigeminy and trigeminy; rare couplets were also recorded. He was given a prescription for quinidine. Two days after starting this medication, Mr. P noticed gastrointestinal symptoms of diarrhea and slight nausea. He was switched to procainamide and experienced no further distress. Ten months after the initiation of this drug, he noticed a return of his "flutter" symptoms and lightheadedness. The Holter monitor now showed frequent couplets and nonsustained ventricular tachycardia. Also, he began complaining of arthralgias and stopped his regular exercise program. Procainamide was discontinued, and he was admitted to the hospital. He underwent exercise thallium testing to rule out the possibility of ischemia-induced ectopy. The test was negative for ischemia; however, dyskinesis of the anterior and anteroapical walls was noted, which was consistent with aneurysm. During subsequent electrophysiologic testing, ventricular tachycardia was provoked and required defibrillation to regain normal sinus rhythm. He was begun on mexiletine and was retested when serum levels were therapeutic. Ventricular tachycardia was no longer inducible, and Mr. P was discharged on mexiletine and told to resume his normal activities and participate in a monitored cardiac rehabilitation program.

Case 4. Critical Care

Mrs. S is a 72-year-old woman who arrived in the emergency department with mild symptoms of fatigue, shortness of breath, and recent (1-day) history of diaphoresis and nausea. An anterior wall myocardial infarction (MI) was diagnosed, but Mrs. S denies ever experiencing chest pain.

Her past medical history includes two silent MIs, insulin-dependent diabetes mellitus for 22 years, obesity, cigarette abuse, sedentary lifestyle, arthritis, and cataracts (right worse than left). Mrs. S is a widow and lives in a second-floor apartment. Her son lives on the first floor, and he is trying to convince his mother to move downstairs.

On day 3 after admission, Mrs. S developed severe respiratory distress and was transferred to the critical care unit for management of pulmonary edema and congestive heart failure. Her Inderal was discontinued, and she was started on oxygen, intravenous morphine, and furosemide (Lasix). Her cardiac output dropped, consistent with cardiogenic shock. Invasive monitoring allowed hemodynamic observation as intravenous dobutamine and nitroglycerin were added to her pharmacologic regimen. Potassium was given orally. Her symptoms resolved; however, it took 5 days to wean her from intravenous support and onto oral medications. She left the critical care unit on oxygen, Isordil, digitalis, Lasix, and an ACE inhibitor. After 6 days of symptom-free, graded ambulation, Mrs. S was transferred to a rehabilitation facility for further endurance training. A cardiac catheterization was postponed until she gained strength or became symptomatic.

Summary

- Drugs have primary effects, secondary effects, and side effects.
- Selectivity means that when a certain concentration of the drug exists, the drug is preferentially attracted to one group or subgroup of receptors.
- An agonist (drug) is one that facilitates activity within a cell; an antagonist (drug) inhibits agonist activity.
- Triple therapy for coronary artery disease involves the use of beta blockers, calcium-channel blockers, and nitrates.
- New groups of beta adrenergic blocking medications are being used cautiously when the ejection fraction is less than 35%.
- Pharmacologic management of heart failure includes the use of diuretics, positive inotropes, venodilators, arteriodilators, calcium-channel blockers, ACE inhibitors, and, in severe failure, morphine.
- Digoxin toxicity is relatively common and may include nausea, arrhythmias, and light sensitivity.
- Abnormal cardiac impulse formation or conduction can be treated by altering cell membrane permeability to specific ions (e.g., sodium, calcium).
- Although exercise may be responsible for production of arrhythmias, an electrolyte imbalance or toxic levels of antiarrhythmic drugs may also be responsible.
- Drugs used to treat hypertension act by altering kidney, autonomic nervous system, and peripheral vessel activity to reduce circulating volume, promote vasodilation, and inhibit vasoconstriction and cardiac inotropy.
- Diuretics can predispose the exercising individual to hypotension or arrhythmias owing to volume reduction or electrolyte disturbances, respectively.
- Cardiac drugs used in critical care settings typically act by altering the sympathetic and parasympathetic nervous systems and are used cautiously with hemodynamic monitoring.
- Although patients of all ages can be treated with most cardiac drugs, an awareness of the unique alterations in pharmacokinetics in the very young or the elderly patient is essential.
- Drug management for hyperlipoproteinemia is influenced by the type of lipid dysfunction present.

- Rebound hypoglycemia may occur hours after exercise-induced hypoglycemia.

References

1. Katzung BG. Introduction. In: Katzung BG (ed). Basic and Clinical Pharmacology. 4th ed. East Norwalk, Conn, Appleton & Lange, 1989.
2. Ross EM, Gilman AG. Pharmacodynamics: Mechanisms of drug action and the relationship between drug concentration and effect. In: Gilman AG, Goodman LS, Rall TW, Murad F (eds). Goodman and Gilman's The Pharmacologic Basis of Therapeutics. 7th ed. New York, Macmillan, 1985, p 35.
3. Benet LZ. Pharmacokinetics: Absorption, distribution and elimination. In: Katzung BG (ed). Basic and Clinical Pharmacology. 4th ed. East Norwalk, Conn, Appleton & Lange, 1989, p 29.
4. Blaschke TF, Nies AS, Mamelok RD. Principles of therapeutics. In: Gilman AG, Goodman LS, Rall TW, Murad F (eds). Goodman and Gilman's The Pharmacologic Basis of Therapeutics. 7th ed. New York, Macmillan, 1985, pp 50–53.
5. Opie LH, Gersh BJ. Antithrombotic agents: Platelet inhibitors, anticoagulants, and fibrinolytics. In: Opie LH (ed). Drugs for the Heart. 2nd ed. Philadelphia, WB Saunders, 1987, p 163.
6. Conley CL. Hemostasis. In: Mountcastle VB. Medical Physiology. 13th ed. St. Louis, CV Mosby, 1974, p 1040.
7. Hoffman BB. Adrenoceptor-blocking drugs. In: Katzung BG (ed). Basic and Clinical Pharmacology. 4th ed. East Norwalk, Conn, Appleton & Lange, 1989, p 112.
8. Opie LH, Sonnenblick EH, et al. Beta-blocking agents. In: Opie LH (ed). Drugs for the Heart. 2nd ed. Philadelphia, WB Saunders, 1987, p 9.
9. Needleman P, Corr PB, Johnson EM. Drugs used for the treatment of angina: Organic nitrates, calcium channel blockers, and beta-adrenergic antagonists. In: Gilman AG, Goodman LS, Rall TW, Murad F (eds). Goodman and Gilman's The Pharmacologic Basis of Therapeutics. 7th ed. New York, Macmillan, 1985, pp 808–810.
10. Dec GW, O'Gara PT, Curfman GD. Acute myocardial infarction. In: Rakel R (ed). Conn's Current Therapy 1990. Philadelphia, WB Saunders, 1990, p 266.
11. O'Gara PT, Dec WG, Curfman GD. Acute myocardial infarction. In: Rakel R (ed). Conn's Current Therapy 1991. Philadelphia, WB Saunders, 1991.
12. Cannon C. New treatment strategies for the management of acute myocardial infarction. In: The New Era of Reperfusion (Physician edition). Expanding the Treatment Paradigm for Acute Myocardial Infarction in GP IIb/IIIa Inhibitors. Excerpta Medica Inc., Bellemeade, NJ, March 1999, Vol. 3, No. 1, p 4.
13. Francis GS. Congestive heart failure. In: Rakel R (ed). Conn's Current Therapy 1990. Philadelphia, WB Saunders, 1990, p 242.
14. Packer M, Carver JR, Rodeheffer RJ. Effect of oral milrinone on mortality in severe chronic heart failure. N Engl J Med 325:1468–1475, 1991.
15. Rose BD. Pathogenesis of essential hypertension. In: Rose BD. Pathophysiology of Renal Disease. 2nd ed. New York, McGraw-Hill, 1987, pp 475–476.
16. The SOLVD Investigators. Effect of enalapril on mortality and the development of heart failure in asymptomatic patients with reduced left ventricular ejection fraction. N Engl J Med 327:685–691, 1992.
17. Pfeffer MA, et al. Effects of captopril on mortality and morbidity with left ventricular dysfunction after myocardial infarction. N Engl J Med 327:669–677, 1992.
18. Hondeghen L, Mason J. Agents used in cardiac arrhythmias. In: Katzung BG (ed). Basic and Clinical Pharmacology. 4th ed. Appleton & Lange, East Norwalk, Conn, Appleton & Lange, 1989.
19. Katzung B, Scheinman M. Drugs used in cardiac arrhythmias. In: Katzung BG (ed). Clinical Pharmacology. East Norwalk, Conn, Appleton & Lange, 1988–1989.
20. Zsoter T. Pharmacotherapy of hypertension. In: Kalant H, Roschlau W, Sellers E. Principles of Medical Pharmacology. 4th ed. New York, Oxford University Press, 1985.
21. Benowitz M, Bourne H. Anti-hypertensive agents. In: Katzung BG (ed). Basic and Clinical Pharmacology. 4th ed. East Norwalk, Conn, Appleton & Lange, 1989.
22. Weir MR. Angiotensin II receptor antagonists: A new class of antihypertensive agents. Am Fam Physician 53(2):589–594. 1996.
23. Schaeffer EJ. Hyperlipoproteinemia. In: Rakel R (ed). Conn's Current Therapy 1990. Philadelphia, WB Saunders, 1990.
24. Katzung B, Parmley W. Cardiac glycosides and other drugs used in congestive heart failure. In: Katzung BG (ed). Basic and Clinical Pharmacology. 4th ed. East Norwalk, Conn, Appleton & Lange, 1989.
25. Albert J, Rippe J. Manual of Cardiovascular Diagnosis and Therapy. 3rd ed. Boston, Little, Brown, 1988.
26. Textbook of Advanced Cardiac Life Support. Dallas, American Heart Association, 1987.
27. Sullivan G, Korman L. Drug-associated confusional states in older persons. In: Chaprone DJ (ed). Pharmacology and the Aged Revisited. Topics Geriatr Rehab, 8:4, June 1993; pp 21–23.
28. Notterman D. Pediatric pharmacology. In: Chernow B (ed). Essentials of Critical Care Pharmacology. 2nd ed. Baltimore, Williams & Wilkins, 1989.
29. MacLeod S, Radde I. Textbook of Pediatric Clinical Pharmacology. Littleton, Mass, PSG Publishing Company, 1985.
30. Copeland J. Teaching conference in clinical cardiology. University of Miami, School of Medicine, February 19–22, 1991.
31. Salmon S. Immunopharmacology. In: Katzung BG (ed). Basic and Clinical Pharmacology. 4th ed. East Norwalk, Conn, Appleton & Lange, 1989.

Suggested Readings

Andries E, Stroobandt R (ed). International Congress Series 724, Amsterdam Proceedings of the Workshop on Cardiac Arrhythmias (Mallorca, October 18–19, 1985), Excerpta Medica, 1986.

Chernow B (ed). Essentials of Critical Care Pharmacology. 2nd ed. Baltimore, Williams & Wilkins, 1989.

Chung E. Manual of Cardiac Arrhythmias. Stoneham, Mass, Butterworth-Heinemann, 1986.

Conn PM, Gebhardt GF. Essentials of Pharmacology. Philadelphia, FA Davis, 1989.

Dunagan MR. Manual of Medical Therapeutics. 26th ed. Boston, Little, Brown, 1989.

Gilman AG, Goodman LS, Rall TW, Murad F (eds). Goodman and Gilman's The Pharmacological Basis of Therapeutics. 7th ed. New York, Macmillan, 1985.

Hahn AB, Barkin RL, Oestreich SJ. Pharmacology in Nursing. 15th ed. St. Louis, CV Mosby, 1982.

Harvey AM, Johns RJ, McKusick VA, et al. Principles and Practice of Medicine. 22nd ed. East Norwalk, Conn, Appleton & Lange, 1988.

Kalant H, Roschlau W, Sellers E. Principles of Medical Pharmacology. 4th ed. New York, Oxford University Press, 1985.

Katzung BG (ed). Basic and Clinical Pharmacology. 4th ed. East Norwalk, Conn, Appleton & Lange, 1989.

Learning to Live Well with Diabetes. Minneapolis, DCI Publishing, 1987.

MacLeod S, Radde I. Textbook of Pediatric Clinical Pharmacology. Littleton, Mass, PSG Publishing Company, 1985.

Mountcastle VB. Medical Physiology. 13th ed. St. Louis, CV Mosby, 1974.

Opie LH. Drugs for the Heart. 2nd ed. Philadelphia, WB Saunders, 1987.

Rakel R (ed). Conn's Current Therapy 1991. Philadelphia, WB Saunders, 1991.

Simonson W. Medications and the Elderly. Rockville, Md, Aspen Systems Corporation, 1984.

Sokolow M, McIlroy M, Cheitlin M. Clinical Cardiology. 5th ed. East Norwalk, Conn, Appleton & Lange, 1990.

West JB. Physiological Basis of Medical Practice. 11th ed. Baltimore, Williams & Wilkins, 1985.

15

Pulmonary Medications

Lawrence Cahalin
H. Steven Sadowsky

Introduction
Bronchomotor Tone
Principles of Bronchodilator Therapy
  Medications That Promote Bronchodilation
  Nonsteroidal Anti-inflammatory Agents
  Adrenergic and Cholinergic Receptors
  Sympathomimetic Agents
  Sympatholytic Agents
  Parasympatholytic Agents
  Methylxanthines
  Ancillary Pulmonary Medications
  Decongestants

Antihistamines
Antitussives
Mucokinetics
Respiratory Stimulants and Depressants
Paralyzing Agents
Antimicrobial Agents
Other Agents
The Effects of Pulmonary Medications on Exercise
Case Studies
Summary

INTRODUCTION

Any pulmonary medication is prescribed to achieve one or more of the following four basic goals: (1) promotion of bronchodilation and/or relief of bronchoconstriction; (2) facilitation of the removal of secretions from the lungs; (3) improvement of alveolar ventilation and/or oxygenation; and (4) optimization of the breathing pattern.[1-6] The relative importance of each of these goals depends on the specific disease process and the resultant respiratory problem(s). As a consequence, pulmonary-active medications are grouped in accordance with their principal desired effect: bronchodilators, anti-inflammatory agents, decongestants, antihistamines, antitussives, mucokinetics, respiratory stimulants and depressants, paralyzing drugs, and antimicrobial agents.

Bronchodilators are the most frequently used drugs in the treatment of pulmonary disease.[4, 5] Therefore, they will be considered before the other drug groups. However, a brief discussion of the mechanisms of bronchoconstriction, or airway narrowing, is first presented to facilitate an understanding of the actions of bronchodilator drugs. The bronchial smooth muscle fibers of the lungs involuntarily constrict in response to various types of irritation. The resultant bronchoconstriction plays a major role in the pathophysiology of most obstructive pulmonary diseases. Bronchoconstriction can be attributed to any, or all, of three primary pathologic factors: abnormal bronchomotor tone (bronchospasm), inflammation, and mechanical obstruction. With the elimination of overt mechanical obstruction, the control of bronchomotor tone and inflammation become the components

587

of airway management for patients with pulmonary disease. Only after constricted airways are dilated can mucociliary transport, removal of secretions, and subsequent alveolar ventilation and oxygenation take place.[7]

BRONCHOMOTOR TONE

Normal **bronchomotor tone,** an equilibrium point between constrictive and dilational stimuli, is the result of a balance between **adrenergic** and **cholinergic** influences (Fig. 15–1).[8–11] When something (i.e., disease, allergy) disrupts this balance, **bronchospasm** results. The characteristic findings in acute bronchospasm are mucus production, vascular engorgement, and submucosal inflammatory edema. The mechanisms of bronchospasm are most clearly demonstrated when asthma is used as a model. In asthma, an imbalance in autonomic nervous system (ANS) activity causes a predominant parasympathetic influence, increasing bron-

chomotor tone and resulting in narrowing of bronchial and bronchiolar passages.[12]

Other receptors in the connective tissues of the airways (e.g., mast cells) and the blood are also stimulated to release mediator substances. This response is called **inflammation,** and it plays a central role in the production of bronchospasm in the vast majority of respiratory disorders.[13–15] The mediator substances originate from the plasma, adjacent cells, or from the damaged tissue, and are associated with at least eight major events: (1) changes in vascular flow and caliber, (2) changes in vascular permeability, (3) leukocytic (e.g., neutrophils, monocytes, eosinophils, lymphocytes, and basophils) exudation, (4) clustering of leukocytes along the capillary endothelial cells at the site of injury—margination, (5) adherence of the leukocytes to the endothelial surface at the site of injury—sticking, (6) leukocytic insinuation between endothelial cells—emigration, (7) unidirectional migration of polymorphonuclear leukocytes from the bloodstream to the site of injury in response to released attractants—chemotaxis, and (8) phago-

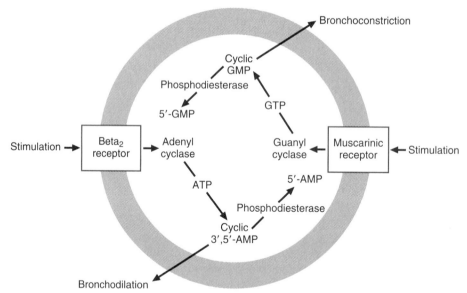

Figure 15–1. Normal bronchomotor tone is the result of a balance between adrenergic and cholinergic influences mediated through the intracellular nucleotides cyclic adenosine 3′,5′-monophosphate (cyclic AMP) and cyclic guanosine monophosphate (cyclic GMP). Adrenergic stimulation of the appropriate receptor catalyzes (via adenyl cyclase) the conversion of adenosine triphosphate (ATP) to cyclic AMP, eliciting relaxation of the affected bronchial smooth muscle. Cyclic AMP is metabolized by phosphodiesterase. Cholinergic stimulation of the appropriate receptor catalyzes (via guanyl cyclase) the conversion of guanosine triphosphate (GTP) to cyclic GMP, eliciting contraction of the affected bronchial smooth muscle. Cyclic GMP is metabolized by phosphodiesterase.

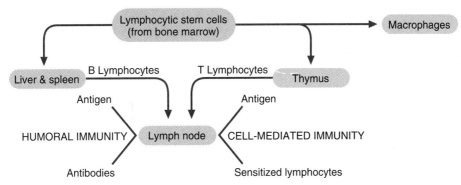

Figure 15–2. In acquired immunity the formation of antibodies (immunoglobulins) results from the interaction of antigens with B lymphocytes and initiates the humoral immune response. The formation of lymphokines results from the interaction of antigens with T lymphocytes and initiates the cell-mediated immune response.

cytosis.[13, 16, 17] Although macrophages, leukocytes, and neutrophils assist in the elimination of invading pathogens by means of phagocytosis, it is the action of the lymphocytes that is probably most significant.[18, 19]

Invading organisms (e.g., bacteria) or other irritants that elicit an immune response are referred to as **allergens** or **antigens.** Antigens stimulate the different types of lymphocytes stored in the lymph nodes to produce two mediator substances: antibodies or sensitized lymphocytes (Fig. 15–2). **Antibodies** are produced by the interaction of antigens and B lymphocytes in a process referred to as humoral immunity. Antibodies are also called **immunoglobulins,** because many reside in the gammaglobulin fraction of the blood. Antibodies are generally grouped into five major classes: IgA, IgE, IgG, IgM, and IgD; the first four of these have been identified in respiratory secretions.[20] Sensitized lymphocytes (also called **lymphokines**) are produced through the interaction of antigens with **T lymphocytes** in a process referred to as **cell-mediated immunity.**

Lymphokines are responsible for a variety of immunologic actions, including the activation of macrophages (by the production and release of macrophage-activating factor), inhibition of leukocyte migration (by the production and release of *leukocyte inhibitory factor*), and destruction of susceptible target cells (*lymphotoxic effect*).[21]

The humoral immunologic response causes the release of chemical mediators from mast cells and leukocytes—a **type I sensitivity reaction.** This immediate reaction is apparently related to IgE anti-body activity and occurs within 10 to 20 minutes. The cell-mediated immunologic response takes approximately 48 hours to develop, and is most likely due to the macrophagic release of specific enzymes that produce inflammation—type IV sensitivity reaction. Type I inflammatory reactions are treated with rapidly acting agents such as corticosteroids, and type IV reactions can be treated with less rapidly acting agents, which may have less profound side effects.

PRINCIPLES OF BRONCHODILATOR THERAPY

The primary goal of bronchodilator therapy is to influence the autonomic nervous system via two opposing nucleotides: **cyclic adenosine monophosphate** (cAMP) and **cyclic guanosine monophosphate** (cGMP) (Fig. 15–3). Cyclic adenosine monophosphate facilitates smooth muscle relaxation and inhibits mast cell degranulation, causing bronchodilation. Cyclic guanosine monophosphate facilitates smooth muscle contraction and may enhance mast cell release of histamine and other mediators to cause **bronchoconstriction.** Within the lungs, the effects of cAMP and/or cGMP can be attributed to either of the following:

• Cholinergic stimulation—muscarinic receptor stimulation, which increases cGMP and enhances bronchoconstriction

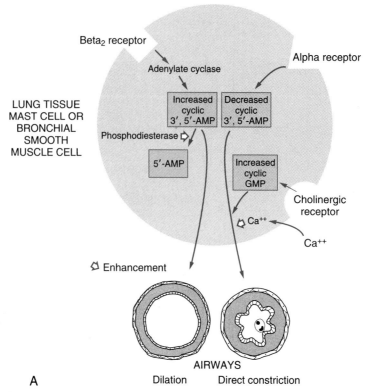

Figure 15-3. *A,* Factors influencing adrenergic and cholinergic mediation of bronchomotor tone.

• Adrenergic stimulation—beta$_2$ receptor stimulation, which produces an increase in cAMP and bronchodilation; alpha$_1$ receptor stimulation, which results in a decrease in cAMP, and facilitates bronchoconstriction.[22, 23]

The effect of parasympathetic activity (heart rate slowing, bronchial constriction, and increased exocrine gland secretion) can be deleterious to a patient with pulmonary disease. To avoid such parasympathetic activity, autonomic-active agents are often used in the pharmacologic treatment of patients with pulmonary disease. Beta-adrenergic agonists, some prostaglandins, corticosteroids (although not technically bronchodilators), and methylxanthines may be given to increase cAMP and thereby promote bronchodilation. Alpha-adrenergic antagonists, corticosteroids, cholinergic antagonists, and cromolyn or nedocromil may be given to inhibit cGMP or enhance cAMP.

Because asthma is the model being used for bronchoconstriction, we will rely upon the recommendations promulgated by the National Asthma Education and Prevention Program and the Na-

Table 15-1.

Pharmacotherapy for the Treatment of Bronchoconstriction

Anti-inflammatory agents
  Corticosteroids
  Cromolyn
  Nedocromil

Bronchodilators
  Anticholinergics
  Beta$_2$ agonists
  Methylxanthines/phosphodiesterase inhibitors
  Nonselective beta agonists

Antihistamines

Immunosuppressives

Antileukotrienes
  Leukotriene receptor antagonists
  5-Lipoxygenase inhibitors

Platelet-activating factor antagonists

Potassium-channel agonists

Prostaglandin inhibitors
  Prostaglandin receptor antagonists
  Thromboxane A$_2$ synthetase inhibitors

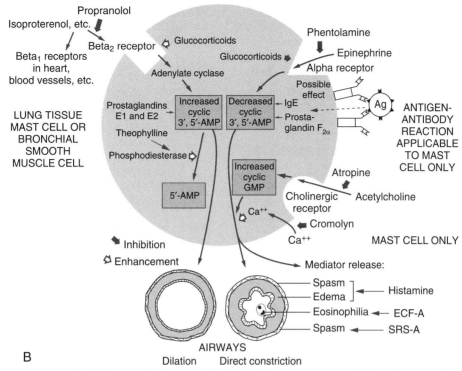

Figure 15–3 Continued. *B*, Pharmacologic control of bronchomotor tone and the allergen-induced release of chemical mediators. Stimulation of beta$_2$ receptors by sympathomimetic agents (e.g., isoproterenol) facilitates dilation. Glucocorticoids, methylxanthines (e.g., theophylline), and some prostaglandins enhance the bronchodilator effect of beta$_2$ adrenergic stimulation. However, glucocorticoids and alpha sympatholytic drugs (e.g., phentolamine) inhibit the alpha-adrenergic contribution to bronchoconstriction. Similarly, parasympatholytics (e.g., atropine) inhibit cholinergic bronchoconstrictive influences. Cromolyn retards the release of mediators by inhibiting calcium ion movement into unstable mast cells, thereby preventing bronchoconstriction. (Adapted from Townley RG. Pharmacologic blocks to mediator release: Clinical application. Adv Asthma Allergy 2:7, 1975.)

tional Institutes of Health in describing the medications used to control bronchoconstriction.[24] The principal drug groups recommended by the National Heart Lung and Blood Institute are listed in Table 15–1 and discussed in the following section.

Medications That Promote Bronchodilation

Corticosteroids

Although **corticosteroids** are not typically regarded as primary bronchodilating agents, bronchoconstriction is essentially an inflammatory response. Corticosteroids are known to suppress the process of IgE-mediated bronchoconstriction and to block or inhibit a variety of mediator substances.[25, 26] Corticosteroids have the following general effects

which contribute to the enhancement of bronchial intraluminal diameter:[6, 23, 27]

- Inhibition of the migration of leukocytes and mast cells
- Reduction of stickiness and margination of polymorphonuclear leukocytes
- Potentiation of catecholamine activity
- Reduction of tissue stores of histamine and other mediators
- Suppression of kinin activity, resulting in constriction of the microvasculature
- Stabilization of mast cell membranes
- Reduction of phosphodiesterase activity

It is because of their profound anti-inflammatory actions that corticosteroids are considered by many to be the drugs of first choice for both the long-term and quick relief of asthma.

Although it influences all medications, the

route of administration of corticosteroids is of particular importance because of the tremendous impact it plays in the incidence of side effects—the more localized the area of administration, the less likely the chance of systemic reaction. During episodes of severe bronchoconstriction, corticosteroids are usually administered intravenously. However, for prolonged use, an oral or inhalational route of administration is used.[27] The inhalational route is preferred because it is associated with fewer side effects.

Most of the adverse effects of corticosteroid therapy are dosage-dependent and take a few days or weeks to manifest themselves. However, some side effects are unavoidable; reactions span the spectrum from merely unpleasant to dangerous. The primary side effects associated with steroid use include: immunosuppression, gastrointestinal disturbance, emotional lability (vacillation between euphoria and depression), insomnia, osteoporosis, retardation of growth, muscle weakness and atrophy (particularly of pelvic and shoulder girdle musculature), hyperglycemia, sodium and water retention, and cushingoid effects.[6, 23, 27] The most often recommended steroids for long-term and quick relief are listed in Table 15–2.

Nonsteroidal Anti-inflammatory Agents

Research in England in the 1960s on an extract of a Mediterranean plant resulted in the discovery of *cromolyn sodium,* which is known by the brand name Intal. More recently, a newer, but very similar, nonsteroidal anti-inflammatory agent, **nedocromil sodium (Tilade)**, has been introduced.[28, 29] Cromolyn and nedocromil are used prophylactically in cases of chronic asthma because they prevent the immediate hypersensitivity reaction (also known as type I reaction). Recall that the immediate hypersensitivity reaction is controlled by mast

Table 15–2.
Long-Term Control and Quick-Relief Steroids

Long-term control medications
  Inhaled: generic names (brand names)
    Beclomethasone (Beclovent, Vanceril)
    Budesonide (Pulmocort, Turbuhaler)
    Flunisolide (AeroBid)
    Fluticasone (Flovent)
    Triamcinolone (Azmacort)
  Oral agents
    Methylprednisolone (Medrol)
    Prednisone (Prednisone, Deltasone, Orasone, Liquid Pred, Prednisone Intensol)
    Prednisolone (Prelone, Pediapred)
Quick-relief medications (oral or intravenous)
  Methylprednisolone (Medrol)
  Prednisone (Prednisone, Deltasone, Orasone, Liquid Pred, Prednisone Intensol)
  Prednisolone (Prelone, Pediapred)

cells via the release of specific mediators (i.e., histamine, lymphokines, bradykinin, among many others) that produce bronchoconstriction and a variety of other signs and symptoms (e.g., mucus secretion, mucosal swelling, and dyspnea). Although cromolyn and nedocromil do not prevent the activation of mast cells and the subsequent release of specific mediators that results from the coupling of IgE with an allergen,[6] they can prevent the late phase reaction in an acute asthma episode (which can cause severe airway obstruction 4 to 6 hours after initial bronchoconstriction).[30, 31] Thus, although cromolyn and nedocromil have no effect upon the mediators released from the antigen-antibody reaction of an acute asthma attack, they prevent later bronchoconstriction by impairing the release of mediator.[30, 31] Both cromolyn and nedocromil have few side effects, the most common being dry mouth and throat and possible airway irritation. Although these drugs are unlikely to eliminate the use of inhaled corticosteroids in patients with more significant obstructive airway disease, they have potentially beneficial steroid-sparing effects.

Adrenergic and Cholinergic Receptors

Medications that stimulate the adrenergic receptors are frequently referred to as **sympathomimet-**

Clinical Note: Inhaled Steroids
The side effects of inhaled steroids appear to be negligible, but are currently under study. Research is needed to validate this clinical observation. One study has implied a possible long-term side effect may be the increased incidence of cataracts.

ics (adrenergic), and those that inhibit adrenergic receptors are referred to as **sympatholytics** (antiadrenergic). Similarly, medications that stimulate the cholinergic receptors are referred to as **parasympathomimetics** (cholinergic), and those that inhibit cholinergic receptors are called **parasympatholytics** (anticholinergic). The actions and adverse effects of the principal bronchodilators, specifically the autonomic active agents (adrenergic sympathomimetics and parasympatholytics) and methylxanthines, will be reviewed next.

Sympathomimetic Agents

Sympathomimetic drugs may be selective or nonselective in their activity. Selective medications react with specific receptors, and nonselective medications react with several receptors. As with all drugs, the response elicited by sympathomimetic agents depends upon the relative intensity of the receptor reaction, the route of administration, and the dosage of the particular drug.[3, 6, 23]

- Alpha receptors are distributed within peripheral and bronchial smooth muscle, the myocardium, and mucosal blood vessels, but they are most abundant in the peripheral smooth muscles.
- Beta$_1$ receptors are more abundant in cardiac tissue, although they are also present in mucosal blood vessels.
- Beta$_2$ receptors predominate in the bronchial smooth muscles but are also found in peripheral smooth muscle and skeletal muscle.

Epinephrine (adrenaline) and *ephedrine* typify the general, nonselective sympathomimetics. Epinephrine has a short duration of action, demonstrating moderate alpha receptor activity, strong beta$_1$ receptor activity, and moderate beta$_2$ receptor activity.[3, 6, 23] Ephedrine has a long duration of action, exhibiting mild alpha receptor activity and moderate beta$_1$ and beta$_2$ activity. Thus, in the treatment of bronchoconstriction, peripheral vascular constriction and accelerated cardiac responses may result from the alpha- and beta$_1$-receptor stimulation. Other adverse reactions include agitation, sweating, headache, and nausea. It should be noted that the route by which a particular medication is administered significantly influences the extent of any adverse reactions.[3, 6, 23] For example, sympathomimetic medications administered by an

Clinical Note: Intramuscular Epinephrine

Intramuscular epinephrine is the drug of choice for treating acute bronchospasm as well as acute anaphylactic reaction because of its quick short-acting response.

inhalational route produce less profound deleterious side effects than when they are administered systemically.

Clearly, drugs that elicit no alpha-receptor activity and a more specific beta$_2$-receptor activity would be desirable for bronchodilator therapy. Unfortunately, however, no purely beta$_2$-specific sympathomimetic medications have been identified. Selective stimulation of beta$_2$ receptors is preferable, because beta$_2$-specific agents would affect the lungs without affecting the heart. Beta$_2$-specific agents produce bronchiolar dilatation by relaxing the bronchial smooth muscle through facilitation of increased cAMP levels. The recommended beta$_2$ agonists can be considered in terms of being either long- or short-acting (Table 15–3). Although the adverse effects of the currently available beta$_2$-specific sympathomimetics are similar to, but usually less profound than, those of the nonspecific beta-receptor sympathomimetics, the severity of them is related to the dosage of the drug administered. The adverse effects that are associated with beta sympathomimetic medications include tremor, palpitations, headache, nervousness, dizziness, nausea, and hypertension. In addition, nonspecific beta sympathomimetic drugs may also elicit inotropic (enhanced myocardial contractility) and chronotropic (enhanced heart rate) effects.

Table 15–3.
Long-Term and Short-Term Beta$_2$ Agonists

Long-acting
   Salmeterol (Serevent, inhaled)
   Albuterol (Volmax, Proventil Repetabs)
Short-acting
   Albuterol (Airet, inhaled, Proventil, Ventolin)
   Bitolterol (Tornalate)
   Pirbuterol (Maxair)
   Terbutaline (Brethaire, Brethine tablet, Bricanyl tablet)

Sympatholytic Agents

Because alpha adrenoreceptor stimulation produces both vasoconstriction and bronchoconstriction, the pharmacologic reduction of alpha-adrenergic activity via alpha-adrenoceptor antagonists is certainly warranted for patients with pulmonary disease. Alpha-receptor sympatholytic action inhibits the decrease of cAMP associated with an antigen-antibody reaction, allowing bronchodilation to occur. The most common side effects associated with alpha-receptor sympatholytic administration are nausea and dizziness.[3, 6, 23]

Parasympatholytic Agents

The lungs receive a very rich supply of parasympathetic innervation through the vagus nerve.[32] The role of parasympatholytic agents is similar to that of alpha sympatholytics in that it is the "lytic" action (inhibitory effect) that produces the desired effect of bronchodilation.[6] Blocking parasympathetic stimulation prevents an increase in cGMP, thereby producing a relative increase in the amount of cAMP and promoting bronchial smooth muscle relaxation. The agent most commonly used for this purpose was the muscarinic antagonist *atropine.* However, because atropine is readily absorbed into the systemic circulation, it is frequently associated with adverse reactions, including CNS stimulation with low doses or depression with high doses; delirium; hallucinations; and decreased gastrointestinal activity.[3, 6, 23] The drug *ipratropium* (Atrovent) is administered by inhalation and therefore is not absorbed as well into the systemic circulation; consequently, it is associated with fewer side effects.[33]

Methylxanthines

The intracellular level of cAMP can be enhanced if the process of its degradation by the enzyme phosphodiesterase (PDE) can be inhibited. By blocking the inactivation of cAMP, bronchodilation is facilitated. The group of drugs that most significantly inhibits phosphodiesterase is the **methylxanthines.**[3, 6, 23] Methylxanthines are also believed to facilitate bronchodilation by means of prostaglandin inhibition, adenosine receptor blockade, enhancement of endogenous catecholamine levels, inhibition of cGMP, and enhancement of the translocation of intracellular calcium.[3, 6, 23] Although findings are still inconclusive, a body of evidence suggests these actions enhance diaphragmatic contractility, reduce patient complaints of dyspnea, and improve exercise tolerance and gas exchange.[34-37] The most commonly used methylxanthines are *theophylline* (Bronkodyl, Theo-Dur, Slo-phyllin) and *aminophylline* (Aminophyllin, cardophyllin), which are associated with a variety of side effects, including increased myocardial work load, heightened susceptibility to ventricular and supraventricular dysrhythmias, and possibly diuresis. The identification and functional characterization of different phosphodiesterase isoenzymes have led to the development of various isoenzyme-selective inhibitors as potential antiasthma drugs. Considering the distribution of isoenzymes in target tissues, with high activity of PDE3 and PDE4 in airway smooth muscle and inflammatory cells, selective inhibitors of these isoenzymes may add to the therapy of chronic airflow obstruction. The development of "second generation" selective drugs has produced more promising clinical results not only for the treatment of bronchial asthma but also for the treatment of chronic obstructive pulmonary disease.[38] Protease inhibitors and inhibitors of neutrophil elastase, cathepsins, and matrix metalloproteases are now in clinical development, and offer great potential as new anti-inflammatory treatments.[39]

Ancillary Pulmonary Medications

In addition to bronchodilators, several other drug groups are frequently used in the treatment of respiratory disorders: decongestants, antihistamines, antitussives, mucokinetics, respiratory stimulants and depressants, paralyzing drugs, and antimicrobial agents. The drug grouping may provide clues regarding the nature of the problem for which it was taken, or vice versa. For example, a patient experiencing mucosal edema may complain of feeling "stuffed up" and may be taking an over-the-counter decongestant or antihistamine.

Decongestants

The common cold, allergies, and many respiratory infections have in common the symptoms of "runny nose and stuffy head." **Decongestants** are used to treat this upper airway mucosal edema and discharge. The most common decongestants are alpha-adrenergic sympathomimetics, specifically $alpha_1$ agonists.[40, 41] These medications stimulate vasoconstriction by binding with the $alpha_1$ receptors in the blood vessels of the mucosal lining of the upper airway. The desired result is a decreased congestion in the upper airways.

Decongestants are frequently combined with other ingredients (e.g., antihistamines) as constituents of commercially available, nonprescription, over-the-counter preparations (Table 15–4). When used appropriately, these medications can be safe and effective. However, if a patient has a specific sensitivity or if the decongestant medication is improperly used, adverse effects may arise. Primary side effects include headache, dizziness, nausea, nervousness, hypertension, and cardiac irregularities (e.g., palpitations).

Antihistamines

Treatment of the respiratory allergic responses associated with seasonal allergies (e.g., hayfever) is one of the most common uses of **antihistamines.** Histamines play a role in the modulation of neural

Table 15–4.
Common Decongestants

DRUG GENERIC (BRAND) NAME	ROUTE OF ADMINISTRATION
Ephedrine (Primatene Tablets*)	Oral
Epinephrine (Primatene Mist)	Nasal spray
Oxymetazoline (Neo-Synephrine 12-Hour)	Nasal spray
Phenylephrine (Neo-Synephrine)	Nasal spray
Phenylpropanolamine (Triaminic,* Contac*)	Oral
Pseudoephedrine (Sudafed)	Oral

*Decongestant combined with other ingredients.

Table 15–5.
Common Antihistamines

DRUG GENERIC (BRAND) NAME	ROUTE OF ADMINISTRATION
Brompheniramine (Dimetapp*)	Oral
Chlorpheniramine (Chlor-Trimeton,* Sudafed,* Coricidin*)	Oral
Dexbrompheniramine (Drixoral*)	Oral
Dimenhydrinate (Dramamine)	Oral
Diphenhydramine (Benadryl)	Oral
Pheniramine (Triaminic*)	Oral
Phenyltoloxamine (Sinutab*)	Oral
Triprolidine (Actifed*)	Oral

* Antihistamine combined with other ingredients.

activity within the central nervous system and the regulation of gastric secretion by means of two types of receptors: H_1 and H_2 **receptors,** respectively.[23] The H_1 receptors, primarily located in vascular, respiratory, and gastrointestinal smooth muscle, are specifically targeted for blockade by antihistamines in the treatment of asthma.[42] H_1-antagonist drugs decrease the mucosal congestion, irritation, and discharge caused by inhaled allergens. Antihistamines may also reduce the coughing and sneezing often associated with common colds.

Some of the antihistamines commonly used to treat the symptoms of hayfever and other hayfever-like allergies are listed in Table 15–5. Antihistamines are frequently combined with other ingredients, such as alpha-adrenergic sympathomimetics. The adverse effects most often attributable to antihistamines include sedation, fatigue, dizziness, blurred vision, loss of coordination, and gastrointestinal distress.

Antitussives

The cough is such a common and troublesome symptom that there are more prescription drugs available for the treatment of coughs than for any other symptom.[43] Used to suppress the ineffective, dry hacking cough associated with minor throat irritations and the common cold, **antitussive agents** act to correct the irritation or block the receptors, or to increase the threshold of the cough center in the brain. They are generally indicated for only short-term use and are not indicated for coughs due to retained secretions.

Antitussives may be classified as topical anesthetics (e.g., *benzonatate*, Tessalon), non-narcotics (e.g., *dextromethorphan*, Congespirin for Children, Mediquell, Pertussin) and narcotics (e.g., *codeine, morphine*); they are frequently combined with other ingredients and are offered under many brand names. The primary adverse effect of antitussive agents is sedation. However, gastrointestinal distress and dizziness may also occur. Common antitussives are listed in Table 15–6.

Mucokinetics

Drugs that promote the mobilization and removal of secretions from the respiratory tract are called **mucokinetic agents.** There are four basic types of mucokinetic agents: mucolytics, expectorants, wetting agents, and surface-active agents.

Mucolytic drugs disrupt the chemical bonds in mucoid and purulent secretions, decreasing the viscosity of the mucus and promoting expectoration. Administered by inhalation or direct intratracheal instillation, *acetylcysteine* (Mucomyst) is the principal mucolytic drug used today. Acetylcys-

teine's primary adverse effects include mucosal irritation, coughing, bronchospasm (especially in asthmatics), and nausea.

Expectorants increase the production of respiratory secretions, thus facilitating their ejection from the respiratory tract. Several expectorant drugs are available, among them are *guaifenesin* (Anti-Tuss, Robitussin), *potassium iodide,* and *ammonium chloride.* These drugs are often combined with others and are available by many trade names (e.g., Contac Cough and Sore Throat Formula, Triminicol Multi-Symptom Cold). Although expectorants are widely used outside the United States, and are sold over the counter in this country, there has been an ongoing debate over their efficacy.[44] Nonetheless, in an acute care setting, expectorants are often administered as an adjunct to vigorous bronchial hygiene techniques.

By humidifying and lubricating secretions, **wetting agents** make expectoration easier for the patient. The diluent of choice is half normal saline (0.45% NaCl), delivered by either continuous aerosol or intermittent ultrasonic nebulization. However, sterile water is sometimes administered via a nebulizer as an airway irritant to induce coughing and facilitate the expectoration of sputum for subsequent laboratory testing.

Surface-active agents may stabilize aerosol droplets and thereby enhance their efficacy as carrier vehicles for nebulized drugs. However, the usefulness of these agents is debatable.[6, 23, 27]

Respiratory Stimulants and Depressants

Any agent that increases the output of the central respiratory centers may be considered a **respiratory stimulant.** Certainly, noxious stimuli, such as pain or verbal exhortation, may result in CNS excitation and thus elicit enhanced respiratory center activity. Medications, such as sympathomimetics and methylxanthines, also stimulate respiratory center activity and induce an increase in ventilation. Drugs that have a specific ability to cause central excitation with subsequently enhanced respiratory center activity are called **analeptics.** Unfortunately, analeptic drugs elicit dose-dependent levels of central stimulation that can ultimately result in convulsions. Therefore, the clinical use of ana-

Table 15–6.
Common Antitussives

DRUG GENERIC (BRAND) NAME	CLASSIFICATION/ ACTION
Benzonatate (Tessalon)	Local anesthetic
Codeine* (many brand names)	Increases threshold in cough center
Dextromethorphan* (many brand names)	Increases threshold in cough center
Diphenhydramine (Benadryl)	Antihistamine
Hydrocodone (Triaminic Expectorant DH)	Increases threshold in cough center

*Frequently combined with other ingredients (i.e., expectorants, decongestants).

Clinical Note: Beta-Blocking Medication and Bronchospasm

Caution should be taken with patients who have a history of bronchospasm or asthma and who are taking beta-blocking medications. Some beta-blocking medications may actually have a slight effect on beta$_2$ receptors, blocking beta$_2$ stimulation. As you recall, beta$_2$ stimulation induces smooth muscle relaxation or bronchodilation in the lungs. Patients taking these medications may demonstrate exercise-induced bronchospasm secondary to the medication's side effects. The bronchospasm does decrease or disappear when these medications are stopped, however.

is contributing to an increased work of breathing and hindering mechanical ventilation. The tranquilizer *haloperidol* (Haldol) may be prescribed for spontaneously breathing patients to control agitation because it has less respiratory depressant action than other tranquilizers or sedatives.[49] Many of the drugs used in the treatment of psychiatric disorders have varying degrees of sedative effect, depressing the central nervous system and possibly leading to respiratory depression in some patients. Some antipsychotic drugs are associated with significant parasympatholytic effects, causing symptoms such as bronchoconstriction, dry mouth, blurred vision, constipation, and urinary retention.

leptic medications is not without controversy, but few would argue that when respiratory failure has been aggravated by an injudicious intervention (e.g., oxygen, narcotics), respiratory stimulants serve a purpose.[6, 23, 27]

Because it stimulates respiration more than it activates the cortical or spinal neurons, *doxapram* is one of the most widely accepted analeptics.[45] Administered intravenously, it is used to prevent a rise in Pa$_{CO_2}$ with oxygen therapy in acute ventilatory failure.[46] It is also used in high-risk postoperative patients to prevent respiratory depression.[47, 48]

Some drugs (e.g., sedatives, tranquilizers) are, to varying degrees, **respiratory depressants.** In general, patients with pulmonary disease should avoid the use of sedatives because they suppress the ventilatory drive. However, in some instances intravenous *morphine* or *diazepam* (Valium) is given to mechanically ventilated patients if anxiety or agitation

Paralyzing Agents

Although tranquilizers can relieve muscle spasm, they do not prevent volitional muscle activity; and in order to completely ablate muscular tone during general anesthesia, the level of anesthesia must be profound—a situation that is not wholly desirable. Therefore, anesthetists and anesthesiologists usually opt for lighter general anesthesia in conjunction with muscle paralyzing agents to produce the desired degree of immobilization. Paralyzing agents are also used to facilitate endotracheal intubation, or to control laryngeal spasm; treat diseases that cause neuromuscular hyperactivity (e.g., tetanus, severe intractable seizure activity); and occasionally to prevent struggling, fighting, or excessive tachypnea in patients being mechanically ventilated. Table 15–7 presents the neuromuscular blocking agents frequently used clinically.

Table 15–7.

Common Neuromuscular Blocking Agents

DRUG GENERIC (BRAND) NAME	TYPE	USUAL DURATION OF EFFECT	ADVERSE REACTIONS
d-Tubocurarine (curare, Tubadil, Tubarine)	Nondepolarizing	Typically 45 to 90 minutes	Hyper- or hypotension, brady- or tachycardia
Pancuronium (Pavulon)	Nondepolarizing	Up to 50 minutes	Mild hypertension, mild tachycardia
Succinylcholine (Suxamethonium, Anectine)	Depolarizing	About 5 minutes	Vagal and sympathetic stimulation; associated fasciculations may cause muscle pain

Antimicrobial Agents

Drugs used to combat small, unicellular organisms (e.g., bacteria, viruses) that invade the body are often called **antimicrobial agents** or **antibiotics.** There are numerous pathogenic organisms, so it is quite likely that many patients receiving physical therapy will be taking one or more antimicrobial drugs. Unfortunately, the majority of antimicrobial agents may be as toxic to the host cells as to the infecting organisms.[23, 27] The commonly used antimicrobial agents (Table 15–8) act by inhibiting cell wall synthesis and function (e.g., the penicillins, the cephalosporins, polypeptides, the antifungal polyenes, the monobactams), protein synthesis (e.g., aminoglycosides, the macrolides, the tetracyclines, the lincomycins), or nucleotide formation (e.g., *rifampin, isoniazid*). Antibacterial drugs may be classified as **bactericidal** (killing or destroying bacteria) or **bacteriostatic** (limiting growth and proliferation of bacteria). The bactericidal or bacteriostatic characteristics of a drug may depend upon the dosage of the drug—some drugs (e.g., erythromycin) are bacteriostatic at low doses and bactericidal at higher doses.

Penicillins are a mainstay in the treatment of respiratory infections. The semisynthetic penicillins have a broader spectrum of antibacterial activity than the natural penicillins.[23, 27] The principal drawback to the use of penicillins is hypersensitivity, which manifests itself as skin rashes, hives, bronchoconstriction, or even anaphylactic reaction. Monobactams are a new class of synthetic antibiotics. These drugs are effective against gram-negative and gram-positive aerobes and anaerobes.

Cephalosporins are generally considered as alternatives to the penicillins, when penicillins are not tolerated by the patient or when they are ineffective. First-generation cephalosporins are used in the treatment of gram-positive cocci and some gram-negative bacteria; second-generation cephalosporins are similar in effectiveness against gram-positive cocci, and are generally thought to be more effective against gram-negative bacteria; third-generation cephalosporins are effective against the greatest number of gram-negative bacteria, but are of limited effectiveness against gram-positive cocci. Cephalosporins may elicit stomach cramps, diarrhea, nausea, and vomiting, and some patients may exhibit hypersensitivity reactions similar to those of penicillins.

Aminoglycoside drugs have a wide spectrum of antibacterial activity; they are active against many aerobic gram-negative bacteria, against some aerobic gram-positive bacteria, and against many anaerobic bacteria.[6, 23, 27] Unfortunately, this wide spectrum of activity is associated with some toxicity. Nephrotoxicity and ototoxicity are the primary toxic manifestations, especially in patients with particular susceptibility (elderly, patients with liver or renal failure). The erythromycins also exhibit a broad spectrum of antibacterial activity, being effective against many gram-positive and some gram-negative bacteria.[6, 23, 27] The most common side effect of erythromycin administration is gastrointestinal distress (stomach cramps, nausea, vomiting, and diarrhea). When the tetracyclines were first introduced, they were effective against many gram-positive and gram-negative bacteria, as well as organisms such as *Chlamydia, Rickettsia,* and *Spirochaeta.* However, because tetracyclines are generally bacteriostatic, many bacterial strains have developed resistance to tetracycline and its derivatives.[6, 23, 27]

There are not many effective drugs for the treatment of viruses in humans. However, research into this area of pharmacology is in a period of explosive discovery. Interferons represent just one of the areas of potential pharmacologic and physiologic benefit; advancements with vaccines are another. Fungal and protozoal infections have historically been associated with tropical and subtropical environments, or with lesser developed areas of the world where sanitation and hygiene are inadequate. The incidence of these infections has become prevalent because immunoinsufficiency, either acquired (AIDS) or induced (after organ transplantation), is more widespread. Therefore, the use of antifungal and antiprotozoal agents is becoming more common.

It is often very difficult to establish the causative agent in an acute pulmonary infection because transoral sputum is often contaminated, yielding mixtures of multiple organisms on culture. Nevertheless, the organisms *Streptococcus pneumoniae* and *Haemophilus influenzae* are generally thought to be the primary causative agents of infection of the respiratory mucosa in patients with chronic obstructive pulmonary dysfunction.[50] Precise diagnosis generally requires that sputum samples are obtained by transtracheal aspiration, bronchoscopy, or transpulmonary aspiration.

Table 15-8.
Common Antimicrobial Medications

GROUP	DRUG NAME	BRAND NAME	INDICATION FOR SPECIFIC ANTIMICROBIAL USE
Aminoglycosides*	Amikacin	Amikin	
	Gentamicin	Apogen, Garamycin	
	Kanamycin	Kantrex, Klebcil	
	Netilimicin	Netromycin	
	Streptomycin		
	Tobramycin	Nebcin	
Cephalosporins†			
First generation	Cefadroxil	Duricef, Ultracef	
	Cefazolin	Ancef, Kefzol	
	Cephalexin	Keflex	
Second generation	Cefaclor	Ceclor	
	Cefamandole	Mandol	
	Cefonicid	Monocid	
	Ceforanide	Percef	
	Cefotetan	Cefotan	
Third generation	Cefoperazone	Cefobid	
	Cefotaxime	Claforan	
	Cefoxitin	Mefoxin	
	Ceftazidime	Fortaz, Tazicef	
	Ceftibuten	Cedax	
Fourth generation	Cefepime	Maxipime	
	Cefpirome	Cefrom	
Macrolides	Erythromycin	ERYC, E-Mycin, Ilosone, EES, Pediamycin, Ilotycin, Erythrocin, Erypar, Ethril	
	Troleanomycin	TAO	
Monobactams	Aztreonam	Azactam	
	Loracarbef	Lorabid	
Lincomycins	Clindamycin	Cleocin	
	Lincomycin	Linocin	
Penicillins			
Natural penicillins	Penicillin G	Bicillin, Crysticillin, Permapen, etc.	
	Penicillin V	V-Cillin, Pen-Vee, Pnapar VK, etc.	
Penicillinase-resistant penicillins	Cloxacillin	Cloxapen, Tegopen	
	Dicloxacillin	Dynapen, Pathocil	
	Methicillin	Staphcillin	
	Nafcillin	Unipen	
	Oxacillin	Bactocil, Prostaphlin	
Aminopenicillins	Amoxicillin	Amoxil, Polymox	
	Ampicillin	Amcill, Omnipen, Polycillin, etc.	
	Bacampicillin	Spectrobid	
Wide-spectrum penicillins	Azlocillin	Azlin	
	Carbenicillin	Geocillin, Geopen, Pyopen	
	Mezlocillin	Mexlin	
	Piperacillin	Pipracil	
	Ticarcillin	Ticar	

Table continued on following page

Table 15–8.
Common Antimicrobial Medications Continued

GROUP	DRUG NAME	BRAND NAME	INDICATION FOR SPECIFIC ANTIMICROBIAL USE
Quinolones	Ciprofloxacin	Cipro	
	Lomefloxacin	Maxaquin	
	Ofloxacin	Floxin	
Sulfonamides	Sulfadiazine	Silvadene	
	Sulfamethoxazole	Gantanol, Methoxanol	
	Sulfisoxazole	Gantrisin	
Tetracyclines	Chlortetracycline	Aureomycin	
	Doxycycline	Doxychel, Vibramycin, etc.	
	Oxytetracycline	Terramycin	
	Tetracycline	Achromycin V, Sumycin, etc.	
Others	Aminosalicylic acid	PAS, Teebacin	
	Bacitracin	Bacitracin ointment	
	Chloramphenicol	Chloromycetin, Amphicol, etc.	
	Cycloserine	Seromycin	
	Sulfamethoxazole/ Trimethoprim	Bactrim, Septra	
	Vancomycin	Vancocin IV, Vancoled	
Anti-tuberculosis drugs	Capreomycin	Capastat	
	Isoniazid	INH, Nydrazid, etc.	
	Pyrazinamide	PZA	
Antiviral drugs	Acyclovir	Zovirax	Herpes (especially simplex-related) infections
	Amantidine	Symadine, Symmetrel	Influenza A infections
	Ribavirin	Tribavirin, Virazole	Respiratory syncytial infections
	Vidarabine	Vira-A	Herpes simplex, cytomegalovirus, varicella zoster infections
	Zidovudine	Retrovir	To slow HIV progression
Antifungal drugs	Amphotericin B	Fungizone	Aspergillosis, blastomycosis, candidiasis, coccidiomycosis, cryptococcosis, histoplasmosis
	Flucytosine	Ancobon	Candidiasis, cryptococcosis, aspergillosis
	Nystatin	Mycostatin, Nilstat	Oropharyngeal candidiasis
Antiprotozoal drugs	Chloroquine	Aralen	Malaria
	Hydroxychloroquine	Plaquenil	Malaria
	Metronidazole	Flagyl	Amebiasis, giardiasis, trichomoniasis
	Pentamidine	Pentam	*Pneumocystis carinii*

*Often used as supplements to the penicillins.
†Cephalosporins generally serve as alternatives to penicillins if they prove ineffective or are poorly tolerated by the patient.

Other Agents

Oxygen should be considered a drug when it is breathed in concentrations higher than those found in atmospheric air. Regardless of its etiology, arterial hypoxemia (partial pressure of oxygen in arterial blood, Pa_{O_2}, less than 60 mm Hg) is the most common indication for oxygen therapy. The therapeutic administration of oxygen can elevate the arterial oxygen tension and increase the arterial oxygen content (which shifts the oxyhemoglobin dissociation curve to the right), improving peripheral tissue oxygenation. Additionally, the constriction of the central pulmonary vascular beds that is associated with hypoxia can be reduced.[51]

Supplemental oxygen is most commonly administered via nasal cannula at flow rates between 1 and 6 L/minute. Systems for such low gas flow rates are generally prescribed on the assumption that the patient is breathing at a relatively constant rate and depth (minute ventilation). However, when breathing patterns deviate from the norm, patients cannot be assured of receiving the intended FI_{O_2} (fraction of inspired oxygen). Therefore, when higher gas flow rates are indicated (e.g., respiratory rate greater than 30 per minute), or more accurate titrations of FI_{O_2} are required, oxygen is typically delivered by any one of several types of moderate- and high-flow face masks (providing oxygen concentrations of 40 to 60% or more).[52] Care must always be exercised so as to avoid the potential for depression of the hypoxic drive to breathe in patients with chronically elevated Pa_{CO_2} (partial pressure of carbon dioxide in arterial blood) levels (primarily patients with COPD).[53, 54]

When used judiciously, oxygen therapy has few side effects. However, depending upon the oxygen concentration and its duration of administration, oxygen toxicity can occur. In general, the pathologic changes in the lungs associated with oxygen toxicity can be described in three phases: exudative, proliferative, and recovery.[55-57] In the exudative phase, damage to the alveolar-capillary membrane results in an increased permeability to water, electrolytes, and protein. Secondarily, the capillaries become plugged with platelets and the interstitium is invaded by polymorphonuclear leukocytes. As lung damage progresses, the inflammatory response is intensified. In the proliferative phase, fibroblasts and type II epithelial cells proliferate in conjunction with interstitial collagen deposition. The recovery phase may result in complete healing or areas of fibrosis.

Since the accidental discovery, in 1980, of the important role the vascular endothelium plays in the regulation of vascular smooth muscle tone, the identification of **endothelium-derived relaxing factor** (EDRF) in 1982, and the later discovery in 1986 that EDRF was indistinguishable from **nitric oxide** (NO), numerous articles regarding the actions and effects of NO have been published.[58-61]

Nitric oxide is widely distributed in the body and plays an important role in the regulation of the circulation. In the body, NO is derived from L-arginine in a reaction catalyzed by NO synthase. Once produced, NO diffuses to the vascular smooth muscle cells where it activates the enzyme guanylate cyclase, leading to increased cGMP levels, and to vascular smooth muscle relaxation. Other potential therapeutic roles of NO include the treatment of endotoxic shock, adult respiratory distress syndrome, and hypertension in various disease states such as atherosclerosis and chronic renal failure.[62-64]

Although the side effects of NO are not completely understood, the marked oxidizing effects of nitrogen dioxide (NO_2—the product of NO and oxygen) are known to (1) decrease alveolar permeability, (2) decrease Pa_{O_2} and DL_{CO}, (3) cause pulmonary edema, (4) cause loss of cilia and disintegration of bronchiolar epithelium, and (5) decrease pulmonary function tests (i.e., FEV_1).[65] The few studies investigating the toxic effects of NO have shown that at concentrations of NO greater than 15 to 20 ppm, Pa_{O_2} decreased 7 to 8 mm Hg, and airway resistance increased.[55, 66, 67]

THE EFFECTS OF PULMONARY MEDICATIONS ON EXERCISE

As indicated earlier, the vast majority of pulmonary medications are used to promote bronchodilation and improve alveolar ventilation and oxygenation.

These effects should improve an individual's ability to exercise and more effectively develop training effects. However, because of the side effects of many pulmonary medications, exercise tolerance and the normal adaptations to habitual exercise conditioning may be retarded. This section is not presented to discourage the use of these medications or exercise training; rather, it should highlight the important role exercise has for patients with pulmonary disease who are taking one or more pulmonary medications.

Habitual exercise performed at the proper intensity, duration, and frequency typically elicits both peripheral and central physiologic adaptations. The central adaptations include (1) improved ventilatory efficiency and (2) improved cardiac performance.[68] Peripheral adaptations include (1) an increase in the number and size of mitochondria, (2) improved extraction of oxygen from circulating blood by the exercising muscles, (3) increased muscle strength, (4) increased mitochondrial enzymatic activity, (5) proliferation of capillaries, (6) an increase in the mean transit time of blood through muscle capillaries, (7) a lowering of peripheral vascular resistance, and (8) an increased arteriovenous oxygen difference.[69–72] Moreover, these central and peripheral adaptations produce (1) a reduction in resting and submaximal heart rates, blood pressure, respiratory rate, and rating of perceived exertion (e.g., Borg scale); (2) improved skeletal muscle and coronary blood flow; (3) increased exercise-induced lipolysis and translocation of lactate from muscle cells to the blood; (4) improved oxygen consumption (lower levels of oxygen during submaximal exercise and higher levels at maximal exercise) and physical work capacity.[73–77]

Unfortunately, many of the favorable effects associated with habitual exercise are markedly delayed or absent in patients with pulmonary disease. In addition, many of the medications routinely used in the treatment of pulmonary disease mask or impede the beneficial effects of exercise. In particular, corticosteroids exhibit several deleterious effects on exercise performance and bodily function. The major deleterious manifestations of corticosteroids include cataracts, diabetes, peptic ulcers, emotional lability, ecchymoses, edema, osteoporosis, weight gain with cushingoid appearance, skeletal muscle myopathy (occurring in the proximal and possibly other muscle groups), and atrophy of type IIb muscle fibers.[6, 27, 78–81] It is of particular concern for patients with pulmonary disease that steroid myopathy and muscular atrophy have not only been identified in the peripheral skeletal muscles but also in the muscle fibers of the diaphragm.[82, 83] The impact of corticosteroids and other pulmonary medications on selected parameters associated with exercise performance is summarized in Table 15–9.

All the untoward effects associated with corticosteroids are significantly dosage-dependent. Moreover, the deleterious side effects of corticosteroids may be reduced in their severity, or forestalled, with the implementation of a regular aerobic exercise regimen and proper nutritional support.[84, 85] In fact, when anabolic steroids are employed in conjunction with corticosteroid therapy and exercise, trained patients with severe pulmonary disease have exhibited increased fat-free mass and improved ventilatory muscle strength and endurance in comparison with patients receiving only corticosteroids.[86, 87]

Because one of the major objectives of pharmacologic intervention and exercise therapy is the improvement of a patient's ability to breathe at rest and during activity, it is important to understand the impact of obstructive and restrictive pulmonary diseases on the pattern of breathing. Making this task difficult, however, is the fact that the exercise-related breathing patterns of patients with obstructive lung diseases have been described as falling somewhere between two extremes: rapid and shallow or slow and deep.[88–90] This apparent lack of agreement stems from the fact that patients with obstructive lung disease must rely to a greater extent upon breathing frequency to augment minute ventilation, because their tidal volumes tend to be significantly smaller than normal as a result of the disease process. As a consequence, patients with obstructive lung disease reach their maximum minute ventilation at lower workloads than do asymptomatic individuals. Patients with obstructive pulmonary diseases are also hampered by a greater degree of alveolar and terminal respiratory unit hyperinflation compared with asymptomatic persons. This leads to larger residual volumes and smaller tidal volumes, further decreasing efficiency and increasing the work of breathing. It seems that the greater the severity

Table 15–9.

Potential Effect of Pulmonary Medications on Selected Variables at Rest and During Exercise

DRUG	HR	BP	RR	Sa_{O_2}	$\dot{V}O_{2\,max}$	RPE	EXERCISE DURATION	MAXIMAL WORKLOAD	SKELETAL MUSCLE Mass	SKELETAL MUSCLE Lipid Metabolism	SKELETAL MUSCLE Glucose Metabolism	SKELETAL MUSCLE Protein Metabolism
Sympathomimetics												
Beta$_2$-specific	⇑	⇑	⇔	⇑	⇑	⇓	⇑	⇑	⇔	?	?	?
Nonspecific	⇑	⇑	⇔	⇑	⇑	⇓	⇑	⇑	⇔	?	?	?
Sympatholytics	⇓	⇓	⇔	⇑	⇓	⇓	⇓	⇓	⇔	?	⇓	?
Parasympatholytics	⇑	⇔	⇑	⇑	⇑	⇓	⇕	⇕	⇔	⇕	⇑	?
Methylxanthines	⇑	⇔	⇔	⇑	⇑	⇓	⇑	⇑	⇔	⇑	⇓	?
Cromolyn sodium	⇔	⇔	⇔	⇑	⇑	⇓	⇔	⇔	⇕	?	⇕	?
Corticosteroids	⇕⇓	⇕⇓	⇕⇓	⇑	⇑	⇓	⇕⇓	⇕⇓	⇕⇓	⇕⇓	⇓	⇕⇓
Oxygen	⇓	⇓	⇓	⇑	⇑	⇓	⇑	⇑	⇔	⇑	?	⇓

Key: HR = heart rate, BP = blood pressure, RR = respiratory rate, Sa_{O_2} = arterial oxygen saturation, $\dot{V}O_{2\,max}$ = maximum oxygen consumption rate, RPE = rating of perceived exertion; ⇑ = increased response, ⇓ = decreased response; ⇕ = either increased or decreased response, ⇔ = no significant effect, ? = questionable effect.

of the obstructive lung disease (i.e., the lower the FEV_1), the longer it takes to achieve an increase in tidal volume.

Although patients with asthma and cystic fibrosis may demonstrate different pathologic changes in the lung, the pattern of breathing during exercise is similar to that used by patients with chronic bronchitic and emphysemic obstructive lung disease.[91] It also appears that the exercise-related pattern of breathing exhibited by patients with restrictive lung disease is similar to that of patients with obstructive lung disease. Patients with restrictive lung disease appear to increase minute ventilation only minimally during exercise, and as a result, there is a decrease in the total breathing cycle time due to a subsequent decrease in inspiratory time and a concomitant increase in inspiratory flow. Because there is less opportunity to increase tidal volume and a greater degree of pulmonary hypertension in patients with restrictive lung disease, exercise tends to be terminated prematurely due to marked oxygen desaturation and dyspnea. Thus, like the patient with obstructive lung disease, the patient with restrictive lung disease tries to increase minute ventilation by increasing breathing frequency, but only slightly increases tidal volume.[73, 92]

The appropriate and judicious use of supplemental oxygen can improve the metabolic activity and work capacity of skeletal muscle, as well as the breathing pattern, of patients with pulmonary disease who are hypoxic. Additionally, the use of **bilevel positive airway pressure** (BiPAP,* a noninvasive ventilatory assistance device providing supplemental oxygen and positive airway pressure during both inspiration and expiration) at rest and during exercise has been shown to significantly increase arterial oxygen saturation levels and decrease the respiratory rates of patients with end-stage lung disease.[93, 94] Careful prescription and titration of medications, as well as appropriate monitoring of the cardiorespiratory responses at rest and during exercise, can permit individuals with lung disease to participate to a greater extent in activities of daily living and exercise training programs.

---

*Respironics, Inc., Pittsburgh, PA 15213.

CASE STUDIES

Case 1

An 89-year-old white woman was admitted to the hospital with complaints of shortness of breath, productive sputum, and nausea. Up to 2 weeks prior to admission, patient was independently active in the community and around her own home. However, 3 days prior to admission, the patient required a walker to get around due to weakness, shortness of breath. She developed a cough 3 weeks prior to admission and had been diagnosed by the physician as having an upper respiratory tract infection and was being treated with Biaxin. The sputum cleared, but the cough persisted. When the patient was brought to the hospital she was diagnosed with mild congestive heart failure. She was started on diuretics and digoxin was continued. While she was in ICU her daughter noticed an increase in thick, gray-yellow sputum. She also had postnasal drip and abdominal discomfort, but denied indigestion. Other complaints included low back pain with radicular signs thought to be aggravated by her coughing. Currently she is on 3 L supplemental O_2.

Social history: The patient lives alone, but has a very supportive, concerned family. She denies smoking or alcohol use.

Past medical history:
    Cholecystectomy, 1993
    Polynephritis
    Atrial fibrillation
    Congestive heart failure
    Arteriosclerotic cardiovascular disease
    Hypertensive cardiovascular disease
Medications:
    Ascorbic acid, 500 mg po bid
    Biaxin (clarithromycin), 250 mg po bid
    Fosamax (alendronate sodium), 10 mg every morning
    Lasix (furosemide), 80 mg po q12h
    Prilosec (omeprazole), 20 mg po q4h or when needed
    Lanoxin, 125 mg po
    Ativan (lorazepam), prn
    Azmacort inhaler (triamcinolone acetonide), qd
    Phenergan with codeine, 5 to 10 mL po q4–6h, prn cough

Case 2

The patient is a 66-year-old white woman morbidly obese, with a chief complaint of low back pain and a lower extremity weakness. She is an ex-smoker who quit 10 years ago, but smoked for 40 years, 2 pack/day habit.
Diagnosis:
  Spinal stenosis; presurgical evaluation
  Lower extremity weakness
  Bronchial asthma: severe for last 5 years

Medications:
Lasix (furosemide), 40 mg bid
Chlorpheniramine, 4 mg bid
Verapamil, 80 mg bid
Albuterol, 4 mg bid
Proventil inhaler, 4 puffs q4h
Beclovent inhaler, 3 puffs q4h
Metolazone, 5 mg tiw
Servant inhaler, 2 puffs bid
Buspar, 10 mg bid
Potassium, 3 in am, 2 in pm
Slo-bid (theophylline) 200 mg, 2 in am, 2 in pm
 The patient's exercise is significantly limited
secondary to shortness of breath. Also, she is an excessive talker, which increases her shortness of breath during exercise.

Summary

This chapter covered the principal groups of drugs used in the treatment of pulmonary dysfunction and their potential effects on exercise performance. The principal points that were addressed include the following:

- Normal bronchomotor tone is the result of a balance between the influences of the sympathetic and parasympathetic divisions of the autonomic nervous system.
- Bronchoconstriction is the result of abnormal bronchomotor tone (bronchospasm), inflammation, or mechanical obstruction.
- The primary goal of bronchodilator therapy is to manipulate the influences of the autonomic nervous system via two opposing nucleotides: cAMP and cGMP.
- Decongestants are used to treat the mucosal edema and increased mucus production often associated with common colds, allergies, and many respiratory infections.
- Antihistamines are often used alone, or combined with other ingredients, to control the production of mucus and the mucosal edema and irritation commonly associated with respiratory allergic responses.
- Antitussives are used to suppress the ineffective, dry hacking cough associated with minor throat irritations and the common cold.
- Mucokinetics promote the mobilization and removal of secretions from the respiratory tract.
- Analeptics are used to stimulate the central nervous system and enhance respiratory center activity.

- Paralyzing agents are used to ensure immobility in patients during surgical procedures, to facilitate endotracheal intubation, and to reduce the work of breathing in some mechanically ventilated patients.
- Antimicrobial agents are used to combat microorganisms that invade the body, either by killing them or by limiting their growth and proliferation.
- Oxygen is considered a drug when it is administered in concentrations higher than those found in the atmospheric air.
- Nitric oxide is used for the treatment of pulmonary hypertension.
- Careful prescription and titration of medications, as well as appropriate monitoring of the cardiorespiratory responses at rest and during exercise, can permit individuals with lung disease to participate to a greater extent in activities of daily living and exercise training programs.

References

1. Respiratory pharmacology. Clin Chest Med 7:311–518, 1986.
2. Ziment I, Popa V. Respiratory pharmacology. Clin Chest Med 7: 313–329, 1986.
3. III Baltic Meeting on Pharmacology. Physiology and Pharmacology of the Respiratory System. Symposium proceedings. Copenhagen, Denmark, August 15–16, 1992. Pharmacol Toxicol 72:1–55, 1993.
4. Drain CB, Robinson SE. The pharmacology of respiratory disorders related to anesthesia. Clin Forum Nurse Anesth 7: 193–199, 1996.
5. Leff AR. Pulmonary and critical care pharmacology and therapeutics. New York, McGraw-Hill, 1996.
6. Rau JL. Respiratory Care Pharmacology. 5th ed. St. Louis, C.V. Mosby, 1998.
7. Deitmer T. Physiology and pathology of the mucociliary system: Special regards to mucociliary transport in malignant lesions of the human larynx. Adv Otorhinolaryngol 43: 1–136, 1989.
8. Marek W. Chronobiology of the bronchial system. Pneumologie 51(suppl 2):430–439, 1997.
9. Morrison JF, Pearson SB. The effect of the circadian rhythm of vagal activity on bronchomotor tone in asthma. Br J Clin Pharmacol 28:545–549, 1989.
10. Leff AR. Endogenous regulation of bronchomotor tone. Am Rev Respir Dis 137:1198–1216, 1988.
11. Widdicombe JG. Pulmonary and respiratory tract receptors. J Exp Biol 100:41–57, 1982.
12. van der Velden VH, Hulsmann AR. Autonomic innervation of human airways: Structure, function, and pathophysiology in asthma. Neuroimmunomodulation 6:145–159, 1999.
13. Pearlman DS. Pathophysiology of the inflammatory response. J Allergy Clin Immunol 104:S132–S137, 1999.

14. Bjornsdottir US, Cypcar DM. Asthma: An inflammatory mediator soup. Allergy 54:55–61, 1999.
15. Carter PM, Heinly TL, Yates SW, Lieberman PL. Asthma: The irreversible airways disease. J Investig Allergol Clin Immunol 7:566–571, 1997.
16. Rossi GL, Olivieri D. Does the mast cell still have a key role in asthma? Chest 112:523–529, 1997.
17. Marney SR Jr. Pathophysiology of reactive airway disease and sinusitis. Ann Otol Rhinol Laryngol 105:98–100, 1996.
18. Leung DY. Molecular basis of allergic diseases. Mol Genet Metab 63:157–167, 1998.
19. Wills-Karp M. Immunologic basis of antigen-induced airway hyperresponsiveness. Annu Rev Immunol 17:255–281, 1999.
20. Chin JE, Hatfield CA, Winterrowd GE, et al. Preclinical evaluation of anti-inflammatory activities of the novel pyrrolopyrimidine PNU-142731A, a potential treatment for asthma. J Pharmacol Exp Ther 290:188–195, 1999.
21. Oda N, Yamashita N, Minoguchi K, et al. Long-term analysis of allergen-specific T cell clones from patients with asthma treated with allergen rush immunotherapy. Cell Immunol 190:43–50, 1998.
22. Dent G, Giembycz MA. Phosphodiesterase inhibitors: Lily the Pink's medicinal compound for asthma? Thorax 51: 647–649, 1996.
23. Dahan A, vanBeek JHGM. Physiology and Pharmacology of Cardio-respiratory Control. Boston: Kluwer Academic, 1998.
24. NHLBI. Guidelines for the diagnosis and management of asthma: Expert panel report 2. In: NIH publication no. 98-4051 ed. Bethesda, Md.: U.S. Dept. of Health and Human Services, Public Health Service, National Institutes of Health, National Heart Lung and Blood Insitute, 1997.
25. Kelly HW. Comparative potency and clinical efficacy of inhaled corticosteroids. Respir Care Clin North Am 5:537–553, 1999.
26. Cave A, Arlett P, Lee E. Inhaled and nasal corticosteroids: Factors affecting the risks of systemic adverse effects. Pharmacol Ther 83:153–179, 1999.
27. Ciccone CD. Pharmacology in rehabilitation. In: Contemporary Perspectives in Rehabilitation. 2nd ed. Philadelphia, FA Davis, 1996.
28. Krawiec ME, Wenzel SE. Inhaled nonsteroidal anti-inflammatory medications in the treatment of asthma. Respir Care Clin North Am 5:555–574, 1999.
29. Haahtela T. Advances in pharmacotherapy of asthma. Curr Probl Dermatol 28:135–152, 1999.
30. Aswania OA, Corlett SA, Chrystyn H. Relative bioavailability of sodium cromoglycate to the lung following inhalation, using urinary excretion. Br J Clin Pharmacol 47:613–618, 1999.
31. Furukawa C, Atkinson D, Forster TJ, et al. Controlled trial of two formulations of cromolyn sodium in the treatment of asthmatic patients > or = 12 years of age. Intal Study Group. Chest 116:65–72, 1999.
32. Sparrow MP, Weichselbaum M, McCray PB. Development of the innervation and airway smooth muscle in human fetal lung. Am J Respir Cell Molec Biol 20:550–560, 1999.
33. Lu CC. Bronchodilator therapy for chronic obstructive pulmonary disease. Respirology 2:317–322, 1997.
34. Gauthier AP, Yan S, Sliwinski P, Macklem PT. Effects of fatigue, fiber length, and aminophylline on human diaphragm contractility. Am J Respir Crit Care Med 152:204–210, 1995.
35. Krzanowski JJ, Polson JB. Mechanism of action of methylxanthines in asthma. J Allergy Clin Immunol 82:143–145, 1988.
36. Murciano D, Aubier M, Curran Y, Pariente R. Action of aminophylline on the strength of contraction of the dia phragm in patients with chronic obstructive respiratory insufficiency. Presse Med 16:1628–1630, 1987.
37. Church MK, Featherstone RL, Cushley MJ, et al. Relationships between adenosine, cyclic nucleotides, and xanthines in asthma. J Allergy Clin Immunol 78:670–675, 1986.
38. Schmidt D, Dent G, Rabe KF. Selective phosphodiesterase inhibitors for the treatment of bronchial asthma and chronic obstructive pulmonary disease. Clin Exp Allergy 29 (suppl 2):99–109, 1999.
39. Barnes PJ. Novel approaches and targets for treatment of chronic obstructive pulmonary disease. Am J Respir Crit Care Med 160:S72–S79, 1999.
40. Fireman P. Pathophysiology and pharmacotherapy of common upper respiratory diseases. Pharmacotherapy 13:101S–109S; 143S–146S, 1993.
41. Hornby PJ, Abrahams TP. Pulmonary pharmacology. Clin Obstet Gynecol 39:17–35, 1996.
42. Slater JW, Zechnich AD, Haxby DG. Second-generation antihistamines: A comparative review. Drugs 57:31–47, 1999.
43. Zemp E, Elsasser S, Schindler C, et al. Long-term ambient air pollution and respiratory symptoms in adults (SAPALDIA study). The SAPALDIA Team. Am J Respir Crit Care Med 159:1257–1266, 1999.
44. Agrawal M. OTC cold, cough and allergy products: More choice or more confusion? J Hosp Mark 13:79–86, 1999.
45. Casaburi R. Pharmacological modulators of respiratory control. Monaldi Arch Chest Dis 53:287–293, 1998.
46. Kerr HD. Doxapram in hypercapnic chronic obstructive pulmonary disease with respiratory failure. J Emerg Med 15: 513–515, 1997.
47. Bjork L, Arborelius M Jr, Renck H, Rosberg B. Doxapram improves pulmonary function after upper abdominal surgery. Acta Anaesthesiol Scand 37:181–188, 1993.
48. Huon C, Rey E, Mussat P, et al. Low-dose doxapram for treatment of apnoea following early weaning in very low birthweight infants: A randomized, double-blind study. Acta Paediatr 87:1180–1184, 1998.
49. Kersten LD. Comprehensive Respiratory Nursing: A Decision-Making Approach. Philadelphia, WB Saunders, 1989, p 864.
50. Sethi S. Infectious exacerbations of chronic bronchitis: Diagnosis and management [see comments]. J Antimicrob Chemother 43 (suppl A): 97–105, 1999.
51. Hillier SC, Graham JA, Hanger CC, et al. Hypoxic vasoconstriction in pulmonary arterioles and venules. J Appl Physiol 82:1084–1090, 1997.
52. Burkhart JE Jr, Stoller JK. Oxygen and aerosolized drug delivery: Matching the device to the patient. Cleve Clin J Med 65:200–208, 1998.
53. Hida W. Role of ventilatory drive in asthma and chronic obstructive pulmonary disease. Curr Opin Pulm Med 5:339–343, 1999.
54. Dunn WF, Nelson SB, Hubmayr RD. Oxygen-induced hypercarbia in obstructive pulmonary disease. Am Rev Respir Dis 144:526–530, 1991.
55. Capellier G, Maupoil V, Boussat S, et al. Oxygen toxicity and tolerance. Minerva Anestesiol 65:388–392, 1999.
56. Beckett WS, Wong ND. Effect of normobaric hyperoxia on airways of normal subjects. J Appl Physiol 64:1683–1687, 1988.
57. Bryan CL, Jenkinson SG. Oxygen toxicity. Clin Chest Med 9:141–152, 1988.
58. Barst RJ. Diagnosis and treatment of pulmonary artery hypertension. Curr Opin Pediatr 8:512–519, 1996.
59. Weitzenblum E, Kessler R, Oswald M, Fraisse P. Medical treatment of pulmonary hypertension in chronic lung disease. Eur Respir J 7:148–152, 1994.

60. Roger N, Barbera JA, Roca J, et al. Nitric oxide inhalation during exercise in chronic obstructive pulmonary disease. Am J Respir Crit Care Med 156:800–806, 1997.

61. Wanstall JC, Jeffery TK. Recognition and management of pulmonary hypertension. Drugs 56:989–1007, 1998.

62. Shah AM, Prendergast BD, Grocott-Mason R, et al. The influence of endothelium-derived nitric oxide on myocardial contractile function. Int J Cardiol 50:225–231, 1995.

63. Paulus WJ, Kastner S, Pujadas P, et al. Left ventricular contractile effects of inducible nitric oxide synthase in the human allograft. Circulation 96:3436–3442, 1997.

64. Watkins DN, Jenkins IR, Rankin JM, Clarke GM. Inhaled nitric oxide in severe acute respiratory failure—Its use in intensive care and description of a delivery system [see comments]. Anaesth Intensive Care 21:861–866, 1993.

65. Rossaint R, Busch T, Falke K. Nitric oxide inhalation therapy in acute respiratory distress syndrome: Intended effects and possible side effects. Methods Enzymol 269:442–453, 1996.

66. Okamoto K, Hamaguchi M, Kukita I, et al. Efficacy of inhaled nitric oxide in children with ARDS. Chest 114:827–833, 1998.

67. Young JD, Dyar O, Xiong L, Howell S. Methaemoglobin production in normal adults inhaling low concentrations of nitric oxide. Intensive Care Med 20:581–584, 1994.

68. Maltais F, LeBlanc P, Jobin J, et al. Intensity of training and physiologic adaptation in patients with chronic obstructive pulmonary disease. Am J Respir Crit Care Med 155:555–561, 1997.

69. Paterson DH, Cunningham DA. The gas transporting systems: Limits and modifications with age and training. Can J Appl Physiol 24:28–40, 1999.

70. Hata K, Hata T, Miyazaki K, et al. Effect of regular aerobic exercise on cerebrovascular tone in young women. J Ultrasound Med 17:133–136, 1998.

71. Aoyagi Y, McLellan TM, Shephard RJ. Interactions of physical training and heat acclimation. The thermophysiology of exercising in a hot climate. Sports Med 23:173–210, 1997.

72. Ades PA, Waldmann ML, Meyer WL, et al. Skeletal muscle and cardiovascular adaptations to exercise conditioning in older coronary patients. Circulation 94:323–330, 1996.

73. Casaburi R, Porszasz J, Burns MR, et al. Physiologic benefits of exercise training in rehabilitation of patients with severe chronic obstructive pulmonary disease. Am J Respir Crit Care Med 155:1541–1551, 1997.

74. Oldridge N. Cardiac rehabilitation in the elderly. Aging (Milano) 10:273–283, 1998.

75. Cress ME, Buchner DM, Questad KA, et al. Exercise: Effects on physical functional performance in independent older adults. J Gerontol A Biol Sci Med Sci 54:M242–M248, 1999.

76. Gulmans VA, de Meer K, Brackel HJ, et al. Outpatient exercise training in children with cystic fibrosis: Physiological effects, perceived competence, and acceptability. Pediatr Pulmonol 28:39–46, 1999.

77. Fuchs-Climent D, Le Gallais D, Varray A, et al. Quality of life and exercise tolerance in chronic obstructive pulmonary disease: Effects of a short and intensive inpatient rehabilitation program. Am J Phys Med Rehabil 78:330–335, 1999.

78. Berger I, Argaman Z, Schwartz SB, et al. Efficacy of corticosteroids in acute bronchiolitis: Short-term and long-term follow-up. Pediatr Pulmonol 26:162–166, 1998.

79. Oermann CM, Sockrider MM, Konstan MW. The use of anti-inflammatory medications in cystic fibrosis: Trends and physician attitudes. Chest 115:1053–1058, 1999.

80. Chay OM, Goh A, Lim WH, et al. Effects of inhaled corticosteroid on bone turnover in children with bronchial asthma. Respirology 4:63–67, 1999.

81. Malo JL, Cartier A, Ghezzo H, et al. Skin bruising, adrenal function and markers of bone metabolism in asthmatics using inhaled beclomethasone and fluticasone. Eur Respir J 13:993–998, 1999.

82. van Balkom RH, van der Heijden HF, van Herwaarden CL, Dekhuijzen PN. Corticosteroid-induced myopathy of the respiratory muscles. Neth J Med 45:114–122, 1994.

83. Decramer M, Stas KJ. Corticosteroid-induced myopathy involving respiratory muscles in patients with chronic obstructive pulmonary disease or asthma. Am Rev Respir Dis 146:800–802, 1992.

84. LaPier TK. Glucocorticoid-induced muscle atrophy. The role of exercise in treatment and prevention. J Cardiopulm Rehabil 17:76–84, 1997.

85. Braith RW, Welsch MA, Mills RM Jr, et al. Resistance exercise prevents glucocorticoid-induced myopathy in heart transplant recipients. Med Sci Sports Exerc 30:483–489, 1998.

86. Creutzberg EC, Schols AM. Anabolic steroids. Curr Opin Clin Nutr Metab Care 2:243–253, 1999.

87. Schols AM, Slangen J, Volovics L, Wouters EF. Weight loss is a reversible factor in the prognosis of chronic obstructive pulmonary disease. Am J Respir Crit Care Med 157:1791–1797, 1998.

88. Orenstein DM, Nixon PA. Exercise performance and breathing patterns in cystic fibrosis: Male-female differences and influence of resting pulmonary function. Pediatr Pulmonol 10:101–105, 1991.

89. Benditt JO, Wood DE, McCool FD, et al. Changes in breathing and ventilatory muscle recruitment patterns induced by lung volume reduction surgery. Am J Respir Crit Care Med 155:279–284, 1997.

90. Chung F, Dean E, Ross J. Cardiopulmonary responses of middle-aged men without cardiopulmonary disease to steady-rate positive and negative work performed on a cycle ergometer. Phys Ther 79:476–487, 1999.

91. Vaz Fragoso CA, Clark T, Kotch A. The tidal volume response to incremental exercise in COPD. Chest 103:1438–1441, 1993.

92. O'Donnell DE. Chau LKL, Webb KA. Qualitative aspects of exertional dyspnea in patients with interstitial lung disease. J Appl Physiol 84:2000–2009, 1998.

93. Renston JP, DiMarco AF, Supinski GS. Respiratory muscle rest using nasal BiPAP ventilation in patients with stable severe COPD. Chest 105:1053–1060, 1994.

94. Kleopa KA, Sherman M, Neal B, et al. BiPAP improves survival and rate of pulmonary function decline in patients with ALS. J Neurol Sci 164:82–88, 1999.

6

Cardiopulmonary Assessment and Intervention

16

Assessment Procedures

Ellen A. Hillegass

INTRODUCTION

Optimal rehabilitation depends on a thorough assessment of the entire patient to evaluate the extent of dysfunction that may affect future performance. In this chapter, the evaluative procedures used to provide information regarding specific cardiopulmonary system diseases are described. While performing the initial assessment, objective information can be obtained from a thorough review of the medical record, an interview with the patient,

and an evaluation of the patient at rest (including observation and inspection, palpation, auscultation, **mediate percussion,** general muscle strength, and joint range of motion) and during activity. In addition, the physical therapist must also have a good understanding of other therapeutic regimens and concomitant problems and be able to recognize them. On conclusion of the evaluation, the therapist should be able to interpret the evaluative findings appropriately to make a decision regarding therapeutic interventions.

610

MEDICAL CHART REVIEW

The purpose of the medical chart review is to extract pertinent information to develop a database on the patient. Based on the information obtained, the physical therapist performs the appropriate physical assessment and develops an optimal treatment plan. The therapist should focus the review of the medical record by identifying the following significant information:

- Diagnosis and date of event
- Symptoms on admission and after the patient's admission
- Other significant medical problems in the past medical history
- Current medications
- Risk factors for cardiovascular and pulmonary disease
- Relevant social history, including smoking, alcohol and drug use, lifestyle, support mechanisms
- Clinical laboratory data
- Radiologic studies
- Oxygen therapy and other respiratory treatment
- Surgical procedures
- Other therapeutic regimens
- Electrocardiogram and telemetry monitoring
- Pulmonary function tests
- Arterial blood gases
- Cardiac catheterization data
- Other diagnostic tests
- Vital signs
- Hospital course since admission, particularly in the patient with cardiac injury to determine whether it has been a complicated or an uncomplicated course
- Occupational history
- Home environment assessment

Diagnosis and Date of Event

The physical therapist needs to know and understand the primary diagnosis as well as any additional diagnoses made since the hospital admission or referral to rehabilitation to determine the appropriateness of treatment and the need for monitoring of the patient's responses. Often a patient's primary diagnosis may have been the reason for admission (e.g., a fractured hip), yet a secondary diagnosis may be the reason for referral for physi-

cal therapy (e.g., pneumonia postoperatively). Any diagnosis that begins "Rule out ——" requires a thorough review of the chart to see if the diagnosis was confirmed or rejected.

The date of the event is significant, because it determines the acuteness of the situation. The date of the primary event or diagnosis is often documented in the physician's history and physical examination report; however, the date of the secondary diagnosis or subsequent events may be discovered by reviewing the physician's progress notes or orders.

Symptoms

Both cardiovascular and pulmonary symptoms need to be evaluated. Cardiac ischemic symptoms are those that occur anywhere above the waist; they are typically expressed on, or exacerbated by, exertion and are relieved with rest. These symptoms may be described differently by each patient. Classically, any discomfort, such as chest pain, tightness or pressure, shortness of breath, palpitations, indigestion, and burning, should be considered a cardiac symptom unless cardiac dysfunction has been ruled out. Reviewing the patient's symptoms on admission and during hospitalization provides the therapist with an awareness of those symptoms that are to be assessed as cardiac or noncardiac. During activity the therapist may be trying to reproduce those symptoms as well as observe for new ones. Ischemic-related symptoms may also be present in other vasculature of the body, and they, too, should be assessed.

Classic pulmonary symptoms are described as shortness of breath, dyspnea on exertion, audible wheezing, cough, increased work of breathing, and sputum production. The severity of the symptoms as well as the means of reproducing these symptoms are important to identify. Changes in these symptoms (e.g., worsening of symptoms versus improvement) assist the therapist in developing a plan of care that meets the patient's changing needs.

Other Medical Problems and Past Medical History

The patient's past medical history, including other medical problems, may have a bearing on the evaluation or the plan of treatment proposed by the therapist. Diagnoses other than cardiovascular and pulmonary may include orthopedic, neurologic, psychological, or **integumentary,** and these diagnoses may affect the optimal treatment plan proposed. For example, an attempt to increase the activity level of a patient with a history of rheumatoid arthritis may be limited by an orthopedic (joint) dysfunction rather than by a cardiovascular or pulmonary condition.

Medications

The medications the patient is currently taking are usually listed in the chart (often in the physician's orders). In the inpatient setting, a comprehensive listing can be found on the nurse's medication chart. Knowledge of the patient's medications can provide information about the patient's present or recent past medical history and may include clues regarding treatment for hypertension, heart failure, angina, bronchospasm, infection, and the like.

Because certain medications may affect the patient's responses to exercise, the physical therapist must become familiar with the broad categories of cardiac and pulmonary medications, understand the indications for their use, and know their general side effects. For further discussion of medications and their indications and side effects see Chapters 14 and 15.

Risk Factors for Heart Disease

From the history and physical examination, one usually can determine whether the patient has any of the following major risk factors for heart disease[1].

- Hypertension
- Smoking
- An elevated serum cholesterol or a diet high in cholesterol
- A family history of heart disease
- Stress
- A sedentary lifestyle
- Older age
- Male gender
- Obesity
- Diabetes

An awareness of the patient's risk factors enables the therapist to develop realistic goals for the pa-

tient's long-term treatment, to identify other rehabilitation team members to whom the patient should be referred, and most important, to decide on precautions to increased activity, depending on the risk for heart disease. Detailed information on the risk factors can be obtained from Chapter 3.

Relevant Social History

Self-abusive social habits, such as excessive drinking of alcohol, smoking, and use of illicit drugs, can affect the cardiopulmonary system and could affect rehabilitation. Therefore, knowledge of the patient's habits, including the length of time involved in the habit and the degree of intake, is an important component of the evaluation. Some of this information can be obtained from the history and physical examination, but often this information is obtained from the patient or the family.

Heavy alcohol consumption has been associated with the development of **cardiomyopathy,** and long-term cigarette smoking has been associated with the development of chronic obstructive lung disease. Drug use is one habit that may not be readily acknowledged but that may be suspected from the individual's behavior (e.g., extreme nervousness), history of sleeplessness, muscle twitching, anorexia, and nasal irritation. For example, cocaine has serious effects on the cardiovascular system, particularly on the coronary arteries. Cocaine is known to cause severe coronary artery spasm and in some cases can precipitate acute myocardial infarction.[2-4] Cocaine use (especially crack cocaine) has been associated with an increased incidence of severe arrhythmias and in some cases sudden death.

The physician or other medical personnel treating the patient may be unaware of the patient's heavy alcohol consumption or drug addiction. Either of these conditions could prove to be an extreme problem early in the patient's hospitalization because of the symptoms and side effects of sudden withdrawal from these substances.

Clinical Laboratory Data

Laboratory data provide important objective information regarding the clinical status of the patient with cardiopulmonary dysfunction. The seriousness of the dysfunction may also be inferred from the magnitude of deviation of the values from normal. The laboratory data specific to the patient with cardiopulmonary dysfunction include the values for cardiac enzymes (creatine phosphokinase, lactate dehydrogenase, aspartate aminotransferase), blood lipids (cholesterol and triglycerides), complete blood cell count (specifically hemoglobin, hematocrit, white blood cell count), arterial blood gases, and culture and sensitivity, as well as the results of **coagulation** studies, electrolyte screening panels, and glucose tolerance tests. These are discussed in greater detail in Chapters 8 and 10.

Radiologic Studies

In most situations the therapist reviews the radiologic report and not the actual study films. The radiologic reports that are routinely reviewed for patients with cardiopulmonary dysfunction include chest radiographs, **computed tomography** (CT) scan, **magnetic resonance imaging** (MRI), and **scintigraphy.**

The chest radiographs provide a general static assessment of pathologic conditions of the lungs and chest wall, including changes in functional lung space, pleural space, chest wall configuration, presence of fluid, heart size, and vascularization of the lungs. Information about the extent of heart failure or cardiomyopathy as well as pneumonia, restrictive lung disease, pleural effusion, and the like can be obtained from the chest radiograph.

In addition to baseline chest radiographs, patients with heart failure and acute pulmonary dysfunction can be followed with serial radiographs to monitor disease progression, effectiveness of treatment, or both. Therefore, it is important to note the date of the radiograph (particularly if the patient's status is fluctuating). Also the orientation of the chest radiograph is important to identify. The ideal chest radiograph is a posteroanterior (PA) film taken at a distance of approximately 6 feet with the patient in an upright position and performing a maximal inspiration. Portable equipment utilizing the anteroposterior (AP) orientation is used to take chest films of patients who are too sick or unstable to be transported to the radiology department for a standard PA film. The quality of the film taken with portable equipment and using the AP orientation is generally poorer than a PA film owing to the position of the patient and the patient's inability to cooperate or to perform a maximal inspiration. The therapist should keep these limitations in mind when evaluating the findings of a portable AP chest radiograph.

Oxygen Therapy and Other Respiratory Treatment

The use of supplemental oxygen should be noted along with its method of delivery (e.g., nasal cannula, face mask, **tracheostomy** collar, blow-by ventilator, or mechanical ventilator). The physical therapist must also know the amount of oxygen being delivered (e.g., 60% via mask or 2 L via cannula). This information should be correlated with arterial blood gas analysis or hemoglobin saturation data to determine if the patient is adequately oxygenated before beginning any therapy. Depending on the arterial blood gas or oxygen saturation information, the therapist may need to use oxygen or to increase the amount of oxygen while exercising the patient (e.g., during formal exercise, activities of daily living, gait). Any patient with a resting PO_2 of less than 60 mm Hg on room air or an oxygen percentage saturation of less than 90% should be considered for supplemental oxygen. If a patient has a low PO_2 but one not below 60 mm Hg on room air or a low PO_2 on oxygen, the patient may require supplemental oxygen with exercise to prevent hypoxemia during exercise. Chapter 10 presents a method of assessing the degree of **hypoxemia** when patients are receiving supplemental oxygen.

Other respiratory treatments (e.g., aerosols, bronchodilator treatments, inspirometers) that are prescribed should be noted because these treatments can improve the patient's exercise performance if they are administered before exercise; however, they may also be extremely fatiguing to the patient and may necessitate limitations on activity immediately following treatment. The necessity for the coordination of physical therapy and respiratory treatments to optimize rehabilitation should be readily apparent. If the patient is being ventilated mechanically, the mode of ventilatory assistance, the set rate, the set volume, the peak inspiratory pressure, the fraction of inspired oxygen, the spontaneous rate, and the like should be identified. A full description of ventilators is found in Chapter 10.

Surgical Procedures

An understanding of specific surgical approaches and procedures, as well as a knowledge of the anatomy of the chest wall, is integral to the chart review process. Knowledge of the approach or procedure may be helpful in defining the physical therapy diagnosis and extent of the problem and in identifying limitations or precautions to any therapeutic procedures being planned. (See Chapter 11.)

It is important to understand the number of and placement of the bypass grafts as well as any complications that occurred during the procedure (e.g., whether a pacemaker was inserted) in patients who have undergone coronary artery bypass surgery. For the patient who has undergone bypass surgery with numerous vessels requiring bypass grafts or requiring left main or left main equivalent bypass, one might assume that the patient was more limited in activity before surgery. With extensive disease, patients usually have more symptoms with activity and may have had restrictions with low levels of exertion. In addition, the patient who experiences complications (such as a perioperative myocardial infarction or stroke) during or following the surgery usually has a slower recovery and may require increased activity supervision and may make slower progress.

In the patient who has undergone pulmonary surgery, the amount of lung tissue that was operated on is significant to note (e.g., **wedge resection, lobectomy,** or **pneumonectomy**), as well as the location of the incision. The greater the amount of lung tissue that was removed, the smaller the amount of lung space is available (one would expect) to actively diffuse oxygen and carbon dioxide and therefore the greater the impairment in performance of activities.

Other Therapeutic Regimens

As a result of the patient's primary or secondary diagnoses or subsequent surgical procedures, additional therapeutic interventions could have an impact on the proposed treatment. Identification of these interventions (e.g., pacemaker implantation, intravenous or intra-arterial drug administration, **parenteral nutrition,** electrolyte replacement, or bedrest limitations) helps the physical therapist develop an appropriate treatment plan with appropriate precautions.

Electrocardiogram and Serial Monitoring

The electrocardiogram (ECG) provides valuable information regarding the state of the heart muscle and the rhythm of the heart. The ECG is used to define previous as well as current myocardial injury, hypertrophy of the heart muscle, pericardial involvement, or delays in the generation of the depolarization impulse. Serial ECG monitoring provides a historic record of the patient's cardiac injury and rhythm disturbances and allows the correlation of the history of rhythm disturbances with changes in medications or medical status. Details of the ECG and rhythm disturbances are discussed in Chapter 9.

Pulmonary Function Tests

A pulmonary function test (PFT) is an essential component of the assessment process because abnormal PFTs indicate the effects of the pathologic condition and may provide clues regarding the patient's motivation. Measurement of PFTs is done via spirometry. Pulmonary function tests can measure static and dynamic properties of the chest and lungs as well as gas exchange. Static measurements assess the lung volumes and capacities (e.g., tidal volume, vital capacity, inspiratory reserve volume) and determine mechanical abnormalities, whereas dynamic measurements provide data on the flow rates of air moving in and out of the lungs. The dynamic properties reflect the nonelastic components of the pulmonary system and include the forced expiratory flows and volumes.

Values for PFTs are used primarily to identify a baseline of pulmonary dysfunction, as well as to follow the progression of altered respiratory mechanics in chronic lung and musculoskeletal diseases. Chapter 10 explains PFTs in greater detail.

Values for PFTs may be described as abnormal owing to the static values (volumes and capacities), the dynamic values (flow volumes and rates), or both. When patients demonstrate decreased volumes and capacities, they are exhibiting restrictive lung dysfunction. They therefore have less lung space for active diffusion of oxygen into the circulatory system and carbon dioxide out of the system. Patients with decreased dynamic values often have limitations on exercise owing to an inability to actively move large volumes of air rapidly. Treatment planning requires modifications, possibly including supplemental oxygen for patients with extremely low lung volumes or bronchodilator medication before exercise for patients with decreased flow rates or volumes.

Arterial Blood Gases

Arterial blood gases are a measurement of the acid-base and oxygenation status of patients via arterial blood sampling. Blood gas determinations can identify the effectiveness of a treatment designed to improve airway clearance and ventilation. Therefore, serial arterial blood gases are often measured to provide feedback on the therapeutic regimen to the medical personnel. Arterial blood gases are discussed in greater detail in Chapter 10.

Cardiac Catheterization Data

Cardiac catheterization, which is an invasive diagnostic procedure, provides information about the anatomy of the coronary arteries and can provide a dynamic assessment of the cardiac muscle. In addition, information on hemodynamic measurement (e.g., estimates of ejection fraction or systolic and diastolic pressures) as well as valvular function can be obtained. Cardiac catheterizations are performed to visualize the cardiac dysfunction and to assist in the decision-making process regarding medical versus surgical management. Repeat cardiac catheterizations also provide information on the progression or, in rare cases, regression of coronary disease or valvular dysfunction. See Chapter 8 for more detailed information.

Vital Signs

Daily recordings of vital signs are often kept in the graphics section of the chart. Vital signs such as heart rate, temperature, blood pressure, and respiration are important to review for trends as well as for the establishment of a baseline. For example, pulmonary patients with infection who are being monitored for improvement can be followed by checking temperature and in some cases respirations and heart rate. Hypertension and treatment for hypertension can be monitored daily by viewing the blood pressure recordings (keeping in mind that these have been recorded at rest and usually in the supine position).

Hospital Course

A thorough review of the medical record, including physicians' and other caregivers' notes, and the order sheets should reveal pertinent information regarding the patient's clinical course since admission. For example, patients with serious complications within the first 4 days of a myocardial infarction have a higher incidence of later serious complications or death. Criteria for a complicated postmyocardial infarction hospital course as defined by McNeer and coworkers include the following[5]:

• Ventricular tachycardia and fibrillation
• Atrial flutter or fibrillation
• Second- or third-degree atrioventricular (AV) block
• Persistent sinus tachycardia (above 100 beats per minute)
• Persistent systolic hypotension (below 90 mm Hg)
• Pulmonary edema
• Cardiogenic shock
• Persistent angina or extension of infarction

Patients who are characterized as "uncomplicated" have significantly lower morbidity and mortality rates following their initial cardiac events. A prolonged or complicated hospital course can affect an individual's activity progression owing to the effects of inactivity or bedrest.

Occupation

Identifying the type of work the patient currently performs allows for the setting of realistic goals and for developing a plan for return to work, if possible. For example, a patient who has experienced a massive complicated myocardial infarction may not be an appropriate candidate for returning to a job requiring heavy lifting and may need a referral for **vocational rehabilitation.** The earlier the referral is made, the less the chance of financial or emotional distress. In addition, if a patient requires job modifications or will be delayed in returning to work, referrals can be made to appropriate team members to assist the employer in making the changes necessary or to assist the patient with financial planning.

Home Environment and Family Situation

A supportive family is important to the success of the rehabilitation of any patient. A support system can improve a patient's ability to respond to disease, whereas a negative home environment can deter the patient's rehabilitation.[6] In addition, if the patient requires a great deal of care, the family's ability to supply this care and its financial resources should be assessed. Early assessment of the family situation and home environment as well as involvement of the family in the patient's rehabilitation provides for optimal transition to home.

INTERVIEW WITH THE PATIENT AND THE FAMILY

After a thorough chart review, the interview with the patient and the family is the next step in the physical therapist's initial evaluation. The purpose of this interview is to gather important information about the patient's present complaint, history of medical problems, report of symptoms, risk factors, perception and understanding of the problem, family situation, and goals for rehabilitation (both occupational and leisure).

Important components of the interview are the establishment of effective communication and rapport with the patient and family. Simple, open-ended questions using language easily understood by the patient and family should elicit the answers needed. For example, the therapist might ask, "What did your discomfort feel like when you were admitted to the hospital?" or "How long have you had this breathing problem?" Listening is essential for learning about the patient's problems, as well as the patient's understanding of and reaction to them. The therapist must remember that a patient with pulmonary dysfunction may have difficulty with phonation owing to shortness of breath and may have to take breaths frequently between words. Table 16–1 provides some sample descriptors and questions for assessing cardiac symptoms.

PHYSICAL EXAMINATION

The physical examination is the third step in the initial evaluation of the patient. The physical examination requires the physical therapist to use the skills of inspection, palpation, percussion, auscultation, and activity evaluation when appropriate.

Inspection

Inspection (observation) is a key component in the assessment of *any* patient, but it is extremely important in patients with cardiopulmonary dysfunction. The patient's physical appearance may

Table 16–1 Differentiation of Nonanginal Discomforts from Angina	
STABLE ANGINA	**NONANGINAL DISCOMFORT (CHEST WALL PAIN)**
1. Relieved by nitroglycerin (30 seconds to 1 minute)	1. Nitroglycerin generally has no effect
2. Comes on at the same heart rate and blood pressure and is relieved by rest (lasts only a few minutes)	2. Occurs any time; lasts for hours
3. Not palpable	3. Muscle soreness, joint soreness, evoked by palpation or deep breaths
4. Associated with feelings of doom, cold sweats, shortness of breath	4. Minimal additional symptoms
5. Often seen with ST-segment depression	5. No ST-segment depression

Source: Irwin SI, Techlin JS. Cardiopulmonary Physical Therapy. 2nd ed. St. Louis, CV Mosby, 1990, p 124.

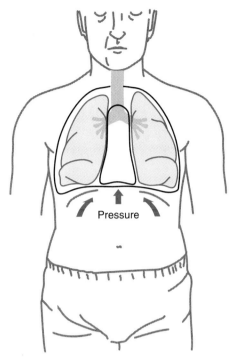

Figure 16–1. The increased size of the abdomen in obesity (or pregnancy) restricts the full downward movement of the diaphragm during inspiration and restricts lung tissue at rest, therefore creating a restrictive effect on the lung.

change slightly as the clinical state changes. Recognition of these slight changes is essential to the day-to-day management and therapeutic treatment of patients with cardiopulmonary dysfunction. Inspection should be performed in a systematic manner, starting with the head and proceeding caudally (until the therapist has developed a degree of proficiency). In addition to the general appearance, the other specific areas that should be noted on inspection include facial expression, effort to breathe through nose or mouth, the neck, the chest in both a resting and a dynamic situation, **phonation**, cough and **sputum** production, posture and positioning, and finally the extremities.

General Appearance

The patient's level of consciousness, body type, posture and positioning, skin tone, and need for external monitoring or support equipment should be considered in an assessment of "general appearance". Obviously, a patient's level of consciousness (e.g., alert, agitated, confused, semico-

matose, comatose) may have a direct impact on whether the treatment plan is understood. A comatose patient may require constant attention for positioning and prevention of pulmonary dysfunction, whereas a confused patient may not be able to follow a therapist's instructions without help. Observation of body type (e.g., obese, normal, **cachectic**) is a routine aspect of assessment that gives an indirect measure of nutrition and in some cases an indication of level of exercise tolerance. For example, a patient who is markedly obese may demonstrate a decreased exercise tolerance and an increased work of breathing owing to the restrictive effects of an excessively large abdomen pushing against the diaphragm (Fig. 16–1). By contrast, cachectic patients may also demonstrate a decreased exercise tolerance and an increased work of breathing with exercise because of weakness from muscle wasting.

Body posture and position should also be assessed to determine their impact on the pulmonary system. Kyphosis and **scoliosis** are two postures that functionally limit vital capacity and may therefore affect exercise tolerance. In addition, if a patient is assuming the **professorial position** (leaning forward on knees or on some object; Fig. 16–2) and demonstrating increased effort with

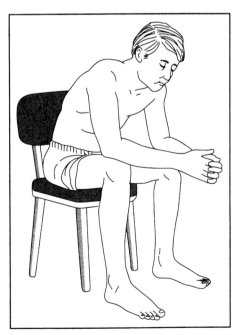

Figure 16–2. The professorial position provides stabilization of the thorax and arms to increase the effectiveness of accessory muscles during breathing.

breathing and increased use of accessory muscles, one might begin to assume the patient has chronic obstructive disease. Most patients with cardiopulmonary dysfunction cannot tolerate lying on a bed with the head flat and often are found lying either in the semi-Fowler's position in bed (Fig. 16–3) or sitting over the side of the bed or in a chair.

Skin tone may indicate the general level of oxygenation and perfusion of the periphery. An individual who has a general **cyanotic** look (bluish color most noticeably at lips and fingernail beds) may have a low PO$_2$ and may be in need of supplemental oxygen.

Finally, the presence of all equipment used in managing the patient, including monitoring or support equipment, should be noted. In addition, an assessment should be made of whether the equipment is being used correctly by the patient. For example, a patient who requires supplemental oxygen may be breathing through the mouth and therefore not inhaling the oxygen appropriately. As a result, the patient may be in a confused state, which can result in an unstable clinical situation. This patient's general appearance may be cyanotic, when in fact the most recent blood gas values recorded on the chart with the patient on the oxygen are normal. However, if the patient forgot to put the oxygen mask on or happened to pull the mask off because of "feelings of suffocation" and became confused and agitated as well as cyanotic, the acute change the therapist may note on entering the patient's room may be reversed by simply observing that the oxygen is not being used appropriately. Quick action by the therapist may solve this unstable clinical situation. In addition, the use of a cardiac monitor, pulmonary artery

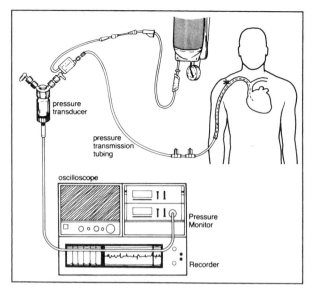

Figure 16–4. The setup for pulmonary artery monitoring. (Redrawn from Darovic GO. Hemodynamic Monitoring. Philadelphia, WB Saunders, 1987, p 85.)

catheter, or **intra-aortic balloon pump** indicates a more seriously ill patient who may have rhythm or hemodynamic disturbances (Fig. 16–4).

Facial Characteristics

Facial expression and effort to breathe are two characteristics that can be observed easily; both give important information for the clinical evaluation of the patient. Facial expressions of distress or fatigue may indicate a need for change in the therapeutic treatment. Facial signs of distress include nasal flaring, sweating, paleness, and focused or enlarged pupils. The effort to breathe can be evaluated not only by the facial expression of distress, but also by the degree of work put forth from the musculature of the face and neck and the movement of the lips to breathe. Pursed-lip breathing is a clinical sign of chronic obstructive lung disease, is performed to alleviate the trapping of air in the lungs, and is characterized by the patient breathing out against lips that are mostly closed and shaped in a circular fashion (Fig. 16–5).

Evaluation of the Neck

The activity of the neck musculature during breathing and the appearance of the jugular veins

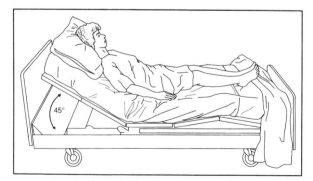

Figure 16–3. Semi-Fowler's position. Patients with cardiopulmonary dysfunction often require the head of the bed elevated.

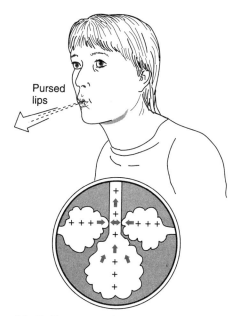

Figure 16-5. Demonstration of pursed-lip breathing and its effects in patients with emphysema. The weakened bronchiole airways are kept open by the effects of positive pressure created by the pursed lips during expiration.

should be a part of the standard patient assessment. The presence of hypertrophy or adaptive shortening of the sternocleidomastoid muscles may indicate a chronic pulmonary condition. (The sternocleidomastoid muscle is a very important accessory respiratory muscle that often hypertrophies when used excessively for breathing; Fig. 16–6). In addition, because of a chronic forward-bent posture of the head and trunk typically assumed to improve the efficiency of the breathing effort, the sternocleidomastoid muscle may adaptively shorten, and the clavicles may appear more prominent. Breathing efforts during activity may elicit more work from the neck accessory muscles to lift the chest wall up and assist in breathing during rest.

The presence of **jugular venous distention** should be assessed with the patient sitting or recumbent in bed with the head elevated at least 45 degrees. Jugular venous distention is said to be present if the veins distend above the level of the clavicles. It is an indication of increased volume in the venous system and may be an early sign of right-sided heart failure (cor pulmonale) (Fig. 16–7). In addition, the patient may have left-sided heart failure (congestive heart failure), but this distinction requires auscultation of the lungs, arte-

rial pressure measurements, and possibly a chest radiograph.

Evaluation of the Chest: Resting and Dynamic

The resting chest is evaluated for its symmetry, configuration, rib angles, and intercostal spaces and musculature. Checking symmetry between sides and comparing anteroposterior (AP) and transverse diameters provide information regarding the chronicity of the cardiopulmonary dysfunction as well as any present pathologic condition. For example, a patient with chronic obstructive disease may have a hyperinflated chest, which increases the AP diameter (more barrel-like). The normal AP diameter is one half the size of the transverse diameter. In the chronically hyperinflated chest wall, the AP diameter may be equal to the transverse diameter (Fig. 16–8). An individual with scoliosis has asymmetry from side to side when observed from either the front or the back.

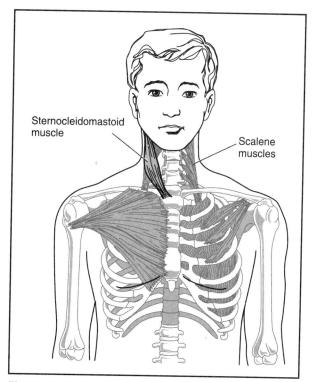

Figure 16-6. The sternocleidomastoid muscles often hypertrophy in chronic obstructive pulmonary disease owing to increased work of the accessory muscles to assist with breathing.

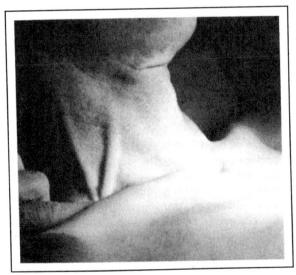

Figure 16-7. Jugular venous distention. (From Daily EK, Schroeder JP. Techniques in Bedside Hemodynamic Monitoring. 2nd ed. St. Louis, CV Mosby, 1981.)

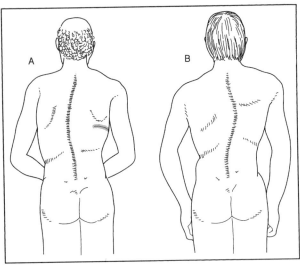

Figure 16-9. *A,* Splinting postthoracic surgery (on right), demonstrating thoracic asymmetry. *B,* Thoracic asymmetry found with scoliosis.

Scoliosis also rotates the lungs as the scoliotic curve progresses throughout life. In addition, an individual who undergoes thoracic surgery with a lateral incision may have developed asymmetry due to pain and splinting or due to actual lung or rib loss from the surgical procedure (Fig. 16–9). Sym-

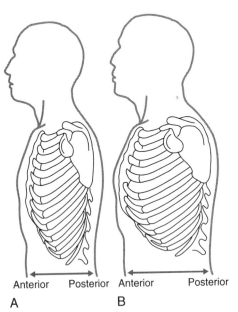

Figure 16-8. *A,* A normal anteroposterior (AP) diameter. *B,* The increased AP diameter in a chronically hyperinflated chest.

metry of the chest wall is also assessed dynamically with palpation of the spinous processes, ribs, and clavicles, comparing the motion from side to side and from top to bottom, anteriorly, laterally, and posteriorly.

Some congenital defects such as **pectus excavatum** (funnel chest) or **pectus carinatum** (pigeon chest) are important to observe, although they often have little effect on pulmonary function unless they are a severe deformity (Fig. 16–10). Pectus excavatum can have an impact on the cardiac function. Rib angles and intercostal spaces should be observed for abnormalities that might suggest the presence of chronic disease. Normally, rib angles measure less than 90 degrees (Fig. 16–11), and they attach to the vertebrae at approximately 45-degree angles. The intercostal spaces are normally broader posteriorly than anteriorly, but chronic hyperinflation causes the rib angles to increase and the intercostal spaces to become broader anteriorly. Consequently, an increased stretch is placed on the diaphragm muscle, and it adapts by becoming flatter and thus less effective (Fig. 16–11).

Other respiratory accessory muscles may hypertrophy as a result of chronic obstructive pulmonary disease because of the demand placed on them owing to the diminished capacity of the diaphragm muscle. The scalenes, trapezius, and inter-

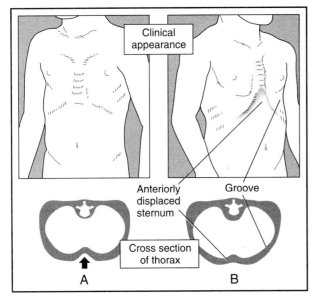

Figure 16–10. Congenital thoracic defects. *A,* Pectus excavatum (funnel chest), characterized by depression in the lower portion of the sternum. *B,* Pectus carinatum (pigeon chest), characterized by a displaced anterior chest and increased anteroposterior diameter.

costals work harder than normal when their contribution to normal resting or exercise breathing is increased. Ultimately, the muscles make adaptive changes to the increased workloads by becoming hypertrophied.

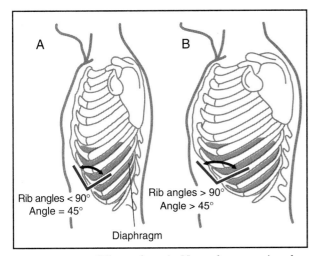

Figure 16–11. Rib angles. *A,* Normal: measuring less than 90 degrees and attaching at the vertebrae at approximately a 45-degree angle. *B,* Abnormal: rib angles greater than 90 degrees and attaching to the vertebrae with angles greater than 45 degrees in the hyperinflated chest. Also note that the position of the diaphragm is flattened.

Clinical Note: Dynamic Breathing Assessment

Patients with rigid chest walls or the diagnosis of diffuse pulmonary fibrosis usually demonstrate a complete lack of lateral costal expansion. Therefore, the chest wall goes up and down, but there is no outward expansion.

Just as the resting chest wall must be evaluated, so must the dynamic or moving chest wall. Observations of breathing patterns, rates, inspiratory to expiratory ratios, and symmetry of chest wall motion must all be made. Abnormal breathing patterns should be noted with descriptive terminology, as is presented in Table 16–2. The normal adult respiratory rate is 10 to 20 breaths per minute and can be assessed by counting the respirations for 1 full minute. Observation and palpation of the moving chest are the recommended methods, but one problem with assessing the respiratory rate is the fact that patients are often aware that respirations are being counted, and therefore they may subconsciously alter the rate.

The ratio of inspiration to expiration during the normal breathing cycle is an important consideration. The normal inspiration-to-expiration ratio is 1:2; however, in individuals with chronic obstructive pulmonary diseases, particularly with asthmatics, the ratio may be reduced to 1:4 owing to their inability to get rid of air in the lungs. Also, the pattern of breathing should be noted: *paradoxical breathing* occurs because of an impairment of the respiratory center's control over breathing (often found in chronic respiratory disease or neurologic insult). An example of paradoxical breathing is the individual with chronic obstructive pulmonary disease and air entrapment who must actively contract the abdominal musculature during expiration to decrease the air trapped in the lungs. The same sort of paradoxical breathing is found in an infant in respiratory distress.

Phonation, Cough, and Cough Production

Evaluation of a patient's speech also is an assessment of shortness of breath at rest. When speech is interrupted for breath, an individual is de-

Table 16–2

Breathing Patterns Commonly Encountered in the Assessment of Patients with Respiratory Problems

PATTERN OF BREATHING	DESCRIPTION
Apnea	Absence of ventilation
Fish-mouth	Apnea with concomitant mouth opening and closing; associated with neck extension and bradypnea
Eupnea	Normal rate, normal depth, regular rhythm
Bradypnea	Slow rate, shallow or normal depth, regular rhythm; associated with drug overdose
Tachypnea	Fast rate, shallow depth, regular rhythm; associated with restrictive lung disease
Hyperpnea	Normal rate, increased depth, regular rhythm
Cheyne-Stokes (periodic)	Increasing then decreasing depth, period of apnea interspersed; somewhat regular rhythm; associated with critically ill patients
Biot's	Slow rate, shallow depth, apneic periods, irregular rhythm; associated with central nervous system disorders like meningitis
Apneustic	Slow rate, deep inspiration followed by apnea, irregular rhythm; associated with brainstem disorders
Prolonged expiration	Fast inspiration, slow and prolonged expiration yet normal rate, depth, and regular rhythm; associated with obstructive lung disease
Orthopnea	Difficulty breathing in postures other than erect
Hyperventilation	Fast rate, increased depth, regular rhythm; results in decreased arterial carbon dioxide, tension; called "Kussmaul breathing" in metabolic acidosis; also associated with central nervous system disorders like encephalitis
Psychogenic dyspnea	Normal rate, regular intervals of sighing; associated with anxiety
Dyspnea	Rapid rate, shallow depth, regular rhythm; associated with accessory muscle activity
Doorstop	Normal rate and rhythm; characterized by abrupt cessation of inspiration when restriction is encountered; associated with pleurisy

Source: Irwin SI, Techlin JS. Cardiopulmonary Physical Therapy. 2nd ed. St. Louis, CV Mosby, 1990, p 286.

scribed as having dyspnea of phonation. Confusion exists in the literature as well as in the clinic, because shortness of breath and dyspnea are often used interchangeably. The definition of dyspnea is "the patient's subjective report of discomfort with breathing." Shortness of breath is thus the actual symptom observed. Therefore, the description of **dyspnea** of phonation is made by identifying how many words can be expressed before the next breath. For example, one-word dyspnea would mean that speech is interrupted for a breath between every word. Voice control can also be used to assess shortness of breath as well as strength of the musculature used in speaking and breathing, because poor voice control often indicates weak musculature in both breathing and speaking.

The strength of the patient's cough needs to be assessed, as well as the production of any secretions from the cough (if they are present). Several characteristics of the cough are essential to evaluate, including the effectiveness of the cough (strength, depth, and length of cough). For example, an individual with weak respiratory accessory muscles (e.g., one who has a high spinal cord injury) would have a very weak and therefore ineffective cough. In addition, an individual with **bronchospasm** may have a very long, drawn out **spasmodic cough** that is just as ineffective.

The secretions should be assessed and described with regard to quantity, color, smell, and consistency (Table 16–3). Normally, persons may raise 100 mL of mucus (clear to white) per day and not notice it.

In addition to the sputum odor, the individual's breath odor should be assessed. Foul-smelling breath may indicate an anaerobic infection of the mouth or respiratory tract, whereas an acetone breath may indicate diabetic **ketoacidosis.**

Table 16-3

Guidelines for Evaluating Cough

COUGH CHARACTERISTICS	ASSOCIATED FEATURES	INTERPRETATION
Nonspecific	Sore throat, runny nose, runny eyes	Acute lung infection; tracheo-bronchitis
Productive	Preceded by an earlier, painful, nonproductive cough associated with an upper respiratory infection	Lobar pneumonia
Dry or productive	Acute bronchitis	Bronchopneumonia
Paroxysmal; mucoid or blood-stained sputum	Flulike syndrome	*Mycoplasma* or viral pneumonia
Purulent sputum	Sputum formerly mucoid	Acute exacerbation of chronic bronchitis
Productive for more than 3 months consecutively and for at least 2 years		Chronic bronchitis
Foul-smelling, copious, layered purulent sputum	Long-standing problem	Bronchiectasis
Blood-tinged sputum	Month long	Tuberculosis or fungal infection
Persistent, nonproductive		Pneumonitis, interstitial fibrosis, pulmonary infiltrates
Persistent, minimally productive	Smoking history, injected pharynx	"Smoker's cough"
Nonspecific; minimal hemoptysis	Long standing	Neoplastic disease
Nonproductive	Long standing; dyspnea	Mediastinal neoplasm
Brassy		Aortic aneurysm
Violent cough	Sudden; onset at the same time as signs of asphyxia; localized wheezing	Aspiration of foreign body
Frothy sputum	Worsens in supine position; dyspnea	Heart failure, pulmonary edema
Hemoptysis	Sudden; simultaneous dyspnea; pleural effusion	Pulmonary infarct

Source: Adapted from Fishman AP. Pulmonary Disease and Disorders. Vol. 1. New York, McGraw-Hill, 1980.

Appearance of Extremities

Observation of the fingers and toes and the calves of the legs should indicate whether long-term problems with circulation and oxygenation are present. **Digital clubbing** of the fingers and toes indicates chronic tissue hypoxia and is found in many instances of hypoxemia-producing disease (Fig. 16-12). Cyanosis (blueness) of the nail beds may also indicate cardiopulmonary dysfunction, but cyanosis can be an indication of decreased circulation to these areas because of cold, vasospasm, peripheral vascular disease, or decreased cardiac output. The calves of the legs should be observed for skin color changes of blue or purple. This may be indicative of peripheral vascular insufficiency.

Auscultation of the Lungs

Auscultation is an evaluation technique used to confirm the findings of chart assessment and inspection as well as to rule out other cardiopulmonary dysfunction. Auscultation is also an excellent tool for reassessment of an individual's ventilation following treatment techniques to improve bronchial hygiene or regional ventilation.

Auscultation requires appropriate equipment (the stethoscope) as well as appropriate instructions to the patient and proper positioning. It is recommended that the physical therapist invest in a personal stethoscope, because stethoscopes fit different people in different ways owing to the types, sizes, and positions of the earpieces. The most appropriate choice is a stethoscope that

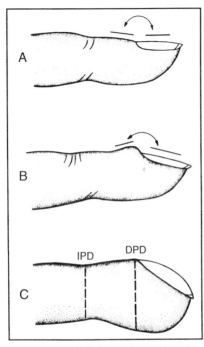

Figure 16–12. Normal digit configuration (*A*) and digital clubbing (*B*). Note that the angle between the nail and the proximal skin exceeds 180 degrees. *C,* Also note that the distal phalangeal depth (DPD) is greater than the interphalangeal depth (IPD). (From Wilkins RL, Krider SJ. Clinical Assessment in Respiratory Care, St. Louis, CV Mosby, 1985.)

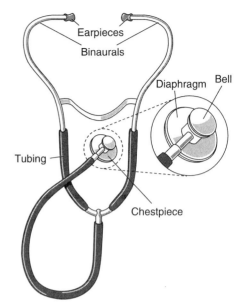

Figure 16–13. A stethoscope, showing the diaphragm (flattened side) and the bell.

comes with adjustable earpieces, with adequate but not excessive tubing, and with both a diaphragm (the flat side) and a bell, including a valve to turn toward either the diaphragm or the bell. Auscultation of lung sounds is performed with the diaphragm of the stethoscope preferably in a quiet environment (Fig. 16–13). Auscultation of heart sounds requires both the diaphragm and the bell and, again, a quiet environment.

For auscultation of the lung sounds, the optimal position is for the patient to be sitting to permit auscultation of the entire lung space, including both the anterior and posterior chest wall. In addition, optimal auscultation involves removal of bed clothes to expose the bare skin while the individual breathes deeply through an open mouth. Unfortunately, some of the more seriously ill patients can neither tolerate the sitting position at the time of initial visit nor perform adequate deep breaths for auscultation.

Auscultation should be performed over the entire lung space, with at least one breath auscul-

tated in each bronchopulmonary segment. The intensity, pitch, and quality of the breath sounds should be compared between right and left and in the craniocaudal direction. Auscultation should be performed in a systematic manner, anteriorly and then posteriorly (or vice versa) (Fig. 16–14). Precautions that should be taken during auscultation are the following:

- Prevent the patient from falling if weak or if poor balance is noted.
- Prevent the patient from becoming dizzy secondary to hyperventilation by auscultating slowly between pulmonary segments.
- Maintain appropriate draping of the patient, particularly females.

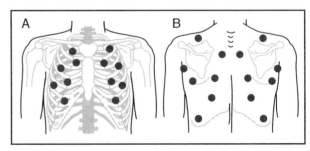

Figure 16–14. One method of auscultating the chest. *A,* The chest. *B,* The back. (Redrawn from Buckingham EB. A Primer of Clinical Diagnosis. 2nd ed. New York, Harper & Row, 1979.)

- If auscultation reveals very faint or distant sounds, remind the patient to take deep breaths and to breathe in and out through the mouth so that a recheck can be done.

Lung Sound Definitions

Disagreement exists regarding the terms used to identify the auscultated lung sounds.[7] Nonetheless, lung sounds may be divided into two types: normal breath sounds and **adventitious breath sounds.** Normal breath sounds are the normal noises of breathing that can be heard with a stethoscope. They are described as vesicular and are soft, low-pitched sounds heard primarily during inspiration. During expiration low, vesicular sounds are minimal and occur only during the initial one third of exhalation. Expiratory sounds flow directly from inspiratory sounds, without a break in the sounds.

Different breath sounds are auscultated over different portions of the tracheobronchial tree,

which are also normal. **Bronchial breath sounds,** described as tubular sounds, are loud, high-pitched sounds with approximately equal inspiratory and expiratory duration. Also a pause occurs between the inspiratory and expiratory components. A third type of "normal" breath sound is heard over the junction of the mainstem bronchi with the segmental bronchi, called bronchovesicular. **Bronchovesicular breath sounds** are a softer version of bronchial sounds but differ only in that they are continuous between inspiration and expiration. Posteriorly the bronchovesicular sounds are normally heard only between the scapulae (Fig. 16–15). Table 16–4 provides a list of errors of auscultation to avoid.

These normal sounds are produced from the turbulence of airflow in the airways. The belief is that the inspiratory component of vesicular sounds is produced regionally within each lung and possibly within each lobe.[8] The expiratory component is believed to be produced in the larger airways. The fact that airflow is directed away from the

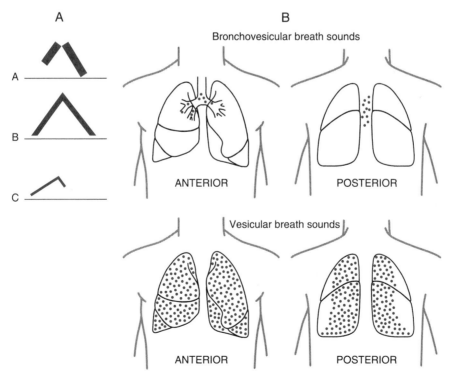

Figure 16–15. *A,* Breath sound diagrams: normal tracheobronchial (A); bronchovesicular (B): vesicular (C) breath sounds. The upstroke represents inspiration and the downstroke expiration. The thickness of the line indicates intensity. *B,* The positions on the anterior and posterior chest walls at which normal vesicular and bronchovesicular breath sounds are identified. (Redrawn from Wilkins RL, Hodgkin JE, Lopez B. Lung Sounds: A Practical Guide. St. Louis, CV Mosby, 1988.)

Table 16–4
Errors of Auscultation to Avoid

ERRORS	CORRECT TECHNIQUE
Listening to breath sounds through the patient's gown	Placing bell or diaphragm directly against the chest wall
Allowing tubing to rub against bed rails or patient's gown	Keeping tubing free from contact with any objects during auscultation
Attempting to auscultate in a noisy room	Turning television or radio off
Interpreting chest hair sounds as adventitious lung sounds	Wetting chest hair before auscultation if thick
Auscultating only the "convenient" areas	Asking alert patient to sit up; rolling comatose patient onto side to auscultate posterior lobes

chest wall during expiration might explain the fading away of the sound during expiration and the reason why only approximately the first third of expiration can be heard.

A pathologic condition in the lungs can change the transmission of the sounds. An increase in lung tissue density causes increased sound transmission. This is the reason one may hear bronchial breath sounds in areas other than the mainstem bronchi when a pathologic condition that causes **consolidation** exists. A decrease in lung tissue density, as in the emphysematous lung, would cause decreased sound transmission. Decreased sound transmission also occurs if only shallow breaths are taken or if distance of transmission between the airways and the stethoscope is increased (as in obesity, pleural effusion, or barrel chest).

When a pathologic condition of the lung is suspected because of increased or decreased transmission sounds, then further evaluative measures must be taken. **Egophony, bronchophony,** and **whispering pectoriloquy** are three techniques to further evaluate the abnormal transmission of sound. Asking a patient to say "99" or "E," or to whisper are three techniques that can be employed to assess the abnormally transmitted sounds. Egophony is demonstrated when a patient is asked to say "E" aloud, but the sound that is auscultated over the chest is "A." Bronchophony is demonstrated when a patient is asked to say "99," and the words are auscultated clearly over the entire chest. Whispering pectoriloquy is evident when a patient is asked to whisper, and the whispered words are clearly and distinctly heard through the stethoscope. The relative strengths of each of the sounds auscultated when using these techniques suggest

the degree of consolidation or hyperinflation of the underlying lung; stronger, louder sounds are heard in the presence of consolidative pathology, whereas weaker, softer sounds are heard in the presence of hyperinflation.

Adventitious Lung Sounds. Adventitious lung sounds are the abnormal noises heard only with a stethoscope. These can be divided into two categories: *continuous* and *discontinuous* lung sounds. The American Thoracic Society and the American College of Chest Physicians Ad Hoc Subcommittee on Pulmonary Nomenclature (ATS-ACCP) further clarified the continuous sounds as *wheezes* (previously defined as *rhonchi*) and the discontinuous adventitious lung sounds as *crackles* (previously called *rales*).[9]

Wheezes. **Wheezes** are continuous adventitious lung sounds with a constant pitch and varying duration. These sounds are most frequently heard on exhalation and are associated with airway obstruction. Some clinicians still advocate using the term **rhonchi** to describe low-pitched continuous adventitious lung sounds. The ATS-ACCP, however, recommends referring to all continuous adventitious sounds as wheezes and specifying whether they are high-pitched or low-pitched. When describing the wheeze it is extremely important to document the time of its occurrence (inspiration or expiration) because this may help to differentiate pathologic conditions.

Wheezes on expiration are most common and are often associated with airway constriction as is found in bronchospasm or when secretions are narrowing the airway. The wheeze on inspiration is not very common and indicates a more severe obstruction of the airway.[10] Wheezes may diminish or change in pitch as a result of bronchodilator treat-

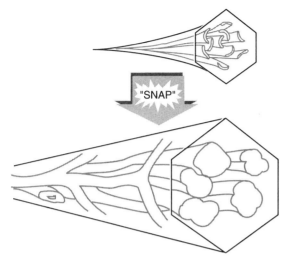

"SNAP"

Figure 16–16. Sudden reexpansion of collapsed peripheral airways. (Redrawn from Murphy RLH. Lung sounds. Basics of respiratory disease. Vol. 8, No. 4, Am Thor Soc, 1980.)

ments. The monophonic, continuous adventitious sound heard over the upper airways of a patient with upper airway obstruction (as when a peanut is lodged in a bronchus or when epiglottic interference occurs) is called **stridor** and differs from the normal wheeze in intensity and pitch.

Crackles. **Crackles** are discontinuous adventitious lung sounds that sound like brief bursts of popping bubbles. Crackles are more commonly heard during inspiration and may be associated with restrictive or obstructive respiratory disorders because they can be produced via several mechanisms.[10–12] They may result from the sudden opening of closed airways[8–14] (Fig. 16–16) or as the result of the movement of secretions during inspiration and expiration.[15] Some clinicians still use the term **rales** for what are now called crackles.

Peripheral airways can collapse owing to atelectasis, pulmonary edema, fibrosis, or compression from pleural effusion, and often crackles auscultated with these pathologic conditions are in the latter half of inspiration. Crackles occurring in the early half of inspiration often result from the popping open of more proximal airways.[14] The closure of proximal airways may result from the weakening of bronchial and broncheolar support structures as occurs in the latter stages of chronic obstructive pathologic diseases such as bronchitis or emphysema. Crackles due to the movement of fluid or secretions within the lungs are often described as

low-pitched and may be found on either inspiration or expiration or both.

Pleural Rub. Another abnormal sound that should be checked by auscultation in the lower lateral chest areas (both right and left) is a **pleural (friction) rub,** which may be an indication of pleural inflammation. The pleural rub sounds like two pieces of leather or sandpaper rubbing together, and it occurs with each inspiration and expiration.[10]

Evaluation of breath sounds via auscultation should be systematic, beginning with an initial description as vesicular, bronchovesicular, bronchial, diminished, or absent. With bronchial and bronchovesicular sounds found in peripheral lung tissue, further definitive techniques such as egophony, bronchophony, and whispering pectoriloquy should be employed. If adventitious sounds are heard, they first must be defined as continuous or discontinuous. Following this distinction, descriptors such as pitch, intensity, duration, and portion of the respiratory cycle in which they occur should be used to further define the sounds. On completion of the auscultatory assessment, the therapist can interpret the sounds with regard to what they may indicate (Table 16–5).

Auscultation of the Heart

Auscultation of heart sounds requires a quiet environment and a stethoscope with a diaphragm and bell. The diaphragm is placed firmly on the skin and is used to auscultate initially the topographic areas on the chest wall, identifying high-pitched sounds. The bell accentuates lower frequency

> ### Clinical Note: Auscultation of Heart Sounds
>
> Auscultation of heart sounds is a clinical skill that can be learned only by practice with auscultation on individuals with different heart sounds. The entry-level practitioner should not be expected to be competent in auscultation of *all* heart sounds. However, an entry-level practitioner should be able to perform a competent systematic auscultation of the heart and be able to note normal heart sounds and blatantly abnormal heart sounds (e.g., loud murmurs and loud atrial or ventricular gallops).

Table 16–5

Guidelines for the Documentation and Interpretation of Auscultated Sounds

TYPE OF SOUND	NOMENCLATURE	INTERPRETATION
Breath sound	Normal	Normal, air-filled lung
	Decreased	Hyperinflation in chronic obstructive pulmonary disease
		Hypoinflation in acute lung disease, e.g., atelectasis, pneumothorax, pleural effusion
	Absent	Pleural effusion
		Pneumothorax
		Severe hyperinflation
		Obesity
	Bronchial	Consolidation
		Atelectasis with adjacent patent airway
	Crackles	Secretions, if biphasic
		Deflation, if monophasic
	Wheezes	Diffuse airway obstruction, if polyphonic
		Localized stenosis, if monophonic
Voice sound	Normal	Normal, air-filled lung
	Decreased	Atelectasis
		Pleural effusion
		Pneumothorax
	Increased	Consolidation
		Pulmonary fibrosis
Extrapulmonary adventitious sounds	Crunch	Mediastinal emphysema
	Pleural rub	Pleural inflammation or reaction
	Pericardial rub	Pericardial inflammation

Source: Irwin SI, Techlin JS. Cardiopulmonary Physical Therapy. 2nd ed. St. Louis, CV Mosby, 1990, p 289.

sounds, including **atrial** and **ventricular gallops,** filtering out the high-pitched sounds. Care must be taken to place the bell lightly on the skin and not to press firmly, because increased pressure causes the skin to act like a diaphragm so that low-frequency sounds cannot be heard.

Auscultation of the heart requires selective listening for each component of the cardiac cycle while placing the stethoscope over the five main topographic areas for auscultation (Fig. 16–17). The five areas where sounds are best heard are

- The **aortic area:** auscultated best in the second intercostal space close to the sternum on the right of the sternum
- The **pulmonary area:** auscultated best at the second intercostal space to the left of the sternum
- The **third left intercostal space:** murmurs of both aortic and pulmonary origin are best heard here
- The **tricuspid area:** located at the lower left sternal border, approximately the fourth to fifth intercostal space

- The **mitral area (apex of heart):** located in the fifth left intercostal space, medial to the midclavicular line

As with breath sounds, auscultation of heart sounds should be performed in a systematic manner, such as by beginning at the aortic area and listening to both the first and second heart sounds. When listening to the sounds, the intensity and timing, as well as any splitting, extra sounds, or murmurs should be noted. The intensity varies according to the proximity to the valve and chest wall.

The first heart sound, S_1 (the *lub* of the lub-dub), is associated with the closure of the mitral and tricuspid valves and corresponds with the onset of ventricular systole. The S_1 sound is normally louder and longer and lower pitched when auscultated at the apex or even in the tricuspid region.

The second heart sound, S_2 (the *dub* of lub-dub), is associated with the closure of the aortic and pulmonary valves and corresponds with the start of ventricular diastole. The second sound has

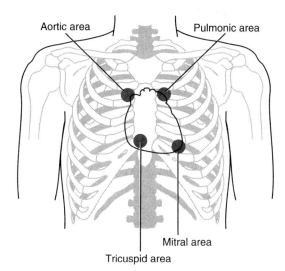

Figure 16–17. Areas to auscultate for sounds generated from the aortic, pulmonary (pulmonic), tricuspid, and mitral valves. In the normal heart, the mitral area is the apical pulse point and the point of maximal impulse. (Redrawn from Leatham A. Introduction to the Examination of the Cardiovascular System. 2nd ed. Oxford, Oxford University Press, 1979, p 20. By permission of Oxford University Press.)

greatest intensity when auscultated at the aortic or pulmonary regions.

Transient splitting of the first or second sound may be noted during inspiration. Splitting of the S_1 is best heard over the tricuspid region, whereas splitting of the S_2 is heard more readily over the pulmonary region. Both splitting sounds are considered to be normal and are indicative of slight timing differences between closure of the left heart valves and the right heart valves.

Abnormal Heart Sounds

Third Heart Sound. A third heart sound (S_3) occurs early in diastole while the ventricle is rapidly filling (immediately following S_2 and sounding like lub-dub-*dub*). The S_3 sound is low-pitched and must be auscultated with the bell of the stethoscope. Auscultation is often best performed with the patient lying on the left side so that the apex of the heart is closest to the chest wall. When an S_3 is heard in healthy children or young adults, it is considered to be normal and is called a *physiologic* third heart sound. When an S_3 is auscultated

in an older, physically inactive person or in the presence of heart disease, it typically indicates a loss of ventricular compliance (failure), often called a *ventricular gallop*. In patients with suspected ventricular dysfunction, the clinician should search carefully for the presence of a ventricular gallop because it is a key diagnostic sign for congestive heart failure.

Fourth Heart Sound. The fourth heart sound (S_4) occurs late in diastole (just before S_1 and sounding like *la*-lub-dub) and is associated with atrial contraction. S_4 is also a low-pitched sound best heard with the bell of the stethoscope. S_4, otherwise known as the *atrial gallop* sound, is not normal and is associated with an increased resistance to ventricular filling. An S_4 is commonly heard in individuals with hypertensive cardiac disease, coronary artery disease, or pulmonary disease and is also commonly found in individuals with a history of myocardial infarction or coronary artery bypass surgery.

Murmurs

Murmurs can be very complex and difficult to understand for the entry-level practitioner. However, there are three broad classifications of murmurs that can help one understand the mechanism of the murmurs:

- Murmurs caused by high rates of flow either through normal or abnormal valves
- Murmurs caused by forward flow through a constricted (stenotic) or deformed valve or by flow into a dilated vessel or chamber
- Murmurs caused by backward flow through a valve (regurgitation).[16]

Murmurs are classified according to their timing, quality, intensity, pitch, location, and radiation. In addition, murmurs are classified by the position of the patient in which the murmur is best heard and by the part of the respiratory cycle in which it is best heard.

Systolic and Diastolic Murmurs. Systolic murmurs are the most common and may be caused by either ejection or regurgitation. These murmurs are heard between S_1 and S_2 and are best described as a "swishing" sound associated with S_1 (instead of hearing lub-dub, one usually hears "*lush*-dub"). One of the most classic systolic murmurs is associated with aortic stenosis. The murmur heard is a high-pitched murmur, best heard at the right sternal border, second intercostal space, frequently radiating to the neck and the carotid arteries.

Systolic murmurs may be produced from other forms of valvular dysfunction, including congenital defects of the atria and ventricles. In addition, diastolic murmurs, although uncommon, may occur. These murmurs are heard immediately following the S_2 and diminish in intensity quickly. Pathologic conditions associated with these murmurs include aortic and pulmonary regurgitation and mitral stenosis.

Another common murmur is associated with mitral valve dysfunction and is called *mitral valve prolapse*. Mitral valve prolapse is a common and benign valvular dysfunction often found in females. When abnormalities exist with the chordae tendineae (as with papillary muscle rupture after a myocardial infarction or with mitral valve prolapse), clicking sounds in the middle of ventricular systole may be heard. These are referred to as *midsystolic clicks*.[17] Further discussion of murmurs is beyond the scope of this text because it is beyond the level of the entry-level practitioner.

Pericardial Friction Rub. An abnormal sound associated with each beat of the heart is known as a pericardial friction rub. It is the sign of pericardial inflammation (pericarditis). Auscultation for a pericardial friction rub is best performed with the patient in the supine position with the therapist listening over the third or fourth intercostal space along the anterior axillary line. The pericardial friction rub sounds like a "creak" with each beat and has also been described as a "leathery" sound, as if two pieces of leather were being rubbed together.[17]

Palpation

Palpation is an assessment technique employed to refine the information previously gathered from the chart review, inspection, and auscultation. The purpose of palpation is to evaluate the mediastinum (for tracheal shift), chest motion, chest wall pain, fremitus, muscle activity of the chest wall and diaphragm, and circulatory status.

The Mediastinum (Tracheal Position)

Evaluation of the mediastinum assesses tracheal shift that is due to disproportionate intrathoracic pressures or lung volumes between the two sides of the thorax. The contents of the thorax may shift toward the affected side when the lung volume or intrathoracic pressure on that side is decreased. This can happen following a lobectomy or pneumonectomy or a large degree of atelectasis. The content of the thorax may shift to the unaffected side (the contralateral side) when there is increased pressure on the same side, as happens in a pleural effusion, a tumor, or an untreated pneumothorax.

Palpation for such shifts is performed while the patient is sitting upright with the neck flexed slightly to allow relaxation of the sternocleidomastoid muscles, and the chin should be positioned in the midline. Palpation proceeds with the tip of the index finger being placed in the suprasternal notch, first medially to the left sternoclavicular joint, and pushed inward toward the cervical spine. Then the index finger is placed medial to the right sternoclavicular joint and pushed inward toward the cervical spine (Fig. 16–18).

When a significant shift to the unaffected side occurs, aggressive treatment is usually indicated. If the shift is due to a pneumothorax, a chest tube is usually inserted immediately. In the case of the

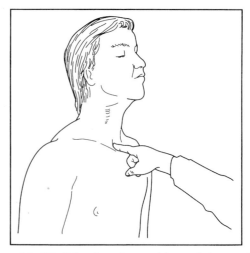

Figure 16–18. Palpation for position of the mediastinum to evaluate for tracheal deviation.

large pleural effusion, a thoracentesis may be performed to drain the fluid or to evaluate the contents of the fluid or both. When the shift goes to the affected side in the patient after a lobectomy or pneumonectomy, the patient should be cautioned against lying on the affected side, because this would only increase the **mediastinal shift**.

Chest Motion

Palpation is performed segmentally to compare the chest wall motion over the upper, middle, and lower lobes while the patient is breathing quietly and while breathing deeply. The important components of the evaluation include the amount of movement of the hands, the presence or absence of symmetry of movement, and the timing of the movement (Figs. 16–19 to 16–21).

The upper chest wall expansion is evaluated by the therapist placing the palms of the hands anteriorly over the chest wall from the fourth rib upward. The fingers should be stretched upward and over the trapezius, and the thumbs should be placed together along the midline of the chest. The skin on the patient's chest may need to be mobilized to position the palms down with the thumbs touching. The patient should be asked to take a maximal inspiration, and the therapist's hands should be relaxed so that they move with the chest wall. Notation of the extent of movement and the symmetry of the movement is important (see Fig. 16–19). Chest wall motion over the right middle lobe and lingula segments of the left upper lobe is evaluated by the therapist placing

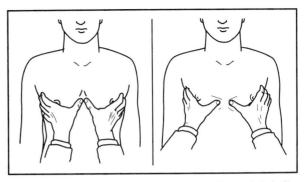

Figure 16–20. Palpation of right middle and left lingula lobe motion. (Redrawn from Cherniack RM, Cherniack L. Respiration in Health and Disease. 2nd ed. Philadelphia, WB Saunders, 1972.)

the fingers laterally and over posterior axillary folds, with the palms pressed firmly on the anterior chest wall. The skin is then drawn medially until the thumbs meet at the midline. The patient should take a maximal inspiration with the therapist's hands gliding with the movement of the lobes underneath. Again, extent of movement and symmetry of movement should be documented (see Fig. 16–20).

The lower chest wall expansion is evaluated with the patient's back toward the therapist, and the therapist's fingers wrapped around the anterior axillary fold. The skin is then drawn medially until the tips of the thumbs meet at the spinal column. While a maximal inspiration is performed by the patient, the therapist should allow the hands to glide with the movement of the rib cage, and the extent of the movement as well as the symmetry should be documented (see Fig. 16–21).

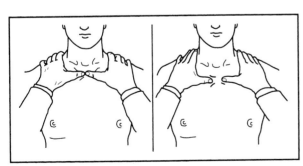

Figure 16–19. Palpation of upper lobe motion. (Redrawn from Cherniack RM, Cherniack L. Respiration in Health and Disease. 2nd ed. Philadelphia, WB Saunders, 1972.)

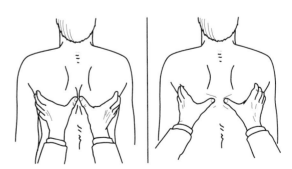

Figure 16–21. Palpation of lower lobe motion. (Redrawn from Cherniack RM, Cherniack L. Respiration in Health and Disease. 2nd ed. Philadelphia, WB Saunders, 1972.)

Evaluation of Fremitus

Fremitus is defined as the vibration that is produced by the voice or by the presence of secretions in the airways and is transmitted to the chest wall and palpated by the hand. Palpation of fremitus is performed with the palms of the hands placed lightly on the chest wall while the patient repeats some word, such as "99," to distinguish normal vocal fremitus from the abnormal fremitus produced by secretions. Normally palpation reveals a uniform vibration throughout the entire chest wall. Increased fremitus is palpated in the presence of an increase in secretions in a particular area. Decreased fremitus indicates an increase in air in the particular area. Palpation of fremitus is especially important when auscultation has defined an area of decreased breath sounds that may be an area of consolidation resulting from secretions. When fremitus is increased, the suspicion of consolidation is supported.

Evaluation of Muscle Activity of Chest Wall and Diaphragm

Palpation is an excellent tool to evaluate the amount of accessory muscle activity used during quiet breathing. By palpating the accessory muscles, in particular the scalenes and the trapezii, an assessment of the amount of work of breathing may be made (Fig. 16-22). In addition, the extent of the diaphragmatic contribution can be assessed with the patient in the supine position (Fig.

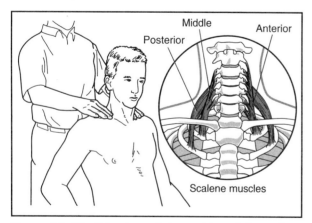

Figure 16-22. Palpation of the activity of the scalene muscles during quiet breathing.

16-23). Normal quiet breathing is mostly performed by the diaphragm, with equal and upward motion of the lower rib cage. Palpation of the anterior chest wall with the thumbs over the costal margins and thumb tips meeting at the xiphoid gives the most accurate assessment of the extent of diaphragmatic activity. With a deep inspiration the hands should travel equally apart, total circumferential diameter increasing by at least 2 to 3 inches. The extent of movement is an important part of the assessment of diaphragmatic excursion. For example, an individual with significant chronic obstructive lung disease might exhibit increased muscle activity of the respiratory accessory muscles and decreased diaphragmatic contribution to quiet breathing.

Chest Wall Pain or Discomfort

Palpation may also be performed to evaluate chest wall discomfort and should include all areas of the chest wall: anterior, posterior, and lateral regions of the thorax. Patients may often develop musculoskeletal pain from bedrest and inactivity, which are frequently associated with diseases of the cardiopulmonary system. Musculoskeletal pain must be differentiated from anginal pain; palpation is an extremely useful tool to distinguish between the two. If chest pain is increased with deep inspiration or if it is increased or reproduced by direct point palpation, it is less likely to be of cardiac origin than of skeletal muscle origin. If a patient reports chest pain during the patient interview and can point to the exact area of pain, then palpation should be done to assess whether this pain is of musculoskeletal origin.

Evaluation of Circulation

Pulses throughout the extremities should be palpated during the initial evaluation because of the diffuse nature of atherosclerotic disease (see Chapter 3). Identification of the risk factors and symptoms of arterial disease is a component of the history that assists in the assessment of arterial disease. Ischemic pain appears in the soft tissue served by the artery that is diseased. In addition to history taking, visual inspection for trophic changes (hair loss, muscle atrophy, dry skin, and

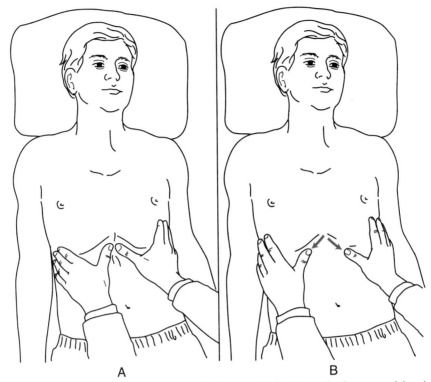

Figure 16–23. Palpation of diaphragmatic motion. *A,* At rest. *B,* At the end of a normal inspiration. (Redrawn from Cherniack RM, Cherniack L. Respiration in Health and Disease. 2nd ed. Philadelphia, WB Saunders, 1972.)

in some cases dry gangrene or ulcers) is a valuable evaluation tool, particularly for examining individuals with moderate to severe arterial occlusion. Blood flow tests provide additional information about the degree of occlusion in the extremities. A reactive hyperemia test may be performed by sharply elevating the limbs to produce blanching. Blanching is more rapid in the partially or severely occluded extremity than in the normal extremity. In addition, palpation of pulses and skin temperature can be performed to assess perfusion of the extremities and the head and neck. Patients with diabetes or peripheral vascular disease often have diminished pulses, particularly in the hands and feet. In addition, individuals with right-sided heart failure and bilateral peripheral edema demonstrate diminished pulses in the foot and ankle. The following is a list of locations for pulse palpation:

- Brachial artery
- Radial artery
- Carotid artery
- Femoral artery

- Popliteal artery (palpated using the fingers of both hands)
- Posterior tibial artery
- Dorsalis pedis artery

The quality of the pulse should be noted, and a comparison should be made to the pulses of the opposite extremity to determine unilateral or individual differences. Pulse palpation may be difficult to quantify and does have a degree of unreliability from one clinician to the next. As a result, pulse palpation is now often supplemented by noninvasive techniques to measure blood flow such as **Doppler velocimetry.** Doppler velocimetry is particularly useful in identifying individuals with asymptomatic arterial disease or those whose pulses are severely obliterated.[18]

Mediate Percussion

Mediate percussion is the final component of the chest examination and is performed to further evaluate any abnormal findings, especially changes

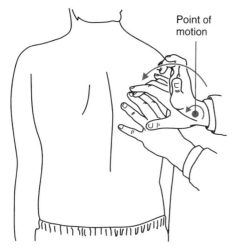

Figure 16-24. The technique for mediate percussion.

in lung density. In addition, percussion is also useful to evaluate the extent of diaphragmatic excursion.

Percussion is performed with the middle finger of one hand placed flat on the chest wall along the intercostal space between two ribs (usually the nondominant hand), while all other fingers are lifted off the chest wall. The other hand is positioned with the wrist in dorsiflexion, acting like a fulcrum, and the hand moving forward and back in rapid succession with the tip of the middle finger striking the nondominant middle finger on the chest wall (Fig. 16-24). Percussion usually proceeds in a cephalocaudal direction and back and forth between the left and right sides, anteriorly and posteriorly.

Three types of sounds are typically produced with percussion. A normal sound is when normal lung tissue is percussed and normal **resonance** is produced. A dull sound is produced with percussion over the liver or other dense tissue (as occurs with consolidation or tumors) and is described as a "thud." The student can reproduce the dull sound by percussing on a bare thigh. A tympanic sound is loud, long, and hollow and may be heard over an empty stomach or a hyperinflated chest. Figure 16-25 shows the areas of normal, tympanic, and dull sounds on a chest. Figure 16-26 demonstrates the systematic technique for evaluation of lung density.

Diaphragmatic excursion can also be assessed by percussion. The patient must be in a seated position with the back exposed to evaluate diaphragmatic excursion. Percussion from the apex of the lungs to the bases of the lungs is performed while a patient is quietly breathing and a line measuring the point of demarcation between resonance to dullness is drawn on the left side and the right. After these lines are drawn, the therapist asks the patient to take a maximal inspiration and to hold this breath. At this time, the therapist continues percussion from the line downward to determine where the new point of dullness to resonance is located and draws a second line. The distance between the lines is the distance of diaphragmatic excursion. Normal excursion is 3 to 5 cm but may be extremely decreased in the patient with chronic obstructive lung disease because of hyperinflation of the chest and a flattened diaphragm (Fig. 16-27).

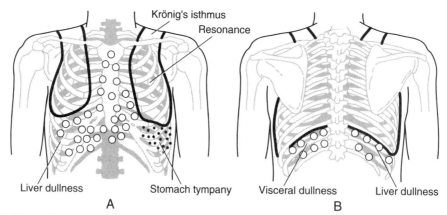

Figure 16-25. Normal resonance pattern of the chest. *A*, Anteriorly. *B*, Posteriorly. Also shown are areas of dullness (*circles*) and tympanic areas (*small dots*). (Redrawn from Irwin SI, Techlin JS. Cardiopulmonary Physical Therapy. 2nd ed. St. Louis, CV Mosby, 1990.)

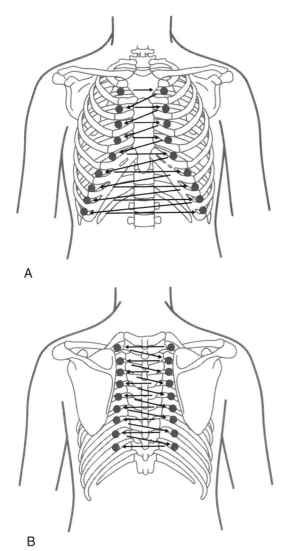

A

B

Figure 16–26. The systematic technique for evaluation of lung density anteriorly (*A*) and posteriorly (*B*).

Activity Evaluation

Following the chest wall examination, the therapist is ready to perform an initial evaluation of the patient's responses to exercise. The activity evaluation (or self-care assessment) is an assessment of the patient's responses to the following situations: rest (supine), sitting, standing, some type of activity of daily living (e.g., dressing lower or upper extremities, combing hair, brushing teeth), and ambulation of some distance; in some cases, **Valsalva's maneuver** is also performed (Fig. 16–28).

For patients recently recovering from a myocardial infarction, the evaluation discussed previously should be performed as soon as the patient is able to get out of bed. This often occurs as early as 1 to 2 days after an uncomplicated myocardial infarction. If the patient has not experienced a myocardial infarction but has some sort of cardiovascular or pulmonary dysfunction, this assessment is made as soon as the patient is considered stable. Patients receiving mechanical ventilatory assistance can perform these activities while still on the ventilator.

During the activity evaluation, the patient's heart rate and rhythm (via ECG telemetry if possible), blood pressure, and symptoms should be monitored with all activities (and O_2 saturation, if applicable). Heart and lung sounds should be measured before each activity and *immediately* following the last activity. The responses should be recorded and interpreted throughout the entire evaluation. The evaluation is terminated at any time during the assessment that an abnormal response is identified if such response makes continuing the evaluation inappropriate or unsafe. On conclusion of the activities evaluation, an individu-

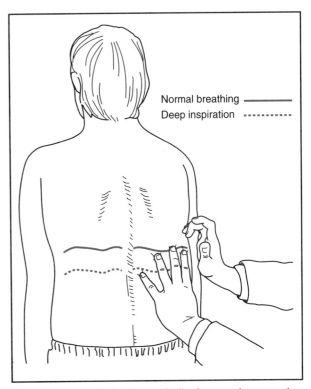

Normal breathing ——————
Deep inspiration - - - - - - - - - -

Figure 16–27. Evaluation of diaphragmatic excursion (normal, 3 to 5 cm); normal breathing (*solid line*), deep inspiration (*broken line*).

SELF-CARE ASSESSMENT

Department of Physical Therapy and Rehabilitation
Cardiac Rehabilitation Program

Patient name _____

Hospital no. _____

Medications _____

O_2 Saturation _____

　　Pre-activity _____

　　With activity_____

Risk factors　　HBP _____　　Family history _____　　Obesity _____

　　　　　　　Smoking _____　　Diabetes _____　　Stress/hostility/anger_____

　　　　　　　Cholesterol levels _____　　Age _____　　Sedentary _____　　Other _____

	HR	BP
Rest (supine)		
Sitting		
Standing		
Activities of daily living		
Ambulation		
Valsalva maneuver		

ECG strips

_____

INTERPRETATION

Therapist _____　　Date _____

Figure 16–28. Self-care assessment form.

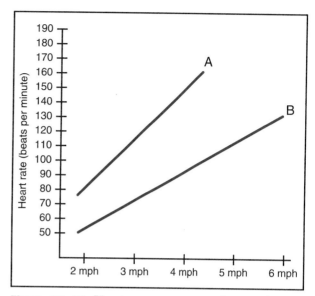

Figure 16–29. Heart rate response to increased workload in a normal sedentary individual (A) versus a trained individual (B).

alized program of progressive monitored ambulation is initiated if the responses were assessed as safe and appropriate. Studies have shown that the heart rate, blood pressure, and ECG responses with ambulation during the activities evaluation strongly correlate with the responses that occur with the patient's daily monitored ambulation program.[19]

Heart Rate Measurement

The heart rate can be measured via palpation and is usually done via the radial pulse; it can also be measured from the ECG, either directly from a digital reading or from a recording of a 6-second ECG strip. Although an ECG recording may be more accurate, the palpation method may be more common in the clinic owing to the lack of availability of ECG equipment. Heart rhythm (the presence or absence of rhythm disturbances) can also be evaluated if palpated continuously for at least 1 minute but is more accurately recorded via the ECG. See Chapter 9 for heart rate measurement on ECG and arrhythmia definitions.

The heart rate should be recorded with all activity, but the important factor is the heart rate *response* to activity. The normal heart rate response to any exertion is a gradual rise with an increase in work. If the individual is well trained (partici-

pates regularly in an aerobic exercise activity), the rate of heart rate rise is much more blunted (Fig. 16–29).

In a patient taking certain cardiac medications, specifically beta-blocking medications, a **blunted** (slower rate of rise and lower peak) **heart rate response** to exercise is anticipated and considered normal. The slower rate of rise aspect of the response is similar to that exhibited by highly trained individuals who also demonstrate a very gradual rate of rise in heart rate with increased work.

In addition, the heart rate achieved with activity should be compared with the predicted maximal heart rate. The predicted maximal heart rate of an individual is related to age. One method of determining the predicted maximal rate is to subtract the patient's age from 220 (220 − age). However, this method is known to underestimate the maximal heart rate in well-trained and in elderly persons. For these patients, the following two formulas are recommended: for males, $205 - \frac{1}{2}$ age; for females, $225 -$ age.[20] Therefore, if an individual were performing near maximal capacity, it is reasonable to expect the measured maximal heart rate to approximate predicted maximal heart rate. Normally, in the acute care setting, patients should not be working anywhere near maximal heart rate.

> ### Clinical Note: Palpation of Arrhythmias
>
> If a *decrease* in heart rate is palpated with activity, this may be due to an increase in arrhythmias that are palpated as pauses. Check telemetry recordings for arrhythmias. An increase in PVCs with activity is an abnormal response to activity.

Abnormal heart rate responses are of three types: a very rapid rise in heart rate with increased workload, a very flat rate of rise (bradycardic response), and a decrease in palpated heart rate. Patients who demonstrate a rapid rise in heart rate generally have one of two problems: severe deconditioning or a cardiovascular condition that is limiting the stroke volume. Patients who are not taking cardiac medications and who demonstrate a very flat rate of rise in heart rate are believed to have underlying cardiovascular disease. Also, individuals who have a decrease in palpated heart rate are not actually showing a true decreased heart rate but rather a decrease in palpable heart rate. If an ECG telemetry unit were available, these individuals should be monitored, because the palpable decrease in heart rate indicates an increase in arrhythmias (probably ventricular). When premature ectopic beats arise in the heart, they can often be palpated as a skip or pause in the pulse. When an increased number of pauses are palpated, it might appear to the therapist palpating the pulse that the heart rate actually decreased with exercise, when in reality the number of arrhythmias increased. If the pauses as well as the palpable beats were counted, one might not see a decrease in heart rate with exercise but rather an increase in heart rate with exercise. So, in reality, the heart rate does not decrease with exercise, but the palpated heart rate may *appear* to decrease if the number of arrhythmias increase. An increase in arrhythmias with exercise is also considered to be an abnormal response to exercise (see Heart Rhythm).

Heart Rhythm

Heart rhythm can be palpated to assess regularity during exercise, but the interpretation of any specific rhythm disturbance cannot be made without ECG monitoring. Numerous patients, with and without cardiopulmonary dysfunction, have arrhythmias, so physical therapists must be able to identify commonly observed basic and life-threatening arrhythmias as well as be able to assess the severity of these arrhythmias to make appropriate clinical decisions. Arrhythmias are discussed in Chapter 9.

Heart rhythm should remain regular with exercise; however, if an individual has arrhythmias at rest, the normal response would be a lack of change in the frequency or type of arrhythmia with an increase in activity. If a change occurs with increased activity, four factors should be considered in the clinical decision-making process: (1) whether the arrhythmias represent a new finding, (2) whether the arrhythmias are benign or life-threatening, (3) whether the patient's pharmacologic regimen may be producing the arrhythmias, and (4) the severity of the symptoms associated with the arrhythmias. Clinically, patients with occasional arrhythmias may not demonstrate serious arrhythmias with increased activity; in fact, arrhythmias may decrease or disappear with activity (as in sinus arrhythmia). In addition, arrhythmias may be well controlled by medication when the patient is at rest but not when the patient becomes active. A serious problem exists when a patient develops symptoms because of an arrhythmia or when the arrhythmia changes in character to become life threatening. Individuals who demonstrate an increasing frequency of premature ventricular ectopy with activity have been shown to have more serious coronary artery disease (two- and three-vessel disease) than individuals who do not.[21] In addition, patients who demonstrate premature ventricular ectopy at rest that disappears with activity have also been shown to have an increased incidence of coronary disease.[22]

Clinically, disturbances in heart rhythm should, at least, be monitored during an initial evaluation by means of direct palpation. When patients are known to have rhythm disturbances (either by direct palpation or history), further efforts should include ECG monitoring during activity and evaluating symptoms with the arrhythmias.

Blood Pressure Measurement

Arterial blood pressure is a general indicator of the function of the heart as a pump. The arterial

Table 16-6

Definition of Resting Blood Pressure

	NORMAL	BORDERLINE	HYPERTENSIVE
Systolic (mm Hg)	<140	140–150	>150
Diastolic (mm Hg)	<90	90–100	>100

Source: American Heart Association Guidelines.

blood pressure is defined as the *systolic* pressure (pressure exerted against the arteries during the ejection cycle) and *diastolic* pressure (pressure exerted against the arteries during rest). Factors affecting blood pressure include cardiac output, peripheral resistance, distensibility of the arteries (vasomotor tone), volume of blood in the system, viscosity of the blood, and neural input.

Normal blood pressure in the aorta and arteries is defined as less than 140 mm Hg systolic and less than 90 mm Hg diastolic. Table 16-6 includes guidelines from the American Heart Association for normal, borderline, and hypertensive blood pressure. Blood pressure can be measured directly by means of indwelling arterial catheterization using a catheter inserted into an artery (as done in laboratory or critical care situations) or indirectly using a **sphygmomanometer.** Blood pressures are usually taken on the upper arm with the distal margin of the cuff approximately 3 cm above the antecubital fossa. Palpation is performed to locate the brachial artery pulse. This is the location for auscultation of the blood pressure. Following inflation of the cuff, auscultation of the first audible sound designates the systolic pressure, whereas the diastolic pressure is the value when the sounds become muffled.

The blood pressure may vary between extremities, with change of position, and with any type of activity. The changes between like extremities may reflect uneven peripheral resistance due to either differences in vasomotor tone or arterial occlusion. Changes in blood pressure with body position may reflect the influences of the vasomotor tone, the venous return, or the hydrostatic effects of gravity,

or a combination of all three. Blood pressure changes associated with activity typically reflect the amount of work the heart must do to meet the metabolic demands of the activity.

Accuracy in measurement is critical to the correct interpretation of the blood pressure. Problems arise in the accurate measurement of blood pressure with activity when a therapist is not using good technique. When a patient stops performing an activity, the direct metabolic demands decrease while the muscle activity that assists in the return of the venous blood stops. As a result, the blood pressure may drop rapidly (within 15 seconds).[22] Therefore, it is essential that the physical therapist be competent in blood pressure measurement and knowledgeable regarding normal blood pressure responses to exertion in addition to being able to identify and react to abnormal responses.

Evaluation of Oxygen Saturation

Patients with heart failure, pulmonary hypertension, or pulmonary disease should be evaluated for activity tolerance by monitoring heart rate, blood pressure, symptoms, and oxygen saturation. A pulse oximeter is used to assess oxygen saturation of hemoglobin, which has a normal range of 98 to 100% (saturation of Hb). The portable pulse oximeter compares the signals received and calculates the degree of oxyhemoglobin saturation based on

Clinical Note: Portable Automatic Blood Pressure Cuffs

Portable automatic blood pressure cuffs are often used in the hospital. This equipment is not always accurate with multiple use.

Clinical Note: Assessing Blood Pressure and Heart Rate During Activity

It is essential to monitor both blood pressure and heart rate during activity rather than making these assessments after activity because blood pressure can drop within 15 seconds of returning to rest. Heart rate and systolic blood pressure are the key determinants of myocardial oxygen demand.

the intensity of the signal received. Normal response to activity is for the O_2 saturation to remain in the normal range. However, patients with chronic pulmonary dysfunction or congestive heart failure often desaturate their oxygen from hemoglobin with activity. Caution should be taken with patients who desaturate with activity below 90%. Exercise should not be continued if oxygen saturation drops to 86% or below. See Chapter 10 for further information.

Normal Responses

To understand normal responses to exercise, it is important to recognize that two key factors affect the blood pressure response: cardiac output and peripheral vascular resistance. Generally, with increased work, the cardiac output increases and the peripheral vascular resistance decreases as a result of (1) the **hypothalamic** response to increased body temperature and (2) the local effects of hydrogen ions, heat, decreased availability of oxygen, and increased carbon dioxide production on the arterioles. Thus, there is a normal increase in systolic blood pressure with increasing levels of exertion. It is important to note that adult females tend to demonstrate a slower rate of rise in the systolic pressure during exertion in contrast to adult males.

The normal diastolic response is a maximum of 10 mm Hg increase or decrease from the resting value because of the adaptive dilation of the peripheral vascular bed that occurs with exercise (Fig. 16–30). Younger persons and trained athletes may demonstrate a progressive decrease in diastolic pressure during exercise as a result of the increased peripheral vasodilation. Therefore, a fall in diastolic pressure greater than the 10 mm Hg can be considered a normal response in this population but not in older, untrained individuals.

The normal systolic and diastolic blood pressure responses to endurance activity (when an individual maintains a constant submaximal workload) are to remain constant or even to decrease slightly. This indicates that the body has achieved a steady state condition and that the central and peripheral mechanisms that adjust the blood pressure (e.g., cardiac output and peripheral vascular resistance) have accommodated to the workload.

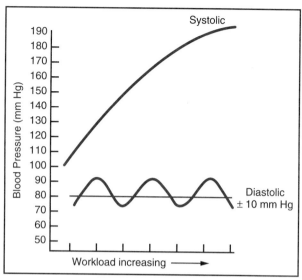

Figure 16–30. The systolic blood pressure gradually rises with a gradual increase in workload. The diastolic blood pressure should change very little (± 10 mm Hg) with an increase in workload. (Redrawn from Scully R, Barnes ML. Physical Therapy. Philadelphia, JB Lippincott, 1989.)

Abnormal Responses

If one knows and understands the normal blood pressure responses to exercise, then identifying abnormal responses is simplified. Abnormalities can exist with the systolic or diastolic response or both. The abnormal responses are first defined, and then the mechanism of action and clinical implications are described.

Abnormal Systolic Responses. There are three abnormal systolic blood pressure responses to activity that are described in the literature: hypertensive, hypotensive, and blunted or flat. A hypertensive blood pressure response is one in which an individual who is normotensive at rest exhibits an abnormally high systolic blood pressure for a given level of exertion. This type of response has been associated with an increased risk for the future development of hypertension at rest. Furthermore, this response should be distinguished from that found in an individual who is hypertensive at rest yet exhibits a normally increasing systolic blood pressure during increasing levels of exertion.[23] Although the mechanism for the hypertensive blood pressure response is not fully understood, it may be related to the following: an increased plasma concentration of **catecholamines,** an increased resistance to blood flow arising from peripheral vascular occlusive disease, or an abnormal centrally mediated resting vasomotor tone.

Exertional systolic hypotension is described as a normally rising systolic pressure at submaximal levels, followed by a sudden progressive decrease in systolic blood pressure in the face of increasing workload (Fig. 16–31); it has been highly correlated with pathologic cardiac conditions.[24] Individuals with exertional hypotension often demonstrate coronary perfusion defects on exercise thallium tests and severe coronary disease, poor ventricular function, or both as documented by coronary angiography.[24]

A blunted blood pressure response is defined as a slight increase in systolic blood pressure at low levels of exertion with a failure to rise with increasing levels of work. This definition applies only to those individuals who are not receiving pharmacologic intervention that might affect blood pressure. Failure to reach a systolic blood pressure in excess of 130 mm Hg at maximal effort in the absence of any medication that restricts the blood pressure is associated with a high risk for future sudden death.[25] However, this is equivalent to the blunted response that is seen in individuals who are receiving beta-adrenergic antagonists as part of a therapeutic pharmacologic regimen. When these medications are prescribed, the blunted blood pressure response is expected and considered normal.

A hypotensive or blunted blood pressure response indicates that either the cardiac output is failing to meet the demands of the body or that the peripheral vascular resistance is rapidly decreasing. Evidence in the literature suggests that hypotensive or blunted blood pressure responses are most often due to a failing cardiac output.[26, 27] Because the cardiac output is directly dependent on stroke volume and heart rate, if the stroke volume is unable to increase appropriately for a given level of work, any increase in cardiac output arises solely as the result of an increase in the heart rate. In this situation, the blood pressure may rise slightly or may remain flat. Unfortunately, because of the concomitant increase in myocardial oxygen demand that accompanies an increase in heart rate, the heart is unable to maintain an increased cardiac output for any significant period of time, which results in a falling blood pressure.

When an individual is performing endurance exercise (of greater than 3 to 5 minutes in duration), a continuous rise in systolic blood pressure is considered an abnormal response. Persons who demonstrate an abnormal blood pressure response during endurance exercise typically have one of two conditions: either a high degree of ventricular wall dysfunction or a dysfunction in the ability of myocardial tissue to extract oxygen from the circulatory system.

Clinical Implications. Patients who demonstrate abnormal blood pressure responses during exercise typically suffer from coronary artery disease (e.g., have a history of angioplasty, angina, coronary bypass surgery, or myocardial infarction), moderate to severe aortic valvular stenosis, or other cardiac muscle dysfunction.[28–29]

The assessment of peak blood pressure as well as the interpretation of the blood pressure response during activity is an essential component of the initial and continuing evaluation of every patient. Although restrictions on any activity might be unnecessary, patients with abnormal systolic blood pressure responses should be monitored closely during typical activities and especially during new exertional activities. In addition, the treatment or exercise prescription may require alterations in duration, intensity, or both. Some activities may require supervision so that the patient can perform the activity safely. Also, the patients themselves should be educated regarding their specific limitations and the signs and symp-

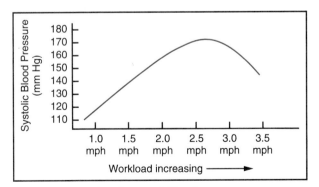

Figure 16–31. An abnormal blood pressure response to an increase in workload. Greater than 2.5 mph workload caused the systolic blood pressure to decrease continually, demonstrating a failure of the heart muscle to meet the demands. (Redrawn from Scully R, Barnes ML. Physical Therapy. Philadelphia, JB Lippincott, 1989.)

toms of overexertion when performing any activities.

Abnormal Diastolic Responses. As stated previously, a normal diastolic blood pressure response is one in which a change is no greater than 10 mm Hg: an abnormal diastolic blood pressure response would be either an increase or decrease of more than 10 mm Hg (in an untrained or older population). In addition, a sustained elevation of the diastolic blood pressure during the recovery phase of activity is considered to be abnormal.[30]

The mechanism behind the progressive rise in diastolic blood pressure is thought to be a response to the need for an increased driving pressure in the coronary arteries, which is necessary to overcome the increased resistance to flow within the coronary arteries. When blood flow through the coronary arteries is decreased below the level needed to meet the demand of the myocardium as a result of either increased vascular tone or vascular occlusion, a stimulus is created for an increased driving pressure to make the blood flow through the resistant arteries.[30] Despite the lack of research-based documentation regarding this abnormality, the physical therapist should be aware of the normal anticipated physiologic response and therefore be very sensitive to a progressive rise in diastolic pressure, interpreting this as an abnormal response. Patients who demonstrate a progressive rise in diastolic pressure usually have numerous risk factors for heart disease, are deemed high risk for or already have coronary artery disease, or have a previous history of coronary angioplasty or bypass surgery. Patients with hypertensive heart disease and compensated heart failure may also demonstrate this abnormal response.

Other Symptoms of Cardiovascular Inadequacy

The other symptoms associated with cardiovascular inadequacy are more difficult to interpret and therefore more difficult to treat. Angina, shortness of breath, and **palpitations** are the most common symptoms of patients with cardiopulmonary dysfunction. The other classic symptoms to be aware of are dizziness, **pallor,** and fatigue. The therapist, therefore, must have a thorough understanding of how to assess these symptoms.

Angina. **Angina** is a discomfort found anywhere above the waist but more likely in the chest, neck, or jaw and is typically described using terms such as dull ache, tightness, fullness, burning, pressure, indigestion, or neck or jaw discomfort. *Classic (or stable) angina* is brought on by exertion or emotional upset and at times by eating; it is relieved by either rest or nitroglycerin. Angina and other chest wall or neurologic complaints are differentiated by the activity that reproduces the discomfort. Angina is reproducible only by increasing myocardial oxygen consumption (as in activity or emotion), whereas musculoskeletal pain can be reproduced by palpation or deep inspiration and expiration, and neurologic pain may follow a dermatome and exist all the time.

There are six types of "chest pain" that make the differential diagnosis of angina difficult, however. Two of these situations relate to angina and include **variant angina** (as found in the pure form called **Prinzmetal's angina**) and **preinfarction angina.**

Variant Angina. Variant angina, defined as angina produced from vasospasm of the coronary arteries in the absence of occlusive disease (i.e., the arteries are free of disease), is called Prinzmetal's angina. Individuals who experience vasospasm often develop resting chest pain, making the classic definition of angina inappropriate.[31] In the case of variant angina, an individual is more likely to have discomfort that is due to emotional upset or inspiration of cold air.

Variant angina usually responds to nitroglycerin and is typically diagnosed when nitroglycerin is found to be effective or when other long-term pharmacologic therapy is found effective. Calcium-channel blockers are typically the long-term pharmacologic choice for the treatment of variant angina. These drugs retard the uptake of the calcium in the cells and therefore inhibit smooth muscle contraction of the arterial walls (see Chapters 2 and 14).

> **Clinical Note: Shortness of Breath with Coronary Artery Disease**
>
> Older women and diabetic patients with coronary artery disease do not complain of the typical chest tightness with exertion, but rather shortness of breath. This shortness of breath goes away slowly (or "eases") with rest.

Preinfarction Angina. Preinfarction angina is defined as *unstable* angina; it occurs at rest and worsens with activity. An individual may or may not have had symptoms of classic angina before experiencing the intense and constant pain of preinfarction angina. This condition is one that requires immediate medical treatment to prevent full transmural infarction.

Although the description of angina may vary from individual to individual, the description remains constant for each individual. Therefore, once the therapist concludes that the symptoms being described constitute angina, then the patient's terms used to describe the angina should be remembered and used in all future assessments of symptoms. The other four types of chest pain in addition to angina are **pericarditis,** mitral valve dysfunction, bronchospasm, and esophageal spasm.

Pericarditis. Pericarditis is an inflammation of the pericardial sac that surrounds the heart and may actually result in a restriction of cardiac output. Patients who are suspected of having pericardial pain should be referred for immediate medical treatment and discontinued from exertional activities until the pericarditis subsides. Pericarditis produces a chest pain symptom that is constant and sharp and is described as intense and "stabbing." Pericarditis pain usually does not increase with activity but may remain constant 24 hours per day and is very intense. Associated fever and fatigue may also occur with the stabbing pain, as well as ECG changes.[32] Pericardial pain is a common symptom following coronary artery bypass surgery and occurs occasionally in the early phase following a myocardial infarction. Treatment usually includes anti-inflammatory medications.

Mitral Valve Dysfunction. Individuals with mitral valve dysfunction (mitral valve prolapse or mitral valve regurgitation) may demonstrate classic angina with exertion yet lack a suspicious risk factor profile. They tend to be younger and are free of cardiovascular occlusive disease. Auscultation of heart sounds usually reveals a systolic murmur or click. Echocardiography usually identifies mitral valve dysfunction. The angina pain from mitral valve dysfunction arises from the diminished blood flow resulting from the subsequent decreased cardiac output.[33]

Bronchospasm. Some patients experience exercise-induced bronchospasm, which can manifest itself as chest wall tightness or discomfort, or both, with exertion. Differentiation of exercise-induced bronchospasm from exertional angina is performed by assessing the individual's degree of difficulty in breathing. An individual experiencing exercise-induced bronchospasm usually demonstrates a greatly increased work of breathing as well as an extreme effort to take the next breath.

Esophageal Spasm. Esophageal spasm or inflammation may produce a midsternal pain that is mistaken for angina.[34] Diffuse esophageal spasm is usually idiopathic and produces a chest pain with dysphagia. Esophageal spasm is suspected when the chest discomfort develops with eating and can be diagnosed with esophageal manometry or with barium swallow. Treatment for this type of chest pain includes medication to decrease the acid reflux into the esophagus, sublingual nitroglycerin, and calcium-channel blockers.[35]

Shortness of Breath. Shortness of breath is one of the other common symptoms found in patients with cardiopulmonary dysfunction. Shortness of breath may be due to several different physiologic mechanisms, including the equivalent of angina in individuals who cannot perceive chest pain or discomfort, as in the diabetic with peripheral neuropathy. Shortness of breath may also be due to limited cardiovascular reserve in patients with coronary disease or cardiac muscle dysfunction; pulmonary disease with limited ventilatory reserve, diffusion, or arterial oxygen-carrying capacity; and finally physiologic limitations in an individual's oxygen transport system when shortness of breath occurs during exercise. When shortness of breath does develop during the assessment, these mechanisms need to be evaluated to determine the cause of the shortness of breath and to make appropriate clinical decisions regarding progression of activity.

Palpitations. Palpitations are a common complaint of patients with cardiopulmonary dysfunction. Palpitations usually indicate arrhythmias.[36] Palpitations must be evaluated to determine the seriousness of any rhythm disturbances as well as the cause of any symptoms. Evaluation usually involves 24-hour Holter monitoring.

Dizziness. Dizziness can have several origins, including the vestibular system, vision, medications, blood pressure, and cardiac output. Dizziness is a symptom that must be evaluated with reference to the activity that produces it and then compared with the blood pressure response. If an individual becomes dizzy on standing and a blood pressure drop is noted, the condition is described as orthostatic hypotension. However, if the patient complains of dizziness with an increase in activity and a blood pressure drop is noted, this patient is defined as having exertional hypotension. Clinical decision making therefore depends on the constellation of symptoms presented by the patient and the effect the associated dizziness has on his or her activity.

Fatigue. Fatigue may also have several origins, including depression, general deconditioning, pharmacologic management and side effects, and physiologic limitation, as seen in the individual with cardiac muscle dysfunction. Therefore, fatigue should never be the only symptom the therapist uses to make a clinical decision regarding exercise prescription or progression. The cause of the fatigue may need to be investigated further if it is the only symptom limiting activity and all other responses are normal.

Monitored Activity

On completion of the full cardiopulmonary assessment, including chest examination and activity evaluation, a decision is made regarding the patient's treatment. Acute care treatment procedures are discussed in Chapter 17. However, the therapist must always remember that each treatment session becomes an assessment, particularly of responses to the treatment. Therefore, each treatment session is, in essence, a monitored activity session, requiring constant reevaluation and assessment as to the significance of the clinical findings.

CASE STUDIES

Case 1

A 72-year-old woman who contracted poliomyelitis in 1948 fell in her retirement home apartment, fracturing the proximal left femur. She was found immediately because she used her emergency call cord in her apartment.

The patient underwent open reduction internal fixation with spinal anesthesia 3 days earlier, and the physician has just ordered physical therapy for out of bed activities and ambulation with a walker.

The chart review revealed the following:

- A 54-year history of smoking approximately 1.5 to 2 packs per day
- No history of hypertension, family history of heart disease, or other major medical problems (patient had been ambulatory with wheeled tripod walker and lives alone)
- Laboratory study results within normal limits
- Chest radiograph demonstrates hyperinflated chest with few patchy areas of infiltrate in both bases

In the interview, the patient reported that she is in a lot of pain. She plans to return to extended care at the retirement home until she is able to take care of herself.

The physical examination revealed the following:

- General appearance: slight grayish color; thin, slightly underweight
- Neck: observation of hypertrophy of sternocleidomastoid muscles bilaterally; forward head, and sits in bed with the head of the bed elevated to 60 degrees
- Chest: Upward movement of chest with every breath; patient is observed to have increased accessory muscle use, increased AP diameter, and increased respiratory rate
- Phonation, cough, and cough production: patient is observed to have moist, nonproductive, ineffective cough; phonation requires breaths between words in sentence; extremities have mild clubbing, gray-blue color with tobacco stains
- Auscultation: decreased breath sounds auscultated with coarse wheezing and wet rales on expiration in bilateral bases but slightly cleared with a cough; auscultation of the heart demonstrates loud atrial gallop with rapid heartbeat
- Palpation: decreased chest wall motion palpated throughout, with palpable fremitus in bilateral bases; increased accessory muscle use including sternocleidomastoid and scalenes, with decreased diaphragmatic excursion; good pulses throughout, except bilateral dorsalis pedis
- Percussion: mild dullness to percussion noted in bases
- Activity evaluation: patient was evaluated in supine-to-sit position only; patient could not tolerate standing owing to increased pain in left lower extremity and dizziness
- Vital signs: heart rate 100 (supine), 120 (sitting); blood pressure 110/70 (supine), 90/66 (sitting)

These findings from the cardiopulmonary assessment demonstrate an elderly female with a long-term history of smoking and signs of chronic obstructive pulmonary disease in addition to the hip fracture. She is at extreme risk for pneumonia. Also, the patient has a problem with orthostatic hypotension as evidenced by her vital signs. The chronic obstructive pulmonary disease and the present pulmonary condition (e.g., infiltrates in bases, retained secretions), as well as the orthostatic hypotension, will affect her activity progression. These need to be addressed.

Case 2

The patient is a 58-year-old woman, admitted with a diagnosis of arthritis in the right knee, who underwent a total knee replacement. The patient's past medical history includes treatment for hypertension (Tenormin, 100 mg/day), adult onset diabetes (controlled with oral insulin), and rheumatic fever as a child. Recently she has had very limited activity because of the painful right knee. The patient is markedly obese.

Since surgery the right knee has been in a continuous passive motion apparatus, but the patient has been limited to bedrest owing to numerous postoperative complications, including infections and nonhealing of the incision. The nurses are unable to get the patient out of bed owing to her weight and complaints of dizziness. The physician has ordered gait training with a walker with toe-touch weight-bearing status.

In the interview, the patient reported that she feels weak since being in bed after surgery. Her plans are to return home to her apartment. She lives alone.

The physical examination revealed the following:

- Inspection: patient is markedly obese with good general appearance; right knee has large bandage with dark pink skin surrounding the bandage and increased edema on right
- Auscultation: reveals normal heart sounds, diminished breath sounds throughout, with crackles on inspiration throughout the bases; nonproductive dry cough
- Palpation: no abnormalities with chest motion, although diaphragmatic excursion appears limited; pulses are intact and normal throughout; patient is sensitive to touch around the right knee
- Activity evaluation: patient requires the maximal assistance of two people (one person to move the right lower extremity) to transfer from a supine to a sitting position and the maximal assistance of two people to raise her to a standing position holding onto walker
- Vital signs: heart rate 66 (supine), 72 (sitting), 80 (standing); blood pressure 108/70 (supine), 90/66 (sitting), 80/60 (standing); patient complained of extreme dizziness with 60 seconds of standing and returned to sitting position

Patient's blood pressure response and symptoms are the major limiting factors to progression. Her weakness from bedrest and her obesity are additional factors. In addition, with the patient's history of hypertension and the current medications she is taking for hypertension, her physician should be notified before she resumes activity. Her medication may be affecting her blood pressure response to the upright position and subsequently blocking the heart rate rise.

Case 3

The patient is a 32-year-old man who was admitted to the intensive care unit with a diagnosis of bilateral lower lobe pneumonia and was placed on a mechanical ventilator on assist-control mode. The patient had seen his physician for a chronically elevated temperature and night sweats 1 week before admission.

The chart review revealed no history of smoking. The chest radiograph demonstrated diffuse patchy infiltrates throughout the interstitium bilaterally. The physician has given orders for increased bed mobility and range of motion and out of bed activities.

The physical examination revealed the following:

- Inspection: The patient is on a volume-assist mode ventilator, alert but pale and cachectic in appearance; he appears to be in no distress at present but does initiate coughing spasmodically when his position is changed; atrophy of lower and upper extremities is apparent on observation; respiration rate is approximately 30 breaths per minute with ventilator assistance.
- Auscultation reveals crackles throughout both bases, lingula, and right middle lobe; heart sounds are normal but very rapid.
- Palpation: patient has a normal chest motion and an absence of fremitus but excessive accessory muscle use; no pain elicited on palpation of the chest; circulation evaluation demonstrated normal pulses bilaterally throughout.
- Activity evaluation: patient required the assistance of one person to roll to the side and sit up in bed and move his legs over the side of the bed.
- Vital signs: heart rate 108 (supine), 130 (sitting over side); blood pressure 110/70 (supine), 120/76 (sitting over side); no symptoms were reported, but patient appeared to increase respiration rate with sitting and complained of fatigue after sitting for a few minutes.

The patient's weakness and decreased ventilatory capacity are limiting his progress. Breathing exercises to work on increasing the depth of ventilation, strengthening, and energy conservation are recommended. Intolerance to activity is also limiting him. Progression of activity should be slow and monitored.

Suspect AIDS (autoimmune deficiency syndrome) as a possible diagnosis in this case (age, severity of pneumonia, symptoms of night sweats and elevated temperatures, and diffuse infiltrates on chest x-ray). Take precautions for any body secretions and fluids. Secretion management is often not indicated in patients with AIDS and pneumonia (Pneumocystis carinii) because secretions originate at the alveolar/capillary membrane.

Summary

- A thorough evaluation of the patient is essential for optimal treatment.
- Included in the cardiopulmonary assessment is a thorough chart review to identify past medical history, diagnostic studies, and current medical status.

- The physical therapist must remember that although the chart should have all the necessary information about the patient, the optimal situation is one that allows the acquisition of pertinent information directly from the patient.
- The patient interview can shed new light on the chart information, or it can provide a completely different picture.
- Performing a physical examination of the patient provides the most accurate information regarding the patient's current cardiopulmonary status.
- The physical examination includes a thorough inspection, auscultation, palpation, percussion, and activity evaluation.
- Based on the initial assessment, a plan of treatment or exercise prescription can be developed for optimal rehabilitation.
- The assessment must be ongoing, and components of the physical examination need to be performed on a daily basis to assess the patient's status with increased activity.
- Reevaluation is just as important for the patient's progression of activity as is the initial assessment.

References

1. Kannel WB, Castelli WP, Gordon T, et al. Serum cholesterol, liproproteins, and the risk of coronary heart disease: The Framingham study. Ann Intern Med 24:1, 1971.
2. Laposata EA. Cocaine induced heart disease: Mechanisms and pathology. J Thorac Imaging 6(1):68–75, 1991.
3. Rezkalla SH, Hale S, Kloner RA. Cocaine induced heart diseases. Am Heart J 120(6):1403–1408, 1990.
4. Morris DC. Cocaine heart disease. Hosp Pract [Off] 26(9):83–92, 1991.
5. McNeer JF, Wallace AG, Wagner GS, et al. The course of acute myocardial infarction. Circulation 51:410, 1975.
6. Steinhart MJ. Depression and chronic fatigue in the patient with heart disease. Prim Care 18(2):309–325, 1991.
7. Wilkins RL. Dexter JR, Murphy RL Jr, DelBono EA. Lung sound nomenclature survey. Chest 98(4):886–889, 1990.
8. Kramin SS. Determination of the site of production of respiratory sounds by subtraction phonopneumography. Am Rev Respir Dis 122:303, 1980.
9. American College of CP & ATS Joint Committee on Pulmonary Nomenclature. Pulmonary terms and symbols. Chest 67:583, 1975.
10. Wilkins RL, Hodgkin JE, Lopez B. Lung Sounds: A Practical Guide. St. Louis, CV Mosby, 1988.
11. Piirila P, Sovijarvi AR, Kaisla T, et al. Crackles in patients with fibrosing alveolitis, bronchiectasis, COPD and heart failure. Chest 99(5):1076–1083, 1991.
12. Nath AR, Capel LH. Inspiratory crackles and the mechanical events of breathing. Thorax 29:695, 1974.
13. Forgacs P. The functional basis of pulmonary sounds. Chest 73:399, 1978.
14. Nath AR, Capel LH. Inspiratory crackles—Early and late. Thorax 29:223, 1974.
15. Murphy RLH. Discontinuous adventitious lung sounds. Semin Respir Med 6:210, 1985.
16. Ravin A. Auscultation of the Heart. Chicago, Year Book Medical Publishers, 1968.
17. Luisada AA, Portaluppi F. The Heart Sounds: New Facts and Their Clinical Applications. New York, Praeger Publishers, 1982.
18. Criqui MH, Fronek A, Klauber MR. The sensitivity, specificity and predictive value of traditional clinical evidence of peripheral arterial disease: Results from noninvasive testing in a defined population. Circulation 71(3):516–522, 1985.
19. Butler SM. Phase one cardiac rehabilitation: The role of functional evaluation in patient progression. Master's thesis. Atlanta, Emory University, 1983.
20. Cooper KH. The Aerobics Way. New York, Bantam Books, 1981.
21. Pleskot M, Pidrman V, Tilser P, et al. (Programmed ventricular stimulation in the evaluation of the clinical significance of premature ventricular contractions). Vnitr Lek 37(6):548–556, 1991.
22. Henachel A, De La Vega F, Taylor HL. Simultaneous direct and indirect blood pressure measurements in man at rest and work. J Appl Physiol 6:506, 1954.
23. Dlin RA, Hanne N, Silverberg DS, et al. Followup of normotensive men with exaggerated blood pressure response to exercise. Am Heart J 106(2):316, 1983.
24. Hakki A, Munley BM, Hadjimiltiades J. Determinants of abnormal blood pressure response to exercise in coronary artery disease. Am J Cardiol 57:71, 1986.
25. Bruce RA, DeRouen T, Peterson DR, et al. Noninvasive predictors of sudden death in men with coronary heart disease. Am J Cardiol 39:833, 1977.
26. Frenneaux MP, Counihan PJ, Caforior AL, et al. Abnormal blood pressure response during exercise in hypertrophic cardiomyopathy. Circulation 82(6):1995–2002, 1990.
27. Pavlovic M. (Decrease in systolic blood pressure during physical exertion in stress tests). Srp Arh Celok Lek 117(11–12):777–786, 1989.
28. Cavan D, O'Donnell MJ, Parkes A, et al. Abnormal blood pressure response to exercise in normoalbuminuric insulin dependent diabetic patients. J Hum Hypertens 5(1):21–26, 1991.
29. Guerrera G, Melina D, Colivicchi F, et al. Abnormal blood pressure response to exercise in borderline hypertension. A two year follow-up study. Am J Hypertens 4(3, pt 1):271–273, 1991.
30. Guyton AC, Jones CE, Coleman TG. Circulatory Physiology: Cardiac Output and Its Regulation. Philadelphia, WB Saunders, 1973.
31. Maseri A, Crea F, Kaski JC, Crake T. Mechanisms of angina pectoris in syndrome X. J Am Coll Cardiol 17:499, 1991.
32. Phillips RE, Feeney MK. The Cardiac Rhythms: A Systematic Approach to Interpretation. Philadelphia, WB Saunders, 1990.
33. Albert MA, Mukerji V, Sabeti M, et al. Mitral valve prolapse, panic disorder, and chest pain. Med Clin North Am 75(5):1119–1133, 1991.
34. Rakel RE. Conn's Current Therapy. Philadelphia, WB Saunders, 1991, pp 424–425.
35. Nevens F, Janssens J, Piessens J, et al. Prospective study on prevalence of esophageal chest pain in patients referred on an elective basis to a cardiac unit for suspected myocardial ischemia. Dig Dis Sci 36(2):229, 1991.
36. Cohen M, Michel TH. Cardiopulmonary Symptoms in Physical Therapy Practice. New York, Churchill Livingstone, 1988.

## 17

Treatment of Acute Cardiopulmonary Conditions

Alexandra Sciaky, Jill Stockford, and Erica Nixon

INTRODUCTION

In physical therapy, sound clinical decision making regarding treatment is based on the physiologic evaluation of the patient. Physical therapists treating patients with acute cardiopulmonary dysfunctions have a unique challenge in that they must integrate frequent, dynamic pathophysiologic changes into their treatment progressions. Acute cardiopulmonary dysfunction can be defined as a disease or state in which the patient's oxygen transport system fails to meet the immediate demands placed on it.[1] Such failure may result in significant periods of bedrest for the patient and the associated adverse effects (Table 17–1). Symptoms indicative of the failure may or may not be present. Patient assessment is clearly described in Chapter 16. The overall objective of this chapter is to provide the clinician with an understanding of treatment interventions, indications for treatment, and issues pertinent to clinical decision making in the care of acutely ill cardiopulmonary patients.

As medical treatment in acute care continues to advance, the acuity level of hospitalized patients continues to rise. Patients are surviving illnesses and events today that would have caused their demise only 10 years ago.[2] The 1990's trend toward managed care in the United States is also having a profound impact on acute care practice. This impact includes shortened length of hospital stay, use of intravenous (IV) therapy and mechanical ventilation in the home, and a decrease in the ratio of physical therapists to physical therapy assistants being hired to treat patients. These changes create new pressures and responsibilities for the physical therapist treating acutely ill patients. The physical therapist has become a key decision maker in determining the most appropriate discharge destination (home, nursing home, subacute unit, rehabilitation unit) for hospital patients. The shortened length of stay means the physical therapist must prioritize not only which patients to treat first but which treatments to do first on a given patient. Careful prioritization is necessary to meet the patient's immediate needs in a short period of time. Addressing the pulmonary needs of the patient is generally the physical therapist's first priority. It might be difficult, for example, for a patient with excessive bronchial secretions to perform mobility exercises and maintain adequate oxygen saturation levels during the activity. This chapter describes the cardiopulmonary treatment techniques that are typically utilized by physical therapists in an acute care hospital. The indications, contraindications, and precautions will be provided and the treatment progression and goals will be discussed.

AIRWAY CLEARANCE TECHNIQUES

Airway clearance techniques are defined as manual or mechanical procedures that facilitate clearance of secretions from the airways. The techniques include postural drainage, percussion, vibration, cough techniques, **manual hyperinflation,** and airway suctioning. The indications for airway clearance techniques are impaired mucociliary transport or an ineffective cough. The clinician can facilitate these mechanisms by using one or more airway clearance techniques with acutely ill patients. Consideration of the pathophysiology and symptoms, the stability of the medical status of the patient, and the patient's adherence to the technique(s) are all important factors in choosing an optimal airway clearance treatment plan. Adherence to hospital infection control policies and procedures is critical to maintain the safety of caregivers and patients. Body substance precautions such as gowns, masks, gloves, and goggles apply to the performance of airway clearance techniques.

Patient assessment before, during, and after treatment provides the clinician with important information by which to judge the patient's tolerance and the treatment's effectiveness. In addition to gathering the necessary equipment and assistance to perform the treatment, airway clearance

---

Table 17–1

Clinical Systemic Effects of Immobilization

Cardiovascular system
  Increased basal heart rate
  Decreased maximal heart rate
  Decreased maximal oxygen uptake
  Orthostatic hypotension
  Increased venous thrombosis risk
  Decreased total blood volume
  Decreased hemoglobin concentration
Respiratory system
  Decreased vital capacity
  Decreased residual volume
  Decreased Pa_{O_2}
  Impaired ability to clear secretions
  Increased ventilation-perfusion mismatch
Musculoskeletal system
  Decreased strength
  Decreased girth
  Decreased efficiency of contraction
  Joint contractures
  Decubitus ulcers
Central nervous system
  Emotional and behavioral disturbances
  Intellectual deficit
  Altered sensation
Metabolic system
  Hypercalcemia
  Osteoporosis

Table 17-2

Precautions and Relative Contraindications for Postural Drainage

PRECAUTIONS	RELATIVE CONTRAINDICATIONS
Pulmonary edema	Increased intracranial pressure
Hemoptysis	Hemodynamically unstable
Massive obesity	Recent esophageal anastomosis
Large pleural effusion	Recent spinal fusion or injury
Massive ascites	Recent head trauma
	Diaphragmatic hernia
	Recent eye surgery

techniques should be performed before or at least 30 minutes following the end of a meal or tube feeding. **Continuous tube feedings** should be interrupted and the patient's stomach checked for residual feeding that might be aspirated during the treatment.[3] Optimal pain control allows the patient to have the greatest comfort and offer fullest cooperation with the treatment. Inhaled bronchodilator medications given prior to airway clearance treatments enhance the overall treatment outcome. Inhaled antibiotic medications, however, will have better deposition into the lung if they are given following the airway clearance treatment. The clinician should also take care to observe proper body mechanics while performing airway clearance techniques to avoid self-injury. The goals of airway clearance techniques are to optimize airway patency, increase ventilation and perfusion matching, promote alveolar expansion and ventilation, and increase gas exchange.[4-6] Treatment duration and frequency are based on pulmonary reevaluation at each session. Often family members or other caregivers will be trained to continue the airway clearance techniques following hospital discharge. In this case the clinician should provide written instructions including techniques, duration, frequency, and precautions as well as personal demonstration of the desired treatment. Treatment is discontinued when the goals have been met or the patient can independently perform his own airway clearance techniques.

Postural Drainage

Postural drainage (PD) is the assumption of one or more body positions that allow gravity to drain secretions from each of the patient's lung segments.[7] In each position the segmental bronchus of the area to be drained is perpendicular to the floor (Fig. 17–1). These positions can be modified when a patient presents with a condition that qualifies as a precaution or relative contraindication to treatment (Table 17–2). A modified position to treat the lateral segment of the right lower lobe would be the left sidelying position with the bed flat rather than in the Trendelenburg position, for example.

Positioning the patient requires the use of an adjustable bed, pillows or blanket rolls, and enough personnel to assist in moving the patient safely. Tissues, a sputum cup, airway suctioning equipment, and **body substance barriers** should be available in order to collect any secretions that are produced. Postural drainage may be used exclusively or in combination with other airway clearance techniques. If PD is used exclusively, each position should be maintained for 5 to 10 minutes or longer, if tolerated.[8] The clinical approach to timing percussion and vibration during postural drainage is clinical evaluation and utilization of the techniques until the secretions clear.[9] Precautions and relative contraindications for percussion and vibration may be found in Table 17–3.

Priority should be given to treating the most affected lung segments first, and the patient should be encouraged to take deep breaths in the PD position and cough (or be suctioned) between

Table 17-3

Precautions and Relative Contraindications for Percussion and Vibration

PRECAUTIONS	RELATIVE CONTRAINDICATIONS
Uncontrolled bronchospasm	Hemoptysis
Osteoporosis	Untreated tension pneumothorax
Rib fractures	Platelet count below 20,000 per mm^3
Metastatic cancer to ribs	Unstable hemodynamic status
Tumor obstruction of airway	Open wounds, burns in the thoracic area
Anxiety	Pulmonary embolism
Coagulopathy	Subcutaneous emphysema
Convulsive or seizure disorder	Recent skin grafts or flaps on thorax
Recent pacemaker placement	

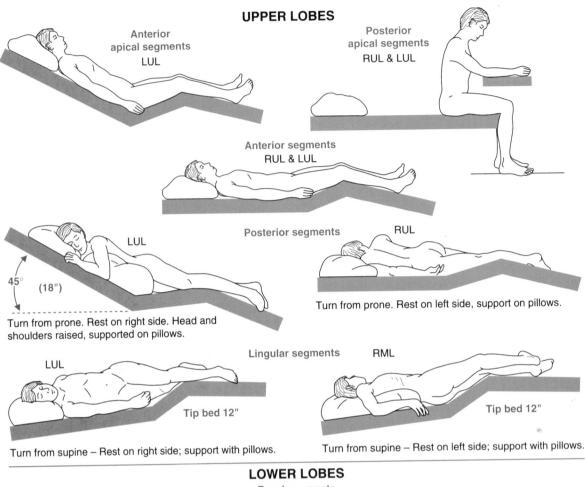

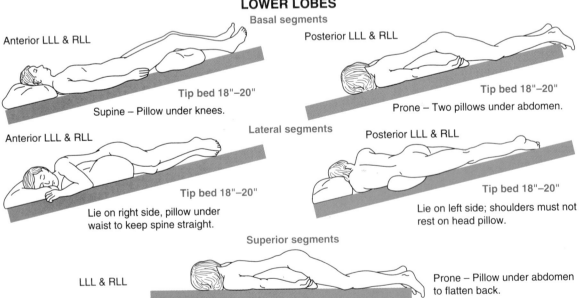

Figure 17-1. The twelve postural drainage positions. LLL, Left lower lobe; RUL, right upper lobe; LUL, left upper lobe; RLL, right lower lobe; RML, right middle lobe. (From White, GC. Basic Clinical Competencies for Respiratory Care: An Integrated Approach. Albany, NY, Delmar Publishers, 1988. Reproduced by permission.)

positions as secretions mobilize. The number of PD positions tolerated per treatment session will vary with each patient. If the patient can tolerate only two or three positions in a session, it is recommended that the clinician vary the PD positions in subsequent sessions in order to drain all affected lung segments. PD positioning may also be coordinated with other procedures such as bathing, turning schedules for skin protection, or changing the bed linen. Signs of treatment intolerance include increased shortness of breath, anxiety, nausea, dizziness, hypertension, and bronchospasm.

Percussion

Chest percussion aimed at loosening retained secretions can be performed manually or with a mechanical device. Manual percussion consists of a rhythmical clapping with cupped hands over the affected lung segment[10] (Fig. 17–2). Air is trapped between each cupped hand and the patient's chest with each clap. A hollow thumping sound should be produced. Slapping sounds indicate poor technique and may cause discomfort for the patient. For caregivers unable to cup their hands, soft plastic percussor cups are available to be held in the hands and tapped over the patient's chest. Caregivers may also reduce their own fatigue by using a mechanical percussor, as mechanical percussion has been found to be similar in effectiveness to manual percussion.[11] Electrically or pneumatically powered percussion devices (Fig. 17–3) can enable patients to treat themselves independently as

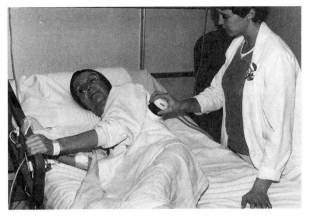

Figure 17–3. Example of mechanical percussor in use.

their medical condition improves. Patients continue to need assistance with treating the posterior lung fields, however.

According to Downs, during manual percussion the hand is cupped with the fingers and thumb adducted.[12] The hands are clapped over the thorax while the wrists and elbows remain relaxed.[12] Percussion is performed during inspiration and expiration. The hands essentially "fall" on the chest in an even, steady rhythm between 100 and 480 times per minute. The amount of force need not be excessive and should be adjusted to promote patient comfort. Bony prominences such as the spinous processes of the vertebrae and the clavicles as well as surgical incisions and medical appliances should be avoided while performing percussion. Precautions and relative contraindications for percussion and vibration are listed in Table 17–3.

Vibration

Vibration is an airway clearance technique that can be performed manually or with a mechanical device. As with percussion, vibration is utilized in postural drainage positions to clear secretions from the affected lung segments. In performing vibration, the palmar aspect of the clinician's hands are in full contact with the patient's chest wall, or one hand may be partially or fully overlapping the other (Fig. 17–4). At the end of a deep inspiration, the clinician exerts pressure on the patient's chest wall and gently oscillates it through the end of expiration. Manual vibration frequency has been reported to be 12 to 20 Hz.[13] This is

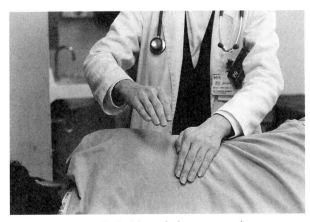

Figure 17–2. Manual chest percussion.

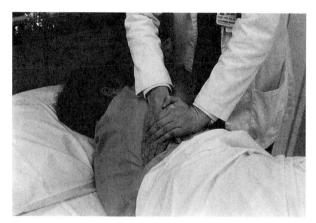

Figure 17-4. Hand placement for chest vibration.

repeated until secretions are mobilized. Vibration may be a useful alternative to percussion in acutely ill patients with chest wall discomfort or pain. The clinician may assess depth and pattern of breathing during manual vibration. The pressure on the thorax exerted during vibration on expiration often causes a volume of air to be expired that is greater than what is expired during tidal breathing. This may encourage a deeper than tidal inspiration to follow and support a more effective cough.

Cough Techniques and Assists

In the acute care setting, patients generally exhibit two types of cough: voluntary and reflex. An **effective cough** consists of four stages. The first stage entails an inspiration greater than tidal volume. Adequate inspiratory volumes for an effective cough are noted to be at least 60% of the patient's predicted vital capacity.[9] The second stage is the closure of the glottis. In the third stage the abdominal and intercostal muscles contract, producing positive intrathoracic pressure. The fourth stage consists of the sudden opening of the glottis and the forceful expulsion of the inspired air. This forceful airstream is designed to carry any materi-

als in its path up and out through the trachea to the mouth for expectoration.

Successful treatment of the acutely ill patient with excessive bronchial secretions includes removal, as well as mobilization, of the secretions. Assessment of cough effectiveness by the physical therapist is vital in determining the amount and type of intervention the patient will need for adequate removal of secretions. According to Massery, an effective cough should maximize the function of each of the preceding four stages.[14] Therefore, the patient should exhibit a deep inspiration combined with trunk extension, a momentary hold, and then a series of sharp expirations while the trunk moves into flexion. Any absence or deficiency in this sequence of events is likely to result in an ineffective cough. This condition can lead to retained secretions and, if left untreated, can progress to atelectasis, hypoxemia, and potentially respiratory failure. For acutely ill patients with reduced cough effectiveness and the ability to follow instructions, the first line of intervention is positioning and teaching proper coughing technique. Massery[14] recommends the following:

- Position the patient to allow for trunk extension and flexion
- Maximize the inspiratory phase via verbal cues, positioning, and active arm movements
- Improve the inspiratory hold by giving verbal cues and by positioning
- Maximize intrathoracic and intraabdominal pressures with muscle contractions or trunk movement
- Orient the patient to respective timing and trunk movements for expulsion

Surgical patients will need to be instructed in how to **splint** their incision by applying pressure over it with a pillow or blanket roll during the expiratory phase of the cough. If pain is inhibiting the patient's ability to perform proper coughing techniques, pain medication should be encouraged and timed with treatment.

In addition to proper technique for an individual cough, therapists can employ combinations of coughing, huffing, and breathing exercises to afford the most desirable result, given the patient's condition and ability to participate. Huffing is a forced expiratory technique without glottal closure. An example of breathing exercises used for airway clearance is the active cycle of breathing.

Clinical Note: Use of Vibration

In acutely ill patients with limited ability to follow instruction (i.e., "take a deep breath"), vibration may help facilitate deep breathing.

Active Cycle of Breathing

The **active cycle of breathing (ACB)** consists of a series of maneuvers performed by the patient to emphasize independence in secretion clearance and thoracic expansion. Pryor[15] showed that this **forced expiratory technique** is as effective as airway clearance techniques performed by a therapist or caregiver. The cycle is as follows:

1. Breathing control: The patient performs diaphragmatic breathing at normal tidal volume for 5 to 10 seconds.
2. Thoracic expansion exercises: In a postural drainage position the patient performs deep inhalation with relaxed exhalation at vital capacity range. This inhalation can be coupled with or without percussion during exhalation.
3. Breathing control for 5 to 10 seconds.
4. Thoracic expansion exercises repeated three to four times.
5. Breathing control for 5 to 10 seconds.
6. Forced expiratory technique: The patient performs one to two huffs at mid to low lung volumes. The patient is to concentrate on abdominal contraction to help force the air out. The glottis should remain open during the huffing.
7. Breathing control for 5 to 10 seconds.

Precaution for this technique includes splinting for postoperative incisions. **Hyperactive airways** may become irritated with the deep breathing and huffing. Administration of inhaled bronchodilators prior to ACB may be helpful.

Manual Hyperinflation and Suctioning

Airway suctioning is performed routinely for intubated patients to facilitate the removal of secretions and to stimulate the cough reflex. Airway suctioning is indicated for patients with artificial airways who have excess pulmonary secretions and the inability to clear the secretions from the airway. If physical therapists reserve airway suctioning for those secretions that the patient is unable to clear from the airway independently, rehabilitation of cough effectiveness can be initiated prior to extubation. Patients with **artificial airways** can be instructed in huffing and cough assist techniques

to enable them to progress to an effective cough, with the exception of glottal closure. Endotracheal and tracheal tubes prevent glottal closure from entering into the intubated patient's attempts to clear secretions. Deep inspiration may be difficult for the intubated patient, in which case lung inflation by means of a manual resuscitator bag may be used.

The frequency of suctioning is determined by the amount of secretions produced in the airway. It is important to remember that the suction catheter can reach only to the level of the mainstem bronchi. Therefore, when lung secretions are retained in the small airways, postural drainage with percussion and/or vibration should be utilized to mobilize the secretions centrally, prior to suctioning. The fundamental steps of the suctioning procedure are as follows:

1. Administer supplemental oxygen to the patient via **manual resuscitator bag** or mechanical ventilator to increase arterial oxygenation. (Fig. 17–5).
2. Monitor oxygen saturation with a pulse oximeter. Document drops in oxygen saturation below 90% and continue bagging with 100% O_2 until saturation is above 90% before continuing.
3. Adjust the pressure on the suction apparatus to 100 to 150 mm Hg, as needed.
4. Connect the vent end of the catheter to the suction tubing.
5. Don sterile gloves. Remove the catheter packaging without causing contamination; maintain

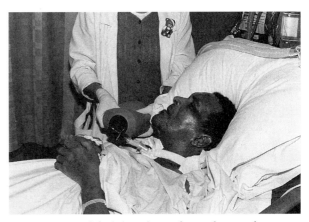

Figure 17–5. Administration of supplemental oxygen via manual resuscitator bag.

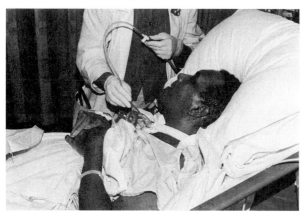

Figure 17–6. Insertion of sterile catheter into tracheal tube.

sterility of any part of the catheter that will touch the patient's trachea.

6. Disconnect the patient from the ventilator or oxygen source.
7. Give five to ten breaths via manual resuscitator bag.
8. Quickly and gently insert the catheter into the tracheal tube without applying suction (Fig. 17–6). The diameter of the catheter should be no larger than one half of the diameter of the airway.
9. Stop advancing the catheter once gentle resistance is met at the level of the carina or one of the mainstem bronchi. Apply suction by placing a finger over the catheter vent.
10. Then, while applying suction, withdraw the catheter slowly, rotating the catheter to optimize the exposure of the side holes to the secretions.

Clinical Note: Indications for Suctioning

For patients who are able to exhale forcefully, the least invasive method of assisted airway clearance is preferable, with suctioning to be reserved as a last resort. To stimulate a cough, first attempt positioning, then active coughing or huffing. If this is not effective, attempt inspiratory facilitation with chest wall stretching or manual bagging. Lavage, or instillation of sterile saline solution to the airway, can be used in an attempt to stimulate a reflexive cough. If none of these less invasive techniques is effective, then suctioning is indicated to clear the airway of secretions.

---

11. Reconnect the patient to the oxygen source and reinflate the patient's lungs with the manual resuscitator bag or the ventilator for five to ten breaths.
12. Repeat steps 6 through 9 until the airway is cleared of secretions, the patient is too fatigued to continue, or intolerance develops.

WEANING FROM MECHANICAL VENTILATION

Intubation and mechanical ventilation are required for most patients with acute respiratory failure. One of the main goals for these patients is to return to spontaneous breathing. The process of discontinuing mechanical ventilation is called weaning. Mechanical ventilation is a means of ensuring adequate gas exchange in a patient who is unable to do so without external support.[16] The benefits of weaning from mechanical ventilation in an expedient manner include minimizing iatrogenic complications, minimizing the duration of ICU stay, and preventing atrophy of the inspiratory muscles.[17]

Weaning Criteria

The process of weaning begins with determining whether or not the patient meets a set of criteria. The factors listed in this section have been shown to indicate that the patient is a candidate to begin the weaning process.[18] The primary consideration for beginning the weaning process is resolution or relative resolution of the initial event or disease that led to acute respiratory failure. The patient's status should be maximized in regard to nutrition, metabolic stability, fluid and electrolyte balance, **hemodynamic stability,** and cardiac function. The patient should be afebrile and must demonstrate an improving or stable chest x-ray, and respiratory secretions should be manageable. Preferably the patient is alert and cooperative, but at the minimum he should be initiating breaths spontaneously. The patient should be psychologically ready for the weaning process. Specific respiratory parameters include the following:

- Adequate gas exchange with FI_{O_2} less than 50% and Sa_{O_2} greater than 90% with a PEEP (positive end-expiratory pressure) of less than 5 cm H_2O.
- Negative inspiratory force of 20 to 30 cm H_2O.
- The ratio of respiratory rate to tidal volume (RR/VT) less than 105, with respiratory rate less than 35 breaths per minute. This ratio is an indicator of rapid shallow breathing and has been found to be the most accurate predictor of weaning failure.[19]
- Minute ventilation (VE = respiratory rate × tidal volume) less than 15 L/minute.

During the wean, the patient will be monitored for respiratory rate, depth and pattern, ABG (arterial blood gas) values, pulse oximetry, cardiac rate and rhythm, and mental status changes. The wean attempt will be terminated with any of the following signs of **respiratory distress:**[16–18]

- Respiratory rate over 35 breaths per minute
- Appearance of paradoxical breathing pattern, use of accessory muscles of respiration, or dyspnea
- Desaturation with Sa_{O_2} less than 90%, any decrease of Pa_{O_2}, or increase in Pa_{CO_2} of 5 mm Hg as monitored by ABG values, especially in the presence of acidosis with a pH less than 7.30
- Change in heart rate over 20 beats per minute, a change in blood pressure over 20 mm Hg, angina, cyanosis, or cardiac arrhythmias
- Change in level of consciousness

Methods of Weaning

Common methods of weaning currently utilized include intermittent mandatory ventilation (IMV), timed spontaneous breathing periods using a **T-piece,** and pressure support ventilation (PSV). Dries[20] indicated superior outcomes with pressure support and T-piece weans in comparison to IMV weans.[20] With IMV, weaning is gradually achieved as the number of ventilator preset breaths is gradually decreased and the patient is progressively more responsible for breathing spontaneously. With a T-piece wean, the patient breathes spontaneously on supplemental O_2 for progressively longer periods of time. PSV augments the patient's inspiratory effort with pressure assistance. Weaning using this method gradually reduces the amount of pressure provided to assist the patient during spontaneous breathing.

Treatment Considerations

Physical therapy interventions facilitate the weaning process by optimizing airway clearance and pulmonary function. Balancing the patient's energy expenditure during the weaning process with the added energy required for performing functional mobility activities or exercise is a challenge for the physical therapist. Communication between therapist, patient, and clinical care team is critical to the success of the weaning process for patients requiring prolonged mechanical ventilation (more than 5 days).

Developing a communication system with the patient is usually difficult, as most often mechanical ventilation interrupts the patient's verbal communication. In addition, many ICU patients have weakness and decreased coordination associated with critical illness which precludes the use of written communication. Further impairing communication is the presence of an oral endotracheal tube which interferes with lip reading. Simple means of communication such as eye blinks or head nods for answering to yes and no questions may be utilized, or available gestures and facial expressions can be a way for the patient to communicate needs. Whatever methods are deemed effective must be utilized consistently to further enhance reliability of communication, and they must be reinforced by all staff.

Once communication is established, tools for assessing dyspnea can be utilized. The simplest method for assessment is a yes or no question: Are you short of breath? This can be further qualified by using a numerical scale, similar to a pain scale, rating dyspnea from 0 to 10, with 0 indicating no shortness of breath, and 10 indicating the worst imaginable shortness of breath.[21] Dyspnea is a clinical manifestation of work of breathing. Although dyspnea during the weaning process may not necessarily be correlated with decreasing respiratory function, it can be directly related to anxiety experienced by the patient, which in itself may lead to weaning failure.[22, 23] The importance of emotional support and calm reassurance combined with positive feedback in facilitating the weaning process cannot be overemphasized.[16]

Airway clearance techniques discussed earlier in this chapter are also an important part of the weaning process. These techniques should be employed prior to the patient's specific weaning trials if presence of excessive secretions are impeding a successful wean. During weaning, these techniques remain a priority to assist in continued success with spontaneous breathing.

Biofeedback for increasing tidal volume and relaxation have been shown to reduce weaning time.[24] Breathing exercises, as discussed later in this chapter, including manual hand placement on the abdomen for recruitment of the diaphragm, can be utilized in conjunction with watching the tidal volume monitor on the ventilator. The biofeedback screen can be positioned to give the patient visual feedback from inspiratory efforts. Breathing exercises with encouragement of slow, deep breaths can be used to normalize the breathing pattern and to keep the respiratory rate within preset limits.

Inspiratory resistance training has been demonstrated to improve respiratory muscle strength and endurance in patients with respiratory failure and has facilitated increased weaning success. Adrich[25] demonstrated substantially lower mortality rates in the group weaned from mechanical ventilation.

Mechanical advantage of the diaphragm muscle can be optimized by attention to positioning.[26] Creating a more normal length-tension relationship may be useful and can be achieved with manual facilitation of the diaphragm. This positioning will decrease the work of breathing and facilitate an efficient breathing pattern. Optimal positioning for the patient will vary with different individuals, with options including dangling at the edge of the bed, sitting in a chair, reverse Trendelenburg's position and semi- to high Fowler's position (see following discussion under Positioning)[17].

Optimizing communication with other health care professionals—namely, the nurse, respiratory therapist, and physician—during the weaning process is imperative for coordination of care. Timing of the physical therapy treatment is essential for optimizing patient success and meeting functional goals. This may mean that physical therapy is not indicated just prior to, during, or after a wean attempt in order to allow rest and minimal environmental stimuli. In contrast, the therapist may be urgently contacted to assist with positioning just prior to weaning, relaxation or breathing exercises during a wean, or airway clearance techniques before, during, or after a wean to facilitate management of secretions.

POSITIONING

Therapeutic Positioning Techniques and Ventilatory Movement Strategies

Employing therapeutic positioning techniques and ventilatory movement strategies can assist with the progression from dependence to independence in mobility and breathing.[27] The techniques involve selecting positions to assist the patient with efficient, diaphragmatic breathing patterns. The techniques are indicated for patients who have weakness of the diaphragm, are unable to correctly use the diaphragm for efficient inspiration, or who have inhibition of the diaphragm muscle due to pain. The training can begin in the intensive care unit during range of motion (ROM) activities. To facilitate inspiratory effort, the therapist instructs the patient to breathe in during shoulder flexion, abduction, and external rotation along with an upward eye gaze. The opposite is true during exhalation; the therapist uses shoulder extension, adduction, and internal rotation with downward eye gaze. In addition, a posterior pelvic tilt position will encourage a diaphragmatic breathing pattern and optimize the length-tension relationship of the diaphragm. The patient should be encouraged to progress this technique to active shoulder ROM coupled with the breathing patterns previously described.

As the patient progresses from partial to full participation in therapy sessions, the therapist can use these positioning concepts during functional mobility activities (ventilatory movement strategies). While performing bed mobility, the patient is instructed to breathe out during rolling, and inhale as he or she extends the trunk to sit. This breathing pattern is used because trunk extension

---

Clinical Note: Range of Motion

Range of motion activities are tailored to the patient's level of participation. If a patient cannot participate, then passive range of motion is performed. As the patient's ability to participate improves, then active-assisted range of motion is used and progressed to active range of motion. The last step is to add resistance, either manually or with small weights.

coincides with inspiration as trunk flexion does with exhalation. The progression of these techniques can be applied to transfers, ambulation, and stair climbing. The patient is instructed to breathe out when leaning forward to stand, and then to inhale when extending into the standing position. Orthopedic (fractures or dislocations) and vascular (deep-vein thrombosis, presence of invasive lines and monitors) dysfunctions require precautionary measures. If the patient has a central intravenous line, a peripheral intravenous line directly over a joint surface, or an intra-aortic balloon pump, then extreme ROM positions are to be avoided in the joint beneath the catheters.

The position of the body greatly influences ventilation and respiration. As an acutely ill patient lies supine in a hospital bed, gravity will cause secretions to pool in the posterior aspects of the lungs. The supine position can reduce functional residual volume by up to 50%.[28, 29] Positioning the patient in sidelying can reduce the pressure on the sacrum and other posterior bony prominences as well as assist in lung expansion and secretion removal. The therapist can perform this activity with the help of another person, or independently if necessary, depending on the size and the participation level of the patient. The therapist needs to use correct body mechanics during positioning of the patient. The following are step-by-step instructions for turning an intensive care patient onto the left side.

- Vital signs are monitored continuously during patient positioning.
- While the patient is still in the supine position, move the patient to the right side of the bed. It is advisable to use a draw sheet to avoid shearing forces on the patient's skin.
- Arrange all tubes, lines, and cords so they will not be kinked or pulled during the rolling. Allow for adequate length.
- If the patient is requiring the use of a ventilator, make sure that the endotracheal tube is secured with tape or the tracheostomy in held in place with cloth ties. The ventilator tubing should be emptied of residual water to prevent accidental lavage.
- Place the patient's right foot over the left (unless orthopedic precautions dictate otherwise), and place a pillow between the knees.
- Gently roll the patient onto the left side using

the draw sheet. This will distribute the force more evenly against the patient's body. If two people are performing the positioning, then one person controls the head and upper trunk, while the other person controls the lower trunk and the legs.

- As the person at the head and trunk continues to hold the patient in the sidelying position with the draw sheet, the other person should place pillows and wedges behind the patient to keep the patient in this sidelying position. If the patient is alert and is strong enough, he or she can hold onto the bedrail while one person adds the external support.
- If the patient is not alert, gently pull the left scapula out once the support has been added. This will prevent the patient from lying on the shoulder and potentially developing skin breakdown.

After the patient is positioned, the therapist can perform airway clearance techniques if indicated. Prone positioning has been shown to assist in mobilizing secretions, and allowing greater volumes of ventilation and increased Pa_{O_2} for the patient with acute respiratory distress syndrome (ARDS).[30] This procedure requires the use of three people. The same first five steps for sidelying positioning are used, with the addition of placing a towel roll for forehead support and a pillow for chest support to where the patient's positioning end point will be. Then, the therapist continues with positioning using these steps.

- One person is positioned at the patient's head, another at the shoulders, and the third at the hip level. The person at the head should coordinate the timing for the roll.
- As the patient is rolled to the prone position, the person at the head is responsible for the integrity of the artificial airway and ventilator tubing, if applicable. If the patient can tolerate

Clinical Note: Final Equipment Check

Before the therapist leaves the room, he or she should check all lines, tubes, and wires to make sure all are functioning as they were prior to the treatment session. All alarms need to be reset if they were silenced during the treatment session.

10 to 20 seconds without mechanical ventilation, disconnection of the ventilator tubing can be made. If this is contraindicated (see Table 17–9), then the person at the patient's head makes sure that no torque is placed on the trachea.[31]

Trendelenburg positioning is optimal for facilitating secretion drainage from the lower lobes of the lungs (Fig. 17–7). It can also be used to increase the blood pressure of a hypotensive patient, but is contraindicated for patients with congestive heart failure or cardiomyopathy. Reverse Trendelenburg position helps reduce hypertension and facilitate the movement of the diaphragm by using gravity to decrease weight of the abdominal contents against it.

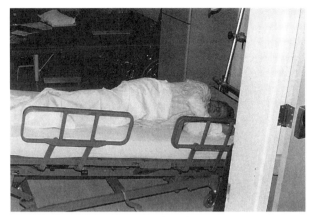

Figure 17–7. Trendelenburg position.

Positioning for Dyspnea Relief

Dyspnea is defined as the sensation of difficult or labored breathing.[32] The patient may experience dyspnea at rest or after a period of activity. The therapist needs to be aware of other potential causes of dyspnea in addition to pulmonary dysfunction. These causes include myocardial ischemia, heart failure, and left ventricular hypertrophy.[32] The therapist should monitor for other signs and symptoms of intolerance to exercise with the occurrence of dyspnea (see Table 17–6). When dyspnea is caused by pulmonary dysfunc-

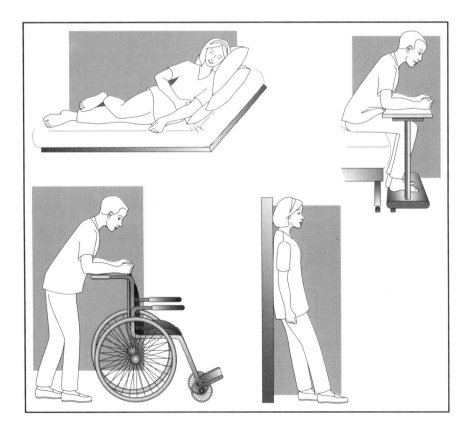

Figure 17–8. Positioning for relief of dyspnea.

tion, a patient may inherently find a position that allows for easier ventilation. With the arms supported, the accessory breathing muscles can act on the rib cage and the thorax, allowing more expansion for inspiration.

The accessory muscles are the sternocleidomastoid, the levators, the scalenes, and the pectoralis major muscles. When the patient leans forward on supported hands, the intra-abdominal pressure rises and thus pushes the diaphragm up in a lengthened position. In view of the improved length-tension relationship, the diaphragm has an increased strength of contraction (Fig. 17–8). The patient often experiences relief of the dyspnea in this position.

BREATHING EXERCISES

Inspiratory Muscle Training

Inspiratory muscle training is indicated for patients who exhibit signs and symptoms of decreased strength or endurance of the diaphragm and intercostal muscles. Signs and symptoms include, but are not limited to, decreased chest expansion, decreased breath sounds, shortness of breath, uncoordinated breathing patterns, bradypnea, and decreased tidal volumes.[33, 34] Patients with respiratory muscle weakness or fatigue may have such diagnoses as COPD, acute spinal cord injury, Guillain-Barré syndrome, amyotrophic lateral sclerosis, poliomyelitis, multiple sclerosis, muscular dystrophy, myasthenia gravis, or ankylosing spondylitis.[34]

The goal of inspiratory muscle training is to increase the ventilatory capacity and decrease dyspnea. An inspiratory muscle training program has two parts: strengthening and endurance training. Each part will have increased or decreased priority according to the needs and medical condition of the patient. Concepts of ventilatory muscle training are the same as those for other skeletal muscle training, incorporating the concepts of overload, specificity, and reversibility.[35] The overload principle applied to endurance muscle training requires low load imposed over longer periods of time. Specificity refers to training the muscles for the function they are to perform, for example, resistance applied to inspiratory versus expiratory mus-

cles. Training effects may be lost over time if training is discontinued.

The first step in any program is to teach the patient (if alert and oriented) the correct way to use the inspiratory muscles to ensure efficient inhalation. Including family members and support system members in the teaching can reinforce the program.

Weakness of a muscle is the inability to generate force against resistance. The length of the muscle affects the force output, as demonstrated in the length-tension curve. In the respiratory system, the strength of the diaphragm and other inspiratory muscles is measured as a function of standard pressure-volume curves.[36] Weakness of the diaphragm will decrease the negative inspiratory pressure generated by the patient, and thereby decrease the volume of air inhaled. Patients with COPD have hyperinflated lungs and a flattening of the diaphragm, which alters the length-tension relationship of this muscle. Fatigue of the inspiratory muscles, particularly of the diaphragm, will result in the failure to meet the demand for adequate alveolar ventilation. Hypoventilation will decrease the arterial partial pressure of oxygen (Pa_{O_2}) and increase the arterial partial pressure of carbon dioxide (Pa_{CO_2}), and can lead to acute respiratory failure.

The diaphragm is made up of all three types of muscle fibers, including **slow-twitch oxidative (SO), fast-twitch oxidative glycolytic (FOG),** and **fast-twitch glycolytic (FG).**[37–39] The adult diaphragm is approximately 55% slow-twitch fibers, compared with about 10% in the infant.[40] Fatigue is related to the SO fibers, whereas weakness is attributed to the FG fibers. When initiating physical therapy treatment, the therapist should realize that all fibers need to be addressed in the cardiopulmonary treatment program. While mechanically supported on a ventilator, the diaphragm can lose 5% of its strength per day.[41] When the patient begins the weaning process, the inspiratory muscles will gain endurance while performing inhalations without the assistance of the ventilator. Endurance training of the diaphragm will increase capillary density, myoglobin content, mitochondrial enzymes, and the concentration of glycogen. Overall, it will increase the proportion of fatigue-resistant slow-twitch fibers.[42, 43] The recommendations include two to three daily sessions of 30 to 60 minutes of deep breathing concentrating on using a diaphragmatic breathing pattern.[44]

An early-stage inspiratory muscle training technique is sniffing. **Sniffing** naturally enlists the diaphragm. With the patient in a comfortable position such as sidelying or reclined, the therapist may assist the patient in placing both hands on the abdominal area to provide proprioceptive feedback. Then, in a relaxed tone of voice, the therapist instructs the patient to sniff quickly through the nose three times with slow, relaxed exhalations. The therapist gives feedback throughout this technique on the quality of sniffing, assessing whether the patient is showing a diaphragmatic breathing pattern. If the patient is able to perform this effectively, the progression of this technique is to reduce the number of sniffs from three down to one at an increasingly slower pace. The goal of this technique is to increase the awareness of correct use of the diaphragm. The technique progression continues until the patient shows the diaphragmatic breathing pattern at a normal rate and depth for all levels of functioning. According to Massery and Frownfelter, there is an 80% success rate with patients affected by primary pulmonary pathologies or neurologic impairments.[45]

Strength training can be performed in a number of different ways, depending on the initial strength of the diaphragm. One method that can be utilized easily for the patient achieving tidal volumes of 500 mL or better is **resisted inhalation.** This can be performed manually by the therapist. The therapist has the patient assume a comfortable position as described earlier to promote diaphragmatic excursion. The therapist gently places the hands just below the rib cage on both sides of the patient's thorax. Before the patient initiates an inspiration, the therapist gives a small amount of resistance to the diaphragm by pushing gently up and in, and continues this pressure through the inspiratory phase. No resistance is given during exhalation. The therapist may also use weights for diaphragmatic strengthening. To evaluate if this is an appropriate method, the therapist first observes to determine if normal diaphragmatic excursion occurs at rest then, with the addition of weights. The patient should be able to breathe comfortably and without accessory muscles for 15 minutes; if the amount of weight is excessive, the pattern of inspiration will become uncoordinated.[46] Several authors suggest that strength training in this manner should include two or three sets of 10 repetitions once or twice a day.[47] However, with either the manual or the weights method, the quality of the contraction needs to be monitored. The patient should not be "pushing" with the abdominal muscles against the resistance, which enhances the exhalation phase of breathing rather than the muscles of inspiration. For a patient with "fair or reduced" diaphragmatic strength (tidal volume less than 500 mL), active breathing exercises are indicated without resistance. A patient with poor strength will find it difficult to exercise with the head of the bed elevated; a supine position will prevent the abdominal contents from pushing up on the diaphragm and limiting its excursion.

Another form of resistive training utilizes specific handheld training devices, such as the P-flex, DHD device, or the Peace Pipe. The resistance is increased by decreasing the radius of the device's airway. The patient inhales through the device at a level that does not cause adverse effects, such as dyspnea or a drop in oxygen saturation, for a 15- to 30-minute session twice per day.[48] When this level is comfortable for the patient, then the resistance is gradually increased.

Chest Wall Stretching

Resistance exercise techniques can also be used with the intercostal muscles. Unilateral costal expansion or bilateral costal exercises address one side or both sides, respectively, of the rib cage and

---

Clinical Note: The Controversy of Inspiratory Muscle Training

Much controversy has surfaced regarding the efficacy of IMT since its introduction into clinical practice. Evidence has been presented both supporting and dismissing IMT as a reliable treatment method. The major discrepancy may exist in the diagnosis for which this treatment is prescribed. A patient with insult to the lung tissue itself—for example, chronic obstructive pulmonary disease (COPD) or adult respiratory distress syndrome (ARDS)—may not tolerate IMT. IMT, which is a strengthening exercise, would increase the demand for oxygen delivery in the diseased lungs. However, a patient with a neuromuscular disease and intact lungs may be more likely to tolerate the increased oxygen demand and derive a benefit.

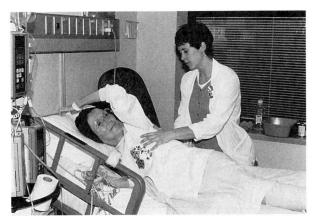

Figure 17–9. Position for applying chest wall stretching.

corresponding intercostal muscles. Unilateral costal expansion exercises may be more useful in the treatment session with a patient who has a large incision from surgery on one side of the thorax. Splinting is a common reaction to incisional and postoperative pain. However, this may lead to decreased expansion on the respective side and prevent full alveolar ventilation. This exercise is most efficiently performed in a sidelying position with the uninvolved side against the bed. The patient brings the arm on the involved side into an abducted position to the level of the head. The therapist gives a stretch before inspiration and continues giving resistance through the inspiratory phase (Fig. 17–9). Hyperexpansion of the lungs as seen in patients with emphysema, asthma, and cystic fibrosis can contribute to increased dyspnea during acute exacerbations. Chest wall stretching performed during exhalations can enhance exhalation and facilitate coughing by temporarily increasing chest wall excursion.

Any contraindications to lying on a particular side need to be acknowledged before using unilateral costal expansion. For example, a patient who has undergone a left partial or whole lung removal may have precautions against lying on the left side. Unilateral costal expansion with resistance is also useful for the patients in the ICU. These patients are often positioned in sidelying for respiratory and integumentary considerations.

Bilateral costal expansion is performed with the patient in a semireclined or sitting position. In this technique, the therapist places both hands on the lateral aspects of the rib cage and gently applies pressure against the ribs during inspiration. The

patient can also be taught to perform this exercise independently.

Deep breathing exercises are indicated for the patient with atelectasis, which is caused by hypoventilation and the collapse of alveoli in the lungs.[44] The use of an incentive spirometer is an effective way to practice diaphragmatic breathing and prevent or reverse atelectasis. Often, it is given to the patient preoperatively so he or she can practice deep breathing. Then after surgery, the patient may be able to perform this technique from memory as the effects of anesthesia start to diminish. The patient is instructed to perform deep breathing exercises with the incentive spirometer ten times every hour to replenish surfactant, which is lost in the presence of atelectasis.[33] The patient needs to be instructed to perform a slow, relaxed breath through the mouthpiece. It is often helpful to have the patient place a hand on the abdominal area to feel the diaphragm working in the correct way. If the patient is having a difficult time performing this technique, the therapist may place a hand over the patient's hand to facilitate the proper technique. Then the therapist should instruct the patient to perform the breathing slowly, with the abdomen rising out during inspiration. The goal is for the patient to be able to use the incentive spirometer independently without proprioceptive or verbal feedback. Alternatively, early mobilization has been shown to be as effective as deep breathing exercises after gallbladder and cardiac bypass surgery.[49–51]

Endurance training of the extremities is another technique that has been explored in an effort to increase ventilatory muscle endurance.

Clinical Note: Why Deep Breathe?

Surfactant production is reduced postoperatively, making patients at risk for serious pulmonary complications such as pneumonia and respiratory failure. Surfactant's role is to reduce surface tension and prevent alveolar collapse (atelectasis). Surfactant is produced by the type II pneumocytes in the alveoli of the lungs. By expanding the alveoli and stretching the type II pneumocytes with deep breaths, surfactant production is stimulated. Deep breathing is the most effective way to prevent alveolar collapse which, without intervention, can lead to more serious postoperative pulmonary complications.

Keens[52] studied pediatric patients with cystic fibrosis and found that upper extremity endurance training did increase the endurance of the ventilatory muscles. However, Belman and Kendregan examined the effects of upper and lower extremity training on ventilatory muscle endurance with adult patients with COPD and found no correlation.[53]

PATIENT EDUCATION

Patient and caregiver education is an integral part of physical therapy treatment in the acute care setting. Patient education has been shown to decrease length of stay,[54] decrease patient anxiety,[55] increase quality of life,[56] increase adherence with medical advice,[57] and increase the patient's participation as an active member of the health care team.[58]

Patient education has been defined as cognitive improvement that results in a positive change in health behavior.[59] This can begin by setting educational goals with the patient or caregivers, and documenting these goals in an objective, measurable, and functional manner. The therapist should discuss these goals with the patient and caregiver to assure they are realistic and applicable. A sample goal for an airway clearance program for a cystic fibrosis patient may be "Patient's caregiver independently completes percussion and postural drainage to assist in airway clearance." The patient's caregiver's independence with the specific techniques can then be observed by the therapist and documented, or verbally assessed if demonstration is not possible. An example of a functional educational goal for exercise with a cardiopulmonary patient might be "Patient independently monitors self with exercise by accurately taking heart rate and stating his functional heart rate limits for rest (70 to 90 beats per minute) and exercise (80 to 120 beats per minute)." If a patient is unable to accurately take his own heart rate, the goal may be, "Patient independently monitors self with exercise using the RPE scale and is able to maintain an exertion level of 13 to 15 during the peak activity period" (see Table 17–17). The accuracy of the patient's reported RPE level can be assessed by correlation with the heart rate taken by the therapist during the peak activity period.

When preparing to teach a patient or caregiver, the physical therapist must assess the learner to determine areas of knowledge to avoid unnecessary duplication, and areas where further education is needed. The learning style should be taken into account, whether it is visual, auditory, or kinesthetic, or a combination of styles. The therapist should inquire of the patient and caregiver expectations for learning and tailor the education to the learner's needs and abilities in several domains.[59] These domains include the following:

- Perceptual. The learner's perceptual needs must be considered in order to assure the ability to receive input and comprehend the material presented. This would include speaking of adequate volume and clarity for learners that are hard of hearing, or providing visual aids such as larger print or personal prescription glasses for visual information.
- Cognitive. If the patient is unable to cognitively comprehend the educational material because of memory deficits, then using repetition or providing written material as a back-up of information may help to compensate. If the patient is still unable to comprehend, then the material should be taught to a caregiver. In general, materials should be written at an eighth grade reading level.
- Motor. If the motor skills are deficient, practice and continued coaching with intrinsic and extrinsic feedback can contribute to motor learning.
- Affective. The affective domain includes a patient or caregiver's attitudes, belief system, and motivation levels. It is more difficult for a patient to learn when not motivated to do so. If teachings threaten cultural or religious beliefs, this conflict may be a detriment to learning.
- Environment. Environmental factors should also be taken into consideration, as it may be difficult for a patient to learn in a noisy environment or while in a position that is uncomfortable or painful.

It is advisable to invest time in planning the implementation of the educational program. Does the patient population or material to be covered lend itself to a group teaching and learning situation? Is it cost effective and practical to do a group teaching? Does the patient or caregiver learn best by reading, watching a demonstration, physically performing the task, or a combination of methods? Make sure to have written and teaching demonstration materials immediately available, if used.

Adherence to exercise programs can create a challenge for the physical therapist. Sluijs, Kok, and van der Zee[60] have suggested that the three main factors contributing to noncompliance are the barriers that patients perceive, lack of positive feedback, and perceived helplessness. Barriers often reported are lack of time, fatigue, pain, lack of motivation, or difficulty fitting exercise into a daily routine. These issues need to be discussed at length with the patient during development of the program so that adjustments can be made to adapt the program to each individual, eliminating as many barriers as possible.[61] This may require compromising, with prescribed frequency from three times per day to one time per day to minimize fatigue and time commitment required. The patient should not feel pain during exercise; if pain is experienced, modification of the program is necessary to eliminate this barrier to adherence. A family member may be recruited as a coach or a partner to help keep the patient motivated to complete the exercise program, or a more structured program such as cardiac or pulmonary rehabilitation programs (see Chapters 18 and 19) can be utilized to promote adherence.

Finally, the therapist should evaluate the effectiveness of the education program.[59] This may be done formally by written or verbal testing, or informally by discussion or observation. If post discharge teaching is indicated, the physical therapist can refer the patient to other health care professionals, to community organizations, or other resources.

Special attention can be focused on preoperative teaching for prevention of pulmonary complications after major surgeries of the thoracic or abdominal cavity.[62-65] The benefits of teaching deep breathing and coughing exercises preoperatively include an increased level of alertness compared with postoperative status, and absence of pain. It is an opportune time to gather baseline data on functional level, discharge options, and social support. However, preoperatively, anxiety levels may be high, which could be a barrier to learning. An example preoperative session is provided here.

EXERCISE

In the acute care setting, patients often have limitations in strength and endurance that prevent optimal functional mobility and efficient breathing patterns. The goal of endurance training in acute care is to maximize the independence and efficiency by which the patient performs ADLs and functional mobility. The indications for mobilization and exercise are listed in Table 17–4. As a patient begins the functional mobility progression, the therapist must remember that the smallest amount of mobilization can cause an abnormal exercise response in some patients, thereby stressing the cardiopulmonary system. Using such parameters as heart rate (HR), systolic and diastolic blood pressure (SBP, DBP), oxygen saturation (Sa_{O_2}), respiratory rate (RR), and electrocardiograms (ECG) gives the therapist important information on how the patient is tolerating the activity. Normal ranges for these physiologic parameters are listed in Table 17–5.

Components of Exercise: Intensity, Duration, Frequency, and Modes

The acute care patient's response to activity or exercise is dependent upon the body's ability to meet the oxygen transport demand. Monitoring cardiopulmonary parameters before, during, and after activity allows the therapist to provide the

---

Clinical Note: Rehabilitation Strategies

Specific strategies may be discussed to help the patient realistically fit the exercise routine into a personal schedule. For example, range-of-motion exercises to regain full mobility can be incorporated into function. To ensure functional shoulder range of motion postoperatively, the patient can be encouraged to emphasize a stretch each time during the day when reaching, such as into a high cabinet. A stretch can also be incorporated when brushing his hair, while also utilizing the mirror for visual feedback. For another example, a postural drainage program can be done while reading, studying, or watching a favorite television program.

Clinical Note: Sample Preoperative Session

"Hello, Mrs. Hunt, I am Erica, from Physical Therapy. I am here to talk with you about your upcoming surgery. First of all, what do you prefer that I call you? Have you ever had physical therapy before?" Here offer a general overview of physical therapy and the purpose of this education session. "I am here to teach you a little bit about what to expect after your surgery and to teach you your responsibilities and expectations of you after the surgery to help prevent postoperative complications. Your main responsibility after the surgery is to do a lot of deep breathing and coughing to keep your lungs healthy. The deep breathing makes sure air is getting to all parts of your lung to prevent collapse and to make it easier to clear secretions. General anesthesia has a depressant effect on your body and makes your respirations slower and more shallow. As soon as you can, begin taking deep breaths." Specific techniques for breathing can be discussed, including diaphragmatic breathing, lateral costal expansion, unilateral expansion, and use of an inspirometer (see Fig. 17–10). Mention to the patient that a written handout that explains these techniques in detail will be provided. "Coughing to clear your lungs is another very important responsibility to prevent the opportunity for pneumonia to develop. The anesthesia has a dehydrating effect, making the mucus thicker and harder to clear. You will also have an abdominal incision, which may make it uncomfortable to cough. Utilize available pain medication and support your incision site with a pillow." Effective technique for coughing can be demonstrated, followed by having the patient demonstrate the technique (see Fig. 17–11). This is an excellent opportunity to assess cough strength. "In addition to deep breathing and coughing, it is also important to learn a few simple exercises for your legs to help maintain muscle tone and circulation." Ankle pumps, quadriceps sets, and gluteal sets can then be taught. "The first day after your surgery we will work together to regain your full range of motion, check your posture, develop a walking program that you can continue at home for fitness, and return to activities of daily living."

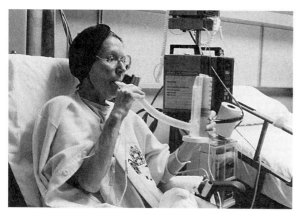

Figure 17–10. Patient using an inspirometer.

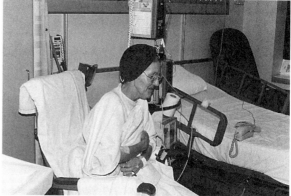

Figure 17–11. Patient supporting incision site with a pillow to maximize comfort.

safest and most effective treatment intervention. In addition to these parameters, signs and symptoms of exercise intolerance that occur during physical therapy treatment indicate that the intervention needs to be stopped or modified. Signs and symptoms of exercise intolerance are listed in Table 17–6. The therapist also needs to be aware of the patient's current medications and their effect on exercise response. A beta adrenergic blocker medication, for example, suppresses the expected heart rate increase with exercise.

Heart rate is most commonly measured at the radial artery in the wrist. However, this may be hard to detect in patients with cardiopulmonary disease, so the carotid or brachial artery can be used, or the therapist can use a stethoscope over the heart. The heart rate should be measured for 30 seconds to 1 minute. Level I cardiac rehabilitation exercise heart rate guidelines are 12 to 24 bpm above resting heart rate, unless the patient is taking beta adrenergic blocking medications.[67] With these medications, heart rates do not in-

Table 17–4

Acute Conditions That Are Indications for Mobilization and Exercise

Alveolar hypoventilation
Pulmonary consolidation
Pulmonary infiltrates
Inflammation of bronchioles and alveoli
Pleural effusions
Acute lung injury and pulmonary edema
Systemic effects of immobilization (see Table
17–1)

From Dean E. Mobilization and exercise. In: Frown-felter D, Dean E. Principles and Practice of Cardiopulmonary Physical Therapy, 3rd ed. St. Louis, Mosby–Year Book, 1996.

Table 17–6

Abnormal Responses to Exercise

Heart rate increases more than 20–30 bpm above
resting heart rate
Heart rate decreases below resting heart rate
Systolic blood pressure increases more than 20–
30 mm Hg above resting level
Systolic blood pressure decreases more than
10 mm Hg below resting level
Oxygen saturation drops below prescribed level
Patient becomes short of breath or respiratory
rate increases to a level not tolerated by the
patient
ECG changes

crease as expected during exercise. Monitoring the rate of perceived exertion (Table 17–6) would be an acceptable alternative in this case.

Blood pressure is measured at the brachial artery with a sphygmomanometer, with the cuff placed $2\frac{1}{2}$ inches above the antecubital space. The bladder of the cuff is placed over the brachial artery and should cover approximately 80% of the patient's upper arm. If the cuff is too narrow, then the blood pressure will read high, and if the cuff is too wide, the blood pressure will read low. The cuff should be at the level of the heart, and the patient's arm should be relaxed.

Blood pressure is expected to rise in direct proportion to the level of exertion performed. A hypertensive response to low level exercise (over 160/90 mm Hg) in the patient who is at least 3 days post-myocardial infarction may be indicative of cardiac ischemia.[68] There should be an increase of 7 to 10 mm Hg for each metabolic equivalent of

Table 17–5

Normal Adult Ranges for Cardiopulmonary Values at Rest

VALUE	NORMAL RANGE
Heart rate	50–100 beats per minute
Systolic blood pressure	85–140 mm Hg
Diastolic blood pressure	40–90 mm Hg
Respiratory rate	12–20 breaths per minute
Oxygen saturation	>95% on $F_{I_{O_2}}$

energy expenditure (MET). Level I cardiac rehabilitation remains in the 1 to 3.5 MET range.[67] The failure of the SBP to rise is a sign of a severe pathologic condition, such as aortic stenosis or poor left ventricular function.[69] Patients with recent coronary artery bypass surgery may also show an abnormal BP response to activity.[68]

Respiratory rate should be measured at rest and during activity. It is best if the patient is not aware of the therapist taking this vital sign. Otherwise, the therapist may not obtain a true reading; the patient may subconsciously or consciously alter the breathing pattern and rate. The respiratory rate should rise proportionally to the work load.

Oxygen saturation (Sa_{O_2}) is measured with a pulse oximeter. The physician should determine a minimum acceptable saturation level that the therapist then uses to determine exercise or functional mobility training and provide titration guidelines, should the patient's Sa_{O_2} level decrease with activity. Typically, the saturation level is to remain between 90 and 94% for acute respiratory problems, with higher minimum levels (96 to 97%) set for acute cardiac conditions. If a patient has supplemental oxygen, the amount of oxygen given must be adequate to keep the saturation at the prescribed minimum level. The physical therapist has the responsibility to monitor this level during activity when oxygen consumption rises (see Fig. 17–12). If the Sa_{O_2} drops below the minimum threshold, the therapist increases the amount of oxygen to keep the saturation in the prescribed range. However, the therapist must also remember that increasing the oxygen may reduce hypoxic drive in

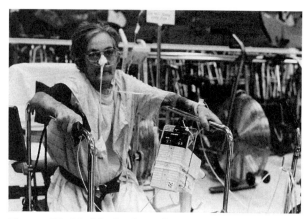

Figure 17–12. Monitoring of oxygen saturation during activity.

patients with chronic obstructive lung disease and the PCO_2 may increase. If the patient is having difficulty maintaining appropriate saturation levels, the therapist should have the patient rest or reduce the intensity or duration of the exercise first and communicate these findings with the patient's physician.

Intensity

Acute care patients' responses to exercise intensity can be measured in several ways. One subjective scale that is used to monitor intensity is the Borg rate of perceived exertion (RPE).[35] The scale is described in Table 17–7. The therapist can monitor exercise intensity by asking the patient to rate the intensity of the activity using the Borg scale. Warm-up and cool-down should remain in the 9 to 11 range, while peak activity should be within the 13 to 15 range. An RPE level of 12 to 13 equals approximately 60% of maximum heart rate and a

level of 16 equals about 85%.[71] A strong correlation exists between RPE, heart rate, and work rate among patients taking beta adrenergic blockers; this group of medications can reduce maximum heart rate by 20 to 30%, making traditional objective methods of interpretation of exercise response ineffective in this patient population.[72]

Levels of shortness of breath can be monitored using the **dyspnea index (DI)**.[73] The following is a description of implementation of the DI. A patient takes a deep breath and then counts to 15 slowly. The number of breaths the patient requires to count to 15 is the dyspnea index. During warm-up and cool-down, it should take the patient with normal lung function 1 to 2 breaths to reach 15, with that rate going up to 3 breaths for the peak activity.

Monitoring the acute care patient for subjective complaints of angina during treatment is important. Angina correlates with ECG changes, including ST-segment depression or elevation. Table 17–8 lists the stages of stable angina. Stable angina appears to occur at a consistent rate pressure product (RPP) during exercise.[68]

Duration

Duration is the amount of time that a patient can tolerate performing a certain activity. The patient's cardiovascular response will help determine the desired duration of activity during the inpatient exercise or mobility session. The therapist may progress a patient from 5 minutes on a lower extremity ergometer to 15 minutes at a time within 3 or 4 days, for example. This can be repeated 2 or 3 times per day as tolerated and should be per-

Table 17–7
Rate of Perceived Exertion

RPE	DESCRIPTION
7	Very, very light
9	Very light
13	Somewhat hard
15	Hard
17	Very hard
19	Very, very hard

From Borg G. Perceived exertion as an indicator of somatic stress. J Rehab Med 2:92–98, 1970.

Table 17–8
Stages of Stable Angina

STAGE	DESCRIPTION
1	Initial perception of discomfort
2	Increase in the intensity of level 1 or the radiation of pain to other areas (jaw, throat, shoulders, arms, or other body parts)
3	Relief is obtained only through cessation of activity
4	Infarction pain

From Atwood JA, Nielsen DH. Scope of cardiac rehabilitation. Phys Ther 65:1812–1819, 1985.

formed six or seven times per week.[67] Patient education is vital in this stage, so that the patient can begin to self-monitor HR, RR, RPE, and DI. Approximately 3 to 4 days after admission for an acute asthma attack, young patients were able to exercise for 5 minutes at 50% VO_2 without a significant change in peak expiratory flow, mean arterial oxygen tension, and mean alveolar-arterial oxygen difference.[74] For acute patients nearing the end of their hospital stay, a 6-minute walk test may be performed. Progress is measured by increases in the distance walked. The patient can also perform this test at home, or possibly at a mall or fitness center, to further assess progress and increase motivation in complying with a home exercise program.

Frequency

Usually, in the acute care patient population, multiple short intervals of exercise followed by rest periods are tolerated better than one long session of exercise on a given day. The therapist may accomplish this by performing airway clearance techniques first in the morning, and then using the afternoon treatment session for functional mobility or other exercises.

Modes of Exercise

Mode refers to the method of exercise or technique that is to be used for training. In the acute care setting most patients have limited exercise capacities because of their medical conditions. Therefore, in order to maximize independence, physical therapists often choose functional activities as the preferred mode of exercise for patients in acute care. Examples of activities that could be

> ### Clinical Note: Using a Walk Test
> In the acute care setting, a patient may not be able to complete a 6-minute walk test. A 3-minute walk test may be used instead, or any period of time can be used, as long as it is used consistently. The objective measure is the distance walked in a specified time, which can then be used to show progress in a patient's level of endurance.

> ### Clinical Note: Congestive Heart Failure
> A patient with decreased venous return, as in congestive heart failure, may need to start an exercise program in a semi-Fowler's position so that venous return is not compromised further by gravity and blood pooling in the lower extremities.

performed in the hospital are bed mobility, standing, transfers, ambulation, stairs, stationary bike, pedal exerciser or restorator, recumbent bike, upper body ergometer, and treadmill.

Functional Mobility Training

Functional mobility training may be initiated as soon as the patient is hemodynamically stable. Before the treatment of a patient in the ICU, however, the therapist should become familiar with the emergency procedures of each individual unit in addition to alarms from ventilators and monitoring devices. A check of the patient's medical status, including laboratory values, x-ray reports, vital signs, last dosage of medications, and past medical/surgical history, is warranted. It has been found that 75% of patients admitted for cerebrovascular disease also have coronary artery disease (CAD), but only 25 to 48% of these patients have a history or prior diagnosis of CAD.[75] Upon entering the patient's room, the therapist should look at positioning and lengths of lines, tubes, and catheters so they can be monitored and protected. Optimally, the therapist will coordinate activities with other disciplines involved with the care of the patient. This arrangement could mean that the therapist will set up a time with the nursing staff the day prior to the start of physical therapy, so that the patient is ready to start at the predetermined time. The goal of functional mobility progression is to have the patient perform as much of the activity as he or she can for as long as possible. The clinical decision making for activity progression is based on the patient's response.

Bed Mobility

Beginning an exercise program often starts at the patient's bedside with the first level of functional mobility, bed mobility. One of the first activities that should be emphasized is bridging. The act of bridging helps with placement and removal of the bedpan, linen changes, and positioning in bed. This activity can be a first step of independence for the patient.

Next, the therapist can have the patient actively assist with rolling. If the therapist is using airway clearance techniques, the therapist can instruct the patient in rolling to position for this technique. Mechanically ventilated, critically ill patients show a 40 to 50% increase in oxygen consumption during chest physical therapy combined with rolling.[76–78] The therapist should bring the bedrail to the most upright position so the patient can use it to assist with the activity.

The patient may then be progressed to sitting at the edge of the bed, or dangling. The therapist should be mindful of proper body mechanics during this stage of functional mobility. The therapist may want the assistance of other staff or may raise the bed up to a level that prevents a forward flexed posture. As the patient is sitting on the edge of the bed, the thorax can move in all planes and the patient has the opportunity to stretch the muscles of the thorax. The patient's tidal volume increases, as well as respiratory rate. Again, the patient's vital signs and response to the activities need continuous monitoring throughout each stage of functional mobility progression.

Transfers and Ambulation

Once the patient is able to sit at the edge of the bed unsupported for 10 minutes and can perform lower extremity ergometry in a sitting position for at least 8 minutes with acceptable responses in vital signs, the patient may progress to standing and ambulating. The use of the four-wheeled walker (Fig. 17–13) allows the patient to walk with support and the availability of a fold-down seat if it is needed. The patient does not need to be extubated to start ambulation training. Contraindications or precautions for advancing functional mobility are listed in Table 17–9.

The patient should be educated on how to use the walker, complete with verbal and visual instructions, as well as demonstration. After the decision has been made that an intubated patient is ready

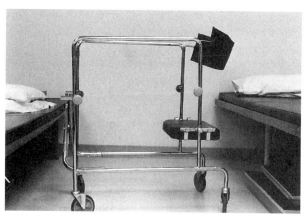

Figure 17–13. Four-wheeled walker for ambulation.

to use the walker, the therapist must arrange for sufficient amounts of assistance. One person needs to assist the patient physically during ambulation while another is responsible for bagging the patient with a self-inflating bag connected to supplemental oxygen. A third person is recommended for pushing intravenous poles and watching for adequate slack on IV lines. A gait belt is warranted for the patient's and the therapist's safety. The therapist should note resting vital signs, including oxygen saturation. Vital signs are monitored frequently, with cessation of activity if warranted by abnormal responses to heart rate, blood pressure, Sa_{O_2}, or fatigue by the patient. The progression of this activity is based on the patient's response.

Once the patient is extubated, the therapist may wish to continue with the wheeled walker, or

Table 17–9
Contraindications or Precautions for Advancing Functional Mobility

Untreated deep-vein thrombosis
Unstable vital signs
Patient not able to follow commands
High ventilatory support (for removing the patient from the ventilator for mobility)
  a. contraindication: PEEP or CPAP > 10 cm H_2O
  b. precautions: PEEP or CPAP > 5 cm H_2O
               PAP > 50 cm H_2O
               minute ventilation > 15 L/min
Other orthopedic, vascular, or neurologic injury that requires alternative bed activities

to progress the patient to a standard walker. The therapist continues to use other personnel according to the level of independence of the patient and the amount of additional IV poles that need to be advanced with the patient. If a patient depends on supplemental oxygen during rest, then oxygen saturation levels need continued monitoring before, during, and after ambulation, with oxygen titration to keep Sa_{O_2} within the recommended range.

As a patient progresses in ambulation, the therapist and the patient work toward goals of increasing ambulation distance and decreasing the levels of assistance. It may be the goal of the patient to ambulate independently without an assistive device or oxygen. The therapist needs to assess whether this is an attainable goal within the acute hospital setting and must determine the patient's course of action to attain these goals.

DISCHARGE PLANNING

With length of hospital stays decreasing dramatically, discharge planning has become a crucial part of treatment in the acute care setting.[79, 80] The role of the acute care physical therapist is shifting and expanding from providing treatment to acting as a consultant, offering recommendations on the patient's current status and rehabilitation potential, discharge destination, activity tolerance, and equipment needs. Anticipating the patient's discharge needs must often be included in the initial physical therapy visit. Because of the increased acuity level of patients being discharged from the acute care setting, an increasing involvement of family members is needed in determining the site for the next level of care. The therapist is often responsible for interpreting information from the patient's performance and the family support system as part of the discharge plan.

During the initial physical therapy evaluation, the patient's current level of function is evaluated and a prognosis is made regarding his or her potential abilities. Determination of the patient's rehabilitation potential has a large bearing on the discharge disposition. This may include preparing the patient for discharge home or for the next level of care, whether that level is acute rehabilitation, subacute rehabilitation, or long-term care. Figure 17–14 offers an example of a decision-making tree for determining discharge destination, taking into consideration accessibility of the home (including number of stairs, presence or absence of a railing, location of bedroom and bathroom, and wheelchair accessibility) and family or social support available. There must be precision in aligning the amount of realistic family or social support available with the amount of assistance the patient requires. This amount of assistance can vary from weekly help with shopping and laundry to 24-hour maximal assistance. Family members will need to be instructed in the level of assistance required by the patient for specific activities of daily living and the home physical therapy program, if needed.

In many acute care settings a discharge planner, often a nurse, has the role of arranging a variety of health support services needed after discharge. This role may include services over a broad spectrum, such as home physical or occupational therapy, home skilled nursing service, home health aides to provide basic care such as bathing, community support services (i.e., meal delivery), and emergency monitoring services for safety checks.

Physical therapists are also involved in securing durable medical equipment to meet a patient's needs. This may include recommending equipment that is ordered by another health care professional, issuing the equipment from department supplies, or contacting a vendor to supply and deliver needed equipment. Insurance coverage is often an integral part of decision making, as is discussion with the patient on what items will be most appropriate.

Because a patient's status may change on a daily basis, this discharge plan must be frequently reassessed and modified according to the patient's improvement or lack thereof. As a result of this ongoing assessment, a crucial responsibility of the therapist is to communicate these updated recommendations to other members of the health care team. It must be remembered at this point that the most important member of the health care team is the patient. The therapist's professional opinions must be discussed with the patient and caregivers, decisions reached, then shared with other members of the health care team.

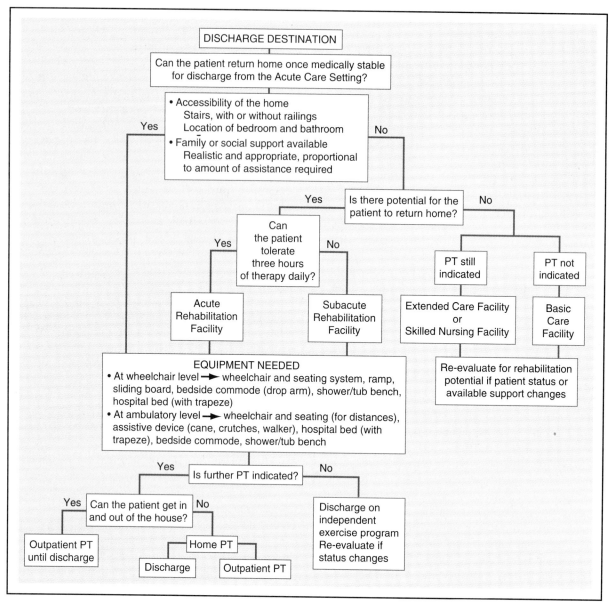

Figure 17-14. Decision tree for discharge planning.

PEDIATRIC CONSIDERATIONS

Whether a physical therapist is providing direct cardiopulmonary care to acutely ill pediatric (neonates, infants, and children) patients or incorporating cardiopulmonary techniques into developmental therapy, a knowledge of cardiopulmonary development and congenital pathology is essential.

Treatment in the pediatric population is directed at problems that arise from developmental abnormalities, prematurity, infection, immunologic deficiencies, trauma, and diseases associated with childhood. Cystic fibrosis, a genetic exocrine gland involvement affecting the pulmonary system, is discussed in Chapter 6. Provision of cardiopulmonary physical therapy in the pediatric population may require postgraduate or specialized training of the physical therapist.

The principles of treatment for pediatric patients with cardiopulmonary dysfunction are the same as for adults, with certain necessary modifications. Pediatric patients also require very close monitoring because of their decreased tolerance for hemodynamic changes and limitations in communicating distress. The purpose of this section is to briefly describe the treatment considerations that are indicated in pediatrics because of body size, physiologic differences, and level of psychological and communicative development. Moerchen and Crane[81] offer a more detailed description of pediatric cardiopulmonary care.

Cardiac dysfunction in pediatric patients is often related to congential heart anomalies, whereas in adults coronary artery disease is most often the source. Surgical intervention in both populations is common. Postoperative physical therapy aims to increase respiration, mobilize secretions, and progress functional mobility.[82] It is important to prevent the deconditioning effects of bedrest postoperatively in children as with adults and to try to mobilize the patient out of bed by the second postoperative day. For children who were able to walk preoperatively, ambulation is possible following extubation once arterial and groin lines have been removed.

Modification of airway clearance techniques for pediatric patients involves positioning the child or infant on the therapist's lap or on pillows and conforming the therapist's hand to the patient's chest. Small hand-held percussors and vibrators are also available. In caring for premature infants, careful evaluation of the risks and benefits of treatment is required due to the infant's limited tolerance to handling. The therapist can minimize stimulation to the infant by coordinating position changes for bronchial drainage with other patient care procedures. The bronchial drainage positions for infants are the same as for adults because fetal development of the bronchial tree is complete at the end of 16 weeks of gestation. The bronchial drainage positions may need to be approximated if the infant becomes hemodynamically unstable. The head-down positions should be avoided if intracranial bleeding is suspected. Infants and small children often need assistance in clearing secretions loosened by bronchial drainage, percussion, or vibration. If the patient is unable to cough effectively, the nasal and oaopharyngeal areas can be suctioned while using supplemental oxygen to prevent desaturation. Older children can be encouraged to huff or cough using toys or games that involve forceful breathing (i.e., pinwheels, blowing bubbles). When working with children in general, the therapist can reduce patient anxiety, generate interest, and build rapport by being creative and making treatment sessions as playful as possible.

A child's acute illness ultimately has an impact on the child's parents, siblings, and extended family. The physical therapist can be helpful in instructing family members about the illness as well as the pertinent physical therapy interventions. Parents and others may feel particularly supported when they are encouraged to learn treatment techniques, such as percussion and bronchial drainage, and to perform them as the patient's medical condition stabilizes. In the case of a child with asthma, for example, family members can become familiar with the signs of an impending asthma attack and help the child minimze its effects. They can do this by calming the child, providing medication (as prescribed), and helping with relaxation and breathing exercises. They can also learn to monitor the child for changes in respiratory rate, intercostal retractions, and cyanosis.[83] Family members can also be helpful to the physical therapist who is trying to understand the child's nonverbal or preverbal communications. Certain facial expressions or gestures may have specific meanings for the child. By sharing this information with the therapist, the family can facilitate better communication between the therapist and the patient.

CASE STUDIES

Case Study 1

Mr. X was admitted to the hospital with a diagnosis of adult respiratory distress syndrome (ARDS) secondary to pneumonia. The quick decline of his oxygen transport system required intubation and mechanical ventilation. He eventually required maximal ventilatory support, and developed bilateral pneumothoraces from high levels of PEEP. The physician's course of action was to administer high levels of steroids to diminish the inflammatory process of the lungs and **Pavulon** to reduce total oxygen demands. The combination of the neuromuscular blocking agent, Pavulon, and the steroid, methylprednisolone, caused profound weakness in this patient. Physical therapy treatment at this point included airway clearance techniques to treat the underlying pneumonia. These techniques included percussion and postural drainage, vibration, suctioning, and chest wall stretching. Alternative positions were indicated because of the patient's intolerance to Trendelenburg positioning; the patient's oxygen saturation dropped to 85% with this position. Once the patient was weaned off the Pavulon, more interactive techniques were incorporated into the treatment sessions. These techniques included diaphragmatic breathing and costal expansion breathing exercises. His muscle grades were 1/5 throughout with the exception of finger flexion, which was given a grade of 2/5. Active and active-assisted strengthening exercises were performed with all four extremities.

The patient was extubated 5 days after the initiation of physical therapy, and 17 days after the start of the steroid trial. His long-term physical therapy goals from a pulmonary standpoint were to be independent in pulmonary hygiene and to maintain oxygen saturations of 90% or greater without supplemental oxygen. Once the patient was extubated, he was able to tolerate longer periods of sitting on the edge of the bed, which assisted with costal expansion and ventilatory volumes.

After his transfer from the intensive care unit (ICU) to the general care floor, the patient performed his physical therapy treatments in the gym. His oxygen saturation dropped slightly with the initiation of isotonic exercises, and he required the use of supplemental oxygen during tilt table treatments to keep his saturation at the level prescribed by the physician. The patient was discharged to an outside rehabilitation center, and after 4 weeks at that facility, was discharged to home. The patient did not require supplemental oxygen, and used a walker to assist with ambulation.

This case study describes physical therapy intervention for a patient with pulmonary dysfunction and severe weakness. Multiple physical therapy techniques were used to advance the patient to an independent pulmonary hygiene status and optimal functional mobility.

Case Study 2

Mrs. V is a 42-year-old woman with a history of rheumatic heart disease who developed mitral stenosis and chronic atrial fibrillation. While sitting down and having dinner with her husband and two children, she started slurring her words. The family noticed that her mouth became "crooked." They called EMS and she was transported to the hospital. She was admitted for a right-sided stroke. She was placed on heparin and Coumadin therapy secondary to findings indicating a clot in the left atrium on echocardiogram. Neurologic findings were as follows: left hemiparesis, flaccid left upper extremity, left foot drop, proximal left lower extremity strength 3/5, right upper and lower extremity strength 4/5. A left ankle-foot orthosis had been applied. On hospital day 7, in the physical therapy clinic, her heart rate (HR) was 110, irregularly irregular, her blood pressure (BP) was 122/64, her respiratory rate (RR) was 22 on room air, and oxygen saturation (Sa_{O_2}) was 93% at rest. Her neurologic findings were the same. After she walked with a quad cane and moderate assist of one person for 50 feet, her response was HR 120, irregularly irregular, BP 132/70, RR 28, Sa_{O_2} 92% on room air. The physical therapist then assisted (moderate) the patient in walking up and down four steps with the quad cane and a railing. The patient's response was HR 182, irregularly irregular, BP 110/58, RR 38, Sa_{O_2} 86% on room air, and she complained of shortness of breath and lightheadedness. The physical therapist stopped the treatment, instructed the patient to sit down in a chair and perform deep breathing exercises. After 3 minutes, the patient's vital signs were HR 118, BP 120/60, RR 24, Sa_{O_2} 91% on room air and her shortness of breath and lightheadedness had resolved. The therapist notified the patient's physician of the patient's response to the activity. The physician ordered oxygen per nasal cannula for the patient, to be titrated to keep her oxygen saturation greater than or equal to 90%.

On subsequent visits, the physical therapist continued to monitor the patient's responses to treatment and used oxygen to maintain the patient's Sa_{O_2} in the prescribed range. On hospital day 12, the patient was able to walk 125 feet with a quad cane and moderate assist of one person and walk up and down four steps with a quad cane, a railing, and minimal assistance of one person. She was able to maintain her oxygen saturations above 90% on room air with these activities. After the physical therapist had consulted with the other members of the acute care team, the patient was discharged to her home with family assistance and outpatient physical therapy visits three times per week.

This case study illustrates the importance of monitoring vital signs, symptoms, and oxygen saturation values during progressive functional mobility treatment of a patient with recent stroke and positive cardiac history. By collecting information relative to the patient's cardiopulmonary response to the treatment, the physical therapist was able to safely and effectively progress the patient through higher levels of activity.

Summary

In acute care settings, physical therapy treatment for patients at any age, with primary or secondary cardiopulmonary dysfunction, is aimed at optimizing the patient's oxygen transport system. Treatment interventions designed to meet this goal include airway clearance techniques, therapeutic positioning, breathing and chest wall exercises, patient education, and functional mobility exercises. Treatment in the pediatric population requires modifications based on body size, physiologic differences, and level of psychological and communicative development. Physical therapists working in acute care have a unique challenge in that they must recognize dynamic pathophysiologic changes in their patients and adapt treatment progressions accordingly. This chapter describes the treatment interventions, identifies their indications and precautions, and emphasizes the importance of monitoring acutely ill patients during treatment. Issues pertinent to prioritizing patient care and planning hospital discharge were also discussed.

- Cardiopulmonary physical therapy treatment in the acute care setting is aimed at correcting or improving the function of the patient's oxygen transport system.
- Physical therapy treatment interventions for acutely ill patients with cardiopulmonary dysfunction include airway clearance techniques, therapeutic positioning, breathing and chest wall exercises, patient education, and functional mobility exercise.
- Patients with multiple medical problems and acute respiratory failure may require prolonged periods of mechanical ventilation. Physical therapy interventions for these patients need to be coordinated with the weaning process in order to balance the patient's energy expenditure for breathing with that which would be required for participation in therapy activities.
- Therapeutic positioning techniques are indicated for patients with diaphragmatic weakness or inefficiency. These techniques facilitate inspiratory effort and assist in ventilation and perfusion matching.
- Monitoring patient tolerance to physical therapy treatment using parameters such as HR, BP, Sa_{O_2}, RR, and ECG is crucial to safe and effective activity progression for acutely ill patients.
- The primary role of the acute care physical therapist is shifting from providing treatment to acting as a consultant, offering recommendations based on the patient's functional status and rehabilitation potential, and assisting with determining discharge destination and equipment needs.
- Treatment in the pediatric population with acute cardiopulmonary dysfunction is directed at problems that arise from developmental abnormalities, prematurity, infection, immunologic deficiencies, trauma, and diseases associated with childhood.

References

1. Dean E. Oxygen transport: The basis for cardiopulmonary physical therapy. In: Frownfelter D, Dean E. Principles and Practice of Cardiopulmonary Physical Therapy. 3rd ed. St. Louis, Mosby–Year Book, 1996, p 3.
2. Welch E, Anastasas M. Critical care, critical choices. PT Magazine 4(3):75–77, 1996.
3. Ciesla N. Postural drainage, positioning, and breathing exercises. In: Mackenzie CF. Chest Physiotherapy in the Intensive Care Unit. 2nd ed. Baltimore, Williams & Wilkins, 1989, p 102.
4. Ciesla ND, Klemic N, Imle PC. Chest physical therapy to the patient with multiple trauma: Two case studies. Phys Ther 61:202–205, 1981.
5. Hammon WE, Martin RJ. Chest physical therapy for acute atelectasis. Phys Ther 61:217–220, 1981.
6. Sutton PP, Pavia D, Bateman JRM, Clarke SW. Chest physiotherapy: A review. Eur J Respir Dis 63:188–201, 1982.
7. Watchie J. Cardiopulmonary Physical Therapy: A Clinical Manual. Philadelphia, WB Saunders, 1995, pp 212–214.
8. Downs AM. Clinical application of airway clearance techniques. In: Frownfelter D, Dean E. Principles and Practice of Cardiopulmonary Physical Therapy. 3rd ed. St. Louis, Mosby–Year Book, 1996, p 343.
9. Massery M, Frownfelter D. Facilitating airway clearance with coughing techniques. In: Frownfelter D, Dean E. Principles and Practice of Cardiopulmonary Physical Therapy. 3rd ed. St. Louis, Mosby–Year Book, 1996, p 369.
10. Imle PC. Physical therapy for patients with cardiac, thoracic, or abdominal conditions following surgery or trauma. In: Irwin T, Tecklin J. Cardiopulmonary Physical Therapy. 3rd ed. St. Louis, Mosby–Year Book, 1995, p 380.
11. Maxwell M, Redmond A: Comparative trial of manual and mechanical percussion technique with gravity assisted bronchial drainage in patients with cystic fibrosis. Arch Dis Childhood 54:542–544, 1979.
12. Downs AM. Clinical application of airway clearance techniques. In: Frownfelter D, Dean E. Principles and Practice of Cardiopulmunary Physical Therapy. 3rd ed. St. Louis, Mosby–Year Book, 1996 p 345.
13. Sutton PP, Lopez-Vidriero MT, Pavia D, et al. Assessment of percussion, vibratory-shaking, and breathing exercises in chest physiotherapy. Eur J Respir Dis 66:147–152, 1985.
14. Massery M, Frownfelter D. Facilitating airway clearance with coughing techniques. In: Frownfelter D, Dean E. Principles and Practice of Cardiopulmonary Physical Therapy. 3rd ed. St. Louis, Mosby–Year Book, 1996, p 369–371.
15. Pryor JA, Webber BA, Hodson ME, Batten JC. Evaluation of the forced expiration technique as an adjunct to postural drainage in treatment of cystic fibrosis. Br J Med 18:417–418, 1979.
16. Henneman EA. The art and science of weaning from mechanical ventilation. Focus Crit Care 18:490–501, 1991.
17. Calhoun CJ, Specht NL. Standardizing the weaning process. ACCN Clin Issues Crit Care Nurs 2:398–404, 1991.
18. Folk L, Kewman S. CCMU protocol for weaning from mechanical ventilation. Policy per Critical Care Medicine Unit, University of Michigan Health Systems, Ann Arbor, 1997.
19. Yang KL, Tobin MJ. A prospective study of indexes predicting the outcome of trials of weaning from mechanical ventilation. N Engl J Med 324:1446–1495, 1991.
20. Dries DJ. Weaning from mechanical ventilation. J Trauma 43:372–384, 1997.

21. Carrieri-Kohlman V. Dyspnea in the weaning patient: Assessment and intervention. AACN Clin Issues Crit Care Nurs 2: 462–473, 1991.
22. Gift AC, Plant SM, Jacox A. Psychologic and physiologic factors related to dyspnea in subjects with chronic obstructive pulmonary disease. Heart Lung 15:595–601, 1986.
23. Knebel A. Describing mood state and dyspnea in mechanically ventilated patients prior to weaning (abstract). Am Rev Respir Dis 141:A412, 1990.
24. Holliday JE, Hyers TM. The reduction of weaning time from mechanical ventilation using tidal volume and relaxation biofeedback. Am Rev Respir Dis 141:1214–1220, 1990.
25. Aldrich TK, Darpel JP, Uhrlass RM, et al. Weaning from mechanical ventilation: Adjunctive use of inspiratory muscle resistive training. Crit Care Med 17:143–147, 1989.
26. Shekleton ME. Respiratory muscle conditioning and the work of breathing: A critical balance in the weaning patient. AACN Clin Issues Crit Care Nurs 2:405–414, 1991.
27. Massery M, Frownfelter D. Facilitating ventilation pattern and breathing strategies. In: Frownfelter D, Dean E. Principles and Practice of Cardiopulmonary Physical Therapy. 3rd ed. St. Louis, Mosby–Year Book, 1996, pp 387–388.
28. Craig DB. Postoperative recovery of pulmonary function. Anesth Analg 60:46–52, 1981.
29. Ray JF, Yost L, Moallem S, et al. Immobility, hypoxemia, and pulmonary arteriovenous shunting. Arch Surg 109:537–541, 1974.
30. Langer M, Mascheroni D, Marcolin R, et al. The prone position in ARDS patients. Chest 94:103–107 1988.
31. Sciaky A. Mobilizing the intensive care unit patient: Pathophysiology and treatment. Phys Ther Pract 3:69–80, 1994.
32. Peel C. The cardiopulmonary system and movement dysfunction Phys Ther 76:448–455, 1996.
33. Shekleton M, Berry JK, Covey MK. Respiratory muscle weakness and training. In: Frownfelter D, Dean E. Principles and Practice of Cardiopulmonary Physical Therapy. 3rd ed. St. Louis, Mosby–Year Book, 1996, p 447.
34. Wolfson MR, Bhutani VK, Shaffer TH. Respiratory muscles. In: Irwin S, Tecklin JS. Cardiopulmonary Physical Therapy. St. Louis, CV Mosby, 1985, pp 386–389.
35. Faulkner JA. New perspectives in training for maximum performance. JAMA 205:741–746, 1968.
36. West JB. Respiratory Physiology. 4th ed. Baltimore, Williams & Wilkins, 1990, pp 87–113.
37. Peter JB, Bernard RJ, Edgerton VR, et al. Metabolic profiles of three fiber types of skeletal muscle in guinea pigs and rabbits. Biochemistry 11:2627–2634, 1972.
38. Gesell R, Atkinson AK, Brown RC. The gradation of the intensity of inspiratory contractions. Am J Physiol 131:659–673, 1941.
39. Iscoe S, Dankoff J, Migicovsky R, Polosa C. Recruitment and discharge frequency of phrenic motoneurons during inspiration. Resp Phys 26:113–128, 1975.
40. Keens TG, Bryan AC, Levison H, Ianuzzo CD. Developmental pattern of muscle fibers types in human ventilatory muscles. J Appl Physiol 44:909–913, 1978.
41. Dantzker DR. Respiratory muscle function. In: Bone RC, George RB, Hudson LD. Acute Respiratory Failure. New York, Churchill Livingstone, 1987, p 49.
42. Gollnick PD, Armstrong RB, Saltin B, et al. Effect of training on enzyme activity and fiber composition of human skeletal muscle. J Appl Physiol 34:107–111, 1973.
43. Holloszy JO, Booth FW. Biochemical adaptations to endurance exercise in muscle. Annu Rev Physiol 38:273–291, 1976.
44. Barach AL. Breathing exercises in pulmonary emphysema and allied chronic respiratory disease. Arch Phys Med Rehab 36:379–390, 1955.
45. Massery M, Frownfelter D. Facilitating ventilation patterns and breathing strategies. In: Frownfelter D, Dean E. Principles and Practice of Cardiopulmonary Physical Therapy. 3rd ed. St. Louis, Mosby–Year Book, 1996, p 393.
46. Adkins HV. Improvement of breathing ability in children with respiratory muscle paralysis. Phys Ther 48:577, 1968.
47. Holtackers TR. Physical rehabilitation of the ventilator-dependent patient. In: Irwin S, Tecklin JS. Cardiopulmonary Physical Therapy. 3rd ed. St. Louis, Mosby–Year Book, 1995, p 480.
48. Watchie J. Cardiopulmonary Physical Therapy: A Clinical Manual. Philadelphia, WB Saunders, 1995, p 206.
49. Jenkins S, Soutar SA, Loukota JM, et al. Physiotherapy after coronary artery surgery: Are breathing exercises necessary? Thorax 44:634–639, 1989.
50. Dull JI, Dull WL. Are maximal inspiratory breathing exercises or incentive spirometry better than early mobilization after cardiac surgery? Phys Ther 63:655–659, 1983.
51. Hallbook T, Lindblad B, Lindroth B, et al. Prophylaxis against pulmonary complications in patients undergoing gallbladder surgery: A comparison between early mobilization, physiotherapy with and without bronchodilation. Ann Chir Gynaecol 73:55–58, 1984.
52. Keens TG, Krastin IRB, Wannamaker EM, et al. Ventilatory muscle endurance training in normal subjects and patients with cysitic fibrosis. Am Rev Respir Dis 116:853–860, 1977.
53. Belman MJ, Kendregan BA. Physical training fails to improve ventilatory muscle endurance in patients with chronic obstructive pulmonary disease. Chest 81:440–443, 1982.
54. Devine E, Cook T. A meta-analysis of effects of psychoeducational interventions on length of post surgical hospital stay. Nurs Res 32:333–339, 1983.
55. O'Rourke A, Lewin B, Whitcross S, Pacey W. The effects of physical exercise training and cardiac education on levels of anxiety and depression in the rehabilitation of CABG patients. Int Disability Stud 12:104–106, 1990.
56. Manzetti JD, Goffman LA, Serreida SM, et al. Exercise, education, and quality of life in lung transplant candidates. J Heart Lung Transplant 13:297–305, 1994.
57. Mazzuca SA. Does patient education in chronic disease have therapeutic value? J Chron Dis 35(7):521–529, 1982.
58. Smith CE. Nurse's increasing responsibility for patient education, In: CE Smith (ed). Patient Education. Nurses in Partnership with Other Health Professionals. Orlando, Grune & Stratton, 1987.
59. Sciaky AJ. Patient education. In: Frownfelter D, Dean E. Principles and Practice of Cardiopulmonary Physical Therapy. 3rd ed. St. Louis, Mosby–Year Book, 1996, p 453–465.
60. Sluijs EM, Kok GJ, van der Zee J. Correlates of exercise compliance in physical therapy. Phys Ther 73:771–786, 1993.
61. Chase L, Elkins JA, Readinger J, Shepard KF. Perceptions of physical therapists toward patient education. Phys Ther 73:787–796, 1993.
62. Dean E, Perlstein MF, Mathews M: Acute sugical conditions. In: Frownfelter D, Dean E. Principles and Practice of Cardiopulmonary Physical Therapy. 3rd ed. St. Louis, Mosby–Year Book, 1996, pp 498–499.
63. Stein M, Cassara EL. Preoperative pulmonary evaluation and therapy for surgery patients. JAMA 211:787–790, 1970.
64. Vraciu JK, Vraciu RA. Effectiveness of breathing exercises in preventing pulmonary complications following open heart surgery. Phys Ther 57:1367–1371, 1977.
65. Kigin CM. Chest physical therapy for the postoperative or traumatic injury patient. Phys Ther 61:1724–1736, 1981.
66. Dean E. Mobilization and exercise. In: Frownfelter D, Dean E. Principles and Practice of Cardiopulmonary Physical Therapy. 3rd ed. St. Louis, Mosby–Year Book, 1996, p 271.

67. Atwood JA, Nielsen DH. Scope of cardiac rehabilitation. Phys Ther 65:1812–1819, 1985.
68. Irwin S. Clinical Manifestations and assessment of ischemic heart disease. Phys Ther 65:1806–1811, 1985.
69. Watchie J. Cardiopulmonary Physical Therapy: A clinical Manual. Philadelphia, WB Saunders, 1995 page 189.
70. Borg G. Perceived exertion as an indicator of somatic stress. J Rehab Med 2:92–98, 1970.
71. Watchie J. Cardiopulmonary Physical Therapy: A Clinical Manual. Philadelphia, WB Saunders, 1995, p 201.
72. Eston RG, Thompson M. Use of ratings of perceived exertion for predicting maximal work rate prescribing exercise intensity in patients taking atenolol. Br J Sports Med 31: 114–119, 1997.
73. Watchie J. Cardiopulmonary Physical Therapy: A Clinical Manual. Philadelphia, WB Saunders, 1995, p 192.
74. Packe GE, Freeman W, Cayton RM. Effects of exercise on gas exchange in patients recovering from acute severe asthma. Thorax 45:262–266, 1990.
75. Watchie J. Cardiopulmonary Physical Therapy: A Clinical Manual. Philadelphia, WB Saunders, 1995, p 147.
76. Weissman C, Kemper M. Stressing the critically ill patient: The cardiopulmonary and metabolic responses to an acute increase in oxygen consumption. J Crit Care 8:100–108, 1993.
77. Weissman C, Kemper M, Damask MC, et al. Effect of routine intensive care interaction on metabolic rate. Chest 86: 815–819, 1984.
78. Weissman C, Kemper M. The oxygen uptake-oxygen delivery relationship during ICU interventions. Chest 99:430–435, 1991.
79. Reynolds JP. LOS: SOS? You could say that managed care is about one thing: Discharge planning. PT Magazine 4:38–46, 1996.
80. Lopopolo RB. The effect of hospital restructuring on the role of physical therapists in acute care. Phys Ther 77:918–936, 1997.
81. Moerchen VA, Crane LD. The neonatal and pediatric patient. In: Frownfelter D, Dean E. Principles and Practice of Cardiopulmonary Physical Therapy. 3rd ed. St. Louis, Mosby–Year Book, 1996, pp 635–667.
82. Johnson B. Postoperative physical therapy in the pediatric cardiac surgery patient. Pediatr Phys Ther 3(1):14–22, Spring 1991.
83. Magee CL. Physical therapy for the child with asthma. Pediatr Phys Ther 3(1):23–28, Spring 1991.

18

Therapeutic Interventions in Cardiac Rehabilitation and Prevention

Ellen A. Hillegass and William C. Temes

INTRODUCTION

Cardiac rehabilitation is a multidisciplinary program of education, exercise, and behavioral change established to assist individuals with heart disease in achieving optimal physical, psychological, and functional status within the limits of their disease. This program includes:

- Education of the patient and family in the recognition, prevention, and treatment of cardiovascular disease
- Amelioration or reduction of risk factors
- Dealing with the psychological factors that influence recovery from heart disease
- Structured, progressive physical activity, either in a rehabilitation setting or home program
- Vocational counseling

This chapter describes the various settings, phases and components of cardiac rehabilitation. It also identifies which patient groups are appropriate candidates for rehabilitation and under what conditions rehabilitation is most beneficial. Case studies exemplifying many of the concepts outlined in this chapter are also presented at the end.

CARDIAC REHABILITATION

The Beginning in Acute Care

In 1952, Levine and Lown demonstrated that early mobilization of the acute coronary patient to activity reduced complications and improved the mortality rate.[1] Since then physicians have increasingly realized the benefits of early rehabilitative measures. Physical conditioning can improve heart rate response, arterial blood pressure response in hypertensive individuals, myocardial oxygen uptake, and maximum cardiac output.[2] In addition, improvements in the peripheral circulation, the pulmonary ventilation, and the autonomic nervous system benefit one's tolerance for work. Accompanying these physical improvements are greater emotional stability and self-esteem.

Early mobilization of stable individuals after a cardiac event has become a well-established practice. The time course of care for coronary disease is changing dramatically owing to early diagnostic testing, new interventions, and the current managed care environment. Although rest is important to the impaired myocardium, optimal improvement of the patient requires redefinition of the degree and duration of rest. No longer is the patient lying in bed for weeks at a time. The average patient who undergoes coronary artery bypass surgery is ambulating on the unit by day 3 at the latest. After myocardial infarction, patients are usually moved out of the intensive care unit and into the stepdown (or telemetry) unit within 24 to 48 hours and are often discharged 1 to 2 days later. Patients are no longer encouraged to seek alternative lifestyles or contemplate early retirement as a result of coronary disease. They are no longer spectators, but rather active participants, and many become more active and healthier in life after a cardiac event than they were before.

The Current Outpatient Center

The cardiac rehabilitation center is the facility in which an interdisciplinary team provides the planned and monitored program to promote physical, psychological, educational, and vocational improvement of the cardiac patient. Ideally, the center has classroom space for group patient education, private counseling facilities, and a library for educational materials. Exercise space should allow freedom of movement for warm-up and cool-down exercises and perhaps should have cameras to monitor patients in hallways and around blind corners. The facility should be easily accessible, pleasant, and clean—qualities that are important to boost morale and to support patient compliance. The facility may also be combined with a sports medicine, pulmonary rehabilitation, or fitness facility to increase use and decrease costs.

CANDIDACY

Traditionally the patient groups referred to cardiac rehabilitation included patients with complicated and uncomplicated myocardial infarction (MI), heart failure, heart transplant, and stable angina and postbypass or valve replacement. Occasionally patients are referred to cardiac rehabilitation after angioplasty.

Beyond the typical postinfarction and coronary bypass groups, the population base for cardiac rehabilitation has grown to include individuals who at one time were thought not to be good candidates for rehabilitation (including individuals with comorbid conditions, poor ejection fraction, cardiomyopathy, and serious arrhythmias). Therapists must be flexible in program planning, must address each patient's needs on an individual basis,

and must provide services through a patient-oriented rather than a program-oriented approach. This is particularly important with the groups identified in Table 18–1.

Individuals who are not considered to be good candidates for rehabilitation include

• Patients who have overt congestive heart failure (see Chapter 4), unstable angina pectoris (chest pain at rest), hemodynamic instability (falling blood pressure with exercise), serious arrhyth-

Table 18–1
Candidacy for Cardiac Rehabilitation

PATIENTS WITH POOR VENTRICULAR FUNCTION

This group includes patients who have had large infarctions and cardiomyopathies and, in general, those who have congestive heart failure. It has been demonstrated by a number of investigators that exercise training is safe for these patients with "sick ventricles." In fact, they may show significant changes in both physical and functional work capacity (perhaps more than other groups) because they usually function at such a low level.[3-6] McNeer defines complications post myocardial infarction which include poor ventricular function, significant ischemia with low level activity, shock and serious arrhythmias.[3] Lee and colleagues reported improvement in mean functional aerobic impairment (decreased from 32% to 24%) along with significantly lower ($p < .01$ and $<.05$, respectively) resting and submaximal heart rates in 25 men with ejection fractions less than 40% who were followed for an average of 18.5 months.[5] Coates and associates demonstrated similar improvement in physical work capacity, rate pressure product, and symptom scores in a group of 11 coronary patients who had very low ejection fractions (mean ejection fraction of 19%).[6] Neither of these studies found that exercise was detrimental to cardiovascular health.

PATIENTS WITH HEALTHY VENTRICLES

With the advent of more aggressive initial intervention (e.g., thrombolytic therapy and percutaneous transluminal coronary angioplasty), the degree of ventricular impairment after cardiac events has been limited substantially. Some individuals with unstable angina pectoris can be admitted to the hospital in the morning, undergo percutaneous transluminal coronary angioplasty the same day, and be discharged within 48 hours. Unfortunately, many patients are left wondering which activities are appropriate and safe and how much exercise is too much. Included in this group with healthy ventricles may be patients who have known coronary artery disease but who have not had a myocardial infarction as well as those who have undergone coronary artery bypass surgery and had no previous myocardial damage.

FOLLOW-UP PATIENTS

A group emerging in the cardiac rehabilitation arena includes those who return to a local hospital after having undergone a technical cardiac procedure at a different facility or regional center. This group consists of patients who underwent cardiac transplantation, implantation of a cardiac defibrillator or another sophisticated procedure.

ELDERLY PATIENTS

An increasingly elderly population that is often more debilitated is being referred for physical conditioning modification programs.

ASYMPTOMATIC AT-RISK PATIENTS

These individuals have no known coronary disease but do demonstrate multiple major or minor risk factors, or both. This group is referred for preventive modes of treatment. Individuals in this group may also include the offspring of patients with coronary artery disease who have elevated cholesterol, a multiple risk factor profile, or both.

mias, conduction defects, or impaired function of other organ systems
- Patients who have uncontrolled hypertension
- Patients who have other disease or illness that precludes exercise
- Apparently healthy individuals (mixing healthy individuals with persons who have heart disease may inhibit the former and frustrate the latter)

Unfortunately, many individuals with coronary disease and heart failure are not referred to or do not attend cardiac rehabilitation even though it would be extremely beneficial. According to the Agency for Health Care Policy and Research (AHCPR) clinical practice guidelines on cardiac rehabilitation, "of the several million patients with coronary disease who are candidates for cardiac rehabilitation services, only 11 to 38% of patients typically participate in cardiac rehabilitation programs."[7] In addition, "an estimated 4.7 million patients with heart failure may also be eligible, but few such patients participate in cardiac rehabilitation."[7]

ADMINISTRATIVE ISSUES IN CARDIAC REHABILITATION

Administrative issues revolve around several major goals of rehabilitation:

1. To prevent the harmful effects of prolonged bedrest when a patient is hospitalized with heart disease.
2. To develop cardiovascular fitness after acute illness, with an emphasis on optimal ability for employment and leisure.
3. To identify patients whose psychological response to cardiac disease may require extra support and additional measures for successful rehabilitation.
4. To initiate a program of secondary prevention of cardiovascular disease aimed at reducing the risks of illness and death as well as improving function and quality of life.
5. To accomplish the preceding goals through interdisciplinary efforts directed at discovering each patient's optimal activity level, diet, and ability to improve unfavorable risk factors.

THE CARDIAC REHABILITATION TEAM

Successful cardiac rehabilitation programs emphasize an interdisciplinary approach with team members contributing to all phases of patient assessment and direct patient care. The number of team members, as well as the role and function of each, may vary from center to center. Some facilities may have one person performing more than one function. In all cases, primary patient care remains the responsibility of the referring physician. Typical members of the cardiac rehabilitation program are found in Table 18–2. In addition, core competencies for cardiac rehabilitation professionals were published by the American Association of Cardiovascular and Pulmonary Rehabilitation and should be reviewed.[8]

Program Components

Because cardiac rehabilitation involves more than exercise, the components of a cardiac rehabilitation program should include all aspects of **secondary prevention** of cardiovascular disease. Exercise training has long been the center of cardiac rehabilitation, yet is only one of several components aimed at reducing risk of illness and death as well as improving function and quality of life. Actual behavior change is necessary for cardiac rehabilitation to be successful. Therefore, because cardiovascular disease involves many factors, a program that assesses the many factors and develops intervention strategies for each one is necessary. Program outcomes are individualized based upon the applicable risk factors that require monitoring and intervention and should be assessed in short-term and long-term follow-up of the patients who have entered the program. See Table 18–3 for program components.

If the cardiac rehabilitation program does not have certain program components on site, a system of referral and follow-up is necessary. This should include a system of assessing goal achievement of desired outcomes for each component and for each participant.

Table 18–2

Members of the Cardiac Rehabilitation Team

MEDICAL DIRECTOR

This individual is a physician who is responsible for the overall effectiveness and safety of the program. The medical director works closely with the program coordinator and other members of the team, being available for consultation, meeting with referring physicians, etc.

PROGRAM COORDINATOR

This individual should be skilled in personnel and team management as the program coordinator oversees all team personnel and facilities. This individual develops and revises policy, procedures, and budgets; selects needed equipment; and is responsible for coordinating and supervising staff. The program coordinator works with other departments or facilities to evaluate the program needs. The person who takes on this role may be a physical therapist, registered nurse, or exercise physiologist, or another appropriate allied health professional with administrative leadership qualities.

EXERCISE TRAINING PROFESSIONAL

This person is a professional who is knowledgeable in exercise physiology, pathology, exercise training techniques, monitoring equipment, arrhythmia recognition, cardiopulmonary resuscitation, and advanced cardiac life support (including defibrillation). Commitment to a healthy lifestyle is necessary because this person is a role model for patients and other staff members. The preparation and training of physical therapists make them the ideal professional group for this position. However, in many programs registered nurses and exercise physiologists fill this role.

DIETITIAN

A professional knowledgeable in nutrition assessment and counseling, a dietitian also is experienced in dietary planning and modification.

BEHAVIOR SPECIALIST

This person must be a professional skilled in behavioral evaluation and counseling techniques who is familiar with coping mechanisms, family patterns of interaction, and available community resources. A psychologist or medical social worker usually fits this position.

VOCATIONAL COUNSELOR

This may be a referral source to the program to assist the individual in a return to work, or in counseling and referral for training for a different career.

Table 18–3

Cardiac Rehabilitation Program Components

RISK FACTOR	ASSESSMENT	TREATMENT
Smoking	Current and past smoking habits	Referral to smoking cessation
Exercise	Exercise habits, weekly calorie expenditure, maximal functional capacity	Exercise prescription for supervised or individual exercise training
Nutrition/lipids	Weight, body fat (body mass index), cholesterol, LDL, and HDL	Nutritional counseling, medical management for elevated cholesterol, weight management
Psychosocial	Stress, hostility, depression	Referral for counseling, group support
Hypertension	Blood pressure, vascular status (pulses, bruits)	Diet, exercise, counseling, and medication, if necessary
Diabetes	Blood glucose fasting blood sugars, urine testing	Diet, exercise, medication (insulin) and diabetic education re: multisystem dysfunction
Menopausal females	Estrogen status, possibly bone density	Dietary evaluation and counseling, estrogen replacement, calcium and other bone-building supplements

Efficacy of Cardiac Rehabilitation

Medically prescribed and supervised exercise as part of a comprehensive rehabilitation program is a well-accepted standard of care throughout the world for cardiac patients, particularly following an acute myocardial infarction or coronary revascularization procedure. The degree of benefit from cardiac rehabilitation programs as documented in the literature varies considerably. However, exercise rehabilitation has made a positive impact on several risk factors, functional capacity, cardiovascular efficiency, and to some degree on cardiac mortality rate.[9]

Risk factors have been shown to be favorably affected by exercise training in individuals with and without cardiac conditions.[10-13] The benefits of exercise training include

- Loss of excess weight or body fat
- Lowering of lipid levels, including total cholesterol and triglycerides
- Elevation of levels of high-density lipoproteins (HDLs)
- Reduction of elevated blood pressure levels
- Improvement in glucose insulin dynamics

Heart rate, systolic blood pressure, and the rate-pressure product are generally lower during submaximal efforts following exercise conditioning, resulting in reduced myocardial oxygen demand.[14, 15] This is particularly important to patients with exertional ischemia. Reported improvements in symptom-limited, maximal oxygen consumption for patients with angina pectoris ranged from 32 to 56%.[14]

Reduction of physical work capacity is thought to be the result of the degree of myocardial damage, myocardial ischemia, or both. Patients with acute myocardial infarction and coronary bypass surgery have been shown to demonstrate significant improvement in aerobic capacity following exercise conditioning, on the order of 11 to 66%. The greatest improvements were found in patients with the lowest initial maximum oxygen consumption levels.[14, 16, 17] The specific cardiovascular adaptations that occur in coronary patients vary depending on the training stimulus and the duration of the program. Eshani and colleagues demonstrated an increase in ejection fraction, stroke vol-ume, and rate pressure product during maximal exercise in post–myocardial infarction patients who were trained at intensities of at least 85% of maximal heart rate for at least 1 year in duration.[18] However, no matter what mechanism or physiologic adaptation takes place in trained coronary patients, an increase of aerobic capacity means increased tolerance for daily life activities consisting of repeated submaximal physical exertion. This translates into a potential for an improved quality of life.

A definitive randomized clinical trial on the independent effect of exercise in prevention of recurrent coronary events in patients recovering from myocardial infarction, coronary bypass surgery, or angina pectoris has not been conducted. The ability of a single study to test the hypothesis that exercise reduces the mortality rate from coronary heart disease would require a randomized trial of more than 4000 patients. The ability to control all the variables in a single study is nearly impossible and certainly improbable. Nonetheless, several reports have attempted to demonstrate a reduced cardiac mortality rate based on combined data from several larger studies (meta-analysis) and have, in fact, shown some interesting trends and statistical significance with a reduction in mortality rate similar to the salvage rate attributed to beta-blocking drugs in clinical trials following a myocardial infarction.[19]

MANAGEMENT AND EVALUATION OF PATIENTS DURING THE ACUTE PHASE

Cardiac rehabilitation is typically organized in progressive phases of programming to meet the specific needs of individuals and their families in their stages of recovery. Phase I is the acute or in-hospital phase, phase II is the outpatient or intensive monitoring, phase III is the training and maintenance phase, and phase IV is reserved for the high-risk patients in a disease prevention program (Table 18–4).

Inpatient cardiac rehabilitation begins when a patient arrives in the telemetry unit, but it may commence at the bedside in the intensive or coronary care unit, especially if the individual has had to remain there for an extended period of time.

Table 18–4

Phases of Cardiac Rehabilitation

PHASE I: ACUTE PHASE OR MONITORING PHASE

Inpatient cardiac rehabilitation begins when the patient is determined to be medically stable following a myocardial infarction, coronary artery bypass surgery, angioplasty, valve repair, or congestive heart failure.

PHASE II: SUBACUTE PHASE OF REHABILITATION OR CONDITIONING PHASE

This initial outpatient phase begins as early as 24 hours after discharge, and lasts up to 6 weeks. Frequency of visits depend on the patient's clinical needs. Patients are monitored by ECG telemetry and are taught the basics of self-monitoring and proper exercise procedure. In addition, secondary prevention of disease by implementation of risk factor reduction is a key component of this phase.

PHASE III: TRAINING OR INTENSIVE REHABILITATION

Patients are usually seen once a week, and extends from the time the patient finishes phase II to indefinitely. Patients exercise in larger groups and continue to progress in their exercise program. Resistance training often begins in this phase.

PHASE IV: ONGOING CONDITIONING (MAINTENANCE) PHASE OR PREVENTION PROGRAM

Candidates for this program are individuals who are at high risk for infarction due to their risk factor profile, as well as those who want to continue to be followed by supervision of trained personnel.

Overall, the goals of inpatient cardiac rehabilitation are to assess for safety to perform activities in the home or the alternative care site after discharge from the hospital, and to increase knowledge of the disease and the management of the disease. In addition, the team members must function cohesively in preparing the patient for discharge so as not to make the instructions too complicated or too simple. Specific goals of inpatient cardiac rehabilitation are as follows:

• Evaluation of individual physiologic responses to self-care and ambulation activities. In the telemetry or step-down unit, patients are usually closely monitored by electrocardiogram (ECG) while at rest. However, the hemodynamic changes that can take place with position change, self-care activities, toileting, and the like are potentially dangerous and usually go unobserved or are not closely monitored.

• Provision of feedback to physicians and nurses regarding the patient's response to activity so that recommendations for activity can be made. The cardiac rehabilitation assessment is worthless unless the results can be applied practically while the patient is in the hospital or preparing for discharge. Information should be shared with all team members.

• Provision of safe guidelines for progression of activity throughout convalescence. A day-to-day reassessment of function, as well as hemodynamic and ECG responses to progressive activity provides further information to the physician. This is especially important because it relates to decisions on medication adjustments and on preparation for discharge. To facilitate the team's effectiveness, an overall activity plan can be used for progression in phase I.

• Provision of patient and family education with reference to disease entity, risk factors and appropriate modification, self-monitoring techniques, and general activity guidelines. It is most important to instill a sense of confidence about what the patient can do safely and what rate of recovery to expect regarding activity.

Initial Assessment

The initial assessment is conducted as soon as possible by each team member involved in the patient's care, usually within a few hours of referral. A quick response is important to the patient who is anticipating resuming activity, as well as to the medical and allied health care team who have only a short amount of time to work with the patient and family during the inpatient stay. The assessment should include a thorough chart review, patient-family interview, physical examination, and self-care and ambulation assessment or screening.

• *Chart review*—to obtain information, a review of pertinent medical history; physician admission report and subsequent chart notes; surgical report, including cardiac catheterization data; medications; laboratory studies (e.g., cardiac enzymes, hemoglobin/hematocrit, lipid analysis); noninvasive studies (e.g., echocardiography, ECG, exercise tests, nuclear studies); nurses notes; physician orders, including those for activity and special instructions for cardiac rehabilitation; and any other pertinent data (e.g., age, home town, insurance provider, height, weight).

• *Patient-family interview*—to gain a subjective description of symptoms and other problems; to assess the risk factor profile (see Table 18–5), diet profile, and patient-family goals; and to guide discharge disposition.

• *Physical examination*—to include assessment of vital signs (e.g., heart rate, blood pressure), auscultation of lung and heart sounds, chest wall inspection and palpation, examination of extremities (peripheral pulses, edema), and gross range of motion and strength.

• *Self-care and ambulation evaluation (activities of daily living [ADL] monitor)*—to monitor the patient's hemodynamic, symptomatic, and ECG response to typical self-care activities. This evaluation is performed one-on-one with a physical therapist and involves the use of a portable ECG monitor so the therapist can observe ECG changes as they occur when the patient becomes mobile (Fig. 18–1). Another option is to have a second person stationed at the central ECG monitors to observe any changes; however, a direct method of communication between therapist and observer must be available. Parameters to be measured during the evaluation include heart rate, blood pressure, ECG, and signs and symptoms. Each parameter is recorded at rest, with activity, immediately after the activity, and 1 to 3 minutes after the activity. Activities may include resting supine, sitting, standing, hygiene and grooming, Valsalva's maneuver (with nonsurgical patients), and lower and upper extremity dressing (Fig. 18–2).

• *Ambulation activity*—to determine, in addition to the physiologic parameters, the patient's balance and coordination, level of independence, and distance traveled relative to normal ambulation velocity. Response to stair climbing should be evaluated before discharge if the patient must

Table 18–5		
Cardiovascular Disease Risk Factor Checklist		
HYPERTENSION	**SMOKING HISTORY**	**HYPERCHOLESTEROLEMIA**
☐ Known high blood pressure prior to hospitalization ☐ Taking antihypertension medications prior to hospitalization ☐ Unknown prior to hospitalization ☐ History of normal BP	☐ Current smoker (>9 cigs/day) ☐ Quit at time of hospitalization ☐ Former smoker ☐ Never smoked	☐ Known elevated cholesterol ☐ Elevated at time of hospitalization ☐ Unknown ☐ Hx of normal chol
Physical activity ☐ Not participated in >3 exercise sessions/wk ☐ Regularly exercises 3/wk	Stress: hostility, anger ☐ Self-reports hx of high stress levels ☐ Self-reports no hx ☐ Others report hx ☐ Demonstrates hostility, anger	Weight ☐ >15 lb overweight ☐ Within normal wt
Family history ☐ Father *and* mother with CAD ☐ Father *or* mother with CAD ☐ Grandparents or uncles/aunts with CAD ☐ No family hx of CAD		
Alcohol or substance use ☐ Self-reports hx of alcohol substance abuse ☐ Presentation suggests hx of substance abuse ☐ No evidence of abuse	Diabetes ☐ Hx of elevated blood sugar or diabetes ☐ Hx of normal blood sugar	Other ☐ Age ☐ Male sex ☐ Menopausal female

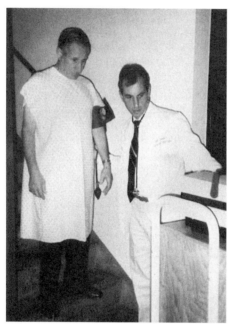

Figure 18-1. Monitoring the electrocardiogram and blood pressure during stair climbing.

negotiate stairs at home and is considered well enough to do so; however, this is not an activity to be performed early in the recovery phase.

Activity Program Guidelines

Indications for an Unmodified Program. Patients who demonstrate appropriate hemodynamic,

ECG, and symptomatic responses to the self-care and ambulation evaluation can have their activity levels increased. The rate of progression is individualized and adjusted to each patient's particular limitation, depending on many clinical and functional factors (e.g., complicated versus uncomplicated course, ventricular function, premorbid functional level, number of days on bedrest, philosophy of the referring physician). The physiologic parameters of heart rate, blood pressure, signs and symptoms, ECG findings, and heart sounds continue to be monitored each session, with the results communicated when possible to the patient's nurse and always documented in the chart. Exercise periods are usually conducted at least once daily, lasting approximately 10 minutes for patients on modified programs and 15 minutes for patients who have no limitations. Intensity of activity should be gauged by more than just heart rate limits and should be based on the patient's clinical status and medication regimen. Historically, heart rate levels up to 120 beats per minute (bpm) or 20 to 30 bpm above the resting rate have been used as guidelines; however, with the wide variety of rate-limiting medications, this method is not appropriate. It is the combination of all factors (hemodynamic, symptoms, and ECG findings) that must be considered in determining specific intensity parameters. Table 18-6 provides the functional classification guide for inpatient activities.

Indications for a Modified Program. Program parameters are modified for persons desig-

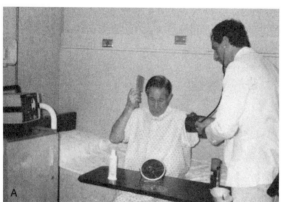
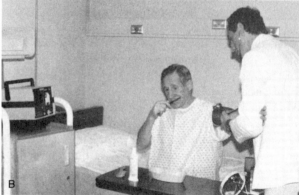

Figure 18-2. The physical therapist monitors blood pressure responses while the patient performs typical activities of daily living.

Table 18–6

Functional Classification Guide for Inpatient Activities

FUNCTIONAL CLASS I	FUNCTIONAL CLASS II	FUNCTIONAL CLASS III	FUNCTIONAL CLASS IV	FUNCTIONAL CLASS V	FUNCTIONAL CLASS VI
Sits up in bed with assistance Does own self-care activities—seated, or may need assistance Stands at bedside with assistance Sits up in chair 15–30 minutes, 2–3 times per day	Sits up in bed independently Stands independently Does own self-care activities in bathroom—seated Walks in room and to bathroom (may need assistance)	Sits and stands independently Does own self-care activities in bathroom, seated or standing Walks in halls with assistance short distances (50–100 ft) as tolerated, up to 3 times per day	Does own self-care and bathes Walks in halls short distances (150–200 ft) with minimal assistance, 3–4 times per day	Walk in halls independently, moderate distances (250–500 ft), 3–4 times per day	Independent ambulation on unit 3–6 times per day vs. as desired

nated as "complicated" for one or more of the following reasons:

- Large infarction clinically, although stable after 2 to 3 days
- Resting tachycardia (100 bpm) or inappropriate heart rate increase with self-care activities
- Blood pressure failing to rise or decreasing with self-care activities
- The ECG revealing more than 6 to 8 premature ventricular complexes per minute or progressive heart block with self-care activities
- Angina or undue fatigue with self-care activities
- Need for prolonged bedrest (more than 4 days)

Indications for Withholding a Program. The following are criteria to exclude patients from participation in the activity program:

- Severe pump failure (as evidenced by shortness of breath, peripheral edema, diaphoresis, or chest x-ray and falling blood pressure response to activity).
- Classification in a high-risk subset, described by
  - Recurrent malignant arrhythmias (ventricular tachycardia, four premature ventricular complexes in a row, ventricular fibrillation)
  - Angina at rest
  - Second- or third-degree heart block
  - Persistent hypotension (less than 90 mm Hg)
  - Rapid atrial rhythm
  - Unstable angina pectoris or change in symptoms in the preceding 24 hours

General Precautions

Before initiating each activity session, the patient's status should be reassessed. There *must* be a review of the patient's chart. The ECG monitor should be checked for any new changes and vital signs; cardiac rhythm, symptoms, and heart and lung sounds need to be rechecked. Activity sessions should not be initiated within 1 hour after meals. This delay allows adequate digestion to occur without increased myocardial oxygen demand. It is also important to avoid isometric exercise, specifically breath holding with exercise, because it may produce dramatic changes in blood pressure and arrhythmias. Table 18–7 provides a sample progressive activity plan for a typical length of stay.

Relative Contraindications to Continuing Exercise

Whenever one of the following occurs, the event should be documented appropriately and the patient's nurse, physician, or both should be contacted immediately.

- Unusual heart rate increase—greater than 50 bpm increase with low-level activity
- Blood pressure indicative of hypertension—ab-

Table 18–7

Progressive Activity for Five-Day Length of Stay

DAY	MET LEVEL	ACTIVITY
Day 1, CCU	1–2	Bedrest until stable, use of bedside commode, out of bed to chair if stable
Day 2, step-down unit	2–3	Sitting warm-ups, walking in room, self-care activities
Days 3–5	2–3	Out of bed as tolerated if stable, walk 5–10 minutes in hall (supervised as needed)
	3–4	Shower with seat, walk 5–10 minutes 2–3 times/day, up/down one half flight of stairs
	3–4	Treadmill walking or up/down full flight of stairs

normally high systolic (greater than 210 mm Hg) or diastolic (greater than 110 mm Hg) pressure

• Drop in systolic blood pressure (greater than 10 mm Hg) with low-level exercise (*not* just a drop in systolic blood pressure with standing)

• Symptoms with activity:
  • Angina (level 1 out of 4)—see index of angina levels (Table 18–8)
  • Undue dyspnea (level 2+/4+)—see dyspnea index (Table 18–8)
  • Excessive fatigue
  • Mental confusion or dizziness
  • Severe leg claudication—level 8/10 on a pain scale of 10

• Signs of pallor, cold sweat, ataxia

• Changing heart sounds with activity—new murmur or ventricular gallop

• An ECG abnormality, including marked ST-segment changes (may be only a single event that requires notification, as well as a sustained event) or serious arrhythmias (development of

coupled premature ventricular complexes or three in a row, second- or third-degree atrioventricular block, or intermittent rate–dependent conduction disturbance).

Other Components of the Acute Phase

The amount and type of information provided to patients and their families depend on a variety of factors, which include ability to follow directions, emotional stability after the cardiac event, patient and family's **readiness to learn,** and basic level of understanding and education. Considering the wealth of information they receive and the usual emotional fragility of the participants, it is best to keep information that patients and their families should retain in a neatly organized packet to which they can refer in the future. The instruc-

Table 18–8

Angina and Dyspnea Rating Scales

5-GRADE ANGINA SCALE	5-GRADE DYSPNEA SCALE	10-GRADE ANGINA/ DYSPNEA SCALE
0 No angina	0 No dyspnea	0 Nothing
1 Light, barely noticeable	1 Mild, noticeable	1 Very slight
2 Moderate, bothersome	2 Mild, some difficulty	2 Slight
3 Severe, very uncomfortable: preinfarction pain	3 Moderate difficulty, but can continue	3 Moderate
4 Most pain ever experienced: infarction pain	4 Severe difficulty, cannot continue	4 Somewhat severe
		5 Severe
		6
		7 Very severe
		8
		9
		10 Very, very severe; maximal

tions should be kept as simple as possible. It is particularly helpful to have the various team members coordinate their educational materials in one packet. Table 18–9 gives a sample clinical pathway for rehabilitation services.

Any education plan should be specific to the individual's needs and particular risk factors. Almost all patients, and especially family members, are concerned about the prognosis of the disease, the foods they can or cannot eat, what to do in an emergency or if chest pain recurs, and what they can or cannot do physically when they get home. Concerns about acceptable activity usually include sexual activity, although many individuals do not verbalize this concern.

It is no one person's responsibility to provide all the information, but rather that of each team member within the particular specialty area. The educational component should include, but not be limited to, discussions about the following:

• The particular disease process and prognosis — usually discussed by the patient's physician and reinforced by nursing and other allied health team members
• The individual's risk factors and recommendations for behavior modification — usually performed by team members relative to their impact on the problem
• General activity guidelines and home exercise prescription — performed by the physical therapist with specific input from the physician
• The role of exercise — performed by the physical therapist and reinforced by other team members
• Medications (especially the use of nitroglycerin) — performed by the physician, nurse, or pharmacist and reinforced by other team members
• Nutrition and prescribed diet — performed by the physician and dietitian
• Self-monitoring techniques — according to the patient's ability (usually based on symptom-limited response because heart rate may be difficult or inappropriate for patients to learn to monitor at this time) and performed by the physician, nurse, and physical therapist
• What to do in an emergency

Audiovisual aids (e.g., videos, books) are helpful for patients and family and may be left with them for a time when they are most alert, rested, and prepared to hear the message being presented. This level of readiness is not always present at the time a team member visits.

Table 18–9
Rehabilitation Services in Typical Clinical Pathway for Uncomplicated Myocardial Infarction

DAY	ACTIVITY	EDUCATION
Day 2, cardiac rehabilitation consultant to assess	Up in chair Bedside commode	Explanation of event Treatment plan
Day 3	Walk 5–10 min in hall Self-care activities	Assess readiness to learn Teach signs/symptoms NTG use Emergency response to symptoms
Day 4	Walk in hall 5–10 min, 3–4/day, assess stairs	Safety factors Do's and Dont's for home activity Introduce Phase II: secondary prevention
Discharge planning		

* Indications for variations in pathway:
    Frailty
    Orthopedic problems
    Cognitive impairment
    Cerebrovascular accident
    Renal insufficiency
    Postoperative bleeding
    Serious arrhythmias
    Pulmonary complications
    Severely impaired left ventricular function

Diet and Nutrition. Individual counseling by the dietitian with input from the attending physician usually begins during the inpatient stay. Specific problem areas such as hyperlipidemia, obesity, diabetes, and sodium restriction need to be addressed on an individual basis. Usually the person who prepares the meals at home wants to spend as much time as possible learning what they should or should not prepare. More specifics on this topic are discussed later in the chapter.

Psychological and Behavioral Rehabilitation. Most patients experience some degree of fear, anxiety, depression, and anger that should be monitored. Psychologists, specialized clinical nurse practitioners, social workers, and others are often available to help patients deal with these problems. However, in day-to-day interactions with therapists, dietitians, and other cardiac rehabilitation team members, patients often more readily trust and look to these individuals for support in dealing with their disability. Patients need to be observed by all team members for any degree of denial or anxiety, which may be demonstrated in a variety of ways, such as anger, irritability, or conflict with different team members. Team members should be alert for patients and family members who have a need for psychological intervention.

Outcome Measures

Because of the limitation of time that a patient has in the hospital, the acute phase of cardiac rehabilitation is limited. Therefore, the outcomes expected are based upon the functional limitations or disabilities of the patient as assessed upon the

Table 18–10

Optimal Outcomes for Patients with Cardiovascular Pump Dysfunction or Failure per APTA Guide to Physical Therapist Practice

FUNCTIONAL LIMITATION/ DISABILITY	PATIENT/CLIENT SATISFACTION	SECONDARY PREVENTION
Health-related quality of life is improved	Access, availability, and services provided are acceptable to patient/client, family, significant others, and caregivers	Risk of functional decline is reduced
Optimal return to role function (worker, student, spouse, grandparent) is achieved	Administrative management of practice is acceptable to patient/client, family, significant others, and caregivers	Risk of impairment or of impairment progression is reduced
Risk of disability associated with cardiovascular pump dysfunction is reduced	Clinical proficiency of physical therapist is acceptable to patient/client, family, significant others, and caregivers	Need for additional physical therapist intervention is decreased
Safety of patient/client and caregivers is increased	Coordination and conformity of care acceptable to patient/client, family, significant others, and caregivers	Level of patient/client adherence to the intervention program is maximized
Self-care and home management activities, including ADL and work (job/school/play) and leisure activities, including instrumental activities of daily living (IADL) are performed safely, efficiently, and at a maximal level of independence with or without devices and equipment	Interpersonal skills of physical therapist are acceptable to patient/client, family, significant others, and caregivers	Patient/client and caregivers are aware of the factors that may indicate need for reexamination or a new episode of care, including changes in the following: caregiver status, community adaptation, leisure or leisure activities, living environment, disease or impairment that may affect function, or home or work (job/school/play) settings
Understanding of personal and environmental factors that promote optimal health status is demonstrated		Professional recommendations are integrated into home, community, work (job/school/play), or leisure environments
Understanding of strategies to prevent further functional limitation and disability is demonstrated		Utilization and cost of health care services are decreased

Source: American Physical Therapy Association. Guide to physical therapist practice. Phys Ther 77:1163–1650, 1997.

initial and any subsequent assessments made by the therapist. The *Guide to Physical Therapist Practice* provides guidelines on optimal outcomes for patients as well as appropriate terminology for documentation based upon the severity of their cardiovascular pump dysfunction.[20] Table 18–10 provides overall outcomes for patients with cardiovascular pump dysfunction and pump failure. Specific outcome measures for the acute phase are given in Table 18–11.

Discharge Planning

Patients and their families usually have little time to prepare for discharge, although discussions typically begin as soon as the patient is stabilized in the intensive care unit. Cardiac rehabilitation team members begin presenting discharge information early rather than waiting until the day of discharge (Fig. 18–3). The planning should include the following:

1. A review of general activity guidelines, exercise prescription, dietary regimen, medications (indications, when to take them, and when to contact the physician), and symptoms to observe with actions to take if they occur.
2. A referral to outpatient cardiac rehabilitation for continued treatment and lifestyle modification, to begin as early as 2 to 3 days after discharge. Patients who are not referred immedi-

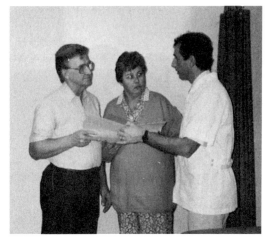

Figure 18–3. The physical therapist reviews discharge recommendations with the patient (*left*) and spouse.

ately and are not given a date or time for return before discharge are less likely to return.
3. A low-level, symptom-limited exercise test for the patient before discharge is preferred; however, some patients return to their physician's office after discharge and have an exercise test performed in the office at that time. The test provides valuable information to the cardiac rehabilitation team in establishing discharge activity guidelines and prescriptions for exercise on return to the outpatient program, although some programs accept patients who are unable to perform an exercise test.

Table 18–11
Specific Outcome Measures Used in Acute Phase of Cardiac Rehabilitation
Self-management of symptoms
Patient/client knowledge of factors associated with condition
Aerobic capacity (or exercise tolerance) or endurance
Ability to perform physical tasks related to self-care and home management
Physiologic response to increased oxygen demand
Strength
Symptoms associated with increased oxygen demand
Level of assistance/supervision required for task performance
Safety
Joint integrity

SECONDARY PREVENTION IN OUTPATIENT CARDIAC REHABILITATION

Exercise Training

Many approaches to outpatient cardiac rehabilitation exist, from large, multidisciplinary team approaches to smaller programs in which one person performs multiple functions. Although there are philosophic differences regarding frequency of activity, mode of exercise, monitoring, and the like, the goals are generally the same. Ideally, the program begins within 48 to 72 hours following discharge from the hospital. Thus, problems that arise early after discharge can be sorted out, questions about care can be answered, and, most important, patients and their families can receive support from the staff and other patients. The goals of outpatient cardiac rehabilitation programs include the following:

- Provision of a flexible, individualized exercise program of the proper intensity to elicit improvement in the patient's cardiovascular fitness without exceeding the safe limits of exercise
- Provision of a program that emphasizes patient education so that the individual can begin to understand the disease and to implement lifestyle changes
- Provision of a program to enhance the confidence of patients with ischemic heart disease in their ability to work at safe, functional levels of activity
- Provision of a program to aid the patient in personal risk factor reduction (secondary prevention) to help prevent new or recurrent cardiovascular complications
- Provision of a program that assists in and accelerates the return to work (most patients who have had an uncomplicated course should be able to return to work within 2 months)
- Promotion of psychological, behavioral, and educational improvement

Program Classification

For purposes of clarity, the initial outpatient period is classified as phase II, the higher level conditioning program as phase III. Phases II and III are often based in a hospital or satellite setting because of the likelihood of dealing with higher risk patients and the potential need for emergency medical services; however, these services can be performed in independent practice settings with appropriate medical support systems. Reimbursement issues may dictate where these programs are carried out. Phase IV or prevention and maintenance programs are often held outside the hospital setting in local YMCAs, or community colleges. Recommendations are made regarding the usual length of time in each phase, but programs should last as long as the patient's symptoms indicate. Often patients terminate the programs due to the termination of the reimbursement.

Home-Based Cardiac Rehabilitation

A substantial number of uncomplicated (low risk) patients with heart disease are considered to be candidates for cardiac rehabilitation but are unable to attend the outpatient program on a regular basis owing to the travel distance. For this group of patients, a different approach should be considered so that they benefit from the structure and support of this program. During the inpatient interview process, the therapist can determine whether at home therapy could be safely performed. Patients considered candidates for the program are given more extensive discharge instructions regarding self-monitoring techniques, exercise guidelines, dietary management, medications, and the like, and are taught to keep an accurate daily activity log. A weekly telephone call is made by a member of the cardiac rehabilitation team to the patient to discuss progress or problems and to provide additional information or materials for program progression.

Some programs also have the capability of having ECG information transmitted over the telephone lines while the patient exercises at home. When the patient returns for follow-up care with the physician or for exercise testing (usually performed 3 to 6 weeks after discharge), a 2 to 3 hour follow-up session is arranged with cardiac rehabilitation team members to review the individual's program. Follow-up telephone calls continue weekly for the next month, and activity logs are sent by the patient every 2 weeks; thereafter, monthly contacts are maintained for up to 6 to 12 months. Studies on this form of rehabilitation versus no program versus supervised exercise programs have been favorable; however, physical work capacity improves most significantly in supervised programs.[21, 22]

Initial Assessment

The objective of the physical evaluation is to assess ventricular function (myocardial reserve, infarct size, or both; presence and severity of ischemia or serious arrhythmia, or both) as it relates to the ramifications of the disease state on the functional abilities of the patient. Components of the initial assessment include

- A thorough medical history
- A patient-family interview
- A physical examination
- An exercise test (see Figs. 18–4 and 18–5)
- A blood chemistry panel

However, as sometimes patients are referred to outpatient rehabilitation without undergoing an inpatient assessment and phase I rehabilitation or have been referred because of a diagnosis of stable angina or who have undergone angioplasty, all patients should undergo an initial assessment upon entry into outpatient rehabilitation. This assessment is discussed in detail in Chapter 16.

General Management Strategies

The maintenance of a safe and effective risk reduction program is paramount in establishing treatment monitoring guidelines. The frequency of monitoring and the degree of direct supervision of an exercise treatment program must be determined for each patient based on prior clinical course (complicated or uncomplicated), exercise

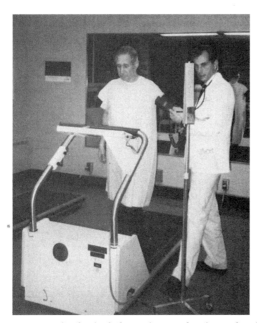

Figure 18–4. A physical therapist conducting a low-level exercise test.

test results, degree of ventricular impairment, initial assessment, and risk stratification (Tables 18–12 and 18–13). For some patients, direct monitoring and close supervision of each exercise session may be required and entirely appropriate for the first several weeks (Table 18–14). However, for the majority of patients who have had a clinically uncomplicated course and an exercise test that was uneventful, or that produced no negative findings, such close supervision and monitoring at each session can be counterproductive, implying more risk than is warranted. A number of studies have shown that the incidence of serious complications in the latter group is quite low. For such patients an effective risk reduction program must concern itself with the development of self-confidence, the motivation for change, the sense of direct involvement of the patient with the management of the exercise program, and the development of skill in self-monitoring.

Some conditions should limit participation in an exercise program. Patients are not considered candidates for a cardiac rehabilitation program when they have

- Unstable status—for example, recurrent ischemic pain, uncompensated congestive heart failure, resting tachycardia (greater than 100 bpm; slightly higher for postoperative patients), severe bradycardia (less than 50 bpm)
- Uncontrolled hypertension
- Other illness or disease that precludes exercise
- Apparently good health (low risk for cardiac disease).

Exercise for the Coronary Patient—An Individualized Plan

A patient's exercise plan should be determined by objective assessment of clinical status, functional capacity, and personal need. What may be good for one person may prove to be detrimental to another. In addition to making a clinical evaluation, the therapist must determine the patient's exercise needs, interests, abilities, and previous habits. The exercise plan should also consider the facilities and equipment that are available as well as the climate and environmental factors that may

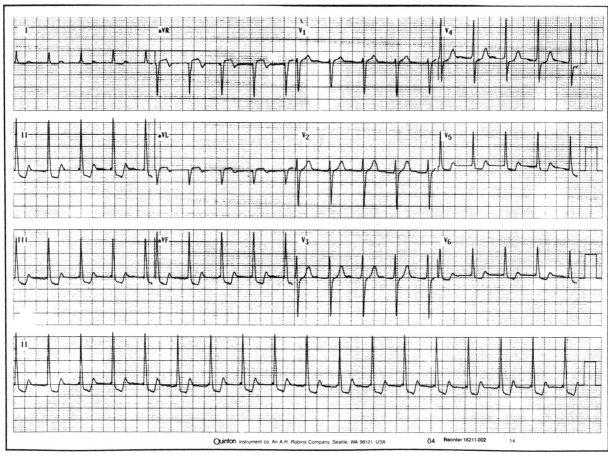

Figure 18-5. Typical 12-lead electrocardiogram tracing. Tracings should be assessed for the presence of significant ischemia.

affect whether the program can be carried out conveniently. These considerations are important in motivating the patient to be compliant with the program.

The Effects of Exercise

The specific demand of habitual physical exercise produces a biochemical change that ultimately enhances the functioning of skeletal muscle and the cardiovascular system. To a large degree the improvement made by the cardiac patient depends on the degree of ventricular impairment and function. Several studies have demonstrated that some coronary patients can, in fact, improve not only the maximal aerobic capacity but the cardiac output as well.[24-27] Even patients with clinically large infarctions and poor ventricular function demon-

strated significant improvement with regard to physical work capacity.[25] There are perhaps even greater functional consequences for them because their reserve is usually so low initially that simple, light household and ADL tasks are very difficult to perform. Persons with less impaired ventricular function (ejection fraction greater than 50%) often do not notice a very substantial difference in exercise tolerance with usual activities unless they are stressed significantly (at which point they would probably slow down or stop).

Exercise training creates change specifically in the muscle groups that are challenged. This fact becomes important in selecting the most appropriate activity to produce the greatest functional gain. Nearly everyone needs to walk some distance. In addition, we all need to use our arms to some degree, some of us more than others. Why is it then that so many cardiac patients ride stationary

Table 18-12
Stratification for Risk of Event (Not Specific Solely to Exercise)

LOWEST RISK	MODERATE RISK	HIGHEST RISK
No significant LV dysfunction (EF > 50%)	Moderately impaired LV function (EF = 40–59%)	Decreased LV function (EF <40%)
No resting or exercise-induced complex dysrhythmia	Signs/symptoms including angina at moderate levels of exercise (5–6.9 METs) or in recovery	Survivor of cardiac arrest or sudden death
Uncomplicated MI; CABG; angioplasty, atherectomy, or stent	Moderate risk is assumed for patients who do not meet the classification of either highest risk or lowest risk.	Complex ventricular dysrhythmia at rest or with exercise
Absence of CHF or signs/symptoms indicating postevent ischemia		MI or cardiac surgery complicated by cardiogenic shock, CHF, and/or signs/symptoms of postprocedure ischemia
Normal hymodynamics with exercise or recovery		Abnormal hemodynamics with exercise (especially flat or decreasing systolic blood pressure or chronotropic incompetence with increasing workload)
Asymptomatic including absence of angina with exertion or recovery		Signs/symptoms including angina pectoris at low levels of exercise (<5.0 METs) or in recovery
Functional capacity ≥7.0 METs*		Functional capacity <5.0 METs*
Absence of clinical depression		Clinically significant depression
Lowest risk classification is assumed when each of the risk factors in the category is present.		Highest risk classification is assumed with the presence of any one of the risk factors included in this category.

*Note: If measured functional capacity is not available, this variable is not considered in the risk stratification process.

Source: American Association of Cardiovascular and Pulmonary Rehabilitation. Guidelines for Cardiac Rehabilitation and Secondary Prevention Programs. 3rd ed. Champaign, IL, Human Kinetics, 1999, Table 4–2, p 45.

(LV = left ventricle, METs = metabolic equivalent table, EF = ejection fraction, CHF = congestive heart failure, MI = myocardial infarction, CABG = coronary artery bypass graft.)

Table 18-13
Additional Medical Therapy to Be Considered in Assessing Level of Risk for Subsequent Events

Lipids	A. If LDL > 100, consider pharmacologic intervention; if HDL < 35, emphasize weight loss and exercise
Antiplatelet	A. Start ASA 80–325 mg qd if not contraindicated B. Manage warfarin to international normalized ration = 2.0–3.5 for post-MI patients
ACE inhibitors	A. Start early post-MI in stable, high-risk patients (anterior MI, Killip class II (S_3 gallop, rales, radiographic CHF) B. Continue indefinitely for all with LV dysfunction (EF < 40%) or symptoms of failure C. Use as needed to manage blood pressure or symptoms in all other patients
Beta-blockers	A. Consider starting in all post-MI patients except those with acute symptomatic heart failure or other contraindications B. Use as needed to manage angina, rhythm, or blood pressure in all other patients
Estrogen replacement	A. Consider estrogen replacement in all postmenopausal women B. Individualize recommendation consistent with other health risks

Source: American Association of Cardiovascular and Pulmonary Rehabilitation. Guidelines for Cardiac Rehabilitation and Secondary Prevention Programs. 3rd ed. Champaign, IL, Human Kinetics, 1999, Table 4–3, p 46.

Table 18–14

Recommendations for ECG Monitoring and Close Supervision During Exercise

Lowest risk	Patients are at the lowest level of risk for complications during exercise. They may be monitored for 6–18 sessions, beginning with continuous ECG monitoring along with close clinical supervision initially, decreasing the intensity of ECG monitoring to intermittent during sessions 8–12. Hemodynamic response to exercise should be normal* and progression of the exercise prescription should be regular† during those sessions. Close clinical supervision, which may include direct supervision of exercise sessions, should continue for at least 30 days after the event.
Moderate risk	Patients are moderate risk for complications during exercise. They may be monitored for 12–24 sessions, initially with continuous ECG monitoring along with close clinical supervision, decreasing the intensity of ECG monitoring to intermittent during latter sessions. Hemodynamic response to exercise should be normal* and progression of the exercise prescription should be regular† during those sessions. Close clinical supervision, which may include direct supervision of exercise sessions, may be required for up to 60–90 days after the event.
Highest risk	Patients are at the highest level of risk for complications during exercise. They may be monitored for 18–24 sessions or more, initially with continuous ECG monitoring along with close clinical supervision, decreasing the intensity of ECG monitoring to intermittent during latter sessions. Hemodynamic response to exercise should be normal* and progression of the exercise prescription should be regular† during those sessions. Close clinical supervision, including direct supervision of exercise sessions, may be required for 90 days or more after the event.

* Normal hemodynamic response as defined by appropriately increasing systolic blood pressure, level or falling diastolic blood pressure, appropriately increasing heart rate, and no symptoms indicating exercise intolerance.

† Regular progression of the exercise prescription is defined by periodic (e.g., daily to weekly) progression of the exercise prescription such that functional capacity is increasing and exercise is well tolerated without undue fatigue.

Source: American Association of Cardiovascular and Pulmonary Rehabilitation. Guidelines for Cardiac Rehabilitation and Secondary Prevention Programs. 3rd ed. Champaign, IL, Human Kinetics, 1999, Table 4–4, p 49.

bicycles? The exercise program should produce changes *specific* to the functional needs of the patient, especially those who have upper extremity demands. Upper extremity testing and training must be incorporated into the patients' plans, particularly if they will be returning to a vocation that requires a significant amount of arm work (e.g., maintenance workers, loggers, carpenters, plumbers).

The effects of conditioning last only as long as the individual continues to exercise. Cardiac patients must understand that exercise must be included as a lifetime process for the results to be lasting.

Types of Exercise: Aerobic and Anaerobic

Aerobic exercise involving moving large muscle groups in a dynamic manner has been shown to produce a substantial benefit in cardiorespiratory endurance. Static or isometric (anaerobic) exercise involving the development of tension but little or no change in muscle length or movement for short periods of time may improve strength but may also produce undesirable responses in the cardiac patient. Isometric exercise may, in fact, impose a pressure load on the left ventricle that is not tolerated well, increasing myocardial demand, especially in patients who have poor ventricular function.[28]

Aerobic forms of exercise can be performed continuously and can produce a training effect at workload intensities of 70% to 85% of maximal heart rate (as low as 40% to 50% in the elderly or in individuals with severe ventricular dysfunction) or 50% to 85% of maximal oxygen consumption.[9] Duration and frequency of exercise are also key elements in determining the correct formula for training.

Intensity. Training intensity is the key element in the exercise prescription for an individual starting an aerobic exercise program because if exertion is too intense, training can be compromised, hazardous, or both (Tables 18–15 and 18–16).

Table 18-15
Abnormal Responses to Exercise

Exercise hypertension
Systolic—greater than 240 mm Hg
Diastolic—greater than 110 mm Hg, or until controlled

Systolic hypotension (greater than 20 mm Hg drop from upright resting blood pressure)

Unusual heart rate response—too rapid an increase, failure to increase, or a decrease with exercise

Symptoms
Significant anginal response
Undue dyspnea
Excessive fatigue
Mental confusion or dizziness
Severe leg claudication

Signs
Pallor
Cold sweat
Ataxia
New murmur
Pulmonary rales
Onset of significant third heart sound

ECG abnormalities
Serious arrhythmias
Second- or third-degree heart block
Onset of right or left bundle branch block
Acute ST changes

Source: Guidelines for Cardiac Rehabilitation Centers. 2nd ed. Los Angeles, American Heart Association, 1982.

Heart rate is often a reliable indicator of myocardial and total oxygen requirement during exercise. Heart rate responses are commonly used to quantify and monitor endurance training.

Formulas used to predict appropriate training heart rates have been used in planning exercise programs for healthy individuals and for some patient groups, including those with coronary artery disease (Fig. 18-6). The commonly accepted range of training heart rate is 70% to 85% of maximal heart rate or 50% to 85% of maximal oxygen consumption.[30, 31] The effects of beta blockers, calcium-channel blockers, surgical intervention, and pacemakers, among others, make it improbable that these methods would be accurate for cardiac patients who need more precise and effective measurements. Beta blockers and some calcium-channel blockers decrease resting and exercising heart rate response. However, neither

A $PMHR = 220 - AGE$

B $PMHR = 205 - 1/2\ AGE$

C $Target\ HR = (MHR - RHR)(\%) + RHR$

Figure 18-6. Formulas for calculating predicted and target heart rates. Two formulas for the determination of the predicted maximal heart rate (PMHR) are (A) for the general population and (B) for fit individuals older than 40. *Note:* These formulas should not be used when the true maximal heart rate can be determined or the patient is taking medications that would affect the resting and exercise heart rate (e.g., beta-blocking medications). *C,* The formula for determining a target heart rate (HR) using the Karvonen method multiplies the difference between the maximal and resting heart rates by the training percentage.

beta- nor calcium-blocking medications alter the relationship between the percentage of heart rate and the percentage of oxygen consumption.[32] The important implication is that, when exercise testing an individual before beginning exercise training, the individual should be taking the medication that will be used during the training program.

Table 18-16
Upper Limits (Signs and Symptoms) for Exercise Intensity

Peak exercise training heart rate should be set below the heart rate that occurred at the onset of any of the following:
Angina or other symptoms of cardiovascular insufficiency
Plateau or decrease in systolic blood pressure (SBP)
SBP > 240 mm Hg or diastolic BP > 110 mm Hg
Electrocardiographic evidence of ischemia (ST-segment depression)
Increased frequency of ventricular arrhythmias
Ventricular arrhythmias of >6/minute
Exercise electrocardiographic evidence of left ventricular dysfunction
Other significant ECG disturbances (e.g., second- or third-degree AV block, supraventricular tachycardia, exercise-induced atrial fibrillation)
Level 3-4 dyspnea
Other clear signs or symptoms of exertional intolerance

Source: Adapted from ACSM's Guidelines for Graded Exercise Testing and Prescription. 5th ed. Baltimore, Williams & Wilkins, 1995.

The medication should not be discontinued for the exercise test. If medication that affects heart rate is started or discontinued, or if the dosage is significantly altered after the initial test, a repeat exercise test should be performed to define the training heart rate. The key principle in determining a safe and appropriate intensity of exercise for individuals with heart disease is individualizing the prescription of exercise.

The importance of **ventilatory threshold** in exercise prescription has begun to be examined. This measurement, which is determined during metabolic exercise testing, is the level of exercise at which there is a nonlinear increase in the ventilation in relation to oxygen uptake. It is the estimated upper limit of aerobic exercise. Comparing heart rate relationships with the measured oxygen consumption and the ventilatory threshold provides a much more exact measurement of exertion levels and is a preferred noninvasive method of assessing training limitations. This method is particularly helpful in patients who have multisystem dysfunction, such as coronary artery disease with chronic obstructive pulmonary disease, coronary artery disease and diabetes, and ventricular pump dysfunction. In particular, patients on beta blockers and calcium-channel blockers and those with pacemakers would benefit most from this type of assessment. Most testing, however, is done without metabolic analysis of exercise; therefore, a combination of other intensity parameters should be examined in establishing a training heart rate.

Establishing a training heart rate by rating of perceived exertion. This method of measuring heart rate was first introduced in 1962 by Gunnar Borg[33] (Table 18–17). It is a scale of subjective levels of exertion beginning with "very, very light level," and advancing to "very, very hard level." This scale has been adapted several times to make it more easily understood. It has been shown to be a fairly accurate marker in some studies relating it to ventilatory threshold. Using it in conjunction with other markers of ischemia and arrhythmias and relative to maximal heart rate makes this a very valuable tool, especially for the individual who has difficulty in accurately measuring a pulse, such as in the presence of atrial fibrillation.

Establishing training heart rates using signs and symptoms. Patients may initially demonstrate symptoms of ischemia in the form of angina pectoris, dyspnea, or both. This should always be documented in relation to ECG changes and levels of myocardial oxygen consumption (heart rate times blood pressure). Usually this response has made itself evident in the testing laboratory, and precautions or limitations are documented before exercise training begins. However, changes can occur rapidly in this patient population, and it is often the therapist in the exercise area who first identifies this change (see Table 18–16). Levels of angina should be discussed with all patients before beginning exercise, with instructions as to appropriate responses. Cardiac patients are often allowed and even encouraged to exercise up to level 1 (see Table 18–8) as long as they are comfortable and recover well when they cool down. Some patients prefer to use nitroglycerin during exercise when symptoms begin or even during warm-up to prevent the onset of angina. Taking nitroglycerin often allows them to exercise at higher levels of intensity. Heart rate, blood pressure, and ECG changes must be monitored in these patients.[34]

Dyspnea is often another indication of exercise intolerance and may be used as a guide to limit intensity. Coronary patients with a smoking history and perhaps some degree of chronic obstructive pulmonary disease may find this a particularly useful tool to determine intensity (see Table 18–8).

Continuous Aerobic Training. Aerobic training involves three phases of exercise: a warm-up phase, a peak interval phase, and a cool-down

Table 18–17	
Scales for Rating of Perceived Exertion*	
15 GRADE SCALE	**10 GRADE SCALE**
6 No exertion at all	0 Nothing at all
7 Extremely light	
8	0.5 Very, very light
9 Very light	1 Very light
10	
11 Light	2 Light (weak)
12	
13 Somewhat hard	3 Moderate
14	4
15 Hard (heavy)	5 Heavy (strong)
16	6
17 Very hard	7 Very heavy
18	8
19 Extremely hard	9
20 Maximal exertion	10 Very, very heavy (maximal)

*Comparison of the 6–20 scale and the 0–10 scale.

phase. Each phase is important in the cardiac patient population because it allows certain physiologic adaptations to occur for the patient to exercise safely. The warm-up phase usually lasts 5 to 10 minutes and involves a form of stretching routine of the exercising muscles and a period of slower performance of the aerobic activity (e.g., walking before a walk/jog or before jogging). This allows time for the exercising muscles to achieve adequate stretch to the length they will be used during peak exercise, as well as time for the peripheral vasculature and coronary arteries to dilate and carry larger volumes of arterial blood.

The peak interval usually lasts 15 to 45 minutes, depending on the level of conditioning, and is the period when the individual works at training intensity levels. Established parameters should be checked every 10 minutes or less to determine if the individual is exercising at, above, or below expected levels. The cool-down is a period of 5 to 15 minutes after the peak interval, during which time the exercising muscles are slowly brought to rest. Too abrupt an end or a cessation of exercise can reduce the return of blood to the myocardium, creating irritation and increased arrhythmia. Included in the cool-down period should be some stretching exercises for individuals who are extremely deconditioned or who have notable muscular inflexibility.

Resistance Exercise Training. The previous perception of muscle resistance exercise was that it was harmful or of no benefit to cardiac patients; however, the scientific literature did not support this perception. Instead, muscle strengthening programs using resistive weight exercises have become an acceptable component of cardiac rehabilitation for many patients. As resistive exercises improve muscle strength and endurance, these exercises may improve exercise tolerance as well.[35-37] Muscle strengthening and endurance may be important for the return to activities of daily living and leisure and vocational activities in many patients.

Muscle resistive exercises of low weight (approximately 40% of one repetition maximum) and high repetitions have demonstrated lower myocardial oxygen consumption as compared to dynamic exercise and have proven to be safe and efficacious.[38, 39] Careful selection of candidates is imperative. The American Association of Cardiovascular and Pulmonary Rehabilitation (AACVPR) provides guidelines on patient selection for resistive train-

ing[23] (Table 18–18). Once a patient is cleared as a candidate, the patient needs to be monitored (including HR, BP, ECG, and symptoms) during the initial assessment. The initial assessment may involve a one repetition maximum lift (1-RM), a modified 1-RM (90% of expected repetition maximum), isokinetic testing, or a progressive increase in weight loads to tolerance. After the initial assessment, the resistive program should be performed approximately two to three times/week. The American Heart Association (AHA) and the

---

Table 18–18

Patient Considerations for Resistance Exercise Programming*

Although there are no data documenting safety of resistance training after MI, CABG, or PTCA, certain precautions should be taken. Care must be taken to avoid problems associated with sternal wound healing (CABG) and femoral arterial puncture site (PTCA). In addition, avoidance of excessive myocardial work early after MI is essential.

For all cardiac patients, there must be no evidence of

- Symptomatic congestive heart failure
- Uncontrolled arrhythmias
- Severe valvular disease
- Unstable symptoms
- Uncontrolled hypertension

Patients with moderate hypertension (SBP $\geq$ 160 mm Hg or DBP $\geq$ 100 mm Hg) should be referred to appropriate management, but it is not an absolute contraindication for participation in a resistance training program.

Participation in resistance training may begin following

- A minimum of 5 weeks post MI including 3 weeks of continuous program participation
- A minimum of 8 weeks post CABG including 3 weeks of continuous program participation
- A minimum of 2 weeks of consistent participation post PTCA

---

*A resistance exercise program, for the purposes of this table, is defined as one in which patients lift weights 50% or greater than 1-RM. The use of elastic bands, 1- to 3-lb hand weights and light free weights may be initiated in a progressive fashion at immediate outpatient program entry, provided there are no other contraindications.

Source: American Association of Cardiovascular and Pulmonary Rehabilitation. Guidelines for Cardiac Rehabilitation and Secondary Prevention Programs. 3rd ed. Champaign, IL, Human Kinetics, 1999, Table 7–10, p 112.

Table 18-19

Recommendations for Resistance Training

Pretest: To identify the load that should be performed, a 1 repetition maximum (1-RM) should be performed.

Training: Weights should be set at approximately 30–50% of the 1-RM.

Perform one set of 8–10 repetitions for each major muscle group 2–3 times/week with a day of rest between each workout.

Specific considerations during resistance training:

1. Exercise large muscle groups before small muscle groups.
2. Raise weights slowly with controlled movements, and return weights slowly with controlled movements.
3. Exhale during the exertion phase of the lift, inhale during the return to rest position.
4. Increase loads by 5 to 10 lb when 12–15 repetitions can be performed comfortably.
5. Minimize rest periods between exercises if trying to maximize endurance of muscles.
6. Avoid straining; avoid sustained tight gripping; RPE should be between 11 and 13 (on scale of 20).
7. Stop exercise in event of warning signs or symptoms such as dizziness, palpitations, unusual shortness of breath, or angina.

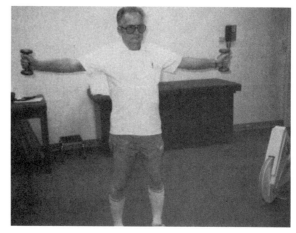

Figure 18-7. This patient is using weights to perform upper extremity exercises.

AACVPR have developed guidelines based upon current literature that recommend a low-intensity program of resistance training for cardiac and older patients[23, 40] (Table 18–19).

Resistive exercise programs can include a variety of options including elastic bands, light hand or cuff weights, free weights or dumbbells, wall pulleys, or weight machines (Figs. 18–7 and 18–8). Table 18–20 lists progressive resistance options.

As the outcome of the resistance program is to return the individual to work, recreational, or daily living activities with less fatigue and less risk of injury, outcome measures should be based upon the limitation assessed. Muscle strength, endurance, and hemodynamic and symptomatic responses to activities should be measured and recorded before and after resistance training sessions.

Circuit Training

Circuit training entails performing a series of activities one after another. At the end of the last activity, one starts from the beginning again and carries on until the entire series has been repeated several times. The advantage is that every individual undergoes a program adjusted to a personal level of fitness. Circuit training can also be performed in a limited space and produces a high degree of motivation.

Flexibility Programs

Activities of daily living, leisure activities, and occupational activities all require an optimal range of motion of joints involved in work; therefore, maintaining or improving range of motion may be an

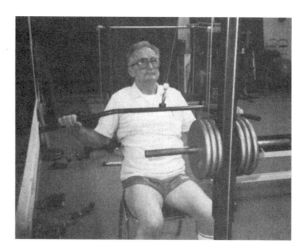

Figure 18-8. This patient is performing a resistance workout as part of a comprehensive cardiac rehabilitation program.

Table 18–20
Options for Progressive Resistance Exercise

Elastic bands (sometimes referred to as Thera-Band)
  Inexpensive
  Variable thickness makes it variable in resistance (different colors are used for different thickness and resistance)
  Progressive resistance can be performed throughout entire range of motion
  Portable; can be carried anywhere

Cuff and hand weights
  Inexpensive
  Variable weight ranges from $\frac{1}{2}$–10 lb
  Portable
  Add to energy cost of activity of walking or other aerobic activity
  Used for progressive resistive exercise as well as increasing energy cost

Free weights: dumbbells and barbells
  Inexpensive
  Variable weights ranging from 1 lb with increments of 1–5 lb
  Dumbbells are handheld; free weight plates are attached on the ends of a barbell
  Used for progressive resistance exercises
  Light dumbbells are portable; heavier weights are not practical to be carried outside rehabilitation center

Wall pulleys
  Relatively inexpensive
  Require little space
  Require some instruction for correct use

Weight machines
  Expensive, requires substantial space
  Used for circuit training or multistation format

important component of the cardiac rehabilitation program. Rehabilitation programs should emphasize proper stretching as part of a warm-up and cool-down, especially of upper and lower trunk, neck, and low back and hip regions. Flexibility exercises should be performed in a slow, controlled manner after the muscle has had an increase in circulation (Fig. 18–9).

Considerations with Exercise Prescription

Most patients entering cardiac rehabilitation programs have not in their recent past been involved in a regular exercise program. Because the large

majority are also in the 40- to 70-year age group, the physical therapist should be concerned about the neuromuscular capability of this patient population. Exercise intensity, especially early on, should consider the patient's relative neuromuscular capability.

Silent ischemia is a phenomenon of changes that can be measured electrocardiographically (ST-segment depression of more than 2 mm lasting longer than 3 min in recovery, T-wave changes, arrhythmias) and hemodynamically (drops in systolic blood pressure and abnormal heart sounds [S_4 gallop] in the absence of angina pectoris). Patients in this group are at high risk for ventricular tachycardia or ventricular fibrillation during exercise training.[41] Exercise intensity must be moni-

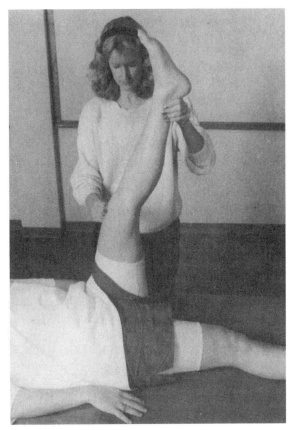

Figure 18–9. Incorporating flexibility exercises into an exercise prescription is important in cardiac rehabilitation. One of the key flexibility exercises involves stretching the hamstring muscle. Hamstring stretching is optimally performed with one leg flat on the table, while the opposite hip is flexed to 90 degrees, starting with the knee bent at 90 degrees. The lower leg (knee to foot) is then passively extended to the end of the passive range while maintaining the pelvis in neutral position.

tored closely and the patient counseled regarding the use of heart rate and rating of perceived exertion in this clinical picture.

Four- Versus Two-Extremity Exercise

Most exercise programs with coronary patients have emphasized dynamic leg exercise; however, activity patterns during daily life are more varied. Many tasks require static or isometric efforts, sometimes in combination with dynamic exercise and often involving more upper than lower extremity efforts. In prescribing exercises for conditioning, it is desirable to impose a large metabolic load on the individual without causing cardiovascular or subjective strain. Spreading the work over greater muscle mass by using arms and legs together may allow a greater load to be tolerated with similar cardiac and subjective strain; however, the ability of the individual with left ventricular dysfunction to tolerate and benefit from this mode of training may vary. Combining upper and lower extremity exercise can produce a higher maximal oxygen consumption than that produced by either body segment alone.[42] A larger actively exercising skeletal muscle mass may explain this finding (Fig. 18–10).

Gutin and colleagues have examined the physiologic response to arm and leg work with special attention to oxygen consumption and ventilatory threshold.[43] They found maximal oxygen consumption and heart rate significantly lower for exercise with arms alone but not for arms and legs combined or legs alone. The ventilatory threshold was significantly higher for arms alone than for legs alone, and even though adding arms to legs did not increase peak physiologic measures, it did not result in the ventilatory threshold occurring at a higher percentage of oxygen consumption. The rate pressure product and rating of perceived exertion were similar for all of these modes. None of the studies comparing two- and four-extremity ergometry included patients with coronary disease.

Emphasis is increasing in exercise and rehabilitation centers on combined arm and leg work (e.g., use of the Schwinn Airdyne ergometer, Nordictrack cross-country ski machines, and hand weights while walking or jogging). In our experi-

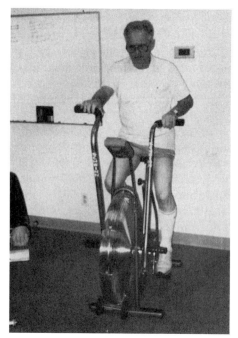

Figure 18–10. This patient is performing a four-extremity exercise.

ence, many coronary patients perceive work performance to be less taxing on four-extremity ergometers than treadmill walking at equivalent rate pressure products and tend to overexercise at unsafe levels. Patients with moderate to poor ventricular function should be monitored closely on this equipment.

Frequency and Duration of Exercise

Just as there is no best method to determine training heart rate, there is no standard exercise duration for all coronary patients. Exercise duration should be individualized and based on several factors:

- Length of disability
- Reduced activity as a result of the acute event
- Premorbid activity level and neuromuscular capability

Individuals who were quite active and who had good to moderate ventricular function usually can tolerate 20 to 30 minutes of exercise within 1 to 2 weeks of beginning the outpatient program, whereas individuals who have sustained considerable ventricular impairment or have a long-standing illness may have difficulty exercising for more than a few minutes before fatigue sets in. These patients usually do best with an intermittent activity program of low intensity, short duration, frequent rest periods, and progressing by systematically reducing periods of rest and increasing periods of exercise. In either case, it is important to remember that the exercising muscle needs time to recover before further activity can be tolerated comfortably. Some patients believe that if 30 minutes of exercise is good, 60 minutes is probably better, and 2 hours better still.

Understanding the way the body recovers from exercise and the need for modified activity patterns and rest periods, especially in phase II, is of utmost importance. Patients should learn that they are just beginning a process that, it is hoped, will last a lifetime and that a slow, systematic approach is not only safer but more enjoyable. The goal is to have the patient reach 45 minutes of continuous aerobic activity, including a warm-up and cooldown period, as soon as the patient can adjust and without exercising beyond the symptom limit. This may take 3 to 6 weeks or longer.

Most patients should be able to tolerate daily exercise. Some patients may find it difficult to maintain the same intensity or duration every day; however, they should be encouraged to work to their prescribed levels at least four times a week for the best conditioning effect. Initially, some patients with less than 20 minutes of exercise tolerance will be asked to work out two times per day and perhaps three times a day if tolerance is 10 minutes or less. Unless a patient is on bed rest or is hospitalized with restricted activity, independent exercise should be possible, even for most high-risk patients, as long as the patient understands how to monitor signs and symptoms and control activity levels. This should be an early lesson to enhance a patient's psychological outlook.

Program Progression

Patients should be taught to pay attention to their bodies' responses to increasing activity and to progress in an orderly fashion based on acceptable evidence of tolerance of the activity (Fig. 18–11). Patients should have their program goals reviewed on a regular basis (at least every 2 weeks initially)

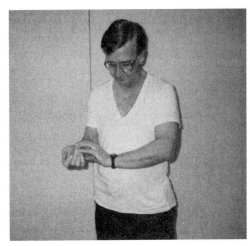

Figure 18–11. This patient is taking his own pulse as part of a self-monitoring instructional session. Patients learn self-monitoring in order to assess the intensity of their exercise session and to be able to progress their activity on their own.

to reestablish guidelines for their exercise program (including contraindications to exercise), and for risk reduction in general. Program progression can take several forms:

- Increasing the *intensity* of exercise
- Increasing the *duration* of exercise
- Changing the *mode* of exercise (e.g., including upper or combined upper and lower extremity exercise)

Many patients in phase II can progress to 85% to 95% or greater of the initial exercise test results, especially if the test was low level, and was stopped before any limiting symptoms appeared. A determination of the patient's safety of progression should be based on a daily observation and reassessment by the therapist. Cardiac bypass patients are often quite limited during the initial few weeks of the program owing to various medical factors, such as a low hemoglobin level and a healing sternum, but they demonstrate a rather quick turnaround and begin to work at much higher levels when these conditions normalize. Upper extremity stretching and strengthening are important with this population in particular and should be included in the exercise program when the sternum is well healed at approximately 6 weeks (Fig. 18–12). Some patients may also develop complications or problems that force them to discontinue their program for a period of time. When they

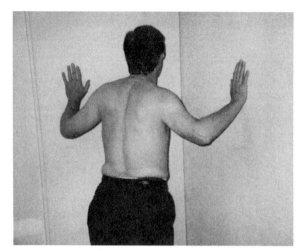

Figure 18-12. This patient is performing postoperative stretching exercises for upper thoracic/pectoral and cervical areas.

resume, they must be cautioned about trying to catch up and progress too quickly. In general, if the individual becomes better conditioned, exercise intensity can be increased without significant increase in heart rate response, symptoms, or ECG changes. Most patients can be expected to increase the peak interval period of exercise by at least 5 minutes a week barring medical complications.

Safety in the Outpatient Cardiac Rehabilitation Setting

Safety in the outpatient cardiac rehabilitation exercise setting must be the top priority for any program. Even with the best precautions, major cardiovascular events may occur, the most frequent of which is sudden cardiac arrest.[9] Selection of appropriate patients who are adequately evaluated and deemed appropriate candidates for training (e.g., under medical supervision outside the program, screened via exercise test before entry to the program); who are cooperative, especially in understanding and use of heart rate and symptoms as limitations in exercise; and who are willing to follow the prescribed medical regimen is of critical importance.

The ability to deal with cardiac arrest and other medical emergencies depends on the immediate response of trained personnel in the exercise area, available emergency equipment, and availability of trained physicians. All professional exercise personnel must be trained to perform immediate ba-

sic cardiac life support in accordance with American Heart Association standards (advanced cardiac life support preferred), including defibrillation. All persons involved with the cardiac rehabilitation program must know their roles and have practice in the various emergency procedures (Tables 18–21 and 18–22).

Most data available demonstrate a relatively low rate for cardiovascular complications during supervised cardiac rehabilitation programs. Van Camp and Peterson's survey of 167 cardiac rehabilitation programs suggests an incidence rate of 8 to 9 per 1 million patient hours of exercise for cardiac arrest, 3 to 4 per 1 million patient hours of exercise for myocardial infarction, and 1.3 per 1 million patient hours for fatalities.[44]

Other precautions with regard to safety in the cardiac rehabilitation setting include

• Avoidance of exercise within 1 to 2 hours after meals
• Avoidance of isometrics and breath holding with exercise
• Adding warm-up and extended cool-off periods of 15 minutes or more with strenuous exercise
• Keeping showers brief and not at a hot or cold temperature (keep legs active)

Other Considerations in Planning Exercise Programs

Altitude

At 3000 feet above sea level and less, most patients find little discomfort exercising; however, above this level, and certainly above 5000 feet, the atmospheric pressure begins to drop, and the body adapts to achieve the same cardiac output by increasing the heart rate. Angina levels may be reached sooner in terms of exercise intensity and physically demanding activity that may not be a problem at sea level. Patients who enjoy skiing (especially cross-country) or who travel to destinations with an elevation above 3500 feet (e.g., Denver, Mexico City) should be counseled about activity guidelines at these levels.

Cold

Cold temperatures cause an increase in peripheral resistance at rest and with exercise. This periph-

Table 18-21
Emergency Procedures for Cardiac Rehabilitation

The following is instituted for persons who demonstrate cardiopulmonary distress and require emergency procedures during cardiac rehabilitation.

A. Nonmonitored patient—Individual who is found unconscious or loses consciousness with no respiration or palpable pulse
  1. Person discovering victim
     a. Assess situation, determine need for CPR
     b. Call for help
     c. Initiate CPR
     d. Remain with patient until relieved
  2. Second person to respond
     a. Call for assistance
     b. Activate the EMS (call 911)
     c. Alert facility, front desk of emergency department, and person to inform medical director
     d. Assist with CPR
  3. Third person to respond
     a. Delivers crash cart to scene of code
  4. Exercise assistants
     a. Assist with CPR
     b. Escort other patients from the area and remain with them
     c. Direct ambulance personnel

If a code is called during cardiac rehabilitation, the cardiac rehabilitation coordinator is in charge of the code procedure. In the coordinator's absence, designated ACLS personnel will assume charge role and initiate ACLS standards of care until the emergency department personnel arrive or the paramedics, if program is held out of hospital.

B. Monitored arrest—The first available staff member who observes the emergency should immediately assess the patient's status and respond by performing the specific procedure that that staff member is authorized to deliver.
    The second available staff member activates the emergency medical system and returns to assist the first rescuer. The third staff member delivers the crash cart to the code site and prepares it for use.
  1. Ventricular tachycardia (losing or lost consciousness), ventricular fibrillation
     a. If observed, administer precordial thump
     b. If no change in rhythm, defibrillate at 400 watts per sec
     c. Wait 10 seconds, check rhythm
     d. If no change, defibrillate again at 400 watts per sec
     e. If no response, initiate CPR
  2. Severe bradycardia, asystole, or other pulmonary emergency—initiate CPR and continue until directed to stop by physician
  3. Severe myocardial ischemia (with persistent symptoms and signs)
     a. Sitting or supine posture, check ECG
     b. Give oxygen and nitroglycerin
     c. Evaluate blood pressure and symptoms
     d. Notify the cardiologist covering the exercise class or the patient's attending physician

Emergency procedures vary according to established hospital and community standards.
CPR, cardiopulmonary resuscitation; EMS, Emergency Medical Service; ACLS, Advanced Cardiac Life Support.

Table 18-22
Basic and Emergency Equipment

BASIC EQUIPMENT	EMERGENCY EQUIPMENT
Blood pressure cuffs and mercury sphygmomanometers (mercury sphygmomanometers are preferred owing to ease of calibration, accuracy, and long-lasting components)	Defibrillator with monitor
Dual-head (bell and diaphragm) stethoscopes	Emergency medications, airway maintenance supplies, artificial respirator, suction machine, and the like (see American Heart Association, Advanced Cardiac Life Support, American College of Sports Medicine Guidelines)
Telemetry monitoring with strip chart recorder	Oxygen and supplies for oxygen administration
Exercise equipment—bicycle ergometers, treadmills, arm ergometers, rowing machines, pulleys, free weights, track, four-extremity ergometers	First aid equipment
Wall clock with second hand	Communication system (telephone)

eral vasoconstriction can subsequently cause an increase in arterial blood pressure and possibly create a situation for earlier ischemic changes with increased myocardial oxygen demands as well as cold-induced vasospasm. Patients exercising outdoors in cold weather should be counseled about the importance of wearing layers of clothing, a wool hat and gloves for body heat retention; and a scarf around the mouth to warm the air; and taking in an adequate amount of fluid despite the lack of noticeable perspiration.

Heat and Humidity

In response to higher temperatures and dilation of peripheral vasculature, heart rate increases to maintain adequate cardiac output. The ability of an individual to perform successfully in hot environments depends on the magnitude of heat, the existing humidity, the movement of air, and the intensity and duration of exercise. The amount of direct exposure as opposed to shade or cloud cover is also a critical factor. One of the primary concerns when exercising in the heat is dehydration. With high sweat rates, the body loses a large volume of water. Because a major portion of the water comes from blood volume, a serious condition exists unless rehydration is accomplished by consuming appropriate fluids (preferably water), both during and after exercise. Again, early symptoms of angina may occur. Avoidance of vigorous exercise or activity in temperatures above 75°F or humidity greater than 65% to 70% is usually recommended. Wearing looser fitting and fewer clothes, protecting the skin by applying a sun screen, exercising at cooler times of the day, and staying in shaded areas as much as possible are recommended. Patients should consult with their physicians before using a steam bath or sauna.

SECONDARY PREVENTION: MANAGEMENT OF RISK FACTORS

Early Intervention

Educating the individual with heart disease about the problem of CAD plays a significant role in preventing further cardiovascular disease and in the rehabilitation process as a whole. Patients and their families must be informed about how to make lifestyle changes and kept up to date on current medical information as it pertains to the disease process. Many changes have occurred in the past 10 years that have had a profound effect on the management of cardiovascular disease, including exercise interventions, dietary modifications, and other lifestyle changes. Once through the crisis stage, and perhaps as early as the first or second day after the event (myocardial infarction, coronary artery bypass graft surgery, or other cardiovascular disorder), patients and their families are most receptive to learning about what they can do to reduce the risk of disease progression. It is at this time that, in addition to being supportive, the health care team (including the physician, nurse, physical therapist, and dietitian) should begin the process of presenting specific information relating to the individual's particular risk factor profile. As patients progress through the hospitalization, small amounts of information in various forms prepare them to make educated choices about their cardiac health.

The Outpatient Setting

A patient's educational background should not be a limiting or predisposing factor in achieving an understanding of the disease and rehabilitative process or risk factor modification. There is no limit to the number of health care professionals, including physicians and nurses, whose level of understanding falls far short of what is necessary to make appropriate "heart healthy" choices. These individuals often need the most guidance and supervision because of the preconceived expectation that they will make all the correct decisions.

Basic education should be provided in both an individual encounter and in a group format. Initially, the patient and the family must understand their particular requirements regarding lifestyle modifications and a specific plan of action. The need to establish a specific time for follow-up should not be overlooked. Frequent checks of the level of understanding and progress being made should be performed by all team members with each visit. If a patient or family member seems to be having difficulty with the plan, for whatever reason, a team member should intervene to determine if goals were set too high, if certain points need to be clarified, or if some other problem mandates attention and program modification (e.g., problems related to the side effect of medications, new symptoms, or psychological problems).

Participation in group education programs is an excellent source of support for patients with similar cardiac diagnoses. Most programs include, and should encourage, spousal or family participation because their concerns and level of understanding play a vital role in the patient's rehabilitation process. Sharing their cardiac experiences helps individuals adjust to their feelings and fears about the present and the future. Skilled, knowledgeable leaders are required for these education programs and should encompass a variety of disciplines because no single individual can address all aspects of care in the depth of expertise required.

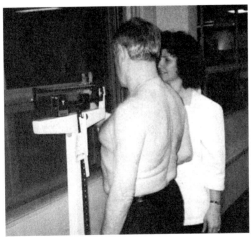

Figure 18-13. The dietitian checks a patient's weight during a cardiac rehabilitation treatment session.

Diet and Nutrition

Dietary management for the cardiac outpatient should be designed to fit that person's specific lipid abnormality, cultural background, and lifestyle. To determine specific needs for intervention, a nutritional assessment should be performed by a dietitian or physical therapist that includes the following anthropometric, biochemical, dietetic, and clinical parameters. Anthropometric parameters include height, weight, weight history, and skinfold measurements (when capable) to help determine the appropriate percentage of body fat. This information is useful in determining ideal weight and may show tendencies of the patient for weight gain or loss (Fig. 18–13). A biochemical analysis includes

- Lipid profile (total serum cholesterol, HDL cholesterol, low-density lipoprotein [LDL] cholesterol, very low density lipoprotein [VLDL] cholesterol, and triglycerides)
- Electrolyte panel (Na^+ and K^+)
- Complete blood cell count (hemoglobin, hematocrit, white blood cells, and platelets)
- Blood urea nitrogen, creatinine, prealbumin and serum albumin

The lipid profile is helpful when the ratio of total cholesterol to HDL cholesterol is calculated and compared with the data collected in the Framingham study.[45] Total cholesterol values should be evaluated as well as values for LDL and HDL cholesterol, total cholesterol to HDL cholesterol, LDL to HDL cholesterol ratio, apolipoproteins, and triglycerides (Tables 18–23 and 18–24). Optimal values for apolipoproteins are still under investigation. Even with an established normal cholesterol level, the validity of the values obtained during the analysis of lipids is questionable.[46] Much discrepancy has been observed among laboratories when lipids are analyzed.[47]

To decrease the risk of coronary artery disease and its progression, it is necessary to increase levels of HDL and decrease levels of LDL cholesterol, total cholesterol, and triglycerides. Studies indicate that for each 1% decrease in total cholesterol there is a corresponding 2% decrease in the risk of developing coronary disease.[48, 49] Lipids may be altered through many methods, some of which offer better results than others (Table 18–25). There are many causes of hyperlipidemia, each of which must be identified and treated. If one method to alter lipids fails, other methods are available.

A complete blood cell count helps to identify patients, especially postoperative patients, who may be limited functionally because of poor oxygen-carrying capacity of the blood cells. Electrolyte panels determine deficiencies or abnormalities in other systems or organs.

Table 18–23

Lipid Values Indicative of Higher Risk

Total cholesterol (mg/dL)	>220	20–29 yr old
(>75th percentile)	>220	30–39 yr old
	>240	40 yr or older
Low-density lipoprotein	>100	
(LDL) (mg/dL)	>175	extremely high risk
High-density lipoprotein	<35	
(HDL) (mg/dL)		
LDL:HDL	3:1	
Triglycerides (mg/dL)	>250	

Source: Data from Lowering blood cholesterol to prevent heart disease. JAMA 253:2080–2090, 1985; Brown WV, Ginsberg H, Karmally W. Diet and the decrease of coronary heart disease. Am J Cardiol 54:27C–29C, 1984; Castelli WP, Garrison RD, Wilson PWF, et al. Incidence of coronary heart disease and lipoprotein cholesterol levels: The Framingham study. JAMA 256:2835–2838, 1986; Heiss G. Are triglycerides a risk factor for ischemic heart disease? An appraisal of evidence. Perspectives in Lipid Disorders 2:15–19, 1985.

Weight Loss

Obesity is a significant risk factor for coronary artery disease, and one reason is the effect that it has on serum lipid levels. Weight loss has been shown to reduce total cholesterol, LDL cholesterol, and triglycerides and to increase HDL cholesterol.[50, 51]

A dietetic or clinical analysis should include a 24-hour recall of food eaten or a 3- to 7-day food diary, and a nutritional history specific for coronary heart disease, including information on the use of fat, types of oils, cholesterol-rich foods, alcohol, caffeine, sucrose, sodium, and fiber. An individual diet prescription can be outlined, utilizing the patient's nutritional history and food preferences as well as estimating caloric needs by considering activity level and basal energy requirements.

Table 18–24

Lipid Management and Recommendations for Intervention

INTERVENTION	RECOMMENDATIONS
Primary goal: LDL < 100 mg/dL	Start AHA Step II Diet in all patients: <30% fat, <7% saturated fat, <200 mg/dL cholesterol

Secondary goals:
HDL > 35 mg/dL
TG < 200 mg/dL
	Assess fasting lipid profile. In post-MI patients, lipid profile may take 4–6 weeks to stabilize. Add drug therapy according to following guide:
	
	LDL < 100 mg/dL: *no* drug therapy
	LDL 100-130 mg/dL: *consider* adding drug therapy to diet listed below
	LDL > 130 mg/dL: *add* drug therapy to diet as listed here:
	  When TG < 200 mg/dL: use statin, resin, niacin
	  When TG 200–400 mg/dL: use stain or niacin
	  When TG > 400 mg/dL: use combined drug therapy of niacin, fibrate, statin
	IF LDL goal *not* achieved: use combination drug therapy
	HDL < 35 mg/dL
	  Emphasize weight management and physical activity
	  Advise smoking cessation, if needed, to achieve LDL goals; consider niacin, statin, fibrate

Key: HDL = high-density lipoproteins; LDL = low-density lipoproteins; TG = triglycerides.
Source: Adapted from the American Heart Association Consensus Panel Statement: Preventing Heart Attack and Death, 1995.

Table 18–25

A Comparison of the Various Methods to Alter Lipids: Effects

METHODS	TOTAL CHOLESTEROL	LDL	HDL	TRIGLYCERIDES
Diet low in cholesterol and saturated fat, high in polyunsaturated fat	−16 to −30% (−27 to −58 mg/dL) (−12 mg/dL per 100 mg/dL decrease in dietary cholesterol)	−38% (−45 mg/dL)	0 to −33% (−6 mg/dL)	−13%
Fish consumption	−8 to −57% (88 mg/dL)	−15% (−17 to −26 mg/dL)	+4 to +18%	−35 to −79% (−237 mg/dL)
Monounsaturated fats	−13 to −18%	−21%	—	—
Increased intake of beans, wheat, oats, and other grains	−10 to −30%	−14 to −24%	−5.6 to −12.7%	−8 to −41%
Vegetarian or modified vegetarian diet	−30 to −58 mg/dL	−20 to −45 mg/dL	−4 to −7 mg/dL	−27 mg/dL
Weight loss	−5.5 to −57 mg/dL	−11.1 to −13 mg/dL	+2.3 to +5 mg/dL	−21.5 to −503 mg/dL
≤ Two cups of coffee/day	−20 mg/dL	−20 mg/dL	—	−10 to −20%
Exercise	−10 to −39.2 mg/dL (−16.4%)	−5 to −8 mg/dL (−13%)	+1.2 to +14 mg/dL (0 to +25%)	−15.8 to −131 mg/dL (−45%)
Smoking cessation	−3.45 to −23 mg/dL	—	+2 to +6 mg/dL	—
Stress reduction	−29 to −47 mg/dL (−4 to −35%)	—	−8 mg/dL	−29 mg/dL
Lipid-lowering drugs	−28 to −48%	−24 to −42%	−9 to +21%	−5.8 to −18.4%

Source: Cahalin LP. A comparison of various methods to alter lipids. Cardiopulmonary Phys Ther 1:5, 1990.

Psychosocial Recovery

Readjustment after a cardiac event can be influenced by the degree of anxiety, depression, or denial each patient manifests on recovery from the acute stage. The more pronounced the symptoms at this point, the poorer the rehabilitation potential. Some of the scientific literature discusses the detrimental effects of depression, hopelessness, social isolation, and acute mental stress on the recovery process and risk of progression of disease.[52–57] The patients' perceptions of their health status are also influenced by previous experience; premorbid health misconceptions; and body concerns, especially an increased awareness of the chest region. According to the AACVPR guidelines, several risk factors for psychosocial adjustment following a cardiac event have been identified (Table 18–26).

The support of the cardiac rehabilitation team and other patients can be a significant factor in reversing this state. Some patients need extra support and education, but exaggerated attention to the disease may be harmful to others. Fostering adequate communication and good relationships with patients promotes recovery by precluding misunderstandings and correcting patients' misperceptions of their state of health. Relatives, neighbors, and friends should be made aware of the goals of the active rehabilitation program. Information must be provided to counteract restrictive attitudes that can lead to psychological invalidism.

During this readjustment period, the patient increases self-confidence and improves self-image while learning an individual response to increasing levels of activity. Sexual activity is still of great interest in the age groups in which heart disease is prevalent. There may be problems due to physical load, effect of medications, or even fear of per-

Table 18–26

Risk Factors for Adjustment Difficulties in Cardiac Patients

Patients with a combination of the following characteristics should be considered at higher risk for adjustment difficulties necessitating additional evaluation and support:

Patients who live alone
Patients who are not married and do not have a confidant
Patients who are recently divorced or widowed
Patients who are socially isolated
Patients from multiproblem families
Patients with low incomes
Patients who smoke
Patients who are obese
Patients who have multiple chronic illnesses
Patients without spiritual or religious comfort
Patients who have impaired cognitive functioning
Patients who have cultural or religious values that conflict with a philosophy of self-reliance and optimism

formance. It is therefore worthwhile to focus on this point in discussions with both the patient and the partner (see Fig. 18–14).

It has been suggested that adequate social support is an important ingredient in recovery from the crisis of acute illness. Mumford and colleagues found that informational and emotional support to hospitalized heart patients can reduce their length of stay.[58] Successful rehabilitation and re-

turn to a productive lifestyle are of interest from the standpoint of both economic benefit and improved quality of life. Another study addresses problems and interventions germane to heart patients. In a controlled study of 46 patients who had experienced a myocardial infarction, researchers found that educational and counseling interventions produced better outcomes in measures of psychological dysfunction, unhealthy lifestyle, and dependence on health care than did educational interventions alone.[59] Successful adjustment has been shown to have a positive impact on medical recommendations, return to work, and morbidity and mortality rates.[60–63] Social support literature is often vague about what specific ingredients or processes within supportive relationships lead to positive health outcomes. In a study of disaster survivors, Murphy addresses this issue and proposes that self-efficacy may be a key variable.[64] Self-efficacy is defined as the individual's expectation of capability to execute a specific behavior. The presence of supportive others seems to increase self-confidence in one's ability to carry out specific behavior. Self-efficacy theory also suggests that levels of self-efficacy can be enhanced by increasing social support generally and by breaking down the specific denied behavior into small manageable steps, which is referred to as goal scaling.[65] According to Southard, the majority of patients recovering from cardiac events have not had their psychosocial needs addressed or optimally treated in both the inpatient and outpatient settings.[66] Therefore, the AACVPR recommends certain guidelines (Table 18–27) in regard to psychosocial concerns of the cardiac rehabilitation patient.

Compliance

A major problem in all cardiac rehabilitation programs regardless of type or structure is compliance. Although the data are variable, only 20% to 50% of participants continue to exercise after 1 year.[67] The factors that promote poor compliance are rather complex and may include duration of rehabilitation, regimen complexity, nature of side effects, presence of symptoms, and social and environmental factors, as well as factors related to the therapist, such as patient-therapist interaction. Another key factor is physician encouragement, sup-

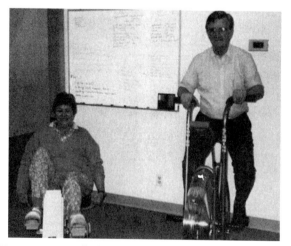

Figure 18–14. Patient (*right*) and spouse enjoying an exercise session together.

Table 18–27
Assessment and Outcomes Related to Psychosocial Concerns

ASSESSMENT

Staff should identify clinical significant levels of psychosocial distress using a combination of clinical interview and psychosocial screening instruments at program entry, exit, and periodic follow-up

OUTCOMES

Clinical: The patient should experience emotional well-being as evidenced by the absence of

1. Psychosocial distress indicated by clinically significant levels of depression, social isolation, anxiety, anger, hostility
2. Drug dependency
3. Excessive psychophysiologic arousal

Behavioral: Program services should enhance the patient's ability to

1. Describe the recovery and rehabilitation process
2. Develop realistic health-related expectations
3. Assume responsibility for behavior change
4. Demonstrate problem-solving capabilities
5. Engage in physical exercise, meditation, and other relaxation techniques
6. Demonstrate effective use of other cognitive-behavioral stress management skills
7. Obtain effective social support
8. Comply with psychotropic medications if prescribed
9. Reduce or eliminate alcohol, tobacco, caffeine usage, or other nonprescription psychoactive drugs
10. Return to meaningful social, vocational, and avocational roles

Source: American Association of Cardiovascular and Pulmonary Rehabilitation. Guidelines for Cardiac Rehabilitation and Secondary Prevention Programs. 3rd ed. Champaign, IL, Human Kinetics, 1999, Guideline 28, p 116.

port, and effectiveness in the role of cardiac rehabilitation team leader.

Programs should include mechanisms to combat recidivism. Strategies generally involve education and behavioral measures, as well as attempts to remove barriers to participation. Such barriers begin with the convenience factor. Location, time of day, and facility amenities are among the determinants of convenience to the patient. Few pa-

tients will travel more than 10 miles to participate in an exercise program, especially if it is not in the same geographic area as their work. Programs should be scheduled to be convenient for employed and retired persons. Facilities and amenities, particularly parking and locker rooms, are other factors in the perception of convenience to the patient.[68]

The rehabilitation team plays a vital role in the long-term compliance of the patient. Strong leadership, enthusiasm, and development of a good relationship between therapist and patient can reinforce and motivate appropriate lifestyle change. The process begins with obtaining a history of the patient's previous exercise habits, health beliefs, and perceptions of the need to make lifestyle changes. This helps in setting reasonable goals and in identifying potential problems. Special efforts should be made to improve patients' satisfaction with the care and attention they receive. At the same time their concept of self-management should be reinforced by encouraging them to take responsibility for their own health actions and providing techniques for self-monitoring, such as the rating of perceived exertion and heart rate limits. Patients can thus obtain more immediate feedback, which, in turn, becomes a powerful source of reinforcement for maintaining the exercise habit. Involving the family as much as possible, including allowing spouses to exercise with patients, is encouraged.

Outcome Measurement

According to the AHCPR's summary of the scientific literature on cardiac rehabilitation, the most substantial results of cardiac rehabilitation services are identified in Table 18–28. In addition, the

Table 18–28
Substantial Benefits of Cardiac Rehabilitation

Improvement in exercise tolerance
Improvement in symptoms
Improvement in blood lipids
Reduction in cigarette smoking
Improvement in psychosocial well-being and reduction of stress
Reduction in mortality rate

Factors Not Affected by Cardiac Rehabilitation Exercise Training Alone

Body weight (when exercise training was a sole intervention)
Rates of nonfatal reinfarction
Development of coronary collateral circulation
Regression or limitation of progression of angiographically documented coronary atherosclerosis (when exercise training was a sole intervention)
Ventricular ejection fraction and regional wall motion abnormalities
Occurrence of cardiac arrhythmias

- Blood pressure (at rest and with activity)
- Exercise tolerance
- Symptoms (at rest and with various activities)
- Psychological well-being
- Quality of life
- Morbidity
- Mortality

Table 18-30 provides the three outcome domains that should be monitored (health, clinical, and behavioral) as well as examples of specific measures for each domain.

Follow-up Assessment

Routine follow-up assessment by each team member should be performed and discussed with the patient at least twice a month during the subacute and intensive rehabilitation phases. At this time each team member should review the progress made by the patient since entering the program and any problems (risk factors) that still need to be modified. New short-term goals and changes in the program should be established as patients increase their exercise performance and are cleared to resume various activities, for example, returning

measures that were *not* strongly affected by cardiac rehabilitation, and in particular the exercise training, include those factors in Table 18-29. Therefore, specific outcome measures that can be utilized in a multidiscipline outpatient cardiac rehabilitation include:

- Lipid changes
- Smoking cessation
- Body weight

Outcomes: Three Domains with Their Corresponding Categories

BEHAVIORAL	CLINICAL	HEALTH
Diet	Physical	Morbidity
		Future events
		MI
		CABG
		Angioplasty
		New angina
		Serious arrhythmias
Weight management	Weight	
Exercise	Blood pressure	Mortality
Smoking cessation	Lipids	
Stress reduction	Functional capacity	Quality of life
Recognition of signs/symptoms	Blood nicotine levels	
Medical management	Oxygenation, O_2 saturation	
	Symptom management	
	Psychosocial	
	Return to vocation/leisure	
	Psychological status	
	Medical utilization	
	Hospitalizations	
	Medication	
	Physician/ER visits	

to work. A copy of these assessments must be forwarded to the attending physician, who remains the primary physician throughout.

Criteria for Discharge

When to discharge a patient from any program is a difficult decision to make, probably more so for cardiac patients because they are making lifelong changes, some of which require long-term support mechanisms from the appropriate sources. It is not easy for the patient and spouse to maintain a continuous awareness of the requirements of the program, and self-motivation is often hard. However, reimbursement agencies are requesting definitions of discharge criteria, and perhaps they are correct in trying to identify the point at which the individual is considered to have completed the rehabilitation phase of recovery. Therefore, rehabilitation goals and plans must be outcome-oriented. Some key points for discharge (adapted from the Guide to Physical Therapist Practice)[20] include the following:

- The anticipated goals and the desired outcomes have been achieved.
- Patient/client declines to continue intervention.
- Patient/client is unable to continue to progress toward goals because of medical or psychosocial complications.
- Failure to make reasonable progress toward goals, owing to
  - Nonadherence to the home program
  - Failure to attend scheduled appointments
  - Lack of willingness or ability to participate in the program

Records and Documentation

Records provide a method of retrieving information, evaluating the value and validity of the rehabilitation process, and analyzing cost effectiveness and quality assurance. Records should be kept thoroughly and accurately, subject to periodic analysis, and include

- Attending physician referral and authorization for treatment
- Copies of pertinent medical data: results of ECG, echocardiogram, exercise tests, other noninvasive

tests, cardiac catheterization report, results of cardiac surgery, and report from attending physician
- Initial cardiac rehabilitation evaluation summary and goals listed by team members
- Regular progress notes from each session that summarize the patient's performance, including resting and exercise heart rates, resting and exercise blood pressures, signs and symptoms, workload, peak interval time, ECG results, and any other pertinent data (e.g., medication changes, physician appointments, environmental conditions)
- Monthly reports to attending physician as summarized by the medical director, program coordinator, and staff
- Monthly log records—copies of patient's home records (e.g., exercise log, weight record, diet diary)
- Discharge summary, including progress the patient has made regarding functional changes; physiologic and psychological changes; risk factor modifications achieved and those still needing further attention; compliance with home program; reasons for limited change, if that is the case; recommendations for follow-up testing or counseling; and reason the patient is being discharged

Medical and Legal Considerations

At times, certain legal and insurance considerations assume a very significant role in the rehabilitation of the cardiac patient. Possible legal problems stem from two aspects of this program:

- Adverse effects of medically prescribed exercise testing and fitness conditioning
- Consideration of disability pension and insurance benefits that may influence the patient's motivation to return to work and may affect the attitude of an employer toward a person with "a heart problem"

Exercise testing and recommendations to patients in the conditioning program by a physician constitute medical treatment. All medical personnel must be continuously alert to those aspects of testing and training that are eventually dangerous to each individual. They must pay special attention to recognize indications and contraindications to be sure that a thorough pre-exercise screening examination has been performed, that the exercise sessions are properly supervised and monitored, and that exercise is terminated when potentially dangerous situations arise. There must be adequate advance preparation for and training in emergency procedures in accordance with generally accepted medical standards. Patients also must be fully informed of the potential benefits, risks, and hazards associated with exercise conditioning programs and be given an opportunity to ask questions and withdraw from treatment without jeopardy of future medical care so that the informed consent document can be classified as legally valid. In addition, when a physician authorizes a return to work for the patient, the physician must understand the duties and potential hazards of the work for which clearance is being given.

Charges to Patients and Third-Party Carriers

Cardiac rehabilitation is not a major income producer in most facilities. In fact, cardiac rehabilitation often has difficulty breaking even in many settings in which both direct and indirect costs are factored, the latter being difficult to budget. Cardiac rehabilitation is considered by many administrations to be part of the total picture of cardiology care (product line) and can, to some degree, be carried by other subdepartments, given the positive influence a quality cardiac care program can have on the hospital and the community. The business structure and nature of each program and the overhead expenses dictate how fees are established. During the 1990s dramatic changes in health care management and subsequently health care reimbursement took place. As a result of a changing health care environment, personnel in the program should stay current with changes in health care costs and health care reimbursement. Specifically, personnel should verify each individual's policy, level of reimbursement and number of rehabilitation sessions covered by each plan. Private health care plans change regularly as they are being bought and sold by other agencies, there-

fore, each enrollee should be assessed for health care plan, and a telephone number to contact the insurance company to verify cardiac rehabilitation reimbursement. Some health maintenance organizations (HMOs) have contracts with specific institutions and may cover only six sessions of outpatient rehabilitation, whereas all inpatient care is covered. Sometimes these organizations require a letter to the medical director of the HMO to explain the seriousness of the patient's condition asking for greater than six sessions to be covered.

As of 1997, Medicare provided for cardiac rehabilitation for up to 12 weeks or 36 visits of an approved outpatient cardiac rehabilitation program for individuals with a diagnosis of acute myocardial infarction (within the preceding 12 months), who have undergone coronary bypass surgery, or who have stable angina pectoris and are considered to have a medical need for cardiac rehabilitation. Because a growing percentage of the cardiac patient population is covered by Medicare, it is important to have the program certified by Medicare. Many other insurance carriers follow Medicare's lead in coverage and, as Medicare changes, they will probably follow.

Medicare's additional requirements include that a designated area for the rehabilitation be established, a physician and cardiopulmonary emergency equipment must be readily available, and that staffing must consist of qualified personnel. Table 18–31 gives Medicare guidelines for obtaining reimbursement. Blue Cross–Blue Shield coverage varies considerably from state to state; however, the national policy is to support and provide some degree of coverage.

Patient education is felt to be the role of the physician and is not reimbursed. State-aid agencies rarely cover cardiac rehabilitation services. Nutrition counseling is rarely reimbursed as a separate service. Reimbursement for exercise testing depends on the policy; however, it is usually reimbursed as a procedure when ordered by the physician before commencing rehabilitation.

It is important to the financial success of the program to be familiar with reimbursement rates, company policies, and limitations in coverage of insurance companies in the area for inpatient and outpatient cardiac rehabilitation. Policies regarding treatment of uninsured or uncovered services must be established and understood by all team

Table 18-31

Medicare Guidelines for Reimbursement and Fee-for-Services Payment

PROFESSIONAL STAFF SHOULD:

Obtain a signed physician order from the referring physician with appropriate Medicare diagnosis code for establishing medical necessity.

Obtain the *Physician's Current Procedural Terminology* (known as the CPT-4 Code Book), which is a listing of all outpatient procedures applied within the services of medicine. Review the established numerical code for each procedure. As part of the 1998 CPT-4 Code Book, the following two codes are appropriate to the program:

93797—physician services for outpatient program without continuous ECG monitoring (The 92797 code is subject to regional interpretation and is not accepted by all intermediaries.)

93798—physician services for outpatient program with continuous ECG monitoring

Identify the appropriate diagnosis code that must accompany the procedure charge. The diagnosis code is obtained in two steps: (1) the physician must denote the diagnosis on referral, and (2) the diagnosis is coded using the *International Classification of Diseases* also called the ICD-9 Code Book. Current acceptable diagnoses and codes for reimbursement are as follows:

Stable angina	413.9
CABG	414 and then V45.81
Anterolateral MI	410.02
Anterior AMI	410.12
Inferior lateral AMI	410.22
Inferior AMI	410.42
Lateral AMI	410.52
Unspecified AMI site	410.92

Where required, obtain preadmission or precertification for services, recording

Insurance policy, managed care plan, and coverage benefits

Appropriate contact person

Precertification confirmation, notation of number of visits, time of service, copayments, and amount of reimbursement

Source: American Association of Cardiovascular and Pulmonary Rehabilitation. Guidelines for Cardiac Rehabilitation and Secondary Prevention Programs. 3rd ed. Champaign, IL, Human Kinetics, 1999, Table 9–5, p 193.

members and explained to the patient and family before commencing the rehabilitation program. Each individual should also be familiar with the program charges for each phase. Some programs take the position that it is the patient's responsibility to find out whether a particular insurance company covers cardiac rehabilitation. Having someone who can answer basic questions about insurance coverage can be helpful when the patient and family are going through a stressful time.

Special Patient Populations

The prescription of exercise for special patient populations requires the integration of clinical information and exercise physiology. The need for an appropriate exercise prescription in patients with noncardiac disease has been documented; however, patients with multiple system dysfunction may require special attention. The more we learn about exercise and disease, the more we find an influence of one on the other. Women, children, and the elderly are distinct groups that also may require a different approach with cardiac rehabilitation. Therefore, the following sections provide additional information to consider when working with these populations.

Patients with Peripheral Vascular Disease

Peripheral vascular disease is a fairly common disorder among individuals with coronary artery disease. The limiting factor to exercise is claudication—angina-like pain usually in the buttocks, the calf of one or both lower extremities, or both. Much like angina, claudication is related to exertional level. Exercise training has demonstrated significant functional improvement with reduction of symptoms at equivalent workloads.[69, 70] Patients must be tolerant of working to various levels of discomfort, and the supervising therapist should use a symptom-limited approach with varying modes of exercise. One mode should include walking because it is the most functional and usually limited activity for the individual to perform. Cigarette smokers must also agree to a smoking cessation program if they are serious about reducing their risk of disease progression.

Patients with Chronic Obstructive Pulmonary Disease

Many patients with coronary disease have a long-standing history of cigarette smoking with some degree of obstructive airway disease. Some individuals may be taking medications (e.g., theophylline) that are known to induce supraventricular arrhythmia with activity. Dyspnea levels, discussed earlier in this chapter (see Intensity), are most effective for determining an appropriate exercise intensity level. For patients with chronic obstructive pulmonary disease, pursed-lip breathing may enhance exercise performance because it helps control ventilation and oxygenation by reducing respiratory rate and increasing tidal volume, and improving ventilation of previously underventilated areas. Use of upper extremity support with exercise, such as holding the bars of treadmills, stationary bikes, and rolling walkers, may assist the patient in stabilizing accessory muscles for improved ventilation. In more severe cases, supplemental oxygen may be of benefit. Blood saturation levels with exercise should be monitored, but preferably with arterial blood gases. Pulse oximetry is the minimal amount of monitoring. The supervising therapist should pay close attention to clinical signs of desaturation (e.g., blue nail beds and overall change in coloration). Additional information on pulmonary rehabilitation is found in Chapter 19.

Clinical Note: Beta-blocking Medications and Dyspnea

Caution should be taken with patients who have COPD and who are taking beta-blocking medications, specifically nonselective beta blockers (e.g., Inderal). These medications block sympathetic stimulation to the $beta_1$ receptors in the heart as well as the $beta_2$ receptors found in the smooth muscles of the bronchi. The result of blocked $beta_2$ receptors can be bronchoconstriction, resulting in an increase in dyspnea. Because this increase in dyspnea *may* occur with some $beta_1$ selective drugs, evaluation of dyspnea is a critical component during exercise (particularly auscultation for wheezing with exercise).

Patients with Diabetes Mellitus

Diabetes is a risk factor for coronary disease, and diabetic patients are three times more likely to have coronary artery disease than nondiabetics.[71] In addition, type II diabetes (noninsulin-dependent type, which includes 80% to 90% of all diabetics) is associated with obesity. Research on the effect of exercise on the lives of patients with type II diabetes has been promising, demonstrating improvements in insulin activity and glucose tolerance, potential reductions in dosage and need of insulin or oral hypoglycemic medications, and reduction of body fat.[72] Patients should be cautious and aware of signs and symptoms of hypoglycemic episodes that can occur during or after the exercise session. Just before starting an exercise session each day, the patient should obtain a pre-exercise blood glucose reading. This reading is in addition to that for the daily fasting blood glucose value. If the pre-exercise blood glucose value is between 100 and 300 mg/dL, the person can engage in exercise. Because of the enhancement of insulin sensitivity with exercise, persons with diabetes should abstain from exercise during the peak activity of their insulin. If the pre-exercise value is equal to or greater than 300 mg/dL, exercise may induce a rise in blood glucose rather than a decline. Because of the major role of glucose as a fuel for exercise, there may not be enough energy to sustain the exercise if the pre-exercise blood glucose level is equal to or less than 100 mg/dL. The person may become hypoglycemic. Some form of simple carbohydrate (e.g., juice, sugar, glucose) should be kept in the exercise area in case of such an emergency.

As with anyone who exercises, persons with diabetes should begin the session with a 5- to 10-minute warm-up, which includes stretching and light calisthenics. At the end of the session, time must be allotted for a cool-down session. The exercise prescription for a person with diabetes is similar to the nondiabetic. Because of the postexercise recovery phase, a person may have a decrease in blood glucose values for up to 24 hours. Persons with diabetes must be told that on days they do not engage in exercise their blood glucose values may be higher. See Chapter 7 for more information on diabetes.

Clinical Note: Hypoglycemic Symptoms

Similarly, individuals who are diabetic and on beta-blocking medications should be monitored closely when initiating or progressing their exercise prescription. When an individual becomes hypoglycemic the sympathetic nervous system produces a systemic response, including tremors, rapid heart rate, and lightheadedness, which are warning signs to increase sugar intake immediately. Beta-blocking medications block the sympathetic response to hypoglycemia, thereby blocking all the warning signs as well.

Patients Who Have Had a Cerebrovascular Accident

Some individuals present to the cardiac rehabilitation program with impaired ventricular function, having previously sustained a cerebrovascular accident. They therefore have special medical and physical needs. Common sequelae of cerebrovascular accidents include weakness or neglect of one or more extremities, problems in communication, cognitive-perceptual dysfunction, and dysphagia.[73] Inability to exercise weakened muscles or ones with excessive tone for prolonged periods may necessitate exercise of short duration. Despite unilateral limb dysfunction, the use of four-extremity ergometers such as the Schwinn Airdyne may allow for greater intensity of exercise. Blood pressure and heart rate responses to isometric and to upper and lower extremity ergometry have been found to be no greater in those who have had cerebrovascular accidents than in an age-matched control group[74]; however, with four-extremity ergometry and impaired ventricular function these patients are extremely important to monitor. The supervising therapist should be attuned especially to symptoms that exercising patients may have but cannot easily express because of a communication disorder.

Patients with Renal Disease

Patients with end-stage renal disease can benefit significantly from regular exercise training, although they may not exhibit the same responses to exercise as the patients usually seen in the cardiac rehabilitation program. Exercise tolerance in patients on hemodialysis has been found to be significantly below normal.[75, 76] This low tolerance is probably due to lower arterial oxygen content because of

- Lower hematocrit and hemoglobin values for oxygen transport
- Altered stroke volume affected by the disease or its treatment
- Peripheral factors as a result of autonomic dysfunction and metabolic acidosis

Exercise training has been found to increase physical work capacity, increase HDL cholesterol levels, and increase hematocrit values in this group. Improvements in glucose tolerance, blood pressure control, and physiologic profiles—important risk factors for heart disease—also result from exercise training.[77] Exercise sessions should be scheduled according to the patient's condition before and after dialysis and the time requirements of the treatment. Often the day before and the day of dialysis are the patient's weakest days. Intermittent exercise, with work-to-rest ratios of 1:2 or 1:1, may be appropriate initially, although most patients can gradually increase to 30 to 45 minutes of continuous exercise over time. Training heart rates are difficult to use because of variable heart rate response, medication schedule, and physiologic changes that occur in these patients from day to day depending on their dialysis schedule. The Borg perceived exertion scale works well in evaluating these patients (see Table 18–17).

Heart Disease and Women

Coronary artery disease is the leading killer of women and kills more women than *all* cancers combined.[78] Studies report that coronary artery disease is underdiagnosed and undertreated in women as compared to men.[79] This finding is related to the fact that women present a different clinical picture, and therefore present a different challenge to both primary and secondary prevention programs. Women are usually older (an average of 10 years older) than men when first presentation of the disease occurs and present with different symptoms; they are more likely to complain of abdominal pain, nausea, fatigue, or short-ness of breath.[80, 81] Women also are less likely than men to be referred for diagnostic tests and intervention. The sensitivity and specificity of diagnostic testing for coronary artery disease differ in women, especially in exercise testing.[80, 82] Certain diagnostic tests, particularly exercise echocardiography and exercise thallium sestamibi testing offer more prognostic information than exercise testing alone.[83, 84] Long-term survival rates are similar for men and women after coronary artery disease procedures (angioplasty and CABG surgery), however, the mortality rate is higher in women at the time of the actual procedure.[80, 85–87]

Certainly cardiac rehabilitation is a recommended treatment following any cardiac procedure or acute injury, but limited information exists on compliance with cardiac rehabilitation in women.[88] Studies including women have shown improvements after cardiac rehabilitation similar to those in men with regard to risk factor modification, exercise training, and psychosocial and vocational counseling.[89–92] However, women are less likely than men to enroll in cardiac rehabilitation,[93] and their drop-out rates are higher than men.[94] In programs in which women are brought together for exercise and education sessions separately from the men, compliance to rehabilitation has not been a problem. Therefore, separate times for women may be a recommendation to encourage compliance.

Pediatric Programs

As children with congenital cardiovascular disorders survive into their adult years, it becomes increasingly important to evaluate, train, and advise them and their families in activity and exercise prescription guidelines. Cardiac rehabilitation for children after cardiac surgery is emerging as an area of considerable interest. The Children's Hospital National Medical Center in Washington, D.C., has established a 12-week training program focusing on this specialty in an environment similar to that used in an elementary and secondary physical education class.[95] It is led by experienced physical education teachers who have expertise in current methodology and techniques of physical education and by other staff members, including exercise specialists and a pediatric cardiologist.

Parents and siblings are encouraged to participate in the activity component of the program. These programs have demonstrated significant improvement in the child's physical work capacity as well as improved social interactions.

Cardiac rehabilitation in children should be provided to patients with repaired complex congenital diseases who have functional or psychosocial problems with the disease. The purpose of these programs are to improve exercise efficiency, aerobic capacity, and quality of life, as well as to reduce the incidence of sudden death and enable young individuals to participate safely and effectively in sports. Upon survey of international centers, very few actually treat pediatric cases. Of those who were surveyed, the chief outcome of these programs demonstrated increased exercise capacity, increased cardiac output at rest and with peak exercise, increased O_2 uptake, increased exercise test duration, and improved quality of life.[96]

Screening of children for cardiovascular risk has become a topic of interest and some controversy. The American Academy of Pediatrics recommends screening children with a family history of premature coronary artery disease or hyperlipidemia; others support mass screenings of all children because some research has shown as many as two thirds of the children with elevated cholesterol levels would go undetected by use of the Academy's recommendations.[97, 98] Several studies have noted a stronger relationship between several risk factors such as exercise and serum lipids and glucose intolerance and weight-height and skinfold thickness.[99] Advocates of mass screening also encourage aggressive early management of hyperlipidemia in this population and point to school-based interventions as the best means of reaching the greatest number of children.[100]

The Elderly Coronary Patient

Most elderly cardiac patients who have not exercised in their recent past probably have low expectations and possibly negative attitudes toward the rehabilitation process, participating only because their physicians told them they should. These same individuals may show the most improvement functionally. Exercise can promote a sense of well-being and heighten self-esteem, both of which are essential to independent living.

Regular physical activity can modify known coronary risk factors in the elderly. In a study of elderly Japanese men in Hawaii, higher levels of physical activity were associated with higher serum HDL and lower triglyceride levels.[101] Likewise, elderly athletic men have been shown to have higher HDL levels and lower total cholesterol–to-HDL ratios than elderly sedentary men.[102]

Many elderly patients present with multiple joint and musculoskeletal limitations. Therefore, a thorough mechanical assessment should be performed before initiating any exercise program. To achieve the greatest success early in the program and to diminish patient discouragement because "it hurts too much," light calisthenics and stretching exercises should be employed. Jarring activities such as jogging should be minimized to avoid musculoskeletal injury. Swimming is an excellent exercise; however, some weight-bearing activity should be encouraged, especially for women, to forestall the adverse effects of osteoporosis. A cool-down period is especially important for the elderly following aerobic activity and should actually be of slightly longer duration for adequate recovery. Frequency of exercise may need to be limited to every other day to give the musculoskeletal system a chance to rest.

PRIMARY PREVENTION

Cardiac rehabilitation for individuals with coronary artery disease might not be necessary for many individuals if primary prevention of the disease existed (active intervention for risk factors that cause coronary artery disease). Therefore, primary prevention is an important component of wellness and rehabilitation programs that should be incorporated in all programs. Candidates for a primary prevention are those individuals who are at moderate or high risk of developing coronary artery disease (prior to manifestation of the disease) and those with family histories of heart disease.

When presenting the need for primary prevention programs one needs only to look at the statistics regarding the prevalence of modifiable risk factors in the current population.[103–106] Cigarette smoking is the number one most preventable cause of disease, disability, and death in the United States today.[103] Over half of all adult Americans have a blood cholesterol level of over 200 mg/dL.[106] One in four adult Americans have hypertension.[104] In addition, there is a large proportion of the population in the United States that leads a sedentary lifestyle, despite the fact that epidemiologic studies have documented evidence demonstrating that regular physical activity protects against the development and progression of several chronic diseases. Obesity, identified as an important risk factor for both men and women, appears to interact with or amplify the effects of other risk factors, although the mechanisms are unknown. Obesity has increased over the past 20 years, and statistics state that 47 million adult Americans are overweight, therefore making this risk factor a serious health problem.[105] Primary prevention programs therefore have a large target audience.

Two major problems inherent in a primary prevention program are compliance (especially long term) and lack of payment for services by medical insurance companies. Also, the expected outcome of a primary prevention program is a lack of manifestation of the disease, which is a difficult outcome to measure for an individual. This often creates a situation of denial or "it won't happen to me" attitude, which interferes with continual motivation and subsequently compliance. In addition, when medical insurance companies do not reimburse payment for services, individuals are less likely to continue to pay for services. Therefore, similar statistics as reported in the fitness literature regarding compliance and long-term commitment to diet, exercise training, and behavior modification would be applicable to this population.[106]

Although research is somewhat limited in long-term outcomes of primary prevention programs, scientific literature does support the reduction of risk factors as a result of a primary prevention program.[103–106] Risk factors that are affected by a primary prevention program include reduction of total cholesterol to HDL ratio, reduction in LDL cholesterol, improvement in aerobic capacity and exercise tolerance, reduction in weight, reduction in resting blood pressure in hypertensive individuals, improved glucose tolerance and insulin sensitivity, improved feeling of well-being, and improved tolerance to stressful situations. Therefore, the components of a primary prevention program should include:

- Development of an aerobic exercise prescription
- Dietary counseling for those with diabetes, weight management problems, and elevated cholesterol
- Stress management or biofeedback
- Smoking cessation
- Pharmacologic management for blood pressure, diabetes, or hypercholesterolemia

Primary prevention programs should be implemented at the work site, fitness centers, senior citizen centers, and primary physician's offices as well as the cardiac rehabilitation centers. As most primary prevention programs are not reimbursed from medical insurance, individual fee for service or monthly payment plans may motivate more participation in these programs. Until the time that scientific and clinical outcomes demonstrate the efficacy of such programs, primary prevention will not be reimbursed under health care plans. Encouragement by primary physicians also increases involvement in a program. Centers that provide these services should therefore be documenting both short-term and long-term (morbidity, mortality rates) outcomes for possible inclusion in medical insurance reimbursement plans in the future.

CASE STUDIES

Case 1. Effect of Cardiac Rehabilitation on a Young Patient with Idiopathic Cardiomyopathy

Clinical History

On September 15, 1996, JS, a 22-year-old man, was admitted to the hospital from his doctor's office following a work-up for progressive dyspnea and orthopnea of 10 days' duration. The chest radiograph demonstrated cardiomegaly with pulmonary vascular engorgement and pulmonary venous hypertension. The ECG demonstrated left axis deviation, left ventricular hypertrophy, and diffuse Q waves anteriorly and inferiorly. Echocardiography demonstrated a dilated left ventricle with severe generalized hypokinesis and an estimated ejection fraction of 15% to 17%. On admission, his resting heart rate was 120 bpm, blood pressure 132/102 mm Hg, and respiratory rate 28; he had a loud S_3 heart sound, and S_4 on auscultation.

JS was diagnosed as having a dilated cardiomyopathy of unknown origin, and he received conservative treatment for congestive heart failure, including high doses of furosemide (Lasix, 80 to 120 mg), captopril, continuous oxygen, and establishment of a 1-g sodium diet. He was placed on strict bedrest and made a rather miraculous recovery during the next 7 days.

Cardiac Rehabilitation

On September 22, JS was referred to cardiac rehabilitation for monitoring during low-level activity, beginning with getting out of bed and into a chair. During the next several days his program was slowly advanced to include ADLs and progressive ambulation. He tolerated low-level activity well and had appropriate physiologic responses; however, it became difficult to restrain his activity as he began to feel stronger. Repeat echocardiography on September 29 still demonstrated severe left ventricular hypokinesis, not quite as sluggish, with an estimated ejection fraction of 20% to 25%. On September 30, JS was discharged from the hospital to his grandmother's house and given a 2-g sodium diet and very low-level activity guidelines. He was told not to exceed household ambulation and to avoid climbing stairs.

JS was a 6-foot 1-inch, well-built auto mechanic who lived in a second-floor apartment with his girlfriend. He had smoked cigarettes since he was 14 years old and consumed 4 to 6 cans of beer per day. He weighed 205 lb on admission to the hospital and diuresed 17 lb before his discharge.

Outpatient Program

JS underwent low-level treadmill testing on October 4 and began outpatient cardiac rehabilitation on October 6. Treadmill test results were very good considering his clinical status and degree of left ventricular dysfunction (see Exercise Tests). His training program results during the first 6 months were also very impressive.

Training Program

Date	Initial	1 month	2 months	3 months	6 months
Time (peak int)	3 × 5 min	5-20-5	5-30-5	5-30-5	5-40-5
Training heart rate (bpm)	120–126	132–138	132–144	132–150	150
Workload (treadmill, mph)	2	2.5–3.0	3.0	3.4	4–5
Weight (lb)	190	192	188	194	196

JS moved back to his apartment in January 1997 and returned to part-time employment in April 1997, again working on cars. In May 1997 JS stopped coming to cardiac rehabilitation although we did keep in touch with him by telephone. He reported that he was doing well and complying with his home exercise program and dietary regimen; however, he refused to come in for a follow-up visit. In November 1997, JS was readmitted to the hospital's intensive care unit in overt congestive heart failure, his weight 211 lb. Over the next 10 days he gradually improved. Nonetheless, the physician decided to have him evaluated for heart transplant at the University Hospital. Following a work-up by the heart transplant team, JS was declared to be a good candidate for transplantation; however, because of his limited finances and the scarcity of donor organs, JS was placed on a potential recipient list, and he was discharged home with high doses of Lasix, captopril, and digoxin, guidelines for low-level activity, and a beeper to signal when a donor organ was received. In the meantime, he was referred back to the cardiac rehabilitation program, where he worked closely with the rehabilitation team, especially with the dietitian, who helped JS and his girlfriend adopt a reasonable low-sodium diet plan.

As time progressed, JS demonstrated significant progress with his program. Four months after evaluation for cardiac transplantation, he decided to take himself off the list of potential recipients. Recent repeat echocardiography demonstrated marked global hypokinesis; however, in comparison with previous studies, left ventricular systolic function appeared to have improved. JS remains compliant with his home program of exercise and strict low-sodium diet and is reassessed regularly (at least monthly) in the phase IV program. His weight fluctuates within 6 pounds, and he is back in school studying computer programming.

Exercise Tests

Date	Initial	12/96	5/97	8/98	9/99
Protocol	Balke 2	Balke 3	Bruce	Bruce	Bruce
Time (min)	10	9	9	10	11
Heart rate (bpm)	87–170	89–187	90–185	66–188	74–186
Mean blood pressure (mm Hg)	146/96	178/70	180/80	176/84	180/90
ECG	PACs	PAC, PVCs	PVCs	PVCs	PVCs
$\dot{V}O_{2\,max}$ (mL/kg/min)	18.8 (39%)	26.7 (56%)	24.4 (52%)	22.7 (48%)	26.2 (56%)
Heart rate at ventilatory threshold (bpm)	136	145	150	165	160
Weight (lb)	189	191	194	192	187

Case 2. Effect of Cardiac Rehabilitation on an Individual with an Uncomplicated Myocardial Infarction and Percutaneous Transluminal Coronary Angioplasty

Clinical History

JH was a 51-year-old glazier when admitted to the emergency department on January 16, 1997, with a 2-hour duration of substernal discomfort after playing a vigorous game of basketball with his two sons. He had no previous history of chest discomfort; however, he had noticed some recent shortness of breath on the job. Echocardiography performed in the emergency department confirmed early ECG changes of anteroseptal infarction with a small area of akinesis. He was admitted to the intensive care unit and taken to the cardiac catheterization laboratory the next day for angiography. Selective coronary catheterization demonstrated proximal and mid left anterior descending artery (LAD) lesions of 80%, 75% to 80% lesions in the obtuse marginal branch of the circumflex, and a normal right coronary artery. It was decided to perform a percutaneous transluminal coronary angioplasty procedure on the 2 LAD lesions, which was done successfully with resultant 30% proximal stenosis. JH was placed on calcium antagonists (nifedipine 10 mg, three times a day) and was returned to the intensive care unit for the next 48 hours before being moved to the stepdown unit. Repeat echocardiography on January 20 confirmed a small area of anteroseptal akinesis with good ventricular function.

Cardiac Rehabilitation

On January 20 JH was referred to cardiac rehabilitation for evaluation of appropriate activity guidelines. He demonstrated appropriate response to ADLs and ambulation except for slight tachycardia of 132 bpm with ambulation; however, no other symptoms or ECG changes occurred, and blood pressure response was appropriate.

JH's risk factor profile looked pretty good. He had a history of hypertension for the past 5 years that was controlled by diet; a family history of heart disease, with his father having had a myocardial infarction; and a slight problem with his weight (6 feet 6 inches, 230 lb). His hobbies included fishing and watching sports, which are relatively sedentary. He was seen twice daily by the cardiac rehabilitation team for monitored ambulation, function on the stairs, and counseling by the dietitian; he was given discharge guidelines by the rehabilitation team. He also underwent a low-level treadmill test before discharge on January 22.

JH entered phase II of the cardiac rehabilitation program on January 24 and began a progressive ambulation training program at training heart rates of 126 to 138 and/or systolic blood pressure to 180, diastolic to 90. Unfortunately, his diastolic blood pressure was hard to maintain below 100, and it was elected to increase his nifedipine. JH's training program and exercise test results follow:

Training Program

Date	Initial	3 months	6 months	year 1	year 2	year 3
Time	5-20-5	5-45-5	5-60-5	5-60-5	5-60-5	5-60-5
Training heart rate (bpm)	126–132	140–150	150	150	150	150
Workload (treadmill and jogging)	3 mph (TM)	4–5 mph (TM)	9-min mile	8-min mile	7.5-min mile	7.5-min mile
Weight (lb)	227	214	220	210	206	205

Exercise Tests

Date	Initial	5/97	6/98	4/99
Protocol	Mod. Bruce	Bruce	Bruce	Bruce
Time (min)	9	12	13	13.5
Heart rate (bpm)	78–152	72–145	63–146	48–155
Mean blood pressure (mm Hg)	190/100	240/112	230/96	204/88
$VO_{2\,max}$ (mL/kg/min)	Not tested	36.5	39.3	42.4
Heart rate at ventilatory threshold (bpm)	Not tested	128	123	130

JH returned to work within 4 weeks after his myocardial infarction and to full activity by week 6. Of significance is the continued improvement of his physical work capacity, lower resting heart rate, and improved blood pressure response. JH has participated in many 10-km races and recently ran a sub 40-minute race. His wife and children have become avid exercisers as well.

Case 3. Effect of Cardiac Rehabilitation on an Individual Who Had a Complicated Myocardial Infarction Course (Moderate Risk)

Clinical History

RK is a 63-year-old man who recently (4 months ago) retired from more than 30 years as a health and physical education instructor. He had no history of heart disease, chest pain, or shortness of breath with activity. He did have mild hypertension (systolic 160s, diastolic 80s) that was documented for the past 5 years, which was not treated medically. Other risk factors included a positive family history (mother and father having died of heart disease in their late 60s and a younger brother who had undergone coronary artery bypass graft surgery 2 years earlier at the age of 52). On October 12, 1997, he was admitted to the emergency department with a 1-hour history of chest pain. The ECG demonstrated evidence of acute injury pattern in the anterior leads. He was taken immediately to the cardiac catheterization laboratory where he was found to have a total occlusion of the mid LAD, a mid circumflex lesion of 50%, and a normal right coronary artery. A percutaneous transluminal coronary angioplasty was performed successfully (100% decreased to 40%) at that time. He spent the next 72 hours recovering in the intensive care unit with rhythm disturbances, including atrial fibrillation and multifocal premature ventricular complexes. Cardiac medications included low doses of verapamil.

Cardiac Rehabilitation

After being moved to the stepdown unit, cardiac rehabilitation was initiated on October 16 with instruction to move the patient slowly and assess cardiac rhythm. During self-care monitoring, he demonstrated several abnormal responses:

1. Resting heart rate: 98 supine, 110 sitting, 120 standing, 162 ADL (brushing teeth) at bedside
2. Blood pressure: 110/70 supine, 100/70 sitting, 90/60 standing, 85/50 ADL
3. Symptoms: fatigue and lightheadedness reported with ADLs
4. ECG: initially sinus rhythm, then atrial flutter (2:1) and atrial fibrillation with ADLs

Self-care monitoring was terminated, and RK returned to bed where his heart rate returned to the 90s, his symptoms improved, and his blood pressure returned to 110/70. His cardiologist was notified immediately of his poor response to low-level activity, so the verapamil dosage was increased and digoxin was added. Later that same day self-care monitoring was repeated, the results of which were an appropriate response to ADLs and ambulation of 600 feet.

RK progressed well the next 2 days with appropriate ECG and physiologic responses to activity, but on October 19, he notified nursing of right-sided chest pain at rest with accompanying hemoptysis. A lung scan revealed probable pulmonary embolus, and a chest radiograph demonstrated a moderate-sized pleural effusion. He was immediately started on anticoagulants (heparin) and was put on bedrest over the next few days until a chest radiograph confirmed clearing and his chest discomfort resolved some 72 hours later. Before his discharge on October 25, he underwent a low-level treadmill test and completed 4 minutes using a Bruce protocol, achieving a maximal heart rate of 100 and a maximal systolic blood pressure of 154 with multifocal premature ventricular complexes (fewer than 6 per minute). No clinical or ECG changes indicated the presence of ischemia, and the test was stopped because of dyspnea and fatigue. Discharge guidelines were based on dyspnea levels (not to exceed 2+/4+) or an RPE level of 12 with any activity.

Outpatient Program

On October 27, RK returned to the hospital to begin phase II of the cardiac rehabilitation program. He reported no problems the first 2 days at home and tolerated low-level activity as prescribed. His program progression during the first 4 weeks (seen twice a week) was unremarkable, and he progressed to 25 minutes of continuous ambulation at a training heart rate of 96 bpm. At that time, however, his rhythm had changed from sinus to junctional, and he began having more frequent episodes of supraventricular tachycardia to rates of 160 to 180 bpm, along with multifocal pre-

mature ventricular contractions with occasional coupling. In addition, he experienced occasional bouts of lightheadedness not associated with position change or exercise. His cardiologist was notified, and he elected to increase his dosage of verapamil and add disopyramide phosphate (Norpace; antiarrhythmic).

He was scheduled for a thallium treadmill test in 1 week. However, 48 hours later, RK was brought to the emergency department with severe chest pain. He was taken immediately to the cardiac catheterization laboratory where it was determined that the original mid LAD lesion had narrowed again. It was redilated successfully and RK was taken to the intensive care unit, where he was monitored closely for the next 48 hours.

Before discharge he underwent a thallium treadmill test, and metabolic data were also collected (see Exercise Tests). The thallium test demonstrated a small area of stress-induced ischemia of the anteroapical segment of the left ventricle.

RK returned to phase II for 2 more weeks and then moved to phase III, during which his program was slowly graduated to include 40 minutes of continuous ambulation at a training heart rate of 90 to 96 bpm, light weight training, and use of a four-extremity ergometer (Schwinn Airdyne). His home program included 15 minutes of warm-up stretching exercises (he placed a great deal of emphasis on flexibility owing to an old back problem), 35 to 45 minutes of fast walking or aerobics, and 10 to 15 minutes of cool-down exercises. He also did a series of exercises with 3- to 5-lb free weights for upper body conditioning. RK underwent repeat metabolic treadmill testing following completion of phase III and again 1 year later after participating in phase IV (see Exercise Tests). Of particular interest, besides improvement in physical work capacity, is the higher ventilatory threshold heart rates relative to maximal heart rates. Of significance is the increased total time, lower resting heart rate, higher systolic blood pressure with exercise, and improved ECG response at maximal exercise. RK continues to do well despite bouts with supraventricular arrhythmia.

Exercise Tests

Date	10/25/97	12/3/97	4/7/98	6/16/99
Protocol	Bruce	Bruce	Bruce	Bruce
Time (min)	4.0	7.0	10.0	11.5
Heart rate (bpm)	58–108	57–122	49–133	47–128
Mean blood pressure (mm Hg)	154/68	152/72	176/82	188/84
ECG	1 mm ST ↓	1.5 mm ST ↓	1.5 mm ST ↓	<1 mm ST ↓
$VO_{2\,max}$ (mL/kg/min)		16.8	19.6	23.4
Heart rate at ventilatory threshold (bpm)		90	100	108
Weight (lb)		152	155	159
RPE at ventilatory threshold		14	13	12

Case 4. Effect of Cardiac Rehabilitation for a Patient Who Had a Myocardial Infarction Followed by Coronary Bypass Surgery

Clinical History

BS was a 40-year-old college administrator at the time of his admission to the hospital from the emergency department on January 20, 1996, following several episodes of nocturnal chest pain, nausea, and vomiting. He also had one episode of chest pain with nausea and vomiting the previous day while walking up a hill. In the emergency department his ECG tracing was suggestive of an old anteroseptal infarction and anterolateral ischemia. His creatine phosphokinase value on admission rose to a maximum of 452 μ/ml (N = <150). BS had been a 1-pack-a-day smoker since he was 19. He had a history of mild hypertension that had not been treated and was physically inactive and overweight at 5 feet 11 inches and 192 lb. His brother had elevated blood sugar levels and was on medication; otherwise, there was no family history of heart disease. On admission BS's blood cholesterol level was 270, triglycerides 204, HDL 23, and LDL 149.

Cardiac catheterization, which was performed on January 22, demonstrated a minimal impairment of left ventricular function inferiorly, a proximal LAD stenosis of 70%, a very large circumflex artery with 90% stenosis proximally, and a right coronary artery stenosis of 100% with retrograde filling of the posterior descending branch from collaterals of the left coronary system. On January 24, he underwent three-vessel bypass surgery, which included using the internal mammary ar-

tery as a graft to bypass the LAD lesion and two vein grafts to the obtuse marginal branch of the circumflex and posterior descending branches. Following a good postoperative recovery, which included phase I cardiac rehabilitation started on day 2 after the operation, and an appropriate response to progressive activity, he was discharged home 6 days after his surgery.

Outpatient Rehabilitation

BS was an ideal candidate for cardiac rehabilitation. He was well motivated, had three major and four minor risk factors, and experienced minimal ventricular dysfunction. Three days after discharge from the hospital, BS started phase II cardiac rehabilitation. He received an orientation to the program and began ambulation on the treadmill for 15 minutes at low level (2 mph, 0% grade) during his first visit. He was then referred for his initial low-level treadmill test (see Exercise Tests).

BS obviously made significant improvement in physical work capacity and in all exercise test parameters. Most noteworthy is a progressively lower resting heart rate, lower diastolic blood pressure values, and higher heart rate response before reaching ventilatory threshold. Most impressive is the change in BS's risk profile within 1 year after bypass surgery:

- Smoking—stopped
- Elevated cholesterol—normalized
- Hypertension—normalized
- Overweight—normalized
- Sedentary—became more active
- Stress—although hard to assess, BS reports that he now takes time to do the things he knew he should have been doing and enjoys life to the fullest.

Training Program

Date	Initial	3 mo	6 mo	yr 1	yr 2
Time	5-15-5	5-40-5	5-50-5	10-60-5	10-60-70-5
Training heart rate (bpm)	120	132–144	150	150	150+
Workload (treadmill, jogging)	2 mph	walk/jog	10-min mile	8-min mile	7.5-min mile
Weight (lb)	193	181	175	166	167

Lipid Values

Cholesterol	204	225	185	197	152
Triglycerides	158	117	77	46	97
HDL	23	32	45	43	55
Chol: HDL ratio	8.9:1	7:1	4:1	4.6:1	2.8:1
LDL	149	168	125	145	77

Exercise Tests

Date	2/2/96	4/5/96	11/11/96	5/9/97
Protocol	Mod. Bruce	Bruce	Bruce	Bruce
Time (min)	9	11	15	15
Heart rate (bpm)	75–135	80–188	62–177	54–178
Mean blood pressure (mm Hg)	150/80	180/96	190/90	190/80

			Premature atrial complexes	Occasional premature ventricular complexes
ECG				
$\dot{V}O_{2\,max}$ (mL/kg/min)	Not tested	Not tested	39.14 (108% N)	42.18 (114% N)
Heart rate at ventilatory threshold (bpm)			145–150	160
RPE at ventilatory threshold			12	12

Summary

- A growing number of patient populations are identified as appropriate candidates for exercise training.
- Longer duration and higher levels of intensity may produce the greatest change in exercise performance and risk factors across all patient populations.
- Stratification of patients as low, moderate, and high risk is an important element in the rehabilitation process to maintain a safe environment for all patients and to assist individuals who need a higher degree of support.
- Ways must be sought to keep individuals motivated to continue with their risk reduction programs.
- Programs that are patient-oriented instead of facility-oriented are most successful.
- Physical therapists should be acutely aware of the cardiovascular implications of the problems of all patient populations, especially when treating the elderly.
- One future problem to be confronted in cardiac rehabilitation is that of ensuring adequate reimbursement for all patients who choose to participate. This may in turn help to improve long-term patient compliance.

References

1. Levine SA, Lown B. "Armchair" treatment of acute coronary thrombosis. JAMA 148:1365, 1952.
2. Leon AS, Certo C, Comoss, P, et al. Position paper of the American Association of Cardiovascular and Pulmonary Rehabilitation: Scientific evidence of the value of cardiac rehabilitation services with emphasis on patients following myocardial infarction—section I: Exercise conditioning component. J Cardiopulmonary Rehab 10:79–87, 1990.
3. McNeer JF, Wallace AG, Wagner GS, et al. The course of acute myocardial infarction: Feasibility of early discharge of the uncomplicated patient. Circulation 51:410, 1975.
4. Maskin C, Reddy H, Gulanick M, Perez L. Exercise training in chronic heart failure: Improvement in cardiac performance and maximum oxygen uptake. Circulation 74(suppl II):310, 1986.
5. Lee AP, Ice R, Blessey R, San Marco ME. Long-term effects of physical training on coronary patients with impaired ventricular function. Circulation 60:1519–1526, 1979.
6. Coates AJ, Adamopoulos S, Meyer TE, et al. Effects of physical training in chronic heart failure. Lancet 335(8681):63–66, 1990.
7. Wenger NK, Froelicher ES, Smith LK, et al. Cardiac Rehabilitation. Clinical Practice Guideline No. 17. Rockville, MD, US Department of Health and Human Services, Public Health Service, Agency for Health Care Policy and Research, and the National Heart, Lung and Blood Institute. AHCPR Publication No. 96-0672, October 1995.
8. Southard DR, Certo C, Comoss P, et al. Core competencies for cardiac rehabilitation professionals. J Cardiopulmonary Rehabil 14:87–92, 1994.
9. Wenger NK, Hellerstein HK. Rehabilitation of the Coronary Patient. New York, John Wiley & Sons, 1984.
10. Garrow JS. Effects of exercise on obesity. Acta Med Scand 711(suppl):67–74, 1986.
11. Haskell WL. The influence of exercise training on plasma lipids and lipoproteins in health and disease. Acta Med Scand 711(suppl):25–38, 1986.
12. Hagberg JM, Seals DR. Exercise training and hypertension. Acta Med Scand 711(suppl):131–136, 1986.
13. Holloszy JO, Schultz J, Kusnierkiewicz J, et al. Glucose tolerance and insulin resistance. Acta Med Scand 711(suppl):67–73, 1986.
14. Clausen JP. Circulatory adjustments to dynamic exercise and physical training in normal subjects and in patients with coronary artery disease. In: Sonnenblick EH, Lesch M (eds). Exercise and the Heart. New York, Grune & Stratton, 1977, pp 39–75.
15. Detry J-MR, Rousseau M, Vandenbroucke G, et al. Increased arteriovenous oxygen difference after physical training in coronary heart disease. Circulation 64:109–118, 1971.
16. Pollack ML, Wilmore JH. Exercise in Health and Disease: Evaluation and Prescription for Prevention and Rehabilitation. 2nd ed. Philadelphia, WB Saunders, 1990, pp 1–750.
17. Thompson PD. The benefits and risks of exercise training in patients with chronic coronary artery disease. JAMA 259:1537–1540, 1988.
18. Ehsani AA, Biello DR, Schultz J, et al. Improvement of left ventricular contractile function in patients with coronary artery disease. Circulation 74:350–388, 1986.
19. May GS, Eberlein KA, Furberg CD, et al. Secondary prevention after myocardial infarction: A review of long term trials. Prog Cardiovasc Dis 24:331–362, 1982.
20. American Physical Therapy Association. Guide to Physical Therapist Practice. Phys Ther 77:1163–1650, 1997.
21. Heath GW, Malorey PM, Fure CW. Group exercise versus home exercise in coronary artery bypass graft patients:

Effects on physical activity. J Cardiopulmonary Rehab 7: 190–195, 1987.

22. DeBusk RF, Haskell WL, Miller NH, et al. Medically directed at-home rehabilitation soon after clinically uncomplicated acute myocardial infarction. A new model for patient care. Am J Cardiol 55:251–257, 1985.

23. American Association of Cardiovascular and Pulmonary Rehabilitation. Guidelines for Cardiac Rehabilitation and Secondary Prevention Programs. 3rd ed. Champaign, IL, Human Kinetics, 1999.

24. Froelicher V, Jensen D, Genter F, et al. A randomized trial of exercise training in patients with coronary heart disease. JAMA 252:1291–1297, 1984.

25. Conn EH, Williams RS, Wallace AG. Exercise responses before and after physical conditioning in patients with severely depressed left ventricular function. Am J Cardiol 49: 296–300, 1982.

26. Arvan S. Exercise performance of the high risk acute myocardial infarction patient after cardiac rehabilitation. Am J Cardiol 62(4):197–201, 1988.

27. Sullivan MJ, Cobb FR. The anaerobic threshold in chronic heart failure. Relation to blood lactate, ventilatory basis, reproducibility and response to exercise training. Circulation 81(suppl 2)II:47–58, 1990.

28. Naughton JP, Hellerstein HK. Exercise Testing and Exercise Training in Coronary Heart Disease. New York, Academic Press, 1973.

29. American College of Sports Medicine. ACSM's Guidelines for Exercise Testing and Prescription. 5th ed. Baltimore, Williams & Wilkins, 1995.

30. Goldberg L, Elliott DL, Kuehl KS, et al. Assessment of exercise intensity formulas by use of ventilatory threshold. Chest 94:95–98, 1988.

31. Gibbons E. The influence of anaerobic threshold in exercise prescription. Sports Med 27:357–361, 1987.

32. Dwyer J, Bybee R. Heart rate indices of the anaerobic threshold. Med Sci Sports Exerc 15:72–76, 1983.

33. Borg C, Linderholm H. Perceived exertion and pulse rate during graded exercise in various age groups. Acta Med Scand (suppl) 472:194–206, 1967.

34. Ades PA, Grunvald MH, Weiss RM, Hanson JS. Usefulness of myocardial ischemia as a predictor of training effect with cardiac rehabilitation after acute myocardial infarction or coronary artery bypass graft. Am J Cardiol 63(15): 1032–1036, 1989.

35. Keleman MH. Resistance training safety and essential guidelines for cardiac and coronary prone patients. Med Sci Sports Exerc 21:675–677, 1989.

36. McCartney N, McKelvie RS, Haslam DR, Jones NL. Usefulness of weightlifting training in improving strength and maximal power output on coronary artery disease. Am J Cardiol 12:254–260, 1991.

37. Steward KJ. Resistance training effects on strength and cardiovascular endurance in cardiac and coronary prone patients. Med Sci Sports Exerc 21:678–682, 1989.

38. DeBusk RF, Valdez R, Houston N, Haskell W. Cardiovascular responses to dynamic and static effort soon after myocardial infarction: Application to occupational assessment. Circulation 58:368–375, 1978.

39. Sparling P, Cantwell JD. Strength training guidelines for cardiac patients. Physician Sportsmed 17:190–196, 1989.

40. American Heart Association. Exercise Standards: A statement for healthcare professionals. Circulation 91:580–615, 1995.

41. Hossack VF, Hartwick R. Cardiac arrest associated with supervised cardiac rehabilitation. J Cardiopulmonary Rehab 2:402–408, 1982.

42. Bergh V, Kamstrup L, Ekblom B. Maximal oxygen uptake during exercise with various combinations of arm and leg work. J Appl Physiol 41:191–196, 1976.

43. Gutin B, Ang EK, Torrey MA. Cardiorespiratory and subjective responses to incremental and constant load ergometry with arms and legs. Arch Phys Med Rehabil 69:510–513, 1988.

44. Van Camp SP, Peterson RA. Cardiorespiratory complications of outpatient cardiac rehabilitation programs. JAMA 256(9):1160–1163, 1986.

45. Kannel WB, Castelli WP, Gordon T, et al. Serum cholesterol lipoproteins and risk of coronary heart diseases: The Framingham study. Ann Intern Med 74:1–12, 1971.

46. Lowering blood cholesterol to prevent heart disease. JAMA 253:2080–2090, 1985.

47. Blank DW, Hoeg JM, Kroll MH, et al. The method of determination must be considered in interpreting blood cholesterol levels. JAMA 256:2867–2870, 1986.

48. Lipid Research Clinics Program: The Lipid Research Clinics Coronary Primary Prevention Trial Results I. Reduction in incidence of coronary heart disease. JAMA 251:351–364, 1984.

49. Lipid Research Clinics Program: The Lipid Research Clinics Coronary Primary Prevention Trial Results II. The relationship of reduction in incidence of coronary heart disease to cholesterol lowering. JAMA 251:365–374, 1984.

50. Wood PD, Stefanick ML, Dreon DM, et al. Changes in plasma lipoproteins in overweight men during weight loss through dieting as compared with exercise. N Engl J Med 319:1173–1179, 1988.

51. Tran ZV, Weltman A. Differential effects of exercise on serum lipid and lipoprotein levels seen with changes in body weight. A meta-analysis. JAMA 254:919–924, 1985.

52. Allison TG, Williams DE, Miller TD, et al. Medical and economic costs of psychologic distress in patients with coronary artery disease. Mayo Clinic Proc 70:734–742, 1995.

53. Case RB, Moss AJ, Case N, et al. Living alone after myocardial infarction: Impact of prognosis. JAMA 117:1003–1009, 1992.

54. Everson SA, Goldberg DE, Kaplan GA, et al. Hopelessness and risk of mortality and incidence of myocardial infarction and cancer. Psychosom Med 58:113–121, 1996.

55. Frasure-Smith N, Lesperance F, Talajic M. Depression and 18-month prognosis after myocardial infarction. Circulation 91:999–1005, 1995.

56. Rozanski A, Bairey CN, Krantz DS, et al. Mental stress and the induction of silent myocardial ischemia in patients with coronary artery disease. N Engl J Med 311:552–559, 1984.

57. Wenger NK. In hospital exercise rehabilitation after myocardial infarction and myocardial revascularization: Physiologic basis, methodology, and results. In: NK Wenger, HK Hellerstein (eds). Rehabilitation of the Coronary Patient. 3rd ed. New York, Churchill Livingstone, 1992.

58. Mumford E, Schlessinger H, Glass G. The effects of psychological intervention on recovery from surgery and heart attacks: An analysis of the literature. Am J Public Health 72(2):141–151, 1982.

59. Oldenburg B, Perkins R, Andrews G. Controlled trial of psychological intervention in myocardial infarction. J Consult Clin Psychol 53:852–859, 1985.

60. Amery A, Birkenhager W, Brixko P, et al. Mortality and morbidity results from the European Working Party on high blood pressure in the elderly trial. Lancet 1:1349–1354, 1985.

61. Berkman L, Syme SL. Social networks, host resistance and

mortality: A nine-year follow-up study of Alameda County residents. Am J Epidemiol 109:186–204, 1979.

62. Cooper CL, Faragher ED, Bray CL, Ramsdale DR: The significance of psychosocial factors in predicting coronary disease in patients with valvular heart disease. Soc Sci Med 20:315–318, 1985.

63. Oldridge NB, Guyatt G, Jones N, et al. Effects on quality of life with comprehensive rehabilitation after acute myocardial infarction. Am J Cardiol 67:1084–1089, 1991.

64. Murphy S. Self efficacy and social support-mediators of stress on mental health following a natural disorder. West J Nurs Res 9(1):58–87, 1987.

65. Strecher V, McEvoy B, Becker M, Rosenstock I. The role of self efficacy in achieving behavior changes. Health Educ Q 13(1):73–91, 1986.

66. Southard DR, Broyden R. Psychosocial services in cardiac rehabilitation: A status report. J Cardiopulmonary Rehabil 10:255–263, 1990.

67. Oldridge NB. Cardiac rehabilitation exercise programme. Compliance and compliance-enhancing strategies. Sports Med 6(1):42–55, 1988.

68. Pashkow F, Pashkow P, Schafer M, Ferguson C. Successful Cardiac Rehabilitation. Loveland, Colo, The Heartwatchers Press, 1988.

69. Mannarino E, Pasqualini L, Menna M, et al. Effects of physical training on peripheral vascular disease: A controlled study. Angiology 40(1):5–10, 1989.

70. Johnson EC, Vogles WF, Atterbom HA, et al. Effects of exercise training on common femoral artery blood flow in patients with intermittent claudication. Circulation 80(5pt2):III59–72, 1989.

71. Kannel WB, McGee DL. Diabetes and cardiovascular risk factors: The Framingham study. Circulation 59:8, 1979.

72. American Diabetes Association. The Physicians Guide to Type II Diabetes (NIDMM): Diagnosis and Treatment. New York, American Diabetes Association, 1984.

73. Fowler RS, Fordyce WE. Strokes: Why Do They Behave That Way? Dallas, Texas, American Heart Association, 1974.

74. Monga TN, DeForge DA, Williams J, Wolfe LA. Cardiovascular responses to acute exercise in patients with cerebrovascular accidents. Arch Phys Med Rehabil 69:937–940, 1988.

75. Painter P, Hanson P. A model for clinical exercise prescription: Application to hemodialysis patients. J Cardiopulmonary Rehab 7:177–189, 1987.

76. Painter P, Messer-Rehale D, Hanson P, et al. Exercise capacity in hemodialysis, CAPD and renal transplant patients. Nephron 42:47–51, 1986.

77. Christie I, Pewen W. A 12 week trial of exercise training in patients on continuous ambulatory peritoneal dialysis (unpublished).

78. American Heart Association. 1992 Heart and Stroke Facts. Washington, DC, Am Heart Assoc, 1997.

79. Redberg RF. Coronary artery disease in women: Understanding the diagnostic and management pitfalls. Medscape Women's Health 3(5), 1998.

80. Limacher MC. Exercise and rehabilitation in women: Indications and outcomes. Cardiol Clin 16(1):27–36, 1998.

81. Brezinka V, Kitrel F. Psychosocial factors of coronary heart disease in women: A review. Soc Sci Med 42(10):1351–1365, 1996.

82. Weiner D, Ryan T, McCabe C, et al. Exercise stress testing: Correlations among history of angina, ST segment response and prevalence of coronary artery disease in the Coronary Artery Surgery Study. N Engl J Med 301:230–235, 1979.

83. Taillefer R, DePuey EG, Udelson JE, et al. Comparative diagnostic accuracy of T1-201 and Tc-99m sestamibi SPECT imaging (perfusion and ECG-gated Spect) in detecting coronary artery disease in women. J Am Coll Cardiol 29(1):69–77, 1997.

84. Sawada S, Ryan T, Fineberg N. Exercise echocardiographic detection of coronary artery disease in women. J Am Coll Cardiol 14:1440–1447, 1989.

85. Fisher L, Kennedy J, Davis K, et al. Association of sex, physical size and operative mortality after coronary artery bypass in the Coronary Artery Surgery Study (CASS). J Thorac Cardiovasc Surg 84:334–341, 1981.

86. Khan SS, Nessim S, Gray R, et al. Increased mortality of women in coronary artery bypass surgery: Evidence for referral bias. Ann Intern Med 112(8):561–567, 1990.

87. Cowley MJ, Mullin SM, Kelsey SF, et al. Sex differences in early and long-term results of coronary angioplasty in the NHLB PTCA registry. Circulation 71:90–97, 1985.

88. Ginzel AR. Women's compliance with cardiac rehabilitation programs. Prog Cardiovasc Nurs 11(1):30–35, 1996.

89. Balady GJ, Fletcher BJ, Froelicher ES, et al. Cardiac rehabilitation programs. A statement for healthcare professionals from the American Heart Association. Circulation 90:1602–1610, 1994.

90. Pashkow FJ. Cardiac rehabilitation: Not just exercise anymore. Cleve Clin J Med 63(2):116–123, 1996.

91. Carhart RL Jr, Ades PA. Gender differences in cardiac rehabilitation. Cardiol Clin 116(1):37–43, 1998.

92. Lieberman L, Meana M, Stewart D. Cardiac rehabilitation: Gender differences in factors influencing participation. J Womens Health 7(6):717–723, 1998.

93. Thomas RJ, Miller NH, Lamendola C, et al. National survey on gender differences in cardiac rehabilitation programs: Patient characteristics and enrollment patterns. J Cardiopulm Rehabil 16:402–412, 1996.

94. Cannistra LB, Balady GJ, O'Malley CJ, et al. Comparison of the clinical profile and outcome of women and men in cardiac rehabilitation. Am J Cardiol 69:1274–1279, 1992.

95. Tomassoni TL, Galioto FM, Vaccaro P, et al. The pediatric cardiac rehabilitation program at Children's Hospital National Medical Center, Washington, D.C. J Cardiopulmonary Rehab 7:259–262, 1987.

96. Calzori A, Pastore E, Biodi G. Cardiac rehabilitation in children: Interdisciplinary approach. Minerva Pediatr 49(12):559–565, 1997.

97. American Academy of Pediatrics. Position statement on cholesterol screening. Pediatrics 83:141–142, 1989.

98. Blessey R, Blessey S. Hypercholesterolemia in children: Is it a problem requiring intervention? Cardiopulmonary Phys Ther J 1:10–12, 1990.

99. Srinivasan SR. Biological determinants of serum lipoprotein. In: Berenson G (ed). Causation of Cardiovascular Risk Factors in Children. New York, Raven Press, 1986, pp 83–129.

100. Walter HJ, Hofman A, Vaughan RD, et al. Modification of risk factors for coronary heart disease: Five year results of a school based intervention trial. N Engl J Med 318:1093–1100, 1988.

101. Seals DR, Allen WK, Hurley BF, et al. Elevated high density lipoprotein cholesterol levels in older endurance athletes. Am J Cardiol 54:390–393, 1984.

102. Lampman RM. Evaluating and prescribing exercise for elderly patients. Geriatrics 42(8):63–65, 1987.

103. US Government Printing Office. Reducing the Health Consequences of Smoking: 25 Years of Progress. Washington, DC, Government Printing Office, 1989.

104. National High Blood Pressure Education Program of the National Institutes of Health, National Heart Lung and Blood Institute. The Sixth Report of the Joint National Committee on Detection, Evaluation, and Treatment of High Blood Pressure. NIH Publication 98-1080, 1997.

105. St. Jeor ST, Brownell KD, Atkinson RL. American Heart Association Prevention Conference III: Obesity. Circulation 88:1392–1397, 1993.

106. Gotto AM. Lipid lowering, regression, and coronary events. Circulation 92:646–656, 1995.

## 19

Pulmonary Rehabilitation

Rhonda N. Barr

HISTORICAL PERSPECTIVE

Rehabilitation programs for patients with chronic obstructive pulmonary disease (COPD) have existed for more than 25 years. The American College of Chest Physicians in 1974 defined pulmonary rehabilitation and described aspects of care for patients with respiratory impairments. These were incorporated into an official position statement by the American Thoracic Society in 1981.[1] Even though COPD is one of the leading causes of illness and death in the United States,[2, 3] pulmonary rehabilitation programs have only of late achieved recognition and acceptance comparable to rehabilitation programs for patients with cardiovascular, neuromuscular, or musculoskeletal disorders. The American Thoracic Society position paper and most of the research available address the benefits of rehabilitation for patients with COPD while neglecting rehabilitation outcomes for patients with other chronic respiratory diseases such as restrictive lung diseases, spinal and chest deformities, neuromuscular conditions that lead to respiratory failure, pulmonary vascular diseases, and those that affect the very obese.

Although some outcomes of pulmonary rehabilitation programs are well documented,[4] others are still a matter of controversy (Table 19–1). Most of the early research in the area of pulmonary rehabilitation focused on the lack of improvement, as documented by pulmonary function testing, or the failure to reverse the natural progression of the disease process. Steadily deteriorating function and eventual death despite intervention has been until

Table 19–1	
Outcomes of Pulmonary Rehabilitation	
OUTCOMES OF IMPROVEMENT	**OUTCOMES WITHOUT ACCEPTED IMPROVEMENTS**
Symptom-limited exercise capacity[8-28]	Lung function[12-14, 16-18, 20-27, 32]
Functional level (ADL)[10, 15, 16, 21-23, 26, 29]	Heart function[12, 19, 20, 25]
Respiratory symptoms[10, 15, 21, 22, 24-26, 29-31]	Maximal aerobic capacity[10, 12, 24]
Respiratory muscle function[14, 16, 32]	Mortality rate[29]
Psychological status[10, 22, 29]	
Quality of life[10, 12, 24, 26, 29, 33]	
Frequency of hospitalization[21, 22, 29, 34]	

relatively recent years the accepted fate of patients with COPD. Consequently, rehabilitation intervention had been considered palliative, and **third-party payers** have often severely limited the benefits paid for pulmonary rehabilitation. These factors have hampered the growth of rehabilitation services for pulmonary patients.

Despite these adversities, many successful pulmonary rehabilitation programs exist. The need for early detection and treatment of respiratory dysfunction is widely accepted. Many cardiac rehabilitation programs have increased their scope to include patients with other chronic diseases, such as respiratory diseases. Rehabilitation research is now emphasizing functional and quality-of-life outcomes (see Table 19–1) as measures of efficacy instead of changes in physiologic parameters. This trend supports the benefits that pulmonary specialists have claimed for rehabilitation.

Many rehabilitation principles can be generalized to all patient populations, including pulmonary rehabilitation patients: the need for multidisciplinary programming; goals aimed at restoring optimal physical and psychological functioning; and components of exercise, education and counseling. Disease-specific aspects of rehabilitation include

• Education
• Medical management
• Physiologic and symptomatic limitations to physical effort

In this chapter, goals for rehabilitation of the pulmonary patient, the structure of pulmonary rehabilitation programs, and physical therapy strategies are presented.

GOALS OF PULMONARY REHABILITATION

Although the overall goals of a pulmonary rehabilitation program can be very general and applicable to a wide range of patients, the goals for an individual must be very specific and pertinent to the individual's lifestyle, needs, and interests. This is possible only after a thorough evaluation of the patient's disease state and clinical course, a patient-family interview, and a physical examination.

The rehabilitation personnel should assist the patient in identifying realistic goals that can be described in behavioral terms and measured as outcomes for rehabilitation. They should be goals that can make the most impact on daily life. If they are small goals, that are easily attainable and can be maintained over a long period of time, they will be the most realistic and life enhancing.

Examples of unrealistic goals are to eliminate dyspnea, to have a normal lifestyle, or to be able to discontinue supplemental oxygen use. More realistic would be goals of learning and implementing strategies to relieve dyspnea, increasing activity tolerance, and improving oxygen saturation levels during activity.

How successfully program goals are attained during pulmonary rehabilitation are described as "outcomes." For each general program goal listed below, some possible outcome measures are suggested. Detailed information on outcomes for cardiopulmonary rehabilitation are found in several sources.[5-7]

• Improvement in health-related behaviors: The patient will stop tobacco use, stop drug or alcohol misuse, and comply with medical and rehabilitation treatments. Outcome measures for this area of change include behavioral surveys, patient diaries, and other self-report tools, as well as carbon monoxide levels for tobacco use.[6]

- Improvement in clinical symptoms and progression of disease: The patient will be able to effectively mobilize respiratory secretions, employ strategies to relieve symptoms of dyspnea and cough, recognize early signs of the need for medical intervention, decrease the frequency and severity of respiratory exacerbations, and obtain optimal oxygen saturation throughout the day and night. Outcomes for this area include those in the clinical domain: cost of medical care, frequency and length of hospital stays, pulse oximetry measurements, stability of pulmonary function tests, dyspnea ratings, and questionnaires.[6, 7]

- Improvement in function and daily activity tolerance: The patient will gain sufficient strength, flexibility, and endurance to accomplish identified activities of daily living (ADL) and requirements of employment and recreational tasks; and will learn to employ strategies to manipulate the environment to maximize physical functioning. Outcomes related to this area of improvement include those in the clinical and health status domains: graded exercise tests, timed walk tests, timed ADL tests, return to work, functional status, and quality-of-life questionnaires.[6, 7]

- Improvement in nutritional status: The patient will obtain and maintain optimal body weight and composition, demonstrate adequate growth and physical maturation, or both. Outcomes in the clinical domain are body weight, body mass index, waist circumference, and nutrition related laboratory values (albumin, protein). Behavioral domain outcomes related to nutritional improvement include diet questionnaires and food diaries.[6]

- Improvement in mood, confidence, self-esteem, and self-efficacy: The patient will become independent in all areas of care, know how to contact appropriate resources for assistance, develop adequate psychosocial support, and improve overall well-being. In the clinical domain several questionnaires are related to psychosocial functioning. The health status domain includes many quality-of-life measures, some which are related specifically to people with pulmonary disease.[6, 7]

STRUCTURE OF PULMONARY REHABILITATION PROGRAMS

Pulmonary rehabilitation programs vary widely in their overall structure. Programs are offered in an inpatient rehabilitation or subacute facility, as an outpatient program in a hospital or freestanding clinic, or in the patient's home. Each setting has its advantages and disadvantages in terms of convenience for patients, cost of delivering services, resources available, and socialization opportunities. Benefits associated with pulmonary rehabilitation have been demonstrated in each setting, but there is no agreement on which setting offers the best value.

For some programs, pulmonary rehabilitation begins during an acute hospitalization, at which time appropriate candidates for outpatient rehabilitation can be identified, patient education and support can be initiated, and the response to activity and exercise can be evaluated. Treatment is aimed at reducing immobility and maintaining function during the hospitalization. All components of pulmonary rehabilitation can begin during the acute inpatient program, within the limits of patient tolerance and medical condition.

Despite the variability in the structure of pulmonary rehabilitation programs, there are some accepted recommendations for the qualifications of personnel, program components, and patient candidacy.[1, 4, 5, 35]

Pulmonary Rehabilitation Personnel

The specific professionals involved in pulmonary rehabilitation vary from program to program. Their particular qualifications and interests are more important than the professional degrees they hold. Optimally, the core of the pulmonary rehabilitation program team consists of at least three to four rehabilitation specialists with varied experience and academic backgrounds. Additional professionals may consult with patients on an "as needed" basis or serve as program advisers to meet the needs of a diverse patient population.

The Patient

The patient with pulmonary disease participating in the pulmonary rehabilitation program, the patient's spouse or family, and the primary care provider play a central role on the team. The patient must be empowered to lead the rehabilitation process with the assistance and guidance of the rehabilitation professionals. This may be difficult for some patients who have taken a passive role in their own treatment, and for families who have become caretakers. Individualized and family counseling may be indicated for those who are unable to assume the responsibility of this role.

The Medical Director

The medical director should be a physician who is a **pulmonologist.** He or she directs the rehabilitation program in matters of overall policy, procedures, and medical care, including specialized diagnostic tests and medical treatments for pulmonary diseases.

The Program Director

The program director is the administrator or coordinator of services. This person is the team leader, directing day-to-day functions of the pulmonary rehabilitation program according to the established policies and procedures. A diverse background in respiratory care and in education and administration are necessary for this individual. The program director is often a nurse, respiratory therapist, or physical therapist. In smaller programs, the program director also provides direct patient care services.

Other Team Members

Other team members may include a variety of specialists who can assume the leadership in the areas of exercise, respiratory care, education, counseling or behavior management, pharmacology, nutrition, recreation, and vocational training.

Program Components

According to the position papers of the American Thoracic Society and the American Association of Cardiovascular and Pulmonary Rehabilitation[4] on pulmonary rehabilitation[1] and other sources,[15, 36-38] a comprehensive pulmonary rehabilitation program should incorporate the following components

- Exercise and functional training
- Education/patient training
- Psychosocial management

Although a physical therapist may participate in any or all of these pulmonary rehabilitation program components, traditionally the physical therapist makes the greatest contributions in the areas of pulmonary care, exercise, and functional training and education.

In addition to treatments for airway clearance and relief of dyspnea the management of chronic hypoxemia is important. Patients need to be assessed for supplemental oxygen requirements during activity and sleep. Although this is part of the overall medical care of the patient, under the direction of the patient's personal physician, the rehabilitation program will support the patient's use and understanding of oxygen therapy. By evaluating the patient's hypoxemic response to the exercise component of the program, recommendations for changes in oxygen dosage or delivery systems may at times be necessary.

Exercise and Functional Training

Instruction in energy conservation, pacing, and the use of adaptive equipment may be necessary to optimize the patient's ability to carry out usual daily activities for home, work, and recreation. Exercise to improve strength, flexibility, and cardiopulmonary endurance, including respiratory

---

American Association of Cardiovascular and Pulmonary Rehabilitation

One of the best resources for finding programs within the state or another state is the American Association of Cardiovascular and Pulmonary Rehabilitation (AACVPR) or the Internet.

muscle training, is a major component of rehabilitation. Specific guidelines for exercise for the pulmonary patient are addressed later in this chapter.

Education and Patient Training

Patient and family education are often provided in a group classroom format to facilitate questions and discussion. Topics may include anatomy and pathophysiology of disease, medical management, early detection and treatment of acute illness, use and misuse of oxygen, and practical solutions to incorporating diet reform and activity into daily lives. Patient training involves the transfer of knowledge and skill in performing treatment techniques. Some of these include respiratory treatment techniques for clearing accumulated pulmonary secretions and relieving dyspnea such as

- Bronchial drainage
- Breathing techniques
- Cough facilitation
- Postures to improve breathing
- Relaxation techniques
- Bronchodilators
- Respiratory assistance devices to rest the breathing muscles at night or during exercise[39-45]

It is very important to try a variety of procedures while the patient is in the rehabilitation setting to evaluate which are most effective for the patient and can be instituted in the home environment. Patients whose production of mucus is **copious** may require two to four respiratory treatments each day, whereas other patients may require treatment only during an acute illness. These procedures are described in more detail in Chapter 17 and later in this chapter under Physical Therapy Management.

Psychosocial Management

Psychosocial management is an integral component of pulmonary rehabilitation because chronic disease places stress on the whole family. Coping strategies, stress reduction and management techniques, and support systems are necessary.[36, 46, 47] Behavioral strategies for facilitating lifestyle changes and compliance with treatments should be incorporated to improve the outcome of rehabilitation. Patients may also need financial assistance, vocational rehabilitation services, or both.

Patient Candidacy

Ideally, any person with a primary or secondary pulmonary disease or anyone at risk for the development of pulmonary disease could be a candidate for rehabilitation (Table 19–2). Such a broad definition of candidacy would include very large numbers of people. The high cost of health care prohibits the inclusion of all potential rehabilitation candidates. Therefore, realistic priorities must be set so that the available health care dollars can be allocated to those who can derive the most benefit from them. Too frequently these priorities are determined by third-party payers. Generally, candidates for rehabilitation must meet the follow-

Table 19–2
Conditions That Produce Candidates for Pulmonary Rehabilitation

OBSTRUCTIVE DISEASES	RESTRICTIVE DISEASES	EXPOSURE TO RISKS FOR COPD	CHEST WALL DEFECTS	PULMONARY VASCULAR CONDITIONS	OTHER
Emphysema Bronchitis Bronchiectasis Cystic fibrosis Alpha-antitrypsin deficiency Asthma	Idiopathic pulmonary fibrosis Sarcoidosis Asbestosis Silicosis Adult respiratory distress syndrome	Cigarette smoking Occupational exposure Air pollution Infections of the lungs Impaired immune defenses	Neuromuscular weakness Chest deformities Obesity Spinal deformities Chest surgery	Pulmonary emboli Idiopathic, occlusive conditions Pulmonary hypertension	Pre-lung transplant Post-lung transplant

> **Clinical Note: Early Referrals for Pulmonary Rehabilitation**
>
> Physicians often need to be reminded or encouraged to refer patients *early* for pulmonary rehabilitation as they may not see a patient as a candidate until the patient's pulmonary function is *severely* affected.

ing criteria: a diagnosed respiratory disease and documented functional limitations. There are regional differences in reimbursement patterns for rehabilitation services. In some areas, patients are required to obtain approval from third-party payers before they can enter rehabilitation programs.

All patients with respiratory symptoms of wheezing, coughing, or dyspnea, with or without abnormal spirometry, and those who are identified as at risk for the development of COPD need medical therapeutic intervention and preventive care.[3] This care usually includes a recommendation of smoking cessation, immunizations and vaccinations, and prescription of appropriate medication and oxygen, if needed.[15, 36, 39–43] Comprehensive rehabilitation services are usually reserved for those with moderate to moderately severe COPD.[4] However, even patients with very advanced disease who are extremely limited by respiratory symptoms can demonstrate important functional gains and should not be excluded from rehabilitation programs.[10]

PHYSICAL THERAPY MANAGEMENT

Because of regional differences in practice patterns, the role of the physical therapist in pulmonary rehabilitation varies widely among programs. Some programs do not have a physical therapist at all, whereas others consult with a physical therapist only for patients with complicated diagnoses, such as those who have musculoskeletal or neuromuscular conditions in addition to pulmonary disease.

Ideally, the physical therapist has expertise in evaluating and treating patients with a wide variety of pulmonary conditions, and is involved in all components of the program. In addition to leading exercise sessions, the physical therapist may

also provide educational sessions, smoking cessation programs, weight control or reduction programs, and stress management and relaxation training. The physical therapist may also evaluate the patient's performance in rehabilitation by monitoring progress, assessing outcomes, and participating in quality improvement projects.

PATIENT EVALUATION PROCEDURES

In this section, information on patient evaluation, treatment, and follow-up are reviewed to facilitate the development of the physical therapist in assuming a significant role in pulmonary rehabilitation. A more comprehensive guide for examination, evaluation, intervention, and outcomes is described in "The Cardiopulmonary Preferred Practice Patterns" in the *Guide to Physical Therapist Practice.*[48]

A patient referred to a pulmonary rehabilitation program should be receiving regular medical care from a personal physician. Diagnostic testing should be completed and all medical conditions considered as stable prior to beginning the rehabilitation program.[4, 49]

The physical therapist should evaluate each pulmonary rehabilitation candidate by completing a chart review of medical conditions and laboratory and other test results, interviewing the patient, and performing a physical examination, including an assessment of activity tolerance.

Chart Review

The chart should be reviewed for the current pulmonary diagnosis and all diagnostic and laboratory testing that has established the diagnosis, prognosis, and stage of disease. This may include, but is not limited to, pulmonary function testing, chest roentgenogram, arterial blood gas analysis, electrocardiogram, blood counts, and blood chemistry. In addition, all treatments related to the disease should be identified, such as surgical interventions, oral and inhaled medication, oxygen therapy, assisted ventilation therapy, and artificial airways.

In addition to pulmonary conditions, the chart should be reviewed for other medical diagnoses that need to be addressed during rehabilitation. These diagnoses include cardiac disease, diabetes, hypertension, peripheral vascular disease, lipid disorders, arthritis, and cancer, or any chronic condition that may interfere with activity tolerance and function. Pertinent family history may indicate the patient's risk for developing some chronic conditions such as hypertension, diabetes, and cardiac disease.

The information obtained in the chart review will assist the physical therapist in setting individualized goals and treatments, monitoring for adverse responses, providing appropriate education and counseling, or initiating referrals to other professionals, if indicated.

Patient Interview

The physical therapist can gather additional information from the patient and spouse or family during an interview. Specific information to be obtained should be identified prior to the interview so that it is effective, efficient, and complete. To facilitate this process, interview questions may be standardized for all participants. Questions may solicit information regarding:

- Use of tobacco, alcohol, and nonprescription drugs
- Usual activity level, including employment, recreation, and home
- Regularity of exercise, including availability of equipment at home
- Symptoms that limit activity, rated for severity and frequency
- Compliance with prescribed medication and treatments
- Support from family and friends
- History of environmental exposures and sensitivities (including passive smoke)
- Goals for participating in the rehabilitation program

Several standardized patient questionnaires are available to assist in obtaining information and to provide a measure of how pulmonary disease has affected quality of life. These questionnaires, when used repeatedly over time, are important tools for documenting outcomes associated with participation in pulmonary rehabilitation.[6]

Patient Examination

The patient examination may include a battery of tests and measurements that yield a description of function or physical capacity. These test results will provide information on which to base patient-specific rehabilitation goals and treatments. They also provide a baseline measurement for comparison with repeated testing and for documentation of changes as a result of rehabilitation.

- Body weight and height (body mass index), girth (waist-to-hip ratio) or composition (skinfold measurements) assessment: Patients may have nutritional problems that need addressing to promote health and function. Excess weight contributes to higher energy demands and ventilation requirements. Therefore, weight loss may be a rehabilitation goal. Patients who are underweight must have adequate nutrition and calories to build strength and endurance. Either condition would indicate a need for dietary intervention.
- Chest evaluation (auscultation, cough assessment, inspection of breathing pattern): Patients who, on examination, demonstrate lung secretion retention or an ineffective cough may benefit from airway clearance techniques. Those who demonstrate bronchial wheezing may benefit from a trial of bronchodilator therapy. Patients with increased use of respiratory accessory muscles at rest or with activity may benefit from instruction in relaxation and paced breathing techniques.
- Musculoskeletal examination (joint function, strength, posture): Patients undergoing pulmonary rehabilitation are often older, lead sedentary lifestyles, and have a multitude of joint dysfunction and pain, postural deviations, and strength deficiencies from inactivity. The physical therapist should adequately address the need for exercise programming that will correct deficiencies that contribute to the dysfunction and minimize aggravation of musculoskeletal symptoms.
- Activity assessment (functional tasks, exercise testing): The evaluation of a patient's capacity to perform standardized functional tasks (ADL or timed walk tests) or formal ergometric testing

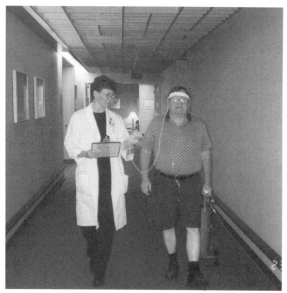

Figure 19–1. Timed walked test. The physical therapist monitors the pulse and oxygen saturation changes continuously with the pulse oximeter.

(Fig. 19–1) traditionally provides the information from which to derive an exercise prescription. The activity assessment should include tests that provide documentation of functional limitations, formulation of safe and effective training parameters, and identification of specific functional goals. Patient goals may include increasing aerobic capacity, improving endurance for sustained activity, or enhancing skills for specific tasks to maximize efficiency. Tests that are typically included in a pulmonary rehabilitation program are summarized in Table 19–3.

TREATMENT INTERVENTION

Pulmonary Care

The physiologic basis for treatment and descriptions of pulmonary hygiene (airway clearance)

Table 19–3
Summary of Standardized Functional and Exercise Tolerance Tests Utilized in Pulmonary Rehabilitation Programs

TEST	DATA OBTAINED	APPLICATION
Symptom-limited maximum tests (progressive multistaged)[49, 50] Treadmill testing Leg cycle ergometry Arm cycle ergometry	Peak work (estimated METs), maximum heart rate and blood pressure, oxygen saturation, symptom and exertion ratings, ECG changes (possible peak oxygen consumption and minute ventilation)	Test defines maximum aerobic work capacity and safe training parameters, and screens for cardiac problems; most useful for patients with mild, moderate and moderately severe lung disease
Single-staged endurance tests[49, 50] Treadmill testing Leg cycle ergometry Arm cycle ergometry	Steady-state heart rate and blood pressure, symptom and exertion ratings, oxygen saturation and endurance time at a selected submaximal workload (TM or cycle).	Defines endurance limitations in patients with moderate to severe pulmonary disease that are unable to reach or maintain aerobic training intensities
Functional timed walk tests 12-minute walk test[51–53] 6-minute walk test[52, 54, 55]	Distance walked, rest time, average walking velocity, heart rate, blood pressure, symptom and exertion ratings, and oxygen saturation during self-selected walking speeds	Defines walking performance for functional community ambulation requirements; useful for evaluating patients unable to use exercise equipment, or with severe pulmonary limitations
Physical performance test[56–58]	Time required to complete simulated or actual ADL tasks; symptom rating, oxygen saturation during typical ADL	Applicable to patients with severe lung disease and the elderly
Timed get up and go test[54, 59]	Time to complete test, ability to perform test safely	Applicable to patients with severe lung disease and the elderly; correlated with risk for falls

techniques are reviewed in Chapter 17. The main emphasis of pulmonary care in the rehabilitation setting is the removal of excessive secretions that obstruct airways, cause ventilatory defects and bothersome symptoms of cough, and possibly lead to an increased incidence of respiratory infections and deterioration of lung function.[60-63] This is especially important for patients who have chronic, copious, or thick pulmonary secretions, such as those with cystic fibrosis, bronchiectasis, and chronic bronchitis.[46] Patients with severe neuromuscular weakness of the respiratory muscles may also benefit from airway clearance techniques because acute pulmonary infections often cause respiratory failure in this patient group.[64-67]

Following a thorough evaluation, the physical therapist should employ treatment techniques that offer the best therapeutic results and are most convenient for the patient to continue at home. It is essential to offer the patient and family a variety of treatment options to enhance compliance.[68] Treatment modifications may be necessary if the patient does not have assistance at home. Modifications that may allow for self-treatment include the following:

- Changes in bronchial drainage positions to facilitate the ease of assuming the appropriate position independently and comfortably. Firm foam wedges or cushions may be used to assume the **Trendelenburg position.**
- If percussion or vibration is necessary for complete airway clearance and adequate assistance is not available, then **palm cups, mechanical percussors,**[69] or a self-administered, high-frequency **chest compression system** can be employed instead.[70, 71]
- Performance of a series of deep breathing exercises, forced expirations, and coughing or use of devices that provide intermittent positive expiratory pressure may be adequate without **bronchial drainage.**[72-78] The breathing and coughing exercises may be done after bronchodilator treatments, first thing in the morning to remove the secretions that have accumulated overnight, or before and after each exercise session.
- Sustained exercise, if tolerated by the patient, can have very beneficial airway-clearing effects.[79-81]

Pulmonary rehabilitation should include assessing the patient's ability to perform treatments in-dependently and effectively. The short-term effects of these treatments, such as improved breath sounds, volume of pulmonary secretions produced, and subjective improvements in breathing ability, are important to monitor immediately after treatments. Long-term benefits that are monitored over the rehabilitation period may include

- Maintenance of baseline pulmonary function
- Reduced frequency of respiratory exacerbations
- Decreased number and length of hospitalizations

Functional Training

Functional training is especially important for patients who have end-stage disease or significant symptoms of weakness, fatigue, or severe dyspnea that limit activities. Treatment goals include

- Adapting the environment to improve the ease of performing activities of daily living
- Altering the performance of tasks to decrease energy costs
- Incorporating methods to relieve symptoms associated with activity

Essential to rehabilitation is the reversal of deconditioning to improve the patient's ability to do work. However, once the disease has progressed to the point that a patient is unable to sustain a training exercise load, then functional activity training and energy conservation become major components of rehabilitation.[46, 10, 82]

Environmental Modifications

Identification of the activities of daily living that are most problematic for the patient is the first step in modifying the environment. Once identified, the areas in the home in which these activities are performed should be evaluated for modification. Adaptations are usually necessary in the bathroom, bedroom, and kitchen. Basic concepts include

- Providing work areas with supported seating of appropriate height for tasks done on a counter or table
- Placing equipment that is used most often in convenient locations so that bending, reaching, and lifting are minimized

- Locating a table or counter at work stations on which one can slide heavy items instead of lifting and carrying them
- Locating chairs at appropriate places when rests are needed, such as on the landing of stairs or beside the bathtub
- Using adaptive equipment to simplify tasks and improve comfort, for instance, a bath seat and hand-held shower head, a wheeled cart for transporting laundry or items for the dinner table, a set of grab bars or booster seats to get up from a toilet or a low chair, a wheeled walker and hospital bed if necessary
- Improving ventilation for the bathroom, kitchen, or other areas in which fumes, dust, smoke, or steam may cause respiratory symptoms

Task Modification

Tasks can be modified by including energy conservation techniques. Basic concepts include

- Slowing down the pace
- Minimizing large body movements such as moving the body weight up and down
- Setting priorities and organizing activities to minimize wasted movement
- Planning appropriate amounts of time to complete the task, including breaks for rest

Each activity can be broken down into smaller tasks and analyzed with regard to the most energy-efficient method to complete it.

Relief of Dyspnea

Simple procedures to minimize and relieve shortness of breath during activities of daily living can become incorporated into the functional training. Controlling the breathing pattern, altering pos-

Clinical Note: Bending Movements

Bending over at the waist, from either a standing or a sitting position, should be limited because a Valsalva maneuver actually occurs, making the patient more breathless and raising the blood pressure.

Clinical Note: Dyspnea Monitoring

Dyspnea monitoring is an essential training component in all functional training. Patients should be taught to measure their dyspnea level with all tasks of daily living as well as any other activities they perform.

tures to improve respiratory muscle function, and using relaxation techniques are some key principles of treatment.

An important principle in relieving dyspnea is that the patient should maintain an uninterrupted breathing pattern by avoiding breath holding, **Valsalva's maneuver,** or unnecessary talking during the task. Pursed-lip breathing may be useful for patients with obstructive lung disease whenever an increase in breathing effort is noticed. This naturally slows down respirations and decreases minute ventilation, relieving dyspnea in some patients.[46, 83, 84] Exhalations through pursed lips during lifting, pushing, or pulling activities prevents breath holding and straining.

Patients with restrictive interstitial lung disease experience greater work of breathing when taking slower, deeper breaths owing to the increased elastic resistance in their respiratory systems. During effort, these patients demonstrate rapid, shallow breathing, which is more energy-efficient for them.[85, 86] With either obstructive or restrictive pulmonary dysfunction, patients naturally assume a breathing pattern that requires the least energy and delays respiratory muscle fatigue.[87-91]

Breathing retraining or teaching the patient to use a specific breathing strategy that is not automatic is a controversial component of pulmonary rehabilitation. Even if successfully retrained for a new breathing pattern, the patient is likely to maintain it only with conscious effort and to resume a natural breathing pattern when attention is diverted to a task. In addition, the patient often finds the new breathing pattern fatiguing or uncomfortable.[46, 91, 92]

Many patients with severe COPD have diaphragms flattened by lung hyperinflation. A leaning-forward position may offer postural relief from dyspnea by improving the function of a flattened diaphragm. This position increases the intra-abdominal pressure and pushes the diaphragm up into the thorax and into a more optimal position for contraction.[93-95] Leaning forward with upper extremity support (Fig. 19–2) has the additional benefit of fixing the distal attachments of respiratory accessory muscles (e.g., pectoralis major or sternocleidomastoid) and allowing the thoracic attachments to pull the chest into inspiration.[93] Supported leaning-forward postures along with a comfortable, controlled breathing pattern may be used between efforts to help relieve shortness of breath.

Relaxation of nonrespiratory muscles is another breathing technique that may decrease wasted energy consumption and hasten relief of dyspnea. Contraction-relaxation techniques or **autogenic** (mental imaging) **relaxation** can be employed for this purpose. In some cases, biofeedback may help the patient learn to relax specific muscle groups. By teaching the patient control of the relaxation response and breathing pattern, the anxiety associated with dyspnea can be reduced.[47, 96]

Physiologic monitoring during functional training should be employed to ensure the safety and appropriateness of the exercises. Heart rate, blood pressure, respiratory rate, pulse oximetry, and dyspnea or effort scales, such as the **Borg scale** (Tables 19–4 and 19–5), are essential responses to monitor. The activity can be described in terms of intensity (percentage of maximum heart rate or degree of effort), duration (minutes of continuous or intermittent work), and frequency or number of repetitions of the activity carried out. Any symptoms (e.g., shortness of breath, fatigue, palpitations, chest discomfort) or a decrease of 3% to 5% on pulse oximetry should be noted. If the patient's level of desaturation is consistently below 88% on pulse oximetry, the physician should be contacted to prescribe supplemental oxygen or to increase the dosage of oxygen already in use.[15, 41, 42, 97]

Table 19–4
Dyspnea Scale

+1   Mild, noticeable to patient but not observer
+2   Mild, some difficulty, noticeable to observer
+3   Moderate difficulty, but can continue
+4   Severe difficulty, patient cannot continue

Source: American College of Sports Medicine. Guidelines for Exercise Testing and Precription. 4th ed. Philadelphia, Lea & Febiger, 1991. Reprinted with permission.

Table 19–5
Ratings of Perceived Exertion Scale

RATING	INTERPRETATION
6	
7	Very, very light
8	
9	Very light
10	
11	Fairly light
12	
13	Somewhat hard
14	
15	Hard
16	
17	Very hard
18	
19	Very, very hard
20	

Source: Borg G. Psychophysical basis of perceived exertion. Med Sci Sport Exerc 14[5]:377–381, 1982. © American College of Sports Medicine.

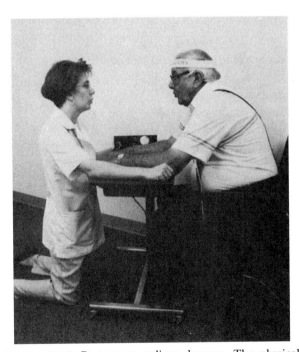

Figure 19–2. Postures to relieve dyspnea. The physical therapist is instructing the patient in sitting in the leaning-forward position, using a table for upper extremity support, and doing pursed-lip breathing. The pulse oximeter with a forehead transducer, held securely with a headband, is used to monitor changes with the treatment technique.

The physical therapist may advance functional training by

- Decreasing physical assistance offered to the patient in performing a task
- Decreasing the time to complete tasks
- Decreasing the time or frequency of rest periods
- Decreasing the dependence on adaptive equipment

The ultimate goal is for the patient to be able to perform the necessary activities of daily living within a functional time frame, with as much independence as possible, and without desaturation, undue fatigue, or shortness of breath.

Progress in rehabilitation can be documented using a variety of measures, such as the quantity of work performed or the decrease in heart rate, respiratory rate, perceived exertion, or symptoms during performance of the functional task. Such changes seem to indicate that the patient is more efficient at performing the task. Improvement can also be documented by observing the patient apply the treatment concepts to new tasks or environments. Standardized timed ADL tests or questionnaires that focus on functional abilities and quality of life offer outcome measures for functional training.

Physical Conditioning

The goals of physical conditioning exercises are aimed at increasing cardiorespiratory endurance, maximal work capacity, strength, flexibility, and respiratory muscle function. Because it is not always possible to work on all these areas at once, especially if the patient is very debilitated or deconditioned, priorities should be set for individualized goals based on the needs of the patient. It is optimal to prescribe exercises that accomplish more than one goal at a time and emphasize functional gains, such as increasing cardiorespiratory endurance for walking.

> ### Clinical Note: Coexisting Illness
> Caution should be taken with all patients who have coexisting conditions, especially when the coexisting illness is heart disease. See precautions and exercise guidelines in Chapter 18.

Because exercise performance varies with the severity of disease, a discussion of the patient with mild, moderate, and severe respiratory disease is presented. Several classifications for describing clinical status are available, most of which use a combination of pulmonary function tests, symptoms, and exercise tolerance.[49, 98, 99]

Patients with Mild Lung Disease

Patients with mild lung disease usually have shortness of breath only with relatively heavy exercise, such as climbing hills and stairs, but may be asymptomatic with usual daily activities. Because respiratory symptoms are very mild, they do not often present to the physician for treatment of lung disease. The only indicating signs of mild disease may be symptoms with extreme effort, a chronic cough or sputum production, or a history of smoking or occupational exposure. Identifying the presence of lung disease at this early stage may be possible only through routine employment screenings and annual physical examinations.

Spirometry testing of the patient with mild disease shows values within 70% to 85% of predicted values for vital capacity (VC) and forced expiratory volume in 1 second (FEV_1). Ventilatory responses to exercise are normal and with sufficient ventilatory reserves during maximum effort. Arterial blood gas values are normal or with slight reductions in arterial oxygen levels.

Exercise for patients with mild disease can be prescribed using testing and training protocols that would be used for a normal population. Because exercise intensities associated with physiologic conditioning of the aerobic system should be easily attainable, the patient should do very well on an independent training program, and formal rehabilitation is not usually indicated.

Patients with Moderate Lung Disease

Patients with moderate lung disease usually present with an acute exacerbation of their disease or worsening symptoms of shortness of breath with normal daily activities. These patients may have shown a pattern of restricting or modifying their activity level to prevent respiratory symptoms. Still, they may attribute their symptoms to normal aging, to being out of shape or overweight, or to a smoking habit. Many seem to believe that their symptoms would be resolved with simple changes in lifestyle.

An episode of acute pneumonia or pulmonary complications following an elective surgery may be the appropriate time to identify the patient with moderate lung disease and initiate treatment. If the patient is rehabilitated at this stage of the disease process, further pulmonary complications may be prevented.

The patient with moderate lung disease has a VC and an FEV_1 between 55% and 70% of predicted values and an exercise tolerance that is limited by ventilation. That is, the ventilatory reserves are exhausted at peak exercise loads. The patient becomes short of breath with usual activities of daily living and with a moderate to fast walking pace (approximately 3 to 4 METs). Mild to moderate hypoxemia may be present at rest and may either improve or worsen with exercise.

Exercise tolerance evaluations for patients with moderate lung disease can be performed using progressive exercise protocols. However, the protocol should start at a very low MET level (1.5 METs) and be advanced by 0.5 MET per stage.[49] Ideally, the electrocardiogram (ECG), blood pressure (BP), heart rate (HR), and pulse oximetry are monitored continuously during the test.[49] Alternatively, a functional 12-minute walking test can be used.[51, 52, 100] See Chapters 8 and 10 for more information on evaluation procedures.

Exercise prescription should be aimed at increasing duration to a submaximum workload that is sufficient to cause physiologic adaptation to effort. An initial training heart rate or workload can be estimated from the point on the exercise test at which the patient became noticeably but mildly dyspneic (level 2 to 3 on the dyspnea scale). The patient should first work to maintain this level for 20 to 30 minutes. Intermittent short bouts of slightly higher workloads can then be introduced gradually.

Because of ventilatory limitations during exercise, the intensity of the exercise and relative heart rate are lower than that usually prescribed for training the normal population. Therefore, the patient should exercise more frequently, at least five to seven times weekly. The total dosage of the exercise stimulus may bring about modest in-

creases in the symptom-limited maximum $\dot{V}O_2$ and decreases in the heart rate and minute ventilation responses to submaximum workloads.[10, 97, 101–103]

If the patient demonstrates arterial desaturation on pulse oximetry during exercise, supplemental oxygen may improve performance.[43] One training goal for some patients may be to reduce the supplemental oxygen dosage gradually, so that eventually only room air is necessary during exercise training. However, the majority of patients who require supplemental oxygen will never attain this goal.

Patients with Severe Lung Disease

Patients with severe lung disease usually are restricted by symptoms of shortness of breath during most daily activities. Even walking at a slow pace is limited. With spirometric testing, patients with severe lung disease demonstrate a VC and an FEV_1 below 55% of predicted values. The patient may require intermittent or continuous oxygen at rest and with activity and may have elevated arterial carbon dioxide levels. Some patients with severe disease show signs of right ventricular dysfunction during exercise, which seems to be related to oxygen desaturation, and improve with supplemental oxygen during exercise.[104]

Patients with severe lung disease require a modified approach to exercise testing. They should be given either low-level intermittent tests, in which they are given rests between work stages, or a steady-state endurance test at a 2 to 3 MET level.[50] Alternatively, a 6-, 3-, or even 2-minute functional walking test may be utilized.[52] Monitoring the patient closely for desaturation and exercise-induced arrhythmias is important during testing procedures. Supplemental oxygen dosages that maintain a saturation value higher than 88% should be identified and prescribed for patients who reach desaturation levels during exercise.[43, 15, 97, 104]

The exercise prescription for patients with severe lung disease should be based on symptom-limited walking speeds and distances. Interval training programs are optimal, with very short exercise bouts and frequent rests initially. The prescription can be advanced gradually by increasing the number of bouts, lengthening the bouts, or decreasing the length of the rest periods. Because the initial training prescription (intensity and duration) is very low, the patient should exercise a minimum of one time per day. As the total exercise duration increases to 20 minutes continuously, the frequency may be reduced to five to seven times per week. Even very *small* gains in exercise tolerance for the patient with severe lung disease can be significant for functional improvements and quality of life.[10, 46, 22, 105, 106]

Patients with severe lung disease need intensive monitoring and supervision, the degree of which depends on the severity of the disease. Therefore, a stratified approach to monitoring during rehabilitation sessions is most appropriate. Patients in the mild disease category may require only monitoring of exercise intensity through heart rate and perceived exertion determinations. Blood pressure, pulse oximetry, and ECG should be monitored only in patients who demonstrate hypertension or hypoxemia or who also have cardiac disease.[15, 107, 108]

Patients in the moderate disease category should be monitored more frequently with pulse oximetry, heart rate, peak blood pressure, perceived exertion, and rating of severity of symptoms during the first 4 to 6 weeks of rehabilitation. Increased monitoring for patients with moderate disease assists in documenting improvement and establishing higher training workloads as they are tolerated.

Patients in the severe lung disease category need continuous monitoring of pulse oximetry and heart rate and intermittent determinations of blood pressure, dyspnea and exertion scales. Patients with arrhythmias require ECG monitoring.[107, 108] All patients should gradually require less supervision and monitoring as rehabilitation goals are met, and the patient develops independence in self-regulation and monitoring of the exercise intensity, duration, and frequency.

Strengthening

Patients with lung disease often suffer from appetite suppression, weight loss, and wasting of muscle mass.[46, 109–111] For optimal rehabilitation, the patient's nutritional status must be determined regarding its adequacy for meeting the demands of increasing activity levels and replacing lost muscle. Increasing strength and local muscle endurance improves the patient's ability to perform func-

tional activities, decrease local muscle fatigue, and enhance body image.[112]

Lower extremity strengthening can be accomplished through the aerobic training program if cycling, stair climbing, bench stepping, or aerobic dance are used as modes. If level walking is the primary aerobic training mode, very little strengthening occurs unless hill climbing is included. As an alternative, the patient can use resistive weight training equipment, particularly if the equipment allows the patient to remain upright, or assume leaning forward postures to make breathing more comfortable, or both. The program should be started with low resistance and progressed first by increasing repetitions, for example, 3 to 4 sets of 6 to 10 repetitions, before adding additional weight.

Upper body (trunk and upper extremity) training requires more ventilatory work, and patients are more likely to hold their breath, develop asynchronous breathing patterns, and become dyspneic.[113, 114] However, clinical studies have demonstrated that patients with respiratory disorders can train successfully with upper body resistive work, which produces improvements in dyspnea, fatigue, and respiratory muscle function.[11, 12, 32] The strengthening program should start with very light weights (pulleys, TheraBand, wrist weights, weighted wands) and, again, advance first by increasing the number of repetitions. As the patient improves, light free weights or weight machines can be used. A 30-second bout of exercise with several minutes rest between bouts is a useful approach for patients with lung disease. Rotating between machines for upper extremity and lower extremity exercise may also improve tolerance for the strengthening program. Aerobic training modes of arm cranking and leg cycles that include arm work, rowing machines, or cross-country ski machines can also promote upper body strengthening and endurance (Fig. 19–3).

During resistive work, the physical therapist should monitor the breathing pattern, heart rate, blood pressure, and pulse oximetry. The ECG should also be monitored if the patient has cardiovascular disease or demonstrates arrhythmias.

The results of standardized lifting tests or dynamometry or records of the resistive loads tolerated during training are objective ways to demonstrate the outcomes of a strengthening program. Improvement in muscle endurance can be shown by recording the increase in repetitions of an exer-

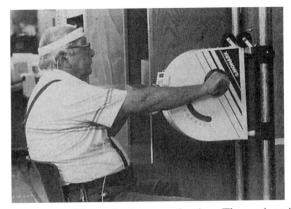

Figure 19–3. Upper body strengthening. The patient is using intermittent arm cranking for both upper extremity strengthening and endurance training. The use of the forehead transducer for the pulse oximeter allows for stable measurements during vigorous arm movements.

cise per unit of time. Lastly, the measured or reported ability of the patient to carry out employment-specific, recreational, or daily activities should be documented.

Flexibility

Most patients with chronic respiratory disease have significant changes in posture and reduced mobility. These changes can be a result of inactivity or structural changes of the chest wall with hyperinflation and hypertrophy of the respiratory muscles. Flexibility exercises should be included to improve posture, increase joint range of motion, decrease stiffness, and prevent injury.

Gentle stretching with full body movements as occurs with dance, yoga, or calisthenics is appropriate for the pulmonary rehabilitation patient, especially if breathing exercises are coordinated with the movements. For instance, movements that bring full shoulder flexion, back extension, and

Clinical Note: Extension Exercises

Extension exercises should be incorporated into the patient's exercise program. Cervical and thoracic extension will improve thoracic expansion and hip extension will prevent hip flexion contractures.

inspiration can be performed together to increase trunk flexibility and facilitate breathing. Exercises with forward-reaching and trunk flexion or with unilateral or bilateral hip and lower trunk flexion may be combined with expiration.

The purpose of combined flexibility and breathing exercises is to teach the patient how body movements can influence and assist or resist ventilation. The flexibility or mobility exercises can be used as a warm-up or cool-down activity for aerobic conditioning or at any time to relieve muscle tension or anxiety.

Monitoring changes in posture, range of motion, and subjective ratings of stiffness can be used to document the effects of a flexibility program. Long-term outcomes of the program may be documented from a reduced incidence of back pain or joint injuries.

Respiratory Muscle Exercise

Exercises for improving respiratory muscle function are an important component of a pulmonary rehabilitation program. The increased work of breathing and chest wall changes that occur with chronic lung disease make respiratory muscle fatigue more likely to occur.[92] The fact that respiratory muscle fatigue is chronic may be significantly related to symptoms of shortness of breath. Two general approaches for improving respiratory muscle function are to

- Rest the muscles with a device to assist breathing at night such as continuous positive airway pressure (CPAP)[39–42]
- Increase the performance capacity of the respiratory muscles through exercise training[115–118]

The work of breathing, or ventilatory work of moving air in and out of the lungs, is increased with most exercise or activity. Aerobic exercise training of the upper or lower extremities or both, that is moderate to high intensity may be an adequate stimulus to improve respiratory muscle endurance.[14, 32, 101] However, it is unlikely that older patients or those who have significant lung disease would be able to sustain high enough intensities to induce these changes.[11, 12, 13]

Training specific respiratory muscles with a resistive breathing device has been shown to improve respiratory muscle function in quadriplegics

> ### Clinical Note: Using Sandbags Over the Diaphragm
>
> According to the literature, sandbags on the abdomen do not actually strengthen the diaphragm. Clinically, patients have been observed to develop poor breathing mechanics if they have been taught diaphragmatic exercises with sandbags on the abdomen.

> ### Clinical Note: Respiratory Muscle Training
>
> Note that when a patient stops a respiratory muscle training program, clinically the benefit of respiratory muscle training stops as well, similar to when individuals stop skeletal muscle training. Therefore, respiratory muscle training needs to be a lifelong training program, or the benefits are diminished. Respiratory muscle training has also been used in patients with congestive heart failure with good success if they continue their training program.

and in patients with COPD.[119, 127] However, the presence of a carryover effect of improved respiratory muscle function to improved exercise tolerance, decreased dyspnea, and improved maximal work capacity has not been proved.[122, 123, 125–127] At least theoretically, the patient should be able to withstand more ventilatory work with less respiratory muscle fatigue so that exercise and pulmonary exacerbations are better tolerated.

For training the respiratory muscles, the patient is required to breathe against an added resistive load. This is accomplished by using one of several devices on the market that increases airway resistance (Fig. 19–4). The initial training prescription should include a resistance of 25% to 35% of the maximal negative inspiratory pressure measured at functional residual volume, a duration of up to 15 minutes, and a frequency of twice daily.[125–127] Alternatively, the patient can be started at an arbitrarily low resistance, that is, one that can be sustained for 15 minutes without fatigue, dyspnea, or oxygen desaturation. If the patient can complete

two 15 minute sessions with a 20-minute rest between bouts, then the resistance can be increased to the next higher setting.[127]

Although most of the clinical studies on the efficacy of respiratory muscle training have included only patients with COPD or quadriplegia as subjects, the treatment may be applicable to other patient groups in whom respiratory muscle weakness or fatigability is demonstrated: those who have neuromuscular syndromes, thoracic wall deformities such as kyphoscoliosis, and restrictive pulmonary diseases and those who are morbidly obese.

Outcomes of respiratory muscle training can be documented by recording increases in the training resistance and maximal inspiratory pressures. A change in the patient's breathing strategy (flow rate, breathing rate, and depth) may alter the effective resistive load. Therefore, these factors need to be controlled during training and evaluation sessions.[125–127] Reported improvements in dyspnea and the ability to carry out activities of daily living are potential outcomes of respiratory muscle training.

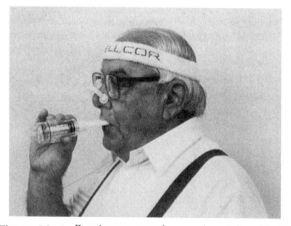

Figure 19–4. Respiratory muscle exercise. A hand-held, single-patient use respiratory muscle exerciser is employed to offer added airway resistance and increase respiratory muscle strength and endurance.

CASE STUDIES

Case 1. The Patient with Chronic Restrictive Pulmonary Disease

CB is a 40-year-old woman with kyphoscoliosis, morbid obesity, chronic hypoventilation, and sleep apnea. Because of sleep deprivation at night, the patient experiences excessive daytime sleepiness. She has been treated with supplemental oxygen by nasal cannula, 1 L/minute, and continuous positive airway pressure at night. She was also referred to pulmonary rehabilitation to improve her exercise tolerance and to reduce her weight and percentage of body fat.

Tests

Chest roentgenogram:	Obesity, spinal deformity, no acute disease
Arterial blood gas (on room air):	Pa_{O_2}, 55; Pa_{CO_2}, 60; pH, 7.39; HCO_3^-, 36; base excess 10 (hypoxemia with mixed respiratory acidosis and metabolic alkalosis; compensated)
Electrocardiogram (rest, 12-lead):	normal sinus rhythm, left ventricular hypertrophy
Echocardiogram:	Mild left ventricular hypertrophy, left ventricular ejection fraction (LVEF), 78%; right ventricular ejection fraction (RVEF), 54%
Pulmonary function tests:	VC, 0.8 L, FEV_1, 0.78 L; maximum voluntary ventilation (MVV), 24 L/min (severe restrictive lung disease)

Physical Therapy Evaluation

1. Patient interview: CB complained of right lower extremity pain at night and leg and foot pain and shortness of breath during walking. She reported being most comfortable pushing a cart while walking and could walk less than one block at a time. She had been confined to her home primarily, going out with assistance only. She wished to be able to go to the store or to a friend's house independently, to get off oxygen if possible, and to be less short of breath. She also wanted to be able to do some of her own housework and to climb stairs.

2. Resting evaluation: Relaxed breathing pattern on oxygen at 1 L/minute by nasal prongs. Very short stature, very obese, and with a marked kyphoscoliosis. While sitting: heart rate (HR), 67 bpm; blood pressure (BP), 110/78 mm Hg; respiratory rate (RR), 20; oxygen saturation (SO_2), 97%.

3. Cardiovascular evaluation: Test protocol was a single-stage walk at self-selected velocity on the treadmill: the treadmill speed was 2.5 mph, and the grade was 0%. CB walked a total of 2.0 minutes, stopping with shortness of breath. Peak HR, 101 bpm; BP, 124/80; RR, 42; SO_2, 75%; minute ventilation (V_E), 18 L/minute; rating of perceived exertion (RPE), 15. The patient recovered, returning to her baseline HR and So_2 within 1.0 to 1.5 minutes. She was able to repeat the same workload three more times. Her total exercise time was 7.5 minutes, and her total rest time was 6 minutes.

   Upper extremity endurance test (upper extremity ergometer): At less than 5 watts at 50 rpm, the patient was able to exercise for less than 1 minute.

She stopped with shortness of breath and arm fatigue. Peak HR, 96; BP, 130/84; So_2, 78%; RR, 45; V_E, 20.2; RPE, 17. CB recovered to her baseline within 2 minutes.

4. Functional evaluation: During a 6-minute walking test, CB walked 625 feet with three rest stops. She climbed up and down six steps in 3 minutes with two rest periods. She was limited by leg pain and shortness of breath. Peak HR, 105; BP, 118/80; RR, 45; So_2, 80%; RPE, 15 with walking and 17 with stair climbing.

Rehabilitation Goals

- Lose approximately 50 kg (110 lb) of body weight over the next 6 to 12 months or about 8 to 16 kg (12–24 lbs) in the next 6 to 8 weeks.
- Increase endurance to 2.0 to 2.5 mph (walking) and to 20 to 40 minutes.
- Increase endurance for arm work to 5 watts for 10 minutes.
- Increase walking distance to more than 1000 feet in 6 minutes.
- Increase stair climbing to one flight (12 steps) within 2 minutes.

Training Program

Because the patient consistently became desaturated below 85%, the supplemental oxygen flow rate was increased to 1 to 3 L/minute as needed during exercise sessions (based on protocol). Because weight loss was an important consideration, the exercise load was kept at a low to moderate intensity as tolerated. Increasing the total duration was emphasized to increase the caloric expenditure. Her severe pulmonary limitations made an interval program necessary. Functional activities of walking and stair climbing were the primary mode of training to accomplish the patient's identified goals.

Exercise Prescription

Modes:	Hall walking and treadmill walking, stair climbing, stationary cycling, and upper extremity ergometry
Intensity:	2.5 to 2.8 METs or a self-selected pace
Duration:	2-minute bouts with 2-minute rests; progress to 5-minute bouts with 1-minute rests as tolerated
Frequency:	Twice a day in physical therapy, once independently (three times a day total)

Monitoring and Ongoing Evaluations

Measured each session:	Workload, total exercise duration (minutes), total rest time, peak HR, RR, RPE, pulse oximetry, and signs and symptoms of exercise intolerance

| Measured with increases in work intensity: | Peak V̇E, BP, and breathing pattern |
| Measured weekly for documenting outcomes: | Total body weight; ability to do activities of daily living independently, ability to self-monitor exercise performance, patient satisfaction; and subjective ratings of progress in symptoms, functional progress, and ability to sleep |

Rehabilitation Outcomes

CB was discharged after 8 weeks of inpatient rehabilitation, during which she increased her exercise tolerance from a 2.8 MET level to 4 METs and her exercise duration from 6 minutes to 45 minutes. She lost a total of 20 kg (44 lb) of body weight and became independent in all activities of daily living and in carrying out her exercise program. She required 1 to 2 L of supplemental oxygen during her training sessions but could go portions of the day without oxygen. CB reported that she was feeling more confident in her abilities and that she was sleeping better during the night with less sleepiness during the day.

Case 2. The Patient with Cystic Fibrosis

SS is a 9-year-old girl with cystic fibrosis who is followed on an outpatient basis in the cystic fibrosis center, every 3 months. She has moderate COPD and pancreatic insufficiency as a result of her cystic fibrosis. For the past 4 years, SS has required hospitalization to treat pulmonary exacerbations with intravenous antibiotics and chest physical therapy. She has recently had a permanent central line placed for home antibiotic therapy. She also underwent jejunostomy for supplemental feedings at night. Current medications include methylprednisolone (Medrol), theophylline (Slo-bid), albuterol (metered-dose inhaler), oral dicloxacillin, and pancrelipase (Pancrease).

Tests

Chest roentgenogram:	Bilateral hyperinflated lungs with peribronchial cuffing and chronic infiltrative changes; central line extends into the proximal aspect of the right atrium
Pulmonary function tests (pre- and post-bronchodilator):	FVC, 1.40/1.63 L; FEV$_1$, 0.79/1.03 L/minute; FEV$_1$/FVC, 56/63%
Clinical microbiology report:	Sputum quantification: 105,000,000 colony-forming units per mL of Pseudomonas aeruginosa

Physical Therapy Evaluation

1. Patient interview: SS stated that she had been feeling pretty well and attended school regularly. She occasionally has a cold that increases her cough and mucus production. She reported no problems in doing her home treatments but has been less energetic lately. SS has had some problems in physical education class because her teacher makes her sit down when she starts to cough. Her sports interests include skating, biking, and gymnastics and swimming in the summer.

2. Respiratory evaluation: SS's breathing pattern was slightly tachypneic (24 breaths per minute). A barrel chest and nail clubbing were evident, as were bilateral upper lobes with coarse inspiratory rales. Her cough was strong, effective, and productive of 5 to 10 mL of thick, tan mucus.

3. Cardiovascular evaluation: Using a Bruce treadmill protocol, the following measurements were taken: resting HR, 127 bpm; resting So$_2$, 94%; peak HR, 180 bpm; peak So$_2$, 90%; peak METs, 10.0; peak RPE, 18. The reason for termination was leg fatigue and shortness of breath. Interpretation of results: Normal cardiovascular exercise response to 85% of age-predicted maximal heart rate; mild desaturation (4%) at peak exercise. SS's exercise tolerance was in the 25th percentile of the normal population for her age and sex.

Rehabilitation Goals

- Clearing of pulmonary rales on auscultation
- Decrease symptoms of cough and fatigue
- Improve leg strength and muscle endurance
- Increase exercise tolerance to the 50th percentile
- Increase participation in physical education class

Rehabilitation Program

1. Pulmonary treatments: SS and her mother have been performing postural drainage with percussion twice daily (before breakfast and at bedtime). SS's mother has been assisting with treatments, using a palm cup for percussion. Lower and middle lobes have been emphasized. SS coughed well after treatment at each position and cleared mucus easily. She uses her albuterol inhaler before each treatment. Her treatment techniques were superior.

    Modifications in SS's pulmonary treatment regimen were as follows: Postural drainage positions for the upper lobes were reviewed. SS was shown how to do self-percussion for these positions. In addition, she was instructed in the forced expiratory maneuver to be performed for 5 minutes before physical education class and exercise. She was also issued and instructed in the operation of a positive expiratory pressure (PEP) mask, which was to be used independently after school each day. Her mother was shown how to use a stethoscope for monitoring breath sounds before and after pulmonary treatments.

2. Exercise training program: SS was encouraged to continue her gymnastics for whole body strengthen-

ing and flexibility training. Also for leg strengthening and endurance, she was instructed to continue her biking and to choose routes with an incline. Climbing stairs two at a time and jumping rope were other modes of leg strengthening.

Cardiovascular training guidelines were kept simple and emphasized her recreation. Running games (e.g., kickball, tag, dodgeball), biking, swimming, or jumping rope were listed as possible conditioning modes. She was instructed to exercise at an RPE rating of 13 to 15 or at a pace that induced breathing with moderate effort and coughing, a duration of 20 to 30 minutes without significant rest breaks, and a frequency of daily. She was also issued and instructed in the use of a dance videotape for children to be substituted for her regular exercise on rainy days or to supplement her conditioning play.

In addition, a letter with information on cystic fibrosis and treatment for pulmonary disease was sent to her physical education teacher, with a request for assistance in meeting SS's goals.

Monitoring and Measurements

Measured at each session:	Breath sounds, especially of the upper lobes, and volume of mucus produced were to be recorded by SS or her mother with each postural drainage treatment, or at least 3 days per week. A chart of her exercises was given to SS to record the activity, the length of play conditioning in minutes, the rating of perceived exertion, and the amount of mucus produced. She was encouraged to fill in this chart each evening and to bring it with her to her next physical therapy evaluation session.
Measured every 3 months:	At each follow-up evaluation, SS was monitored for changes in exercise tolerance, improved pulmonary function test results and breath sounds, ability to participate in school and play, compliance with home instructions, and growth in height and body weight.
Measured yearly:	The frequency of hospitalization and use of home antibiotics, school attendance, and changes in chest roentgenogram were evaluated annually.

Rehabilitation Outcomes

According to her home records, which she brought to the 3-month return visit, SS was compliant with her postural drainage sessions 80% of the time. She also maintained her exercise program an average of 5 days per week. She was able to demonstrate her postural drainage positions and percussion of the upper lobes and her forced cough technique with satisfaction. Her breath sounds were somewhat improved, with fine to medium rales in the upper lobes.

SS reported an improvement in her ability to participate in school physical education class and a better understanding of her coughing by her teacher.

On exercise testing, SS increased her peak work to 11.8 METs (25th to 50th percentile), with a maximal HR of 195 bpm, a peak RPE of 19, and pulse oximetry of 94%. She no longer demonstrated any desaturation with maximal exercise. The test was terminated with leg fatigue and no shortness of breath. Pulmonary function tests were unchanged, and she had gained about 2 kg of weight.

Case 3. The Patient with Emphysema

WS is a 48-year-old man with a history of progressive severe COPD and cor pulmonale. He was evaluated by the pulmonary medicine department and was thought to be a good candidate for lung transplantation. He was referred to the pulmonary rehabilitation program to obtain an evaluation of his current physical capabilities and to increase his exercise tolerance and strength before transplantation.

WS is on the following supplements and medications: oxygen, 1.5 L/minute at night, and phenytoin (Dilantin) for a history of seizures.

Tests

Chest roentgenogram:	Hyperinflated lungs, with flattened diaphragms; increased anteroposterior diameter and bullous changes in the bases of the lungs. The pulmonary arteries appeared large.
Pulmonary function tests:	VC, 1.67 L (39% predicted); inspiratory capacity, 1.22 L (43% predicted); total lung capacity, 9.15 L (133% predicted); FEV_1, 0.55 L (15% predicted); FEV_1/VC, 33%; MVV, 35 L/min (25% predicted); DL_{CO}, 22 mL/mm Hg/min (69% predicted)

Resting ECG:	Normal sinus rhythm, with occasional supraventricular premature complexes; poor R wave progression
Hematology profile:	White blood cell count, 6.2; red blood cell count, 5.5; hemoglobin, 16.1; hematocrit, 49%; platelets, 262,000; reticulocytes, 0.3
Arterial blood gas:	Pa_{O_2}, 56 mm Hg; Pa_{CO_2}, 45 mm Hg; pH, 7.37; HCO_3^-, 28; So_2, 92% (on room air, at rest)
Cardiopulmonary exercise test (performed on a cycle ergometer):	Resting heart rate, 92 bpm; resting blood pressure, 169/106; peak heart rate, 138 bpm; peak blood pressure, 220/113; maximum Vo_2, 0.86 L/min or 3.2 METs; maximum V_E, 34 L/min. Arterial blood gases: Pa_{O_2}, 45; Pa_{CO_2}, 53; pH, 7.32; So_2, 80%. ECG, no changes in arrhythmia or ST segments. Test terminated with grade 4 dyspnea.

Interpretation: exercise capacity severely limited by ventilation deficits, with respiratory acidosis and arterial oxygen desaturation at peak exercise. Also resting and exercise hypertension.

Physical Therapy Evaluation

1. Patient interview: WS is currently working full time as an assistant director of a mental health center. His work tasks are primarily sedentary but include walking from a parking lot to the building, approximately a half-block walk. Other activities are some very light gardening, photography, traveling, and reading. He uses meditation and biofeedback for relaxation training. He is married and has two grown children. Family and friends are supportive.

   WS reported symptoms of severe dyspnea that limit his activities of daily living, primarily shaving, showering, and dressing. Also he is unable to climb even one flight of stairs or walk more than one block without resting for relief of dyspnea. He wears his supplemental oxygen only at night. He has become quite limited in his ability to continue his current hobbies. He reported an interest in conditioning to improve his chances for a positive outcome of the lung transplantation.

2. Respiratory evaluation: WS's breathing pattern was moderately distressed at rest, with tachypnea (rate 28) and use of inspiratory accessory muscles. A barrel chest was noted. His breath sounds were decreased throughout, without adventitious sounds, and his cough was dry and nonproductive. The maximum negative inspiratory force was -48 cm H_2O; breathing endurance time at a load of -12 cm H_2O (25% max) was 5 minutes, limited by dyspnea.

3. Functional evaluation: Activities of daily living that require upper body and arm movement were the most difficult for WS to complete. During the assessment of shaving and dressing skills, he demonstrated increased dyspnea when his arms were held at face level for longer than 1 minute, when his arms were raised overhead, or when he leaned forward to reach his feet. During effort, he frequently held his breath and grunted on expiration. His pulse increased to 108 bpm, and pulse oximetry decreased to 88%. Time to complete each task was also recorded.

4. Cardiovascular endurance: WS's 6-minute walk test results were as follows: resting HR, 92 bpm; resting BP, 152/96; resting So_2, 92% (room air); peak HR, 121 bpm; peak BP, 198/102; peak So_2, 82%; recovery time to return to baseline, 4 minutes; distance walked, 620 feet, with 3 stops for rest; peak RPE, 17; dyspnea rating, $+3$; V_E, 28 L at peak exercise (80% MVV).

Rehabilitation Goals

- Increase walking endurance and distance
- Reduce dyspnea, if possible
- Increase tolerance for activities of daily living
- Improve respiratory muscle function
- Maintain or improve general health for upcoming surgery

Rehabilitation Program

1. Respiratory muscle training: WS was started at the lowest resistance setting (approximately -12 cm H_2O) for 5 minutes, twice daily at home. He was instructed to increase the duration by 1 to 2 minutes every 3 to 4 days as tolerated, until he reached 15 minutes. The resistance setting would then be increased gradually, as determined during weekly reassessments.

2. Exercise training: WS was started on a walking program at home and exercised on the treadmill and bicycle ergometer during the rehabilitation sessions. He was begun on an intermittent exercise training program, with incorporation of dyspnea relief skills. Emphasis was placed on pacing and control of a continuous breathing pattern while increasing the total exercise duration. Also, WS was placed on 1 to 3 L/min of oxygen during his training session to keep the So_2 above 88%.

Modes:	Walking, treadmill, bicycling
Intensity:	RPE, 15; dyspnea, 2 to 3; HR 110 to 120 bpm; 2.0 to 2.5 METs; V_E, 25 L
Duration:	2-minute exercise; 2-minute rests; 4 to 5 bouts
Frequency:	Daily

Monitoring: HR, BP, pulse oximetry, RPE, and dyspnea rating.

3. Upper body training: WS was started on upper body calisthenics using an unweighted wand. Initially, two to three repetitions were performed on each exercise, which included overhead and reaching-forward movements with breathing techniques incorporated into the exercise. Repetitions were increased gradually to 20, then light weights were added in 0.25-lb increments. In addition, ball-handling exercises were performed with the rehabilitation group.

Measurements and Ongoing Evaluations

Measured at each session:	At each rehabilitation session, the patient was assessed for total walking time and distance, oxygen dosage, and So_2 at peak exercise. Resistance setting and duration of respiratory training, repetitions of upper body exercises, and maximum weight of resistance were also measured.
Measured weekly:	Measurements of maximal negative inspiratory force and endurance time at 25% maximum resistance, 6-minute walking distance, and compliance with home programs were assessed weekly.

Rehabilitation Outcomes

WS increased his walking distance to 1150 feet in 6 minutes and his maximal negative inspiratory force to −62 cm H_2O. His upper body endurance increased to 20 repetitions of exercise, using 2 lb. He also modified his activities of daily living with pacing and organizing so that he was less dyspneic. He completed his formal rehabilitation but continues to return for monthly reevaluations of his status and changes in his treatments until his lung transplantation.

Summary

• Rehabilitation intervention has been considered maintenance activity, and third-party payers have often severely limited the benefits paid for pulmonary rehabilitation.

• Rehabilitation research is currently emphasizing functional outcomes as measures of efficacy instead of changes in physiologic parameters.

• Goals for an individual must be very specific and pertinent to that individual's lifestyle, needs, and interests.

• Any person with a primary or secondary pulmonary disease or anyone at risk for the development of pulmonary disease is a potential candidate for rehabilitation.

• Candidates for rehabilitation must meet the following criteria: a diagnosed respiratory disease and documented functional limitations.

• A comprehensive pulmonary rehabilitation program should include exercise and functional training, education and patient training and psychosocial management.

• After an assessment is made, therapeutic intervention often includes prescription of medication and possibly oxygen, preventive care such as immunizations and vaccinations, smoking cessation, avoidance of environmental irritants, adequate hydration, and proper nutrition including weight control.

• Respiratory treatment techniques for clearing accumulated pulmonary secretions and relieving dyspnea include bronchial drainage, breathing techniques, cough facilitation, postures to improve breathing, relaxation techniques, bronchodilators, and the use of respiratory assistance devices to rest the breathing muscles at night or during exercise.

• The main emphasis of pulmonary care in the rehabilitation setting is the removal of excessive secretions that obstruct airways and cause ventilatory defects, cause bothersome symptoms of cough, and possibly lead to an increased incidence of respiratory infections and deterioration of lung function.

• Treatment goals include adapting the environment to improve the ease of performing activities of daily living, altering the performance of tasks to decrease energy costs, and incorporating methods to relieve symptoms associated with activity.

• Identification of the activities of daily living that are most problematic for the patient is the first step in modifying the environment. Once identified, the areas in the home in which these activities are performed need to be evaluated for modification.

- An important concept in relieving dyspnea is that the patient continues an uninterrupted breathing pattern by avoiding breath holding, Valsalva's maneuvers, or unnecessary talking during the task.
- Patients with restrictive interstitial lung disease experience greater work of breathing when taking slower, deeper breaths because of the increased elastic resistance in their respiratory system.
- Relaxation of nonrespiratory muscles is another breathing technique that may decrease wasted energy and hasten relief of dyspnea.
- Patients with severe lung disease require a modified approach to exercise testing. Tests should either be low-level intermittent tests, in which the patient is given rests between work stages, or a steady-state endurance test at a 2 to 3 MET level.
- Patients in the moderate disease category should be monitored more frequently with pulse oximetry and for peak heart rate and blood pressure. Ratings of effort and symptoms are also needed during the first 4 to 6 weeks of rehabilitation.
- Patients in the severe lung disease category need continuous monitoring of pulse oximetry and heart rate, with intermittent monitoring of blood pressure, dyspnea, and exertion scales. Some patients with arrhythmias require ECG monitoring.
- Patients with lung disease often have appetite suppression, weight loss, and wasting of muscle mass.
- Upper body (trunk and upper extremity) training requires more ventilatory work, and the patient is more likely to breath hold, develop an asynchronous breathing pattern, and become dyspneic.
- Most patients with chronic respiratory disease have significant changes in posture and reduced mobility.
- Two general approaches for improving respiratory muscle function are to rest the muscles with an assisted breathing device at night or to increase the performance capacity of the respiratory muscles through exercise training.
- For training the respiratory muscles, the patient is required to breathe against an added resistive load. The initial training prescription should include a resistance of 25 to 35 % of the maximal negative inspiratory pressure measured at functional residual volume, a duration of up to 15 minutes, and a frequency of twice daily.

References

1. American Thoracic Society. Pulmonary rehabilitation: Official American Thoracic Society position statement. Am Rev Respir Dis 124:663–666, 1981.
2. Task Force Report: Epidemiology of respiratory diseases. US Department of Health and Human Services, Public Health Service. National Institutes of Health, Publication 81-2019, pp 13–25, 156–158, 1980.
3. Higgins M. Epidemiology of COPD, state of the art. Chest 85(6 suppl):3S–6S, 1984
4. Ries AL. Position paper of the American Association of Cardiovascular and Pulmonary Rehabilitation. Scientific basis of pulmonary rehabilitation. J Cardiopulmonary Rehabil 10(11):418–441, 1990.
5. Connors G, Hilling L (ed). Guidelines for Pulmonary Rehabilitation Programs. 2nd ed. American Association of Cardiovascular and Pulmonary Rehabilitation. Champaign, IL, Human Kinetics, 1993.
6. Pashkow P. Outcomes in cardiopulmonary rehabilitation. Phys Ther 76(6):643–656, 1996.
7. Dean E. Preferred practice patterns in cardiopulmonary physical therapy: A guide to physiologic measures. Cardiopulmonary Phys Ther J 10(4):124–134, 1999.
8. Haggerty MC, Stockdale-Wooley R, ZuWallack R. Functional status in pulmonary rehabilitation participants. J Cardiopulmonary Rehabil 19(1):35:42, 1998.
9. Scherer YK, Schnieder LE. The effect of a pulmonary rehabilitation program on self-efficacy, perception of dyspnea, and physical endurance. Heart Lung 26(1):14–22, 1997.
10. Niederman MS, Clemente PH, Fein AM, et al. Benefits of a multidisciplinary pulmonary rehabilitation program: Improvements are independent of lung function. Chest 19(4):798–804, 1988.
11. Ries AL, Ellis B, Hawkins RW. Upper extremity exercise training in chronic obstructive pulmonary disease. Chest 93(4):688–692, 1988.
12. Lake FR, Henderson K, Brifta T, et al. Upper-limb and lower-limb exercise training in patients with chronic airflow obstruction. Chest 97(5):1077–1082, 1990.
13. Belman MJ, Kendregan BA. Physical training fails to improve ventilatory muscle endurance in patients with chronic obstructive pulmonary disease. Chest 81(4):440–443, 1982.
14. Orenstein DM, Franklin BA, Doershuk CF, et al. Exercise conditioning and cardiorespiratory fitness in cystic fibrosis. Chest 80(4):392–398, 1981.
15. Moser KM, Bokinsky G, Savage RT, et al. Results of a comprehensive rehabilitation program: Physiologic and functional effects on patients with chronic obstructive pulmonary disease. Arch Intern Med 140:1596–1601, 1980.
16. Bass H, Whitcomb JF, Forman R. Exercise training: Therapy for patients with chronic obstructive pulmonary disease. Chest 57(2):116–121, 1970.
17. Swerts P, Kretzers L, Terpstra-Linderman E, et al. Exercise reconditioning in the rehabilitation of patients with chronic obstructive pulmonary disease: A short- and long-term analysis. Arch Phys Med Rehabil 71:570–573, 1990.
18. Vyas MN, Banister EW, Morton JW, et al. Response to exercises in patients with chronic airway obstruction: Effects of exercise training. Am Rev Respir Dis 103:390–399, 1971.
19. Degre S, Sergysels R, Measin R, et al. Hemodynamic responses to physical training in patients with chronic lung disease. Am Rev Respir Dis 110:395–402, 1974.
20. Chester EF, Belman MJ, Bahler RC, et al. Multidisciplinary

treatment of chronic pulmonary insufficiency. Chest 72(6): 695–702, 1977.

21. Foster S, Thomas HM. Pulmonary rehabilitation in lung disease other than chronic obstructive pulmonary disease. Am Rev Respir Dis 141:601–604, 1990.

22. Brundin, A. Physical training in severe chronic obstructive lung disease. Scand J Respir Dis 55:25–36, 1974.

23. Holden DA, Stelmach KD, Curtis PS, et al. The impact of a rehabilitation program on functional status of patients with chronic lung disease. Respir Care 35(4):332–341, 1990.

24. McGavin CR, Gupta SP, Lloyd EL, et al. Physical rehabilitation for the chronic bronchitic: Results of a controlled trial of exercises in the home. Thorax 32:307–311, 1977.

25. Mertens DJ, Shephard RJ, Kavanagh T. Long-term exercise therapy for chronic obstructive lung disease. Respiration 35:96–107, 1978.

26. Sinclair DJM, Ingram CG. Controlled trial of supervised exercise training in chronic bronchitis. Br Med J 280:519–521, 1980.

27. Unger LM, Moser KM, Hansen P. Selection of an exercise program for patients with chronic obstructive pulmonary disease. Heart Lung 9(1):68–76, 1980.

28. Ries AL, Archibald CJ. Endurance exercise training at maximal targets in patients with chronic obstructive pulmonary disease. J Cardiopulmonary Rehabil 7:594–601, 1987.

29. Sahn SA, Nett LM, Petty TL. Ten year follow-up of a comprehensive rehabilitation program for severe COPD, Chest 77(suppl 2):311–314, 1980.

30. Reardon J, Awad E, Normandin E, et al. The effect of comprehensive outpatient pulmonary rehabilitation on dyspnea. Chest 1059(4):2046–2052, 1994.

31. Ramirez-Venegas A, Ward JL, Olmstead EM, et al. Effect of exercise training on dyspnea measures in patients with chronic obstructive pulmonary disease. J Cardiopulmonary Rehabil 17(2):103–109, 1997.

32. Keens TG, Krastins RB, Wannamaker EM, et al. Ventilatory muscle endurance training in normal subjects and patients with cystic fibrosis. Am Rev Respir Dis 116:853–860, 1977.

33. Wijkstra PJ, ten Vergert EM, van Altena R, et al. Long term benefits of rehabilitation at home on quality of life and exercise tolerance in patients with chronic obstructive pulmonary disease. Thorax 50(8):824–828, 1995.

34. Hudson LD, Tyler M, Petty TL. Hospitalization needs during an outpatient rehabilitation program for severe chronic airway obstruction. Chest 70(5):606–610, 1976.

35. Lacasse Y, Guyatt GH, Goldstein RS. The components of a respiratory rehabilitation program: A systematic overview. Chest 111(4): 1077–1088, 1997.

36. Lertzman MM, Cherniack RM. Rehabilitation of patients with COPD. Am Rev Respir Dis 114:1145–1165, 1976.

37. Hudson LD, Pierson DJ. Rehabilitation of patients with chronic obstructive pulmonary disease. Med Clin North Am 65:629–644, 1981.

38. Hodgkin JE, Balchurn OJ, Kass I, et al. Chronic obstructive airway diseases: Current concepts in diagnosis and comprehensive care. JAMA 232:1243–1260, 1975.

39. Scano G, Gigliotti PF, Duranti R, et al. Changes in ventilatory muscle function with negative pressure ventilation in patients with severe COPD. Chest 97:322–327, 1990.

40. Goldstein RS, DeRosie JA, Avendano MA, et al. Influence of noninvasive position pressure ventilation on inspiratory muscles. Chest 99:408–415, 1991.

41. Cropp A, Marco AF. Effects of intermittent negative pressure ventilation in respiratory muscle function in patients with severe chronic obstructive pulmonary disease. Am Rev Respir Dis 135:1056–1061, 1987.

42. Zibrak JD, Hill NS, Federman EC, et al. Evaluation of intermittent long-term negative pressure ventilation in patients with severe chronic obstructive pulmonary disease. Am Rev Respir Dis 138:1515–1518, 1988.

43. O'Donnell DE, Sani R, Younes M. Improvement in exercise endurance in patients with chronic airflow limitation using continuous positive airway pressure. Am Rev Respir Dis 138:1510–1514, 1988.

44. O'Donnell DE, Sani R. Giesbrecht G, et al. Effect of continuous positive airway pressure on respiration sensation in patients with chronic obstructive pulmonary disease during submaximal exercise. Am Rev Respir Dis 138:1185–1191, 1988.

45. Mahler DA, O'Donnell DE. Alternative modes of exercise training for pulmonary patients. J Cardiopulmonary Rehabil 11:58–63, 1991.

46. Paine R, Make BJ. Pulmonary rehabilitation for the elderly. Clin Geriatr Med 2:313–335, 1986.

47. Dudley DL, Glaser EM, Jorgenson BN, et al. Psychosocial concomitants to rehabilitation in chronic obstructive pulmonary disease. Part 2. Psychosocial treatment. Chest 77(4):544–551, 1980.

48. American Physical Therapy Association. Guide to Physical Therapist Practice. Alexandria, VA, APTA, 1997.

49. American College of Sports Medicine. Guidelines for Exercise Testing and Prescription. 4th ed. Philadelphia, Lea & Febiger, 1991.

50. Wasserman K, Hansen JE, Due DY, Whipp BJ. Protocols for exercise testing. In: Principles of Exercise Testing and Interpretation. Philadelphia, Lea & Febiger, 1986, Chap. 5.

51. McGavin CR, Gupta SP, McHardy GJR. Twelve minute walking test for assessing disability in chronic bronchitis, Br Med J I:822–823, 1976.

52. Butland RJA, Pany JA, Gross ER, et al. Two-, six-, and 12-minute walking tests in respiratory disease. Br Med J 284: 1607–1608, 1982.

53. Bernstein ML, Despars JA, Singh NP, et al. Reanalysis of the 12-minute walk in patients with chronic obstructive pulmonary disease. Chest 105(1):163–167, 1994.

54. Menard-Rothe MS, Sobush DC, Bousamra M, et al. Self-selected walking velocity for functional ambulation in patients with end-stage emphysema. J Cardiopulmonary Rehabil 17:85–91, 1997.

55. Cahalin L, Pappagianopoulos P, Prevost S, et al. The relationship of the 6-min walk test to maximal oxygen consumption in transplant candidates with end-stage lung disease. Chest 108(2):452–459, 1995.

56. Reuben DB, Sui AL. An objective measure of physical function of elderly outpatients. J Am Geriatr Soc 38:1105–1112, 1990.

57. Rozzini R, Giovanni B, et al. Physical performance test and activities of daily living scales in the assessment of health status in elderly people. J Am Geriatr Soc 41:1109–1113, 1993.

58. Wells CL, Whitney SL. The reliability of the physical performance test in the clinical setting for patients with end stage lung disease and lung transplant recipients. Cardiopulmonary Phys Ther 7(4):9–11, 1996.

59. Podsiadlo D, Richardson S. The timed "Up and Go": A test of basic functional mobility for frail elderly persons. J Am Geriatr Soc 2:142–148, 1991.

60. Wanner A. The role of mucus in chronic obstructive pulmonary disease. Chest 92(2):11S–15S, 1990.

61. Desmond KJ, Schwenk WF, Thomas E, et al. Immediate and long-term effects of chest physiotherapy in patients with cystic fibrosis. J Pediatr 103:538–631, 1983.

62. Tecklin JS, Holsclaw DS. Evaluation of bronchial drainage in patients with cystic fibrosis. Phys Ther 55(10):1081–1084, 1975.

63. Selsby D, Jones JG. Some physiological and clinical aspects of chest physiotherapy. Br J Anaesth 64:621–631, 1990.
64. Carter RE. Respiratory aspects of spinal cord injury management. Paraplegia 25:262–266, 1987.
65. Mansel JK, Norman JR. Respiratory complications and management of spinal cord injuries. Chest 97:1446–1452, 1990.
66. Alvarez SE, Peterson M, Lansford BR. Respiratory treatment of the adult patient with spinal cord injury. Phys Ther 61(12):1737–1745, 1981.
67. Beigofsky EH. Respiratory failure in disorders of the thoracic cage. Am Rev Respir Dis 119:643–666, 1979.
68. Muszynski-Kwan AT, Perlman R, Rivington-Law BA. Compliance with and effectiveness of chest physio-therapy in cystic fibrosis: A review. Physiotherapy Canada 40(1):28–32, 1988.
69. Maxwell M, Redmond A. Comparative trial of manual and mechanical percussion technique with gravity-assisted bronchial drainage in patients with cystic fibrosis. Arch Dis Child 54:542–544, 1979.
70. Hansen LG, Warwick WJ. High-frequency chest compression system to aid in clearance of mucus from the lung. Biomed Instrum Technol 24:289–294, 1990.
71. Warwick WJ, Hansen LG. The long-term effect of high-frequency chest compression therapy on pulmonary complications of cystic fibrosis. Pediatr Pulmonol 11:265–271, 1991.
72. Rossman CM, Waldes R, Sampson D, et al. Effect of chest physiotherapy on the removal of mucus in patients with cystic fibrosis. Am Rev Respir Dis 126:131–135, 1982.
73. DeBoeck C, Zinman R. Cough versus chest physiotherapy. A Rev Respir Dis 129:182–184, 1984.
74. Sutton PP, Lopez-Vidriero MT, Pavia D, et al. Assessment of percussion, vibratory-shaking and breathing exercises in chest physiotherapy. Eur J Respir Dis 66:147–152, 1985.
75. Verboon JML, Bakker W, Sterk PJ. The value of the forced expiration technique with and without postural drainage in adults with cystic fibrosis. Eur J Respir Dis 69:169–174, 1986.
76. Van Hengstum M, Festen J, Bearskens C, et al. Conventional physiotherapy and forced expiration manoeuvres have similar effects on tracheobronchial clearance. Eur Respir J 1:758–761, 1988.
77. Falk M, Kelstrup M, Andersen JB, et al. Improving the ketchup bottle method with positive expiratory pressure, PEP, in cystic fibrosis. Eur J Respir Dis 65:423–432, 1984.
78. Oberwaldner B, Evans JC, Zach MS. Forced expirations against a variable resistance: A new chest physiotherapy method in cystic fibrosis. Pediatr Pulmonol 2:358–367, 1986.
79. Oldenburg FA, Dolovica MB, Montgomery JM, et al. Effects of postural drainage, exercise, and cough on mucus clearance in chronic bronchitis. Am Rev Respir Dis 120:739–745, 1979.
80. Zach MS, Oberwaldner B, Hausler F. Cystic fibrosis: Physical exercise versus chest physiotherapy. Arch Dis Child 57:587–589, 1982.
81. Salh W, Bilton D, Dodd M, et al. Effect of exercise and physiotherapy in aiding sputum expectoration in adults with cystic fibrosis. Thorax 44:1006–1008, 1989.
82. Hodgkin JE. Pulmonary rehabilitation. Clin Chest Med 11(3):447–454, 1990.
83. Mueller RE, Petty TL, Filley GF. Ventilation and arterial blood gas changes induced by pursed lips breathing. J Appl Physiol 28(6):784–789, 1970.
84. Paul G, Eldridge F, Mitchell J, et al. Some effects of slowing respiration rate in chronic emphysema and bronchitis. J Appl Physiol 21(3):877–882, 1966.
85. Chung F, Dean E. Pathophysiology and cardiorespiratory consequences of interstitial lung disease: Review and clinical implications. Phys Ther 69(11):956–966, 1989.
86. Jones JL, Killian KJ, Summers E, et al. Inspiratory muscle forces and endurance in maximum resistive loading. J Appl Physiol 58:1608–1621, 1985.
87. Meerhaeghe AV, Scano G, Sergysels R, et al. Respiratory drive and ventilatory pattern during exercise in interstitial lung disease. Bull Eur Physiopathol Respir 17:15–26, 1981.
88. Bradley GW, Crawford R. Regulation of breathing during exercise in normal subjects and in chronic lung disease. Clin Sci Mol Med 51:575–582, 1976.
89. Grassino A. A rationale for training respiratory muscles. Int Rehabil Med 6:175–1984.
90. Bellemare F, Grassino A. Force reserve of the diaphragm in patients with COPD. J Appl Physiol 55:8–15, 1983.
91. Dodd DS, Brancatisano T, Engel LA. Chest wall mechanics during exercise in patients with severe chronic air flow obstruction. Am Rev Respir Dis 129:33–38, 1984.
92. Roussos C. Respiratory muscle fatigue and ventilatory failure. Chest 97 (suppl 3):89S–96S, 1990.
93. Sharp JT, Drutz WS, Molsan T, et al. Postural relief of dyspnea in severe chronic obstructive pulmonary disease. Am Rev Respir Dis 122:201–211, 1980.
94. Druz WS, Sharp JT. Electrical and mechanical activity of the diaphragm accompanying body position in severe chronic obstructive pulmonary disease. Am Rev Respir Dis 125:275–280, 1982.
95. Delgado HR, Braun SR, Skatrud JB, et al. Chest wall and abdominal motion during exercise in patients with chronic obstructive pulmonary disease. Am Rev Respir Dis 125:200–205, 1982.
96. Dudley DL, Glaser EM, Jorgenson BN, et al. Psychosocial concomitants to rehabilitation in chronic obstructive pulmonary disease. Part I. Psychosocial and psychological considerations. Chest 77(3):413–420, 1980.
97. Belman MJ. Exercise in chronic obstructive pulmonary disease. Clin Chest Med 7(4):585–596, 1986.
98. Harber P. Alternative partial respiratory disability rating schemes. Am Rev Respir Dis 134:481–487, 1986.
99. Engelberg AL (ed). Guides to the Evaluation of Permanent Impairment. 3rd ed. Chicago, American Medical Association, 1988.
100. Upton CJ, Tyrrell JC, Hiller EJ. Two minute walking distance in cystic fibrosis. Arch Dis Child 63:1444–1448, 1988.
101. Gimenez M. Exercise training in patients with chronic airways obstruction. Eur Respir J 2(suppl 7):611S–617S), 1989.
102. Casaburi R, Wasserman K, Patessio A, et al. A new perspective in pulmonary rehabilitation: Anaerobic threshold as a discriminant in training. Eur Respir J 2(suppl 7):618S–623S, 1989.
103. Carter R, Coast JR, Idell S. Exercise training in patients with chronic obstructive pulmonary disease. Med Sci Sports Exerc 24(3):281–291, 1992.
104. MacNu W, Morgan AD, Wathen CG, et al. Right ventricular performance during exercise in chronic obstructive pulmonary disease: The effects of oxygen. Respiration 48:206–215, 1985.
105. Kaplan RM, Atkins CJ, Timms R. Validity of a quality of well-being scale as an outcome measure in chronic obstructive pulmonary disease. J Chron Dis 37(2):85–95, 1984.
106. Orenstein DM, Nixon PA, Ross EA, et al. The quality of well-being in cystic fibrosis. Chest 95:344-347, 1989.
107. Cheong TKH, Magder S, Shapiro S, et al. Cardiac arrhyth-

mias during exercise in severe chronic obstructive pulmonary disease. Chest 97:973–977, 1990.
108. Incalzi RA, Pistelli R, Fuso L, et al. Cardiac arrhythmias and left ventricular function in respiratory failure from chronic obstructive pulmonary disease. Chest 97:1092–1097, 1990.
109. Hunter AMB, Carey MA, Larsh HW. The nutritional status of patients with chronic obstructive pulmonary disease. A Rev Respir Dis 124:376–381, 1981.
110. Marcotte JE, Canny GJ, Grisdale R, et al. Effects of nutritional status on exercise performance in advanced cystic fibrosis. Chest 90(3):375–379, 1986.
111. Donahoe M, Roders RM. Nutritional assessment and support in chronic obstructive pulmonary disease. Clin Chest Med 11(3):487–495, 1990.
112. Strauss GD, Osher A, Wang CI, et al. Variable weight training in cystic fibrosis. Chest 92(2):273–276, 1987.
113. Tangri S, Woolf CR. The breathing pattern in chronic obstructive lung disease during the performance of some common daily activities. Chest 63:126–127, 1973.
114. Celli BR, Rassulo J, Make BJ. Dyasynchronous breathing during arm but not leg exercise in patients with chronic airflow obstruction. N Engl J Med 3:14(23):1485–1489, 1986.
115. Martin JG. Clinical intervention in chronic respiratory failure. Chest 97(suppl 3):105S–109S, 1990.
116. Shaffer TH, Wolfson MR, Bhutani VK. Respiratory muscle functions, assessment, and training. Phys Ther 61(12):1711–1723, 1981.
117. Grassino A. A rationale for training respiratory muscles. Int Rehabil Med 6:175–178, 1984.
118. Roussos C, Macklem PT. The respiratory muscles. N Engl J Med 307(13):786–797, 1982.
119. Leith DE, Bradley M. Ventilatory muscle strength and endurance training. J Appl Physiol 41(4):508–516, 1976.
120. Gross D, Ladd HW, Riley EJ, et al. The effect of training on strength and endurance of the diaphragm in quadriplegia. Am J Med 68:27–35, 1980.
121. Pardy RL, Rivington RN, Despas PJ, et al. The effects of inspiratory muscle training on exercise performance in chronic airflow limitation. Am Rev Respir Dis 123:426–433, 1981.
122. Belman MJ, Mittman C. Ventilatory muscle training improves exercise capacity in chronic obstructive pulmonary disease patiens. Am Rev Respir Dis 121:273–280, 1980.
123. Levine S, Weiser P, Gillen J. Evaluation of a ventilatory muscle endurance training program in the rehabilitation of patients with chronic obstructive pulmonary disease. Am Rev Respir Dis 133(3):400–406, 1986.
124. Belman MJ. Shadmehr R. Targeted resistive ventilatory muscle training in chronic obstructive pulmonary disease. J Appl Physiol 65(6):2726–2735, 1988.
125. Larson JL, Kim MJ, Sharp JT, et al. Inspiratory muscle training with a pressure threshold breathing device in patients with chronic obstructive pulmonary disease. Am Rev Respir Dis 138:689–696, 1988.
126. Harver A, Mahler DA, Daubenspeck JA. Targeted inspiratory muscle training improves respiratory muscle function and reduces dyspnea in patiens with chronic obstructive pulmonary disease. Ann Intern Med 111:117–124, 1989.
127. Flynn MG, Barter CE, Nosworthy JC, et al. Threshold pressure training, breathing pattern, and exercise performance in chronic airflow obstruction. Chest 95(3):535–540, 1989.

20

Outcome Measures: Reimbursement Issues and Documentation

Peg Pashkow

INTRODUCTION

Physical therapists (PTs) are skilled at assessing patients' impairments, functional limitations, and disabilities as well as the results of interventions. They are also skilled at reevaluation and refinement of the plan of care. But in order to survive in today's health care system, PTs must be prepared to evaluate patient outcomes considering a broader set of variables, translate data into meaningful clinical information, and use this information to develop and refine clinical practice guidelines.

Cardiopulmonary rehabilitation is an interdisciplinary intervention that includes professionals such as physicians, nurses, respiratory therapists, physical and occupational therapists, psychologists, dietitians, and exercise physiologists (see Chapters

18 and 19). This team of players works together to help each patient reach the best possible outcomes, similar to the teamwork that is common in physical rehabilitation. The measurement of these outcomes is the subject of this chapter.

OUTCOMES DEFINED

Outcomes have been defined as those changes, either favorable or adverse, in the actual or potential health status of persons, groups, or communities that can be attributed to prior or concurrent care.[1] While focusing on providing an effective, quality plan of care, therapists acknowledge that multiple patient factors affect outcomes. Table 20–1 (factors affecting patient outcomes) lists both clinical and nonclinical factors, which in ad-

Table 20–1	
Factors Affecting Patient Outcomes	
CLINICAL FACTORS	NONCLINICAL FACTORS
Principal diagnosis, severity	Health-related quality of life
Acute clinical stability	Cultural, ethnic, and socioeconomic attributes, beliefs, and behaviors
Comorbidity, severity	Patient attitudes and preferences
Physical functional status	Psychological, cognitive, and psychosocial functioning
Age, sex	

Table 20–2	
Diversity of Patient Outcomes	
CLINICAL FACTORS	NONCLINICAL FACTORS
Severity of principal diagnosis	Health-related quality of life
Acute clinical stability	Resource utilization
Comorbidity, severity	Costs of care
Complications, iatrogenic illness	Satisfaction
Physical functional status	
Survival	

dition to the intervention as well as random events result in multiple possible outcomes noted in Table 20–2 (diversity of patient outcomes). When interpreting outcome data, it is important to recognize and differentiate confounding factors before making inferences about clinical effectiveness.

A method frequently used to condense the multitude of outcomes is to divide them into primary and secondary outcomes. The primary outcome, health, includes health status, functional status, and well-being. Health status, assessed by evaluating morbidity and mortality rates, is generally reserved for large clinical trials in which the sample size is sufficient to demonstrate statistical significance. Functional status is the ability to engage in important everyday behaviors physically, psychologically, and socially and should not be confused with functional capacity, which is a clinical measure. Functional status and well-being, measured by evaluating quality of life, can be assessed in any rehabilitation program.

Quality of life is the multifactorial, functional effect of an illness and its consequent therapy upon a patient.[2] Quality of life must be measured

from the patient's perspective, to reflect the importance and effect of the patient's beliefs, values, and judgments on the results of the intervention.[3] A positive outcome on quality of life is demonstrated by patient-reported improvement in physical, emotional, and social functioning, as well as improvement in general well-being.

Secondary outcomes include the multiple clinical and behavioral variables important to the patient with cardiopulmonary dysfunction. Economic and satisfaction variables important to the cardiopulmonary program are a part of these outcomes. Some clinical measures of importance include functional capacity, lipid levels, smoking status, blood pressure, glucose levels, measures of obesity and body fat, and frequency and intensity of angina and dyspnea. Because of the ability to standardize and objectively measure clinical factors, these outcomes historically have been the primary focus in our documentation and outcome measurement.

Behavioral outcomes assess the changes in lifestyle that may be the result of education efforts in cardiopulmonary rehabilitation. These outcomes include symptom management, adherence to exercise and medication regimens, smoking cessation, diet management, and stress management.

By documenting the utilization of key health care resources, economic outcomes (a surrogate

Clinical Note: Confounding Factors

When interpreting outcome data, it is important to recognize and differentiate confounding factors before making inferences about clinical effectiveness.

Clinical Note: Quality of Life

Quality of life is the multifactorial, functional effect of an illness and its consequent therapy upon a patient.[2]

for cost effectiveness) can be reported. These resources include the number of hospital days, emergency department visits, physician office visits, rehabilitation visits, medication changes and compliance, and the cost of these. Patient satisfaction is historically assessed by hospital marketing departments and is now required by the Joint Commission on Accreditation of Healthcare Organizations (JCAHO) for hospital accreditation. A standardized questionnaire can assess satisfaction with regard to the issues of access, facility, reception, billing, program components, and staff. Although clinical, behavioral, and economic and satisfaction variables have a significant impact on health outcomes, they are secondary to primary health outcomes.

IMPORTANCE OF MEASURING OUTCOMES

There are a number of important reasons for individual programs to measure outcomes, including to demonstrate accountability, to improve clinical and management decision making for optimal care delivery, for research, and as incentives. Although research has substantiated the efficacy of the intervention in controlled studies, it is the responsibility of individual rehabilitation programs to demonstrate effectiveness in their clinical setting. Measuring and sharing this outcome information demonstrates accountability to the patients, referring physicians, staff, administrators, and payers.

Since 1993, the JCAHO has encouraged outcome measurement as an important form of evaluation leading to continuous improvement, and since 1998, it has been required. The second edition of the *Guidelines for Cardiac Rehabilitation Program*,[4] published by the American Association of Cardiovascular and Pulmonary Rehabilitation (AACVPR), advises that documentation must include records of expected and observed treatment outcomes.

Clinical Note: Outcome Information

Measuring and sharing outcome information demonstrates accountability to patients, referring physicians, staff, administrators, and payers.

Clinical Note: Outcome Data and Decision Making

Management decision making is enhanced when outcome data lead to the formulation of new protocols, reeducation of practitioners, and redistribution of program resources to improve care delivery.

Outcome data can be used to relate variations in patient outcomes to variations in patient care and to identify opportunities for improvement. In this way, outcome measurement helps in clinical decision making by helping clinicians, patients, and payers evaluate the expected risks and benefits of alternative treatments. Studies by drug companies and actuarial tables by insurers have always provided information assisting in clinical decision making and determining what the payer would cover because of proven efficacy. Today, the agency that accredits managed care organizations, the National Committee for Quality Assurance (NCQA), requires that these organizations utilize outcome data to predict risks and guide service delivery.

As managers are challenged to improve clinical value in relation to costs of care,[5] good outcome data, once analyzed and interpreted, can guide service delivery, such as assessment, diagnosis, treatment, determining staff needs, and allocating program resources. Management decision making is enhanced when outcome data lead to the formulation of new protocols, reeducation of practitioners, and redistribution of program resources to improve care delivery.

Historically, collecting outcome data has been left to the realm of research. Standardized methods applied in clinical trials are also important to data collection for outcome measurement in the clinical setting. By standardizing methods of data collection, the medical record becomes more clear, concise, and accurate. This facilitates the collection, merging, analysis, and interpretation of data for the PT, and provides information conducive for research and possible publication.

Outcome measurement also provides incentives to staff who want to see the results of their labor, to patients who have adhered to lifestyle changes, to referring physicians and administrators who are accountable to both patient and payer, and to payers, who need to see proven efficacy and a positive bottom line to fund the services.

The AACVPR Outcome Committee in 1995 suggested that a minimum of at least one health, one clinical, and one behavioral outcome be measured.[6] Outcome measurement is among the requirements for AACVPR program certification. States such as North and South Carolina, which license rehabilitation programs, require outcomes to be tracked to maintain licensure. In 1998, the JCAHO required that hospitals periodically submit results of at least two outcome measures for a minimum of 20% of their population served.[7] The number of measures is expected to increase in the future, as is the percentage of the population in-

cluded. Physical therapists should stay informed of the latest standards, guidelines, and requirements.

SELECTION OF DATA TO MEASURE

Data are considered essential when the information can be quantified and evaluated for change over time and the findings may be changed by interventions. Staff, administration, patients, payers, physicians, and others have special interests that help to determine what data will be documented. The worksheet in Figure 20–1 can help identify a program's areas of focus to help determine what data should be collected.

QUICK SURVEY

Type of rehabilitation program: Cardiac   Pulmonary   Cardiopulmonary   _____# new patients per week
Do you offer dietary counseling?   Yes   No   Group   Individual
By Dietitian, RN, Ex Specialist, Other _____
Do you measure change in dietary habits?   Yes   No
By Diet Habit Survey, Quick Check, Block Food Questionnaire, Weight   Other _____
Do you offer stress management?   Yes   No   Group   Individual
By Psychologist, RN, Ex Specialist, Other _____
Do you measure change in stress, depression, hostility, anxiety?   Yes   No
By Beck Depression, Geriatric Depression Scale, SCL 90-R, State Trait Anxiety,
   Cook Medley Hostility, Other _____
Do you discuss medications and compliance with medication regimen?   Yes   No   Group   Individual
By RN, Pharmacist, Ex Specialist, Physician, other _____   _____
Do you offer smoke cessation classes?   Yes   No   Offer other options? _____
Do you measure change in smoking status?   Yes   No   Self report   Nicotine level   Other _____
Do you measure   Body fat,   Waist-hip ratio,   BMI,   Weight
Do you record lipid profiles?   Yes   No   Data available for _____% of patients
Do you get results from your own testing, hospital lab, physician office, other? _____
Do you get results at entry?   At exit?   At 6 months?   At 1 year?   Other _____
Do most of your patients have a GXT prior to entry?   At exit?   At one year?   Other measure of ex capacity
_____

Do you inquire about return to work and work status (full time, part time, retired, NA)?   Yes   No
Are you measuring quality of life?   Yes   No   *Circle those used*
   MOS SF-36   Rand 36-Item   HSQ   CRQ   QLMI
   Dartmouth COOP   SGRQ   Seattle Angina Questionnaire
   SIP   PFSS   LHFQ
   IEQ   PFSDQ   Ferrans and Powers
   Nottingham Health Survey   Other _____   Other _____
Do patients complete a satisfaction survey?   Yes   No
Do you record medical utilization?   Hospital days   ER visits   Other _____
Do you know the cost per patient for the rehab program?   Yes   No   _____% of patients in managed care

Do you collect this data in a computer? Spreadsheet   Database   Other _____
Do you analyze your data for Administration   Staff   Payers   Physicians   Patients   Other _____

Figure 20–1. This Quick Survey can help identify the outcomes important in a program.

It is imperative that the measurement instruments utilized to quantify and evaluate change be both valid and reliable. Validity is the extent to which an instrument measures the characteristics that it is intended to measure. Validity refers to the appropriateness, meaningfulness, and usefulness of a measure as well as the justifiability of the inferences that can be drawn from the data and the measurements. Reliability is the degree to which an instrument and its protocol are free from random error, such that its resulting scores are stable and consistent or reproducible when properly administered under similar circumstances. Tables listing some valid and reliable instruments for measuring outcomes are found in Table 20–3.

Physical therapists practicing in cardiopulmonary settings collect demographic and outcome data at the time of the initial evaluation and then on a daily basis as they reevaluate, treat, and record their patient's condition. Such data are generally clinical in nature and include heart rate, blood pressure, oxygen saturation, symptoms, and activity levels in METs or functional terms. Additionally, cardiopulmonary physical therapists record behavioral outcomes data to evaluate the impact of counseling and instruction as well as the patient's ability to adhere to healthy lifestyle practices. Methods utilized include exercise and diet diaries, stress management observation, and specific questioning regarding compliance with medication regimens and smoking cessation. For this data to be included in a structured outcome project, the clinician need only adhere to a standardized method of documentation.

Demographic data are needed so that when analyzing outcome data, in addition to large populations of patients, cohorts of patients with similar characteristics can be studied. Some examples of demographic data to record are:

• Age
• Gender
• Race
• Marital status

Clinical Note: Demographic Data

Demographic data are needed so that when analyzing outcome data, cohorts of patients with similar characteristics can be studied.

• Primary diagnosis (with date)
• Comorbidities
• Surgeries and other interventions with date
• Medications with dose and frequency
• Referring physician
• Payer

Examples of clinical and behavioral data, regularly measured by cardiopulmonary clinicians or easily accessed through the patient's chart, include:

• Weight, BMI, percentage of body fat, or waist-hip ratio
• Resting heart rate and blood pressure
• Lipid levels
• Glucose level
• Exercise capacity
• Symptoms
• Employment status
• Utilization of health care services
• Cardiac risk factor changes
• Exercise habits
• Smoking habits

In follow-up, the preceding list of clinical and behavioral measures should be augmented with the documentation of utilization of health care to report on economic outcomes, such as:

• Hospital days
• Emergency room visits
• Physician office visits
• Medication changes and compliance
• Cost of rehabilitation
• Time for rehabilitation, including drive time

No instrument for collecting this type of data has been validated and published at this time. Rehabilitation programs that collect this data do so by asking the patient in an interview (in person or by phone) or by questionnaire. A sample of questions from the UCSD Health Care Utilization Questionnaire being employed as part of the California Pulmonary Rehabilitation Collaborative Project, an outcome study conducted at the University of California at San Diego, inquires:

During the past 3 months:

How many visits did you make to the physician, osteopath, or nurse practitioner?
How many telephone calls did you make to your doctor or doctor's staff?
How many days were you in the hospital as an inpatient?

Text continued on page 35

Table 20–3

Comparison of Measurement Instruments

MEASUREMENT INSTRUMENT	ACRONYM	ITEMS	SELF	TIME PER PT(MIN)	TIME PER STAFF (MIN)	PARAMETERS MEASURED
General Quality of Life Measures						
Medical Outcomes Study Short Form[8]	SF-36	36	Yes	5 to 10	5	Physical, psychological, and social functioning
RAND 36-item Health Survey 1.0	RAND 36					
Nottingham Health Profile[9]	NHP	45	Yes	10	10	Energy, pain, emotion, sleep, mobility, social isolation and ADL
Sickness Impact Profile[10, 11]	SIP	136	Yes	30	20	Physical, psychosocial, and 5 independent factors
Quality of Well-Being Scale[12]	QWB	18–62	No	10–15	20	Mobility, physical activity, social activity, self care and symptoms
Illness Effects Questionnaire[13]	IEQ	20	Yes	20	25	Biological, psychological and social aspects
Dartmouth Primary Care Cooperative Information[14]	COOP	9 charts	Yes	5–7	5–7	Physical, emotional and social role function, pain, overall health, health change and social support
DUKE Health Profiles—Revised[15]		17	Yes	2–4	3	Health and dysfunction
Multidimensional Health Locus of Control Inventory[16]	MHLOC	18	Yes	2–4	Unknown	Perceived control over health and health care
Quality of Life Systemic Inventory[17]	QLSI	30	No	45	60	The gap between patient's condition and goal for 30 life domains prioritized by patient
Symptom Questionnaire[18]		92	Yes	2–5	10–15	Depression, anxiety, somatic complaints and anger-hostility
Cardiac Specific Quality of Life Measures						
Minnesota Living with Heart Failure Questionnaire[19]	LHFQ	21	Yes	10–15	3–5	Physical, socioeconomic, and psychological impairment
Outcomes Institute Angina Type Specification[20]	MOS-Angina	14	Yes	2–3	5–8	Patient outcome questions, with additional physician questions based on patient's course of care

Table continued on following page

Table 20–3

Comparison of Measurement Instruments Continued

MEASUREMENT INSTRUMENT	ACRONYM	ITEMS	SELF	TIME PER PT(MIN)	TIME PER STAFF (MIN)	PARAMETERS MEASURED
Cardiac Specific Quality of Life Measures Continued						
Quality of Life after Myocardial Infarction[21]	QLMI	26	No	10	Trace	Physical limitations (symptoms, restrictions) and emotional function (confidence, self-esteem, and emotions)
MacNew Quality of Life after Myocardial Infarction[22]	MacNew QLMI	27	Yes			Physical, emotional, and social domains (modified from QLMI)
Ferrans and Powers Quality of Life Index-Version[23]	QLI	72	Yes	10	15–30	Health and functioning, cardiac, socioeconomic, psychological/spiritual, and family
Seattle Angina Questionnaire[24]	SAQ	19	Yes	3–4		Physical limitations, angina stability, angina frequency, treatment satisfaction, and disease perception
Pulmonary Specific Quality of Life Measures						
Chronic Respiratory Disease Questionnaire[25]	CRQ	20	No	25–30	35	Dyspnea, fatigue, emotional function, and feeling of mastery over disease
St. George's Respiratory Questionnaire[26]	SGRQ	76	Yes	15	10	Symptoms, activity, and impact of disease
Pulmonary Functional Status Scale[27]	PFSS	56	Yes	15–30	10–25	ADL in respiratory patients
Pulmonary Functional Status and Dyspnea Questionnaire[28]	PFSDQ	164	Yes	15	15	ADL and dyspnea
Living with Asthma Questionnaire[29]		68	Yes	20	20	Quality of life in patients with asthma
Functional Activity and Exercise Related Measures						
The New York Heart Association functional classification[30]	NYHA	4	No	NA	1	Physical activity performance
The Specific Activity Scale[31]		5	No	5	1	Activities of daily living
Baseline Dyspnea Index/Transitional Dyspnea Index[32]		15	No	5–10	5–10	Functional impairment, magnitude of task, magnitude of effort
Duke Activity Scale Index[33]		12	Yes	5	2	Functional status

Table 20-3

Comparison of Measurement Instruments Continued

MEASUREMENT INSTRUMENT	ACRONYM	ITEMS	SELF	TIME PER PT(MIN)	TIME PER STAFF (MIN)	PARAMETERS MEASURED
Functional Activity and Exercise Related Measures Continued						
Borg Scale[34, 35]		NA	No	Seconds	Seconds	Perceived exertion
Visual analogue scale[36]		NA	No	Seconds	1	Severity of dyspnea during exercise
Maximal and Submaximal Progressive Multistage Exercise Test[37]	GXT	NA	No	45–60	45–60	Changes in exercise capacity
6- or 12-minute walk[38, 39]		NA	No	20–30	20–30	Exercise endurance
Human Activity Profile (formerly ADAPT)[40]	HAP	105	Yes	15–30	20–50	Activity level (Formerly ADAPT)
Functional Status Questionnaire[41]	FSQ	34	Yes	15	3–5	Physical, psychological, social, and role function in ambulatory patients
Psychological Measures						
Hopkins Symptom Checklist—Revised[42]	SCL-90-R	90	Yes	20	30*	Nine subscales, such as somatization, depression, anxiety, and hostility
Minnesota Multiphasic Personality Inventory-2[43]	MMPI	567	Yes	180	60*	Depression, anxiety, psychosis, personality disorders
Cook-Medley Hostility Inventory[44]		50	Yes	15	15*	Hostility
Buss Durkey Hostility Inventory[45]						Hostility
Beck Depression Inventory[46]	BDI	21	Yes	5–10	15*	Depression, mood state
Center for Epidemiological Studies Depression Inventory[47]	CES-D	20	Yes	10	15	Depression, mood state
State-Trait Anxiety Inventory[48]	STAI	40	Yes	20	5*	Anxiety
COPD Self Efficacy Scale[49]		34	Yes	5–10	30*	Confidence level
COPE Inventory[50]	COPE	52	Yes	20	20*	Different ways in which people respond to stress
Jenkins Activity Survey[51]	JAS	20	Yes	20	15*	Four common components of type A behavior
Profile of Mood States[52]	POMS	65	Yes	15	20*	Various mood states (e.g., tension, anger, depression, confusion)

Table continued on following page

Table 20–3

Comparison of Measurement Instruments Continued

MEASUREMENT INSTRUMENT	ACRONYM	ITEMS	SELF	TIME PER PT(MIN)	TIME PER STAFF (MIN)	PARAMETERS MEASURED
Psychological Measures Continued						
Cardiac Depression Scale[53]	CDS	26	Yes	10	40	Depression
Face Scale[54]		20	No	2	2*	Mood
Psychological General Well-Being Index[55]	PGWB	22	Yes	15	25*	Both negative (depression, anxiety) and positive (vitality, health) mood states
Ways of Coping Questionnaire[56]		NA	Yes	10	20	Thoughts and actions that people use to handle stressful situations
Sociological Measures						
Marital Adjustment Scale[56]	MAS	16	Yes	5	5	Marital adjustment
MOS Social Support Survey[57]		20	Yes	10	5	Four functional support scales
Psychosocial Adjustment to Illness[58]		45	Yes	15	10	Coping with illness or handicap
Other Health Related Behavior Measures						
Harvard-Willett Food Frequency Questionnaire[59]		116	Yes	45–60	†	Type, quantity, and frequency of food ingested
Block Food Questionnaire[60]		128	No	30–45	45	Calories, fat, fiber, protein, carbohydrates, linoleic/oleic acids, vitamins, minerals
Diet Habit Survey[61]		32	Yes	30	20–30	Cholesterol, saturated fat intake, complex carbohydrates, salt
Quick Check (Quantitative)[62]		74	Yes	15	3–5	Fat, saturated fat, cholesterol
Health Knowledge Test[63]		40	Yes	15–20	5–10	Knowledge of disease management skills in pulmonary patients
Cardiac Knowledge Questionnaire[64]		55	Yes			Knowledge of cardiovascular system and coronary heart disease, lifestyle change issues, and perceptions of severity/prognosis

Key: Under "Self," yes = self-administered, no = structured interview. Under Time per Pt is time in minutes for patient to complete questionnaire. Time per Staff refers to time in minutes for staff to administer, score, and interpret questionnaire.

* Psychologist must interpret.

† Must be mailed out for computer scoring.

Source: Adapted from Pashkow P, Ades PA, Emery CF, et al. Outcome measurement in cardiac and pulmonary rehabilitation. J Cardiopulm Rehabil 15(6):397–398, 1995; with permission from Lippincott-Raven. Adapted from Pashkow P. Outcomes in cardiopulmonary rehabilitation. Phys Ther 76(6):647, 649, 1996; with permission from the American Physical Therapy Association.

Clinical Note: Data Collection

To maintain efficiency, collect only necessary data and use all data that are collected.

How many times did you use an ambulance?

How many miles do you travel to obtain your medical care?

Finally, because it is also important to measure outcomes from the patient's point of view, quality of life (QOL) should be measured. Measuring quality of life is new to most clinicians. There are many valid and reliable instruments available, and a variety of them are described in the tables found in Figure 20–1. Resources for administration, collection, and interpretation of data must be considered when selecting which or how many instruments can be used. Instruments that are easy on the respondent and staff in that they can be scored and interpreted quickly and efficiently are best. Standardized, self-report questionnaires are most popular and efficient. Many hospitals administer generic QOL questionnaires to all their patients receiving both inpatient and outpatient care and have established protocols for administration, scoring, and tracking for comparisons over time. The cardiopulmonary rehabilitation staff should access, review, and utilize this data when available and then determine whether additional disease-specific QOL information is needed and feasible to obtain. Table 20–4 lists the benefits of both generic and disease-specific quality of life instruments.

METHODOLOGY

When implementing a system for outcome measurement, the following important operational steps must be addressed:

- Procedures are standardized, including staff in the process
- Data collection forms and databases are used for documentation
- Frequency of data collection is defined
- Data are collected and merged
- Data are analyzed and interpreted
- Findings are distributed

Staff members need instruction in the outcomes process including the importance and benefits of strict adherence to standardized methods as well as the protocol. Compliance with the outcome process must be complete and comprehensive in order to generate unbiased data. Conclusions about an outcome may be erroneous if the staff measures outcomes differently or records data only occasionally or incompletely. Data collection is the responsibility of each clinician, but the process of compiling data for reports often is assigned to just one or two persons. All clinicians need relevant outcome data to assess the benefit of their interventions[66] and to demonstrate accountability for the expense of care.[67]

The perception that measuring outcome data is labor intensive and tedious has made it an unwelcome force to confront at a time when rehabilitation professionals are being asked to justify the cost of their time. Clinicians fear that outcomes of patients that do not meet expected norms may cost them professionally and financially. To improve participation in standardized documentation, administrators and managers need to identify and address issues and attitudes that might compromise participation.[67] Russek and colleagues[67] studied 220 clinicians, 71% of whom were physical therapists, and identified five factors that are obstacles to outcome assessment. These factors are inconvenience, acceptance of operational definitions, automation, paperwork, and training.

Table 20–4

Benefits of Generic and Disease-Specific Instruments

GENERIC QOL INSTRUMENTS	DISEASE-SPECIFIC QOL INSTRUMENTS
Apply to heterogeneous population	Responsive to a specific population with same disease or condition
Allow cross-population comparisons (compare with other chronic diseases)	Focus on problematic areas for a given population
Address multiple issues related to limitations in health status (e.g., comorbidities, age)	Address issues related to clinical manifestations of a disorder

Establishing a system that streamlines documentation and facilitates relevant outcome measurement can help overcome obstacles to measurement. Staff should be included in deciding the outcomes to be tracked and the methodology to be used. Once the outcome data points have been well defined, the most efficient and accurate data source should be determined. Sources of data include quality of life questionnaires and medical records for laboratory data and insurance. Once the clinical data needed has been identified, the data collection should be integrated within the initial evaluation, interim status notes, and discharge notes. See Figure 20–2 for an example of a form that the staff at one hospital designed. The ongoing archiving or journaling of data serves to track short- and long-term outcomes. To maintain efficiency, collect only data needed and use all data collected.

A well-designed, menu-driven computer database system can standardize and streamline the process of documentation. It reduces problems with accuracy, legibility, spelling, and grammar. Compared to a paper system, a computerized program also allows easy and timely access to a considerable amount of data. Regardless of the system employed, data elements have to be carefully defined with allowable values described so that, whether collected and keyed into a computer or documented on paper, data are consistent and valid for use in the later steps of consolidating, comparing, and analyzing data. Missing or erroneous data elements cost time and, if not corrected, can sacrifice the validity of the conclusions. Systems that allow real-time data entry are most conducive to providing individualized comparative reports in a timely fashion. Timely information is important to clinicians who need this information to make clinical decisions and to communicate with patients, physicians, and payers.

The timing and frequency of data collection must be well defined, because changes in data that have been collected too early or too late may not be related to the intervention. Suggested times for data collection are on admission, at discharge, and 6 months, 1 year, and 2 years after care. Some payers are asking for outcome data about their clients halfway through a cardiac or pulmonary rehabilitation program to be assured that the intervention is having the expected results before authorizing payment for the remainder of the program. Case managers, who may be physical therapists, may assist in the follow-up data collection, depending on the organization's determination of responsibility. Data collected in follow-up may be obtained over the phone, from mailed questionnaires, or in personal interviews.

Once the process begins, data must be collected continuously and then concurrently or periodically submitted into a database for aggregation and analysis. A number of vendors sell computer software database systems for the collection, merging, retrieval, analysis, and reporting of patient and program outcomes. Some have programs specifically written for the cardiopulmonary population. Resources are listed in Table 20–5.

Many organizations have implemented a hospital-wide, automated, data-gathering system, often called a medical information system (MIS). It is unlikely, though, that all information in the organization is integrated into this system. In fact, it has been reported that of all the information in a medical record, half comes from various computer-generated reports, rather than one integrated MIS. Examples found in cardiopulmonary patient charts might include a spirometry report, a graded exercise test, an echocardiography report, and a catherization report. The so-called "electronic patient record," which would allow the transfer of all data from different health service providers, regardless of location, into one system has been proposed for the future, but because all hardware and software will need to be compatible and all providers must be willing to share information, this type of system may not be available for a number of years.

Another option for data collection, aggregation, and reporting is to join a commercial computerized database service. Some of these services allow a clinic to fax or scan forms that staff members or patients have completed, and others provide software so the data may be entered and reports generated on site or sent by modem or electronic transfer to a central data collection center. Some are highly sophisticated and require the input of numerous data elements, yet others are more limited in scope. Each clinic or rehabilitation program should determine what system best meets their needs, budget, and focus.

Text continued on page 42

PATIENT INFORMATION

NAME		AGE	
PHONE NO.		DOB	
M.D.	SSAN		
DIAGNOSIS		EF	
OTHER			
ALLERGIES		LIVING WILL	
ENTRY DATE		EXIT DATE	

MEDICAL RECORDS

☐ H&P   ☐ PART INFO   ☐ DIET CONSULT _____ _____

☐ DC   ☐ EX CONSENT   ☐ PSYCH CONSULT _____ _____

☐ 12 LEAD

☐ REFERRAL   ☐ RELEASE   ☐ RPTS TO M.D. _____ _____

PATIENT ASSESSMENT

Risk Factors

☐ HIGH BP	☐ FAMILY HISTORY
☐ HIGH CHOL	☐ OBESITY
☐ SMOKING	☐ HIGH STRESS
☐ DIABETES	☐ SEDENTARY LIFESTYLE

HISTORY

☐ LUNG DISEASE	☐ CHF
☐ VALVE DISEASE	☐ ARRHYTHMIAS
☐ RENAL DISEASE	☐ THYROID
☐ LIVER DISEASE	☐ GI DISORDERS
☐ VASCULAR DISEASE	☐ OTHER:

PHYSICAL ASSESSMENT

Blood Pressure	HEART SOUNDS
LEFT ARM	LUNG SOUNDS
RIGHT ARM	Surgical Sites
STANDING	LEGS
EDEMA	CHEST

MUSCULOSKELETAL ASSESSMENT

AROM	FLEXIBILITY
STRENGTH	ARTHRITIS
BALANCE	OTHER:

MEDICATIONS

SIGNATURE	DATE

RISK STRATIFICATION

Low Risk

☐ NO COMPLEX ARRHYTHMIAS

☐ NO MYOCARDIAL ISCHEMIA   ☐ EF > 49%

☐ UNCOMPLICATED COURSE

☐ VO2 MAX > 6 METS POST 3 WEEKS

Intermediate Risk

☐ EF 31-49%   ☐ FAILURE TO COMPLY

☐ VO2 MAX < 6 METS POST 3 WEEKS

☐ MYOCARDIAL ISCHEMIA: 1-2 MM ST SEG DEPRESSION, ANGINA

☐ UNCONTROLLED RISK FACTORS

High Risk

☐ EF < 31% ☐ COMPLEX VENTRICULAR ARRHYTHMIAS

☐ SURVIVOR OF SUDDEN CARDIAC DEATH

☐ DECREASE IN SBP OF > 15 MM HG OR FAILURE TO RISE WITH EXERCISE

☐ MI, COMPLICATED WITH CHF, SHOCK, OR COMPLEX ARRHYTHMIAS

☐ SEVERE CAD AND MYOCARDIAL ISCHEMIA >2 MM ST SEG DEP

☐ OTHER:

EXERCISE PRESCRIPTION

GXT DATE		
PROTOCOL		
METS		
TIME		
RESULTS		
REST HR/BP		
MAX HR/BP		
HR RESERVE		
HR RANGE		
TRAINING	RPE 12-14	RPE 12-14
MET RANGE		
MODE	☐ WALK	☐ WALK
	☐ CYCLE	☐ CYCLE
	☐ ARM	☐ ARM
FREQUENCY	3 X WEEK	
DURATION	30-40 MIN	

SIGNATURES

DATE	DATE
DATE	DATE

Figure 20–2(1). Sample form for collecting patient data for outcome tracking. (Courtesy of Teri Redmond, RN, MS in Cardiac Rehabilitation at Transylvania Community Hospital, Brevard, NC.)

PARTICIPANT'						DATE:
FOCUS		IDEAL	ENTRY	EXIT	GOAL	PATIENT INFORMATION
TOBACCO	USAGE	STOP				Smoking is a major risk factor for heart disease. It damages artery linings, making them susceptible to plaque build-up. Smoking only 4 cigarettes a day increases your risk by 50%. Second-hand smoke can be lethal.
BLOOD PRESSURE		<140/ 90				Keeping blood pressure (BP) low is protective to the heart and arteries. Levels remaining at 140/90 (or above) generally are considered to increase your risk.
DIET HABIT SURVEY	TOTAL CHOL	<200				Scores above 220 for men and 190 for women are recommended. These scores refer to a diet less than 25% fat. Refer to dietitian's recommendations.
	SAT FAT	< 8%				
	FAT	<25%				
	SODIUM	<2,300				
LIPIDS						Cholesterol is one of the main components of plaque that clogs up arteries. Total cholesterol should be <200, but <180 is ideal. The higher the HDL, the better (45+ is ideal; <35 is high risk). If you divide cholesterol by HDL, the ratio should be <4.0. The LDL (or the bad stuff) ideally should be <100. Triglycerides refer to fat in the blood (<160 is ideal; >250 is moderate risk, and >500 is high risk. These can be improved by exercise, weight loss, limiting alcohol intake, and avoiding excess sugar.
	DATE					
	CHOL	< 200				
	HDL-GOOD	>45				
	RATIO	< 4.0				
	LDL-BAD	<100				
	TRIG	<160				
DIABETES	GLUCOSE	< 110				Increased blood sugars damage artery linings making them susceptible to plaque build-up. Exercise, weight loss, and eating healthy may help to control blood sugars.
OBESITY	WEIGHT					Excess weight makes your heart work harder. A low-fat diet and daily exercise are the primary means to reduce weight. Slow weight loss of 1-2 pounds per week is recommended. 1/2% of body fat per. month is a good target Ideal body fat for men is < 19%, and < 25% for women.
	HEIGHT					
	BODY FAT					
	SKINFOLDS					
STRESS	SCALE					Being under a lot of stress (especially hostile outbursts, anger, and irritability) are linked highly to heart disease. Most people need to learn how to relax.
QUALITY OF LIFE	OVERALL	>25				This score relates how satisfied you are with your quality of life. The scale ranges from 0-30. Scores below 25 relate to a poor quality of life. Hopefully, as time goes on, these areas will improve. If not, discuss your areas of concern with a professional.
	HLTH/	>25				
	SOCIO-ECON	>25				
	PSYCH-SPIR	>25				
	FAMILY	>25				
EXERCISE	6-MIN					Your exercise prescription is as follows: Frequency:4-6 times per week; Intensity: Heart-Rate Range _____. Time: 30-40 minutes. One training effect of exercise is a decreased resting heart rate. This means the heart has become a more efficient pump.
	RPE					
	REST HR					
	EXERCISE HR					
	STRESS TEST					
	METS RESULTS					
GENDER						Males experience heart disease earlier; women catch up after menopause. Hormone replacement should be considered for post-menopausal women.
VOCATIONAL	BACK TO WORK		☐ YES ☐ NO	☐ YES ☐ NO		
PARTICIPANT SIGNATURE						
STAFF SIGNATURE					DATE SIGNED	

Figure 20–2(2). *Continued*

PARTICIPANT					KEY: E Explanation W:Written Material V:Verbalizes Understanding T:Inadequate Understanding N=No
INIT PLAN/EDUCATION	**METH**	**EVAL**	**DATE**	**INIT**	**PROGRESS**
ASSESS WILLINGNESS TO QUIT	E				
PROVIDE LIST OF PROGRAMS AVAILABLE	W				
INFORM PT NOT TO SMOKE 2 HRS < EXER	E				
ASSESS COMPLIANCE FREQUENTLY	E				
DANGERS OF SMOKING	WE				
MONITOR BP FREQ; NOTIFY M.D. OF CHG					
NO EXERCISE IF >200/110; STOP IF >220/115					
PATHOPHYSIOLOGY OF HTN	WE				
BENEFITS OF OTHER LIFESTYLE CHANGES	WE				
DIET CONSULT-HEART HEALTHY DIET					
FOOD LABELS	WE				
LOW SODIUM	WE				
HIGH FIBER	WE				
FOOD-DRUG INTERACTION	WE				
LIPIDS ENTRY REVIEW WITH PT	E				
EXIT REVIEW WITH PT	E				
ASSESS COMPLIANCE TO DIETARY PLAN	E				
PATHOPHYSIOLOGY OF HYPERLIPIDEMIA	E				
VITAMIN E, FOLATE					
DIET CONSULT	E				
REVIEW LIPID MEDICATION PRN	WE				
BENEFITS OF EXERCISE	E				
OTHER LIFESTYLE MODIFICATIONS:	E				
AVOID ALCOHOL, EXCESS SUGAR, AND					
SMOKING					
PRE/POST BLOOD GLUCOSE TILL WNL					
NO EXERCISE IF <60 OR >300; NOTIFY M.D.					
CHO SUPPLEMENT AVAILABLE					
DIET CONSULT: DIABETIC DIET	WE				
GUIDELINES FOR EXERCISE & DIABETES	WE				
S&S SYMPTOMS OF HYPO-/HYPER-GLYCEMIA	WE				
MONITOR WEEKLY WEIGHTS					WEIGHT: 1 2 3 4 5 6
EXER RX LOW-INTEN ,LONG-DUR, LOW IMPACT	E				WEIGHT: 7 8 9 10 11 12
ASSESS BODY FAT INITIALLY AND EXIT	E				
PROVIDE SUPPORT AND ENCOURAGEMENT	E				
DIET CONSULT ON GRADUAL WEIGHT LOSS	WE				
PSYCH CONSULT & FOLLOW-UP					☐ STRESS MANAGEMENT
STRESS MANAGEMENT CLASSES	E				☐ RELAXATION
BOOKS:					☐ SELF-EFFICACY
PROVIDE SUPPORT AND ENCOURAGEMENT					☐ BEHAVIOR MODIFICATION
DEPRESSION/ANGER	WE				☐ COMMUNICATION
REVIEW PRE-TEST SCORE	E				
REVIEW POST-TEST SCORE	E				
CARDIAC EXERCISE PRESCRIPTION 3 X WEEK					
REVIEW EXERCISE EQUIPMENT	E				
EXERCISE GUIDELINES	EW				
BENEFITS OF EXERCISE	EW				
HOME EXERCISE					
TAKE OWN PULSE					
STATE TARGET HR RANGE					
DISCHARGE PLANS	EW				
BENEFITS OF HORMONE REPLACEMENT	EW				INITIALS SIGNATURE DATE
WITH WOMEN					
ENCOURAGE RETURN TO WORK	E				
ASSESS RESPONSE TO WORK	E				
VOCATIONAL REHABILITATION PRN					
OTHER EDUCATION: ☐ CHF	WE				
☐ HEART, A&P, PATHO, S&S TO RPT	WE				
☐ MEDS/NITRO	WE				
☐ CARDIAC INTERVENTIONS	WE				
☐ SEXUAL ACTIVITY	WE				

Figure 20–2(3). *Continued*

PARTICIPANT	PROGRESS RECORD: NONE	PHYSICIAN:

ENTRY NOTE AND PLAN:

FOUR WEEKS PROGRESS:

EIGHT WEEKS PROGRESS:

TWELVE WEEKS PROGRESS:

NUTRITIONAL:

GOALS	NOTES AND PROGRESS

PLAN

PSYCHOLOGICAL:

VOCATIONAL:

Please call if I can be of further assistance. Thank you for the referral.

Figure 20–2(4). *Continued*

Table 20–5

Resources and Additional References

RESOURCES FOR OUTCOME INSTRUMENTS

Outcomes Committee of the American Association of Cardiovascular and Pulmonary Rehabilitation, *Outcome Tools Resource Guide,* 1995 (with current updates)
AACVPR
7600 Terrace Avenue, Suite 203
Middleton, WI 53562
Phone: (608) 831-6989
Fax (608) 831-5122
Internet site: http://www.aacvpr.org

QualityMetric, Inc.
John E. Ware, PhD
640 George Washington Highway
Lincoln, RI 02865
Phone: (401) 334-8800
Fax: (401) 334-8801
Internet site: http://www.amihealthy.com/

Medical Outcomes Study (MOS) SF–36
Medical Outcomes Trust
15 Court Square, Suite 400
Boston, MA 02108
Phone: (617) 523-7336, extension 202
Fax: (617) 523-7322
Internet site: http://www.outcomes-trust.org

Rand 36-Item Health Survey 1.0 (identically worded SF-36 questions; scoring differs)
Ron Hays at RAND
1700 Main Street
PO Box 2138
Santa Monica, CA 90407-2138
Phone: (310) 393-0411

HSQ, Health Status Questionnaire (39 questions, the complete SF-36 with 3 questions added relating to depression)
Stratis Health Outcomes Institute
2901 Metro Drive, Suite 400
Bloomington, MN 55425-1525
Phone: (952) 854-3306
Fax: (952) 853-8503
Internet site: http://www.stratishealth.org

Cole B, Finch E, Gowland C, Mayo N. Physical Rehabilitation Outcomes Measures, 1994
Canadian Physiotherapy Association National Office
2345 Yonge Street, Suite 410
Toronto, Ontario M4P 2E3
Phone: (416) 932-1888 or (800) 387-8679
Fax: (416) 932-9708
Internet site: http://www.physiotherapy.ca

OUTCOME SOFTWARE and SERVICES with CARDIOVASCULAR PRODUCTS

HeartWatchers International, Inc.
PO Box 39185
Solon, OH 44139-9185
Phone/fax: (800) 315-4022
Internet site: http://www.heartwatchers.com

Lumedx (formerly Seattle Systems) National Cardiovascular Management Database
2101 Webster Street, Suite 1690
Oakland, CA 94612
Phone: (510) 419-1000 or (800) 966-0699; Fax: (510) 419-3699
Internet site: http://www.lumedx.com

FOTO (Focus On Therapeutic Outcomes, Inc.)
PO Box 11444
Knoxville, TN 37939
Phone: (800) 482-3686 or (423) 450-9699; Fax: (423) 450-9484
Internet site: http://www.fotoinc.com

ADDITIONAL REFERENCES

American Physical Therapy Association's Task Force on Standards for Measurement in Physical Therapy. Standards for tests and measurements in physical therapy practice. Phys Ther 71(8): 589–622; 1991.

Guyatt G, Jaeschke R, Feeny D, Patrick D. Measurements in clinical trials: Choosing the right approach. In: Spiker B (ed). Quality of Life and Pharmacoeconomics in Clinical Trials. Philadelphia, Lippincott-Raven, 1996, pp 41–48.

Johnston MV, Keith RA, Hinderer SR. Measurement standards for interdisciplinary medical rehabilitation. Arch Phys Med Rehabil 73:s3–s23, 1992.

Lauer MS, Fortin DF. Databases in cardiology. In: Topol EJ (ed). Textbook of Cardiovascular Medicine. Philadelphia, Lippincott-Raven, 1988, pp 1083–1106.

Oldridge N. Outcome assessment in cardiac rehabilitation: Health-related quality of life and economic evaluation. J Cardiopulm Rehabil 17: 179–194, 1997.

The Commission on Accreditation of Rehabilitation Facilities has created a list of questions to ask when selecting external outcome data system products and services.[68]

Measures and Data Sets

1. What descriptive elements are included (patient characteristics, referral sources)?
2. What information about processes of care is included (treatments, programs)?
3. What outcome measures and data elements are included?
4. What domains of outcome measurement are included in the tools and data elements?
5. Are standardized measures included in the data set?
6. What validity and reliability assessments have been conducted on the measures? What are the findings?
7. Are there accommodations for user-specified fields?

Data Collection and Submission

1. Is there a pooled database to which users submit data?
2. What is the data collection format (forms, software)?
3. How are the data transmitted to the pooled database?
4. What is the frequency of data transmission?
5. What are the specifications for inclusion of cases in the pooled database?
6. How much time is necessary to complete data elements (measures, other data items)?
7. Are there certain specific individuals identified who must complete data for submission (patient, family, clinicians)?

Reporting

1. What reports are provided to subscribers? Content?
2. What is the turnaround time between data submission to receiving the report?
3. Are special reports available? Cost? Process? Timing?
4. Can organizations produce their own reports?
5. Can organizations receive their own data in a database format for the organization's manipulation and analysis?

Comparative and Predictive Information

1. Who participates in the comparison base for any pooled database?
2. What information do subscribers receive to describe the comparison base (types, sizes, location of providers)?
3. What data elements are included in the comparison summaries?
4. Are any predictions made (expected length of stay, outcomes)? If so, how are they calculated?

References for cardiovascular data management services and software are listed in Table 20–5.

Careful analysis and interpretation are critical components of outcome measurement. Few departments and hospital organizations have staff with the analytic skills necessary to guide them in aggregating their data into meaningful data sets for analysis. Therefore, the expertise of someone who knows statistical methods should be enlisted. If there is no one in the organization, a consultant should be enlisted. Nearby universities or colleges may have faculty or graduate students to serve as a resource. Data should not be presented without the minimum of mean and standard deviations.

In addition, adjustment for risk for different subgroups helps discern confounding factors affecting outcomes. Because patients with the same diagnosis have different levels of severity, comorbidities, age, values, and multiple other factors that influence their outcomes, they cannot be classified as one group with the same outcome. There is a need to statistically adjust the analyses of their outcomes, which is best handled by someone knowledgeable in basic statistics so that the interpretation will be accurate.

Distribution of the findings should be done once the data have been analyzed and interpreted. Recipients of this information include staff, case managers, administration, the marketing department, physicians and other referral sources, accreditation agencies, and payers, from managed care organizations to Medicare and Medicaid. Reports they receive should be graphic, clear, and concise, providing information for each of them to use to make their decisions related to the care provided.

Figure 20–3 illustrates a quarterly outcome "Report Card" from the Cardiac Rehabilitation and Prevention Program at Butterworth Health System in Grand Rapids, Michigan.

USE OF OUTCOME INFORMATION

Management

The rationale for looking at our outcomes is driven by accrediting agencies, payers, marketing,

Pathway: Cardiac Rehabilitation and Prevention   **October 1997**

This report is prepared pursuant to but not limited to (P.A. 368 of 1978). This report is a review function and as such is confidential and shall be used only for the purpose provided by law and shall not be a public record and shall not be available for court subpoena.

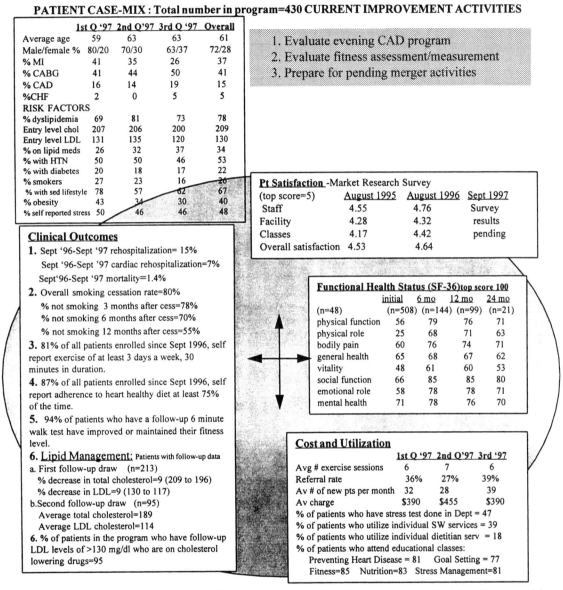

PATIENT CASE-MIX : Total number in program=430 CURRENT IMPROVEMENT ACTIVITIES

	1st Q '97	2nd Q'97	3rd Q '97	Overall
Average age	59	63	63	61
Male/female %	80/20	70/30	63/37	72/28
% MI	41	35	26	37
% CABG	41	44	50	41
% CAD	16	14	19	15
%CHF	2	0	5	5
RISK FACTORS				
% dyslipidemia	69	81	73	78
Entry level chol	207	206	200	209
Entry level LDL	131	135	120	130
% on lipid meds	26	32	37	34
% with HTN	50	50	46	53
% with diabetes	20	18	17	22
% smokers	27	23	16	26
% with sed lifestyle	78	57	62	67
% obesity	43	34	30	40
% self reported stress	50	46	46	48

1. Evaluate evening CAD program
2. Evaluate fitness assessment/measurement
3. Prepare for pending merger activities

Clinical Outcomes

1. Sept '96-Sept '97 rehospitalization= 15%

   Sept '96-Sept '97 cardiac rehospitalization=7%

   Sept'96-Sept '97 mortality=1.4%

2. Overall smoking cessation rate=80%

   % not smoking 3 months after cess=78%

   % not smoking 6 months after cess=70%

   % not smoking 12 months after cess=55%

3. 81% of all patients enrolled since Sept 1996, self report exercise of at least 3 days a week, 30 minutes in duration.

4. 87% of all patients enrolled since Sept 1996, self report adherence to heart healthy diet at least 75% of the time.

5. 94% of patients who have a follow-up 6 minute walk test have improved or maintained their fitness level.

6. Lipid Management: Patients with follow-up data

a. First follow-up draw   (n=213)

   % decrease in total cholesterol=9 (209 to 196)

   % decrease in LDL=9 (130 to 117)

b.Second follow-up draw   (n=95)

   Average total cholesterol=189

   Average LDL cholesterol=114

6. % of patients in the program who have follow-up LDL levels of >130 mg/dl who are on cholesterol lowering drugs=95

Pt Satisfaction -Market Research Survey

(top score=5)	August 1995	August 1996	Sept 1997
Staff	4.55	4.76	Survey
Facility	4.28	4.32	results
Classes	4.17	4.42	pending
Overall satisfaction	4.53	4.64	

Functional Health Status (SF-36) top score 100

	initial	6 mo	12 mo	24 mo
(n=48)	(n=508)	(n=144)	(n=99)	(n=21)
physical function	56	79	76	71
physical role	25	68	71	63
bodily pain	60	76	74	71
general health	65	68	67	62
vitality	48	61	60	53
social function	66	85	85	80
emotional role	58	78	78	71
mental health	71	78	76	70

Cost and Utilization

	1st Q '97	2nd Q'97	3rd '97
Avg # exercise sessions	6	7	6
Referral rate	36%	27%	39%
Av # of new pts per month	32	28	39
Av charge	$390	$455	$390

% of patients who have stress test done in Dept = 47

% of patients who utilize individual SW services = 39

% of patients who utilize individual dietitian serv = 18

% of patients who attend educational classes:

   Preventing Heart Disease = 81   Goal Setting = 77

   Fitness=85   Nutrition=83   Stress Management=81

Figure 20-3. Example of a Cardiac Rehabilitation and Prevention Program Report Card for Outcomes Management. (Courtesy of Butterworth Health System, Grand Rapids, MI.)

and administration, each of whom want to benchmark the profession. This process of **benchmarking,** the ability to compare oneself with an acceptable industry-wide standard or to make comparisons with other rehabilitation programs within a corporation, region, state, or nation, provides an opportunity to learn. This process also provides a method by which the profession can be judged. Although not new to physical therapists who have worked in physical medicine settings, this is new for the cardiac and pulmonary rehabilitation setting. State and regional organizations are establishing systems to compare their outcomes and identify "best practices" to improve their operations and protocols. Clinicians are wise to participate in projects aimed at establishing benchmarks.

The emphasis on data today has created an important role for information technology in delivering reliable and effective disease management programs. As care becomes more and more coordinated across the continuum, management is challenged to track data across inpatient and outpatient settings, merging different data collection methods and information systems. Clinicians in cardiopulmonary rehabilitation can contribute by integrating outcome measurement with disease management, establishing a coordinated clinical system.

Accreditation

The JCAHO's description of efficacy is the degree to which the care of the patient has been shown to accomplish the desired or projected outcomes. In order to pass accreditation, evidence should be charted in discharge orders (medical approval to release and final exercise prescription), discharge interview, outcome comparison sheet, and the patient satisfaction questionnaire.[69] JCAHO patient focused functions require that documentation/charting must include important issues of safety, assessment, appropriateness (planning), care of patients, patient education (implementation), and evaluation. Final evaluation of the patient must show effectiveness and continuity of care.

The Joint Commission's Indicator Measurement System (IMSystem) is an indicator-based performance measurement system designed to measure outcomes of health care organizations. Measuring outcomes is a requirement for the accreditation process, although health care organizations are given the option to collect and report their data to the JCAHO through either the IMSystem or other JCAHO-approved systems.

Reimbursement

Outcome information should also be used to enhance the cardiopulmonary rehabilitation program's reimbursement, referrals, census, and compliance, each of which has an impact on the financial security of the program. In successful negotiations with payers, rehabilitation professionals need to demonstrate the results of their programs, not data or references from published articles demonstrating what the potential might be. Outcome information provides the clinician with the ability to demonstrate to payers that the cardiopulmonary rehabilitation program meets the ideal requirements to be included in the contracts for disease management programs. As part of comprehensive cardiovascular and pulmonary disease management, cardiac and pulmonary rehabilitation programs offer support for patient follow-up that provides confidence for payers.

Under the Department of Health and Human Services, the Health Care Financing Administration (HCFA) is the federal agency charged with administering Medicare. Cardiac rehabilitation is currently reimbursed under the Outpatient Prospective Payment System (OPPS). HCFA.gov is a website dedicated to informing the public and provider with current policies through its content and links to other informative websites. Physical therapists are responsible for staying current with the criteria and regulations for proper documentation and billing and with reimbursement of services offered.

CASE STUDIES

Case Study 1

GJB is a 48-year-old man who was referred to cardiac rehabilitation after coronary artery bypass graft (CABG) surgery with sepsis 6/97 requiring postoperative intra-aortic balloon pump (IABP). The CABG followed an anterior myocardial infarction (MI) 6/97. Because of global left ventricular (LV) dysfunction (EF 5 to 10%), he was awaiting orthotopic heart transplant (OHT).

On admission, his chief complaint was generalized weakness, and he stated that apprehension, pain, and dyspnea all contributed to his inactivity. His exercise activity was limited to chair and breathing exercises. His physician advised a low-sodium, low-fat diet. The first page of Figure 20–4, a Patient Summary Report, lists core data, goals, and plan of care. The second page lists baseline outcome data as well as outcome data after completion of the rehabilitation program.

Review of the outcome portion of the Patient Summary Report (page 2 of Figure 20–4) clearly shows the patient's improvement. He has reached his goal to increase strength and endurance and has become inde-

BEST CARE MEDICAL CENTER
CARDIAC REHABILITATION AND WELLNESS
PATIENT SUMMARY REPORT

GJB   **10/21/97**
Patient ID # 10001   Entry: 7/20/97   Exit: 10/21/97

Date of Birth	12/22/1948	Age	48
Social Security Number		Patient ID #	10001
Physicians:			

Risk Stratification:	High

Diagnoses: Date

Primary	CABG	06/01/97
Secondary	CHF	06/05/97
	Hypertension	11/90
	Hyperlipidemia	02/06/94

Medications:

	Drug	Dosage	Frequency
Antiplatelet	Ecotrin	325 mg	qd
Diuretic	Lasix	20 mg	bid
Hypolipidemic agent	Zocor	20 mg	qd
Antianginal agent	Nitro Transderm	0.4 mg/hr	qd
Ace Inhibitor	Captopril	25 mg	tid
Antiarrhythmic agent	Amiodarone	200 mg	qd
Digitalis	Digitoxin	0.125 mg	qod
Other	K-Dur	20 mg	qd
	Pepcid	20 mg	bid

Risk Factors:

Modifiable	Hyperlipidemia
	Sedentary lifestyle
Non-Modifiable	Male

Goals:

	Desired	Change	Goal Date
Short term	↓ Daily fat intake	↓ to <20%	01/01/98
	↑ Exercise time & sessions/week	>30minutes, tiw	12/01/97
Long term	Maintain low fat, low salt diet		
	Exercise regularly		

Plan of Care:

		Date completed
Exercise	Telemetry monitored	10/21/97
	Home Program	ongoing
Diet	Low fat diet	ongoing
	Low salt diet	ongoing
Education	Understanding heart disease	7/24/97
	Understanding medications	7/31/97
	Understanding fats and nutrition	8/7/97

Figure 20-4(1). Sample Patient Outcome Report. (Courtesy of Heart Watchers International, Inc.)

pendent again with ADLs, mobility skills, and ambulation. This is evident in his improved scores in the physical dimensions, as well as in all other dimensions of the quality of life questionnaire. The patient is no longer on the transplant list as a result of his good progress.

Case Study 2

The Cardiac Rehabilitation and Wellness Program at Best Care Medical Center reviewed their Core Program Data and the Clinical Presentation of their patients (Figure 20-5, pages 1 and 2, respectively) to determine

BEST CARE MEDICAL CENTER
CARDIAC REHABILITATION AND WELLNESS
PATIENT SUMMARY REPORT

GJB
Patient ID # 10001

10/21/97
Entry: 7/20/97   Exit: 10/21/97

CLINICAL OUTCOMES	Entry	Exit	Change	GOAL
Functional capacity on GXT	4.1 METs	5.3 METs	29%	5.0 METs
Lipids				
HDL-C	27	30	3	>45
LDL-C	186	170	(16)	<100
Total/HDL	7.5	6.4	(1.1)	<5.0
Triglycerides	300	240	(60)	<150
Blood Pressure				
Systolic blood pressure	90	104		<140
Diastolic blood pressure	72	80		<90
Weight	198	196	(2)	192

HEALTH OUTCOMES	Entry	Exit	Change	
Quality of life SF-36				GOAL: Higher scores indicate improved QOL
Physical functioning	46	58	12	
Bodily Pain	40	58	18	
Role functioning - Physical	45	62	17	
Role functioning - Emotional	44	66	22	
General Health	42	62	20	
Social functioning	50	70	20	
Vitality	46	66	20	
Health Transition	40	63	23	
Mental Health	44	64	20	

BEHAVIORAL OUTCOMES	Entry	Exit	Change	GOALS
Exercise Activity				
Days per week	3	5	2	
Minutes per day	10	30	20	
Diet Habit Survey	179	214	35	Higher score indicates better diet

ECONOMIC OUTCOMES	Entry	Exit	Change	GOAL: A decrease indicates less cost
Employment:	past 3 mos	since entry		
# Days missed due to CAD	50	15	(35)	
Medical Utilization:	past 3 mos	since entry		
# ER visits, due to CAD	2	0	(02)	
# Hospital days, due to CAD	28	0	(28)	
# Unplanned physician visits	4	1	(03)	
# Rehab visits	0	36	36	Intervention

Figure 20–4(2). *Continued*

what outcomes would be most important to their patient population. Because of the high percentage of patients with hyperlipidemia and a sedentary lifestyle, they decided to focus their education in these areas. The results would be measured with lipid levels and the diet habit survey and exercise activity behavior along with a 6-minute walk test. They selected the Medical Outcome Study Short Form 36 (SF-36) to measure quality of life, and used a self-report from the patients for employment and medical utilization information. The Program Outcome Report is seen on page 3 of Figure 20–5.

BEST CARE MEDICAL CENTER
CARDIAC REHABILITATION AND WELLNESS
PROGRAM OUTCOME REPORT
10/21/97

CORE PROGRAM DATA	Number	%
Patients		
Total	60	100
Males	42	70
Females	18	30
Mean Age		
Total	70	
Males	69	
Females	72	
Marital Status		
Married/significant other	42	70
Single	3	5
Divorced	6	10
Widowed	9	15
Risk Stratification Level		
High Risk	13	21.7
Intermediate Risk	35	58.3
Low Risk	12	20.0
Referring Physician		
Ambrose, Edwena	04	6.7
Black, Harold	03	5.0
Daily, Charles	06	10.0
Jefferson, Mary	11	18.3
Mandella, Henrico	08	13.3
Reider, Sandra	01	1.7
Talisman, Stanley	12	20.0
Waggoner, Daniel	15	25.0
Insurance Providers		
Blue Cross/Blue Shield	07	11.7
Kaiser	03	5.0
Medicare HMO	25	41.7
Medicare	21	35.0
Other	04	6.7

Figure 20–5(1). Sample Program Outcome Report. (Courtesy of Heart Watchers International, Inc.)

Results are positive in all areas. More importantly, compared to the last report, when unplanned physician visits and ER visits showed no change, efforts made to improve the patient's symptom control, understanding of disease, and use of medications through changes in educational class content and written materials have reaped excellent results.

Summary

- Outcomes are those changes (favorable or adverse) in actual or potential health status that can be attributed to prior or current care.
- Primary outcomes include health status, func-

BEST CARE MEDICAL CENTER
CARDIAC REHABILITATION AND WELLNESS
PROGRAM OUTCOME REPORT

CLINICAL PRESENTATION   **10/21/1997**

Primary Diagnosis/Intervention	#	%	Secondary Diagnoses/Intervention	#	%
CABG	21	35.0	Asthma	3	5.0
MI	17	28.3	Atrial Fibrillation, chronic	9	15.0
CHF	6	10.0	Atrial Fibrillation, paroxysmal	3	5.0
Stable Angina	5	8.3	CABG	6	10.0
Valvular disease or surgery	3	5.0	CAD	9	15.0
PTCA	3	5.0	Cardiomyopathy	9	15.0
Stent	3	5.0	CHF	15	25.0
Atherectomy	2	3.3	COPD	6	10.0
			CVA	3	5.0
Medication Regimen			Diabetes Mellitus, Type I	5	8.3
ASA	48	80	Diabetes Mellitus, Type II	14	23.3
Hypolipidemic Agents	30	50	Heart Transplantation	1	1.7
Beta Blockers	18	30	Hyperlipidemia	40	66.7
Ace Inhibitors	18	30	Hypertension	30	50.0
			ICD	6	10.0
Risk Factors, Modifiable			MI, old	20	33.3
Hyperlipidemia	42	70.0	Other	1	1.7
Sedentary Lifestyle	42	70.0	Pacemaker	11	18.3
Hypertension	30	50.0	PTCA	30	50.0
Obesity	30	50.0	PVD	12	20.0
Smoking	18	30.0	Renal Failure	6	10.0
Unmanaged Stress	12	20.0	Stable Angina	6	10.0
			Stent	6	9.0
Risk Factors, Unmodifiable			Valvular disease	9	15.0
Family History	30	50.0			
Diabetes	21	35.0			
History of previous CAD	20	33.3			
Female, Post Menopause, no ERT	12	20.0			

Figure 20–5(2). *Continued*

tional status, and well-being. Functional status and well-being are measured by evaluating quality of life.

- Secondary outcomes include the multiple clinical and behavioral variables important to the patient. Some examples of clinical measures include functional capacity, lipid levels, blood pressure, measures of body fat, smoking status, frequency of angina, and dyspnea levels with activity.
- Behavioral variables assess changes in lifestyle, in-

cluding symptom management, adherence to exercise and medication regimen, smoking cessation, and diet intervention.

- Some of the reasons to measure outcomes include demonstration of accountability, improvement in clinical and management decision making, research, and incentive purposes.
- The AACVPR Outcome Committee recommends a minimum of at least one health, one clinical, and one behavioral outcome be measured.
- Data to be collected should be quantified and

BEST CARE MEDICAL CENTER
CARDIAC REHABILITATION AND WELLNESS
PROGRAM OUTCOME REPORT
10/21/1997

CLINICAL OUTCOMES	ENTRY	EXIT	Δ	6MO	Δ	1YR	Δ
6 minute walk test (ft)	1310	1560	250				
Weight (lbs)	188	186	(02)				
Blood Pressure							
Systolic BP>140	138	136	(02)				
Diastolic BP >90	76	77	01				
Lipids							
HDL-C	32	37	05				
LDL-C	172	150	(22)				
Total/HDL Ratio	8.1	6.1	(02)				
Triglycerides	270	240	(30)				

BEHAVIORAL OUTCOMES	ENTRY	EXIT	Δ	6MO	Δ	1YR	Δ
Smoking							
Current	18	12	(06)				
Number per day	20	12	(08)				
Former	28	28					
Never	14	14					
Exercise Activity							
Days per week	2	4	2				
Minutes per day	20	30	10				
Diet Habit Survey	179	214	35				

HEALTH OUTCOMES	ENTRY	EXIT	Δ	6MO	Δ	1YR	Δ
Quality of Life (SF-36)							
Bodily Pain	72	78	06				
General Health	68	78	10				
Health Transition	68	79	11				
Mental Health	66	76	10				
Physical Functioning	72	80	08				
Role Functioning – Emotional	67	75	08				
Role Functioning – Physical	73	81	08				
Social Functioning	69	79	10				
Vitality	71	78	07				

ECONOMIC OUTCOMES	ENTRY	EXIT	Δ	6MO	Δ	1YR	Δ
Employment, past 3 months							
# Days work missed, due to CAD	12	1	(11)				
Medical Utilization, past 3mos							
# ER Visits	2	0	(02)				
# Hospital Days	8	0	(08)				
# Unplanned Physician Visits	3	1	(02)				

Figure 20–5(3). *Continued*

evaluated for change over time, especially when any interventions have occurred.

- The measurement instruments utilized must be both valid and reliable. Validity means the tool measures the characteristics that it is intended to measure. Reliability refers to the degree to which

an instrument and its protocol are free from random error and provide reproducible information.

- Establishing a system that streamlines documentation and facilitates relevant outcome measurement can improve that measurement and decrease time spent in measurement.

- The timing and frequency of data collection are important because collecting some variables too early or too late might not demonstrate the change from the intervention.
- Outcome information may be a potential to enhance the program's reimbursement, referrals, census, and compliance, each of which has an impact on the financial security of the program.

References

1. Donabedian A. The methods and findings of quality assessment and monitoring: An illustrated analysis. Ann Arbor, Health Administration Press, 1985.
2. Patrick D, Erickson P. Health Status and Health Policy. Quality of Life in Health Care Evaluation and Resource Allocation. New York, Oxford University Press, 1993.
3. Spilker B. Introduction. In: Spilker B (ed). Quality of Life Assessments in Clinical Trials. New York, Raven Press, 1990, pp 3–9.
4. American Association for Cardiovascular and Pulmonary Rehabilitation. Guidelines for Cardiac Rehabilitation Programs. 3rd ed. Champaign, IL, Human Kinetics, 1998.
5. Nelson E, Greenfield S. Outcomes matter most. J Clin Outcomes Management 1(1):9–10, 1994.
6. Pashkow P, Ades P, Emery C, et al. Outcome measurement in cardiac and pulmonary rehabilitation. J Cardiopulm Rehabil 15:394–405, 1995.
7. Joint Commission on Accreditation of Healthcare Organizations. Oakbrook Terrace, IL, IMSystem General Information. 1997.
8. Stewart A, Hays R, Ware JJ. The MOS short-form general health survey. Reliability and validity in a patient population. Med Care 26:724–735, 1988.
9. Hunt S, McEwen J, McKenna S. A quantitative approach to perceived health. J Epidemiol Community Health 34:281–295, 1980.
10. Gibson B, Gibson J, Bergner M, et al. The sickness impact profile—Development of an outcome measure of health care. Ann Intern Med 65(12):1304–1310, 1975.
11. Bergner M, Bobbitt R, Carter W, et al. The Sickness Impact Profile: Development and final revision of a health status measure. Med Care 19:787–805, 1981.
12. Kaplan R, Atkins C, Timms R. Validity of a quality of well-being scale as an outcome measure in chronic obstructive pulmonary disease. J Chron Dis 37:85–95, 1984.
13. Greenberg G, Peterson R, Heilbronner R. Illness Effects Questionnaire. Philadelphia, PA (unpublished). Psychology Department, Children's Rehabilitation Hospital, Thomas Jefferson University Hospital, 1989.
14. Wasson J, Keller A, Rubenstein L, et al. Benefits and obstacles of health status assessment in ambulatory settings. Med Care 30(5):42–49, 1992.
15. Parkerson GJ, Broadhead W, Tse C-K. The Duke Health Profile: A 17-item measure of health and dysfunction. Med Care 28:1056–1072, 1990.
16. Wallston K, Wallston B. Health locus of control scales. In: Lefcourt H (ed). Research with the Locus of Control Construct. New York, Academic Press, 1981.
17. Dupuis G, Perrault J, Lambany M, et al. A new tool to assess quality of life: The Quality of Life Systemic Inventory. Quality Life Cardiovasc Care Spring:36–40, 1989.
18. Kellner R. Manual of the symptom questionnaire (unpublished). Albuquerque Department of Psychiatry, School of Medicine, No. 87131, 1987.
19. Rector T, Kubo S, Cohn J. Patients' self-assessment of their congestive heart failure. Heart Failure Oct/Nov: 198–209, 1987.
20. Rogers W, Johnstone D, Yusuf S, et al. Quality of life among 5025 patients with left ventricular dysfunction randomized between placebo and enalapril: The study of left ventricular dysfunction. J Am Coll Cardiol 23:393–400, 1994.
21. Oldridge N, Guyatt G, Jones N, et al. Effects on quality of life with comprehensive rehabilitation after acute myocardial infarction. Am J Cardiol 67:1084–1089, 1991.
22. Lim L-Y, Valenti L, Knapp J, et al. A self-administered quality of life questionnaire after acute myocardial infarction. J Clin Epidemiol 46:1249–1256, 1993.
23. Ferrans C, Powers M. Psychometric assessment of the Quality of Life Index. Res Nurs Health 15:29–38, 1992.
24. Spertus J, Winder J, Dewhurst T, et al. Development and evaluation of the Seattle Angina Questionnaire: A new functional status measure for coronary artery disease. J Am Coll Cardiol 25:333–341, 1995.
25. Guyatt G, Berman L, Townsend M, et al. A measure of quality of life for clinical trials in chronic lung disease. Thorax 42:773–778, 1987.
26. Jones P, Quirk F, Baveystock C, Littlejohn P. A self-complete measure of health status for chronic airflow limitation. Am Rev Respir Dis 145:1321–1327, 1992.
27. Weaver T, Narsavage G. Physiological and psychological variables related to functional status in chronic obstructive pulmonary disease. Nurs Res 41:286–291, 1992.
28. Lareau S, Carrieri-Kohlman V, Janson-Bjerklie S, Roos P. Development and testing of the Pulmonary Functional Status and Dyspnea Questionnaire (PFSDQ). Heart Lung 23(3):242–250, 1994.
29. Hyland M. The living with asthma questionnaire. Respir Med 85(suppl B):13–16, 1991.
30. Harvey R, Doyle E, Ellis K, et al. Major changes made by the Criteria Committee of the New York Heart Association. Circulation 49:390, 1974.
31. Goldman L, Hashimoto B, Cook E, et al. Comparative reproducibility and validity of systems for assessing cardiovascular functional class: Advantages of a new Specific Activity Scale. Circulation 64:1227–1234, 1981.
32. Mahler D, Weinberg D, Wells C, Feinstein A. The measurement of dyspnea: Contents, interobserver agreement, and physiologic correlates of two new clinical indexes. Chest 85:751–758, 1984.
33. Hlatky M, Boineau R, Higgenbotham M, et al. A brief self-administered questionnaire to determine functional capacity (The Duke Activity Status Index). Am J Cardiol 64:651–654, 1989.
34. Borg G. Perceived exertion as an indicator of somatic stress. Scand J Rehabil Med 2:92–98, 1970.
35. Borg G. Psychophysical basis of perceived exertion. Med Sci Sports Exerc 14:377–381, 1982.
36. Gift A. Validation of a vertical visual analogue scale as a measure of clinical dyspnea. Rehab Nurse 14:323–325, 1989.
37. American College of Sports Medicine. Guidelines for Graded Exercise Testing and Exercise Prescription. 4th ed. Philadelphia, Lea & Febiger, 1991.
38. Guyatt G, Sullivan M, Thompson P, et al. The 6-minute walk: A new measure of exercise capacity in patients with chronic heart failure. Can Med Assoc J 132:919–923, 1985.

39. Cipkin D, Scriven J, Crake T, Poole-Wilson P. Six minute walking test for assessing exercise capacity in chronic heart failure. BMJ 292:653–655, 1986.
40. Daughton D, Fix A, Kass I, et al. Maximum oxygen consumption and the ADAPT quality of life scale. Arch Phys Med Rehabil 63:620–622, 1982.
41. Jette A, Davies A, Cleary P, et al. The functional status questionnaire: Reliability and validity when used in primary care. J Gen Intern Med 1:143–149, 1986.
42. Derogatis R, Brand R, Jenkins C, et al. SCL-90-R: Administration, Scoring and Procedures Manual II for the R (revised) Version and Other Instruments of the Psychopathology Rating Scale Series. 2nd ed. Towson, MD, Clinic Psychometric Research, 1983.
43. Dahlstrom W, Walsh G, Dahlstrom L. An MMPI Handbook. Clinical Interpretation. Rev. ed. Minneapolis, University of Minnesota, 1975.
44. Cook W, Medley D. Proposed hostility and pharisaic-virtue scales for the MMPI. J Appl Psych 38:414–418, 1954.
45. Buss A, Durkee A. An inventory for assessing different kinds of hostility. J Consult Psych 21:343–349, 1957.
46. Beck A. The Beck Depression Inventory. Philadelphia, Center for Cognitive Therapy, 1978.
47. Radloff L. The CES-D scale: A self-report depression scale for research in the general population. Appl Psychol Measurement 1:385–401, 1977.
48. Spielberger C, Gonsuch R, Luschene R. Manual for the State—Trait Anxiety Inventory. Palo Alto, CA, Consulting Psychologist Press, 1970.
49. Wigel J, Creer T, Kotses H. The COPD Self-Efficacy Scale. Chest 99:1193–1196, 1991.
50. Carver C, Scheier M, Weintraub J. Assessing coping strategies: A theoretically based approach. J Pers Soc Psychol 56:267–283, 1989.
51. Jenkins C, Rosenman R, Friedman M. Development of an objective psychological test for the determination of the coronary prone behavior pattern in employed men. J Chron Dis 20:371–379, 1967.
52. McNair D, Lorr M, Droppleman L. Profile of Mood States. San Diego, Educational and Industrial Testing Service, 1971.
53. Hare D, Davis C. Validation of a new depression scale for cardiac patients in quality of life assessment. Aust NZ J Med 23:630, 1993.
54. Lorish C, Maisiak R. The face scale: A brief, nonverbal method for assessing patient mood. Arthritis Rheum 29(7):906–910, 1986.
55. Wenger N, Mattson M, Furberg C. Assessment of Quality of Life in Clinical Trials of Cardiovascular Therapies. New York, Le Jacq Communications, 1984.
56. Folkman S, Lazarus R. Ways of Coping Questionnaire. J Pers Soc Psychol 48:150–170, 1985.
57. Sherbourne C, Stewart A. The MOS social support survey. Soc Sci Med 32(6):705–714, 1991.
58. Morrow G, Chiarello R, Derogatis L. Psychosocial adjustment to illness scale. Psychol Med 8:605–610, 1978.
59. Willett W, Sampson L, Stampfer M, et al. Reproducibility and validity of a semi-quantitative food frequency questionnaire. Am J Epidemiol 122:51, 1985.
60. Block G, Clifford C, Naughton M, et al. A brief dietary screen for high fat intake. J Nutr Educ 21:199–207, 1989.
61. Connor S, Gustafson J, Sexton G, et al. The diet habit survey: A new method of dietary assessment that relates to plasma cholesterol changes. J Am Dietetic Assoc 92(1):41–47, 1992.
62. Blankenhorn DH, Nessim SA, Johnson RL, et al. Beneficial effects of combined colestipol-niacin therapy on coronary atherosclerosis and coronary venous bypass grafts [published erratum appears in JAMA 259(18):2698, 1988]. JAMA 257(23):3233–3240, 1987.
63. Hopp J, Lee J, Hills R. Development and validation of a pulmonary rehabilitation knowledge test. J Cardiopulm Rehabil 8:15–18, 1989.
64. Maeland J, Havik O. Measuring cardiac health knowledge. Scand J Caring Sci 1:23–31, 1987.
65. Pashkow P. Outcomes in cardiopulmonary rehabilitation. Phys Ther 76(6):643–656, 1996.
66. American Physical Therapy Association. A guide to physical therapist practice. Phys Ther 77(11), 1997.
67. Russek L, Wooden M, Ekedahl S, Bush A. Attitudes toward standardized data collection. Phys Ther 77(7):714–729, 1997.
68. Wilkerson D. Issues in the use of outcomes data system tools and services. Advances on accreditation—Focus on outcomes. Tucson, Commission on Accreditation of Rehabilitation Facilities, 1996.
69. Joint Commission on Accreditation of Healthcare Organizations. 1997 Accreditation Manual for Hospitals. Vol. I. Chicago, JCAHO, 1996.

Glossary

a wave—the rise in the atrial pressure curve caused by the contraction of the atria during atrial systole

abdominal aortic aneurysmectomy (AAA)—localized area of increased aortic diameter in abdominal area; usually atherosclerotic, but may be an extension of a dissection from above in the aorta

ablation procedure—cauterization of the area in the heart that is inducing the arrhythmia

ABO blood group—system of the most common major blood groups A, B, AB, and O; ABO blood group compatibility is essential for blood transfusion

accessory atrioventricular tracts or bundles—the fine terminal branches of the internodal tracts that are postulated to "bypass" the atrioventricular node; their existence and function are controversial

ACE inhibitors—see angiotensin-converting enzyme inhibitors

acebutolol (Sectral)—a beta-adrenoceptor blocking agent

acellular hyaline membrane—a layer of nearly translucent material (formerly eosinophilic) that lines the bronchioles, alveolar ducts, and alveoli of premature infants with respiratory distress

acetylcholine—an acetic acid ester of choline; liberated from the preganglionic and postganglionic endings of parasympathetic fibers and from the preganglionic endings of the sympathetic fibers where it acts as a transmitter on the effector organ; causes cardiac inhibition, vasodilation, gastrointestinal peristalsis, and other parasympathetic effects

acetylcholinesterase—an enzyme that catalyzes the hydrolysis of acetylcholine to form acetic acid and choline

acidemia—a condition of increased hydrogen ion concentration (decreased pH) in the blood

acidosis—a pathologic condition arising from the accumulation of acid in (or loss of base from) the body

acromegaly—an enlargement of the head, face, hands, feet, and internal organs that results from the hypersecretion of growth hormone from an abnormal pituitary gland after maturity

action potential—the rapid sequence of changes in electrical potential that takes place across a cell membrane during depolarization and repolarization

activation gate—the manner in which flux is controlled through an ionic channel in a cell membrane; as the membrane potential becomes less negative, this "gate" opens, allowing ions to pass along the channel

active cycle of breathing (ACB)—a series of maneuvers performed by the patient to clear secretions and increase thoracic expansion

active transport—the utilization of energy to move ions against an electrochemical gradient

acute rejection—presence of preformed antibodies or infiltrates of mononuclear cells leading to myocyte necrosis in a transplanted organ

acute respiratory acidosis—a pathologic condition typified by a lower than normal pH and a higher than normal Pa_{CO_2}

acute ventilatory failure (or acute respiratory failure)—a pathologic condition typified by a pH below 7.30 and a Pa_{CO_2} greater than 50 mmHg

acyclovir (Zovirax)—an antiviral agent that is effective against herpes virus infections

adenosine triphosphate (ATP)—a nucleotide composed of a nitrogenous base, *adenine;* a pentose sugar, *ribose;* and three *phosphate radicals.*

779

The last two phosphate radicals are bound to the main portion of the molecule by so-called *high-energy phosphate bonds,* which may be broken easily to release energy for bodily needs

adenylate cyclase—one of the many catalytic units within a cell that may be activated by G proteins when a receptor site is stimulated; adenylate cyclase catalyzes the conversion of adenosine triphosphate (ATP) to cyclic adenosine monophosphate (cAMP)

adipocytes—fat cells

adipose—of or related to fat

adrenergic—nerve fibers of the sympathetic division of the autonomic nervous system that secrete norepinephrine

adrenoceptors—the sites on an effector organ innervated by postganglionic adrenergic fibers of the sympathetic division of the autonomic nervous system

adult respiratory distress syndrome (ARDS)—syndrome of acute respiratory failure characterized by severe hypoxemia, bilateral pulmonary infiltrates, and decreased lung compliance

advanced cardiac life support (ACLS)—the electrical, pharmacologic, vascular and airway access techniques used to resuscitate or sustain life in addition to those associated with the basic life support measures of cardiopulmonary resuscitation

adventitia—the outermost layer of connective tissue of an artery or vein; tunica adventitia

adventitious breath sounds—abnormal sounds heard during auscultation of the lung fields

aerosol—liquid or solid particles suspended in a gas

aerosol mask—a device used to facilitate the delivery of an aerosol to a patient

afterload—the force against which the muscular wall of the ventricle exerts its contraction

agenesis—an abnormal development or absence of a part

agonist—a drug that interacts with receptors to initiate a response

airway clearance techniques—manual or mechanical procedures that facilitate clearance of secretions from the airways

airway reactivity—the alteration in bronchomotor tone in response to noxious stimuli

airway resistance (R_{aw})—the force opposing the flow of gases during ventilation; results from obstruction or turbulent flow in the upper and lower airways

albumin—one of the most common plasma proteins

alcoholic cardiomyopathy—cardiac muscle disease that is associated with chronic alcohol abuse

aldosterone—a steroid hormone produced in the adrenal cortex; it causes resorption of sodium and excretion of hydrogen and potassium in the distal renal tubules

aldosteronism—an intrinsic disorder of the adrenal cortex that results in the excessive secretion of aldosterone

alkalemia—an increase in the pH of the blood; a decrease in the hydrogen ion concentration of the blood

alkalosis—a pathologic condition arising from the accumulation of base in (or loss of acid from) the body

alkalotic—referring to the condition of alkalosis

allergen—an antigenic substance; a cause of an altered reactivity

allergic angiitis—an inflammation of the small (dermal) blood vessels with polymorphonuclear infiltrate; cutaneous vasculitis

alpha-adrenergic receptor—a subclass of neuroreceptors located at the norepinephrine synapses of the sympathetic (adrenergic) division of the autonomic nervous system; further divided into alpha$_1$ and alpha$_2$ categories

alpha$_1$-acid-glycoprotein—a subgroup of the alpha-globulin fraction of blood; one of the most common plasma proteins

alpha$_1$-antitrypsin deficiency—a genetically determined (autosomal recessive) disorder in which the glycoprotein alpha$_1$-antitrypsin (the major protease inhibitor of human serum) is deficient; persons with the disorder are predisposed to juvenile hepatic cirrhosis and pulmonary emphysema

alpha$_1$ (α_1) receptor—alpha-adrenergic neuroreceptors that are located primarily in the vascular and intestinal smooth muscle, where they elicit contraction or relaxation, respectively

alpha$_2$ (α_2) receptor—alpha-adrenergic neuroreceptors that are located primarily on the presynaptic terminals of certain adrenergic receptors, where they elicit a reduction in norepinephrine release; postsynaptically on fat cells, where they decrease lipolysis; and postsynaptically on certain central nervous system adrenergic receptors, where they elicit a reduction in sympathetic output from the brain stem

alpha sympatholytic—a drug that inhibits alpha-adrenergic receptors of the autonomic nervous system

alteplase recombinant tPA—a tissue plasminogen activator (tPA; Activase)

alveolar-arterial defects—an imperfection or absence of the alveolar/arterial blood supply

alveolar ducts—the part of the respiratory passages that connects the respiratory bronchioles and the alveolar sacs

alveolar hemorrhage—the escape of blood through pulmonary blood vessels into the alveolar spaces

alveolar hyperventilation—increased alveolar ventilation to the extent that arterial carbon dioxide levels are decreased below normal; Pa$_{CO_2}$ less than 30 mm Hg; respiratory alkalemia

alveolar pattern—one of two main roentgenographic patterns; radiopaque confluent densities that may have a localized, diffuse, or centralized distribution depending on the disease process; likened to "fluffy clouds"

alveolar sacs—the terminal dilation of the alveolar ducts

alveolar surfaces—the combined area of the alveoli

alveolar ventilation—the alveolar gas flow

alveolitis—inflammation of the alveoli

alveolus—one of the terminal saclike dilations of the alveolar ducts in the lungs

amantadine (Symadine, Symmetrel)—an antiviral agent; used in the prevention and treatment of influenza A infection (also used in the treatment of parkinsonism)

amenorrhea—the absence of menstruation

aminoglycoside drugs—antibacteria drugs that are active against gram-negative, some gram-positive and anaerobic bacteria

amiodarone (Cordarone)—a coronary vasodilator used in the treatment of symptomatic supraventricular and ventricular arrythmias

amrinone (Inocor)—an inotropic agent with vasodilator action; used in the treatment of congestive heart failure

amyotrophic lateral sclerosis (ALS)—a disease of the motor tracts of the lateral columns and anterior horns of the spinal cord; associated with progressive muscular atrophy and fibrillation and hyperreflexia

anaerobic threshold (AT)—the limit of the ability of the blood to buffer the by-products of anaerobiosis (e.g., lactic acid); the onset of plasma lactate accumulation (OPLA); an indirect measure of an individual's endurance

analeptic—a central nervous system stimulant; used in the treatment of depressed central nervous system function

anatomic dead space volume—the volume of gas that occupies the nonrespiratory conducting airways

anemia—a condition in which the number of red blood cells per cubic millimeter or the volume of packed red blood cells per 100 mL of blood is less than normal (also when the amount of hemoglobin per 100 mL of blood is less than normal); three types of anemias are classified by the mean corpuscular volume as microcytic (small red blood cells), normocytic, or macrocytic (large red blood cells)

aneurysm—a circumscribed dilatation, especially of an artery or a chamber of the heart

angina—angina pectoris

angina pectoris—severe constricting pain in the chest, often radiating from the precordium to the left shoulder and down the arm, due to ischemia of the heart muscle, which is usually caused by coronary disease

angioblastic tissue—the primordial mesenchymal tissue that develops into embryonic blood cells and vascular endothelium

angiogenesis—development of new blood vessels

angiotensin-converting enzyme (ACE)—a dipeptidyl-carboxypeptidase that splits off histidyl-leucine from angiotensin I to form angiotensin II; located in endothelial cells; most of the conversion occurs as blood passes through the lungs

angiotensin-converting enzyme (ACE) inhibitors—a group of antihypertensive drugs that works by inhibiting the action of angiotensin-converting enzyme, thus blocking the conversion of angiotensin I to angiotensin II

angiotensin I—a decapeptide formed by the splitting of the tetradecapeptide angiotensinogen in the presence of renin; physiologically inactive

angiotensin II—a potent vasopressor; an octapeptide formed by the splitting off of histidyl-leucine from angiotensin I, it is the greatest stimulus to the adrenal gland for the production and release of aldosterone

angiotensinogen—a tetradecapeptide formed by the liver (formerly considered to be a portion of the alpha$_2$-globulin fraction of the proteins in the circulating plasma) that is converted to angiotensin I by renin

anisoylated plasminogen streptokinase activator complex (APSAC) (Eminase)—a form of streptokinase to which a methoxybenzene has been added

ankle brachial index (ABI)—a noninvasive test that compares the blood pressure obtained with a Doppler from the dorsalis pedis to the blood pressure from the higher of the two brachial pressures; an ABI of .9 or higher is normal

ankylosing spondylitis—arthritis of the spine, progressing to bony fixation with lipping of the vertebral margins; Marie-Strümpell disease

anorexia nervosa—a psychological disorder in which an individual exhibits an aversion to food owing to an extreme fear of becoming obese

antagonist—a drug that interacts with receptors to block or inhibit a response

anterior basal segmental bronchus—the portion of the tracheobronchial tree arising from the right lower lobe bronchus that is distributed to the anterior basal segment

anterior cardiac veins—three or four small veins receiving blood from the right ventricle

anterior interventricular artery—the anterior interventricular branch of the left coronary artery; left anterior descending artery

anterior interventricular sulcus—a groove on the anterosuperior surface of the heart that marks the location of the interventricular septum

anterior leaflet of the mitral valve—the larger of the two cusps of the mitral valve; it has no basal zone; also called the anteromedial, aortic, or septal leaflet

anterior papillary muscles—arise from the interior border of the moderator band in the right ventricle and from the sternocostal wall of the left ventricle

anterior pulmonary plexus—a network of nerves formed by branches of the vagus nerves and the deep cardiac plexus supplying anterior branches of the bronchi and the pulmonary and bronchial vessels

anterior segmental bronchus—the portion of the tracheobronchial tree arising from the right or left upper lobe bronchus that is distributed to the anterior segment

anterolateral thoracotomy—an incision into the anterolateral aspect of the chest wall

anteromedial basal segmental bronchus—the portion of the tracheobronchial tree arising from the left lower lobe bronchus that is distributed to the anteromedial basal segment

anteroposterior (AP) view—describes the direction of the roentgen ray beam through the patient from anterior to posterior

anthracycline—an antineoplastic agent; a glycoside antibiotic used in the treatment of solid tumors (e.g., breast, ovarian, small cell bronchogenic cancers), it is believed to intercalate between the base pairs of DNA, thus inhibiting its synthesis; cardiac cells are especially sensitive to the chemotoxic effects of anthracycline glycosides

anthracycline toxicity—refers to the two types of cardiotoxicity generally associated with anthracycline: an acute, transient type characterized by abnormal ECG findings (e.g., ST and T wave changes, tachyarrhythmias); and a chronic, cumulative, dose-dependent type characterized by congestive heart failure and cardiorespiratory decompensation

antibiotic—a substance that inhibits the growth of a microorganism; derived from a mold or bacterium

antibody—a class of immunoglobulins that results from an antigenic stimulus

anticholinesterase—a drug that inhibits or inactivates acetylcholinesterase

anticoagulant—an agent that prevents coagulation

antidiuretic hormone (ADH)—a nonpeptide hormone that causes contraction of vascular smooth muscle; vasopressin

antigen—any substance capable of causing the production of antibodies

antigen-antibody reaction—the combination of an antibody with an antigen of the type that initially stimulated the formation of the antibody, causing the agglutination, precipitation, fixation, or phagocytosis of the antigen

antihistamine—a drug that inhibits the action of histamine

antilymphocyte globulin (ALG)—an immunosuppressant; used to suppress the cell-mediated immune response to transplanted tissue (e.g., liver, heart)

antimicrobial—a substance that destroys or prevents the development or action of microbes

antithymocyte globulin (ATG)—an immunosuppressant; used to suppress the cell-mediated immune response to transplanted tissue (e.g., liver, heart)

antitussive—a drug that relieves coughing

aorta—the main trunk of the systemic arterial system arising from the left ventricle

aortic aneurysm—a circumscribed dilation of the aorta

aortic area (space)—the region of the chest (second intercostal space along the right sternal border) where the normal and pathologic sounds made by the aortic valve are traditionally said to be best appreciated

aortic sinuses—three dilations above the attached margins of the cusps of the aortic valve at the root of the aorta

aortic stenosis—a pathologic narrowing of the orifice of the aortic valve

aortic vestibule—the portion of the left ventricle immediately below the aortic orifice

aorticopulmonary septum—the spiral septum formed from the bulbar and truncal ridges that separates the bulbus cordis and the truncus arteriosus into a ventral pulmonary trunk and dorsal aorta

apex of the heart—the conical extremity of the heart formed by the left ventricle

Apgar score—numerical scale (0 to 10) in which 0 to 2 points are assigned to each of five criteria (heart rate, respiratory effort, muscle tone, response to stimulation, and skin color); used in assessment of the status of newborn infants at 1 and 5 minutes following birth

apical segmental bronchus—the portion of the tracheobronchial tree arising from the right upper lobe bronchus that is distributed to the apical segment

apicoposterior segmental bronchus—the portion of the tracheobronchial tree arising from the left upper lobe bronchus that is distributed to the apicoposterior segment

aplasia—abnormal development or congenital absence of an organ or tissue

aplastic anemia—a condition of less than the normal amount of erythrocytes and hemoglobin as a result of defective bone marrow; usually associated with granulocytopenia and thrombocytopenia

Arantius's nodules—nodular, fibrous thickenings at the midpoints of the free edges of the semilunar cusps of the aortic valve

arbutamine—a new pharmacologic agent used for stress testing; this medication increases cardiac contractility as well as the rate of contraction, acting as a catecholamine

arch of the aorta—the curved portion of the aorta between the ascending and descending portions of the aorta

arm ergometry—upper extremity exercise performed on a crank dynamometer

arrhythmia—a loss of rhythm; an irregularity of the heart beat

arrhythmogenic—capable of producing cardiac arrhythmias

arterial catheter—a hollow, tubular device placed intra-arterially to allow the passage of fluid into or out of the artery

arterial duplex ultrasonography—diagnostic test for defining arterial stenoses and occlusions

arteries—blood vessels conveying blood in a direction away from the heart

arteriole—a minute artery with a muscular wall; a terminal artery continuous with the capillary networks

artificial airway—use of an oral or nasal endotracheal tube for short-term artificial ventilation or tracheostomy for long-term artificial ventilation

aryepiglottic folds—the posterior boundary of the laryngeal inlet formed by the ligamentous and muscular fibers between the epiglottis and arytenoid apex

ascending aorta—the first part of the aorta between its origin from the heart and the arch of the aorta

ascites—abnormal accumulation of fluid in the peritoneal cavity

aspartate aminotransferase (AST)—an enzyme released into the blood as the result of myocardial injury; formerly serum glutamic-oxaloacetic transaminase (SGOT)

asphyxia—impaired or absent oxygen and carbon dioxide exchange

aspiration pneumonia—inflammation of the lung parenchyma resulting from the entrance of oral or gastric contents into the bronchi

asplenia—congenital absence of the spleen

assist-control mode—a method of mechanical ventilatory assistance in which a set volume of gas is delivered each time the inspiratory phase is triggered

asthma—bronchoconstriction, mucosal edema, and mucous plugging of the airways in response to some noxious stimulus

Åstrand exercise protocol—a graded exercise test protocol for treadmill or bicycle ergometers; treadmill: constant 5 mph speed; after 3 minutes at 0% grade, the grade is increased 2.5% every 2 minutes; bicycle: constant 50 or 60 rpm, after 3 minutes at 0 W resistance, the resistance is increased by 25 W every 2 minutes

atelectasis—the absence of gas in part or all of a lung; an air sac collapse

atelectatic—relating to atelectasis

atenolol (Tenormin)—a beta-adrenergic blocking agent

atherosclerosis—degeneration and hardening of the walls of arteries and sometimes the valves of the heart

atherosclerotic heart disease—the blockage of coronary blood vessels owing to the formation of atherosclerotic plaque

atherosclerotic occlusive disease—the blockage of blood vessels as the result of atherosclerotic plaque formation

atherosis—lipid deposits in the intima of arteries that produce a yellow swelling on the endothelial surface

ATP—adenosine triphosphate

atria—a chamber or cavity to which are connected several chambers or passageways

atrial fibrillation—rapid twitching of the atrial

walls resulting in lack of atrial contractions and therefore an irregular heart beat

atrial flutter—rapid atrial contraction, usually at rates between 250 and 400 per minute

atrial gallop—the triple cadence of heart sounds heard by auscultation and characterized by an audible sound (fourth heart sound) occurring in late diastole in addition to the normal first and second heart sounds; presystolic gallop

atrial kick—the increased ventricular stroke volume resulting from the priming force of atrial contraction immediately before ventricular contraction

atrial septal defect (ASD)—opening in the septum between the two atria as the result of a failure of the septum primum or secundum to close normally during development

atrial tachycardia—depolarization of the atria at a rate in excess of 100 per minute

atrioventricular canals—the left and right halves of the atrioventricular canal of the heart tube, formed by the union of the dorsal and ventral endocardial cushions

atrioventricular nodal artery—a branch of the right coronary artery proximal to the posterior interventricular artery that supplies the atrioventricular node in 80% of hearts

atrioventricular (AV) node—an accumulation of specialized myocytes located near the ostium of the coronary sinus

atrium—the division of the heart tube between the ventricle and the sinus venosus

atypical chest pain—angina that does not conform to the typical or normal form

auscultatory gap—the fading away, and the reappearance at a lower point, of the sounds that indicate systolic blood pressure; in hypertensive patients this may lead to the recording of falsely low (as much as 25 mm Hg) systolic blood pressure values (it may be avoided by pumping the sphygmomanometer 30 mm Hg beyond palpable systolic pressure)

autoantibody response—the formation of antibodies in response to antigenic constituents of one's own tissue

autogenic relaxation—self-directed lessening of tension

autoimmunity—a condition in which one's own tissues are the object of the immune system

automatic implantable cardiac defibrillator (AICD)—an implanted electrical device that senses irregular cardiac rhythm (ventricular fibrillation) and provides a high-energy shock to terminate the ventricular fibrillation and convert to the patient's normal rhythm

automaticity—a cell's ability to initiate its own depolarization

autonomic dysreflexia (hyperreflexia)—exaggerated autonomic nervous system responses

autonomic nervous system—comprises all the afferent and efferent nerves through which the viscera is innervated

autonomic neuropathy—any disease that affects the autonomic nervous system

autosomal dominant trait—any genetic characteristic transmitted to the exclusion of a contrasting allele

axillary-femoral bypass—a surgical procedure that circumvents flow-limiting stenoses or occlusions of the infrarenal aorta and iliac arteries by creating a tunnel from the axillary artery, beneath the pectoralis major, into the subcutaneous tissue of the lateral chest wall, passing medial to the anterior superior iliac spine to reach the ipsilateral femoral artery; axillofemoral bypass

axillary thoracotomy—an incision into the chest wall in the region of the axilla

azathioprine (Imuran)—an immunosuppressive agent used in organ transplantation; a cytotoxic agent used in the treatment of autoimmune hemolytic anemias, systemic lupus erythematosus, and rheumatoid arthritis

azotemia—retention of nitrogen as the result of some process other than renal failure

Bachmann's bundle—the portion of the specialized conduction system of the heart that is a continuation of the right atrial anterior internodal tract into the left atrium

bactericidal—having the ability to cause the death of bacteria

bacteriostatic—having the ability to inhibit or retard the growth of bacteria

Bainbridge's reflex—an atrial stretch reflex that causes changes in heart rate; it is elicited when the right atrial pressure rises sufficiently to distend the right atrium

Balke's exercise protocol—a graded treadmill exercise test protocol consisting of stages of variable (tester choice) duration with incremental speed and grade change at each stage

baroreceptors—sensory nerve endings in the walls of the auricles of the heart, vena cavae, aortic arch, and carotid sinuses that are sensitive to stretch (resulting from increased pressure from within)

barotrauma—injury caused by too much or too little pressure

basal cells—undifferentiated cells in parts of the airway lined by pseudostratified epithelium; basal cells mature to replace other epithelial types

basal chordae—chordae tendineae that arise directly from the ventricular wall to attach to the basal regions of the leaflets of the valves of the heart

base excess (BE)—a measure of the metabolic acid-base status; if a positive value, a measure of metabolic alkalosis; if a negative value (base deficit), a measure of metabolic acidosis; the amount of acid or alkali that would have to be added per unit volume of whole blood (at 37°C and at a P_{CO_2} of 40 mm Hg) to achieve a pH of 7.40

base of the heart—that portion of the heart bounded by the bifurcation of the pulmonary trunk superiorly, the coronary sulcus inferiorly, the sulcus terminalis on the right, and the oblique vein of the left atrium on the left

basic cardiac life support (BCLS)—the emergency procedures of establishing an airway, providing breathing, and performing cardiac compressions as needed; cardiopulmonary resuscitation (CPR)

Becker muscular dystrophy—a milder allelic variant of Duchenne's muscular dystrophy with more variable clinical manifestations

behavior specialist—a member of a multidisciplinary cardiac or pulmonary rehabilitation team; a mental health professional (e.g., social worker, psychologist)

benchmarking—a process of comparing information with an acceptable industry-wide standard or with other rehabilitation programs

beriberi—a specific type of polyneuropathy resulting principally from a vitamin B_1 deficiency

beta-adrenergic blocker—any substance that results in the selective inhibition of the responses of effector cells to beta-adrenergic stimuli

beta-adrenergic receptor—a specific subclass of neuroreceptor located at the norepinephrine synapses of the sympathetic (adrenergic) division of the autonomic nervous system; further divided into beta$_1$ and beta$_2$ categories

beta blockade—selective inhibition of the responses of effector cells to beta-adrenergic stimuli

beta$_1$ (β_1) receptor—distributed predominantly in cardiac smooth muscle (where they increase heart rate and contractility), kidney (where they increase renin secretion), and fat cells (where they increase lipolysis)

beta$_2$ (β_2) receptor—distributed predominantly in bronchiolar smooth muscle (where they elicit bronchodilation), peripheral and hepatic vascular smooth muscle (where they cause vasodilation), gastrointestinal smooth muscle (where they decrease motility), and skeletal muscle and liver cells (where they cause increased cellular metabolism)

bigeminal—paired; especially, the occurrence of heart beats in pairs

bilateral sequential lung transplantation—double lung transplantation

bioavailability—the physiologic availability of a particular amount of a drug

bioelectrical impedance—the estimation of body composition or changes in volume by measuring the resistance to the flow of electrons (electrical impedance) between two electrodes placed on distant parts of the body

biphasic positive airway pressure (BIPAP)—use of a tightly fitting nasal mask to noninvasively deliver positive airway pressures during inspiration as well as expiration

bipolar pacing system—a type of cardiac pacemaker that employs electrodes that have two poles

biventricular hypertrophy—thickening of the walls of both ventricles of the heart in response to an obstructed outflow

bleb—a sac containing fluid or gas; refers to the coalescent alveolar sacs formed from the destruction of alveolar septa as the result of pulmonary disease (e.g., emphysema)

blood islands—clusters of mesodermal cells on the outer surface of the yolk sac that differentiate into the first blood cells

blood urea nitrogen (BUN)—the most prevalent nonprotein nitrogenous compound in the blood; normally about 10 to 15 mg of urea per 100 mL of blood

blunted heart rate response—a less than anticipated heart rate for the amount of work being performed; flat heart rate response

body mass index (BMI)—calculation derived from body mass and stature computed by dividing body mass (in kg) by height (m²)

body of the sternum—the middle segment of the sternum

body plethysmography—the measurement and recording of changes in volume (usually lung volumes) obtained by placing the body in a chamber that surrounds it completely

body substance barrier—material such as gloves, mask, and isolation gown, that prevents exposure to infected body substances

bone marrow transplantation (BMT)—procedure to replace diseased marrow or to reconstitute marrow following high-dose chemoradiotherapy to eradicate malignancies

Borg scale—a numerical scale of 1 to 10 (or sometimes 6 to 20) for the rating of perceived exertion of exercise

brachiocephalic trunk—the largest branch of the arch of the aorta; innominate artery; gives off the right common carotid and right subclavian arteries

bradycardia—heart rate of less than 60 beats per minute

bretylium tosylate (Bretylol)—a sympatholytic agent that inhibits the release of norepinephrine from nerve endings

bronchial breath sounds—the sounds normally heard over the large bronchi on auscultation of the chest; the inspiration to expiration ratio is typically 1 to 1; an abnormal sound when heard over the peripheral lung tissue

bronchial buds—outgrowths of the primordial bronchus of the fetus from which the bronchi and lungs eventually form

bronchial drainage—the removal of fluids (e.g., secretions) from the bronchi; postural drainage

bronchial glands—mucous and seromucous glands, the secretory units of which lie outside the muscular layer of the bronchi

bronchiectasis—dilation of the bronchial and bronchiolar walls as the result of chronic inflammation or obstruction

bronchioles—a subdivision of the bronchi that are less than 1 mm in diameter and have no cartilage in their walls

bronchiolitis—an inflammation of the bronchioles

bronchoconstriction—a reduction in the luminal caliber of a bronchus or bronchi

bronchogenic carcinoma—squamous or oat cell cancer arising in the mucosa of the bronchi

bronchogram—the radiographic image obtained following the injection of a radiopaque material into the tracheobronchial tree

bronchography—the radiographic examination of the tracheobronchial tree after the injection of a radiopaque material

bronchophony—the increased intensity and clarity of vocal sounds heard over a region of consolidated lung tissue

bronchopneumonia—acute inflammation of the walls of the small bronchi and bronchioles

bronchopulmonary dysplasia (BPD)—chronic pulmonary insufficiency associated with long-term positive-pressure mechanical ventilatory support, especially in premature infants

bronchopulmonary segments—the largest subdivisions of a lobe of the lung; each is fed by a direct branch from a lobar bronchus

bronchoscopy—inspection of the interior of the tracheobronchial tree through a bronchoscope

bronchospasm—involuntary contraction of the smooth muscle of the bronchi and bronchioles

bronchovesicular breath sounds—a mixture of bronchial and vesicular breath sounds normally heard in the region of the mainstem bronchi (anteriorly, in the first and second intercostal spaces; posteriorly, between the scapulae); the duration of the inspiratory and expiratory phases is about equal

Bruce exercise test protocol—a graded treadmill exercise test protocol consisting of stages of 3-minutes' duration with incremental speed (1.7, 2.5, 3.4, 4.3, 5.0, 5.5, 6.0, 6.5 mph) and a grade (2%) change at each stage

brush cells—nonciliated epithelial cells in the trachea that have a distinct luminal border (brush border) of microvilli; probably play a role in absorption

buccal—adjacent to the cheek (wall)

bulbar—relating to the hindbrain (rhombencephalon)

bulbar ridges—the spiral epithelial outgrowths from the walls of the bulbus cordis that combine with the truncal ridges to form the aorticopulmonary septum

bulbous cordis—the division of the heart tube between the truncus arteriosus and the ventricle

bulboventricular loop—the bend formed in the developing heart tube as its length increases more rapidly than that of the surrounding pericardium

bulimia nervosa—a chronic disorder characterized by repeated bouts of eating (bingeing), followed by self-induced vomiting and anorexia

bullous emphysema—the destruction of alveolar septa and the reduction in the number of alveoli, creating thin-walled cavities (bullae)

C-reactive protein—an acute-phase reactant to inflammation, recently related to an increased risk for coronary artery disease

cachectic—relating to cachexia

cachexia—weight loss and wasting as the result of a chronic disease or an emotional disturbance

calcium channel blockers—a group of drugs that work by relaxing the smooth muscle within the arterial walls, resulting in a decreased afterload

calcium pump—a biologic mechanism that uses energy from ATP to actively transport calcium across the cell membrane

capacitance vessels—the large venules and veins that form a large, variable-volume, and low-pressure reservoir

capillaries—the smallest vessels at the junction of the arteriole with the venous vascular beds; resembling a hair; fine; minute; a capillary vessel

capillary stasis—stagnation of blood in the capillaries

captopril (Capoten)—an antihypertensive agent; an angiotension-converting enzyme inhibitor

carbonaceous—containing or composed of carbon

carbonic anhydrase—an enzyme in red blood cells that catalyzes the conversion of carbon dioxide into carbonic acid or vice versa

carboxyhemoglobin—the result of the union of carbon monoxide with hemoglobin

cardiac cirrhosis—the fibrotic reaction that occurs within the liver as the result of prolonged congestive heart failure

cardiac cycle—the period from the beginning of one heart beat to the beginning of the next

cardiac impression—the indentations on the inner surfaces of the lungs that outline the contact areas of the heart

cardiac index—a relative measure of cardiac output based on body size; expressed in terms of volume (L) per area (m²) per unit of time (minute)

cardiac jelly—the noncellular material between the endothelial lining and the myocardial layer of the early embryonic heart

cardiac muscle dysfunction (CMD)—a term that has gained popularity in describing an apparently common finding in patients with heart and lung disease

cardiac notch—a roughly V-shaped depression in the anterior border of the left lung at the level of the fourth costal cartilage

cardiac output—the amount of blood ejected into the aorta each minute

cardiac plexus—the anastomosing network of sympathetic and parasympathetic (vagus) nerves that surround the arch of the aorta and the pulmonary artery before continuing to the atria, ventricles, and coronary vessels

cardiac rehabilitation—a multidisciplinary program designed to assist patients with cardiac disease to achieve their optimal physiologic, psychological, and functional status through the use of education and exercise to decrease the risk of a secondary event

cardiac rehabilitation center—a facility in which cardiac rehabilitation is conducted

cardiac silhouette—the outline of the heart seen on a radiographic image of the chest

cardiac tamponade—compression of the heart resulting from accumulation of fluid within the pericardial sac

cardiogenic—of cardiac origin

cardiogenic area—the region of the coelom of the presomite embryo in which mesenchymal cells begin to migrate and proliferate between the layers of the splanchnic mesoderm and endoderm

cardiogenic cords—strands of mesenchymal cells that develop in the cardiogenic area of the presomite embryo

cardiogenic shock—a condition arising when the blood supply to the body tissues is insufficient because of inadequate cardiac output

cardiomegaly—enlargement of the heart

cardiomyopathy—any disease of the myocardium; a classification of diseases of the myocardium that have no known underlying etiology

cardiomyoplasty—an alternative to heart transplantation, this surgical procedure takes a transformed, fatigue-resistant skeletal muscle (often the latissimus) and wraps it around the patient's heart; this muscle is then electrically stimulated to contract with systole

cardiopulmonary resuscitation (CPR)—see BCLS

Cardioquin—an anti-arrhythmic drug

cardiothymic silhouette—the line of demarcation between the thymus gland and the heart in the superior mediastinum; sometimes visible in radiographic images of the chest

cardiotoxic—having a deleterious or detrimental effect on the action of the heart

cardioversion—the restoration of the normal rhythm of the heart by electrical countershock

carina—the ridge separating the openings of the right and left main bronchi at their junction with the trachea

carotid duplex ultrasonography—a diagnostic procedure to identify plaque, stenoses, and occlusions of internal, common, and external carotid arteries and flow direction in vertebral arteries

carotid endarterectomy—the excision of occluding material (e.g., thrombus) from the carotid artery

carotid massage—the manual rhythmic compression of the carotid sinuses at the bifurcation of the common into the internal and external carotid arteries in an effort to slow the heart rate

carotid sinuses—slight dilatations of the common carotid arteries at their bifurcation into the internal and external carotid arteries that contain baroreceptors; cause slowing of the heart rate, vasodilation, and reduction of blood pressure

catecholamine—pyrocatechol with an alkylamine side chain; examples are epinephrine, norepinephrine, and dopamine; a native stimulant

cathechol-o-methyl transferase (COMT)—the enzyme that catalyzes the degradation of the catecholamines norepinephrine and epinephrine at the synaptic junction

cavitation—the formation of a cavity

cell-mediated immunity—the process in which lymphokines are produced through the interaction of antigens with T-lymphocytes

central fibrous body—a part of the fibroskeleton of the heart located between the annulus of the aortic valve and the atrioventricular annuli; right fibrous trigone

central venous catheter—a hollow, tubular instrument passed through a peripheral vein into the vena cava immediately proximal to the right atrium; used for the measurement of right atrial pressure or the infusion of fluids and medications

centriacinar emphysema—a condition resulting from the destruction of the septal walls of the alveoli surrounding the central terminal bronchioles; centrilobular emphysema

cephalosporins—alternative medications to penicillins; used against gram-positive cocci and some gram-negative cocci

cervical pleura—the serous membrane that covers the uppermost aspect of the lung in the neck

channels—macromolecular protein pathways that cross the lipid bilayer of a cell's membrane

chemoattractant—a hormone or chemical agent that attracts other cells

chemoreceptor reflex—an increase in the depth and rate of ventilation in response to a lack of oxygen; it also influences heart rate

chest compression system—a mechanical device that applies pressure in such a way to decrease the anteroposterior dimension of the body, thus squeezing the contents of the thoracic cage between the vertebrae and the sternum

chest physical therapy (CPT)—a multifaceted area of practice that includes many evaluation and treatment techniques with the goals to improve airway clearance, ventilation, and exercise tolerance; reduce work of breathing; and restore patient to fullest potential

chest radiograph—chest x-ray

chest roentgenogram—chest x-ray

chest x-ray—a radiograph or roentgenogram of the thorax

chest wall stretching—manual techniques applied to the chest wall to improve the flexibility of the chest wall

Cheyne-Stokes respiration—the pattern of breathing with gradual increase in depth and sometimes in rate to a maximum, followed by a decrease resulting in apnea; the cycles ordinarily are 30 seconds to a minute in length; characteristically seen in coma from alteration in the nervous centers of respiration

Chlamydia pneumoniae—obligate intracellular parasites that divide by binary fission and depend on energy from a host cell to survive; found in lung as infection markers

cholinergic—nerve fibers that secrete acetylcholine

cholinoceptors—an alternative name for cholinergic adrenoceptors

chordae tendineae—small, delicate fibrous cords attaching to the leaflets (cusps) of the valves of the heart

chronic airflow obstruction—a blockage or impediment to the flow of air that is of long duration

chronic interstitial lung disease—a disease that affects the connective tissue framework of the lung

chronic obstructive pulmonary disease (COPD)—a general descriptive term used for those diseases in which forced expiratory flow rates are decreased

chronic renal failure (CRF)—an insufficiency or nonperformance of the kidney(s) of long duration

chronotropic—affecting the rate of the rhythm of the heart

chronotropic incompetence—failure of the normal rate regulating mechanisms of the heart

chronotropy—relating to the rate or timing of an event

ciliated cell—the most abundant type of cell found in the bronchial epithelium

circuit—the tubing that connects a mechanical ventilator to a patient's endotracheal or tracheostomy tube

circuit training—an exercise program in which an individual performs a series of activities one after another

circumflex artery—a branch of the left coronary artery that passes to the diaphragmatic surface of the left ventricle

cirrhosis—a progressive liver disease characterized by nodular regeneration, fibrosis, and alteration of hepatic parenchymal structure

Clara's cells—nonciliated epithelial cells that are most prevalent in the terminal airways; Clara's cells are believed to play a secondary role in the production of surfactant

clear region—the middle portion of the valve leaflet of the mitral and tricuspid valves; it is smooth and translucent, receives few chordae, and has a thinner lamina fibrosa than the other parts of the leaflet; clear zone

clearance—removal of a substance from the blood often by renal excretion; measured in mL/min

closing volume—the lung volume at which airway closure begins during expiration: an index of the status of the small airways

clubbing—a proliferative change in the soft tissues of the distal fingers and toes (especially the nail beds), resulting in a broadening of their ends; the nails are abnormally curved

coagulation—the process of clotting, especially of the blood

coagulopathy—any condition that affects coagulability, especially of the blood

coal workers' pneumoconiosis (CWP)—an inflammation, typically leading to fibrosis of the lungs, caused by the inhalation of coal dust

coalescent opacities—the blending or fusing together of opaque regions in a radiographic image

coarctation of the aorta—a deformity of the media of the aorta at the level of the ductus arteriosus that causes stricture or stenosis of the lumen

collagen vascular disease—diverse group of systemic diseases characterized by diffuse abnormalities of the vasculature and inflammatory lesions involving the joints, muscles, and connective tissues

collateral vessels—secondary or accessory branches of blood vessels

colonized—the presence of a group or groups of microorganisms

commensal—pertaining to a relationship between two organisms in which one organism benefits and the other is unharmed

commissural chordae—chordae tendineae that attach at the corners of adjacent valve leaflets (commissures)

commissurotomy—a surgical division of the junction between adjacent cusps of a valve of the heart

common atrioventricular bundle—the collection of specialized myocytes that begins at the atrioventricular node and passes through the annulus of the right atrioventricular valve to the membranous portion of the interventricular septum where it splits into two branches; bundle of His; His-Kent bundle

community-acquired pneumonia—the causative agent is from the general community; viruses being one third of cause, bacteria the other two thirds

compensatory acid-base disorder—a normal or anticipated attempt to restore the acid-base balance that occurs in response to some disruptive factor

compensatory pause—the suspension or delay of myocardial electrical activity that may occur following an extrasystole

compliance (C)—a measure of the distensibility of a material; the reciprocal of elastance

complicated myocardial infarction—a myocardial infarction of such severity that there is evidence of continued ischemia, left ventricular failure, shock, serious arrhythmia or other conduction disturbance, or other serious illness persisting beyond the fourth day after the infarction; constitutes a high-risk subset of patients

computed tomography (CT)—produces a computer-generated cross-sectional image that is derived from the synthesis of roentgen-ray transmission data obtained in several different directions through a given plane

conductivity—the property of transmitting or conveying electrical impulses

consolidation—solidification of a normally aerated portion of a lung due to the presence of cellular exudate in the alveolar spaces

continuous ambulatory peritoneal dialysis (CAPD)—a method for the removal of soluble substances and water by means of the intermittent introduction of a dialysis solution into, and subsequently removal of it from the peritoneal cavity, while an individual carries on normal daily activities

continuous arteriovenous hemofiltration (CAVH)—a method for the removal of soluble substances and water from the blood by filtering arterial blood through a semipermeable membrane (ultrafiltration) and simultaneously reinfusing venous blood

continuous positive airway pressure (CPAP)—an airway maneuver, in spontaneously breathing patients, in which airway pressure is maintained above atmospheric pressure throughout the respiratory cycle (inspiratory and expiratory phases)

continuous subcutaneous insulin infusion (CSII)—a method for the controlled introduction of insulin beneath the skin

continuous tube feeding—nutrition provided through a nasogastric tube

contractility—an ill-defined concept that represents muscular performance at any given preload and afterload

contraindication—a circumstance or condition that, because of associated risk, makes the use of a particular intervention inadvisable

contrast echocardiography—procedure in which a contrast agent is injected intravenously during an echocardiogram to improve the diagnostic accuracy

conus arteriosus—the outflow tract of the right ventricle; infundibulum

copious—present in large quantity

cor pulmonale—right-sided heart failure arising from disease of the lungs; chronic cor pulmonale is characterized by right ventricular hypertrophy; acute cor pulmonale is characterized by right ventricular dilation

coronary angiography—radiographic imaging of the vessels of the heart

coronary artery bypass graft (CABG)—a surgical procedure in which flow-limiting stenoses or occlusions of the coronary arteries are circumvented

coronary artery disease—the presence of a flow-limiting obstruction in the coronary arteries that has not yet produced the signs and symptoms of ischemic myocardial damage

coronary artery spasm—an involuntary constriction of the smooth muscle of the coronary arteries

coronary atherosclerosis—arteriosclerosis characterized by lipid deposits in the intima; irregularly distributed in large and medium-sized arteries of the heart

coronary heart disease (CHD)—the signs and symptoms of ischemic myocardial damage as the result of a flow-limiting obstruction in the coronary arteries

coronary sinus—the left horn of the sinus venosus, forming a short trunk that receives most of the veins of the heart

coronary sulcus—the groove on the outer surfaces of the heart that marks the division between the atria and the ventricles

corticosteroid—a drug having action similar to that of the adrenal cortex

corticosteroid-related myopathy—any abnormal condition that affects the muscular tissues, usually proximal muscles

cortisol—a steroid hormone secreted by the adrenal cortex; hydrocortisone

costal groove of the rib—the groove along the inferior border of the rib dorsally that changes to the internal surface of the rib where it bends

costophrenic angle—the junction of the costal and diaphragmatic pleurae

costovertebral pleura—the serous membrane that lines the ribs and vertebrae

couplet—two consecutive atrial or ventricular extrasystoles; paired extrasystoles

crackles—adventitious breath sounds heard on auscultation of the parenchymal tissues of the lungs when fluid has accumulated in the distal airways or when air sacs are collapsed and partially reopening (during inspiration)

crash cart—slang term describing the container that holds the emergency medications and equipment used as part of advanced cardiac life support techniques

creatine phosphokinase (CPK)—an enzyme that catalyzes the transfer of a high-energy phosphate from phosphocreatinine to ADP; creatine kinase

creatinine—a component of urine and the final product of creatine catabolism

crista terminalis—a muscular ridge that separates the right atrium into two parts

cromolyn sodium (Intal)—a prophylactic anti-asthmatic agent

crush injuries—the damage or wounds that result from being squeezed between two hard objects

cryptogenic fibrosing alveolitis—an alveolar inflammatory process of indeterminate etiology that leads to fibrosis of the lungs

crystalline silicon dioxide—the primary constituent of sand; silica

cuirass—a type of negative pressure mechanical ventilator that covers the anterior surface of the thorax

Cushing's syndrome—a condition that arises from increased adrenocortical secretion of cortisone or as a side effect of steroid therapy; characterized by truncal obesity, moon face, acne, hypertension, decreased carbohydrate tolerance, protein catabolism, hirsutism (especially in females), and psychiatric disturbances; pituitary basophilism

cusps—the leaflets of the heart's valves

cyanosis—a bluish or purplish coloration of the skin and mucous membranes as a result of insufficient oxygenation; when reduced hemoglobin exceeds 5 g per 100 mL of blood

cyanotic—pertaining to cyanosis

cycle ergometer testing—an exercise performed on a stationary bicycle

cyclic adenosine monophosphate (cAMP)—the "second messenger" created by the catalytic interaction of ATP with adenylate cyclase following activation by G proteins at enzymatic receptor sites in the cell surface; one of the primary effects of cAMP is to change the degree of phosphorylation of several enzymes involved in muscle contraction

cyclic guanosine monophosphate (cGMP)—a nucleotide that facilitates smooth muscle contraction and may enhance mast cell release of histamine and other mediators to cause bronchoconstriction

cyclic nucleotide phosphodiesterase—an enzyme that breaks the bonds between the diesterified orthophosphoric acids that constitute the components of nucleic acids

cyclosporine (cyclosporin, cyclosporin A)—an immunosuppressive agent; a cyclic oligopeptide produced by the fungus *Tolypocladium inflatum Gams*

cylindric bronchiectasis—a dilatation, of uniform caliber, of the bronchi and bronchioles that results from chronic inflammation or obstruction

cystic fibrosis—generalized disorder of exocrine gland function; impairs clearance of secretions, especially mucus, and may involve the bowel; an autosomal recessive disorder

cystic lesion—an injury or wound caused by the formation of cysts

cystinuria—the presence of cystine in the urine; results from a defect in renal tubular reabsorption of amino acids, especially cystine

cytomegalovirus (CMV)—a herpetovirus that causes an enlargement of the cells of various organs and the development of characteristic intranuclear inclusion bodies

cytosol—cytoplasm, with the exception of the mitochondria and endoplasmic reticular components

cytosolic—pertaining to cytosol

cytotoxic—destructive to cells

decongestant—an agent that possesses the property of reducing congestion

decreased breath sounds—difficult to hear; caused by reduced inspiration or hyperinflation

decubitus views—refers to radiographic images obtained while the patient is lying down

deep (distal) bronchial veins—an intrapulmonary bronchiolar plexus of veins that communicates freely with the pulmonary veins and eventually coalesces into a single trunk that ends in a main pulmonary vein or in the left atrium

deep cardiac plexus—the dorsal part of the network of nerves that constitutes the cardiac plexus; formed by branches from the cervical and upper thoracic sympathetic ganglia and from the vagus and recurrent laryngeal nerves; located anterior to the tracheal bifurcation, superior to the division of the pulmonary trunk, and posterior to the arch of the aorta

deep chordae—chordae tendineae that attach to the more peripheral aspects of the rough region of a valve leaflet

defibrillate—the act of stopping fibrillation of either atrial or ventricular muscle

defibrillation—cessation of fibrillation of either atrial or ventricular muscle, with restoration of a normal rhythm

defibrillator—anything that stops fibrillation of either atrial or ventricular muscle and restores a normal rhythm

demographic data—descriptive characteristics and traits of populations, such as age, gender, race

demyelinating—refers to the destruction or loss of myelin

depolarization—the loss of a negative charge in the myocardial cells

depressor muscle of the septum of the nose—muscle running from the maxilla above the central incisor tooth to the nasal septum (flares the nostrils)

desaturate—the act of desaturating; an increase in the percentage of total oxygen-binding sites on the hemoglobin molecule that is unfilled

descending aorta—the part of the aorta between the arch and the bifurcation into the iliac arteries; it includes the thoracic and abdominal aortae

diabetes mellitus (DM)—a disease in which carbohydrate utilization is reduced while lipid and protein utilization is enhanced as the result of a relative deficiency in the amount of insulin

diabetic cardiomyopathy—myocardial dysfunction attributable to the effects of diabetes

diagonal artery—the first, and generally largest, of the left anterior ventricular branches of the anterior interventricular (left anterior descending) coronary artery; it sometimes arises directly from the trunk of the left coronary artery

dialysate—the portion of a solution that can pass through a dialyzing membrane; diffusate

dialysis—a form of filtration that separates smaller molecules from larger ones in a solution by placing a semipermeable membrane between the solution and water

diaphoresis—perspiration, often profuse

diaphragm—the musculotendinous dome that forms the floor of the thorax

diaphragmatic paralysis—loss of function of the diaphragm or hemidiaphragm as the result of a disease or injury to the nerve supply

diaphragmatic pleura—the serous membrane lining the diaphragm

diastasis—the late portion of diastole when blood is entering the ventricles slowly and the venous pressure tends to rise

diastole—the period of ventricular relaxation

diastolic blood pressure (DBP)—the lowest arterial blood pressure reached during a given ventricular cycle

diastolic dysfunction or diastolic heart failure—an inability of the ventricles to accept the blood ejected from the atria

diffusing capacity (DL_{CO})—the amount of gas (typically carbon monoxide or oxygen) taken up by the pulmonary capillary blood per unit of time per unit of average pressure gradient between the alveolar gas and the pulmonary capillary blood; expressed in terms of mL/minute/mm Hg

diffusion—the passive tendency of molecules to move from an area of high concentration to an area of lower concentration

digital clubbing—a proliferative change in the soft tissues of the distal fingers and toes (especially the nail beds), resulting in a broadening of their ends; the nails are abnormally curved

digital subtraction angiography—technique to produce an angiogram without directly injecting contrast material into either an artery or heart chamber

digitalis—the dried leaf of *Digitalis purpurea,* a genus of perennial flowering plants that are the main source of cardioactive steroid glycosides used in the treatment of certain heart diseases, especially heart failure

digitoxin (Crystodigin)—one of the primary digitalis-like drugs used in the treatment of congestive heart failure; a secondary derivative of the leaves of *Digitalis purpurea;* it is better absorbed from the gastrointestinal tract than digitalis

digoxin (Lanoxin, Lanoxicaps)—one of the primary digitalis-like drugs used in the treatment of congestive heart failure; a derivative of *Digitalis lanata*

1,25-dihydroxycholecalciferol—the most active known derivative of vitamin D

dilated cardiomyopathy—a disease of the myocardium characterized by ventricular dilatation and cardiac muscle contractile dysfunction

diplopia—double vision; the perception of one object as two objects

dipyridamole (Persantine)—an agent that reduces platelet aggregation and causes coronary vasodilation

directional coronary atherectomy (DCA)—a procedure in which atherosclerotic plaque is removed from the lumen of a coronary artery

dissecting aneurysm—the splitting of an arterial wall by interstitial hemorrhage or by blood that enters from an intimal tear

distributing vessels—the elastic and muscular arteries

distribution—in relation to medication: depends on the circulatory system, the ability of the medication to pass through particular cell membranes, and the permeability of the capillaries; drug binding also a factor

diuresis—the excretion of urine; commonly denotes production of unusually large volumes of urine

dobutamine (Dobutrex)—a synthetic derivative of dopamine; possesses strong inotropic but weak chronotropic properties

dopamine (Intropin)—a neural transmitter substance and an intermediate in the biosynthesis of norepinephrine and epinephrine; used at low dosages to enhance renal perfusion and at high dosages as a vasopressor agent

dopaminergic—relating to those nerves or receptor sites that employ dopamine as their neurotransmitter

Doppler velocimetry—the use of Doppler ultrasonography techniques to determine both direction and velocity of blood flow

double lung transplantation—early technique for lung transplantation using a tracheal anastomosis and a double lung en bloc

doxapram—an analeptic that stimulates respiration more than it activates the cortical or spinal neurons

dromotropic—possessing the ability to influence the conduction velocity of a nerve or muscle fiber

Duchenne muscular dystrophy—a lethal, X-linked recessive disorder of childhood characterized by early onset of progressive, generalized muscle weakness and pseudohypertrophy of certain muscle groups

ductus venosus—the continuation of the umbilical vein through the liver to the inferior vena cava in the fetus

dysarthria—a disturbance of articulation

dysphagia—difficulty in swallowing; aphagia

dyspnea—a subjective difficulty or distress in breathing

dyspnea index (DI)—measurement of the number of breaths the patient requires to count to 15

dyspneic—relating to or suffering from dyspnea

echocardiography—the use of ultrasound in the assessment of the heart and great vessels

ectopic foci—multiple aberrant points of origin; the locations from which abnormal myocardial depolarizations originate

ectopic pacemakers—any center of rhythmic depolarization other than the sinus node

effective cough—four-stage cough consisting of a deep inspiration, glottis closure, abdominal muscle contraction, and forceful exhalation

egophony—an auscultatory finding denoting an increased density of the underlying lung tissue; demonstrated when the vowel sound "e" is spoken but is heard through the stethoscope as "a"

Ehlers-Danlos syndrome—a generalized connective tissue disorder that results from a deficient quality or quantity of collagen; characterized by overelasticity and friability of the skin, hypermobility of the joints, and fragility of the superficial vasculature

ejection fraction (EF)—the portion of the stroke volume pumped from the left ventricle

elastance—a measure of an object's tendency to return to its normal shape after removal of the force that distorted it

elastase—a serum proteinase that hydrolyzes elastin

elastin—a fibrous mucoprotein that constitutes the primary connective tissue protein of elastic structures

electrocardiogram (ECG)—a graphic record of the electrical activity of the heart

electroencephalograph (EEG)—a graphic record of the electrical activity of the brain or the apparatus used to obtain it

electrolyte—any substance that, when placed in solution, conducts and is decomposed by electricity

electromyographic—pertaining to the graphic record of the electrical activity of active muscle or the apparatus used to obtain it

electron beam computed tomography (EBCT)—a noninvasive method to detect and quantify coronary atherosclerosis by detecting coronary calcifications

electron transport chain—the series of oxidation-reduction reactions through which electrons are accepted from reduced compounds and eventually transferred to oxygen, liberating energy and forming water; respiratory chain

electrophysiologic mapping studies (EPS)—diagnostic test to identify the specific area that may be initiating an arrhythmia; arrhythmia is induced and specific medication is then given to attempt to restore normal rhythm

embolectomy—the removal of an embolus

emboli—the plural of embolus; multiple plugs that occlude a vessel; composed of detached thrombus, bacterial mass, vegetation, or other foreign bodies

emphysematous changes—relating to the pathologic alterations arising from emphysema; characterized by undue breathlessness with exertion, abnormal enlargement of the airways distal to the terminal bronchioles, destruction of the walls of the alveoli, and reduction in the number of alveoli

enalapril (Vasotec)—an antihypertensive agent; an angiotensin-converting enzyme inhibitor

encephalopathy—any disease of the brain

end-stage renal disease (ESRD)—any condition that impairs the function of the kidneys to such an extent that the patient exhibits kidney failure, hypertension, excessive glomerular permeability to proteins, and other specific tubular abnormalities

endocardial biopsy—a sample of the endomyocardium taken to determine myocardial rejection in cardiac transplant patients

endocardial cushions—the epithelial outgrowths of the dorsal and ventral walls of the atrioventricular divisions of the heart tube

endocardial fibroelastosis—a congenital disorder characterized by thickening of the endothelium and subendothelial layer of connective tissue of the left ventricle, thickening and malformation of the cardiac valves, and hypertrophy of the heart; endocardial sclerosis

endocardial heart tubes—canalized extensions of the cardiogenic cords that form the primitive lateral hearts where the first contractions occur

endocardial leads—electrical connection, usually of a pacemaker, attached to the innermost epithelial lining of the heart

endocarditis—inflammation of the innermost epithelial lining of the heart

endocardium—the innermost epithelial lining of the heart; formed from the inner endocardial tube

endogenous—a substance produced in the body

endoluminal stent—a thin coil, wire, or thread placed within the lumen of a blood vessel or other tubular structure; used to maintain the patency of an intact but constricted lumen

endothelial-derived contracting factor (EDCF)—a substance released from the endothelial cells of the arterioles; postulated to release calcium ions causing muscle contraction

endothelial-derived relaxation factor (EDRF)—a substance released from the endothelial cells of the arterioles in response to histamine; postulated to remove calcium ions from myosin-ATPase sites, thus returning muscle fibrils to the resting state

endotracheal tube—a flexible, hollow cyclinder inserted nasally or orally into the trachea to provide an airway

enteral—via an intestinal route, referring to one of the routes by which a medication is administered

epicardial lead—electrical connection, usually of a pacemaker, attached to the innermost epithelial lining of the heart

epicardium—the outermost layer of the heart; the visceral layer of the pericardium; formed from the outer layer of the myoepicardial mantle

epinephrine (Adrenalin Chloride)—a sympathomimetic agent; the most potent stimulant of alpha- and beta-adrenergic receptors

ergonovine stimulation—a test of cardiac performance in which a pharmacologic stimulant (ergonovine) is administered to the patient; ergonovine is an alkaloid of ergot used as a stimulant of smooth muscle

erythrocyte sedimentation rate (ESR)—the rate of sedimentation of red blood cells in anticoagulated blood; measured by mixing venous blood with a solution of sodium citrate and allowing it to stand for an hour in a calibrated pipet; an above normal rate (>15 mm for men; >20 mm for women) is associated with anemia or inflammation

erythropoietin—a protein secreted by the kidney that stimulates the formation of red blood cells from bone marrow

eschar—the thick, coagulated crust that forms after a chemical or thermal burn

Escherichia coli—a species of aerobic, facultatively anaerobic bacteria that contains gram-negative rods; occurs normally in the intestines

esophagus—the portion of the foregut that connects the pharynx and the stomach

essential (primary) hypertension—abnormally high blood pressure that has no discernible cause; accounts for approximately 90% of cases of hypertension

eukaryote—a cell containing a membrane-bound nucleus with DNA and RNA chromosomes

Ewing's sarcoma—a malignant neoplasm of the bones of the extremities; endothelial myeloma

exacerbation—an increase in severity of the signs and symptoms of a disease

exchange vessels—the capillaries, sinusoids, and postcapillary venules where the exchange of gases, nutrients, and metabolic products occurs

excitation-contraction coupling—the mechanism by which the action potential causes myofibrillar contraction

exercise prescription—the instruction given to a patient or client regarding the mode, intensity, duration, and frequency of exercise to be performed

exercise testing—monitored, multilevel cardiovascular or pulmonary (or both) evaluation of a patient's responses to controlled stress (exercise)

exercise tolerance—the capacity of the energy systems (both aerobic and anaerobic) combined to perform exercise; also, the components of the oxygen transport system and their capacity to provide oxygen

exocrine glands—the secretory or excretory organs from which the secretions reach a free surface of the body by way of ducts

exogenous—substance produced outside the body

expectorant—anything that promotes bronchial secretion and facilitates its expulsion

expiratory reserve volume (ERV)—the additional volume of air that can be let out beyond the normal tidal exhalation

expiratory retard—an orificial resistance applied during exhalation that permits the ventilatory circuit pressure to drop slowly to atmospheric pressure as the flow of expiratory gas ceases

external elastic lamina—a fenestrated layer of elastic connective tissue that covers the tunica media

external intercostal muscles—11 pair of muscles; each attaching from the inferior border of a rib to the superior border of the rib below; acts to pull the ribs together

extracellular parasite—an organism that lives in and derives nourishment from another organism without invading the host's cells

extracorporeal ultrafiltration—a process by which large molecules are separated from small molecules in a solution outside the body

extrapyramidal—outside or other than the pyramidal (corticospinal) tract

extrinsic asthma—a narrowing of the bronchial airways as the result of an allergic reaction to foreign substances

exudate—any fluid that gradually passes (oozes) out of a body tissue, usually as the result of inflammation

exudative infiltrate—fluid that has permeated or penetrated into the tissues

facioscapulohumeral muscular dystrophy—a genetically transmitted (autosomal dominant inheritance) abnormality of the muscle characterized by wasting of the muscles of the face, shoulder girdle, and arms

facultative parasite—an organism that lives in and derives nourishment from another organism under more than one specific set of environmental factors

false chordae—a fibrous collagenous cord passing from the papillary muscles to one another or to the ventricular walls

false negative result—a test result that erroneously excludes an individual from a particular reference group because of insufficiently stringent testing criteria

false ribs—the five lower ribs on either side of the thorax that do not articulate directly with the sternum

fan-shaped chordae—chordae with radiating branches projecting outward from a single stem to attach to the margins of the interleaflet commissures

fasciculations—involuntary contractions of groups of muscle fibers; a coarser type of muscular contraction than fibrillation

fast-twitch glycolytic (FG) fibers—muscle fibers that have a high capability for electrochemical transmission of action potentials, high activity level of myosin ATPase, and the ability to generate energy rapidly for quick, powerful actions

fast-twitch oxidative glycolytic (FOG) fibers—muscle fibers that have fast shortening speed combined with moderately well-developed capacity for both aerobic and anaerobic energy transfer

fecal impaction—a collection of compressed or hardened feces in the colon or rectum that cannot be moved voluntarily

femoral-popliteal bypass—a surgical procedure in which a vascular prosthesis is placed to bypass an occlusion of the distal femoral artery or proximal popliteal artery, or both

fetid breath—foul-smelling breath

fibrin—a filamentous elastic protein derived from fibrinogen in the presence of thrombin

fibroplastic—producing fibrous tissue

fibrosis—the reactive or preparative process in which fibrous tissue is formed

fibroskeleton of the heart—an intricate, malleable, three-dimensional continuum of dense and membraneous collagen forming the annuli of the principal valvular orifices

fibrous pericardium—outer sac of the pericardial sac consisting of collagenous fibrous tissue

filum coronarium—the anterolateral arm of the mitral annulus

FI_{O_2}—the fraction of inspired oxygen; the portion of an inhaled mixture of gases that is oxygen

first-degree atrioventricular block—an impairment of the normal conduction between the atria and the ventricles; characterized by a prolongation of the P-R interval (atrioventricular conduction time)

first heart sound (S_1)—a sound heard during auscultation of the heart; occurs at the onset of ventricular systole (just preceding the normally palpable pulse in a peripheral artery); produced primarily by closure of the atrioventricular valves

first pass effect—the partial inactivation of a drug as the result of metabolic processes

flux—the number of moles of a substance crossing through a unit area of a membrane per unit time

foam cells—cells that have accumulated or ingested material that dissolves during the tissue preparation, usually lipids; lipophage

focal biliary cirrhosis—damage to hepatic parenchymal cells as the result of bile duct obstruction

foramen ovale—an oval opening in the dorsal part of the septum secundum

foramen secundum—an opening in the dorsal part of the septum primum that forms before the septum fuses with the endocardial cushions

forced expiratory flow, 200–1200 ($FEF_{200-1200}$)—the mean flow rate of gas measured between two expired volumes (200 mL and 1200 mL) during a forced vital capacity maneuver

forced expiratory technique—forceful exhalation techniques such as cough, huff, and active cycle breathing to clear the airways

forced expiratory volume in 1 second (FEV_1)—the maximal volume that can be expired in 1 second, starting from a maximal inspiratory effort

forced midexpiratory flow (FEF_{25-75})—the mean flow rate of gas measured between two expired volumes (25% of FVC and 75% of FVC) during a forced vital capacity maneuver

forced vital capacity (FVC)—the largest volume of gas that can be forcefully exhaled from the lungs after a maximal inspiratory effort

fossa ovalis—an ovoid depression above and to the left of the inferior vena cava orifice on the lower central portion of the septal wall of the right atrium

fourth heart sound (S_4)—a sound heard in late diastole on auscultation over the heart; corresponds with atrial contraction; is rarely heard in normal hearts

Fowler's position—a supine-lying position in which the head of the bed is elevated approximately 2 feet

fractionation—separation of the components of a mixture

Frank-Starling mechanism—the response to increased diastolic volume, in which the ventricular muscle fibers are on a greater stretch and therefore contract more forcefully

free-edge chordae—single strands arising from the papillary muscle and attaching near the middle of the free margin of a valve leaflet

free fatty acids (FFAs)—the product obtained when fatty acids (from the hydrolysis of triglycerides) are bound to proteins in the plasma

fremitus—a vibration imparted to the hand resting on the chest or other part of the body

Friedreich's ataxia—uncoordinated voluntary movement of the extremities, with eventual paralysis, as the result of sclerosis of the lateral and posterior columns of the spinal cord; an autosomal recessive trait; hereditary spinal ataxia

fulminant—suddenly occurring

functional capacity—ability or power to perform necessary activities

functional residual capacity (FRC)—the sum of the expiratory reserve and residual volumes; it is the amount of air remaining in the lungs at the end of a normal tidal exhalation

furosemide (Lasix)—a diuretic agent

ganglioside—a glycosphingolipid (fatty acid derivative) that contains one or more sialic acid residues; found primarily in nerve tissue and in the spleen

gas transport system—the combination of musculoskeletal, cardiovascular, and respiratory systems, which together function to deliver and eliminate gases

globin—the protein molecule of hemoglobin

globular leukocytes—migratory cells of the tracheobronchial epithelia, possibly derived from mast cells; postulated to play a role in the immunologic process

glomerular filtration rate (GFR)—the volume of water filtered out of the plasma through the glomerular capillaries into Bowman's capsule per unit time

glottis—the fissure between the vocal folds; also called the rima glottidis

glucagon—a pancreatic hormone that initiates the release of glycogen from the liver

gluconeogenesis—the formation of glycogen from noncarbohydrates

glucose tolerance test—a test of the liver's ability to absorb and store excess amounts of glucose; normally, after ingestion of 100 g of glucose, the blood sugar level rises and returns to normal within 2 hours; in diabetic patients, the rise is greater and the return to normal is prolonged or absent

glycogenolysis—the hydrolysis of glycogen to glucose

glycosylated hemoglobin (Hb A$_{1c}$)—hemoglobin to which glucose and related monosaccharides bind

GPIIa/IIb glycoprotein inhibitors—antiplatelet agents

graft failure—failure of transplanted tissue to function in the recipient

graft surveillance—a procedure to measure flow through a surgically repaired bypass graft to assess for restenosis

granulation—the formation of very small, rounded connective tissue projections that form on healing surfaces

granulomatosis—any condition characterized by the formation of nodular inflammatory lesions

granulomatous uveitis—an inflammation of the vascular (middle) coat of the eye

Graves' disease—diffuse hyperplasia of the thyroid gland, a form of hyperthyroidism

great cardiac vein—vein that runs from the apex of the heart to the base of the ventricles in the anterior interventricular sulcus, before turning to the left in the coronary sulcus to reach the back of the heart

growth hormone—a protein hormone from the anterior lobe of the pituitary that promotes bodily growth, fat mobilization, and inhibition of glucose utilization; somatotropin

Guillain-Barré syndrome—a neuromuscular disorder characterized by paresthesia of the limbs, muscular weakness or flaccid paralysis; acute idiopathic polyneuritis; etiology is probably immune mediated

H$_1$ receptors—located in vascular, respiratory and gastrointestinal smooth muscle; targeted for blockade by antihistamines

half-life—the time it takes for the plasma concentration of a drug to be reduced to 50% of its peak value

Hamman-Rich syndrome—interstitial fibrosis of the lung, leading to severe right ventricular failure and cor pulmonale

head of the rib—the end of the rib that articulates with the vertebrae

heart-lung transplantation—removal of a patient's heart and two lungs, which are then replaced with donor heart and lungs

heart rate variability—assessment of fluctuations in the heart rate over periods ranging from 2 to 15 minutes with deep breathing exercises; minimal variability with this activity may indicate increased risk of death for patients following myocardial infarction and risk of myocardial infarction

helium dilution method—one of the most commonly used methods for the measurement of static lung volumes

hematocrit—the percentage of the volume of a sample of blood occupied by cells

heme—a ferrous ion covalently bound to four nitrogens on the pyrole groups of a porphyrin ring

hemidiaphragm—one of the two domes of the diaphragm

hemiplegia—paralysis of one side of the body

hemochromatosis—a disorder of iron metabolism

hemodynamic stability—stable heart rate and blood pressure

hemolytic—destructive to blood cells

hemoptysis—expectoration of blood derived from the lungs as a result of pulmonary or bronchial hemorrhage

hemostasis—stagnation of blood; stoppage of bleeding

hemothorax—the presence of blood in the pleural cavity

heparin—an anticoagulant; prevents platelet agglutination and subsequent thrombus formation

hepatic encephalopathy—a complex neuropsychiatric syndrome that complicates advanced liver disease; may manifest as cerebral edema and coma in the acute situation or subtle neurologic dysfunction in the chronic situation

hepatitis—inflammation of the liver; usually in response to a viral infection but may also be from toxic agents

hepatomegaly—abnormally enlarged liver

herpes simplex—a group of infections caused by one of the two types of herpes simplex virus; type 1, the pathogen of herpes simplex in humans; type 2, the cause of genital herpes

heterologous—pertains to a substance derived from an animal of a different species

heterotopic transplantation—the donor heart is anastomosed to the native heart without removal of the native heart

high-density lipoprotein (HDL)—one of the major classes of lipoproteins, containing about 50% protein and much smaller concentrations of phospholipids than either VLDL or LDL; has a flotation fraction (density) between 1.063 and 1.21

high-output congestive heart failure—heart failure resulting from a volume overload

high-risk patient—patients, who by nature of their cardiovascular or pulmonary disease, demonstrate markedly abnormal signs and symptoms during activity

hilus—the point at which the nerves, vessels, and primary bronchi penetrate the parenchyma of each lung

histochemistry—pertaining to the composition of the tissues

histocompatibility complex—the quality of cellular or tissue graft enabling it to be accepted and functional when transplanted to another organism

Hodgkin's disease—a malignant neoplasm of lymphoid cells of uncertain origin; associated with inflammatory infiltration of lymphocytes and eosinophilic leukocytes and fibrosis

Holter monitoring—a technique of long-term recording of ECG activity to screen for arrhythmias or ischemia

Homans' sign—the gastrocnemius muscle is squeezed while the foot is dorsiflexed with force to assess for deep-vein thrombosis

homocysteine—elevated levels of this vitamin/hormone compound increase the risk for coronary artery disease; low levels of folate and vitamin B_6 are related to increased circulating homocysteine

homocystinuria—an autosomal recessive trait resulting in a defect in the enzyme cystathionine synthetase, that when exhibited is characterized by excessive excretion of homocysteine in the urine

homologous—alike in specific ways

horizontal fissure—the secondary groove that separates the middle from the upper lobe of the right lung

huffing—a technique to assist in the expectoration of secretions; a cough assistance technique

humoral—pertaining to any clear fluid or semifluid hyaline anatomic substance

hyaline membrane disease—a disease of the neonate associated with decreased amounts of surfactant characterized by atelectasis and alveolar ducts lined by an eosinophilic membrane

hyaline membrane—an eosinophilic membrane lining the alveolar ducts of infants suffering from respiratory distress syndrome

hydralazine (Apresoline)—a vasodilating antihypertensive agent

hyperactive airways—excessive activity of the bronchioles; increased bronchoconstriction

hyperalimentation—the administration of nutrients beyond the normal minimum requirement

hyperbilirubinemia—an abnormally high amount of bilirubin in the circulating blood, resulting in clinically apparent icterus or jaundice when the concentration is sufficient

hypercapnia—hypercarbia; the presence of an abnormally large amount of carbon dioxide in the circulating blood

hypercholesterolemia—the presence of abnormally large amounts of cholesterol in the circulating blood

hyperglycemia—the presence of abnormally high concentrations of glucose in the circulating blood

hyperinflated—distended beyond the normal extent

hyperkalemia—a greater than normal concentration of potassium ions in the circulating blood that may be due to tissue destruction, renal failure, and Addison's disease; may cause bradycardia with hypotension and changes in the electrocardiogram, including elevating the T wave, and muscle weakness

hyperlipidemia—the presence of an abnormally high level of lipids in the circulating blood; lipemia

hyperlucent lung syndrome—a variant of panacinar (panlobular) emphysema

hypernatremia—an abnormally high concentration of sodium ions in the plasma

hyperosmolality—an increase in the osmotic concentration of a solution

hyperparathyroidism—a condition due to an increase in the secretion of the parathyroid glands; characterized by elevated serum calcium levels and decreased serum phosphorus

hyperplasia—an increase in the number of cells in an organ or tissue; hypertrophy

hyperplastic—pertaining to hyperplasia

hyperreflexia—exaggeration of reflexes

hypersomnolence—a condition of drowsiness approaching coma

hypertension (HTN)—an arterial blood pressure in excess of 140/90 mm Hg (American Heart Association) or 160/95 mm Hg (World Health Organization)

hypertensive heart disease—myocardial dysfunction as a result of abnormally high blood pressure

hyperthyroidism—an abnormality of the thyroid gland in which thyroid hormone secretion is increased

hypertriglyceridemia—a condition in which the triglyceride concentration in the blood is greater than normal

hypertrophic cardiomyopathy—a disease of the myocardium characterized by inappropriate and excessive left ventricular hypertrophy and normal or even enhanced cardiac muscle contractile function

hypertrophy—a general increase in the size or bulk of an organ or tissue, unrelated to tumor formation

hyperuricemia—a greater than normal concentration of uric acid in the blood

hyperventilation—an arterial carbon dioxide level that is below normal as a result of increased alveolar ventilation relative to metabolic carbon dioxide production

hypoadaptive—a failure in the occurrence of expected or anticipated results

hypogammaglobulinemia—a less than normal amount of the gamma fraction of serum globulin

hypokalemia—an abnormally low concentration of potassium ions in the circulating blood

hyponatremia—an abnormally low concentration of sodium ions in the circulating blood

hypophosphatemia—a less than normal concentration of alkaline phosphatase in the blood; hypophosphatasia

hypoplasia—the underdevelopment of an organ or tissue

hyposthenia—weakness

hypothalamic—pertaining to the hypothalamus (the ventromedial region of the diencephalon forming the walls of the ventral portion of the third ventricle); the hypothalamus is intimately involved in autonomic nervous system and endocrine functioning

hypothalamic dysfunction—an abnormal function of the hypothalamus

hypothyroidism—a condition in which the production of thyroid hormone is below normal; characterized by low metabolic rate, tendency for weight gain, somnolence

hypovolemic—pertaining to hypovolemia (decreased amount of blood in the body)

hypoxemia—a condition in which arterial oxygenation is below normal

hypoxia—a condition in which the level of oxygen in the arterial blood or tissue is below normal

idiopathic—of unknown origin

idiopathic congestive cardiomyopathy—a myocardial dysfunction that has no discernible cause

idiopathic hypertrophic subaortic stenosis (IHSS)—an obstruction of the left ventricular outflow tract due to hypertrophy of the left ventricular septum; of unknown origin

idiopathic pulmonary fibrosis—the formation of tissue containing fibroblasts, and the fibers and fibrils they form, in the lungs for no known reason

ileus—obstruction of the intestines, lack of intestinal movement

iliocostalis cervicis muscle—an accessory inspiratory muscle arising from the angles of the upper six ribs, medial to the iliocostalis thoracis, and

inserting into the transverse processes of the fourth, fifth, and sixth cervical vertebrae

iliocostalis lumborum muscle—an accessory inspiratory muscle arising from the sacrum, the iliac crest, and the spinous processes of most of the lumbar and the lower two thoracic vertebrae upward to the lower borders of the last six or seven ribs as far laterally as their angles

iliocostalis muscles—accessory inspiratory muscles that are the most lateral division of the erector spinae group

iliocostalis thoracis muscle—an accessory inspiratory muscle arising from the upper borders of the lower six ribs medial to the insertion of the iliocostalis lumborum up to the upper six ribs

immune system—a complex of interrelated cellular, molecular, and genetic components that provide a defense against foreign organisms or substances and abnormal native cells

immunodeficiency—a condition in which some component of the immune system is lacking

immunoglobulin (Ig)—a protein consisting of two pairs of polypeptide chains, one pair of low molecular weight chains, and one pair of high (relatively) molecular weight chains linked together by disulfide bonds

immunosuppression—the prevention or interference with the development of an immunologic response; use of medications to suppress the immune system of the individual receiving a donated organ to prevent rejection

immunosuppressive—any agent that prevents or interferes with the development of an immunologic response

implantable cardiac defibrillator (ICD)—see AICD

inactivation gate—the chemical (e.g., neurotransmitter) or electrical (e.g., membrane potential) action that closes an ion channel after it has been opened

incentive—a reward attached to a desired goal; used in rehabilitation and department management

incentive spirometer—a flow- or volume-dependent device that is used to facilitate slow, deep, sustained inspiratory efforts in patients who might otherwise be disposed to breathe shallowly

incubator—a container in which controlled environmental conditions (e.g., temperature, pressure, gas composition) may be maintained

infarction—the sudden venous or arterial insufficiency that produces an area of macroscopic necrosis

inferior pulmonary vein—the vein returning blood from right or left lower lobes of the lungs to the left atrium

inferior vena cava—the blood vessel that receives blood from the lower limbs and the greater part of the pelvic and abdominal organs; it begins at the level of the fifth lumbar vertebra on the right side, pierces the diaphragm at the level of the eighth thoracic vertebra, and empties into the back part of the right atrium of the heart

inflammation—a complex of histologic and cytologic reactions that occur in response to an injury or abnormal stimulus caused by a biologic, chemical, or physical agent

infundibulum—the outflow tract of the right ventricle, conus arteriosus

innermost intercostal muscles—11 pairs of muscles, each attaching from the superior border of a rib to the inferior border of the rib above; acts to pull the ribs together

inoculum—the causative agent (microorganism or other material) that is introduced into the body

inotrope—an agent that influences the contractility of muscular tissue

inotropic—influencing the contractility of muscular tissue

inotropy—the characteristic contractile state of muscular tissue

inspiratory capacity (IC)—the sum of the tidal and inspiratory reserve volumes; the maximum amount of air that can be inhaled after a normal tidal exhalation

inspiratory hold—a mechanical ventilatory maneuver in which either the preset pressure or predetermined volume is reached and held for some period of time before exhalation is initiated

inspiratory muscle training (IMT)(also inspiratory resistance training)—training in order to increase ventilatory capacity and reduce dyspnea; the program has two parts—strengthening and endurance training

inspiratory reserve volume (IRV)—the additional volume of air that can be taken into the lungs beyond the normal tidal inhalation

insulin-dependent diabetes mellitus (IDDM)—a metabolic disease that requires insulin therapy in which lipid and protein utilization are increased and carbohydrate utilization is decreased as the result of a relative or absolute insulin deficiency; juvenile diabetes; type I diabetes

integumentary—relating to the covering of a body or body part

interalveolar septum—the tissue between two adjacent alveoli; comprises the alveolar epithelium, the capillary epithelium, and the interstitial space

interatrial atrioventricular tracts or bundles—specialized paths for interatrial conduction of the depolarization wave

interatrial septum—the wall separating the right and left atria

intercostal muscles—the three sets of 11 pairs of muscles occupying the intercostal spaces and connecting the adjoining ribs; external, internal, and innermost intercostal muscles

intercurrent—occurring during the course of an existing process

intermediate cells—may be undifferentiated forms of ciliated or secretory cells in the tracheal epithelium

intermittent claudication—an attack of lamenesis and pain caused by ischemia, chiefly of the calf muscles, that is brought on by walking and is due to atherosclerotic lesions in peripheral arteries

intermittent mandatory ventilation (IMV)—a mode of mechanical ventilatory assistance; the mandatory (preset) ventilator breath is delivered at a preset interval regardless of the phase of the patient's breathing efforts

internal elastic lamina—a fenestrated layer of elastic connective tissue that covers the tunica intima

internal intercostal muscles—11 pairs of muscles, each attaching from the superior border of a rib to the inferior border of the rib above; acts to pull the ribs together

internodal atrioventricular tracts or bundles— specialized conduction pathways between the sinoatrial and atrioventricular nodes

interpolated—to occur, or be inserted, between other things

interstitial pattern—one of two main roentgenographic patterns characterized by interstitial thickening and the formation of thin-walled cystic spaces less than 10 mm in diameter, generally divided into three subcategories (fine, medium, coarse) based on the degree of interstitial thickening and the size of the cystic spaces; reticular pattern

interstitial pneumonitis—an inflammation involving the spaces within an organ or tissue (excluding body spaces or cavities)

interventricular foramen—the opening that separates the interventricular septum from the endocardial cushions

interventricular septum—the septum that develops from the ventricular apex, growing toward the fused dorsal and ventral endocardial cushions, and separating the ventricle into left and right halves

intima—the innermost coat of a vessel, tunica intima

intra-aortic balloon counterpulsation (IABC)—a means of assisting ventricular ejection by reducing aortic pressure just before and during ventricular systole with an intra-aortic balloon pump activated by an automatic mechanism triggered by the ECG

intra-aortic balloon pump (IABP)—a pump connected to a balloon catheter that is inserted into the descending aorta to provide temporary cardiac assistance by means of counterpulsation

intrapleural drainage tube—a hollow cylinder inserted through the chest wall into the pleural space

intrapulmonary shunt—the passage of blood from the right side of the heart through the lungs to the left side of the heart without participation in gas exchange; perfusion in excess of ventilation

intrinsic asthma—a condition of the lungs in which there is widespread bronchial and bronchiolar constriction due to varying degrees of smooth muscle spasm, mucosal edema, and mucous plugging that has no identifiable extrinsic cause

intubated—the condition of having a hollow cylindric device inserted through the nose or mouth into the trachea

intubation—the insertion of a hollow cylindric device through the nose or mouth into the trachea

intussusception—the infolding of one segment of the intestine within another

iron lung—a large, relatively airtight chamber into which a patient is placed with head exposed for mechanical ventilation; used during polio epidemic in 1950s and rarely used today.

irregular emphysema—atypical emphysema

ischemia—a condition of having an inadequate supply of arterial blood

ischemic—relating to ischemia

islets of Langerhans—cellular masses in the interstitial tissue of the pancreas that produce insulin and glucagon

isoenzymes—enzymes that are very similar in catalytic properties but can be differentiated by variations in their physical properties

isoproterenol (Isuprel)—a sympathomimetic beta-receptor stimulant; similar to epinephrine but does not share its vasoconstricting properties

isovolumic contraction—the action of the ventricular muscle fibers in early systole, when they initially increase their tension without shortening and thus without an associated alteration of ventricular volume

isovolumic relaxation—the phase immediately

following aortic valve closure and continuing until the mitral valve opens when ventricular pressure falls below atrial pressure

isthmus—a constriction connecting two larger parts of an organ or other anatomic structure

I-type receptors—stretch receptors in the interstitium of the lung

Jackson-Pratt drain—a flexible silicon rubber suction drain with small intraluminal ridges that prevent its collapse

jaundice—icterus; a yellowish staining of the integument, sclerae, and deeper tissues and the excretions with bile pigment

Joint Commission on Accreditation of Healthcare (JCAHO)—agency that accredits hospitals

jugular venous distension (JVD)—stretching or overfilling of the jugular vein

junctional rhythm—the rhythm of the heart when the atrioventricular node initiates the depolarization wave; nodal rhythm; atrioventricular junctional rhythm

junctional tachycardia—a junctional rhythm in which the heart rate exceeds 100 beats per minute

juxtaglomerular—in close proximity to a renal glomerulus

Kaposi's sarcoma—a multiform malignant neoplasm occurring in the skin, consisting of spindle cells and irregular small vascular spaces

Kawasaki's disease—a polymorphous erythematous febrile disease of unknown origin; characterized by a desquamation of fingers and toes and a furrowing depression of the nails; mucocutaneous lymph node syndrome

Kerley B lines—fine horizontal lines a few centimeters above the costophrenic angle in chest radiographs; postulated to be caused by distention of interlobular lymphatics with edema fluid

ketoacidosis—acidosis resulting from the formation of excessive ketone bodies (a group of ketones containing acetone)

ketogenesis—the production of ketones

ketone—a substance with the carbonyl group linking two carbon atoms

ketosis—a condition (e.g., diabetes, starvation) in which the production of ketone bodies is enhanced

Kohn's pores—interalveolar foramina

Korotkoff's sounds—sounds heard over an artery when pressure over it is reduced during the determination of blood pressure by the auscultatory method

Krebs cycle—tricarboxylic acid cycle; the second stage of carbohydrate breakdown where acetyl-CoA is degraded to carbon dioxide and hydrogen within the mitochondria

Kulchitsky's cells—the rarest type of bronchial epithelial cell; Kulchitsky's cells are neurosecretory cells believed to play a role in the regulation of lobular growth

kyphoscoliosis—a deformity of the spine characterized by excessive flexion and lateral curvature

labetalol (Normodyne, Trandate)—an antihypertensive agent; an alpha- and a beta-adrenergic blocking agent

lactate—a salt or an ester of lactic acid

lactic dehydrogenase (LDH)—an enzyme (actually four) that acts in the oxidation of lactate to pyruvate; the L-isomer transfers H ions to ferricytochrome *c*, and the D-isomer carries H ions to NAD^+

Lambert's canals—collateral interalveolar ducts

Lanoxin—a trade name of digoxin preparation (see *digoxin*)

laryngopharynx—extends from the epiglottis to the inferior border of the cricoid cartilage

laryngospasm—an involuntary muscular contraction that results in closure of the glottic aperture

laryngotracheal diverticulum—the pouch that develops from the laryngotracheal groove as a precursor of the laryngotracheal tube

laryngotracheal groove—the depression in the posterior wall of the pharynx from which the lower larynx and the trachea, bronchi, and lungs eventually develop

laryngotracheal tube—the tube that develops from the laryngotracheal diverticulum as a precursor of the bronchi and lungs

larynx—the organ of voice production; formed from the proximal end of the laryngotracheal tube and the fourth and sixth pairs of branchial arches

lateral basal segmental bronchus—the portion of the tracheobroncheal tree arising from the right or left lower lobe bronchus that is distributed to the lateral basal segment

lateral segmental bronchus—the portion of the tracheobroncheal tree arising from the right middle lobe bronchus that is distributed to the lateral segment

lateral thoracotomy—a surgical incision into the lateral chest wall

latissimus dorsi muscle—an accessory inspiratory muscle arising from the spinous process of the lower six thoracic, the lumbar, and the upper sacral vertebrae; from the posterior aspect of the iliac crest; and slips from the lower three or four ribs to attach to the intertubercular groove of the humerus

leaflet chordae of the anterior leaflet of the mitral valve—specialized variants of rough zone chordae; strut chordae

left atrioventricular orifice—the opening leading from the left atrium into the left ventricle

left atrium—the chamber of the heart that receives blood from the pulmonary veins

left auricle—the small conical projection from the left atrium; remnant of the left portion of the primitive atrium

left bundle branches—the left crus of the atrioventricular (His) bundle of specialized myocytes that ramifies in the subendocardium of the left ventricle; part of the specialized conduction system of the heart

left common carotid artery—arises from the highest part of the arch of the aorta to the left of the brachiocephalic trunk

left coronary artery—originates in the left posterior aortic sinus, passing between the pulmonary trunk and the left auricle, as it proceeds to the atrioventricular sulcus, where it typically divides into two branches: the anterior interventricular (descending) ramus and the circumflex ramus; usually supplies almost all of the left ventricle and atrium and most of the interventricular septum

left coronary plexus—primarily an extension of the left half of the deep part of the cardiac plexus, although it does receive some fibers from the right half; it follows the distribution of the left coronary artery, supplying the left atrium and ventricle

left dominant coronary arterial system—the majority of the blood supply to the heart is provided via the left coronary artery; occurs in about 20% of the population

left fibrous trigone—the part of the fibroskeleton of the heart that is located between the left side of the left annulus of the mitral valve and the aortic annulus

left inferior pulmonary vein—the vein that returns blood from the lower lobe of the left lung to the left atrium

left lateral view—refers to the preferred view for a lateral radiograph of the chest; taken with the left side of the chest against the film cassette

left (obtuse) margin of the heart—the left border of the heart, descending obliquely (convex toward the left) from the left auricle to the cardiac apex; formed mainly by the left ventricle, separates the sternocostal and the left surfaces of the heart

left (pulmonary) surface of the heart—the surface of the heart, consisting almost entirely of the left ventricle, that faces upward, back, and toward the left; it is convex and widest above, narrowing toward the cardiac apex

left marginal artery—a large ventricular branch of the circumflex artery, occurring in about 90% of cases

left marginal vein—one of the larger tributaries to the great cardiac vein; delivers blood from the left ventricle

left pulmonary artery—the left branch of the pulmonary artery distributed to the left lung; runs in front of the descending aorta and the left primary bronchus to the root of the lung

left subclavian artery—the last branch from the arch of the aorta

left superior pulmonary vein—the vein that returns blood from the upper lobe of the left lung to the left atrium

left ventricle—one of the four chambers of the heart; receives arterialized blood from the left atrium, propelling it by contraction of its muscular walls into the aorta

left ventricular assist device (LVAD) or system (LVAS)—permanent support of the systemic circulation for patients who require heart transplants but unable to match with suitable donors; a bridge to transplantation when all other medical interventions are unsuccessful

left ventricular end-diastolic pressure (LVEDP)—the pressure in the left ventricle at the end of the diastolic phase of the cardiac cycle

left ventricular end-diastolic volume (LVEDV)—the volume in the left ventricle at the end of the diastolic phase of the cardiac cycle

leukocytosis—an abnormally large number (usually > 10,000/mm³) of white blood cells

leukopenia—decreased white blood cell count found in bone marrow depression, acute viral infection, alcohol ingestion, and agranulocytosis

leukotriene—a product of arachidonic acid metabolism; postulated to have a role as a mediator in inflammatory and allergic reactions

Levophed (norepinephrine)—a selective beta₁ agonist

lidocaine (Xylocaine)—a local anesthetic with significant antiarrhythmic properties

ligamentum arteriosum—the remains of the ductus arteriosus of the fetus; between the left pulmonary artery and the arch of the aorta

ligamentum teres—the remains of the umbilical vein of the fetus

ligamentum venosum—the remains of the ductus venosus of the fetus

limb-girdle muscular dystrophy—a genetically transmitted (autosomal recessive) progressive abnormality of the muscle that usually begins in the preadolescent period; characterized by enlarged, weakened, and inelastic muscles; commonly affects the pelvic girdle predominantly

limbus marginalis—the line of demarcation between the muscular septum and a thin,

rounded, collagenous area immediately below the right and posterior cusps of the aortic valve

limen nasi—the upper limit of the lower nasal cartilage

lingula—the anteroinferior area of the left upper lobe corresponding to the right middle lobe

lipolysis—the hydrolysis of fat

lipoprotein a (Lpa)—a lipid particle that is strongly associated with atherosclerosis and possibly an independent risk factor for coronary artery disease

lisinopril (Zestril)—an antihypertensive agent; an angiotensin converting enzyme inhibitor

lobar—relating to a lobe (in this case, of a lung)

lobectomy—the excision of a lobe (in this case, of a lung)

lobular bronchiole—the bronchiole that enters the secondary lobules of the lung; each lobular bronchiole gives off about six terminal bronchioles

loop diuretic—one of a group of agents that enhances the excretion of urine; acts by inhibiting sodium and chloride reabsorption not only in the proximal and distal tubules but also in Henle's loop

lordotic view—a posteroanterior or anteroposterior upright radiograph in which the roentgen-ray beam is aimed at an oblique angle

lovastatin—an antihyperlipidemic agent; reduces both normal and elevated serum cholesterol levels

low-density lipoprotein (LDL)—one of the major classes of lipoproteins, having a relatively large molecular weight and containing proportionally less protein and more cholesterol and triglycerides than HDL; has a flotation fraction (density) of between 1.019 and 1.063

low-output congestive heart failure—the description most frequently associated with heart failure; the result of a low cardiac output at rest or during exertion

lower lobe bronchus—the portion of the tracheobronchial tree that gives off the segmental and subsegmental bronchi of the lower lobe of the lung

lung abscess—a circumscribed collection of pus, associated with tissue destruction, within the lung

lung bud—the endodermal origin of the bronchi and lungs in the fetus

lung volume reduction surgery (LVRS)—a surgical procedure aimed at reducing the size of the lungs in patients with emphysema

lunulae—the thin lamina fibrosa on either side of Arantius's nodules of the semilunar cusps of the aortic valve

lymphadenopathy—any disease process that affects the lymph nodes

lymphatic space—a tissue or vessel filled with lymph

lymphocyte—a white blood cell formed in lymphoid tissue throughout the body; a non-native cell found in the mucosa of the tracheobronchial tree

lymphokines—soluble substances that stimulate the activity of monocytes and macrophages; released by sensitized lymphocytes on contact with specific antigens as part of the cellular immune response

lymphoma—a general term for malignant neoplasms of the lymphoid tissues

macrocytic anemia—larger than normal red blood cell volume; found in pernicious anemia, folic acid deficiency, hypothyroidism, and hepatocellular disease

macular—pertaining to a small, discolored patch or spot on the skin that is neither elevated above nor depressed below the surface

magnetic resonance imaging (MRI)—an imaging modality in which the patient's body is placed in a magnetic field and its hydrogen nuclei are excited by radiofrequency pulses at varying angles to the field's axis; nuclear magnetic resonance (NMR)

malaise—a general feeling of discomfort or uneasiness

manual hyperinflation—a greater than normal inflation induced with a manual resuscitator bag

manual resuscitator bag—a self-inflating bag that forces oxygen into the patient when manually compressed

manubrium—the upper segment of the sternum

Marfan's syndrome—a congenital disorder (autosomal dominant) of the mesodermal and ectodermal tissues; characterized by arachnodactyly, excessively long extremities, laxness of the joints, bilateral ectopia lentis, and vascular defects (especially aortic aneurysm)

maximal expiratory flow-volume (MEFV) curve—the expiratory portion of the flow-volume curve generated during a forced expiratory manuever

maximal oxygen consumption ($\dot{V}O_{2\ max}$)—the rate at which oxygen enters the blood from alveolar gas, equal in the steady state to the consumption of oxygen by tissue metabolism throughout the body during maximal exercise; units: milliliters of oxygen (STPD) used per minute

maximum voluntary ventilation (MVV)—the volume of air breathed when an individual breathes as fast and as deeply as possible for a given time (e.g., 12 or 15 seconds)

mean arterial pressure (MAP)—the average pressure within the cardiovascular system throughout the cardiac cycle

mean corpuscular volume (MCV)—blood test that measures red blood cells (RBCs) in terms of individual volume; used to classify anemias; defining the MCV assists in treatment of the cause of the anemia

mechanical percussor—an apparatus used to perform repeated blows or taps to the external chest wall in an effort to mobilize secretions in the underlying lungs

meconium aspiration—the act of sucking into the airways, by the fetus in utero, amniotic fluid contaminated with the first intestinal discharges

meconium ileus—an intestinal obstruction in the newborn following the thickening of meconium due to a lack of trypsin

media—middle; denoting an anatomic structure that is between two other similar structures or that is midway in position

medial basal segmental bronchus—the portion

of the tracheobronchial tree arising from the right lower lobe bronchus that is distributed to the medial basal segment

medial or septal papillary muscles—muscles that are variable in their origin from the wall of the right ventricle

medial segmental bronchus—the portion of the tracheobronchial tree arising from the right middle lobe bronchus that is distributed to the medial segment

medial umbilical ligaments—the remains of the intra-abdominal umbilical arteries of the fetus

median sternotomy—a form of thoracotomy in which the chest wall is entered via a midline incision through the sternum

mediastinal drainage tube—a hollow catheter introduced into the mediastinum to facilitate removal of fluid

mediastinal pleura—the serous membrane overlying the mediastinum

mediastinal shift—a deviation of the mediastinum as the result of an intrathoracic pathologic condition (e.g., movement toward the opposite side of the thoracic cavity due to a tension pneumothorax)

mediastinum—the median portion of the thoracic cavity; divided into superior and inferior divisions

mediastinum, anterior compartment of the inferior division—that portion of the mediastinum bounded by the sternum anteriorly, the pericardium posteriorly, the superior division cranially, and the diaphragm inferiorly; contains the ascending aorta

mediastinum, inferior division—the part of the mediastinum that extends from a line passing from the fourth thoracic vertebra to the lower border of the manubrium downward to the diaphragm; subdivided into anterior, middle, and posterior compartments

mediastinum, middle compartment of the inferior division—that portion of the mediastinum bounded by the pericardium anteriorly and posteriorly, the superior division superiorly, and the

diaphragm inferiorly; contains the heart and great vessels

mediastinum, posterior compartment of the inferior division—that portion of the mediastinum bounded by the bodies of the fifth through the twelfth thoracic vertebrae posteriorly, the pericardium anteriorly, the diaphragm inferiorly, and the superior division cranially; contains the esophagus and thoracic aorta

mediate percussion—the act of tapping on the surface of the chest to evaluate the condition of underlying structures, to identify the resting levels of the hemidiaphragms posteriorly, or to measure diaphragmatic excursion during breathing

medical information system (MIS)—a hospital-wide, automated data-gathering system

membranous septum—a thin, rounded, collagenous area immediately below the right and posterior cusps of the aortic valve in the interventricular septum just below the limbus marginalis

meningioencephalitis—an inflammation of the brain and its membranes

meningitis—an inflammation of the membranes of the brain or spinal cord

mesothelioma—a rare neoplasm derived from the cells lining the pleura and peritoneum

MET (metabolic equivalent)—the cost, in terms of oxygen consumption, of energy expenditure (e.g., 3 to 5 METs for light work; more than 9 METs for heavy work)

metabolic acidosis—decreased arterial plasma pH and bicarbonate concentration as the result of metabolic disease or disturbance

metabolic alkalosis—an increase in the concentration of arterial plasma bicarbonate as the result of metabolic disease or disturbance

metabolic equivalent—see *MET*

metastasis—the spread of a disease process from one part of the body to another

methylxanthines—a class of drugs (e.g., aminophylline) that have diuretic, vasodilator, and cardiac stimulant properties

microatelectasis—the absence of gas in a very small part of the lungs due to resorption of the gas from the alveoli

microcytic anemia—smaller than normal red blood cell size; found in iron deficiency, chronic infections, chronic renal disease, and malignancies

microgallbladder—a very small receptacle on the inferior surface of the liver for the storage of bile

middle cardiac vein—a vein that receives blood from tributaries from both ventricles; runs in the posterior interventricular sulcus

minimally invasive direct coronary artery bypass (MI DCAB)—a surgical procedure involving a small thoracotomy; does not require use of heart-lung bypass machine to perform coronary artery surgery

minoxidil (Loniten)—an antihypertensive agent

minute ventilation ($\dot{V}_E$)—the amount of air moved into or out of the lungs per unit time

mitochondrial enzyme—enzyme (e.g., pyruvate dehydrogenase, lactate dehydrogenase) involved in the exchange and transport of energy within the mitochondrion

mitral area—the region of the chest (at the cardiac apex) where the normal and pathologic sounds made by the mitral valve are traditionally said to be best appreciated

mitral valve prolapse—the excessive retrograde movement of the mitral valve into the left atrium during left ventricular systole

monoamine oxidase (MAO)—an oxidoreductase, containing flavin, that oxidizes amines to aldehydes or ketones, releasing NH_3 and H_2O_2

morphine—the major alkaloid of opium; used as an analgesic, a sedative, and an anxiolytic

mucociliary transport—the action of the cilia in mobilizing the mucus overlying the mucosa of the tracheobronchial tree

mucokinetic—an agent capable of enhancing the mobilization of mucus

mucolytic—an agent capable of dissolving, digesting, or liquefying mucus

mucopolysaccharidoses—a group of lysosomal storage diseases that are characterized by a disorder in metabolism of glycosaminoglycans (mucopolysaccharides)

mucopurulent—containing both mucus and pus

mucous cells—bronchial epithelial cells that secrete mucus; sometimes called *goblet cells*

multifocal—having more than one point of origin

multigated acquisition or angiogram (MUGA) imaging—a process by which a radioisotope is injected as a bolus and allowed to equilibrate within the vasculature, the cardiac cycle is divided into 12 to 28 frames (with the R wave as the reference point), and several hundred cardiac cycles are imaged; radionuclide angiography; gated equilibrium blood-pool imaging

multiple sclerosis—an immune demyelinating disorder of the central nervous system, characterized by remissions and exacerbations of neurologic dysfunction

muscarinic—characterizes the effects of muscarine on cholinergic receptors located at the interfaces between the postganglionic neurons and the effector cells of all parasympathetic terminal synapses and some specialized sympathetic postganglionic cholinergic branches

myalgia—muscular pain

myasthenia gravis—a chronic progressive muscular weakness unaccompanied by atrophy; usually begins in the muscles of the face and throat

Mycobacterium avium-intracellulare—an aerobic, nonmotile bacteria containing gram-positive, acid-fast, straight, or slightly curved rods

Mycobacterium tuberculosis—an aerobic, nonmotile bacteria containing gram-positive, acid-fast, straight or curved rods that cause tuberculosis; tubercle bacillus

myocardial infarction—a local arrest or sudden insufficiency of arterial blood supply that produces a macroscopic area of necrosis in the heart

myocarditis—an inflammation of the muscular walls of the heart

myocardium—the muscular middle layer of tissue

in the heart; formed from the inner layer of the myoepicardial mantle; also used in general reference to the heart as a whole

myocytes—muscle cells

myoepicardial mantle—a thickening of the splanchnic mesenchyme around the outside of the endocardial heart tube

myofibrillar—pertaining to the fine longitudinal fibrils occurring in skeletal or cardiac muscle fibers

myofilaments—the ultramicroscopic threads of filamentous proteins making up myofibrils in striated muscle; thick myofilaments contain myosin, and thin myofilaments contain actin

myogenic—beginning in or starting from muscle

myogenic rhythm—the intrinsic, spontaneous rhythm possessed by each cardiac myocyte

myoglobin—a substance present in muscle that contributes to its color and acts as a storehouse of oxygen

myopathy—any condition or disease that hinders or impairs the function of muscle cells

myotonic muscular dystrophy—a slowly progressive disease, with onset typically in the third decade, inherited by autosomal dominant transmission; characterized by muscular atrophy and generalized weakness, deterioration of vision, lenticular opacities, ptosis, and slurred speech

myxoma—a benign neoplasm derived from connective tissue

nares—nostrils

nasal cannula—a device for the delivery of low-flow supplemental oxygen; generally a tube with two prongs that fit into the nostrils

nasal cavity—the irregularly shaped space bounded by the nares anteriorly, the buccal roof inferiorly, the cranial base superiorly, and the oropharynx posteriorly; divided into three regions: vestibular, olfactory, and respiratory

nasal cavity, olfactory region—the superior nasal concha, the intervening septum and roof of the nasal cavity

nasal cavity, respiratory region—the inferoposterior portion of the nasal cavity bounded by the

olfactory region superiorly, the vestibular region anteriorly, and the posterior nasal apertures posteriorly

nasal cavity, vestibular region (vestibule)—the area extending from the nares backward and upward about two thirds of an inch to the limen nasi

nasal concha—shell-shaped structures projecting into the nasal cavity from the lateral wall toward the medial wall

nasal continuous positive airway pressure (nCPAP)—noninvasive ventilatory support; treatment of choice for sleep apnea

nasal endotracheal tube—a flexible, hollow cylinder, inserted through the nose and into the trachea to provide an airway

nasal pharyngeal airway—a short rubber tube inserted through the nares into the hypopharynx that is used to maintain airway patency

nasal septum—the medial wall that separates the nasal cavity into two chambers

nasalis muscle—the muscle arising lateral to the nasal notch of the maxilla spreading into an aponeurosis from its opposite-side counterpart over the bridge of the nose and an aponeurosis from the procerus, as well as attaching to the alar cartilages (muscle that flares the anterior nasal aperture)

nasopharynx—a continuation of the pharynx, beginning at the posterior nasal apertures, backward and downward

National Emphysema Trial (NET)—multicenter research clinical trial studying the outcomes of lung volume reduction surgery and pulmonary rehabilitation

natriuresis—the urinary excretion of sodium; commonly designates enhanced sodium excretion, which may occur in certain diseases or as a result of the administration of diuretic drugs

natriuretic—a chemical compound that may be used as a means of retarding the tubular reabsorption of sodium ions from glomerular filtrate, thereby resulting in greater amounts of that ion in the urine

Naughton exercise test protocol—a graded treadmill exercise test protocol consisting of stages of variable (tester choice) duration with incremental speed and grade change at each stage

neck of the rib—the portion of the rib that extends from the head to the body or shaft of the rib

necrosis—death of a cell as the result of disease or injury

necrotizing—any pathologic condition that causes the death of cells

nedocromil sodium (Tilade)—nonsteroidal anti-inflammatory agent to prevent immediate hypersensitivity reaction

neonate—a newborn infant; usually refers to the infant in the first 28 days of life

nephron—a portion of the kidney; consists of the renal corpuscle, the proximal convoluted tubule, both limbs of Henle's loop, the distal convoluted tubule, and the collecting tubule

nephrotoxicity—the quality of being toxic to the cells of the kidney

neuroblastoma—a malignant neoplasm that is characterized by immature, poorly differentiated nerve cells of embryonic type

neurogenic—anything that originates in, starts from, or is caused by the nervous system or nerve impulses

neurotoxin—an antibody that causes destruction of ganglion and cortical cells

neurotropic—something that has an affinity for the nervous system

neutropenia—the condition of having too few neutrophils in the circulating blood

nicotinic—characterizes the effect of nicotine on cholinergic receptors found at the junctions between the preganglionic and postganglionic neurons of both branches of the autonomic nervous system and at the neuromuscular junctions of skeletal muscle fibers

nifedipine (Procardia)—a calcium-channel blocking and vasodilating agent

nitrogen washout method—a pulmonary function test used to measure lung volumes and gas distribution within the lungs; the subject breathes 100% oxygen for 7 minutes, and then the concentration of N_2 in the alveolar gas at the end of a forced expiration is measured

nitroglycerin—a vasodilating agent

nitric oxide (NO)—widely distributed in the body; plays role in the regulation of circulation; diffuses to the vascular smooth muscle cells; increases cGMP levels and induces smooth muscle relaxation

nodal myocytes—specialized cardiac muscle cells that contain few myofibrils and an atypical sacrotubular system; primarily located in clusters in both the sinoatrial and atrioventricular nodes; have a faster myogenic rhythm than all other myocytes; have an impulse conduction rate that is slower than Purkinje's cells but faster than transitional or working myocytes

Nomina Anatomica (NA)—the system of anatomic nomenclature adopted by the International Congress of Anatomists

non–Hodgkin's lymphoma—a neoplasm of the lymphoid tissue other than Hodgkin's disease

non–insulin-dependent diabetes mellitus (NIDDM)—a metabolic disease that does not require insulin therapy in which lipid and protein utilization are increased and carbohydrate utilization is decreased as the result of a relative or absolute insulin deficiency; type II diabetes

noncaseating—a type of coagulation necrosis in which the necrotic material contains a mixture of protein and fat (resembling cheese) that is absorbed very slowly; typically occurs in tuberculosis

norepinephrine (Levophed)—a catecholamine hormone that possesses the excitatory actions of epinephrine but has minimal inhibitory effects; it has feeble effects on bronchial smooth muscle and metabolic processes and differs from epinephrine in its cardiovascular action, chiefly vasoconstriction, exerting little effect on cardiac output

normal flora—the population of microorganisms that normally inhabit the internal or external surfaces of healthy individuals

normal sinus rhythm—the cardiac rhythm of depolarization that originates in and proceeds from the sinoatrial node

normocytic (hypochromic) anemia—found in chronic infections, chronic renal disease, malignancies; found in hemorrhage, hemolytic anemia, bone marrow hypoplasia, and splenomegaly

nosocomial—pertains to or originates in the hospital; usually refers to a hospital-acquired infection

obesity—the condition of abnormal amounts of fat in the subcutaneous connective tissues

obesity hypoventilation syndrome—a condition of acidemia and hypercarbia associated with reduced alveolar ventilation secondary to obesity; the chest wall is too heavy to move in the reclined position

obligate intracellular parasite—an organism that must live within the cells of its host to survive

oblique fissure—the main or primary groove separating the upper and middle lobes from the lower lobe of the right lung and the upper and lower lobes of the left lung

oblique sinus—a cul-de-sac formed behind the left atrium by the epicardial coverings of the venae cavae and pulmonary veins

oblique view—a frontal radiograph in which the patient stands diagonally at an angle of 45 to 60 degrees to the film cassette

obliterating bronchitis—an inflammation of the mucosal lining of the bronchi in which the exudate is not expectorated but becomes organized, obliterating the affected bronchial lumen; bronchitis obliterans

obstructive jaundice—the yellowish staining of the skin and sclerae by bile pigments that results from an obstruction to the flow of bile into the duodenum

off-pump coronary artery bypass (OPCAB)—a surgical variation for coronary bypass involving a sternotomy but no cardiopulmonary bypass; surgery is performed on a beating heart

opportunistic infection—the multiplication of parasitic organisms in individuals whose immune systems have become compromised

oral endotracheal tube—a flexible, hollow cylinder that is inserted through the mouth into the trachea to provide an airway

oral pharyngeal airway—a short rubber or plastic device inserted into the mouth to maintain the patency of the airway to the hypopharynx

oropharynx—extends from the pharyngeal isthmus to the upper border of the epiglottis

orthopnea—difficulty breathing in the supine position; requires pillows under the head and shoulders or a sitting position

orthostatic hypotension—the low blood pressure that occurs with rapid changes in upright posture

orthotopic—the normal or usual position

orthotopic heart transplantation—transplantation of the heart in which the native heart is removed and the donor heart is placed in its position

osmolality—the osmotic concentration; the number of osmoles of a solute per kilogram of solvent

ossification—the formation of bone

osteodystrophy—the formation of abnormal or defective bone

osteogenesis imperfecta—a condition of abnormal fragility and plasticity of the bones

osteoporosis—a reduction in the amount of bone or the atrophy of skeletal tissue

outcomes—defined as changes, either favorable or adverse, in the actual or potential health status of persons, groups, or communities that can be attributed to prior or concurrent care

oversew—to close or join with sutures

overshoot—the momentary reversal of membrane potential of a cell during an action potential

oxidative capacity—the potential to combine elements or radicals with oxygen or to lose electrons

oxidative phosphorylation—the formation of high-energy phosphoric bonds from the energy released by the dehydrogenation of various substrates

oximeter—an instrument that determines the oxygen saturation of a blood sample photoelectrically

oxygen hood—a supplemental oxygen delivery device that covers the entire head: generally used in the neonatal setting

oxygen pulse—the volume of oxygen extracted by the peripheral tissues or the volume of oxygen added to the pulmonary blood per heart beat

oxygen saturation—refers to the percentage of hemoglobin that is bound with oxygen

oxygen tent—a supplementary oxygen delivery device that covers the upper torso

oxygen toxicity—the impairment of normal bodily functions (e.g., visual and hearing abnormalities, dyspnea, muscular twitching, anxiety, confusion, incoordination, and convulsions) as a result of breathing concentrations of oxygen that are too high

pacemaker—a device designed to stimulate, by electrical impulses, contraction of the heart muscle

palliative—mitigating; reducing the severity of; denoting a method of treatment of a disease or of its symptoms

pallor—paleness of the skin

palm cup—an adjunctive aid to the performance of chest percussion used in efforts to mobilize excessive pulmonary secretions

palpitation—a pulsation of the heart that is perceptible to the patient

panacinar emphysema—the diffuse, generalized destruction of alveolar structural components

pancarditis—an inflammation of all the structures of the heart

pancreatitis—an inflammation of the pancreas

papillary muscles—projections of cardiac muscle that terminate in the chordae tendineae

paradoxical—other than that which normally occurs

paranasal sinuses—the frontal, ethmoidal, sphenoidal, and maxillary sinuses

paraseptal emphysema—the destruction of alveolar septa and the reduction in the number of alveoli involving the periphery of the pulmonary lobules

parasympathetic nervous system—one of two parts of the autonomic nervous system; the innervation pathway is composed of two motor neurons: the preganglionic neurons compose the visceral efferent nuclei of the brain stem and the lateral columns of the second through fourth sacral segments of the spinal cord; the ganglia are either intramural ganglia within the organ to be innervated or lie nearby; the pre- and postganglionic neural transmitter is traditionally said to be acetylcholine

parasympatholytic—a drug that inhibits cholinergic receptors of the autonomic nervous system

parasympathomimetic—a drug that stimulates cholinergic receptors of the autonomic nervous system

parathyroid hormone—a peptide substance formed in the parathyroid glands that plays a role in calcium deposition and resorption in bone

parenchyma—the specific cells of a gland or organ contained in and supported by the connective tissue framework or stroma

parenteral—via other than an intestinal route; referring to the means by which a medication may be administered (e.g., subcutaneous, intramuscular, intravenous)

parenteral nutrition—the administration of nutritive material by other than an intestinal route; usually via an intravenous or subcutaneous route

paresis—partial or incomplete paralysis

parietal layer—the outer portion of the serous pericardium that is supported by the fibrous pericardium

parietal pleura—the serous membrane that covers the inner surface of the chest wall, the exposed part of the diaphragm and the mediastinum

Parkinson's disease—a syndrome consisting of slowness in the initiation and execution of movement, increased muscle tone, tremor, and impaired postural reflexes

paroxysmal atrial tachycardia (PAT)—recurrent episodes of rapid heart rate (in excess of 100 beats per minute), with abrupt onset and cessation, originating from an ectopic focus in the atria

paroxysmal nocturnal dyspnea (PND)—sudden shortness of breath that awakens an individual in the middle of sleep; the individual needs to sit up to get air

paroxysmal supraventricular tachycardia—recurrent episodes of rapid heart rate (in excess of 100 beats per minute), with abrupt onset and cessation, originating from an ectopic focus in the atria or atrioventricular node

partial expiratory flow volume (PEFV)—a pulmonary function test that may be used to reveal low forced expiratory rates in children

partial thromboplastin time (PTT)—the time it takes for a fibrin clot to form after calcium and a phospholipid have been added to a blood sample; a test of the intrinsic clotting system; activated partial prothrombin time

patent ductus arteriosus (PDA)—a condition in which the vessel that connects the pulmonary artery with the descending aorta in the fetus does not close after birth

pathogenic—anything that causes disease or abnormality

Pavulon (pancuronium bromide)—a neuromuscular blocking agent; often used in the intensive care unit to reduce total oxygen demands

peak expiratory flow (PEF)—the maximum flow of gas at the beginning of a forced expiratory maneuver

peak expiratory flow rate (PEFR)—the highest point on the expiratory curve of a flow-volume loop

pectinate muscles—muscular ridges running across the walls of the auricula of the atria

pectoralis major muscle—an accessory inspiratory muscle arising from the medial third of the clavicle, from the lateral part of the anterior surface of the manubrium and body of the sternum, and from the costal cartilages of the first six ribs to insert onto the lateral lip of the crest of the greater tubercle of the humerus

pectoralis minor muscle—an accessory inspiratory muscle arising from the second to fifth or the third to sixth ribs to insert onto the medial side of the coracoid process

pectus carinatum—a forward projection (much like the keel of a boat) of the sternum; pigeon breast

pectus excavatum—a posterior displacement of the sternum; funnel chest

penetrating wound—trauma that results in disruption of the continuity of the tissue at the surface of the body and extends into the underlying tissue or body cavity

peptic ulcer—a lesion of the alimentary mucosal surface, usually in the stomach or duodenum

percutaneous transluminal coronary angioplasty (PTCA)—a procedure for enlarging the lumen of a narrowed artery; a balloon-tipped catheter is introduced into the artery to be dilated, inflated, and removed

perfusate—the fluid used for perfusion

perfusion—the transporting of dissolved and bound gases to and from the lungs and the cells in the blood

peribronchial—in close proximity to or surrounding a bronchus or the bronchi

pericardectomy—excision of the pericardium

pericardial effusion—the escape of fluid (e.g., vascular fluid) into the pericardial space

pericardial friction rub; pericardial rub—a creaking sound caused by the rubbing together of the inflamed pericardial surfaces as the heart contracts and relaxes

pericardial sac—the fibroserous membrane consisting of mesothelium and submesothelium connective tissue covering the heart and the beginning of the great vessels

pericardial tamponade—a reduction of the venous return to the heart as the result of fluid in the pericardial space

pericardiocentesis—the drainage of fluid from the pericardium by insertion of a hollow needle into the pericardial space

pericarditis—an inflammation of the pericardial sac surrounding the heart

pericardium—the fibroserous membrane covering the heart and the beginning of the great vessels;

forms the boundaries of the anterior, middle, and posterior compartments of the mediastinum

perinatal asphyxia—the impairment or absence of gas exchange (oxygen and carbon dioxide) as the result of ventilatory impairment at any time in the period from the twenty-eighth week of gestation through the seventh day after delivery

peripheral arterial disease (PAD)—an occlusive process involving the peripheral arteries

peripheral neuropathy—any disease involving the peripheral nerves

peripheral vascular disease—any occlusive process involving the vascular beds of the peripheral tissues

peritoneal dialysis—the removal of soluble substances and water from the body by intermittently introducing and removing a dialysate into and from the peritoneal cavity

peritonitis—the inflammation of the peritoneum

persistent fetal circulation—a condition in which the vascular shunts (e.g., foramen ovale, ductus arteriosus) that are present in the fetus fail to close following birth

pertussis—an acute inflammation of the larynx, trachea, and bronchi characterized by recurrent bouts of exhaustive spasmodic coughing that ends in stridor; whooping cough

phagocytosis—the ingestion and digestion of solid substances by cells

pharmacodynamics—the study of the mechanism by which a drug achieves its effect within the body

pharmacokinetics—the study of the movement of a drug within the body; particularly the uptake, distribution, elimination, and transformation of a drug within the body after it has been administered

pharmacologic stress testing—physiologic stress is induced while an individual remains in the resting position by injection of a pharmacologic agent that accelerates the heart beat

pharyngeal isthmus—the space between the free edge of the soft palate and the posterior wall of the pharynx; the juncture of the nasopharynx and oropharynx

pharynx—a musculomembranous tube about 5 to 6 inches long having an upper limit corresponding to the basal surface of the skull; consists of three parts: nasopharynx, oropharynx, and laryngopharynx

phase I cardiac rehabilitation—the program of education and exercise established to assist an individual with heart disease achieve optimal physical and psychological functioning that begins in the acute phase of recovery; typically begins in the coronary critical care unit or the cardiac stepdown unit

phase II cardiac rehabilitation—the program of education, behavioral changes, and exercise established to assist an individual with heart disease achieve optimal physical and psychological functioning that begins in the subacute phase of recovery; typically the initial outpatient phase of rehabilitation

phase III cardiac rehabilitation—the continuing program of education, behavioral changes, and exercise established to assist an individual with heart disease achieve optimal physical and psychological functioning that begins in the acute phase of recovery; typically when intensive, high-intensity rehabilitation occurs

phase IV cardiac rehabilitation—the ongoing or maintenance program of education, behavioral changes, and exercise established to assist an individual with heart disease achieve optimal physical and psychological functioning

phenylalanine-hydroxylase pathway—an intrahepatic intermediary amino acid metabolic pathway

pheochromocytoma—a typically benign neoplasm derived from cells in the adrenal medulla, characterized by the secretion of catecholamines

phonation—the creation of sounds by means of the vocal cords

phosphocreatinine—a compound of creatinine with phosphoric acid; an intermediary energy source, that provides phosphate for the resynthesis of ATP from ADP

phosphodiesterase—an enzyme that splits the phosphodiester bonds of some nucleotides

photophobia—an abnormal sensitivity to or fear of light

physiologic dead space—parts of the lung that are ventilated although they receive no blood supply and therefore cannot participate in gas exchange

pindolol (Visken)—a beta-adrenergic blocking agent used in the treatment of hypertension

plasmapheresis—the removal of whole blood from the body, followed by centrifugal separation into its cellular components and their reinfusion in a saline suspension, thereby reducing the plasma volume without depleting the cell volume

platelet-derived growth factor (PDGF)—a substance derived from platelets that causes the proliferation of endothelial tissue at the site of an arterial sclerotic lesion

plethysmographic tracings—recordings of variations in volume of body parts

pleura—the serous membrane enveloping the lungs and lining the walls of the pleural cavity

pleural abrasion—the excoriation of the mucous membrane of the pleura

pleural effusion—the escape of fluid (e.g., vascular exudate) into the pleural space

pleural pressure—the pressure within the pleural space between the visceral and parietal pleurae

pleural rub—a friction sound created by the rubbing together of the roughened surfaces of the parietal and visceral pleurae

pleural space—the potential space between the parietal and visceral pleura

pleurectomy—the excision of the pleura, usually the parietal pleura

pleurisy—the inflammation of the pleura; pleuritis

pneumatocele—a thin-walled cavity within the lung; characteristic of staphylococcal pneumonia

pneumococcal pneumonia—an inflammation of the lungs due to infection with *Streptococcus pneumoniae* bacteria

pneumoconiosis—an inflammatory fibrosis of the lungs as the result of inhaling dust particles incidental to occupational exposure

***Pneumocystis carinii* pneumonia**—a cystic infection of the lungs caused by the protozoan *Pneumocystis carinii;* pneumocystosis

pneumomediastinum—air within the mediastinal tissues

pneumonectomy—the surgical removal of a single lung

pneumonia—an inflammation of the lungs, particularly as the result of a pathogen

pneumonitis—an inflammation of the lungs

pneumotaxic center—the region of the medulla oblongata concerned with respiration

pneumothorax—air in the pleural cavity

poliomyelitis—an inflammation of the gray matter of the spinal cord

polyarteritis nodosa—an inflammation, with eosinophilic infiltration, of the small or medium-sized arteries

polycythemia—an excessive amount of red corpuscles in the blood

polymyositis—the simultaneous inflammation of several voluntary muscles

polyneuritis—the simultaneous inflammation of several spinal nerves

polyp—any mass of tissue that bulges or projects outward from the normal surface level

porphyrin—four pyrrole groups cyclically linked by methylene bridges

portopulmonary shunting—a potential complication of liver disease

positive end-expiratory pressure (PEEP)—a mechanical ventilatory maneuver in which a thresholdlike resistance applied at the end of exhalation permits the pressure in the ventilator circuit to drop only to a set level above atmospheric pressure

positive expiratory pressure (PEP) mask—a device used to increase the functional residual volume and enhance oxygenation in the treatment of some pulmonary disorders

positive inotropic—the property of being able to enhance the contractility of a muscle

positron emission tomography (PET)—tomographic imaging of tissues formed by tracing the path of photons created by the collision of positrons emitted by a radioactive biochemical (previously administered to the patient) with the electrons normally present in the cells

posterior basal segmental bronchus—the portion of the tracheobronchial tree arising from the right or left lower lobe bronchus that is distributed to the posterior basal segment

posterior interventricular artery—the continuation of the right coronary artery on the posterior surface of the heart

posterior leaflet of the mitral valve—the smaller of the two cusps of the mitral valve; also called the ventricular, mural, or posterolateral leaflet

posterior papillary muscles—muscles that arise at the apical ventriculoseptal juncture in the right ventricle; from the diaphragmatic wall of the left ventricle

posterior pulmonary plexus—a network of nerves formed by branches from the vagus nerves, the deep cardiac plexus and the second and fifth thoracic sympathetic ganglia, and the left recurrent laryngeal nerve supplying posterior branches of the bronchi and the pulmonary and bronchial vessels

posterior segmental bronchus—the portion of the tracheobronchial tree arising from the right upper lobe bronchus that is distributed to the posterior segment

posterior vein of the left ventricle—vein that accompanies the circumflex branch of the left coronary artery across the diaphragmatic surface of the left ventricle

posteroanterior (PA) view—the image produced by the roentgen-ray beam as it passes through the patient from posterior to anterior

posterolateral thoracotomy—a surgical incision into the posterolateral aspect of the chest wall that provides access to the underlying tissues

postperfusion syndrome—a condition of decreased cardiac output in conjunction with other cardiovascular symptoms that arise following the use of a perfusion pump in cardiovascular surgical procedures

postpericardiotomy syndrome—the occurrence, often repeatedly, of the symptoms of pericarditis (with or without febrile episodes) weeks to months after cardiac surgery

postural drainage—the use of gravity to assist or facilitate the removal of fluids or secretions from the lungs by positioning the body in such a manner as to place the involved segment or segments perpendicular to the forces of gravity

postural hypotension—a form of low blood pressure that occurs on the assumption of upright postures; orthostatic hypotension

pravastatin—an antihyperlipidemic agent; acts by inhibiting cholesterol synthesis

prazosin (Minipress)—an antihypertensive agent

prediabetic—a state of potential diabetes mellitus, with normal glucose tolerance but with increased risk of developing diabetes

prednisone—a dehydrogenated analogue of cortisone, having the same uses and actions

preinfarction angina—a severe constricting chest pain, often radiating from the precordium, that frequently precedes a myocardial infarction

preload—the amount of tension on the muscular wall of the ventricle before it contracts

premature atrial complex (PAC, APC)—an extrasystole arising from an ectopic atrial focus that occurs before the usual or expected time of the normal depolarization wave

premature junctional complex—an extrasystole arising from an ectopic atrioventricular nodal focus that occurs before the usual or expected time of the normal depolarization wave

premature ventricular complex (PVC, VPC, VPB)—an extrasystole arising from an ectopic ventricular focus that occurs before the usual or expected time of the normal depolarization wave

preprandial—before a meal

pressor—an agent that enhances vasomotor tone and increases blood pressure

pressoreceptors—pressosensitive; capable of receiving as stimuli changes in pressure, especially in blood pressure

pressure release ventilation—same as BIPAP; a noninvasive method of delivering positive airway pressure during inhalation and exhalation

pressure support ventilation (PSV)—a mode of mechanical ventilatory assistance in which a preselected positive pressure is delivered each time the ventilator is triggered by the patient's spontaneous inspiratory effort

primary acid-base disorder—a disturbance of the normal acid-base balance to which other complications are attributable

primary bronchi—the main bronchi arising from the bifurcation of the trachea; right and left

primary (essential) hypertension—a heterogeneous syndrome; multiple factors contribute to the elevated blood pressure, including cardiac output, systemic vascular resistance, and sodium balance

primitive pulmonary vein—the small venous conduit between the nonfunctioning lungs and the left atrium

Prinzmetal's angina—a form of angina that is not precipitated by cardiac exertion; generally is of longer duration, more severe, and associated with unusual ECG manifestations (e.g., ST-segment elevation) when compared with typical angina pectoris

procainamide (Pronestyl)—an antiarrhythmic agent that depresses the irritability of cardiac muscle; used in the treatment of ventricular arrhythmias

procerus muscle—a small slip of muscle originating as a continuation of the occipitofrontalis and attaching to the fascia covering the lower part of the nasal bone and the upper part of the lateral nasal cartilage (muscle that wrinkles the skin of the nose)

prodromal—an early or premonitory symptom of a disease

professorial position—a standing posture in which the trunk is forward leaning, with the upper body supported on extended arms

progressive systemic sclerosis—a progressive disease characterized by the formation of hyalinized and thickened collagenous fibrous tissues, thickening of the skin and adhesion to the underlying tissues, submucosal fibrosis of the esophagus, pulmonary and myocardial fibrosis, renal vascular changes, Raynaud's phenomenon, atrophy of the soft tissues, and osteoporosis of the distal phalanges; scleroderma

prokaryote—a single-cell organ that lacks nuclear organization, mitotic capacity, or complex organelles

prophylactically—in a manner to prevent disease

propranolol (Inderal)—a beta-adrenergic blocking agent

prostaglandin—a class of physiologically active substances capable of effecting vasodilation, vasoconstriction, stimulation of intestinal or bronchial smooth muscle, uterine stimulation, and lipid metabolism

protein-calorie deficiency—the primary nutritional abnormality contributing to malnutrition

proteinuria—the presence of urinary protein in concentrations greater than 0.3 g in 24-hour urine collection or in concentrations greater than 1 g/L in a random urine collection on two or more occasions

prothrombic—clot forming

prothrombin—a glycoprotein in the blood that is converted to thrombin in the presence of thromboplastin and calcium ions

prothrombin time (PT)—the time it takes for a clot to form after thromboplastin and calcium are added to the blood; the greater the time it takes, the lower the level of prothrombin

pseudohypertrophy—the increase in the size of an organ due to an increase of some tissue other than itself

psittacosis—an infectious disease caused by *Chlamydia psittaci;* characterized by flulike (in mild cases) or bronchopneumonia-like (in severe cases) symptoms

ptosis—the prolapse of an organ or tissue

pulmonary alveoli—the final saclike dilatations of the terminal sacs in the lung

pulmonary area—the region of the chest where

the normal and pathologic sounds made by the pulmonary valve are best appreciated

pulmonary arterial hypertension—a condition of abnormally high pulmonary arterial blood pressure

pulmonary arterioles—the smallest subdivision of the pulmonary arterial tree before the pulmonary capillary bed

pulmonary artery balloon counterpulsation (PABC)—a means of assisting right ventricular ejection by reducing pulmonary artery pressure just before and during ventricular systole with an intrapulmonary-arterial balloon pump activated by an automatic mechanism triggered by the ECG

pulmonary artery catheter—a thin, flexible, flow-directed, balloon-tipped catheter introduced into the pulmonary artery used to monitor cardiovascular pressures

pulmonary artery pressure—the blood pressure in the pulmonary artery

pulmonary artery wedge pressure—the pressure obtained by wedging a flow-directed, balloon-tipped catheter into a small branch of the pulmonary artery so that the flow of blood from behind is blocked and the pressure beyond can be sampled; normally not greater than 12 mm Hg; pulmonary wedge pressure; pulmonary capillary wedge pressure

pulmonary capillaries—an intermeshed network of blood vessels, whose walls consist of a single layer of cells, in the septa and walls of the alveolar ducts and alveoli; the bridge between pulmonary arterioles and venules

pulmonary congestion—the presence of an abnormal amount of fluid in the interstitial spaces of the lungs

pulmonary edema—the accumulation of an excessive amount of fluid in the alveolar spaces of the lungs

pulmonary emboli—a detached piece of thrombus occluding a blood vessel in the lungs

pulmonary fibroplasia—an abnormal increase of nonneoplastic fibrous tissue in the lungs

pulmonary insufficiency—failure of the pulmonic valve to close completely, allowing regurgitation of blood

pulmonary interstitial edema—the presence of an abnormal amount of fluid in the interstitial spaces of the lungs; pulmonary congestion

pulmonary ligament—the extension of the pleural covering below and behind the hilus from the root of the lung

pulmonary perfusion—the pulmonary blood flow

pulmonary stenosis—a narrowing of the pulmonary valvular orifice or the right ventricular outflow tract

pulmonary trunk—the common conduit of the pulmonary artery before its bifurcation into right and left branches

pulmonary vascular resistance (PVR)—pressure (resistance) in the pulmonary vascular system

pulmonary veins—the four veins returning oxygenated blood from the lungs to the left atrium

pulmonic area (space)—the region of the chest (second intercostal space, along the left sternal border) where the normal and pathologic sounds made by the pulmonary valve are traditionally said to be best appreciated

pulmonologist—a physician specializing in pulmonary medicine

pulse oximeter—an instrument that photoelectrically determines the oxygen saturation of arterial blood as it courses through the peripheral arteries with each pulse

pulse volume recordings (PVR)—changes in volume of blood flowing through a limb as measured by plethysmographic tracings to assess for blockage

pulsus alternans—the mechanical alteration of the pulse typified by a regular rhythm and alternating strong and weak pulses; characteristic of significant myocardial disease

pulsus paradoxus—a marked variation in the cardiac stroke volume with respiratory effort, such that the pulse becomes stronger with expiration and weaker with inspiration; characteristic of pericardial effusion or restrictive pericarditis

Purkinje's fibers—the terminal projections of the specialized conduction system of the heart, spread in an interlaced network throughout the endocardium of the ventricles

Purkinje's myocytes—the specialized cardiac muscle cells that are wider and shorter, contain fewer myofibrils and more mitochondria, and have larger intercalated discs than working myocytes; primarily located in terminal branches of the conduction system of the heart; have a myogenic rhythm that is slower than nodal myocytes but faster than working or transitional myocytes; have an impulse conduction rate that is faster than all other myocytes

purulent—containing or forming pus

quadratus lumborum muscle—an accessory inspiratory muscle arising from the iliac crest and transverse processes of the lumbar vertebrae upward to attach to the twelfth rib

quality of life (QOL)—the multifactorial, functional effect of an illness and its consequent therapy upon a patient

quantitative pilocarpine iontophoresis—the introduction of a parasympathetic agent into the tissues by means of an electric current for the purpose of determining the amount of salt in the sweat

quinidine (Cardioquin)—an alkaloid of cinchona, a stereoisomer of quinine; used in the treatment of atrial fibrillation and flutter

R on T phenomenon—the occurrence of an effective premature ventricular depolarization (R wave) during the relative refractory period of the preceding normal complex (T wave)

radioactive nuclide perfusion imaging—radioactive labeled agents used with perfusion imaging to improve the assessment of coronary artery perfusion

radiograph—an x-ray film

radiolucency—the characteristic of being relatively penetrable by x-rays

radiopacity—the condition of being relatively impenetrable by x-rays

rales—an adventitious sound heard on auscultation of breath sounds; characteristically an inspiratory sound; postulated to be caused by the mixing of air with thin secretions in the distal, small airways, or the popping open of collapsed alveoli

rapid-filling phase—the phase that occurs once the mitral valve opens and the ventricular volume begins rising as the ventricle passively fills

rate-pressure product (RPP)—the product of the multiplication of the heart rate by the systolic blood pressure; a parameter used to monitor the onset of angina in some patients

rating of perceived exertion (RPE)—a subjective numerical scale of exercise intensity

Raynaud's phenomenon—the paroxysmal cyanosis of the digits due to contraction of the digital arteries and arterioles

readiness to learn—a principle of adult learning including adequate energy, emotional and physical stability, and awareness of the identified problem or need to learn about the problem

receptor-G protein—guanine nucleotide-binding regulatory proteins (G proteins) are the links between the many different receptors on a cell's surface and their catalytic units or other effectors within the cell

recombinant human vascular endothelial growth factor (VEGF)—a potent angiogenic agent due to its endothelial cell specificity

refractory period—the time following effective myocardial stimulation during which the myocytes fail to respond to a stimulus of threshold intensity

renal failure—the state of insufficiency or nonperformance of the kidneys

renal insufficiency—a decline in the glomerular filtration rate and/or in the tubular function as a consequence of insult to the kidney

renal transplantation—the implantation of a kidney from a compatible donor to restore kidney function in a recipient suffering from renal failure

renin—the enzyme that converts angiotensinogen to angiotensin

reperfusion—the reestablishment of blood flow to a tissue

repolarization—the process of repolarizing the cell, fiber, or membrane after depolarization

residual volume (RV)—the volume of air that

remains in the lungs after a forceful expiratory effort

resistance to flow—the force acting in opposition to the movement of a fluid or gas

resistance vessels—the arterioles and precapillary sphincters that provide peripheral resistance to blood flow

resisted inhalation—a technique of resisting movement of the diaphragm during inhalation for the purpose of increasing the strength of the diaphragm, either by manually resisting or with weights

resistive inspiratory muscle training—a technique of repeatedly inhaling through progressively smaller orifices in an effort to increase the strength and endurance of the inspiratory musculature

resonance—the sound produced by percussing on a part that can vibrate freely

respiration—breathing; taking in of oxygen and throwing off the products of oxidation in the tissues, mainly carbon dioxide and water

respiratory acidosis—inadequate pulmonary ventilation that results in the retention of carbon dioxide and the decrease in blood pH

respiratory alkalosis—hyperventilation that results in an abnormal loss of CO_2 and an increase in blood pH

respiratory bronchioles—the part of the respiratory passages after the terminal bronchioles; the first level at which gas exchange may occur

respiratory center—the region of the medulla oblongata concerned with the control of respiration

respiratory depressant—any agent that acts to reduce the activity of the respiratory center or otherwise retard pulmonary ventilation

respiratory distress—defined as any signs or symptoms of inability to breathe deeply, regularly, and with ease; signs and symptoms includes respiratory rate above 35 breaths per minute, less than 90% Sa_{O_2}, paradoxical breathing, and increased use of accessory muscles

respiratory distress syndrome (RDS)—a condition of acute lung injury from a variety of causes; characterized by interstitial or alveolar edema, or both, and hemorrhage associated with hyaline membrane, proliferation of collagen fibers, and epithelial swelling

respiratory failure—the inability of the respiratory system to ventilate the alveoli

respiratory stimulant—any agent that enhances the activity of the respiratory center

respiratory syncytial virus—a paramyxovirus that forms a multinucleated protoplasmic mass in tissue culture: causes mild respiratory infection in adults but can cause bronchitis and bronchopneumonia in children

resting membrane potential—the electrical potential inside a cell membrane, relative to the extracellular fluid when there is no action potential

restrictive—any condition that limits the normal capacity of an organ system

restrictive cardiomyopathy—a disease of the myocardium characterized by marked endocardial scarring of the ventricles with resulting impaired diastolic filling

restrictive changes—the fibrosis and scarring that are typically associated with restrictive diseases

restrictive lung dysfunction—an abnormal reduction in pulmonary ventilation

reticulation—the formation of a fine network formed by specific structures with cells, formed by cells themselves, or formed by the connective tissue fibers between cells

reticulogranular pattern—a network of granule-like shadows in a radiograph of an infant with infant respiratory distress syndrome (IRDS); the radiographic presentation of IRDS

reticulonodular pattern—a network of nodule-like shadows throughout both lungs; the typical radiographic presentation of idiopathic pulmonary fibrosis

retinopathy—a noninflammatory degenerative disease of the retina

rhabdomyolysis—an acute, fulminating disease that destroys skeletal muscle

rhabdomyosarcoma—a malignant neoplasm derived from skeletal muscle

rheumatoid arthritis (RA)—a systemic disease that affects the connective tissues of the body; characterized by extension of synovial tissue over the articular cartilages with cartilaginous thickening and erosion in multiple joints

rhinorrhea—a discharge from the nasal mucosal lining

rhinovirus—a genus of acid-labile viruses (of which there are more than 100 antigenic types) associated with the common cold in humans and foot-and-mouth disease in cattle

rhonchi—adventitious sounds occurring during inspiration or expiration, heard on auscultation of the lungs, and caused by turbulence created when air passing through the midsized and larger bronchi reaches the secretions in the lumen

rhythmicity—the cadence or pattern of recurrence of a phenomenon

ribavirin (tribavirin, Virazole)—an antiviral agent used to treat respiratory syncytial virus

right anterior ventricular rami—branches to the right ventricle from the right coronary artery

right atrial pressure—the blood pressure in the right atrium

right atrium—the chamber of the heart that receives blood from the venae cavae

right auricle—the small conical projection from the right atrium; remnant of the right portion of the primitive atrium

right bundle branches—offshoots of the right division of His's bundle in the right ventricle

right coronary artery—the artery that arises from the right anterolateral surface of the aorta and passes between the auricular appendage of the right atrium and the pulmonary trunk

right coronary plexus—formed from contributions of both the deep and superficial parts of the cardiac plexus; follows the distribution of the right coronary artery, supplying the right atrium and ventricle

right dominant coronary arterial system—a condition in which the majority of the blood supply to the heart is provided via the right coronary artery; occurs in approximately 50% of the population

right inferior pulmonary vein—the vein that returns blood from the lower lobe of the right lung to the left atrium

right marginal artery—a branch of the right coronary artery

right marginal vein—the vein that receives blood from the right margin of the heart, sometimes emptying directly into the right atrium or joining the small cardiac vein in the coronary sulcus

right pulmonary artery—the right branch of the pulmonary artery distributed to the right lung; runs behind the ascending aorta, superior vena cava, and upper pulmonary vein but in front of the esophagus and right primary bronchus to the root of the lung

right superior pulmonary vein—the vein that returns blood from the upper and middle lobes of the right lung to the left atrium

right (pulmonary) surface—the right side of the heart that is in contact with the right lung

right-to-left shunt—when blood passes from the right to the left side of the heart without participating in gas exchange; intrapulmonary shunt

right ventricle—one of the two lower chambers of the heart

right ventricular hypertrophy—a condition of increased bulk, but not number, of working myocytes in the right ventricle as the result of an increased resistance to right ventricular outflow

rima glottidis—the fissure between the vocal folds commonly called the glottis

rima vestibuli—the fissure between the vestibular folds

roentgenogram—a radiograph x-ray film

rotation—the misalignment of the body with respect to the film cassette, which can distort the image represented in a radiograph

rough zone chordae—chordae that arise from a single stem but split into three filaments: one attaches to the free margin of the leaflet, another attaches to the ventricular aspect of the rough zone of the leaflet, and the third attaches to some intermediate position

rubor dependency test—an assessment procedure of the lower extremity arterial circulation using skin color changes and positional changes

S₁ heart sound—normal "lub" (of "lub-dub") caused by closure of the mitral and tricuspid valves

S₂ heart sound—normal "dub" (of "lub-dub") caused by closure of the pulmonic and aortic valves

S₃ heart sound—abnormal heart sound heard after "lub-dub" ("dub"), indicating ventricular noncompliance except in an athlete

S₄ heart sound—abnormal heart sound heard just before "lub" (of "lub-dub"), often indicating atrial noncompliance

saccular bronchiectasis—a type of chronic dilation of the bronchi or bronchioles that appear to have a pouchlike shape

saccule of the larynx—a small pouch extending upward from the anterior aspect of the sinus of the larynx

salicylic acid (aspirin)—an analgesic and anti-inflammatory agent

sarcoidosis—a systemic granulomatous disease that predominantly affects the lungs with resulting fibrosis

scalene muscles—a group of three muscles (anterior, medial, and posterior scalenes) acting as accessory inspiratory muscles to elevate the first and second ribs

scapuloperoneal myopathy—Emery-Dreifuss muscular dystrophy

scintigraphy—a diagnostic procedure in which a radionuclide is injected intravenously, and a photographic recording of its distribution is made

scleroderma—chronic disorder characterized by progressive collagenous fibrosis of many organs and systems, often beginning with the skin

scoliosis—a condition of lateral curvature of the spine

second-degree atrioventricular block—two types of atrioventricular arrhythmias in which some but not all atrial impulses fail to reach the ventricle, and thus some ventricular depolarizations are dropped; in type I (Wenckebach's), there is progressive lengthening of the atrioventricular conduction time until a ventricular depolarization is dropped; after the dropped cycle the P-R interval returns to normal; in type II, there is a dropped ventricular cycle with or without an alteration in the preceding atrioventricular conduction time

second heart sound (S₂)—the sound created by the closure of the semilunar valves of the heart; signifies the end of ventricular systole

secondary bronchi—the initial divisions off the primary bronchi; the lobar bronchi: three from the right primary bronchus; two from the left primary bronchus

secondary hypertension—a condition of abnormally high blood pressure that is the result of some directly identifiable cause

secondary lobule—an outmoded term describing a functional unit of the lung; anatomically, the secondary lobules contain as many as 50 primary lobules

secondary prevention (of cardiovascular disease)—program components aimed at reducing risk of illness and death after coronary artery disease diagnosis as well as improving function and quality of life

segmental limb pressures—pressure is sequentially inflated in pressure cuffs on thigh, calf, ankle, and transmetatarsal region of foot to localize stenoses or occlusions in peripheral vascular system

selectivity—the ability of a drug to interact with specific receptors on the target tissue and not with other receptors or other tissues

semilunar cusps—the crescentic leaflets of the aortic valve

sensitivity—the probability that, given the presence of a disease, an abnormal test result will indicate the presence of the disease

septomarginal trabecula—the anteroinferior boundary between the inflow and outflow tracts of the right ventricle near the apex

septum primum—the crescent-shaped membrane arising from the dorsocephalic wall of the primitive atrium that initiates the partitioning of the atrium into two chambers; the ends of the septum eventually fuse with the dorsal endocardial cushions of the atrioventricular canal

septum secundum—the crescent-shaped membrane arising from the ventrocranial wall of the atrium on the right side of the septum primum; the ends of the septum reach dorsally toward the sinus venosus

serotype—the antigenic character that distinguishes a subdivision of a species from other strains

serous cavities—hollow spaces filled with serum or a substance having a watery consistency

serous cells—bronchial epithelial cells that secrete mucus

serous pericardium—the inner sac of the pericardial sac consisting of a visceral layer and a parietal layer

serratus anterior muscle—an accessory inspiratory muscle arising from the outer surfaces of the upper eight or nine ribs to attach along the costal aspect of the medial border of the scapula

serratus posterior superior—an accessory inspiratory muscle arising from the lower part of the ligamentum nuchae and the spinous processes of the seventh cervical and the first two or three thoracic vertebrae downward into the upper borders of the second to fourth or fifth ribs

sestamibi—a radioactive perfusion agent used to improve the view of a myocardial perfusion study

shaft of the rib—the central portion of the rib

shock—a state of profound physical depression subsequent to a severe physical injury or impairment

sick sinus syndrome—a condition of continual, chaotic changes in the configuration of the P wave on ECG; characterized by bradycardia alternating with recurrent ectopic extrasystoles and supraventricular tachycardia

sickle cell disease—an anemic disorder of the red blood cells characterized by crescent- or sickle-shaped erythrocytes and by accelerated hemolysis

silent ischemia—a condition of inadequate blood circulation to the myocardium without the typical accompanying signs or symptoms

silhouette sign—a radiographic finding (demonstrated when the normal line of demarcation between two structures is partially or completely obliterated) used to localize lesions within the lung fields

silicosis—a type of pneumoconiosis that results from occupational exposure (over a period of years) to or inhalation of silica dust; characterized by slow, progressive fibrosis of the lungs

simple mask—a type of supplemental oxygen delivery device

single-chain urokinase plasminogen activator (SCU-PA, pro-urokinase)—a proteinase that converts plasminogen to plasmin

single lung transplantation—surgical replacement of one lung with a donor lung using a posterolateral thoracotomy

single-photon emission computed tomography (SPECT)—a noninvasive diagnostic test to detect and quantify myocardial perfusion and contractility defects

sinoatrial (SA) node—the mass of specialized myocytes that normally acts as the "pacemaker" for the specialized conduction system of the heart

sinus arrhythmia—an extrasystole having an ectopic focus within the atrial tissues of the heart (other than the sinoatrial node)

sinus block—failure of an impulse, generated in the sinoatrial node, to get out of the sinoatrial node

sinus bradycardia—a slow heart rate (less than 60 beats per minute) that has its origin in the sinoatrial node

sinus of the larynx—a fusiform recess between the vestibular and vocal folds

sinus venosus—the dilatation of the heart tube inferior to the atrium that is formed by the proximal portions of the veins

sinusoid—a blood channel in certain organs that is lined by reticuloendothelium

six minute walk test—a valid submaximal exercise test useful for assessing exercise tolerance in patients with pulmonary disease or congestive heart failure

sleep apnea—an absence of breathing caused by an upper airway obstruction during sleep

slow twitch oxidative (SO) fibers—muscle fibers that have slow speed of shortening and great reliance on oxidative metabolism; fatigue resistant

small cardiac vein—a vein that receives blood from the back of the right atrium and ventricle; runs between the right atrium and ventricle in the coronary sulcus

small dense LDL—smaller denser LDL particle subtype associated with elevated triglyceride levels; can move into vessel wall faster

sniffing—an early stage inspiratory muscle training technique using the diaphragm muscle

sodium-calcium antiporter—a carrier mechanism that carries sodium and calcium ions through a membrane in opposite directions; the energy for the transport of the ions is derived from the potential energy of the ions being transported

sodium nitroprusside—a potent intravenous antihypertensive agent

sodium-potassium pump—a biochemical mechanism that uses metabolic energy from ATP to achieve the transport of sodium and potassium ions in opposite directions through a membrane

spasmodic cough—an involuntary, uncontrollable sudden explosive forcing of air through the glottis

specificity—the probability that, given the absence of a disease, a normal test result excludes the disease

sphygmomanometer—the instrument used to determine blood pressure

sphygmomanometry—the determination of blood pressure by means of auscultation and a blood pressure cuff (sphygmomanometer)

spinal cord injury—the damage resulting from trauma to the spinal cord

spinocerebellar—refers to all parts of the cerebellum rostral to the primary fissure; corresponds to the region of distribution of the spinocerebellar tracts

spirogram—a tracing or graphic representation of the depth and rapidity of respiratory movements

spirometric measurement—the determination of pulmonary volumes using a spirometer (a counterbalanced cylindric bell sealed by dipping into a trough of water)

splint—protect or guard against pain (e.g., splint an incision)

sputum—expectorated matter; secretions

squamous metaplasia—the transformation of glandular or mucosal epithelium into stratified squamous epithelium

Starling's forces—the force tending to move or retard a substance across a membrane as the result of the differences between hydrostatic and oncotic pressures

Starling's hypothesis—the idea that net filtration through a capillary is proportional to the transmembrane hydrostatic pressure difference minus the transmembrane oncotic pressure difference

static volumes—pulmonary volumes measured at rest without chest wall movement (e.g., residual volume, functional residual volume)

status asthmaticus—severe, prolonged asthma

steatorrhea—the presence of large amounts of fat in the feces

sternocleidomastoid muscle—an accessory inspiratory muscle that arises by two heads (sternal and clavicular) that unite to extend obliquely upward and laterally across the neck to the mastoid process

sternocostal (anterior)—the surface of the heart in contact with the sternum and ribs

sternotomy—a surgical incision through the sternum

sternum—the breast bone; the tripartite flat bone forming the middle part of the anterior chest wall

steroid myopathy—muscle weakness (predominantly proximal muscles) secondary to long-term use of steroids

steroids—a family of chemical substances that make up many hormones and vitamin D

streptokinase (Kabikinase, Streptase)—an extracellular metalloenzyme from hemolytic streptococci that disrupts plasminogen, producing plasmin and causing the liquefaction of fibrin; a potent "clot buster"

stress—refers to the psychological stimuli that impinge on an individual to produce strain or disequilibrium

stress echocardiography—two-dimensional echocardiographic studies during and immediately after exercise to evaluate ischemia-induced wall motion abnormalities noninvasively

stridor—a high-pitched inspiratory or expiratory sound created by an obstruction to air flow, especially an obstruction occurring in the trachea or larynx

stroke volume—the amount of blood ejected from the ventricles with each systolic contraction

strut chordae—the specialized variants of rough zone chordae of the anterior leaflet of the mitral valve; leaflet chordae

subacute—the course of a disease that has moderate severity or duration; denotes a distinction in time between acute and chronic

subendocardial infarction—injury to the subendocardium and adjacent tissue; nontransmural

subepithelial fibrosis—fibrosis occurring beneath the epithelium

sublingual—under the tongue, referring to a parenteral route of a drug administration; also subglossal or hypoglossal

submaximal—denoting less than the maximum potential

submaximal treadmill testing—an exercise protocol with the endpoint being less than the maximal potential

sudden cardiac death—death within 1 hour of the onset of cardiac symptoms; the primary cause being cardiac arrest

sulfonamide diuretic—a sulfa-containing agent that increases the amount of urine excreted

summation effect—the normal blending together of the various densities of the soft tissues that overlie one another in a radiograph

superficial (proximal) bronchial veins—an extrapulmonary plexus of veins that communicates freely with the pulmonary veins, ending on the left in either the left superior intercostal vein or the accessory hemiazygos veins and on the right in the azygos vein

superficial cardiac plexus—the ventral part of the network of nerves that make up the cardiac plexus; formed by a branch from the left superior cervical sympathetic ganglion and the lower of the two cervical cardiac branches of the left vagus nerve; located anterior to the right pulmonary artery, below the arch of the aorta

superior pulmonary veins—the veins that return blood from the left upper, right upper, and middle lobes of the lungs to the left atrium

superior segmental bronchus—the portion of the tracheobronchial tree arising from the right or left lower lobe bronchus that is distributed to the superior segment

superior vena cava—the conduit of blood from the head and neck, upper limbs, and thorax to the right atrium

superior vesical arteries—the remains of the proximal portions of the umbilical arteries of the fetus; supplies the superior portion of the bladder

suppuration—the formation of pus

supravalvular ridges—a linear elevation of tissue in the wall of the aorta that marks the limit of the free borders of the cusps of the aortic valve

supraventricular crest—the boundary between the posteroanterior inflow tract and the anterosuperior outflow tract of the right ventricle

surface-active agent—an agent that acts to reduce the alveolar surface tension

surface tension—the force that results from the interactions of the pressures tending to collapse the alveoli and those tending to expand them

surfactant—a surface-active agent forming a layer over the pulmonary alveolar surfaces that reduces surface tension and alters the relationship between surface tension and surface area, stabilizing alveolar volume

surfactant replacement therapy—an artificial surface-active agent sometimes given to an infant via endotracheal intubation

symbiotic—any intimate relationship between two species

sympathetic nervous system—one of two parts of the autonomic nervous system; the innervation pathway is composed of two motor neurons: the preganglionic neurons comprise the visceral efferent nuclei of the brain stem and the lateral columns of the thoracic and upper two lumbar segments of the spinal cord; the ganglia are the paravertebral ganglia of the sympathetic trunk and the prevertebral ganglia; the preganglionic neural transmitter is traditionally said to be acetylcholine, and the postganglionic transmitter is norepinephrine

sympatholytic—a drug that inhibits adrenergic receptors of the autonomic nervous system

sympathomimetic—a drug that stimulates adrenergic receptors of the autonomic nervous system

synchronized intermittent mandatory ventilation (SIMV)—a mode of mechanical ventilatory assistance; the mandatory (preset) ventilator breath is synchronized with the patient's breathing efforts

syncope—temporary loss of consciousness due to generalized cerebral ischemia

systemic lupus erythematosus (SLE)—a generalized connective tissue disorder, characterized by skin eruptions, arthralgia, leukopenia, visceral lesions, and fever; affects mostly middle-aged females

systole—the period of ventricular contraction

systolic blood pressure (SBP)—the maximum pressure of the blood on the walls of the arteries; occurs near the end of the stroke output of the left ventricle

systolic dysfunction or systolic heart failure—the impaired contraction of the ventricles during systole that produces an inefficient expulsion of blood

systolic murmur—a periodic sound occurring during the systolic phase of the cardiac cycle and heard during auscultation of the heart; usually attributable to mitral or tricuspid regurgitation or to aortic or pulmonary obstruction

T-lymphocytes—specialized cells (lymphocytes) produced by thymus glands; a function in immune reactions

T-piece—large ventilator tubing directly connected to a tracheostomy tube to provide O_2 to patient and possibly some pressure support; usually the last stage in weaning from mechanical ventilation

tachyarrhythmia—rapid irregular heart beat

tachycardia—rapid heart beat (greater than 100 beats/minute)

tachypnea—very rapid breathing; polypnea

tamponade—compression of the heart as the result of fluid accumulating within the pericardial sac

technetium-99m—a radioactive (labeled sestamibi) perfusion agent; used for diagnostic purposes in the cardiac muscles/coronary arteries

tendon of the infundibulum—a fibrous band connecting aortic and pulmonary annuli

tension pneumothorax—the air within the pleural cavity as the result of a communication between the lung and the pleural space in which a valve effect exists; air enters the pleural space on inspiration but is trapped during expiration

terazosin (Hytrin)—an antihypertensive agent; an alpha$_1$-antagonist with actions similar to prazosin but with a longer half-life

terminal bronchioles—the final part of the conducting airways

terminal sacs—the part of the respiratory passages that develops from the alveolar ducts at the end of the canalicular period of lung development; alveolar sacs

tetralogy of Fallot—the most common cyanosis-producing congenital heart defect consisting of pulmonary stenosis, ventricular septal defect, transposition of the aorta, and right ventricular hypertrophy

tetraplegia—paralysis of all four extremities with involvement of the head; quadriplegia

thallium exercise stress test—radionuclear perfusion scintigraphy exercise test in which thallium-201 (a radionuclide) is rapidly injected into the blood at near maximal exercise; either treadmill or bicycle ergometer protocols may be used

thebesian veins—a number of minute veins arising in the walls of the heart, most emptying directly into the atria, but a few ending in the ventricles; smallest cardiac veins

thermodilution method—a means of determining the cardiac output; a cold bolus of saline is injected into the right atrium via the proximal lumen of a flow-directed, thermal-sensitive catheter; the resultant temperature change is sensed by a thermistor near the tip of the catheter located in the pulmonary artery

third-degree (complete) atrioventricular block—the pathologic loss of conduction through the atrioventricular junctional tissues; atrioventricular dissociation in which atrial or sinus foci elicit depolarization of the atria, while an idioventricular focus stimulates the ventricles

third heart sound (S_3)—a weak, low-pitched sound occurring in early diastole, soon after the second heart sound; believed to be caused by vibrations of the poorly compliant ventricular wall as it is distended during filling

third-party payer—the source of reimbursement (e.g., an insurance carrier) for services received (e.g., physical therapy) that is different from the individual who received the services

thoracentesis—insertion of a hollow needle into the pleural cavity to sample or aspirate accumulated fluid

thoracic inlet—the upper margin of the thorax; formed by the first thoracic vertebra posteriorly, the superior border of the manubrium anteriorly, and the first ribs laterally

thoracic outlet—the lower margin of the thorax; formed by the twelfth thoracic vertebra posteri-

orly, the seventh through tenth costal cartilages anteriorly, and the eleventh and twelfth ribs laterally

thoracoabdominal incision—a cut into the abdomen and thorax

thrombin—the enzyme derived from prothrombin (factor II) that converts fibrinogen into fibrin

thrombocytopenia—an abnormally small number of platelets in the blood

thromboembolism—an embolism from a venous thrombus

thrombolysis—the dissolving of a thrombus

thrombophlebitis—the formation of a thrombus as the result of inflammation of a vein

thromboplastin—a substance necessary for the coagulation of blood; catalyzed by calcium, it converts prothrombin to thrombin

thyrotoxicosis—the state produced by excessive quantities of endogenous and exogenous thyroid hormone

tidal volume (V_T)—the volume of air normally inhaled and exhaled with each breath during quiet breathing

tissue plasminogen activator (tPA; Activase)—a genetically engineered thrombolytic agent used in conjunction with heparin for the limitation of infarct size following myocardial infarction due to the blockage of coronary arteries by thrombi

titration—a means of adjusting a drug's dosage by repeatedly increasing or decreasing the dose administered until the desired effect is achieved or the undesired effect is eliminated

Todaro's tendon—a tendonous structure extending from the right fibrous trigone of the heart toward the valve of the inferior vena cava

tomography—a method of body section roentgenography in which the x-ray tube is moved in one direction (usually in an arc)

torsades de pointes—paroxysmal ventricular tachycardia; characterized on ECG by runs of 5 to 20 complexes with an undulating QRS axis that progressively changes direction

total lung capacity (TLC)—the maximum volume

to which the lungs can be expanded; it is the sum of all the pulmonary volumes

total peripheral resistance (TPR)—the force opposing the flow of blood in the systemic circulatory bed; derived by dividing the mean arterial pressure by the cardiac output

trabeculae carneae—irregular muscular ridges or bundles of variable thickness, lining the walls of the ventricles

trachea—the tube extending from the larynx into the lungs; formed from the central portion of the laryngotracheal tube

tracheitis—inflammation of the mucosal lining of the trachea

tracheoesophageal fistula—a congenital abnormality in which the trachea and esophagus freely communicate; frequently associated with esophageal atresia; may also be acquired in later life

tracheostomy—an opening into the trachea; the creation of an opening into the trachea

tracheostomy button—a capped, hollow tube inserted through an opening into the trachea

tracheostomy tube—a curved tube inserted through an opening and projecting into the trachea

transesophageal echocardiography—the use of ultrasound in the investigation of the heart and great vessels and the diagnosis of cardiovascular lesions using a transducer within the esophagus

transitional myocytes—specialized cardiac muscle cells that have a structure similar to regular working myocytes but are less wide; have a myogenic rhythm that is slower than nodal but faster than Purkinje's or working myocytes; have an impulse conduction rate that is faster than working but slower than nodal or Purkinje's myocytes

translation—the motion of an x-ray source parallel to, and at the same distance from, a film cassette that is moved about a target

transmural—across a wall

transmural pressures—the pressure difference across the wall of a container, the difference between the pressure inside and that outside

transmyocardial laser revascularization (TMR)—a treatment for chronic myocardial ischemia involving laser technology to drill holes in the myocardium

transpulmonary pressure—the difference between the pressure of the gas at the mouth (atmospheric pressure) and the pressure within the pleural space (pleural pressure)

transsulfuration pathway—an intrahepatic intermediary amino acid metabolic pathway

transudate—the material that passes through a membrane (e.g., capillary walls, alveoli) as a result of a difference in hydrostatic pressures on either side of the membrane

transverse myelitis—an inflammation of the spinal cord (its complete thickness)

transverse sinus—a cul-de-sac formed by the epicardial coverings of the aorta and the pulmonary trunk

trapezius muscle—an accessory inspiratory muscle, the upper fibers of the trapezius arise from the superior nuchal line on the occiput and the ligamentum nuchae to insert onto the distal third of the clavicle

Trendelenburg position—a supine position with the bed inclined at an angle of 45 degrees so that the hips are higher than the head (head-down position)

Trendelenburg test—used to assess valvular competence of veins

tricarboxylic acid cycle—Krebs cycle

tricuspid space (area)—the region of the chest (fourth and fifth intercostal spaces) where the normal and pathologic sounds made by the tricuspid valve are traditionally said to be best appreciated

triglyceride—a molecule of glycerol bound to three long-chain fatty acid molecules

triplet—three consecutive atrial or ventricular extrasystoles

troponin—a protein molecule attached to the tropomyosin molecule of an actin filament

true chordae—a fibrous collagenous cord spanning the gap between the papillary muscles and the valve leaflets

true ribs—the first seven ribs on either side of

the thorax whose cartilages articulate directly with the sternum

truncal ridges—the spiral epithelial outgrowths from the walls of the truncus arteriosus that combine with the bulbar ridges to form the aorticopulmonary septum

truncus arteriosus—the primitive ascending aorta that opens from both ventricles in the early stages of fetal development

tubercle of the rib—the junction of the neck and the shaft of the rib; an articular portion of tubercle articulates with transverse process of the inferiormost vertebra to which the head is connected

tympany—a low-pitched, drumlike resonance produced by percussing (mediate percussion) the chest wall or other hollow structure

type I (squamous) pneumocytes—the cells covering approximately 93% of the alveolar surface; accounts for about 8.3% of the total cells of the parenchyma of the lungs

type I (Wenckebach's) second-degree block—a progressive lengthening of the P-R interval until a cardiac cycle is dropped; after the dropped cycle the P-R interval is shortened again

type I sensitivity reaction—the release of chemical mediators from mast cells and leukocytes; related to IgE antibody activity

type II (granular) pneumocytes—the cells covering approximately 7% of the alveolar surface; account for about 16% of the total cells comprising the parenchyma of the lungs

type II (Mobitz II) second-degree block—a dropped cardiac cycle with or without alteration in the conduction of preceding intervals

umbilical vein—the vein that returns the blood from the placenta to the fetus

uncompensated metabolic alkalosis—any condition that causes the arterial pH to rise above 7.45 and the partial pressure of bicarbonate to rise above 26mm Hg without eliciting a compensatory alveolar hypoventilation

uncomplicated myocardial infarction—a myocardial infarction in which there is no evidence of continued ischemia, left ventricular failure, shock, serious arrhythmia or other conduction disturbance, or other serious illness persisting beyond the fourth day after the infarction; constitutes a low-risk subset of patients

uncomplicated, high-risk myocardial infarction—a myocardial infarction that is initially considered to be uncomplicated but later manifests poor ventricular function, poor cardiac reserve, or significant ischemia at low levels of exertion; constitutes a moderate-risk subset of patients

unipolar pacing system—a type of cardiac pacemaker

United Network of Organ Sharing (UNOS)—the organization that maintains the waiting list of candidates for transplantation and all their medical data

unstable angina—a constricting chest pain that occurs now at rest when previously it occurred with exertion associated with myocardial ischemia, injury, and necrosis

upper lobe bronchus—that portion of the tracheobronchial tree that gives off the segmental and subsegmental bronchi of the upper lobe of the lung

urea—the chief end-product of amino acid metabolism in the body; excreted in urine

uremia—the excessive concentration of urinary retention products in the blood (e.g., creatinine, uric acid, phenols, guanidine bases, sulfates, phosphates, nitrates, urea, and other nonprotein nitrogenous wastes)

uremic syndrome—the symptoms of renal failure (e.g., water retention and edema, acidosis, excessive concentrations of urinary retention products)

urokinase (abbokinase)—a proteinase that converts plasminogen to plasmin; plasminogen activator

v wave—the rise in the atrial pressure curve near the end of ventricular contraction that results from the gradual accumulation of blood in the atria while the atrioventricular valves are closed during ventricular contraction

Valsalva's maneuver—contraction of the muscles of the abdomen, chest wall, and diaphragm in a forced expiratory effort against the closed glottis

Valsalva's sinuses—three dilations in the aortic wall that correspond to the cusps of the aortic valve

valve leaflets—the cusps of the cardiac valves

valve of the coronary sinus—a semicircular fold of the lining of the right atrium attached to the right and inferior margins of the orifice of the coronary sinus; the remnant of the lower part of the right venous valve of the fetus; thebesian valve

valve of the foramen ovale—a fold of tissue from the margin of the foramen ovale that projects into the left atrium of the fetus; at birth, left atrial blood pressure increases and closes the valve

valve of the inferior vena cava—a crescent-shaped fold attached to the left ventral aspect of the orifice of the inferior vena cava; the remnant of the upper part of the right venous valve of the fetus; eustachian valve

valvular insufficiency—the inadequate closure of one of the valves of the heart, allowing regurgitant flow of blood through the closed valve

valvular stenosis—the narrowing of a valvular orifice

valvuloplasty—the surgical reconstruction of a deformed valve or valve leaflet to relieve an incompetence or stenosis

valvulotomy—a surgical incision through a stenosed valve or valve leaflet to relieve an obstruction

variant angina—atypical angina

varicella zoster—chickenpox; herpes zoster virus

varicose bronchiectasis—the tortuous dilation of the bronchial or bronchiolar airways

vasa vasorum—the blood vessels of the blood vessels; small nutrient blood vessels that supply the larger blood vessels

vascular endothelial growth factor (VEGF)—see recombinant human vascular endothelial growth factor

vascular markings—the shadows produced on a radiographic image of the chest by the pulmonary vasculature

vasculitis—the inflammation of a blood vessel

vasomotor tone (VMT)—the balance between vasoconstriction and dilation

vasopressor—a substance that produces vasoconstriction or an increase in blood pressure

veins—blood vessels carrying blood toward the heart

venography—test to assess for severity of venous insufficiency prior to any surgical intervention

venous filling time test—an assessment of the efficiency of arterial blood flow through capillaries and into veins

venous return—the amount of blood flowing from the veins into the right atrium per minute

ventilation—the replacement of the air or gas in a space by fresh air or gas; movement of gas to and from the alveoli

ventilation-perfusion mismatching—an inequality between the amount of air breathed per unit of time and the amount of blood pumped through the pulmonary vasculature per unit of time; normally a ratio of about 0.8

ventilatory failure—a mechanical inadequacy of the respiratory musculature to move air into and out of the lungs; inability of the lungs to adequately exchange carbon dioxide (Pa_{CO_2} in excess of 50 mm Hg); pulmonary insufficiency

ventilatory reserve—the difference between the amount of air normally breathed (tidal volume) and that which can be maximally breathed (maximal voluntary ventilation)

ventilatory threshold—a measurement determined during exercise testing using a metabolic cart; the level of exercise at which there is a nonlinear increase in the ventilation in relation to oxygen uptakes; also considered to be the estimated upper limit of aerobic exercise

ventricle—the division of the heart tube between the bulbus cordis and the atrium; the lower chamber of the heart

ventricular assistive system (or device)—a mechanical device surgically inserted as a temporary means to improve the pumping of the ventricle while waiting for a donor heart to become available for transplantation

ventricular end-diastolic volume (VEDV)—the volume of blood in the heart ventricles at the end of diastole; just prior to being ejected

ventricular ejection phase—the portion of the cardiac cycle in which blood is driven out of the ventricles

ventricular fibrillation (VF)—a life-threatening arrhythmia originating from an ectopic focus in the ventricles that results in a twitching of individual fibrils, resulting in a lack of cardiac output

ventricular gallop—the triple cadence of heart sounds heard on auscultation and characterized by an audible sound (third heart sound) occurring in early diastole in addition to the normal first and second heart sounds; protodiastolic gallop; "lub-dub-dub"

ventricular septal defect (VSD)—a congenital defect (opening) in the wall between the ventricles; the most prevalent congenital cardiac defect

ventricular tachycardia (VT)—a life-threatening arrhythmia originating from an ectopic focus in the ventricles; ventricular depolarization at a rate in excess of 100 times per minute

ventriculography—the radiographic visualization of the ventricles by the injection of a radiopaque material into them

Venturi mask—a supplemental oxygen delivery device that can be adjusted to deliver a specific fraction of inspired oxygen at relatively high flow rates

venule—a minute vein

verapamil (Calan, Isoptin)—a calcium-channel blocking agent

very low density lipoproteins (VLDL)—one of the major classes of lipoproteins, containing high concentrations of triglycerides and moderate concentrations of cholesterol and phospholipids; has a flotation fraction (density) between 1.006 and 1.019

virus—a group of microbes composed of a protein coat over a central nucleic acid core

visceral—pertaining to the internal organs of the body

visceral pleura—the serous membrane covering the surface of each lung

viscosity—resistance to flow resulting from molecular cohesion

vital capacity (VC)—the sum of the inspiratory reserve, tidal, and expiratory reserve volumes; it is the maximum amount of air that can be exhaled following a maximum inhalation

vocal ligament—a continuation of the cricothyroid ligament

vocational rehabilitation—training, following disease or injury, for an occupation or profession, taking into account the special physical or mental capabilities of the patient

volvulus—an obstruction of the intestine caused by twisting

wandering pacemaker—an abnormal cardiac rhythm in which the site of the controlling focus of depolarization shifts from depolarization to depolarization, usually between the sinus and atrioventricular nodes

warfarin (Coumadin)—an anticoagulant agent that inhibits the formation of prothrombin in the liver

wean—to progressively discontinue artificial ventilation and develop independent breathing

wedge resection—the excision of a wedge-shaped portion of the lung

Wegener's granulomatosis—a rare, progressive, and fatal ulcerative disease of the upper respiratory tract; occurs in young to middle-aged men and is characterized by necrotizing arteritis

Wenckebach (second degree AV Block)—see type 1 second-degree block

wetting agent—a surface-active agent (e.g., surfactant) that forms a monomolecular layer over the pulmonary alveolar surfaces

wheeze—the high-pitched sound made by air passing through narrowed tracheobronchial airways

whispered pectoriloquy—an auscultatory technique; the whispered voice is transmitted through the lungs and chest wall in the same manner as the normal voice; it indicates an increase in the density of the underlying lung tissue

Wilson's disease—exfoliative dermatitis

Wolff-Parkinson-White (W-P-W) syndrome—tachyarrhythmia characterized by a short P-R interval (0.1 second or more) and a prolonged QRS complex; preexcitation syndrome

working myocytes—the cardiac muscle cells that compose the bulk of the heart; to be distinguished from conducting myocytes

xenotransplantation—transplantation of an organ from a different species (e.g., pig organs)

xiphoid process—the lower segment of the sternum

Index

Note: Page numbers in *italics* indicate illustrations; those followed by t indicate tables; and those followed by b indicate boxed material.

Clofibrate, for hyperlipidemia, 570t, 570–571
Clonidine, for hypertension, 566t, 567
Clopidogrel, 550
Closed-circuit method, 433
Closing volumes, age-related increase in, 191
Clot, formation of, 544, *545*
Clotting factors, 544, *545*
Clubbing, 623, *624*
  in bronchiectasis, 272
  in cystic fibrosis, 263
Coagulation, 544, *545*
Coagulation factors, 544, *545*
Coagulation profiles, 338t, 342, 447
Coagulopathy, in congestive heart failure, 142
Coal dust, Caplan's syndrome and, 232
  pneumoconiosis and, 194–195
Cocaine, pulmonary injury from, 252
Coenzyme Q$_{10}$, in congestive heart failure, 144
Cold temperatures, exercise in, 702–703
Colestipol, for hyperlipidemia, 570t, 570–571
Collagen vascular diseases, cardiopulmonary complications in, 307t, 307–311
Collapsed lung. See *Atelectasis.*
Collateral vessels, 91
Commissural chordae, 39
Commissurotomy, 114
Common atrioventricular bundle, 42, 44, *44*
Common carotid artery, left, *32,* 33
Communication, in ventilator weaning, 655
Complete blood cell count (CBC), 338t, 341–342, 342b, 446t, 446–447, 447t
Complete heart block, *405,* 405–406
Compliance, in cardiac rehabilitation, 663, 708–709
  in primary prevention, 717
Compliance (CL), 58, 61, *61,* 184
  age-related decrease in, 190–191
  cardiac, 58
  chest wall. See *Chest wall compliance.*
  in restrictive lung dysfunction, 184, *186,* 186–187
  measurement of, 436
  pulmonary, 58, 61, *61,* 184
    age-related decrease in, 190–191
    for ventilator weaning, 519
    in restrictive lung dysfunction, 184, *186,* 186–187
    measurement of, 436
Compliance curve, 184, *186*
  age-related changes in, 191
Computed tomography (CT), 348, 428
  electron beam, 348–349
  in bronchiectasis, 272
  in emphysema, 280, *280*
  single-photon emission, 348
  with exercise testing, 364
Conducting airways. See also *Airway entries.*
  anatomy of, 19–25, *20–22*

Conduction system, 42–45, *43, 44,* 74–76, *75,* 383–385, *383–385,* 558–560, *559, 560*
Conductivity, cardiac, 381, 382
Congenital heart disease, 116
Congestive atelectasis, 218–219
Congestive heart failure, 106–173. See also *Cardiac muscle dysfunction.*
  arrhythmias and, 110–111
  atrial natriuretic peptide in, 135, *135*
  breathing patterns in, 121, 121b
  cardiomyopathy and, 111–114, 113
  cardiomyoplasty for, 487
  cardiovascular function in, 132t, 132–135, *133, 134*
  case studies of, 159–172
  causes of, 109–119
  classification of, 108–109
  coronary artery disease and, 109–110
  crackles in, 122
  cyanosis in, 126
  dialysis and ultrafiltration for, 148–149
  diastolic, 109
  diet in, 145–146
  diuretics for, 111
  drug therapy for, 146t, 146–148, 487, 551–558, 552–557, 553t
  dyspnea in, 120–121, 138, 138t
    management of, 151–159, 156t. See also *Exercise training.*
  evaluation of, 119–132, 131b
  exercise tolerance in, 126–129
  exercise training in, 151–159. See also *Exercise training.*
  extremity changes in, 126
  functional classification for, 129–132, 130t, 131t
  heart sounds in, 122–123, *123*
  heart transplantation in. See also *Heart transplantation.*
    case study of, 503–504
  hematologic function in, 141, *141*
  high-output, 109
  hypertension and, 109–110
  in diabetes, 297–298
  intra-aortic balloon pump for, 149, *149*
  jugular vein distention in, *124,* 124–125, *125,* 619, *620*
  left ventricular assist devices for, 149–150, *150*
  left-sided, 108
  liver function in, 140b, 140–141, 145
  low-output, 109
  myopathy in, 142–143
  neurohormonal alterations in, 138–140
  orthopnea in, 121
  orthostatic hypotension in, 121
  pancreatic function in, 143–144
  pathophysiology of, 107–108, 132t, 132–145, *133,* 552
  peripheral edema in, 123–124
  prevalence of, 106–107
  psychosocial aspects of, 707–708, 708t, 709t
  pulmonary artery balloon counterpulsation for, 149, *149*

Congestive heart failure *(Continued)*
  pulmonary edema in, 107, 107t, 137–138, 138t, 216–218, *217.* See also *Pulmonary edema.*
  pulsus alternans in, 125
  quality of life in, 129–132, 130t, 131b, 131t
    exercise training and, 152–154, 156t
  radiologic findings in, 119–120
  rales in, 122
  renal function in, 110, 111, 135–137, *136, 137,* 145
  right-sided, 108
  signs and symptoms of, 107, 119, 121–129, 557
    therapy-induced improvement in, 156t
  sinus tachycardia in, 126
  skeletal muscle dysfunction in, 143
  sodium retention in, *136,* 136–137
  stroke volume in, 134, *134*
  surgery for, 150–151
  systolic, 109
  treatment of, 145–151
  ventricular assistive system in, 486–487, *487*
  ventricular end-diastolic volume in, 107, *108*
  vitamin supplements for, 145
  weight gain in, 126
Connective tissue disorders, cardiopulmonary complications in, 311
  restrictive lung dysfunction in, 231–236
Consciousness, assessment of, 617
Consent, for exercise testing, 353, *353*
Consolidation, breath sounds and, 626
Continuous positive airway pressure ventilation, 523, 523b
  exercise training in, 154–155
  nasal, 528, *528*
Contractility, 78, 79, 558–559
  determinants of, 107, *108*
  neurohormonal regulation of, 138–140, *139*
  stroke volume and, 79–80, *80,* 107, *108,* 134, *134*
Contrast echocardiography, 347
Contusion, lung, 241
Conus arteriosus tendon, 40, *40*
Conus ligament, 40, *40*
Cor pulmonale, in chronic obstructive pulmonary disease, 257
  in restrictive lung dysfunction, 188
Coronary artery(ies), anatomy of, *31–33,* 33–34, *89,* 89–90
  blood flow in, *90,* 90–91
  dominance of, 34
  left, *32, 33,* 34
  right, *32, 33,* 33–34
Coronary artery bypass grafting, 457–459, *458, 459*
  case studies of, 473
  graft surveillance in, 371, 372–373
  minimally invasive direct, 458–459
  off-pump, 459
  postoperative complications in, 459b

ISBN 0-7216-7288-4

90069